GE medical book

Jawetz, Melnick & Adelberg's

Medical Microbiology

Twentieth Edition

Geo. F. Brooks, MD
Professor of Laboratory Medicine,
Medicine, and Microbiology and Immunology
Chief, Microbiology Section
Clinical Laboratories,
University of California, San Francisco

Janet S. Butel, PhD
Professor of Virology and Head,
Division of Molecular Virology
Baylor College of Medicine
Houston

L. Nicholas Ornston, PhD
Professor of Biology
Yale University
New Haven

Ernest Jawetz, MD, PhD
Professor of Microbiology and Medicine Emeritus,
University of California, San Francisco

Joseph L. Melnick, PhD
Distinguished Service
Professor of Virology and Epidemiology
Baylor College of Medicine
Houston

Edward A. Adelberg, PhD
Professor of Human Genetics
Yale University School of Medicine
New Haven

Prentice-Hall International Inc.

95 96 97 98 / 10 9 8 7 6 5 4 3 2 1

Prentice Hall International (UK) Limited, *London*
Prentice Hall of Australia Pty. Limited, *Sydney*
Prentice Hall of Canada, Inc., *Toronto*
Prentice Hall Hispanoamericana, S.A., *Mexico*
Prentice Hall of India Private Limited, *New Delhi*
Prentice Hall of Japan, Inc., *Tokyo*
Simon & Schuster Asia Pte. Ltd., *Singapore*
Editora Prentice Hall do Brasil Ltda., *Rio de Janeiro*
Prentice Hall, Englewood Cliffs, *New Jersey*

ISBN: 0-8385-6229-9
ISSN: 1054-2744

Acquisitions Editor: John Dolan
Production Editor: Chris Langan
Senior Art Coordinator: Maggie Belis Darrow

PRINTED IN THE UNITED STATES OF AMERICA

Table of Contents

II. IMMUNOLOGY

III. BACTERIOLOGY

IV. VIROLOGY

PREFACE

Four decades ago, Dr Jack Lange asked Drs Ernest Jawetz, Joseph Melnick, and Edward Adelberg to write a *Review of Medical Microbiology* that would give a "brief, accurate, and up-to-date presentation of those aspects of medical microbiology which are of particular significance in the fields of clinical infections and chemotherapy." Considerable portions of the first edition were devoted to basic science to enhance the understanding of microbiologic principles. Details of technique and procedure and materials of a controversial nature were excluded. These goals for the first edition were pursued also in subsequent editions, and the book became immensely popular by word of mouth between students and from their teachers. Over the years, nearly 1.5 million copies of the book have been published. It has been printed in 13 languages and used by literally millions of students worldwide.

The current twentieth edition of *Jawetz, Melnick & Adelberg's Medical Microbiology* therefore celebrates four decades of bringing scientific progress to students of medicine and other health-related disciplines.

The early editions of the book were written entirely by Drs Jawetz, Melnick, and Adelberg. Later, Dr Donald Heyneman contributed the chapter on parasitology. Drs Geo. F. Brooks, Janet S. Butel, and L. Nicholas Ornston became involved in the book several editions ago, and with the twentieth edition the responsibility for the book has transferred completely to them. With this edition we welcome three new contributors: Dr Stephen A. Morse, who wrote the chapters on Cell Structure and Classification of Bacteria; Dr Roderick Nairn, who wrote the chapter on Immunology; and Dr Jeffrey C. Edman, who wrote the chapter on Mycology.

The primary goals of the first edition have been maintained through the twentieth edition. Extensive revision and updating have been done throughout the book. A new chapter with ten case studies has been added to provide correlation with microbiologic findings. In association with the widespread access to computer-assisted reference systems, the number of specific references has been decreased; recent review papers with extensive bibliographies have been included for students who do not have immediate access to computerized systems. With the twentieth edition, we move to a three-year revision cycle.

The authors and the publishers give special thanks to Dr James Ransom, who edited the first and many of the intervening editions, including this one. We give much credit to him for the high quality, clarity, and consistency of the text.

Geo. F. Brooks
San Francisco
April 1995

Janet S. Butel
Houston

L. Nicholas Ornston
New Haven

The Science of Microbiology 1

BIOLOGIC PRINCIPLES ILLUSTRATED BY MICROBIOLOGY

Nowhere is biologic **diversity** demonstrated more dramatically than by microorganisms, creatures that are not directly visible to the unaided eye. In form and function, be it biochemical property or genetic mechanism, analysis of microorganisms takes us to the limits of biologic understanding. Thus, the need for **originality**—one test of the merit of a scientific **hypothesis**—can be fully met in microbiology. A useful hypothesis should provide a basis for **generalization,** and microbial diversity provides an arena in which this challenge is ever-present.

Prediction, the practical outgrowth of science, is a product created by a blend of technique and theory. **Biochemistry** and **genetics** provide the tools required for analysis of microorganisms. **Microbiology,** in turn, extends the horizons of these scientific disciplines. A biologist might describe such an exchange as **mutualism,** ie, one that benefits all of the contributing parties. In biology, mutualism is called **symbiosis,** a continuing association of different organisms. Should the exchange operate primarily to the benefit of one party, the association is described as **parasitism,** a relationship in which a **host** provides the primary benefit to the parasite. Isolation and characterization of a parasite—eg, a pathogenic bacterium or virus—often requires effective mimicry in the laboratory of the growth environment provided by host cells. This demand sometimes represents a major challenge to the investigator.

The terms "mutualism," "symbiosis," and "parasitism" relate to the science of **ecology,** and the principles of environmental biology are implicit in microbiology. Microorganisms are the products of **evolution,** the biologic consequence of **natural selection** operating upon a vast array of genetically diverse organisms. It is useful to keep the complexity of natural history in mind before generalizing about microorganisms, the most heterogeneous subset of all living creatures.

A major biologic division separates the eukaryotes, organisms containing a membrane-bound nucleus, from prokaryotes, organisms in which DNA is not physically separated from the cytoplasm. As described below and in Chapter 2, further major distinctions can be made between eukaryotes and prokaryotes. Eukaryotes, for example, are distinguished by their relatively large size and by the presence of specialized membrane-bound organelles such as mitochondria.

As described more fully below, microbial eukaryotes are termed **protists,** and within this group the major subdivisions are the **algae,** the **protozoa,** the **fungi,** and the **slime molds.**

Eukaryotes and prokaryotes are organisms because they contain all of the enzymes required for their replication and possess the biologic equipment necessary for the production of metabolic energy. Thus, eukaryotes and prokaryotes stand distinguished from **viruses,** which depend upon host cells for these necessary functions.

VIRUSES

The unique properties of viruses set them apart from living creatures. Heterogeneity among viruses is assured by their dependence upon a host for replication. In a sense, a virus can be regarded as a genetic extension of its host. Host-virus interactions tend to be highly specific, and the biologic range of viruses mirrors the diversity of potential host cells. Further diversity of viruses is exhibited by their broad array of strategies for replication and survival.

A viral particle consists of a nucleic acid molecule, either DNA or RNA, enclosed in a protein coat or capsid. Proteins—frequently glycoproteins—in the capsid determine the specificity of interaction of a virus with its host cell. The capsid protects the nucleic acid and facilitates attachment and penetration of the host cell by the virus. Inside the cell, viral nucleic acid redirects the host's enzymatic machinery to functions associated with replication of the virus. In some cases, genetic information from the virus can be incorporated as DNA into a host chromosome. In other instances, the viral genetic information can serve as a basis for cellular manufacture and release of copies of the virus. This process calls for replication of the viral DNA and production of specific viral proteins. Maturation consists of assembling newly synthesized nucleic acid and protein subunits into mature viral particles which are then liberated into the extracellular environment. Different viruses are known to infect a wide variety of specific plant and animal hosts as well as prokaryotes and at least one eukaryotic alga. Virus-like particles that seem to lack an infectious extracellular phase have been found in fungi as well as in several genera of algae.

A number of transmissible plant diseases are caused by **viroids**—small, single-stranded, covalently closed circular RNA molecules existing as highly base-paired rod-like structures; they do not possess capsids. Their molecular weights are estimated to fall in the range of 75,000–100,000. It is not known whether they are translated in the host into polypeptides or whether they interfere with host functions directly (as RNA); if the former is true, the largest viroid could only be translated into the equivalent of a single polypeptide containing about 55 amino acids. Viroid RNA is replicated by the DNA-dependent RNA polymerase of the plant host; preemption of this enzyme may contribute to viroid pathogenicity.

The RNAs of viroids have been shown to contain inverted repeated base sequences at their termini, a characteristic of transposable elements and retroviruses (see Chapter 7). Thus, it is likely that they have evolved from transposable elements or retroviruses by the deletion of internal sequences.

Scrapie, a degenerative central nervous system disease of sheep, is caused by a filterable agent less than 50 nm in diameter. It is resistant to nucleases and other agents that inactivate nucleic acids but is inactivated by proteases and other agents that react with proteins. The infectious particle has been called a prion; it copurifies with a specific protein, but the presence of nucleic acid within the particle has not been ruled out.

By use of recombinant DNA techniques, the gene encoding the major prion protein has been cloned from hamster brain. The gene—and its corresponding mRNA—is present (and thus expressed) in both normal and scrapie-infected brain tissue. Three competing models exist: (1) Scrapie is a conventional virus with an extremely small nucleic acid genome that has escaped detection; (2) the infectious agent is a small, noncoding RNA molecule that binds to prion protein with high affinity, changing the prion's conformation in a self-propagating manner to a pathologic form; and (3) the prion protein is itself the infectious agent, inducing the synthesis of posttranslational modifying enzymes that convert a normal protein to the pathologic prion form. These models may also apply to the agents of Creutzfeldt-Jakob disease and kuru, which produce very similar diseases in humans.

The general properties of animal viruses pathogenic for humans are described in Chapter 29. Bacterial viruses are described in Chapter 7.

PROKARYOTES

The primary distinguishing characteristics of the prokaryotes are their relatively small size, usually on the order of 1 μm in diameter, and the absence of a nuclear membrane. The DNA of almost all bacteria is a circle with a length of about 1 mm; this is the prokaryotic chromosome. The chromosomal DNA must be folded more than a thousandfold just to fit within the prokaryotic cell membrane. Substantial evidence suggests that the folding may be orderly and may bring specified regions of the DNA into proximity. The specialized region of the cell containing DNA is termed the **nucleoid** and can be visualized by ectron microscopy. Thus, it would be a mistake to conclude that subcellular differentiation, clearly demarcated by membranes in eukaryotes, is lacking in prokaryotes. Indeed, some prokaryotes form membrane-bound subcellular structures with specialized function such as the chromotaphores of photosynthetic bacteria. Such prokaryotic structures differ from eukaryotic counterparts in that the membranes surrounding the specialized region are extensions of the cell membrane.

Prokaryotic Diversity

The small size of the prokaryotic chromosome limits the amount of genetic information it can contain. Reasonable estimates of the number of genes within a typical prokaryote are on the order of 3000, and many of these genes must be dedicated to essential functions such as energy generation, macromolecular synthesis, and cellular replication. Any one prokaryote carries relatively few genes that allow physiologic accommodation of the organism to its environment. The range of potential prokaryotic environments is unimaginably broad, and it follows that the prokaryotic group encompasses a heterogeneous range of specialists, each adapted to a fairly narrowly circumscribed niche.

The range of prokaryotic niches is illustrated by consideration of strategies used for generation of metabolic energy. Light from the sun is the chief source of energy for life. Some prokaryotes such as the purple bacteria convert light energy to metabolic energy in the absence of oxygen production. Other prokaryotes, exemplified by the blue-green bacteria **(cyanobacteria),** produce oxygen that can provide energy through respiration in the absence of light. **Aerobic organisms** depend upon respiration with oxygen for their energy. Some **anaerobic organisms** can use electron acceptors other than oxygen in respiration. Many anaerobes carry out **fermentations** in which energy is derived by metabolic rearrangement of chemical growth substrates. The tremendous chemical range of potential growth substrates for aerobic or anaerobic growth is mirrored in the diversity of prokaryotes that have adapted to their utilization.

Prokaryotic Communities

A useful survival strategy for specialists is to enter into **consortia,** arrangements in which the physiologic characteristics of different organisms contribute to survival of the group as a whole. If the organisms within a physically interconnected community are directly derived from a single cell, the community is a **clone** that may contain up to 10^8 cells. The biology of such a community differs substantially from that of a single cell. For example, the high cell number virtually assures the presence within the clone of at least one cell carrying a variant of any gene on the chromosome. Thus, genetic variability—the wellspring of the evolutionary process called natural selection—is assured within a clone. The high number of cells within clones also is likely to provide physiologic protection to at least some members of the group. Extracellular polysaccharides, for example, may afford protection against potentially lethal agents such as antibiotics or heavy metal ions. Large amounts of polysaccharides produced by the high number of cells within a clone may allow cells within the interior to survive exposure to a lethal agent at a concentration that might kill single cells.

A distinguishing characteristic of prokaryotes is their capacity to exchange small packets of genetic information. This information may be carried on **plasmids,** small and specialized genetic elements that are capable of replication within at least one prokaryotic cell line. In some cases, plasmids may be transferred from one cell to another and thus may carry sets of specialized genetic information through a population. Some plasmids possess a **broad host range** that allows them to convey sets of genes to diverse organisms. Of particular concern are **drug resistance plasmids** that may render diverse bacteria resistant to antibiotic treatment.

The survival strategy of a single prokaryotic cell line may lead to a range of interactions with other organisms. These may include symbiotic relationships illustrated by complex nutritional exchanges among organisms within the human gut. These exchanges benefit both the microorganisms and their human host. Parasitic interactions can be quite deleterious to the host. Advanced symbiosis or parasitism can lead to loss of functions that would allow growth of the symbiont or parasite independent of its host.

The **mycoplasmas,** for example, are parasitic prokaryotes that have lost the ability to form a cell wall. Adaptation of these organisms to their parasitic environment has resulted in incorporation of a substantial quantity of cholesterol into their cell membranes. Cholesterol, not found in other prokaryotes, is assimilated from the metabolic environment provided by the host. Loss of function is exemplified also by obligate intracellular parasites, the **chlamydiae** and **rickettsiae.** These bacteria are extremely small (0.2–0.5 μm in diameter) and depend upon the host cell for many essential metabolites and coenzymes. Some evidence suggests that the host cell may even provide energy in the form of ATP to these bacteria.

The most widely distributed examples of bacterial symbionts appear to be chloroplasts and mitochondria, the energy-yielding organelles of eukaryotes. A substantial body of evidence points to the conclusion that ancestors of these organelles were **endosymbionts,** prokaryotes that established symbiosis within the cell membrane of the ancestral eukaryotic host. The presence of multiple copies of the organelles may have contributed to the relatively large size of eukaryotic cells and to their capacity for specialization, a trait ultimately reflected in the evolution of differentiated multicellular organisms.

Classification of the Prokaryotes

An understanding of any group of organisms requires their **classification.** An appropriate classification system allows a scientist to choose characteristics that allow swift and accurate categorization of a newly encountered organism. The categorization allows prediction of many additional traits shared by other members of the category. In a hospital setting, successful classification of a pathogenic organism may provide the most direct route to its elimination. Classification may also provide a broad understanding of relationships among different organisms, and such information may have great practical value. For example, elimination of a pathogenic organism will be relatively long-lasting if its habitat is occupied by a nonpathogenic variant.

The principles of prokaryotic classification are discussed in Chapter 3. At the outset it should be recognized that any prokaryotic characteristic might serve as a potential criterion for classification. Not all criteria are equally effective in grouping organisms. Possession of DNA, for example, is a useless criterion for distinguishing organisms because all cells contain DNA. The presence of a broad host range plasmid is not a useful criterion because such plasmids may be found in diverse hosts and need not be present all of the time. Useful criteria may be structural, physiologic, biochemical, or genetic. **Spores**—specialized cell structures that may allow survival in extreme environments—are useful structural criteria for classification because well-characterized subsets of bacteria form spores. Some bacterial groups can be effectively subdivided on the basis of their ability to ferment specified carbohydrates. Such criteria may be ineffective when applied to other bacterial groups that may lack any fermentative capability. A biochemical test, the **Gram stain,** is an effective criterion for classification because response to the stain reflects fundamental and complex differences in the bacterial cell surface that divide bacteria into two major groups.

Genetic criteria are increasingly employed in bacterial classification, and many of these advances are made possible by the development of recombinant DNA technology. It is now possible to design DNA probes that swiftly identify organisms carrying specified genetic regions with common ancestry. Comparison of DNA sequences for some genes led to the elucidation of **phylogenetic relationships** among prokaryotes. Ancestral cell lines can be traced, and organisms can be grouped on the basis of their evolutionary affinities. These investigations have led to some striking conclusions. For example, comparison of cytochrome c sequences suggests that all eukaryotes, including humans, arose from one of three different groups of purple photosynthetic bacteria. This conclusion in part explains the evolutionary origin of eukaryotes, but it does not fully take into account the generally accepted view that the eukaryotic cell was derived from the evolutionary merger of different prokaryotic cell lines.

Bacteria & Archaebacteria: the Major Subdivision Within the Prokaryotes

A major success in molecular phylogeny has been the demonstration that prokaryotes fall into two major groups. Most investigations have been directed to one group, the bacteria. The other group, the archaebacteria, has received relatively little attention, in part because many of its representatives are difficult to study in the laboratory. Some archaebacteria, for example, are killed by contact with oxygen, and others grow at temperatures exceeding that of boiling water. Before molecular evidence became available, the major subgroupings of archaebacteria seemed disparate. The methanogens carry out an anaerobic respiration that gives rise to methane; the halophiles demand extremely high salt concentrations for growth; and the thermoacidophiles require high temperature or acidity (or both). It has now been established that these prokaryotes share biochemical traits such as cell wall or membrane components that set the group entirely apart from all other living organisms. An intriguing trait shared by archaebacteria and eukaryotes is the presence of **introns** within genes. The function of introns—segments of DNA that interrupt informational DNA within genes—is not established. What is known is that introns represent a fundamental characteristic shared by the DNA of archaebacteria and eukaryotes. This common trait has led to the suggestion that—just as mitochondria and chloroplasts appear to be evolutionary derivatives of the bacteria—the eukaryotic nucleus may have arisen from an archaebacterial ancestor.

PROTISTS

The "true nucleus" of eukaryotes (from Gr *karyon* "nucleus") is only one of their distinguishing features. The membrane-bound organelles, the microtubules, and the microfilaments of eukaryotes form a complex intracellular structure unlike that found in prokaryotes. The agents of motility for eukaryotic cells are flagella or cilia—complex multistranded structures that do not resemble the flagella of prokaryotes. Gene expression in eukaryotes takes place through a series of events achieving physiologic integration of the nucleus with the endoplasmic reticulum, a structure that has no counterpart in prokaryotes. Eukaryotes are set apart by the organization of their cellular DNA in chromosomes separated by a distinctive mitotic apparatus during cell division.

In general, genetic transfer among eukaryotes depends upon fusion of **haploid gametes** to form a **diploid** cell containing a full set of genes derived from each gamete. The life cycle of many eukaryotes is almost entirely in the diploid state, a form not encountered in prokaryotes. Fusion of gametes to form reproductive progeny is a highly specific event and establishes the basis for eukaryotic **species.** This term can be applied only metaphorically to the prokaryotes, which exchange fragments of DNA through recombination. Taxonomic groupings of eukaryotes frequently are based on shared **morphologic properties,** and it is noteworthy that many taxonomically useful determinants are those associated with reproduction. Almost all successful eukaryotic species are those in which closely related cells, members of the same species, can recombine to form viable offspring. Structures that contribute directly or indirectly to the reproductive event tend to be highly developed and, with minor modifications among closely related species, extensively conserved.

Microbial eukaryotes—**protists**—are members of the four following major groups: algae, protozoa, fungi, and slime molds. It should be noted that these groupings are not necessarily phylogenetic: Closely related organisms may have been categorized separately because underlying biochemical and genetic similarities may not have been recognized.

Algae

The term "algae" has long been used to denote all organisms that produce O_2 as a product of photosynthesis. One major subgroup of these organisms—the blue-green bacteria, or cyanobacteria—are prokaryotic and no longer are termed algae. This classification is reserved exclusively for photosynthetic eukaryotic organisms. All algae contain chlorophyll in the photosynthetic membrane of their subcellular chloroplasts. Many algal species are unicellular microorganisms. Other algae may form extremely large multicellular structures. Kelps of brown algae sometimes are several hundred meters in length. A full description of the algae can be found in Bold HC, Wynne MJ: *Introduction to the Algae: Structure and Reproduction.* Prentice-Hall, 1978. A highly readable account of the properties of algae and other protists is presented in Sagan D, Margulis L: *Garden of Microbial Delights: A Practical Guide to the Subdivisible World.* Harcourt Brace Jovanovich, 1988.

Protozoa

Protozoa are unicellular nonphotosynthetic protists. The most primitive protozoa appear to be flagellated forms that in many respects resemble representatives of the algae. It seems likely that the ancestors of these protozoa were algae that became **heterotrophs:** the nutritional requirements of such organisms are met by organic compounds. Adaptation to a heterotrophic mode of life was sometimes accompanied by loss of chloroplasts, and algae thus gave rise to the closely related protozoa. Similar events have been observed in the laboratory as either mutation or physiologic adaptation has given rise to colorless descendants of algal cells.

From flagellated protozoa appear to have evolved the ameboid and the ciliated types; intermediate forms are known that have flagella at one stage in the life cycle and pseudopodia (characteristic of the ameba) at another stage. A fourth major group of protozoa consists of the sporozoons, parasites with complex life cycles that include a resting or spore stage.

Fungi

The fungi are nonphotosynthetic protists growing as a mass of branching, interlacing filaments ("hyphae") known as a mycelium. Although the hyphae exhibit cross-walls, the cross-walls are perforated and allow free passage of nuclei and cytoplasm. The entire organism is thus a coenocyte (a multinucleated mass of continuous cytoplasm) confined within a series of branching tubes. These tubes, made of polysaccharides such as chitin, are homologous with cell walls. The mycelial forms are called **molds;** a few types, **yeasts,** do not form a mycelium but are easily recognized as fungi by the nature of their sexual reproductive processes and by the presence of transitional forms.

The fungi probably represent an evolutionary offshoot of the protozoa; they are unrelated to the actinomycetes, mycelial bacteria that they superficially resemble. Fungi are subdivided as follows: *Zygomycotina* (the phycomycetes), *Ascomycotina* (the ascomycetes), *Basidiomycotina* (the basidiomycetes), and *Deuteromycotina* (the imperfect fungi).

The evolution of the ascomycetes from the phycomycetes is seen in a transitional group, members of which form a zygote but then transform this directly into an ascus. The basidiomycetes are believed to have evolved in turn from the ascomycetes. The classification of fungi is discussed further in Chapter 45.

Slime Molds

These organisms are characterized by the presence, as a stage in their life cycle, of an ameboid multinucleate mass of cytoplasm call a **plasmodium.** The plasmodium of a slime mold is analogous to the mycelium of a true fungus. Both are coenocytes. In the latter, cytoplasmic flow is confined to the branching network of chitinous tubes, whereas in the former the cytoplasm can flow in all directions. This flow causes the plasmodium to migrate in the direction of its food source, frequently bacteria. In response to a chemical signal, 3′,5′-cyclic AMP (see Chapter 7), the plasmodium, which reaches macroscopic size, differentiates into a stalked body that can produce individual motile cells. These cells, flagellated or ameboid, initiate a new round in the life cycle of the slime mold. The cycle frequently is initiated by sexual fusion of single cells.

The life cycle of the slime molds illustrates a central theme of this chapter: the interdependency of living forms. The growth of slime molds depends upon nutrients provided by bacterial or, in some cases, plant cells. Reproduction of the slime molds via plasmodia can depend upon intercellular recognition and fusion of cells from the same species. Full understanding of a microorganism requires both knowledge of the other organisms with which it coevolved and an appreciation of the range of physiologic responses that may contribute to survival.

REFERENCES

Books

Ainsworth GC, Sussman AS, Sparrow FK (editors): *Fungi: An Advanced Treatise.* 4 vols. Academic Press, 1973.

Barnett JA, Payne RW, Yarrow D (editors): *Yeasts: Characteristics and Identification.* Cambridge Univ Press, 1984.

Bold HC, Wynne MJ: *Introduction to the Algae: Structure and Reproduction.* Prentice-Hall, 1978.

Carlile MJ, Shekel JJ (editors): *Evolution in the Microbial World.* Cambridge Univ Press, 1974.

Diener TO: *Viroids and Viroid Diseases.* Krieger, 1979.

Laskin AI, Lechevalier HA (editors): *CRC Handbook of Microbiology,* 2nd ed. Vol 1: *Bacteria,* 1977; Vol 2: *Fungi, Algae, Protozoa and Viruses,* 1979. CRC Press.

Lederberg J (editor): *Encyclopedia of Microbiology.* 4 vols. Academic Press, 1992.

Levandowsky M, Hutner SH (editors): *Biochemistry and Physiology of Protozoa,* 2nd ed. Academic Press, 1979.

Luria SE et al: *General Virology,* 3rd ed. Wiley, 1978.

Margulis L: *Symbiosis in Cell Evolution: Life and Its Environment on the Early Earth.* Freeman, 1981.

Ragan MA, Chapman DJ: *Biochemical Phylogeny of the Protists.* Academic Press, 1977.

Reisser W (editor): *Algae and Symbiosis: Plants, Animals, Fungi, Viruses, Interactions Explored.* Biopress, 1992.

Sagan D, Margulis L: *Garden of Microbial Delights: A Practical Guide to the Subdivisible World.* Harcourt Brace Jovanovich, 1988.

Sleigh MA: *Protozoa and Other Protists.* Chapman & Hall, 1990.

Stanier RY, Adelberg EA, Ingraham J: *The Microbial World,* 4th ed. Prentice-Hall, 1976.

Woese CR, Wolfe RS (editors): *The Bacteria: A Treatise on Structure and Function.* Vol 8. Academic Press, 1985.

Articles & Reviews

Bruenn JA: Viruslike particles of yeast. Annu Rev Microbiol 1980;34:49.

Diener TO: Viroids: Structure and functions. Science 1979;205:859.

Fox GE et al: The phylogeny of prokaryotes. Science 1980;209:457.

Girard M: The Pasteur Institute's contribution to the field of virology. Annu Rev Microbiol 1988;42:745.

Knoll AH, Barghoorn ES: Precambrian eukaryotic organisms: A reassessment of the evidence. Science 1975; 190:52.

Kolenbrander PE: Intergeneric coaggregation among human oral bacteria and ecology of dental plaque. Annu Rev Microbiol 1989;43:622.

Lake JA et al: Eubacteria, halobacteria, and the origin of photosynthesis: The photocytes. Proc Natl Acad Sci USA 1985;82:3716.

Lemke PA: Viruses of eukaryotic microorganisms. Annu Rev Microbiol 1976;30:105.

Olsen GJ, Woese CR: The winds of (evolutionary) change: Breathing new life into microbiology. J Bacteriol 1994;176:1.

Prusiner SB: Scrapie prions. Annu Rev Microbiol 1989; 43:345.

Raff RA, Mahler HR: The nonsymbiotic origin of mitochondria. Science 1972;177:575.

Robertson HD, Branch AD, Dahlberg JE: Focusing on the nature of the scrapie agent. Cell 1985;40:725.

Rothschild LJ: Protozoa, protista, protoctista: What's in a name. J Hist Biol 1989;22:277.

Schlegel M: Protist evolution and phylogeny as discerned from small subunit ribosomal RNA sequence comparisons. Eur J Protistol 1992;3:207.

Van Valen LM: Algae, proalgae, and eualgae. J Paleontol 1992;66:681.

Wallace DC: Structure and evolution of organelle genomes. Microbiol Rev 1982;46:208.

Woese CR, Magrum LJ, Fox GE: Archaebacteria. J Mol Evol 1978;11:245.

Cell Structure 2

*Stephen A. Morse, MSPH, PhD**

OPTICAL METHODS

The Light Microscope

The resolving power of the light microscope under ideal conditions is about half the wavelength of the light being used. (Resolving power is the distance that must separate two point sources of light if they are to be seen as two distinct images.) With yellow light of a wavelength of 0.4 μm, the smallest separable diameters are thus about 0.2 μm. The useful magnification of a microscope is the magnification that makes visible the smallest resolvable particles. Microscopes used in bacteriology generally employ a 90-power objective lens with a 10-power ocular lens, thus magnifying the specimen 900 times. Particles 0.2 μm in diameter are therefore magnified to about 0.2 mm and so become clearly visible. Further magnification would give no greater resolution of detail and would reduce the visible area (field).

Further improvement in resolving power can be accomplished only by the use of light of shorter wavelengths of about 0.2 μm, thus allowing resolution of particles with diameters of 0.1 μm. Such microscopes, employing quartz lenses and photographic systems, are too expensive and complicated for general use.

The Electron Microscope

The high resolving power of the electron microscope has enabled scientists to observe the detailed structures of prokaryotic and eukaryotic cells. The superior resolution of the electron microscope is due to the fact that electrons have a much shorter wavelength than the photons of white light.

There are two types of electron microscopes in general use: the transmission electron microscope (TEM), which has many features in common with the light microscope; and the scanning electron microscope (SEM). The TEM was the first to be developed and employs a beam of electrons projected from an electron gun and directed or focused by an electromagnetic condenser lens onto a thin specimen. As the electrons strike the specimen, they are differentially scattered by the number and mass of atoms in the specimen; some electrons pass through the specimen and are gathered and focused by an electromagnetic objective lens, which presents an image of the specimen to the projector lens system for further enlargement. The image is visualized by allowing it to impinge on a screen that fluoresces when struck with the electrons. The image can be recorded on photographic film. TEM can resolve particles 0.001 μm apart. Viruses, with diameters of 0.01–0.2 μm, can be easily resolved.

The SEM generally has a lower resolving power than the TEM; however, it is particularly useful for providing three-dimensional images of the surface of microscopic objects. Electrons are focused by means of lenses into a very fine point. The interaction of electrons with the specimen results in the release of different forms of radiation (eg, secondary electrons) from the surface of the material, which can be captured by an appropriate detector, amplified, and then imaged on a television screen.

An important technique in electron microscopy is the use of "shadowing." This involves depositing a thin layer of heavy metal (such as platinum) on the specimen by placing it in the path of a beam of metal ions in a vacuum. The beam is directed at a low angle to the specimen, so that it acquires a "shadow" in the form of an uncoated area on the other side. When an electron beam is then passed through the coated preparation in the electron microscope and a positive print is made from the "negative" image, a three-dimensional effect is achieved (eg, see Figures 2–23, 2–24, and 2–25).

Other important techniques in electron microscopy include the use of ultrathin sections of embedded material; a method of freeze-drying specimens, which prevents the distortion caused by conventional drying procedures; and the use of negative staining with an electron-dense material such as phosphotungstic acid or uranyl salts (eg, Figure 42–1). Without these heavy metal salts, there would not be enough contrast to detect the details of the specimen.

Darkfield Illumination

Darkfield microscopy is frequently performed on the same microscope on which brightfield microscopy is performed. Illumination for darkfield microscopy is

*Director, Division of STD Laboratory Research, National Center for Infectious Diseases, CDC, and Adjunct Professor, Department of Microbiology and Immunology, Emory University School of Medicine.

obtained using a special condenser that both blocks direct light rays and deflects light off a mirror on the side of the condenser at an oblique angle. This creates a "dark field" that contrasts against the highlighted edge of the specimens and results when the oblique rays are reflected from the edge of the specimen upward into the objective of the microscope. This technique is particularly valuable for observing organisms such as *Treponema pallidum,* a spirochete which is less than 0.2 μm in diameter and therefore cannot be observed with direct light (Figure 2–1).

Phase Microscopy

The phase microscope takes advantage of the fact that light waves passing through transparent objects, such as cells, emerge in different phases depending on the properties of the materials though which they pass. A special optical system converts difference in phase into difference in intensity, so that some structures appear darker than others. An important feature is that internal structures are thus differentiated in living cells; with ordinary microscopes, killed and stained preparations must be used.

Autoradiography

If cells that have incorporated radioactive atoms are fixed on a slide, covered with a photographic emulsion, and stored in the dark for a suitable period of time, tracks appear in the developed film emanating from the sites of radioactive disintegration. If the cells are labeled with a weak emitter such as tritium, the tracks are sufficiently short to reveal the position of the radioactive label in cell. The procedure, called autoradiography, has been particularly useful in following the replication of DNA, using tritium-labeled thymidine as a specific tracer. A variation of this method that employs labeled nucleic acid probes is called **in situ hybridization** and has been used to detect the presence of viral, bacterial, and fungal nucleic acid in cells and tissues.

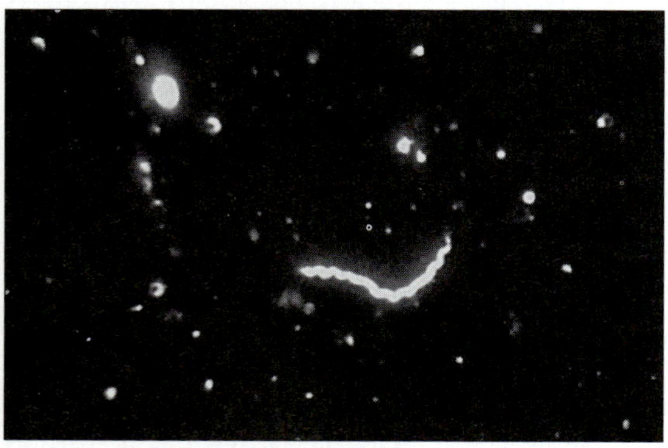

Figure 2–1. Positive darkfield examination. Treponemes are recognized by their characteristic corkscrew-shaped and deliberate forward and backward movement with rotation about the longitudinal axis. (Reproduced, with permission, from Morse SA, Moreland AA, Thompson SE [editors]: *Atlas of Sexually Transmitted Disease.* Gower, 1990.)

EUKARYOTIC CELL STRUCTURE

The Nucleus

The nucleus is bounded by a membrane that is continuous with the endoplasmic reticulum. The nuclear membrane exhibits selective permeability due to pores that permit the exchange of molecules between the nucleus and cytoplasm. The chromosomes of eukaryotic cells contain linear DNA macromolecules arranged as a double helix. They are only visible with a light microscope when the cell is undergoing division and the DNA is in a highly condensed form; at other times, the chromosomes are not condensed and appear as in Figure 2–2. Eukaryotic DNA macromolecules are associated with basic proteins called histones that bind to the DNA by ionic interactions.

Cytoplasmic Structures

The cytoplasm of eukaryotic cells is characterized by the presence of an endoplasmic reticulum, vacuoles, self-reproducing plastids, and an elaborate cytoskeleton composed of microtubules, microfilaments, and intermediate filaments.

The **endoplasmic reticulum** is a network of membrane-bounded channels. In some regions of the endoplasmic reticulum, the membranes are coated with ribosomes; proteins synthesized on these ribosomes pass through the membrane into the channels of the endoplasmic reticulum, through which they can be transported to other parts of the cell. A related structure, the **Golgi apparatus,** pinches off vesicles that can fuse with the cell membrane, releasing the enclosed proteins into the surrounding medium.

The plastids include **mitochondria,** which contain in their membranes the respiratory electron transport system, and **chloroplasts** (in photosynthetic organisms). The plastids contain their own DNA, which codes for some (but not all) of their constituent proteins and transfer RNAs.

The cytoskeleton includes arrays of **microtubules,** which play a role in cytoplasmic membrane function and cell shape as well as forming the mitotic spindle and flagellar components; arrays of actin- and myosin-containing **microfilaments,** which provide the mechanism of ameboid motility; and the **intermediate filaments,** whose function is not known.

Surface Layers

The cytoplasm is enclosed within a plasma membrane composed of protein and phospholipid, similar to the prokaryotic cell membrane illustrated in Figure 2–12. Most animal cells have no other surface layers; however, plant cells have an outer cell wall composed of cellulose. Many eukaryotic microorganisms also

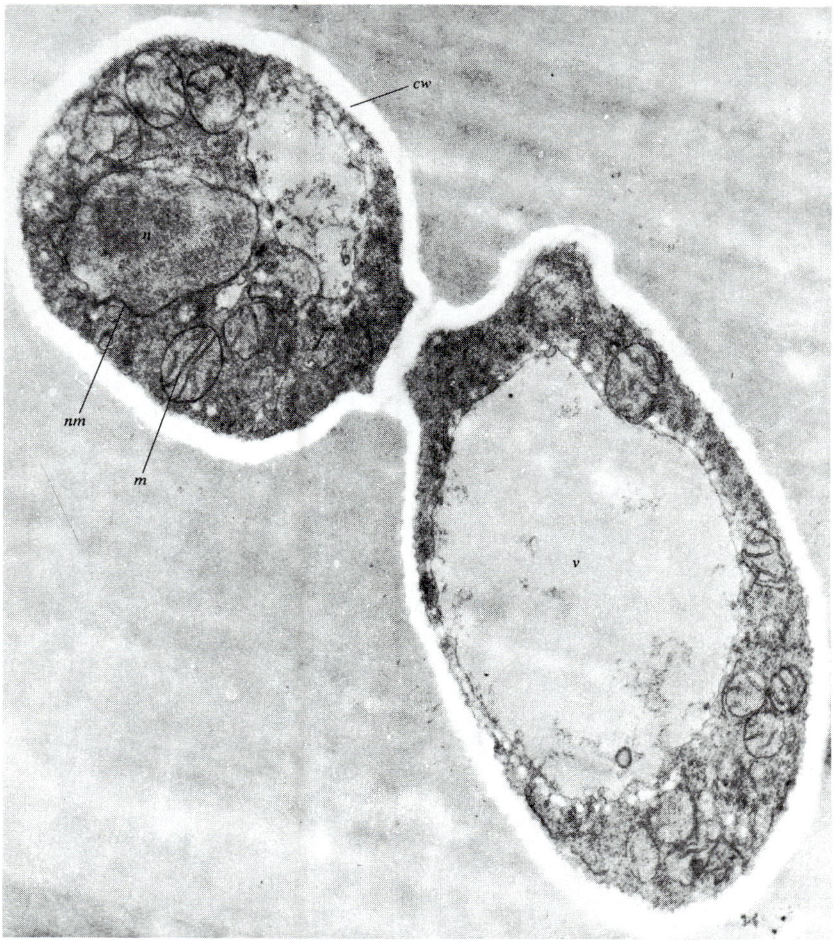

Figure 2–2. Thin section of a eukaryotic cell. A dividing cell of the unicellular yeast *Lipomyces* (17,500 ×). (n, nucleus; nm, nuclear membrane; v, vacuole; m, mitochondrion; cw, cell wall.) Electron micrograph taken by Dr CF Robinow. (Reproduced, with permission, from Stanier RY, Doudoroff M, Adelberg EA: *The Microbial World,* 2nd ed. Copyright © 1963. By permission of Prentice-Hall, Inc., Englewood Cliffs, NJ)

have an outer **cell wall,** which may be composed of a polysaccharide such as cellulose or chitin or may be inorganic, eg, the silica wall of diatoms.

Motility Organelles

Many eukaryotic microorganisms have organelles called **flagella** or **cilia** that move with a wave-like motion to propel the cell through water. Eukaryotic flagella emanate from the polar region of the cell (Figure 2–3), whereas cilia, which are shorter than flagella, surround the cell. Both the flagella and the cilia of eukaryotic cells have the same basic structure and biochemical composition. Both consist of a series of microtubules, hollow protein cylinders composed of a protein called tubulin, surrounded by a membrane. The arrangement of the microtubules is called the "9 + 2 system" because it consists of nine peripheral pairs of microtubules surrounding two single central microtubules (Figure 2–4).

PROKARYOTIC CELL STRUCTURE

The prokaryotic cell is simpler than the eukaryotic cell at every level, with one exception: the cell envelope is more complex.

The Nucleoid

The prokaryotic **nucleoid,** the equivalent of the eukaryotic nucleus, can be seen with the light microscope in stained material (Figure 2–5). It is Feulgen-positive, indicating the presence of DNA. The negatively charged DNA is at least partially neutralized by small polyamines and magnesium ions, but histone-like proteins exist in bacteria and presumably play a role similar to that of histones in eukaryotic chromatin.

Electron micrographs such as Figure 2–6 reveal the absence of a nuclear membrane and a mitotic apparatus. The nuclear region is filled with DNA fibrils. The

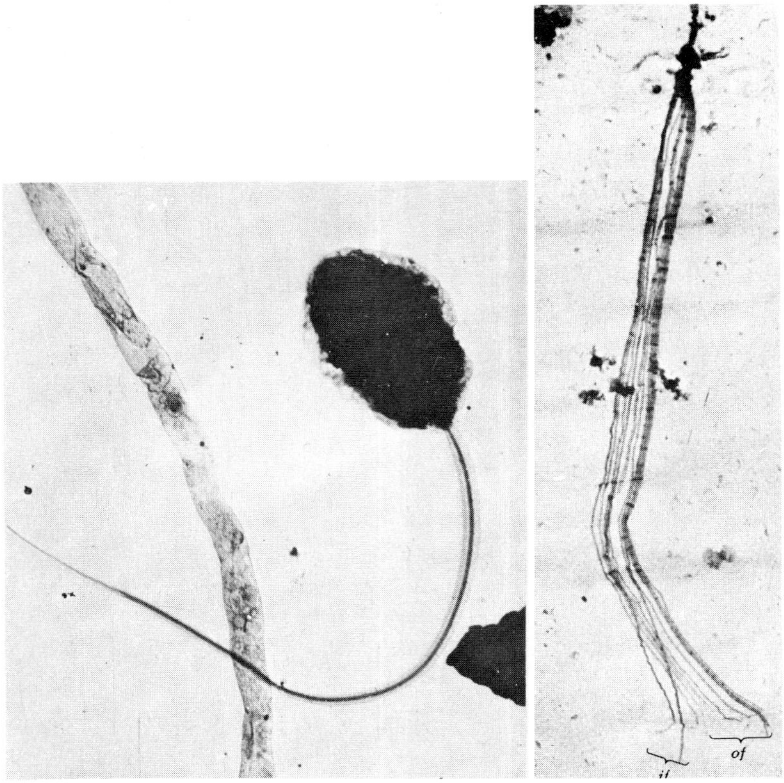

Figure 2–3. Eukaryotic flagella (3000 ×). ***Left:*** A zoospore of the fungus *Allomyces,* with a single flagellum. ***Right:*** A partially disintegrated flagellum of *Allomyces,* showing the two inner fibrils (if) and nine outer fibrils (of). (Courtesy of Manton I et al: J Exp Bot 1952;3:204.)

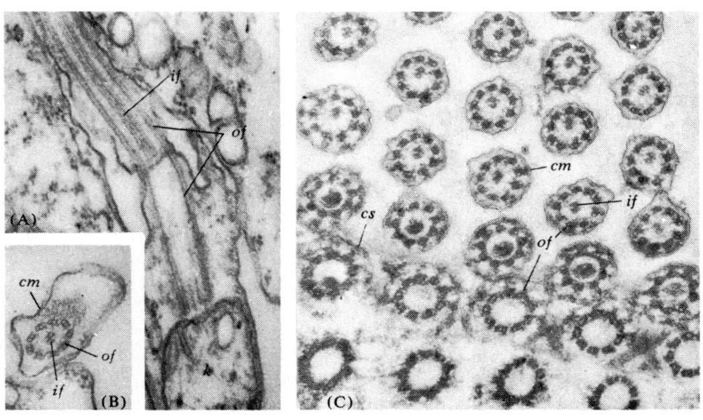

Figure 2–4. Fine structure of eukaryotic flagella and cilia (31,500 ×). ***A:*** Longitudinal section of a flagellum of *Bodo,* a protozoon, showing kinetoplast *(k)* from which extend the outer fibrils *(of).* Note the origin of the inner fibrils *(if)* at the cell surface. ***B:*** Cross section of same flagellum near the surface of the cell, showing outer fibrils *(of),* inner fibrils *(if),* and extension of cell membrane *(cm).* ***C:*** Cross section through surface layer of the ciliate protozoon *Glaucoma,* which cuts across a field of cilia just within the cell membrane (lower half) as well as outside the cell membrane (upper half). (*cs,* cell surface.) Electron micrographs taken by Dr D Pitelka. (Reproduced, with permission, from Stanier RY, Doudoroff M, Adelberg EA: *The Microbial World,* 2nd ed. Copyright © 1963. By permission of Prentice-Hall, Inc., Englewood Cliffs, NJ.)

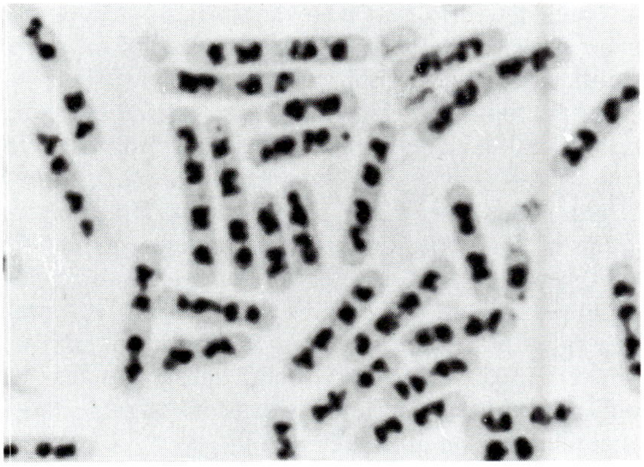

Figure 2–5. Nuclei of *Bacillus cereus* (2500 ×). (Courtesy of Robinow C: Bacteriol Rev 1956;20:207.)

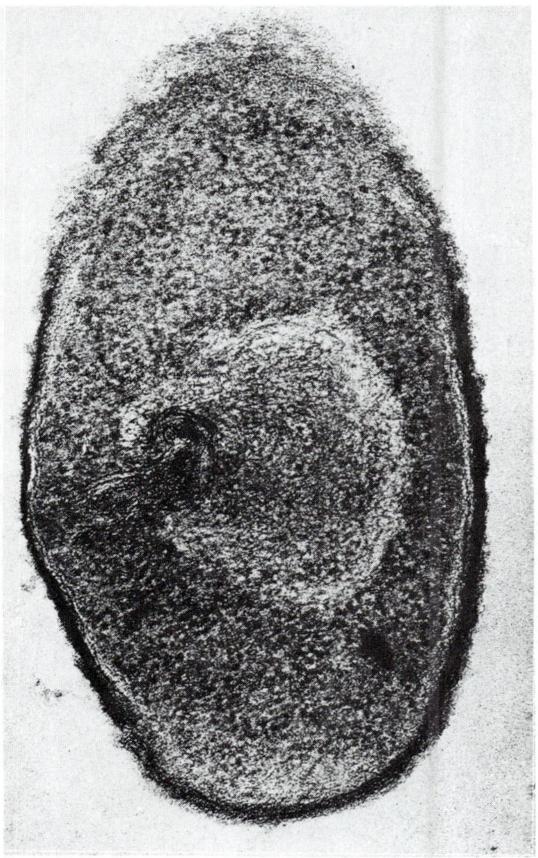

Figure 2–6. Electron micrograph of a thin section of *Bacillus subtilis,* showing the DNA in contact with a mesosome. (Reproduced, with permission, from Ryter A, Jacob F: Membrane et ségrégation nucléaire chez les bactéries. Page 267 of: *Proceedings of the 15th Colloquium on Protides of the Biological Fluids.* Vol 15. Peeters H [editor], 1967.)

nucleoid of bacterial cells has long been considered to consist of a single continuous circular molecule with a molecular weight of approximately 3×10^9. It may thus be considered to be a single, haploid chromosome, approximately 1 mm long in the unfolded state. The number of copies of this chromosome in a cell depends on the stage in the cell cycle; however, when multiple copies are present they are all the same. This classic view of the bacterial chromosome has recently been revised in light of studies using pulsed-field gel electrophoresis to separate large DNA molecules and to distinguish between circular and linear forms. The results of these studies have revealed that some prokaryotes (eg, *Borrelia burgdorferi,* the agent of Lyme disease) have a linear chromosome. Linear chromosomes have also been found in several *Streptomyces* species.

The nucleoid of most bacterial cells can be isolated by gentle lysis followed by centrifugation. The structures thus isolated consist of DNA associated with smaller amounts of RNA, RNA polymerase, and perhaps other proteins. Bacterial DNA, isolated directly on the electron microscope supporting film by gentle lysis of the cells in physiologic salt solution, is seen to have a beaded structure similar to that of eukaryotic chromatin (Figure 2–7).

Examination of serial thin sections through bacterial cells by electron microscopy reveals that the DNA is associated at one point with an invagination of the cytoplasmic membrane called a **mesosome** (Figure 2–6). This attachment is thought to play a role in the separation of the two sister chromosomes following chromosomal replication (see Cell Division, below).

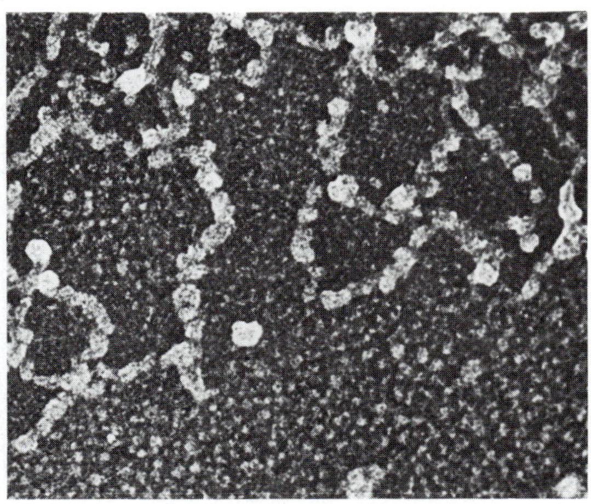

Figure 2–7. Bacteriophage λ DNA prepared by lysing infected cells with lysozyme in NaCl, 150 mmol/L, directly on an electron microscope supporting film. The beaded substructure shows a 13-nm repeating pattern. (Reproduced, with permission, from Griffith JD: Visualization of prokaryotic DNA in a regularly condensed chromatin-like fiber. Proc Natl Acad Sci USA 1976;73:563.)

The genetics and chemistry of the bacterial chromosome are presented in Chapter 4.

Cytoplasmic Structures

Prokaryotic cells lack autonomous plastids, such as mitochondria and chloroplasts; the electron transport enzymes are localized instead in the cytoplasmic membrane. The photosynthetic pigments (carotenoids, bacteriochlorophyll, phycobiliproteins) of photosynthetic bacteria are localized in specialized membrane arrangements that may appear as spherical vesicles or as flattened sheet-like layers underlying the cell membrane. In some cyanobacteria (formerly known as blue-green algae), the photosynthetic membranes often form multilayered structures known as **thylakoids** (Figure 2–8).

Bacteria often store reserve materials in the form of insoluble granules, which are deposited as osmotically inert, neutral polymers. When the source of nitrogen, sulfur, or phosphorus is limited, or when the pH is low, excess carbon in the medium is converted by some bacteria to the polymer **poly-β-hydroxybutyric acid** (Figure 2–9) and by other bacteria to various polymers of glucose such as starch and glycogen. The granules are used as carbon sources when protein and nucleic acid synthesis is resumed. Similarly, certain photosynthetic bacteria oxidize the sulfide from H_2S, producing intracellular granules of elemental **sulfur.** Finally, many bacteria accumulate granules of **polyphosphate,** which are reserves of inorganic phosphate that can be used in the synthesis of ATP. These granules are sometimes termed **volutin granules** or

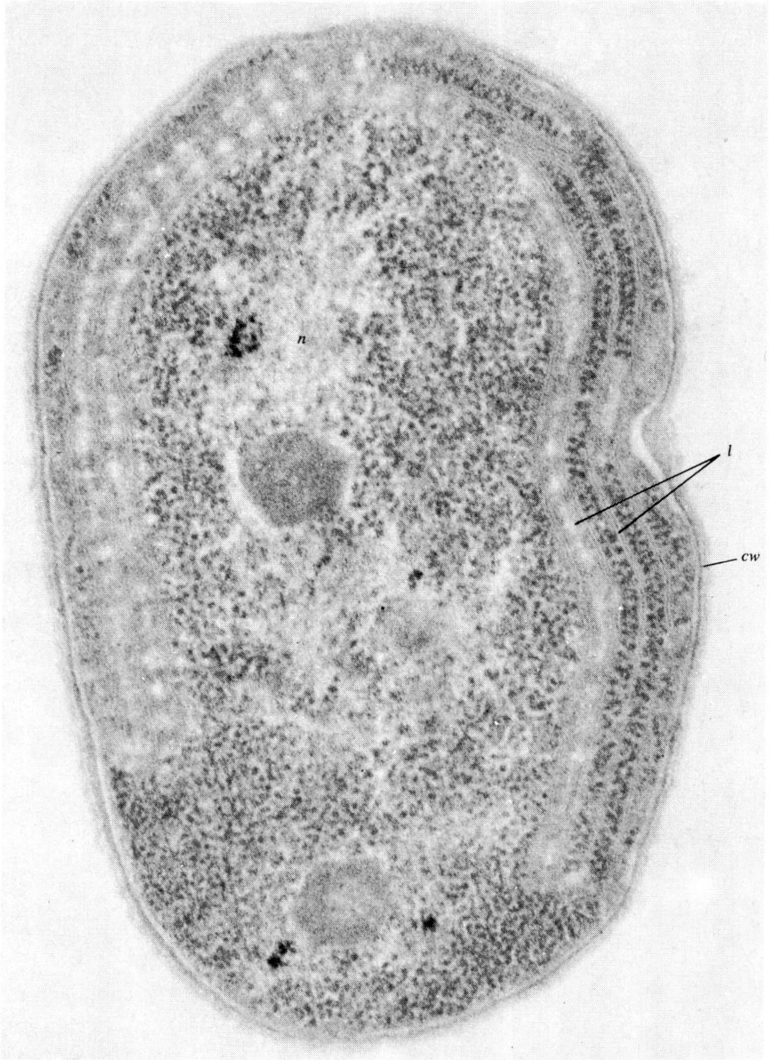

Figure 2–8. Thin section of a cyanobacterium, *Anacystis* (80,500 ×). (*l,* lamellae bearing photosynthetic pigments; *cw,* cell wall; *n,* nuclear region.) (Reprinted by permission of the Rockefeller Institute Press, from Ris H, Singh RN: J Biophys Biochem Cytol 1961;9:63.)

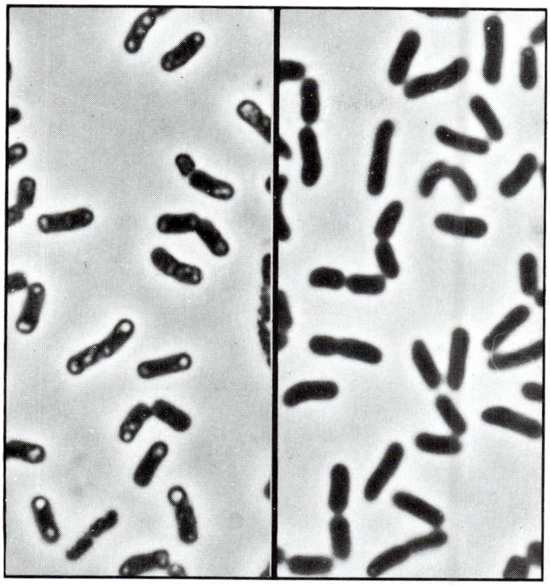

Figure 2–9. Formation and utilization of poly-β-hydroxybutyric acid in *Bacillus megaterium* (1900 ×). ***Left:*** Cells grown on glucose plus acetate, showing granules (light areas). ***Right:*** Cells from the same culture after 24 hours' further incubation in the presence of a nitrogen source but without an exogenous carbon source. The polymer has been completely metabolized. Phase contrast photomicrograph taken by Dr JF Wilkinson. (Reproduced, with permission, from Stanier RY, Doudoroff M, Adelberg EA: *The Microbial World,* 2nd ed. Copyright © 1963. By permission of Prentice-Hall, Inc., Englewood Cliffs, NJ.)

metachromatic granules because they stain red with a blue dye. They are characteristic features of the corynebacteria (Chapter 13).

Microtubular structures, which are characteristics of eukaryotic cells, are generally absent in prokaryotes. In a few instances, however, the electron microscope has revealed bacterial structures that resemble microtubules.

Certain specialized groups of bacteria contain protein-bounded vesicles in their cytoplasm. These include gas vacuoles that control buoyancy in some aquatic bacteria, carboxysomes (containing ribulosebiphosphate carboxylase, the key enzyme of CO_2 fixation) in certain autotrophic bacteria, and magnetosomes (membrane-bound iron granules) that allow certain bacteria to exhibit magnetotaxis (ie, migration or orientation of the cell with respect to the earth's magnetic field).

The Cell Envelope

The layers that surround the prokaryotic cell are referred to collectively as the cell envelope. The structure and organization of the cell envelope differ in gram-positive and gram-negative bacteria; in fact, it is this difference that defines these two major assemblages of bacterial species. Simplified diagrams of the two types of cell envelope are presented in Figure 2–10.

Many bacteria, both gram-positive and gram-negative Eubacteria and Archaeobacteria, possess a two-dimensional paracrystalline, subunit-type lattice of protein or glycoprotein molecules **(S-layer)** as the outermost component of the cell envelope (not shown in Figure 2–10). S-layers are generally composed of a single molecular species. The function of these S-layers is uncertain; in some cases, however, it has been shown to protect the cell from wall-degrading enzymes, from invasion by *Bdellovibrio bacteriovorus* (a predatory bacterium), and from bacteriophages. It also plays a role in the maintenance of cell shape in some species of Archaeobacteria, and it may be involved in cell adhesion to host epidermal surfaces.

A. The Gram-Positive Cell Envelope: The cell envelope of gram-positive cells is relatively simple, consisting of two to three layers: the **cytoplasmic membrane,** a thick **peptidoglycan layer,** and in some bacteria an outer layer called the **capsule.** The structure and function of these layers are described below.

B. The Gram-Negative Cell Envelope: This is a highly complex, multilayered structure (Figure 2–17). The cytoplasmic membrane (called the **inner membrane** in gram-negative bacteria) is surrounded by a single planar sheet of peptidoglycan to which is anchored a complex layer called the **outer membrane.** An outermost capsule may also be present. The space between the inner and outer membrane is called the **periplasmic space.**

The Cytoplasmic Membrane

A. Structure: The bacterial cytoplasmic membrane, also called the cell membrane, is visible in electron micrographs of thin sections (Figure 2–11). It is a typical "unit membrane," composed of phospholipids and proteins; Figure 2–12 illustrates a model of membrane organization. The membranes of prokaryotes are distinguished from those of eukaryotic cells by the absence of sterols, the only exception being mycoplasmas that incorporate sterols, such as cholesterol, into their membranes when growing in sterol-containing media.

Convoluted invaginations of the cytoplasmic membrane form specialized structures called mesosomes (Figure 2–13). There are two types: septal **mesosomes,** which function in the formation of cross-walls during cell division; and lateral mesosomes. The bacterial chromosome (DNA) is attached to a septal mesosome (see Cell Division, below). More extensive invaginations of the cytoplasmic membrane into the cytoplasm are found in bacteria with exceptionally active electron transport systems (eg, photosynthetic and nitrogen-fixing bacteria).

B. Function: The major functions of the cytoplasmic membrane are (1) selective permeability and transport of solutes; (2) electron transport and oxida-

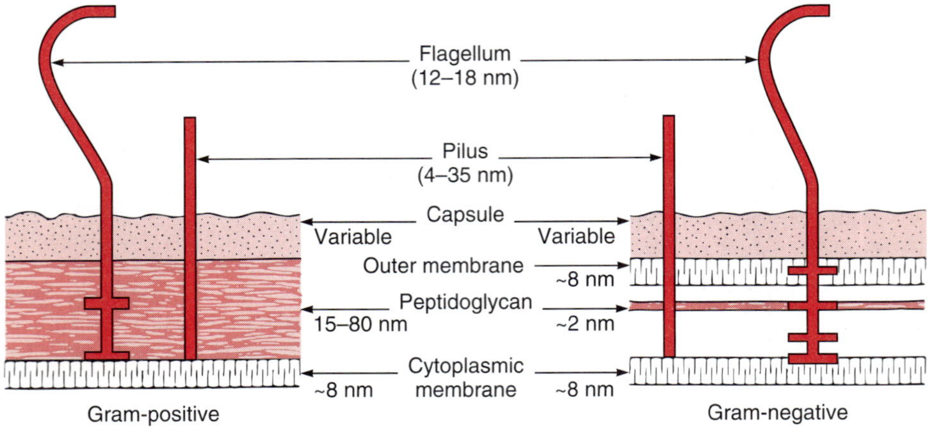

Figure 2–10. Comparison of the structures of gram-positive and gram-negative cell envelopes. The region between the cytoplasmic membrane and the outer membrane of the gram-negative envelope is called the periplasmic space. (Reproduced, with permission, from Ingraham JL, Maaløe O, Neidhardt FC: *Growth of the Bacterial Cell.* Sinauer Associates, 1983.)

tive phosphorylation, in aerobic species; (3) excretion of hydrolytic exoenzymes; (4) bearing the enzymes and carrier molecules that function in the biosynthesis of DNA, cell wall polymers, and membrane lipids; and (5) bearing the receptors and other proteins of the chemotactic and other sensory transduction systems.

At least 50% of the cytoplasmic membrane must be in the semifluid state in order for cell growth to occur. At low temperatures, this is achieved by greatly increased synthesis and incorporation of unsaturated fatty acids.

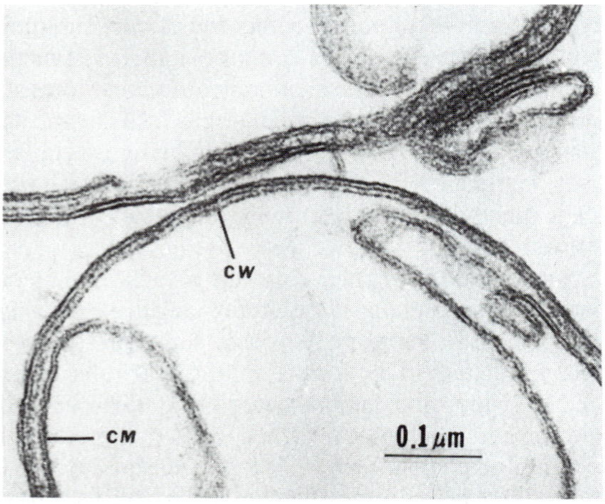

Figure 2–11. The cell membrane. Fragments of the cell membrane (CM) are seen attached to the cell wall (CW) in preparations made from *Escherichia coli.* (Reproduced, with permission, from Schnaitman CA: Solubilization of the cytoplasmic membrane of *Escherichia coli* by Triton X-100. J Bacteriol 1971;108:545.)

1. Permeability and transport–The membrane is both a permeability barrier (lipophobic solutes do not penetrate passively) and a permeability link: Specific protein systems **(permeases)** are present that either facilitate the passive diffusion of specific solutes or catalyze energy-dependent active transport against a gradient.

There are two types of active transport systems: primary and secondary. In primary systems ("pumps"), metabolic energy is used to drive solutes through the membrane against their concentration gradients. In aerobic bacteria, the primary pump is the electron transport system, which uses the energy derived from substrate oxidation to export protons (Chapter 6). As illustrated in Figure 6–32, the exported protons reenter the cell via the membrane ATPase; the energy derived from this ion flow is used by the ATPase to synthesize ATP from ADP plus inorganic phosphate. In anaerobic bacteria, which lack the electron transport system, the system is reversed; proton export takes place through the ATPase at the expense of energy derived from the breakdown of ATP.

In secondary systems, the energy stored in the cation gradients and membrane potential produced by the pumps is used to actively transport solutes, such as amino acids and sugars, into the cell. This is accomplished by cotransport systems: the carrier binds cation and solute, transporting both simultaneously. Since the cation gradient is directed strongly inward, the combined electrochemical gradient drives the solute into the cell against its own concentration gradient.

The cell also has specific protein carriers in the membrane to facilitate the diffusion of certain solutes either into or out of the cell. Thus, if the cell is placed in a medium containing a high concentration of glycerol, it can equilibrate glycerol by facilitated diffusion in the absence of a coupled energy source.

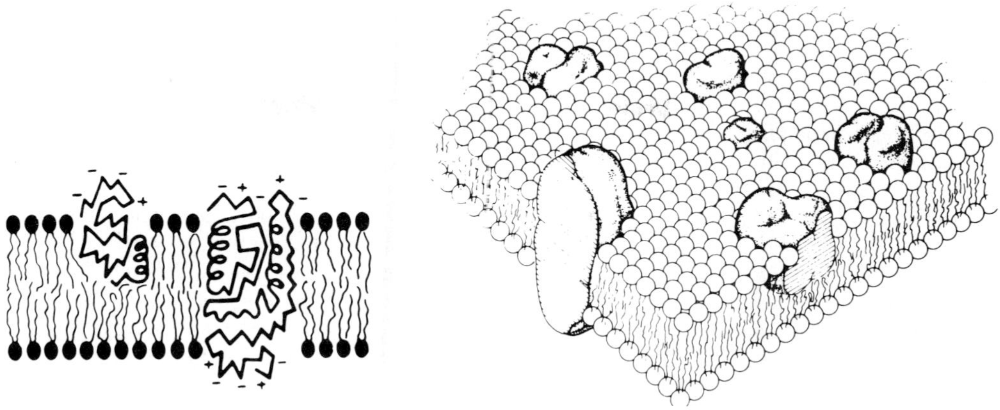

Figure 2–12. A model of membrane structure. Folded polypeptide molecules are visualized as embedded in a phospholipid bilayer, with their hydrophilic regions protruding into the intracellular space, extracellular space, or both. (Reproduced, with permission, from Singer SJ, Nicolson AL: The fluid mosaic model of the structure of cell membranes. Science 1972;175:720. Copyright © 1972 by the American Association for the Advancement of Science.)

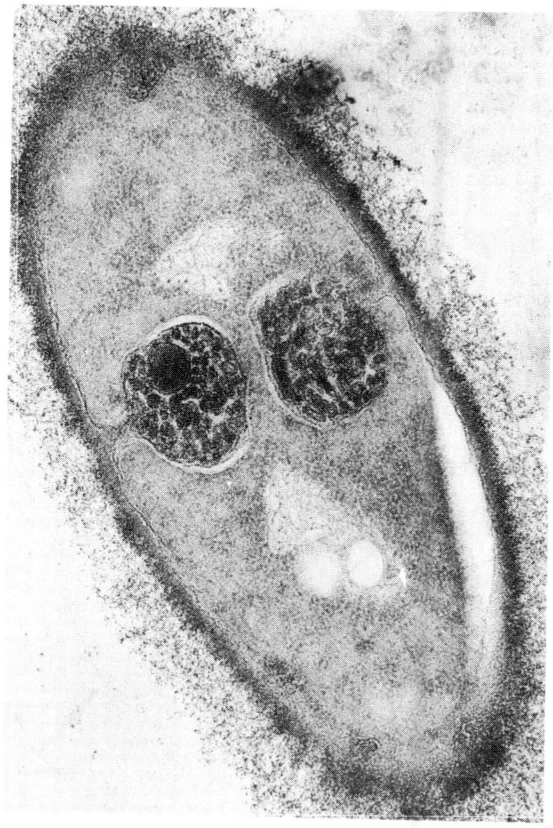

Figure 2–13. Septal mesosomes. A septal mesosome, formed as a concentric fold of the plasma membrane, grows inward. The new transverse septum is seen forming at the base of the concentric mesosome. Cell division will occur by fusion of the membrane layers surrounding the mesosome. (Reproduced, with permission, from Ellar DJ, Lundgren D, Slepecky RA: Fine structure of *Bacillus megaterium* during synchronous growth. J Bacteriol 1967;84:1189.)

In gram-negative bacteria, the transport of many nutrients is facilitated by specific **binding proteins** located in the periplasmic space. The nutrient is first bound to its specific binding protein with a dissociation constant in the range of 10^{-6} to 10^{-7} mol/L; it is then passed to a transport carrier protein of the inner membrane. Such systems are called "shock-sensitive," since osmotic shock (sudden dilution of a cell suspension) damages the outer membrane and allows the binding proteins to leak out.

In addition to true transport, in which a solute is moved across the membrane without change in structure, bacteria use a process called **group translocation** (vectorial metabolism) to effect the net uptake of certain sugars (eg, glucose and mannose), the substrate becoming phosphorylated during the transport process. This process allows bacteria to use their energy resources efficiently by coupling transport with metabolism. In this process, a membrane carrier protein is first phosphorylated in the cytoplasm at the expense of phosphoenolpyruvate; the phosphorylated carrier then binds the free sugar at the exterior membrane face and transports it into the cytoplasm, releasing it as sugar-phosphate. Such systems of sugar transport are called **phosphotransferase systems.**

In *Escherichia coli,* the transport of potassium ion is used to regulate turgor pressure. An increase in external osmolarity at constant K^+ concentration activates the expression of genes coding for a set of K^+ transport proteins and also increases the activity of those proteins.

2. Electron transport and oxidative phosphorylation–The cytochromes and other enzymes and components of the respiratory chain, including certain dehydrogenases, are located in the cytoplasmic membrane. The bacterial cytoplasmic membrane is thus a functional analogue of the mitochondrial membrane—a relationship which has been taken by many biologists to support the theory that mitochondria have evolved from symbiotic bacteria. The mechanism by which ATP generation is coupled to electron transport is discussed in Chapter 6.

3. Excretion of hydrolytic exoenzymes–All organisms that rely on macromolecular organic polymers as a source of nutrients (eg, proteins, polysaccharides, lipids) excrete hydrolytic enzymes that degrade the polymers to subunits small enough to penetrate the cytoplasmic membrane. Higher animals secrete such enzymes into the lumen of the digestive tract; bacteria secrete them directly into the external medium (in the case of gram-positive cells) or into the space (the periplasmic space) between the peptidoglycan layer and the outer membrane of the cell wall in the case of gram-negative bacteria (see The Cell Wall, below). Some gram-negative bacteria such as *Pseudomonas, Erwinia,* and *Serratia* secrete large amounts of proteases, amylases, and pectinases into the extracellular environment. Secreted proteins are synthesized on cytoplasmic ribosomes as preproteins carrying an extra sequence of 15–40 amino acids (most commonly about 20 amino acids) at the amino terminal. This "leader" or "signal" sequence, acting in concert with specific cytoplasmic and membrane proteins, binds the ribosome to the inner face of the cell membrane early in the process of polypeptide synthesis. Translocation through the membrane, initiated by the leader sequence, then takes place; it is not clear whether this occurs simultaneously with chain elongation or late in the process. Following translocation, the leader sequence is cleaved off by a membrane-bound leader peptidase, and the finished protein is released from the membrane in a final step.

Many pathogenic bacteria secrete enzymes (eg, IgA1 protease) and toxins (eg, cholera toxin) by a similar mechanism that are important virulence factors.

4. Biosynthetic functions–The cytoplasmic membrane is the site of the carrier lipids on which the subunits of the cell wall are assembled (see synthesis of cell wall substances in Chapter 6) as well as of the enzymes of cell wall biosynthesis. The enzymes of phospholipid synthesis are also localized in the cytoplasmic membrane. Finally, some proteins of the DNA replicating complex are present at discrete sites in the membrane, presumably in the septal mesosomes to which the DNA is attached.

5. Chemotactic systems–Attractants and repellents bind to specific receptors in the bacterial membrane (see Flagella, below). There are at least 20 different chemoreceptors in the membrane of *E coli,* some of which also function as a first step in the transport process.

C. Antibacterial Agents Affecting the Cell Membrane: Detergents, which contain lipophilic and hydrophilic groups, disrupt cytoplasmic membranes and kill the cell (Chapter 4). One class of antibiotics, the polymyxins, consists of detergent-like cyclic peptides that selectively damage membranes containing phosphatidylethanolamine, a major component of bacterial membranes. A number of antibiotics specifically interfere with biosynthetic functions of the cytoplasmic membranes—eg, nalidixic acid and novobiocin inhibit DNA synthesis, and novobiocin also inhibits teichoic acid synthesis.

A third class of membrane-active agents are the ionophores, compounds that permit rapid diffusion of specific cations through the membrane. Valinomycin, for example, specifically mediates the passage of potassium ions. Some ionophores act by forming hydrophilic pores in the membrane; others act as lipid-soluble ion carriers that behave as though they shuttle back and forth within the membrane. Ionophores can kill cells by discharging the membrane potential, which is essential for oxidative phosphorylation as well as for other membrane-mediated processes; they are not selective for bacteria but act on the membranes of all cells.

The Cell Wall

The layers of the cell envelope lying between the cytoplasmic membrane and the capsule are referred to collectively as the "cell wall." In gram-positive bacteria, the cell wall consists mainly of peptidoglycan and teichoic acids (see below); in gram-negative bacteria, the cell wall includes the peptidoglycan and outer membrane.

The internal osmotic pressure of most bacteria ranges from 5 to 20 atm as a result of solute concentration via active transport. In most environments, this pressure would be sufficient to burst the cell were it not for the presence of a high-tensile-strength cell wall (Figure 2–14). The bacterial cell wall owes its strength to a layer composed of a substance variously referred to as murein, mucopeptide, or **peptidoglycan** (all are synonyms). The structure of peptidoglycan will be discussed below.

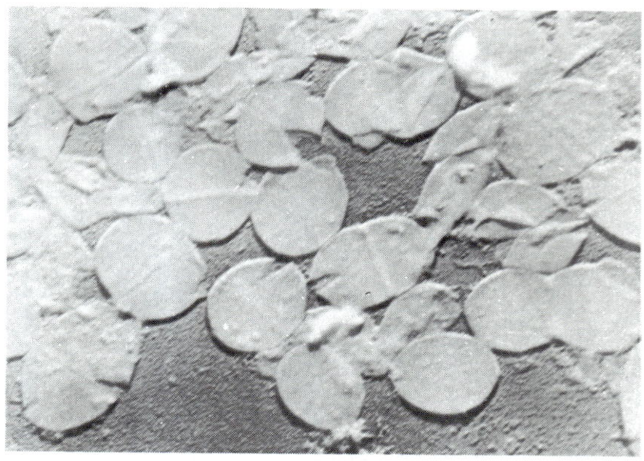

Figure 2–14. Cell walls of *Streptococcus faecalis,* removed from protoplasts by mechanical disintegration and differential centrifugation (11,000 ×). (Courtesy of Salton M, Home R: Biochim Biophys Acta 1951;7:177.)

Bacteria are classified as gram-positive or gram-negative according to their response to the Gram staining procedure. This procedure, named for the histologist Christian Gram, who developed this differential staining procedure in an attempt to stain bacteria in infected tissues. The cells are first stained with crystal violet and iodine and then washed with acetone or alcohol. The latter step decolorizes gram-negative bacteria but not gram-positive bacteria.

The difference between gram-positive and gram-negative bacteria has been shown to reside in the cell wall: gram-positive cells can be decolorized with acetone or alcohol if the cell wall is removed after the staining step but before the washing step. Although the chemical composition of gram-positive and gram-negative walls is now fairly well known (see below), the reason gram-positive walls block the dye-extraction step is still unclear.

In addition to giving osmotic protection, the cell wall plays an essential role in cell division as well as serving as a primer for its own biosynthesis. Various layers of the wall are the sites of major antigenic determinants of the cell surface, and one component—the lipopolysaccharide of gram-negative cell walls—is responsible for the nonspecific endotoxin activity of gram-negative bacteria. The cell wall is, in general, nonselectively permeable; one layer of the gram-negative wall, however—the outer membrane—hinders the passage of relatively large molecules (see below).

The biosynthesis of the cell wall and the antibiotics that interfere with this process are discussed in Chapter 6.

A. The Peptidoglycan Layer: Peptidoglycan is a complex polymer consisting, for the purposes of description, of three parts: a backbone, composed of alternating N-acetylglucosamine and N-acetylmuramic acid; a set of identical tetrapeptide side chains attached to N-acetylmuramic acid; and a set of identical peptide cross-bridges (Figure 2–15). The backbone is the same in all bacterial species; the tetrapeptide side chains and the peptide cross-bridges vary from species to species, those of *Staphylococcus aureus* being illustrated in Figure 2–15. In many gram-negative cell walls, the cross-bridge consists of a direct peptide linkage between the diaminopimelic acid (DAP) amino group of one side chain and the carboxyl group of the terminal D-alanine of a second side chain.

The tetrapeptide side chains of all species, however, have certain important features in common. Most have L-alanine at position 1 (attached to N-acetylmuramic acid); D-glutamate or substituted D-glutamate at position 2; and D-alanine at position 4. Position 3 is the most variable one: Most gram-negative bacteria have diaminopimelic acid at this position, to which is linked the lipoprotein cell wall component discussed below. Gram-positive bacteria may have diaminopimelic acid, L-lysine, or any of several other L-amino acids at position 3.

Diaminopimelic acid is a unique element of prokaryotic cell walls and is the immediate precursor of lysine in the bacterial biosynthesis of that amino acid (Figure 6–23). Bacterial mutants that are blocked prior to diaminopimelic acid in the biosynthetic pathway grow normally when provided with diaminopimelic acid in the medium; when given L-lysine alone, however, they lyse, since they continue to grow but are specifically unable to make new cell wall peptidoglycan.

The fact that all peptidoglycan chains are cross-linked means that each peptidoglycan layer is a single giant molecule. In gram-positive bacteria, there are as many as 40 sheets of peptidoglycan, comprising up to 50% of the cell wall material; in gram-negative bacteria, there appears to be only one or two sheets, comprising 5–10% of the wall material. Bacteria owe their shapes, which are characteristic of particular species, to their cell wall structure.

Several prokaryotic groups, collectively called the archaeobacteria, lack a peptidoglycan layer. In some species within this group, a similar polymer exists containing N-acetyl sugars and three L-amino acids; muramic acid and D-amino acids are absent. In other archaeobacteria, a protein layer is present instead. These organisms also show major differences in their lipids and RNAs (Chapter 1).

B. Special Components of Gram-Positive Cell Walls: Most gram-positive cell walls contain considerable amounts of **teichoic** and **teichuronic acids,** which may account for up to 50% of the dry weight of the wall and 10% of the dry weight of the total cell. In addition, some gram-positive walls may contain polysaccharide molecules.

1. Teichoic and teichuronic acids–These are water-soluble polymers, containing ribitol or glycerol residues joined through phosphodiester linkages and carrying one or more amino acid or sugar substituents (Figure 2–16A). There are two types of teichoic acids: wall teichoic acid, covalently linked to peptidoglycan; and membrane teichoic acid (lipoteichoic acid), covalently linked to membrane glycolipid and concentrated in mesosomes. Some gram-positive species lack wall teichoic acids, but all appear to contain membrane teichoic acids.

The teichoic acids constitute major surface antigens of those gram-positive species that possess them, and their accessibility to antibodies has been taken as evidence that they lie on the outside surface of the peptidoglycan layer. Their activity is often increased, however, by partial digestion of the peptidoglycan; thus, much of the teichoic acid may lie between the cytoplasmic membrane and the peptidoglycan layer, possibly extending upward through pores in the latter (Figure 2–16B). In the pneumococcus *(Streptococcus pneumoniae),* the teichoic acids bear the antigenic determinants called Forssman antigen. In *Streptococcus pyogenes,* lipoteichoic acid is associated with the M protein that protrudes from the cell membrane through

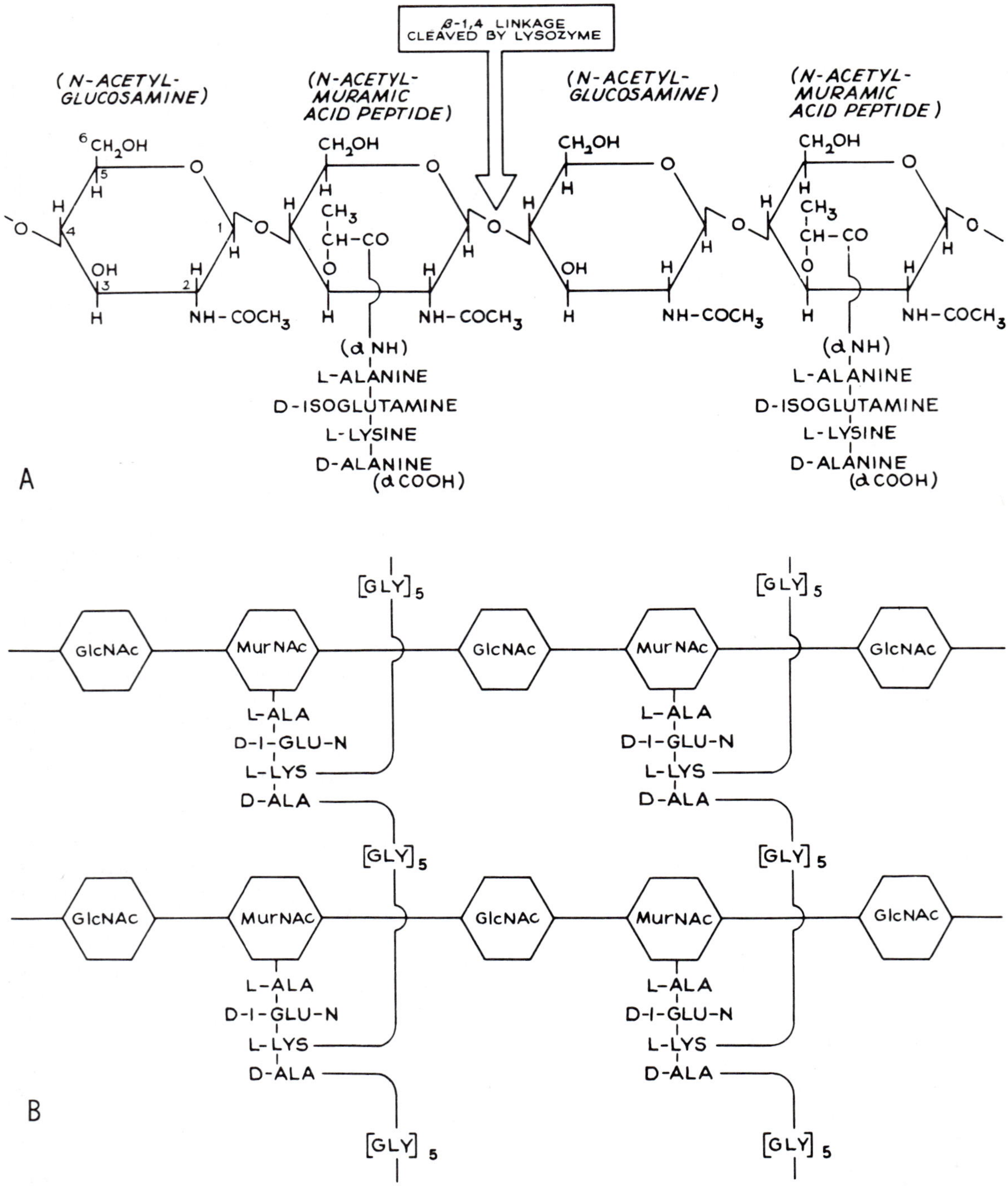

Figure 2–15. ***A:*** A segment of the peptidoglycan of *Staphylococcus aureus*. The backbone of the polymer consists of alternating subunits of N-acetylglucosamine and N-acetylmuramic acid connected by β-1,4 linkages. The muramic acid residues are linked to short peptides, the composition of which varies from one bacterial species to another. In some species, the L-lysine residues are replaced by diaminopimelic acid, an amino acid that is found in nature only in prokaryotic cell walls. Note the D-amino acids, which are also characteristic constituents of prokaryotic cell walls. The peptide chains of the peptidoglycan are cross-linked between parallel polysaccharide backbones, as shown in Fig 2–15B. ***B:*** Schematic representation of the peptidoglycan lattice that is formed by cross-linking. Bridges composed of pentaglycine peptide chains connect the α-carboxyl of the terminal D-alanine residue of one chain with the ε-amino group of the L-lysine residue of the next chain. The nature of the cross-linking bridge varies among different species.

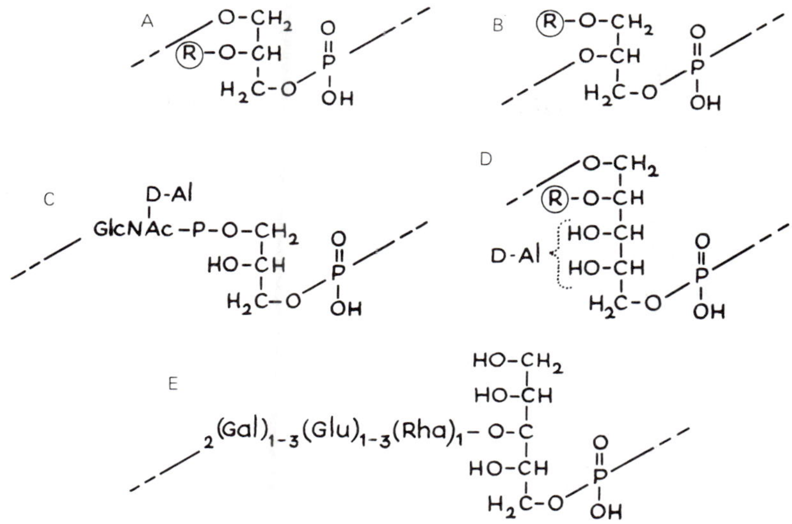

Figure 2–16A. Repeat units of some teichoic acids. ***A:*** Glycerol teichoic acid of *Lactobacillus casei* 7469 (R, D-alanine). ***B:*** Glycerol teichoic acid of *Actinomyces antibioticus* (R, D-alanine). ***C:*** Glycerol teichoic acid of *Staphylococcus lactis* 13. D-Alanine occurs on the 6 position of N-acetylglucosamine. ***D:*** Ribitol teichoic acids of *Bacillus subtilis* (R, glucose) and *Actinomyces streptomycini* (R, succinate). (The D-alanine is attached to position 3 or 4 of ribitol.) ***E:*** Ribitol teichoic acid of the type 6 pneumococcal capsule. (Reproduced with permission, from Stanier RY, Doudoroff M, Adelberg EA: *The Microbial World,* 2nd ed. Copyright © 1963. By permission of Prentice-Hall, Inc., Englewood Cliffs, NJ.)

the peptidoglycan layer. The long molecular M protein together with the lipoteichoic acid form microfibrils that facilitate the attachment of *S pyogenes* to animal cells.

The repeat units of some teichoic acids are shown in Figure 2–16A. The repeat units may be glycerol, joined by 1,3- or 1,2-linkages; ribitol, joined by 1,5-linkages; or more complex units in which glycerol or ribitol is joined to a sugar residue such as glucose, galactose, or N-acetylglucosamine. The chains may be 30 or more repeat units in length, though chain lengths of ten or less are common.

Most teichoic acids contain large amounts of D-alanine, usually attached to position 2 or 3 of glycerol or position 3 or 4 of ribitol. In some of the more complex teichoic acids, however, D-alanine is attached to one of the sugar residues. In addition to D-alanine, other substituents may be attached to the free hydroxyl groups of glycerol and ribitol, eg, glucose, galactose, N-acetylglucosamine, N-acetylgalactosamine, or succinate. A given species may have more than one type of sugar substituent in addition to D-alanine; in such cases, it is not certain whether the different sugars occur on the same or on separate teichoic acid molecules. The composition of the teichoic acid formed by a given bacterial species can vary with the composition of the growth medium.

The function of teichoic acids is still a matter of speculation. The teichoic acids bind magnesium ion and may play a role in the supply of this ion to the cell. They also play a role in the normal functioning of the cell envelope; thus, replacement of choline by ethanolamine as a component of the teichoic acid of pneumococci causes the cells to resist autolysis and to lose the ability to take up transforming DNA (see Chapter 7). Membrane teichoic acids may serve to anchor the wall to the underlying cell membrane.

The teichuronic acids are similar polymers, but the repeat units include sugar acids (such as N-acetylmannosuronic or D-glucosuronic acid) instead of phosphoric acids. They are synthesized in place of teichoic acids when phosphate is limiting.

2. Polysaccharides–The hydrolysis of gram-positive walls has yielded, from certain species, neutral sugars such as mannose, arabinose, galactose, rhamnose, and glucosamine and acidic sugars such as glucuronic acid and mannuronic acid. It has been proposed that these sugars exist as subunits of polysaccharides in the cell wall; the discovery, however, that teichoic and teichuronic acids may contain a variety of sugars (Figure 2–16A) leaves the true origin of these sugars uncertain.

C. Special Components of Gram-Negative Cell Walls: Gram-negative cell walls contain three components that lie outside of the peptidoglycan layer: lipoprotein, outer membrane, and lipopolysaccharide (Figure 2–17).

1. Lipoprotein–Molecules of an unusual **lipoprotein** cross-link the outer membrane and peptidoglycan layers. The lipoprotein contains 57 amino acids, representing repeats of a 15-amino-acid sequence; it is peptide-linked to diaminopimelic acid

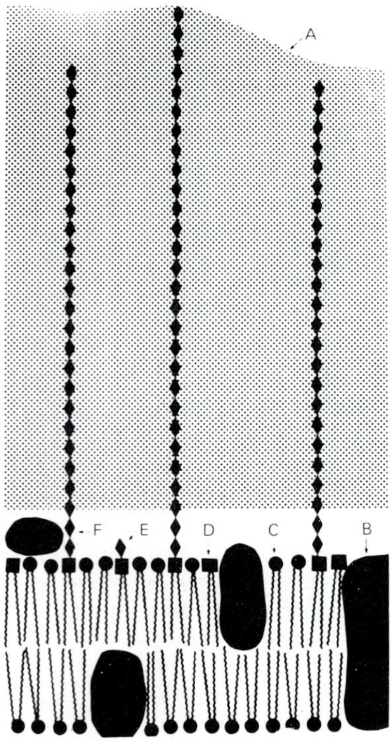

Figure 2–16B. Lipoteichoic acids. A model of the cell wall and membrane of a gram-positive bacterium, showing lipoteichoic acid molecules extending through the cell wall. The wall teichoic acids, covalently linked to muramic acid residues of the peptidoglycan layer, are not shown. (A, cell wall; B, protein; C, phospholipid; D, glycolipid; E, phosphatidyl glycolipid; F, lipoteichoic acid.) (From Van Driel D et al: Cellular location of the lipoteichoic acids of *Lactobacillus fermenti* NCTC 6991 and *Lactobacillus casei* NCTC 6375. J Ultrastruct Res 1971;43:483.)

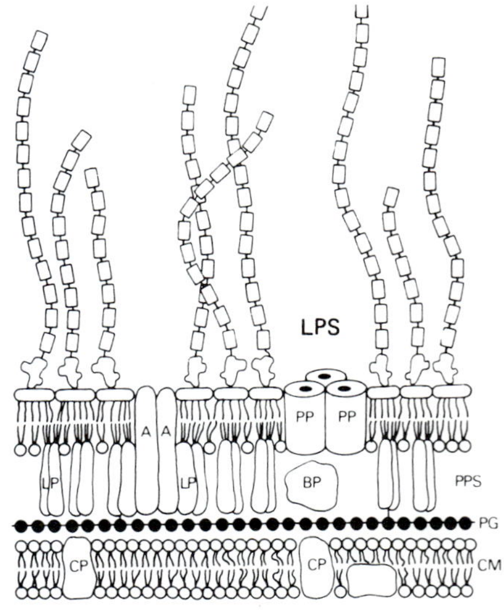

Figure 2–17. Molecular organization of the outer membrane of gram-negative bacteria. (LPS, lipopolysaccharide; A, OmpA protein; PP, pore protein [matrix porin]; LP, lipoprotein; BP, nutrient-binding protein; PPS, periplasmic space; PG, peptidoglycan; CP, carrier protein; CM, cytoplasmic membrane.) (Reproduced, with permission, from Lugtenberg B, Van Alphen LV: Molecular architecture and functioning of the outer membrane of *Escherichia coli* and other gram-negative bacteria. Biochim Biophys Acta 1983;737:51.)

residues of the peptidoglycan tetrapeptide side chains. The lipid component, consisting of a diglyceride thioether linked to a terminal cysteine, is noncovalently inserted in the outer membrane. Lipoprotein is numerically the most abundant protein of gram-negative cells (≈700,000 molecules per cell). Its function (inferred from the behavior of mutants that lack it) is to stabilize the outer membrane and anchor it to the peptidoglycan layer.

2. Outer membrane–The outer membrane is a bilayered structure; its inner leaflet resembles in composition that of the cytoplasmic membrane while the phospholipids of the outer leaflet are replaced by **lipopolysaccharide** (LPS) molecules (see below). As a result, the leaflets of this membrane are asymmetrical, and the properties of this bilayer differ considerably from those of a symmetrical biologic membrane such as the cytoplasmic membrane.

The ability of the outer membrane to exclude hydrophobic molecules is an unusual feature among biologic membranes and serves to protect the cell (in the case of enteric bacteria) from bile salts. Because of its lipid nature, the outer membrane would be expected to exclude hydrophilic molecules as well. However, the outer membrane has special channels, consisting of protein molecules called **porins,** that permit the passive diffusion of low-molecular-weight hydrophilic compounds like sugars, amino acids, and certain ions. Large antibiotic molecules penetrate the outer membrane relatively slowly, which accounts for the relatively high antibiotic resistance of gram-negative bacteria. The permeability of the outer membrane varies widely from one gram-negative species to another; in *Pseudomonas aeruginosa,* for example, which is extremely resistant to antibacterial agents, the outer membrane is 100 times less permeable than that of *E coli.*

The major proteins of the outer membrane, named according to the genes that code for them, have been placed into several functional categories on the basis of mutants in which they are lacking and on the basis of experiments in which purified proteins have been reconstituted into artificial membranes. Porins, exemplified by OmpC, D, and F and PhoE of *E coli* and *Salmonella typhimurium,* are trimeric proteins that penetrate both faces of the outer membrane. They form relatively nonspecific pores that permit the free diffusion of small hydrophilic solutes across the membrane. The porins of different species have different exclusion limits, ranging from molecular weights of about 600 in *E coli* and *S typhimurium* to more than 3000 in *P aeruginosa.*

Members of a second group of outer membrane proteins, which resemble porins in many ways, are exemplified by LamB and Tsx. LamB, an inducible porin that is the receptor for lambda bacteriophage, is responsible for most of the transmembrane diffusion of maltose and maltodextrins; Tsx, the receptor for T6 bacteriophage, is responsible for the transmembrane diffusion of nucleosides and some amino acids. LamB allows some passage of other solutes, however; its relative specificity may reflect weak interactions of solutes with configuration-specific sites within the channel.

The OmpA protein is an abundant protein in the outer membrane. The OmpA protein serves as the receptor for several bacteriophages and also participates in the anchoring of the outer membrane to the peptidoglycan layer; it is also the sex pilus receptor in F-mediated bacterial conjugation (Chapter 7).

The outer membrane also contains a set of less abundant proteins which are involved in the transport of specific molecules such as vitamin B_{12} and iron-siderophore complexes. They show high affinity for their substrates and probably function like the classic carrier transport systems of the inner (cytoplasmic) membrane. The proper function of these proteins requires energy coupled through a protein called TonB. Additional minor proteins include a limited number of enzymes, among them phospholipases and proteases, as well as some penicillin-binding proteins.

The topology of the major proteins of the outer membrane, based on cross-linking studies and analyses of functional relationships, is shown in Figure 2–17. The outer membrane is connected to both the murein layer and the cytoplasmic membrane. The connection with the murein layer is primarily mediated by the outer membrane lipoprotein. About one-third of the lipoprotein molecules are covalently linked to murein and help hold the two structures together. A noncovalent association of some of the porins with the murein layer plays a lesser role in connecting the outer membrane with this structure. Outer membrane proteins are synthesized on ribosomes bound to the cytoplasmic surface of the inner membrane; how they are transferred to the outer membrane is still uncertain, but one hypothesis suggests that transfer occurs at zones of adhesion between the cytoplasmic and outer membranes, which are visible in the electron microscope. These zones of adhesion are also known as "Bayer junctions" after their discoverer; there are about 200 of these junctions per *E coli* cell.

3. Lipopolysaccharide (LPS)–The lipopolysaccharide of gram-negative cell walls consists of a complex lipid, called lipid A, to which is attached a polysaccharide made up of a core and a terminal series of repeat units (Figure 2–18A).

Lipid A consists of phosphorylated glucosamine disaccharide units to which are attached a number of long-chain fatty acids (Figure 2–18B). β-Hydroxymyristic acid, a C_{14} fatty acid, is always present and is unique to this lipid; the other fatty acids, along with substituent groups on the phosphates, vary according to the bacterial species.

The polysaccharide core, shown in Figure 2–18C, is similar in all gram-negative species that have LPS. Each species, however, contains a unique repeat unit, that of *Salmonella newington* being shown in Figure 2–18D. The repeat units are usually linear trisaccharides or branched tetra- or pentasaccharides.

The negatively charged LPS molecules are noncovalently cross-bridged by divalent cations; this stabilizes the membrane and provides a barrier to hydrophobic molecules. Removal of the divalent cations with chelating agents or their displacement by polycationic antibiotics such as polymyxins and aminoglycosides renders the outer membrane permeable to large hydrophobic molecules.

LPS, which is extremely toxic to animals, has been called the **endotoxin** of gram-negative bacteria because it is firmly bound to the cell surface and is released only when the cells are lysed. When LPS is split into lipid A and polysaccharide, all of the toxicity is associated with the former. The polysaccharide, on the other hand, represents a major surface antigen of the bacterial cell—the so-called **O antigen.** Antigenic specificity is conferred by the terminal repeat units, which surround the cell by forming a layer of hydrophilic polysaccharides. The number of possible antigenic types is very great: over 1000 have been recognized in *Salmonella* alone.

LPS is attached to the outer membrane by hydrophobic bonds. It is synthesized on the cytoplasmic membrane and transported to its final exterior position. The presence of LPS is required for the function of many outer membrane proteins.

Not all gram-negative bacteria have outer membrane LPS composed of a variable number of repeated oligosaccharide units (Figure 2–18); the outer membrane glycolipids of bacteria that colonize mucosal surfaces (eg, *Neisseria meningitidis, N gonorrhoeae, Haemophilus influenzae,* and *H ducreyi*) have relatively short, multiantennary (ie, branched) glycans (Figure 2–19). These smaller glycolipids have been compared with the "R-type" truncated LPS structures, which lack O-antigens and are produced by rough mutants of enteric bacteria such as *E coli.* However, their structures more closely resemble those of the glycosphingolipids of mammalian cell membranes, and they are more properly termed **lipooligosaccharides** (LOS). These molecules exhibit extensive antigenic and structural diversity even within a single strain. LOS is an important virulence factor. Epitopes have been identified on LOS which mimic host structures and may enable these organisms to evade the immune response of the host. Some LOS (eg, those from *N gonorrhoeae, N meningitidis,* and *H ducreyi*) have a terminal N-acetyllactosamine (Galβ1-4-GlcNAc)

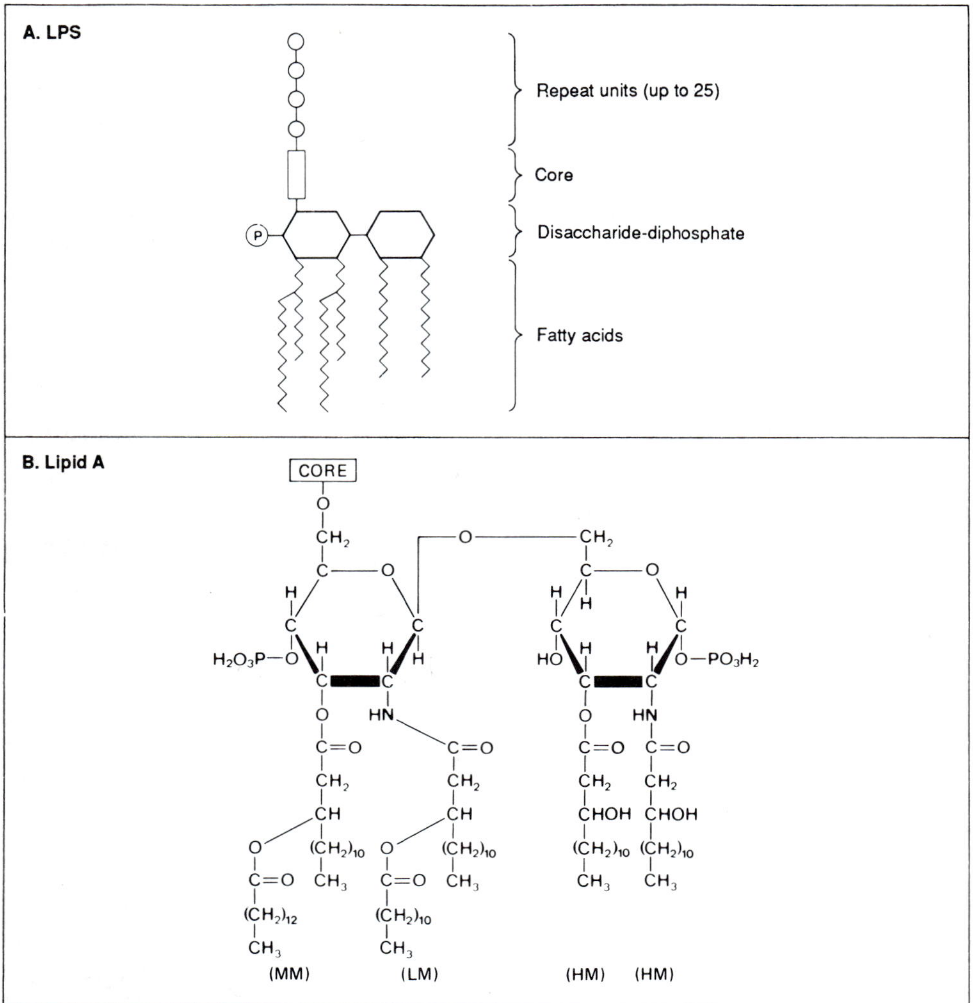

C. Core

Glu-GlcNAc
Gal
Glu-Gal
Hep
Hep-P-P-Eth
KDO
KDO-KDO-P-Eth • N

KDO = Keto-deoxy-octulonate
Hep = L-Glycero-D-mannoheptose
HM = ß-Hydroxymyristic acid (C_{14})
LM = Lauroxymyristic acid
MM = Myristoxymyristic acid
Eth•N = Ethanolamine
Glu = Glucose
GlcNAc = N-Acetylglucosamine
Gal = Galactose

D. Repeat unit

Example: (repeated up to 25 times)

Mannose
Rhamnose
Galactose

Figure 2–18. The lipopolysaccharide (LPS) of the gram-negative cell envelope. ***A:*** A segment of the polymer, showing the arrangements of the major constituents. ***B:*** The structure of lipid A of *Salmonella typhimurium.* ***C:*** The polysaccharide core. ***D:*** A typical repeat unit *(Salmonella newington).* Serologic specificity is determined in part by the type of bond (α or β) between monosaccharide units.

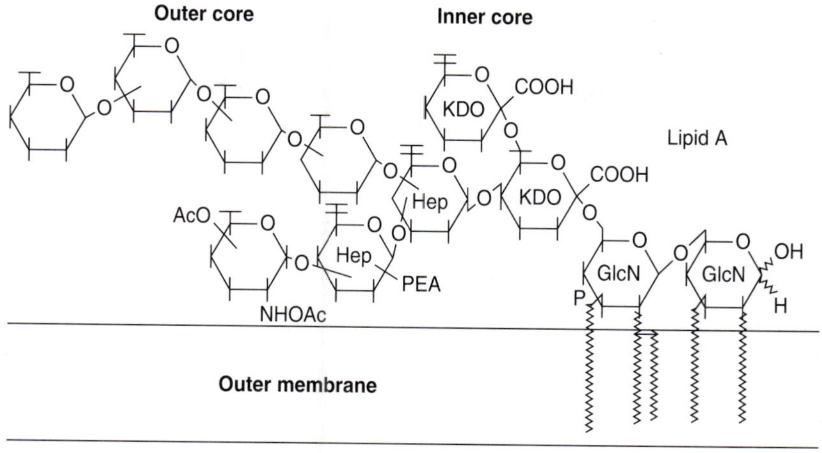

Figure 2–19. Structural model for neisserial lipo-oligosaccharide showing the membrane-associated lipid A and the inner-core and variable outer-core oligosaccharide moieties.

residue which is immunochemically similar to the precursor of the human erythrocyte i antigen. In the presence of a bacterial enzyme called sialyltransferase and a host or bacterial substrate (cytidine monophospho-N-acetylneuraminic acid, CMP-NANA), the N-acetyllactosamine residue in sialylated. This sialylation, which occurs in vivo, provides the organism with the environmental advantages of molecular mimicry of a host antigen and the biologic masking thought to be provided by sialic acids.

4. The periplasmic space–The space between the inner and outer membrane, called the periplasmic space, contains the murein layer and a gel-like solution of proteins. The periplasmic space is approximately 20–40% of the cell volume, which is far from insignificant. The periplasmic proteins include binding proteins for specific substrates (eg, amino acids, sugars, vitamins, and ions), hydrolytic enzymes (eg, alkaline phosphatase and 5′-nucleotidase) that break down nontransportable substrates into transportable ones, and detoxifying enzymes (eg, β-lactamase and aminoglycoside-phosphorylase) that inactivate certain antibiotics. The periplasm also contains high concentrations of highly branched polymers of D-glucose, eight to ten residues long, which are variously substituted with glycerol phosphate and phosphatidylethanolamine residues; some contain O-succinyl esters. These so-called membrane-derived oligosaccharides appear to play a role in osmoregulation, since cells grown in media of low osmolarity increase their synthesis of these compounds 16-fold.

D. Enzymes That Attack Cell Walls: The β1–4 linkage of the peptidoglycan backbone is hydrolyzed by the enzyme **lysozyme,** which is found in animal secretions (tears, saliva, nasal secretions) as well as in egg white. Gram-positive bacteria treated with lysozyme in low-osmotic-strength media lyse; if the osmotic strength of the medium is raised to balance the internal osmotic pressure of the cell, free protoplasts are liberated (Figure 2–20). The outer membrane of

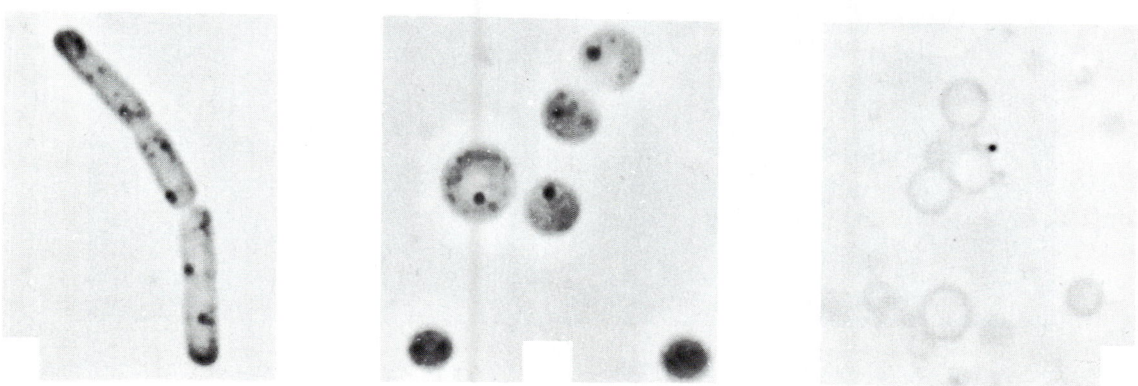

Figure 2–20. *Bacillus megaterium* phase contrast photomicrographs (3000 ×). ***A:*** Before treatment. ***B:*** Protoplasts liberated following treatment with lysozyme and sucrose. ***C:*** After treatment with lysozyme alone; the empty structures are cytoplasmic membranes. (Courtesy of Weibull C: J Bacteriol 1963;66:688.)

the gram-negative cell wall prevents access of lysozyme unless disrupted by an agent such as ethylenediaminetetraacetic acid (EDTA), a chelating agent; in osmotically protected media, cells treated with EDTA-lysozyme form **spheroplasts** that still possess remnants of the complex gram-negative wall, including the outer membrane.

Bacteria themselves possess a number of **autolysins,** hydrolytic enzymes that attack peptidoglycan, including glycosidases, amidases, and peptidases. These enzymes presumably play essential functions in cell growth and division, but their activity is most apparent during the dissolution of dead cells (autolysis).

Enzymes that degrade bacterial cell walls are also found in cells that digest whole bacteria, eg, protozoa and the phagocytic cells of higher animals.

E. Cell Wall Growth: As the protoplast increases in the mass, the cell wall is elongated by the intercalation of newly synthesized subunits into the various wall layers. In streptococci, intercalation into the principal antigen-bearing layer is localized to the equatorial region of the cell wall (Figure 2–21); in some gram-negative bacteria, a process of random intercalation has been inferred, although localized intercalation followed by rapid displacement or turnover could produce the same appearance. In *E coli,* growth of the outer membrane framework takes place exclusively at the cell poles, specialized components such as phage receptors and permeases being inserted randomly into this framework. The peptidoglycan layer of *E coli* appears to grow by randomly located intercalations. In *Bacillus subtilis,* pulse-chase experiments have shown that peptidoglycan and teichoic acids exist in blocks, there being fewer than 12 sites per cell for the insertion of newly synthesized material.

F. Protoplasts, Spheroplasts, and L Forms: Removal of the bacterial wall may be accomplished by hydrolysis with lysozyme or by blocking peptidoglycan biosynthesis with an antibiotic such as penicillin. In osmotically protective media, such treatments liberate **protoplasts** from gram-positive cells and **spheroplasts** (which retain outer membrane and entrapped peptidoglycan) from gram-negative cells.

If such cells are able to grow and divide, they are called **L forms.** L forms are difficult to cultivate and usually require a medium that is solidified with agar as well as having the right osmotic strength. L forms are produced more readily with penicillin than with lysozyme, suggesting the need for residual peptidoglycan.

Some L forms can revert to the normal bacillary form upon removal of the inducing stimulus. Thus, they are able to resume normal cell wall synthesis. Others, however, are stable and never revert. The factor that determines their capacity to revert may again be the presence of residual peptidoglycan, which normally acts as a primer in its own biosynthesis.

Some bacterial species produce L forms spontaneously. The spontaneous or antibiotic-induced formation of L forms in the host may produce chronic infections, the organisms persisting by becoming sequestered in protective regions of the body. Since L-form infections are relatively resistant to antibiotic treatment, they present special problems in chemotherapy. Their reversion to the bacillary form can produce relapses of the overt infection.

Capsule & Glycocalyx

Many bacteria synthesize large amounts of extracellular polymer when growing in their natural environments. With one known exception (the poly-D-glutamic acid capsule of *Bacillus anthracis*), the extracellular material is polysaccharide (Table 2–1). When the polymer forms a condensed, well-defined

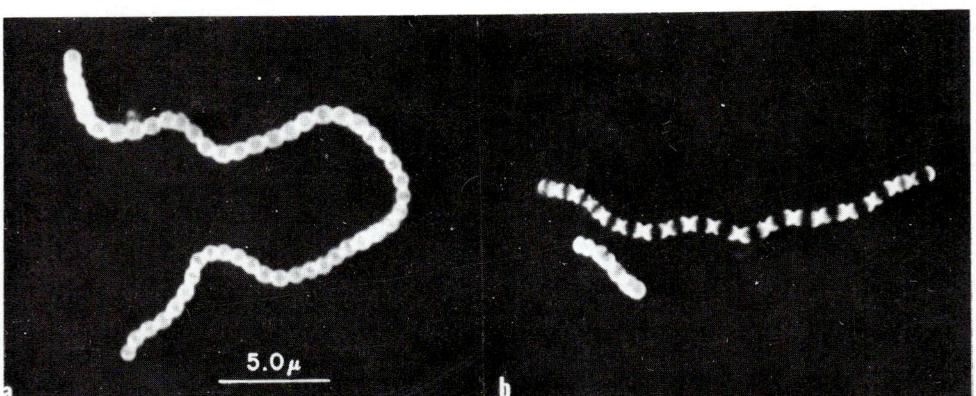

Figure 2–21. Growth of the bacterial cell wall. ***(a)*** Chains of streptococci, stained with fluorescent antibody directed against cell wall antigens. ***(b)*** After 15 minutes' growth in the absence of antibody. New cell wall material, unstained by antibody, has been deposited in the equatorial region of each cell. (Reproduced, with permission, from Cole RM, Hahn JJ: Cell wall replication in *Streptococcus pyogenes.* Science 1962;135:722. Copyright © 1962 by the American Association for the Advancement of Science.)

Table 2–1. Chemical composition of the extracellular polymer in selected bacteria.

Organism	Polymer	Chemical Subunits
Bacillus anthracis	Polypeptide	D-Glutamic acid
Enterobacter aerogenes	Complex polysaccharide	Glucose, fucose, glucuronic acid
Neisseria meningitidis	Homopolymers and heteropolymers, eg,	
	Serogroup A	Partially O-acetylated N-acetylmannosamine-phosphate
	Serogroup B	N-Acetylneuraminic acid (sialic acid)
	Serogroup C	Acetylated sialic acid
	Serogroup 135	Galactose, sialic acid
Streptococcus pneumoniae (pneumococcus)	Complex polysaccharide (many types), eg,	
	Type II	Rhamnose, glucose, glucuronic acid
	Type III	Glucose, glucuronic acid
	Type VI	Galactose, glucose, rhamnose
	Type XIV	Galactose, glucose, N-acetylglucosamine
	Type XVIII	Rhamnose, glucose
Streptococcus pyogenes (group A)	Hyaluronic acid	N-Acetylglucosamine, glucuronic acid
Streptococcus salivarius	Levan	Fructose

layer closely surrounding the cell, it is called the **capsule** (Figure 2–22A); when it forms a loose meshwork of fibrils extending outward from the cell, it is called the **glycocalyx** (Figure 2–22B). In some cases, masses of polymer are formed that appear to be totally detached from the cells but in which cells may be entrapped; in these instances, the extracellular polymer may be referred to simply as a "slime layer." Extracellular polymer is synthesized by enzymes located at the surface of the bacterial cell. *Streptococcus mutans,* for example, uses two enzymes—glucosyl transferase and fructosyl transferase—to synthesize long-chain dextrans (poly-D-glucose) and levans (poly-D-fructose) from sucrose. These polymers are called **homopolymers.** Polymers containing more than one kind of monosaccharide are called **heteropolymers.**

The capsule contributes to the invasiveness of pathogenic bacteria—encapsulated cells are protected from phagocytosis unless they are coated with anticapsular antibody. The glycocalyx plays a role in the adherence of bacteria to surfaces in their environment, including the cells of plant and animal hosts. *S mutans,* for example, owes its capacity to adhere tightly to tooth enamel to its glycocalyx. Bacterial cells of the same or different species become entrapped in the glycocalyx, which forms the layer known as plaque on the tooth surface; acidic products excreted by these bacteria cause dental caries (Chapter 11). The essential role of the glycocalyx in this process—and its formation from sucrose—explains the correlation of dental caries with sucrose consumption by the human population.

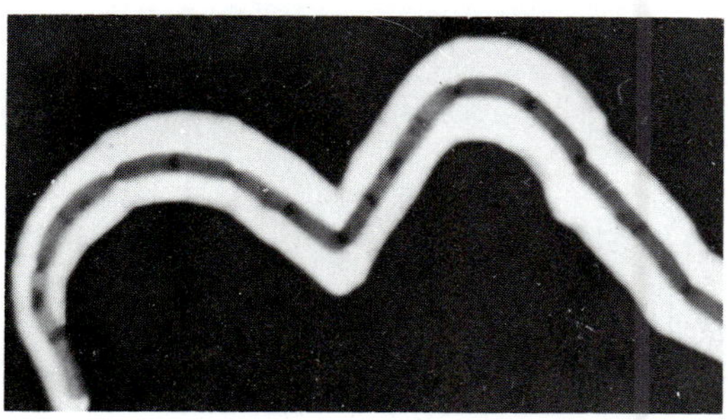

Figure 2–22A. *Bacillus megaterium,* stained by a combination of positive and negative staining (1400 ×). (See section on staining, that follows.) (Courtesy of Welshimer H: J Bacteriol 1953;66:112.)

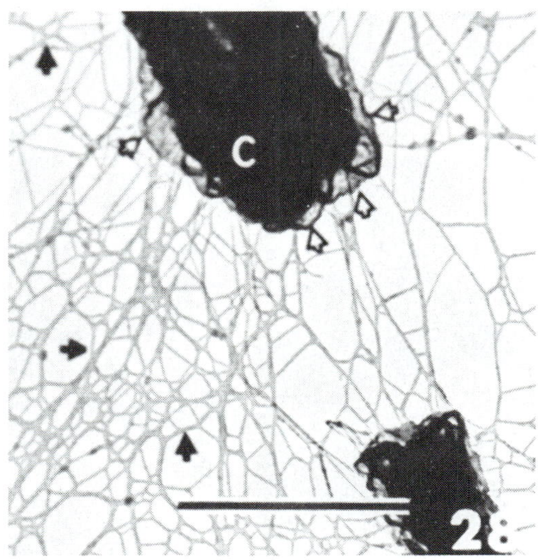

Figure 2–22B. *Klebsiella pneumoniae* cells (C), surrounded by glycocalyx (solid arrows). (Reproduced, with permission, from Cagle GD: Fine structure and distribution of extracellular polymer surrounding selected aerobic bacteria. Can J Microbiol 1975;21:395.)

Flagella

A. Structure: Bacterial flagella are thread-like appendages composed entirely of protein, 12–30 nm in diameter. They are the organs of locomotion for the forms that possess them. Three types of arrangement are known: **monotrichous** (single polar flagellum), **lophotrichous** (multiple polar flagella), and **peritrichous** (flagella distributed over the entire cell). The three types are illustrated in Figures 2–23, 2–24, and 2–25.

A bacterial flagellum is made up of several thousand molecules of a protein subunit called **flagellin.** In a few species (eg, *Caulobacter*), flagella are composed of two types of flagellin, but in most only a single type is found. The flagellum is formed by the aggregation of subunits to form a helical structure. If flagella are removed by mechanically agitating a suspension of bacteria, new flagella are rapidly formed by the synthesis, aggregation, and extrusion of flagellin subunits; motility is restored within 3–6 minutes. The flagellins of different bacterial species presumably differ from one another in primary structure. They are highly antigenic **(H antigens),** and some of the immune responses to infection are directed against these proteins.

The flagellum is attached to the bacterial cell body by a complex structure consisting of a hook and a basal body. The hook is a short curved structure that appears to act as the universal joint between the motor in the basal structure and the flagellum. The basal body bears a set of rings, one pair in gram-positive bacteria and two pairs in gram-negative bacteria. An electron micrograph and interpretative diagrams of the gram-negative structure are shown in Figures 2–26 and 2–27; the rings labeled L and P are absent in gram-positive cells. The complexity of the bacterial flagellum is revealed

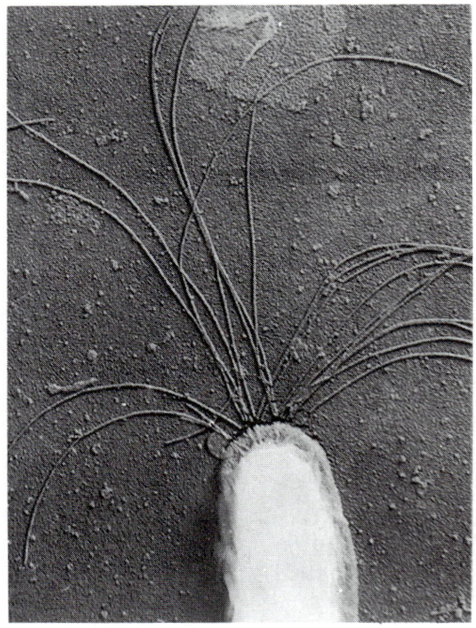

Figure 2–24. Electron micrograph of *Spirillum serpens*, showing lophotrichous flagellation (9000 ×). (Courtesy of van Iterson W: Biochim Biophys Acta 1947;1:527.)

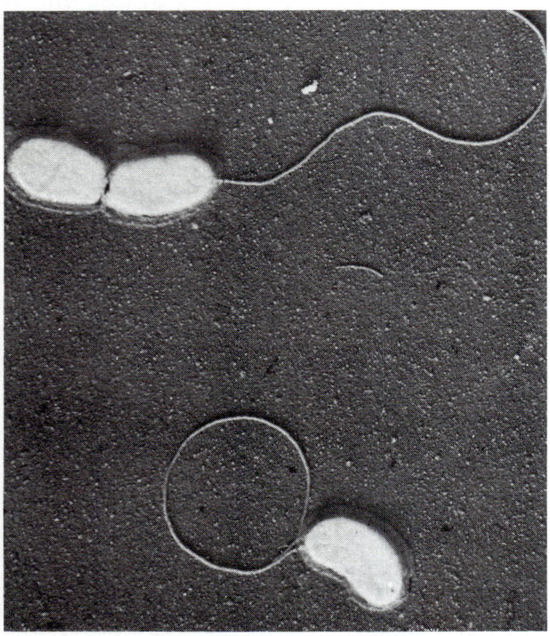

Figure 2–23. *Vibrio metchnikovii*, a monotrichous bacterium (7500 ×). (Courtesy of van Iterson W: Biochim Biophys Acta 1947;1:527.)

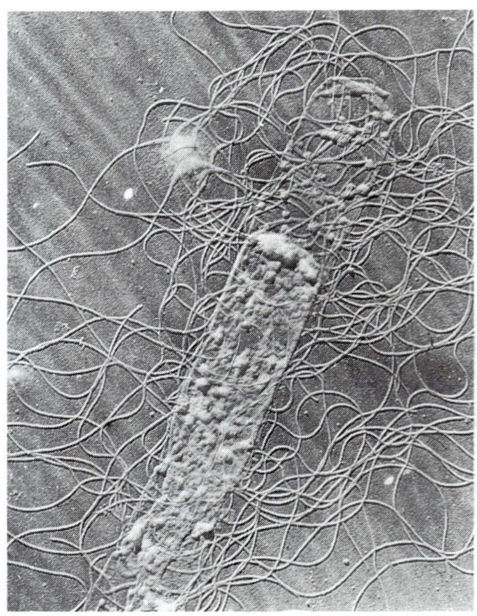

Figure 2–25. Electron micrograph of *Proteus vulgaris*, showing peritrichous flagellation (9000 ×). Note basal granules. (Courtesy of Houwink A, van Iterson W: Biochim Biophys Acta 1950;5:10.)

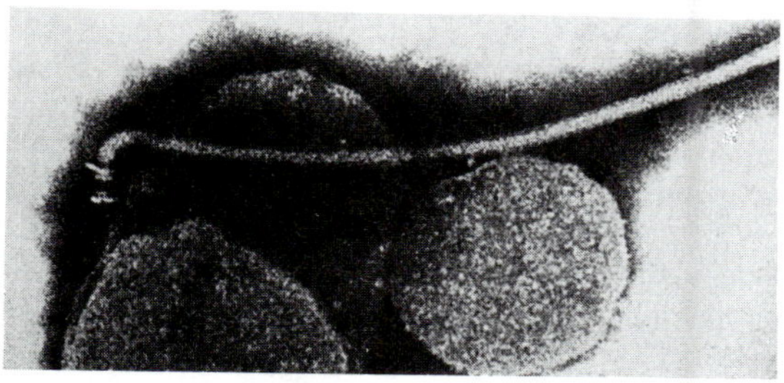

Figure 2–26. Electron micrograph of a negatively stained lysate of *Rhodospirillum molischianum,* showing the basal structure of an isolated flagellum. (Reproduced, with permission, from Cohen-Bazire G, London L: Basal organelles of bacterial flagella. J Bacteriol 1967;94:458.)

by genetic studies, which show that over 40 gene products are involved in its assembly and function.

B. Motility: Bacterial flagella are semirigid helical rotors to which the cell imparts a spinning movement. Rotation is driven by the flow of protons into the cell down the gradient produced by the primary proton pump (see above); in the absence of a metabolic energy source, it can be driven by a proton motive force generated by ionophores. Bacteria living in alkaline environments (alkalophiles) use the energy of the sodium ion gradient—rather than the proton gradient—to drive the flagellar motor.

All of the components of the flagellar motor are located in the cell envelope. Flagella attached to isolated, sealed cell envelopes rotate normally when the medium contains a suitable substrate for respiration or when a proton gradient is artificially established.

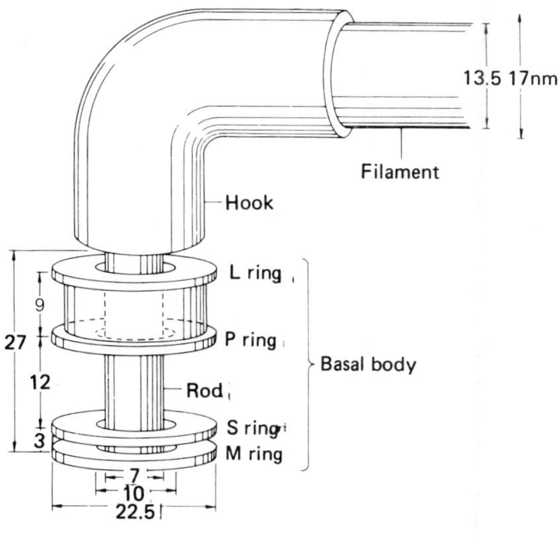

Figure 2–27. Basal structure of the bacterial flagellum. Diagram interpreting the structure seen in Figure 2–24. (Reproduced, with permission, from De Pamphilis ML, Adler J: Fine structure and isolation of the hook-basal body complex of flagella from *Escherichia coli* and *Bacillus subtilis.* J Bacteriol 1971;105:384.)

When a peritrichous bacterium swims, its flagella associate to form a posterior bundle that drives the cell forward in a straight line by counterclockwise rotation. At intervals, the flagella reverse their direction of rotation and momentarily dissociate, causing the cell to tumble until swimming resumes in a new, randomly determined direction. This behavior makes possible the property of **chemotaxis:** A cell that is moving away from the source of a chemical attractant tumbles and reorients itself more frequently than one that is moving toward the attractant, the result being the net movement of the cell toward the source. The presence of a chemical attractant (such as a sugar or an amino acid) is sensed by specific receptors located in the cell membrane (in many cases, the same receptor also participates in membrane transport of that molecule). The bacterial cell is too small to be able to detect the existence of a spatial chemical gradient (ie, a gradient between its two poles); rather, experiments show that it detects temporal gradients, ie, concentrations that decrease with time during which the cell is moving away from the attractant source and increase with time during which the cell is moving toward it.

Some compounds act as repellants rather than attractants. One mechanism by which cells respond to attractants and repellents involves a cGMP-mediated methylation and demethylation of specific proteins in the membrane. Attractants cause a transient inhibition of demethylation of these proteins, while repellents stimulate their demethylation.

The mechanism by which a change in cell behavior is brought about in response to a change in the environment is called **sensory transduction.** Sensory transduction is responsible not only for chemotaxis but also for **aerotaxis** (movement toward the optimal oxygen concentration), **phototaxis** (movement of photosynthetic bacteria toward the light), and **electron acceptor taxis** (movement of respiratory bacteria toward alternative electron acceptors, such as nitrate and fumarate). In these three responses, as in chemotaxis, net movement is determined by regulation of the tumbling response.

Pili (Fimbriae)

Many gram-negative bacteria possess rigid surface appendages called pili (L "hairs") or **fimbriae** (L "fringes"). They are shorter and finer than flagella; like flagella, they are composed of structured protein subunits termed **pilins.** Some pili contain a single type of pilin, others more than one. Minor proteins, located at the tips of pili, are responsible for the attachment properties. Two classes can be distinguished: ordinary pili, which play a role in the adherence of symbiotic bacteria to host cells; and sex pili, which are responsible for the attachment of donor and recipient cells in bacterial conjugation (see Chapter 7). Pili are illustrated in Figure 2–28, in which the sex pili have been coated with phage particles for which they serve as specific receptors. Pilin molecules are arranged helically to form a straight cylinder that does not rotate and lacks a complete basal body.

The virulence of certain pathogenic bacteria depends on the production not only of toxins but also of "colonization antigens," which are now recognized to be ordinary pili that provide the cells with adherent properties. In enteropathogenic *E coli* strains, both the enterotoxins and the colonization antigens (pili) are genetically determined by transmissible plasmids, as discussed in Chapter 7.

In one group of gram-positive cocci, the streptococci, fimbriae are the site of the major surface antigen, the M protein. Lipoteichoic acid, associated with these fimbriae, is responsible for the adherence of group A streptococci to epithelial cells of their hosts.

Pili of different bacteria are antigenically distinct and elicit the formation of antibodies by the host. Antibodies against the pili of one bacterial species will not prevent the attachment of another species. Some bacteria (see Chapter 21), such as *N gonorrhoeae,* are able to make pili of different antigenic types **(antigenic variation)** and thus can still adhere to cells in the presence of antibodies to its original type of pili.

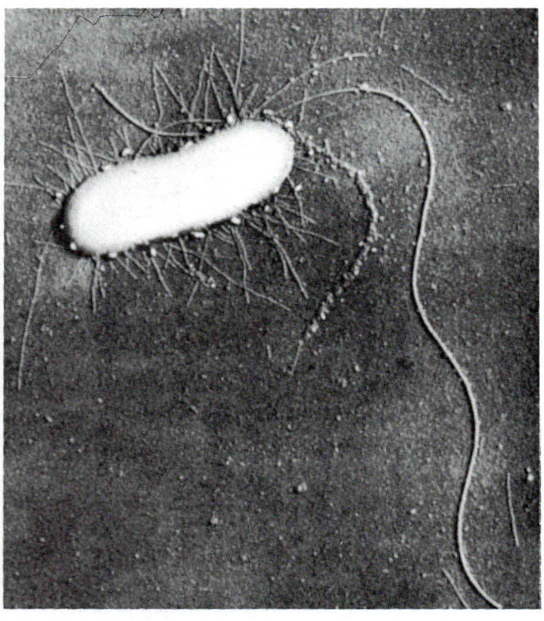

Figure 2–28. Surface appendages of bacteria. Electron micrograph of a cell of *E coli* possessing three types of appendages: ordinary pili (short, straight bristles); a sex pilus (longer, flexible, with phage particles attached); and several flagella (longest, thickest). Diameters: Ordinary pili: 7 nm; sex pili: 8.5 nm; flagella: 25 nm. (Courtesy of J Carnahan and C Brinton.)

Endospores

Members of several bacterial genera are capable of forming endospores (Figure 2–29). The two most common are gram-positive rods: the obligately aerobic genus *Bacillus* and the obligately anaerobic genus *Clostridium.* The other bacteria known to form endospores are the gram-positive coccus *Sporosarcina* and possibly the rickettsial agent of Q fever, *Coxiella burnetii.* These organisms undergo a cycle of differentiation in response to environmental conditions: Under conditions of nutritional depletion, each cell forms a single internal spore that is liberated when the mother cell undergoes autolysis. The spore is a resting cell, highly resistant to desiccation, heat, and chemical agents; when returned to favorable nutritional conditions and activated (see below), the spore germinates to produce a single vegetative cell.

A. Sporulation: The sporulation process begins when nutritional conditions become unfavorable, depletion of the nitrogen or carbon source (or both) being the most significant factor. Sporulation occurs massively in cultures that have terminated exponential growth as a result of such depletion.

Sporulation involves the production of many new structures, enzymes, and metabolites along with the disappearance of many vegetative cell components. These changes represent a true process of **differentiation:** A series of genes whose products determine the formation and final composition of the spore is activated, while another series of genes involved in vegetative cell function is inactivated. These changes involve alterations in the transcriptional specificity of RNA polymerase, which is determined by the association of the polymerase core protein with one or another promoter-specific protein called a sigma factor. Different sigma factors are produced during vegetative growth and sporulation.

The sequence of events in sporulation is highly complex: Differentiation of a vegetative cell of *B subtilis* into an endospore takes about 7 hours under laboratory conditions. Different morphologic and chemical events occur at sequential stages of the process. Seven different stages have been identified. During the process, some bacteria release peptide antibiotics, which may play a role in regulating sporogenesis.

Morphologically, sporulation begins with the formation of an axial filament (Figure 2–30). The process continues with an infolding of the membrane so as to produce a double membrane structure whose facing surfaces correspond to the cell wall-synthesizing surface of the cell envelope. The growing points move progressively toward the pole of the cell so as to engulf the developing spore.

The two spore membranes now engage in the active synthesis of special layers that will form the cell envelope: the **spore wall** and the **cortex,** lying between the facing membranes; and the **coat** and **exosporium,** lying outside the facing membranes. In the newly isolated cytoplasm, or core, many vegetative cell en-

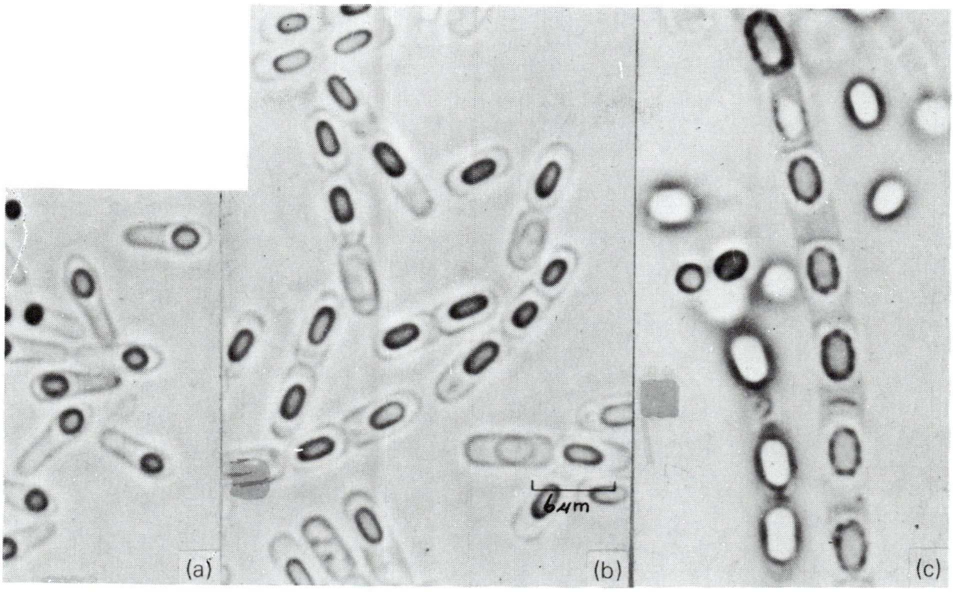

Figure 2–29. Sporulating cells of *Bacillus* species. ***(a):*** Unidentified bacillus from soil. ***(b):*** *B cereus.* ***(c):*** *B megaterium.* (Reproduced, with permission, from Robinow CF, in: Structure. Vol 1 of: *The Bacteria: A Treatise on Structure and Function.* Gunsalus IC, Stanier RY editors. Academic Press, 1960.)

zymes are degraded and are replaced by a set of unique spore constituents. A thin section of a sporulating cell is shown in Figure 2–31.

B. Properties of Endospores:

1. Core–The core is the spore protoplast. It contains a complete nucleus (chromosome), all of the components of the protein-synthesizing apparatus, and an energy-generating system based on glycolysis. Cytochromes are lacking even in aerobic species, the spores of which rely on a shortened electron transport pathway involving flavoproteins. A number of vegetative cell enzymes are increased in amount (eg, alanine racemase), and a number of unique enzymes are formed (eg, dipicolinic acid synthetase). The energy for germination is stored as 3-phosphoglycerate rather than as ATP.

The heat resistance of spores is due in part to their dehydrated state and in part to the presence in the core of large amounts (5–15% of the spore dry weight) of **calcium dipicolinate,** which is formed from an intermediate of the lysine biosynthetic pathway (Figure 6–23). In some way not yet understood, these properties result in the stabilization of the spore enzymes, most of which exhibit normal heat lability when isolated in soluble form.

2. Spore wall–The innermost layer surrounding the inner spore membrane is called the spore wall. It contains normal peptidoglycan and becomes the cell wall of the germinating vegetative cell.

3. Cortex–The cortex is the thickest layer of the spore envelope. It contains an unusual type of peptidoglycan, with many fewer cross-links than are found in cell wall peptidoglycan. Cortex peptidoglycan is extremely sensitive to lysozyme, and its autolysis plays a role in spore germination.

4. Coat–The coat is composed of a keratin-like protein containing many intramolecular disulfide bonds. The impermeability of this layer confers on spores their relative resistance to antibacterial chemical agents.

5. Exosporium–The exosporium is a lipoprotein membrane containing some carbohydrate.

C. Germination: The germination process occurs in three stages: activation, initiation, and outgrowth.

1. Activation–Most endospores cannot germinate immediately after they have formed. But they can germinate after they have rested for several days or are first activated, in a nutritionally rich medium, by one or another agent that damages the spore coat. Among the agents that can overcome spore dormancy are heat, abrasion, acidity, and compounds containing free sulfhydryl groups.

2. Initiation–Once activated, a spore will initiate germination if the environmental conditions are favorable. Different species have evolved receptors that recognize different effectors as signaling a rich medium: thus, initiation is triggered by L-alanine in one species and by adenosine in another. Binding of the effector activates an autolysin that rapidly degrades the cortex peptidoglycan. Water is taken up, calcium dipicolinate is released, and a variety of spore constituents are degraded by hydrolytic enzymes.

3. Outgrowth–Degradation of the cortex and outer layers results in the emergence of a new veg-

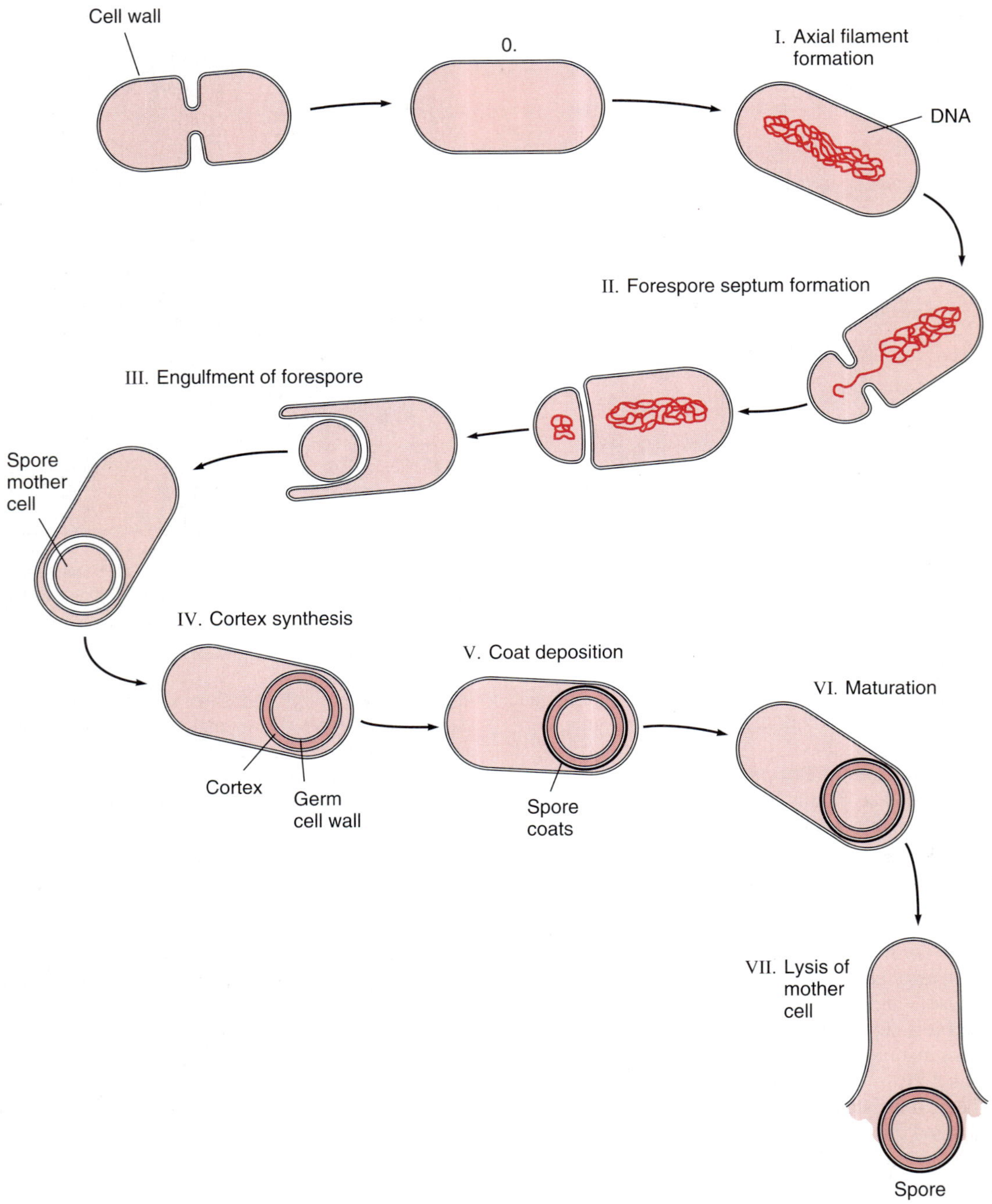

Figure 2–30. The stages of endospore formation. (Reproduced, with permission, from Merrick MJ: Streptomyces. In: Developmental Biology of Procaryotes. Parish JH [editor]. Univ California Press, 1979.)

etative cell consisting of the spore protoplast with its surrounding wall (Figure 2–32). A period of active biosynthesis follows; this period, which terminates in cell division, is called outgrowth. Outgrowth requires a supply of all nutrients essential for cell growth.

STAINING

Stains combine chemically with the bacterial protoplasm; if the cell is not already dead, the staining process itself will kill it. The process is thus a drastic one and may produce artifacts.

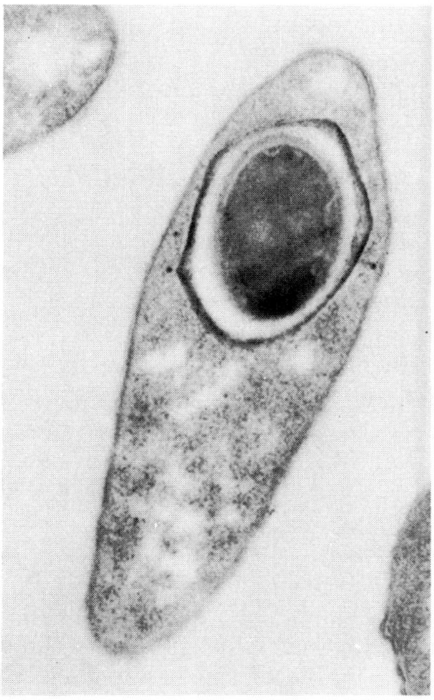

Figure 2–31. Thin section through a sporulating cell of a bacillus (33,000 ×). Electron micrograph taken by Dr CL Hannay. (Reproduced, with permission, from Stanier RY, Doudoroff M, Adelberg EA: *The Microbial World,* 2nd ed. Copyright © 1963. By permission of Prentice-Hall, Inc., Englewood Cliffs, NJ.)

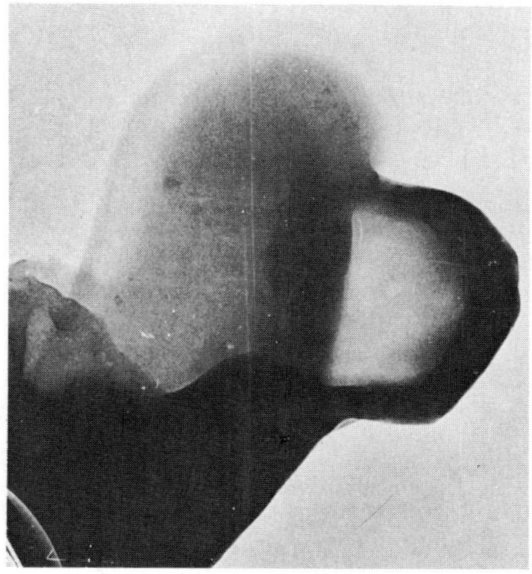

Figure 2–32. Electron micrograph of germinating spore of *Bacillus mycoides.* (Courtesy of Knaysi G, Baker R, Hillier J: J Bacteriol 1947;53:525.)

The commonly used stains are salts. **Basic stains** consist of a colored cation with a colorless anion (eg, methylene blue$^+$ chloride$^-$); **acidic stains** are the reverse (eg, sodium$^+$ eosinate$^-$). Bacterial cells are rich in nucleic acid, bearing negative charges as phosphate groups. These combine with the positively charged basic dyes. Acidic dyes do not stain bacterial cells and hence can be used to stain background material a contrasting color (see Negative Staining, below).

The basic dyes stain bacterial cells uniformly unless the cytoplasmic RNA is destroyed first. Special staining techniques can be used, however, to differentiate flagella, capsules, cell walls, cell membranes, granules, nuclei, and spores.

The Gram Stain

An important taxonomic characteristic of bacteria is their response to Gram's stain. The Gram-staining property appears to be a fundamental one, since the Gram reaction is correlated with many other morphologic properties in phylogenetically related forms (Chapter 3). An organism that is potentially gram-positive may appear so only under a particular set of environmental conditions and in a young culture.

The Gram-staining procedure (see Chapter 47 for details) begins with the application of a basic dye, crystal violet. A solution of iodine is then applied; all bacteria will be stained blue at this point in the procedure. The cells are then treated with alcohol. Gram-positive cells retain the crystal violet-iodine complex, remaining blue; gram-negative cells are completely decolorized by alcohol. As a last step, a counterstain (such as the red dye safranin) is applied so that the decolorized gram-negative cells will take on a contrasting color; the gram-positive cells now appear purple.

The basis of the differential Gram reaction is the structure of the cell wall, as discussed earlier in this chapter.

The Acid-Fast Stain

Acid-fast bacteria are those that retain carbolfuchsin (basic fuchsin dissolved in a phenol-alcohol-water mixture) even when decolorized with hydrochloric acid in alcohol. A smear of cells on a slide is flooded with carbolfuchsin and heated on a steam bath. Following this, the discolorization with acid-alcohol is carried out, and finally a contrasting (blue or green) counterstain is applied. Acid-fast bacteria (mycobacteria and some of the related actinomycetes) appear red; others take on the color of the counterstain.

Negative Staining

This procedure involves staining the background with an acidic dye, leaving the cells contrastingly colorless. The black dye nigrosin is commonly used. This method is used for those cells or structures difficult to stain directly (Figure 2–22A).

The Flagella Stain

Flagella are too fine (12–30 nm in diameter) to be visible in the light microscope. However, their presence and arrangement can be demonstrated by treating the cells with an unstable colloidal suspension of tannic acid salts, causing a heavy precipitate to form on the cell walls and flagella. In this manner, the apparent diameter of the flagella is increased to such an extent that subsequent staining with basic fuchsin makes the flagella visible in the light microscope. Figure 2–33 shows cells stained by this method.

In peritrichous bacteria, the flagella form into bundles during movement, and such bundles may be thick enough to be observed on living cells by darkfield or phase contrast microscopy.

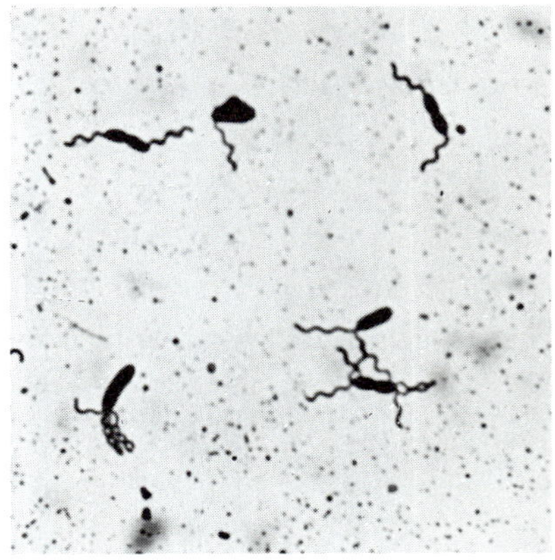

Figure 2–33. Flagella stain of *Pseudomonas* species. (Courtesy of Leifson E: J Bacteriol 1951;62:377.)

The Capsule Stain

Capsules are usually demonstrated by the negative staining procedure or a modification of it (Figure 2–22A). One such "capsule stain" (Welch method) involves treatment with hot crystal violet solution followed by a rinsing with copper sulfate solution. The latter is used to remove excess stain because the conventional washing with water would dissolve the capsule. The copper salt also gives color to the background, with the result that the cell and background appear dark blue and the capsule a much paler blue.

Staining of Nuclei

Nuclei are stainable with the Feulgen stain, which is specific for DNA.

The Spore Stain

Spores are most simply observed as intracellular refractile bodies in unstained cell suspensions or as colorless areas in cells stained by conventional methods. The spore wall is relatively impermeable, but dyes can be made to penetrate it by heating the preparation. The same impermeability then serves to prevent decolorization of the spore by a period of alcohol treatment sufficient to decolorize vegetative cells. The latter can finally be counterstained. Spores are commonly stained with malachite green or carbolfuchsin.

MORPHOLOGIC CHANGES DURING GROWTH

Cell Division

In general, bacteria reproduce by binary fission. Following elongation of the cell, a transverse cell membrane is formed and, subsequently, a new cell wall. In bacteria, the new transverse membrane and wall grow inward from the outer layers, a process in which the septal mesosomes are intimately involved (Figure 2–13). The nuclei, which have doubled in number preceding the division, are distributed equally to the two daughter cells.

Although bacteria lack a mitotic spindle, the transverse membrane is formed in such a way as to separate the two sister chromosomes formed by chromosomal replication. This is accomplished by the attachment of the chromosome to the cell membrane. According to one model, completion of a cycle of DNA replication triggers active membrane synthesis between the sites of attachment of the two sister chromosomes, which are pushed apart by the inward growth of the transverse membrane (Figure 7–4). The deposition of new cell wall material follows, resulting in the elongation and eventual doubling of the cell envelope.

Cell Groupings

If the cells remain temporarily attached following division, certain characteristic groupings result. Depending on the plane of division and the number of divisions through which the cells remain attached, the following may occur in the coccal forms: chains (streptococci), pairs (pneumococci), cubical bundles (sarcinae), or flat plates. Rods may form pairs or chains.

Following fission of some bacteria, characteristic postfission movements occur. For example, a "whipping" motion can bring the cells into parallel positions; repeated division and whipping result in the "palisade" arrangement characteristic of diphtheria bacilli.

Life Cycle Changes

As bacteria progress from the dormant to the actively growing state, certain visible changes take place. The cells tend to become larger, granules disappear, and the protoplasm stains more deeply with basic dyes. When growth slows down again, a gradual change in the reverse direction takes place. Finally, in very old cultures there appear morphologically unusual cells called involution forms. These include filaments, buds, and branched cells, many of which are nonviable.

REFERENCES

Books

Aaronson S: *Chemical Communication at the Microbial Level.* 2 vols. CRC Press, 1982.

Adolph W (editor): *CRC Review on Chromosomes: Eukaryotic, Prokaryotic, and Viral.* CRC Press, 1989.

Balows A et al (editors): *The Prokaryotes,* 2nd ed. *A Handbook on the Biology of Bacteria: Ecophysiology, Isolation, Identification, Applications.* Vols 1, 2, 3, and 4. Springer, 1992.

Beachey EH (editor): *Bacterial Adherence: Receptors and Recognition.* Series B, vol 6. Chapman & Hall, 1980.

Dring GJ, Ellar DJ, Gould GW (editors): *Fundamental and Applied Aspects of Bacterial Spores.* Academic Press, 1985.

Drlica K, Riley M (editors): *The Bacterial Chromosome.* American Society for Microbiology, 1990.

Fuller R, Lovelock DW (editors): *Microbial Ultrastructure: The Use of the Electron Microscope.* Academic Press, 1977.

Goldberger RF (editor): *Molecular Organization and Cell Function.* Vol 2 of: *Biological Regulation and Development.* Plenum Press, 1980.

Hurst A, Gould GW, Dring GJ (editors): *The Bacterial Spore.* Vol 2. Academic Press, 1983.

Inouye M (editor): *Bacterial Outer Membranes: Biogenesis and Functions.* Wiley, 1979.

Martonosi AN (editor): *Enzymes of Biological Membranes,* 2nd ed. Vol 1: *Membrane Structure and Dynamics;* Vol 2: *Biosynthesis and Metabolism;* Vol 3: *Membrane Transport;* Vol 4: *Bioenergetics of Electron and Proton Transport.* Plenum, 1984.

Nanninga N (editor): *Molecular Cytology of* Escherichia coli. Academic Press, 1985.

Neidhardt FC, Ingraham JL, Schaechter M: *Physiology of the Bacteria Cell.* Sinauer, 1990.

Ornston LN, Sokatch JR (editors): *The Bacteria. A Treatise on Structure and Function.* Vol 6: *Bacterial Diversity.* Academic Press, 1978.

Parish JH: *Developmental Biology of Prokaryotes.* Univ California Press, 1979.

Rogers H: *Bacterial Cell Structure.* American Society for Microbiology, 1983.

Rosen BP: *Bacterial Transport.* Marcel Dekker, 1978.

Sokatch JR, Ornston LN: *The Bacteria. A Treatise on Structure and Function.* Vol 7: *Mechanisms of Adaptation.* Academic Press, 1979.

Stanier RY, Rogers HJ (editors): *Relations Between Structure and Function in the Prokaryotic Cell.* Cambridge Univ Press, 1978.

Articles & Reviews

Ames GF: Bacterial periplasmic transport systems: Structure, mechanism, and evolution. Annu Rev Biochem 1986;55:397.

Aronson AI, Fitz-James P: Structure and morphogenesis of the bacterial spore coat. Bacteriol Rev 1976;40:360.

Benz R: Structure and function of porins from gram-negative bacteria. Annu Rev Microbiol 1988;42:359.

Boyd A, Simon M: Bacterial chemotaxis. Annu Rev Physiol 1982;44:501.

Burman LG, Park JT: Molecular model for elongation of the murein sacculus of *Escherichia coli.* Proc Natl Acad Sci USA 1984;81:1844.

Costerton JW, Irvin RT, Cheng KJ: The bacterial glycocalyx in nature and disease. Annu Rev Microbiol 1981; 35:299.

Doetsch RN, Sjoblad RD: Flagellar structure and function in eubacteria. Annu Rev Microbiol 1980;34:69.

Doi RH: Genetic control of sporulation: Annu Rev Genet 1977;11:29.

Elwell LP, Shipley PL: Plasmid-mediated factors associated with virulence of bacteria to animals. Annu Rev Microbiol 1980;34:465.

Giesbrecht P, Wecke J, Reinicke B: One the morphogenesis of the cell wall of staphylococci. Int Rev Cytol 1976;44:225.

Gould GW, Dring GJ: Mechanisms of spore heat resistance. Adv Microb Physiol 1974;11:137.

Greenawalt JW, Whiteside TL: Mesosomes: Membranous bacterial organelles. Bacteriol Rev 1975;39: 405.

Gunn RB: Co- and counter-transport mechanisms in cell membranes. Annu Rev Physiol 1980;42:249.

Henning UL: Determination of cell shape in bacteria. Annu Rev Microbiol 1975;29:45.

Hinnebusch J, Tilly K: Linear plasmids and chromosomes in bacteria. Mol Microbiol 1993;10:917.

Hobot JA et al: Periplasmic gel: New concept resulting from the reinvestigation of bacterial cell envelope ultrastructure by new methods. J Bacteriol 1984;160: 143.

Hultgren SJ et al: Pilus and nonpilus bacterial adhesins: Assembly and function in cell recognition. Cell 1993;73:887.

Kellenberger E: About the organization of condensed and decondensed non-eukaryotic DNA and the concept of vegetative DNA. (A critical review.) Biophys Chem 1987;29:51.

Lo TC: The molecular mechanisms of substrate transport in gram-negative bacteria. Can J Biochem 1979;57: 289.

Lugtenberg B, Van Alphen L: Molecular architecture and functioning of the outer membrane of *Escherichia coli* and other gram-negative bacteria. Biochim Biophys Acta 1983;737:51.

Macnab RM, Aizawa S: Bacterial motility and the bacterial flagellar motor. Annu Rev Biophys Bioeng 1984; 13:51.

Nikaido H: Porins and specific diffusion channels in bacterial outer membranes. J Biol Chem 1994;269:3905.

Pettijohn DE: Prokaryotic DNA in nucleoid structure. CRC Crit Rev Biochem 1976;4:175.

Phillips NJ et al: Structural models of the cell surface lipooligosaccharides of *Neisseria gonorrhoeae* and *Haemophilus influenzae.* Biomed Environ Mass Spectrometry 1990;19:731.

Randall LL, Hardy SJS: Export of protein in bacteria. Microbiol Rev 1984;48:290.

Salton MR, Owen P: Bacterial membrane structure. Annu Rev Microbiol 1976;30:451.

Shively JM: Inclusion bodies of prokaryotes. Annu Rev Microbiol 1974;28:167.

Shockman GD, Barrett JF: Structure, function, and assembly of cell walls of gram-positive bacteria. Annu Rev Microbiol 1983;37:501.

Slater M, Schaechter M: Control of cell division in bacteria. Bacteriol Rev 1974;38:199.

Sleytr UB, Messner P: Crystalline surface layers on bacteria. Annu Rev Microbiol 1983;37:311.

Smith H: Microbial surfaces in relation to pathogenicity. Bacteriol Rev 1977;41:475.

Takayama K, Qureshi N, Mascagni P: Complete structure of lipid A obtained from the lipopolysaccharides of the heptoseless mutant of *Salmonella typhimurium*. J Biol Chem 1983;258:12801.

Taylor BL: Role of proton motive force in sensory transduction in bacteria. Annu Rev Microbiol 1983;37:551.

Vaara M: Agents that increase the permeability of the outer membrane. Microbiol Rev 1992;56:395.

Walsby AE: Gas vesicles. Microbiol Rev 1994;58:94.

Ward JB: Teichoic and teichuronic acids: Biosynthesis, assembly, and location. Microbiol Rev 1981;45:211.

Warth AD: Molecular structure of the bacterial spore. Adv Microb Physiol 1978;17:1.

Wilson DB: Cellular transport mechanisms. Annu Rev Biochem 1978;47:933.

Worcel A, Burgi E: Properties of a membrane-attached form of the folded chromosome of *Escherichia coli*. J Mol Biol 1974;82:91.

Classification of Bacteria 3

*Stephen A. Morse, MSPH, PhD**

DEFINITIONS

Classification, nomenclature, and **identification** are the three separate but interrelated areas of **taxonomy.** Classification can be defined as the arrangement of organisms into taxonomic groups (taxa) on the basis of similarities or relationships. Classification of prokaryotic organisms such as bacteria requires a knowledge obtained by experimental as well as observational techniques, because biochemical, physiologic, genetic, and morphologic properties are often necessary for an adequate description of a taxon. Nomenclature is naming an organism by international rules according to its characteristics. Identification refers to the practical use of a classification scheme: (1) to isolate and distinguish desirable organisms from undesirable ones; (2) to verify the authenticity or special properties of a culture; or, in a clinical setting, (3) to isolate and identify the causative agent of a disease. The latter may permit the selection of pharmacologic treatment specifically directed toward their eradication (Chapter 10). Identification schemes are not classification schemes, though there may be a superficial similarity. An identification scheme for a group of organisms can be devised only after that group has first been classified, ie, recognized as being different from other organisms.

CRITERIA FOR CLASSIFICATION OF BACTERIA

Suitable criteria for purposes of bacterial classification include many of the properties that were described in the preceding chapter. Valuable information can be obtained microscopically by observing cell shape and the presence or absence of specialized structures such as spores or flagella. Staining procedures such as the Gram stain can provide reliable assessment of the nature of cell surfaces. Some bacteria produce characteristic pigments, and others can be differentiated on the basis of their complement of extracellular enzymes; the activity of these proteins often can be detected as zones of clearing surrounding colonies grown in the presence of insoluble substrates (eg, zones of **hemolysis** in agar medium containing red blood cells). Immunologic cross-reaction can give a rapid indication of similar surface structures carried by independently isolated bacteria. Tests such as the oxidase test, which uses an artificial electron acceptor, can be used to distinguish organisms on the basis of the presence of a respiratory enzyme, cytochrome c. Simple biochemical tests can ascertain the presence of characteristic metabolic functions. Criteria leading to successful grouping of some related organisms include measurement of their sensitivity to antibiotics.

All of the foregoing properties are determined, directly or indirectly, by the genes of the examined organisms. Developments in molecular biology now make it possible to investigate the relatedness of genes by determining the ability of DNA from different organisms to cross-hybridize (Chapter 7).

The value of a taxonomic criterion depends upon the biologic group being compared. Traits shared by all or none of the members of a group cannot be used to distinguish its members, but they may define a group (eg, all staphylococci produce the enzyme catalase). In addition, genetic instability can cause some traits to be highly variable within a biologic group or even within a single cell line. For example, antibiotic resistance genes or genes encoding enzymes (lactose utilization, etc) may be carried on **plasmids** (Chapter 7), extrachromosomal genetic elements that may be transferred among unrelated bacteria or that may be lost from a subset of bacterial strains identical in all other respects. Most criteria for classification depend upon growth of the microorganism in the laboratory (Chapter 5). Organisms such as the pathogenic treponemes (Chapter 25) sometimes do not grow in the laboratory, and in these instances techniques that reveal relatedness by measurement of nucleic acid hybridization or by DNA sequence analysis may be of particular value.

*Director, Division of STD Laboratory Research, National Center for Infectious Diseases, CDC, and Adjunct Professor, Department of Microbiology and Immunology, Emory University School of Medicine.

IDENTIFICATION & CLASSIFICATION SYSTEMS

Keys

Keys organize bacterial traits in a manner that permits efficient identification of organisms. The ideal identification system should contain the minimum number of features required for a correct diagnosis. Groups are split into smaller subgroups on the basis of the presence (+) or absence (−) of a diagnostic character. Continuation of the process with different characters guides the investigator to the smallest defined subgroup containing the analyzed organism. In the early stages of this process, organisms may be assigned to subgroups on the basis of characteristics that do not reflect genetic relatedness. It would be perfectly reasonable, for example, for a key to bacteria to include a group such as "bacteria forming red pigments" even though this would include such unrelated forms as *Serratia marcescens* (Chapter 16) and purple photosynthetic bacteria (Chapter 6). These two bacterial assemblages occupy distinct niches and depend upon entirely different forms of energy metabolism. Nevertheless, preliminary grouping of the assemblages would be useful because it would allow an investigator having to identify a red-pigmented culture to immediately narrow the search to relatively few types.

Numerical Taxonomy

Numerical taxonomy (also called computer taxonomy, phenetics, or taxometrics) became widely used in the 1960s. Numerical classification schemes use a large number (frequently 100 or more) of unweighted taxonomically useful characteristics. The computer clusters different strains at selected levels of overall similarity (usually > 80% at the species level) on the basis of the frequency with which they share traits. In addition, numerical classification provides percentage frequencies of positive character states for all strains within each cluster. Such data provide a basis for the construction of a frequency matrix for identification of unknown strains against the defined taxa. Computerized identification has been used to develop diagnostic tests that identify clinically relevant isolates through numerical codes or probabilistic systems.

Phylogenetic Classifications: Toward an Understanding of Evolutionary Relationships Among Bacteria

Phylogenetic classifications are measures of the genetic divergence of different **phyla** (biologic divisions). Close phylogenetic relatedness of two organisms implies that they share a recent ancestor, and the fossil record has made such inferences relatively easy to draw for most representatives of plants and animals. No such record exists for bacteria, and in the absence of molecular evidence, the distinction between convergent and divergent evolution for bacterial traits can be difficult to establish.

The genetic properties of bacteria may allow some genes to be exchanged among distantly related organisms. Furthermore, multiplication of bacteria is almost entirely vegetative, and their mechanisms of genetic exchange rarely involve recombination among large portions of their genomes (Chapter 7). Therefore, the concept of a **species**—the fundamental unit of eukaryotic phylogenies—has an entirely different meaning when applied to bacteria. A eukaryotic species is a biologic group capable of interbreeding to produce viable offspring. A bacterial species is defined as a distinct group of organisms that have certain distinguishing features and generally bear a close resemblance to one another in the more essential features of organization. The decision to circumscribe clusters of organisms within a bacterial species is made by the taxonomist, who may choose to subdivide the group into **biotypes** and to cluster species with genera. Broader groupings such as families may be proposed.

The formal ranks used in the taxonomy of bacteria are listed in Table 3–1. For practical purposes, only the rank of the family, genus, and species are commonly used.

There is considerable genetic diversity among bacteria. Chemical characterization of bacterial DNA revealed a wide range of nucleotide base compositions when DNA from different bacterial sources was compared. The G (guanine) and C (cytosine) compositions of DNA from a single source were always equal, as were the A (adenine) and T (thymine) compositions. These data provided an important clue concerning the base pairing of complementary strands in the physical structure of DNA (Chapter 7). The evidence also showed that the G + C content of closely related bacteria was similar. This was the first indication that the chemical properties of DNA from different organisms could give an indication of their genetic relatedness. Physical studies revealed that the relatedness of DNA from similar organisms could be discerned by measurement of the ability of their chromosomal DNA to cross-hybridize.

DNA sequencing has become a routine laboratory procedure, and comparison of the DNA sequences of

Table 3–1. Taxonomic ranks.

Formal Rank	Example
Kingdom	Prokaryotae
Division	Gracilicutes
Class	Scotobacteria
Order	Eubacteriales
Family	Enterobacteriaceae
Genus	*Escherichia*
Species	*coli*

divergent genes can give a measure of their relatedness. Genes for different functions have diverged at different rates, but in general, the relative rates of divergence are similar. Thus, DNA sequence differences among rapidly diverging genes can be used to ascertain the genetic distance of closely related genes, and sequence differences among slowly diverging genes can be used to measure the relatedness of widely divergent groups of bacteria.

Ribosomes have an essential role in the synthesis of protein. Genes encoding ribosomal RNAs and ribosomal proteins have been highly conserved throughout evolution and have diverged more slowly than other chromosomal genes. Comparison of the nucleotide sequence of 16S ribosomal RNA from a range of biologic sources revealed evolutionary relationships among widely divergent organisms and has led to the elucidation of a new kingdom, the **Archaeobacteria.**

Bergey's Manual of Systematic Bacteriology

The possibility that one might draw inferences about phylogenetic relationships among bacteria is reflected in the organization of the latest edition of *Bergey's Manual of Systematic Bacteriology,* published in four volumes from 1984 through 1989. First published in 1923, the *Manual* is an effort to classify known bacteria and to make this information accessible in the form of a key. A companion volume, published in 1994, *Bergey's Manual of Determinative Bacteriology,* serves as an aid in the identification of those bacteria that have been described and cultured.

In 1980, the International Committee on Systematic Bacteriology published an approved list of bacterial names. This list of about 2500 species replaces a former list that had grown to over 30,000 names; since January 1, 1980, only the new list of names has been considered valid, and the reinstatement of discarded names, the addition of new ones, and other changes require publication in the *International Journal of Systematic Bacteriology.*

Because it is likely that emerging information concerning phylogenetic relationships will lead to further modifications in the organization of bacterial groups within *Bergey's Manual,* its designations must be regarded as provisional.

DESCRIPTION OF THE MAJOR CATEGORIES & GROUPS OF BACTERIA

As discussed in Chapter 2, there are two different groups of prokaryotic organisms: eubacteria and archaeobacteria. Eubacteria contain the more common bacteria, ie, those with which most people are familiar. Archaeobacteria do not produce peptidoglycan, a major difference between them and typical eubacteria. They also differ from eubacteria in that they live in extreme environments (eg, high temperature, high salt, or low pH) and carry out unusual metabolic reactions, such as the formation of methane. A key to the four major categories of bacteria and the groups of bacteria comprising these categories is presented in Table 3–2. The four major categories are based on the character of the cell wall: gram-negative eubacteria that have cell walls, gram-positive eubacteria that have cell walls, eubacteria lacking cell walls, and the archaeobacteria.

Gram-Negative Eubacteria That Have Cell Walls

This is a heterogeneous group of bacteria that have a complex (gram-negative type) cell envelope consisting of an outer membrane, an inner, thin peptidoglycan layer (which contains muramic acid and is present in all but a few organisms that have lost this portion of the cell envelope) and a cytoplasmic membrane. The cell shape (Figure 3–1) may be spherical, oval, straight or curved rods, helical, or filamentous; some of these forms may be sheathed or encapsulated. Reproduction is by binary fission, but some groups reproduce by budding. Fruiting bodies and myxospores may be formed by the myxobacteria. Motility, if present, occurs by means of flagella or by gliding. Members of this category may be **phototrophic** or **nonphototrophic** (Chapter 5) bacteria and include **aerobic, anaerobic, facultatively anaerobic,** and **microaerophilic** species; some members are obligate intracellular parasites.

Gram-Positive Eubacteria That Have Cell Walls

These bacteria have a cell-wall profile of the gram-positive type; cells generally, but not always, stain gram-positive. Cells may be spherical, rods, or filaments (Figure 3–1); the rods and filaments may be nonbranching, or may show true branching. Reproduction is generally by binary fission. Some bacteria in this category produce spores as resting forms (endospores or spores on hyphae). These organisms are generally **chemosynthetic heterotrophs** (Chapter 5) and include aerobic, anaerobic, and facultatively anaerobic species. The groups within this category include simple asporogenous and sporogenous bacteria as well as the structurally complex actinomycetes and their relatives.

Eubacteria Lacking Cell Walls

These are microorganisms that lack cell walls (commonly called **mycoplasmas** and comprise the class Mollicutes) and do not synthesize the precursors of peptidoglycan. They are enclosed by a unit membrane, the plasma membrane (Figure 3–2). They resemble the **L forms** (Chapter 26) that can be generated from many species of bacteria (notably gram-positive eubacteria); unlike L forms, however, mycoplasmas never revert to the walled state, and there are no antigenic relationships between mycoplasmas and eubacterial L forms.

Table 3–2. Major categories and groups of bacteria that cause disease in humans used as an identification scheme in *Bergey's Manual of Determinative Bacteriology,* 9th ed.

Category / Group	Genera
I. Gram-negative eubacteria that have cell walls	
Group 1: The spirochetes	*Treponema*
	Borrelia
	Leptospira
Group 2: Aerobic/microaerophilic, motile helical/vibroid gram-negative bacteria	*Campylobacter*
	Helicobacter
	Spirillum
Group 3: Nonmotile (or rarely motile) curved bacteria	None
Group 4: Gram-negative aerobic/microaerophilic rods and cocci	*Alcaligenes*
	Bordetella
	Brucella
	Francisella
	Legionella
	Moraxella
	Neisseria
	Pseudomonas
	Rochalimaea
	Bacteroides (some species)
Group 5: Facultatively anaerobic gram-negative rods	*Escherichia* (and related coliform bacteria)
	Klebsiella
	Proteus
	Providencia
	Salmonella
	Shigella
	Yersinia
	Vibrio
	Haemophilus
	Pasteurella
Group 6: Gram-negative, anaerobic, straight, curved, and helical rods	*Bacteroides*
	Fusobacterium
	Prevotella
Group 7: Dissimilatory sulfate- or sulfur-reducing bacteria	None
Group 8: Anaerobic gram-negative cocci	None
Group 9: The rickettsiae and chlamydiae	*Rickettsia*
	Coxiella
	Chlamydia
Group 10: Anoxygenic phototrophic bacteria	None
Group 11: Oxygenic phototrophic bacteria	None
Group 12: Aerobic chemolithotrophic bacteria and assorted organisms	None
Group 13: Budding or appendaged bacteria	None
Group 14: Sheathed bacteria	None
Group 15: Nonphotosynthetic, nonfruiting gliding bacteria	*Capnocytophaga*
Group 16: Fruiting gliding bacteria: the myxobacteria	None
II. Gram-positive bacteria that have cell walls	
Group 17: Gram-positive cocci	*Enterococcus*
	Peptostreptococcus
	Staphylococcus
	Streptococcus
Group 18: Endospore-forming gram-positive rods and cocci	*Bacillus*
	Clostridium
Group 19: Regular, nonsporing gram-positive rods	*Erysepelothrix*
	Listeria
Group 20: Irregular, nonsporing gram-positive rods	*Actinomyces*
	Corynebacterium
	Mobiluncus
Group 21: The mycobacteria	*Mycobacterium*
Groups 22–29: Actinomycetes	*Nocardia*
	Streptomyces
	Rhodococcus
III. Cell wall-less eubacteria: The mycoplasmas or mollicutes	
Group 30: Mycoplasmas	*Mycoplasma*
	Ureaplasma
IV. Archaeobacteria	
Group 31: The methanogens	None
Group 32: Archaeal sulfate reducers	None
Group 33: Extremely halophilic archaeobacteria	None
Group 34: Cell wall-less archaeobacteria	None
Group 35: Extremely thermophilic and hyperthermophilic sulfur metabolizers	None

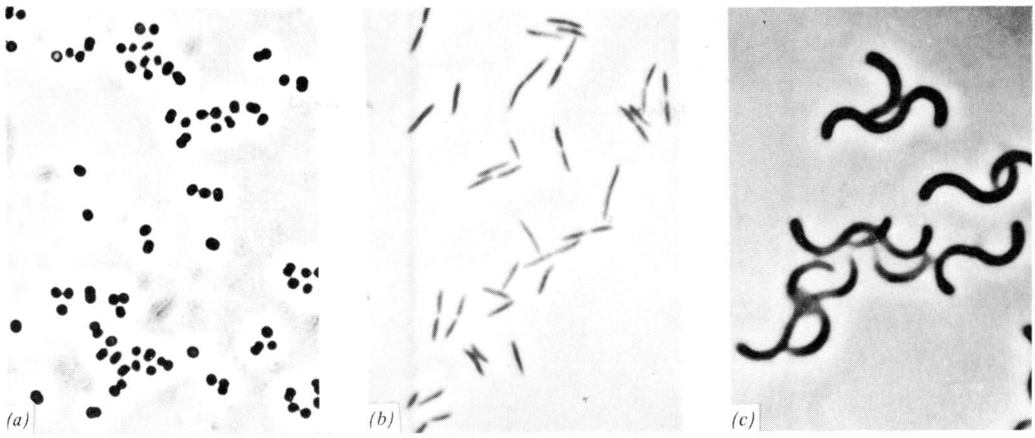

Figure 3–1. The cell shapes that occur among unicellular true bacteria. ***(a)*** Coccus. ***(b)*** Rod. ***(c)*** Spiral. (Phase contrast, 1500 ×.) (Reproduced, with permission, from Stanier RY, Doudoroff M, Adelberg EA: *The Microbial World,* 3rd ed. Copyright © 1970. By permission of Prentice-Hall, Inc., Englewcod Cliffs, NJ.)

Six genera have been designated as mycoplasmas (Chapter 26) on the basis of their habitat and requirement for cholesterol; however, only two genera, contain animal pathogens. Mycoplasmas are highly pleomorphic organisms and range in size from vesicle-like forms to very small (0.2 μm), filtrable forms. Reproduction may be by budding, fragmentation, or binary fission, singly or in combination. Most species require complex medium for growth and tend to form characteristic "fried egg" colonies on solid medium. A unique characteristic of the mollicutes is that some genera require cholesterol for growth; unesterified cholesterol is a unique component of the membranes of both sterol-requiring and -nonrequiring species if present in the medium.

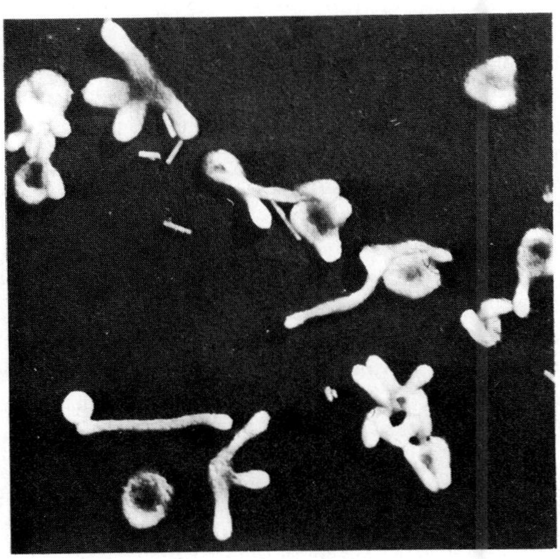

Figure 3–2. Electron micrograph of cells of a member of the *Mycoplasma* group, the agent of bronchopneumonia in the rat (1960 ×). (Reproduced, with permission, from Klieneberger-Nobel E, Cuckow FW: A study of organisms of the pleuropneumonia group by electron microscopy. J Gen Microbiol 1955;12:99.)

The Archaeobacteria

These prokaryotic organisms are predominantly inhabitants of extreme terrestrial and aquatic environments (high salt, high temperature, anaerobic); some are symbionts in the digestive tract of animals. The archaeobacteria consist of aerobic, anaerobic, and facultatively anaerobic organisms that are **chemolithotrophs, heterotrophs,** or **facultative heterotrophs** (Chapter 5). Some species are **mesophiles** while other are capable of growing at temperatures above 100 °C. These hyperthermophilic archaeobacteria are uniquely adapted for growth and multiplication at high temperatures. With few exceptions enzymes isolated from these organism are intrinsically more thermostable than their counterparts from mesophilic organisms. Some of these thermostable enzymes such as the DNA polymerase from *Thermus aquaticus* (Taq polymerase) is an important component of DNA amplification methods such as the polymerase chain reaction (PCR). Archaeobacteria can be distinguished from eubacteria in part by their lack of peptidoglycan cell wall, possession of isoprenoid diether or diglycerol tetraether lipids, and characteristic ribosomal RNA sequences. Archaeobacteria also share some molecular features with eukaryotes (Table 3–3). Cells may have a diversity of shapes, including spherical, spiral, plate- or rod-shaped; unicellular and multicellular forms in filaments or aggregates also occur. Multiplication occurs by either binary fission, budding, constriction, fragmentation, or by unknown mechanisms.

Table 3–3. Some characteristics shared by archaeobacteria and eukaryotic cells which are absent in eubacteria.

Characteristic	Eubacteria	Archaeobacteria, Eukaryotes
Elongation factor-2 (EF-2) contains the amino acid diphthamide and is therefore ADP-ribosylable by diphtheria toxin	No	Yes
The methionyl initiator tRNA is not formylated	No	Yes
Some tRNA genes contain introns	No	Yes
Protein synthesis is inhibited by anisomycin but not by chloramphenicol	No	Yes
DNA-dependent RNA polymerases are multicomponent enzymes and are insensitive to the antibiotics rifampin and streptolydigin	No	Yes

SUBTYPING & ITS APPLICATION

Under certain circumstance (such as an epidemic) it is important to distinguish between strains of a given species or to identify a particular strain. This is called **subtyping;** it is done by examining bacterial isolates for characteristics that allow discrimination below the species level. For any subtyping system to be effective, it must differentiate case from noncase isolates. Classically, subtyping has been accomplished by biotyping, serotyping, antimicrobial susceptibility testing, bacteriophage typing, and bacteriocin typing. For example, more than 130 serogroups of *Vibrio cholerae* have been identified based on antigenic differences in the O polysaccharide of the LPS; however, only the O1 and O139 serogroups are associated with epidemic and pandemic cholera. Within these serogroups, only strains that produce cholera toxin are virulent and cause the disease cholera; nontoxigenic *V cholerae* O1 strains, which are not associated with epidemic cholera, have been isolated from environmental specimens, food and from patients with sporadic diarrhea.

Clonality with respect to isolates of microorganisms from a common-source outbreak is an important concept in the epidemiology of infectious diseases. Exposure to a common source of an etiologic agent has been associated with numerous outbreaks of infections. Generally, these infectious microorganisms are **clonal;** in other words, they are the progeny of a single cell and thus, for all practical purposes, are genetically identical. Thus, subtyping plays an important role in identifying these particular microorganisms. Recent advances in biotechnology have dramatically improved our ability to subtype microorganisms. Hybridoma technology has resulted in the development of monoclonal antibodies against cell surface antigens, which have been used to create highly standardized serology-based subtyping systems. Molecular typing methods, based on the physical characterization of molecules produced by bacteria, increased the discriminatory power of subtyping systems and have made a significant impact on the epidemiology of infectious diseases. Molecular typing methods are often categorized on the basis of the type of macromolecule targeted for subtyping: lipopolysaccharide (LPS)-based methods, protein-based methods, and nucleic acid-based methods. Analysis of LPS by observing banding patterns following sodium dodecyl sulfate polyacrylamide gel electrophoresis (SDS-PAGE) is a relatively simple method for evaluating heterogeneity among strains of gram-negative bacterial species. Detecting the reactivity of monoclonal antibodies with epitopes on LPS is another method for identifying heterogeneity among strains of a given species. Whole-cell and outer membrane protein profiles determined by SDS-PAGE have also been useful for subtyping bacteria

Multilocus enzyme electrophoresis (MLEE), which has been a standard method for investigating eukaryotic population genetics, has also been used to study the genetic diversity and clonal structure of pathogenic microorganisms. MLEE involves the determination of the mobilities of a set of soluble enzymes (usually 15–25 enzymes) by starch gel electrophoresis. Because the rate of migration of a protein during electrophoresis and its net electrostatic charge are determined by its amino acid sequence, mobility variants (referred to as electromorphs or allozymes) of an enzyme are due to amino acid substitutions in the polypeptide sequence, which reflects changes in the DNA sequence encoding the polypeptide. The enzyme-encoding structural genes of *Escherichia coli* exhibit extensive genetic diversity; however, by using MLEE, investigators at the Centers for Disease Control were able to ascertain that strains of *E coli* serotype O157:H7, a recently recognized pathogen associated with outbreaks of hemorrhagic colitis and hemolytic uremic syndrome (Chapter 16), were descended from a clone that is widely distributed in North America.

Developments in nucleic acid isolation, separation, and amplification since 1975 have led to the development of nucleic acid-based subtyping systems. These include plasmid profile analysis, restriction endonuclease analysis, ribotyping, pulsed field gel electrophoresis, PCR amplification and restriction endonuclease digestion of specific genes, arbitrarily primed PCR, and nucleic acid sequence analysis. Plasmid profile analysis was the first, and is technically the simplest, DNA-based technique applied to epidemiologic studies. Plasmids, which are extrachromosomal genetic elements, are isolated from each isolate and then separated by agarose gel electrophoresis to determine their number and size. However, plasmids of identical size but very different sequence or function can exist in many bacteria. Thus, digesting the plasmids with restriction endonucleases and then comparing the number and size of the resulting restriction fragments often provides additional useful information. Plasmid analysis has been shown to be most useful for examining outbreaks that are restricted in time and place (eg, an outbreak in a hospital) and when combined with other subtyping methods.

The use of restriction endonucleases to cleave DNA into discrete fragments is one of the most basic procedures in molecular biology. Restriction endonucleases recognize short DNA sequences (restriction sequence) and they cleave double-stranded DNA within or adjacent to this sequence. Restriction sequences range from 4 to more than 12 bases in length and occur throughout the bacterial chromosome. The short restriction sequences occur more frequently than the longer restriction sequences. Thus, enzyme that recognize the commonly occurring four base-pair restriction sequences will produce more fragments than enzymes that recognize infrequently occurring eight base-pair restriction sequences. Several subtyping methods employ restriction endonuclease digested DNA. The basic method involves digesting DNA with an enzyme that recognizes a frequently occurring restriction site and separating the hundreds of fragments, which range from approximately 0.5 kb to 50 kb in length, by agarose gel electrophoresis followed by visualization under ultraviolet light after staining with ethidium bromide (Figure 3–3). One of the major limitations of this technique is the difficulty in interpreting the complex profiles consisting of hundreds of bands that may be unresolved and overlapping. The use of restriction endonucleases that cut at infrequently occurring restriction sites has circumvented this problem. Digestion of DNA with these enzymes generally results in 5–20 fragments ranging from approximately 10 kb to 800 kb in length. Separation of these large DNA fragments is accomplished by a technique called pulsed field gel electrophoresis, which requires specialized equipment. Theoretically, all bacterial isolates are typeable by this method. Its advantage is that the restriction profile consists of a few well-resolved bands representing the entire bacterial chromosome in a single gel.

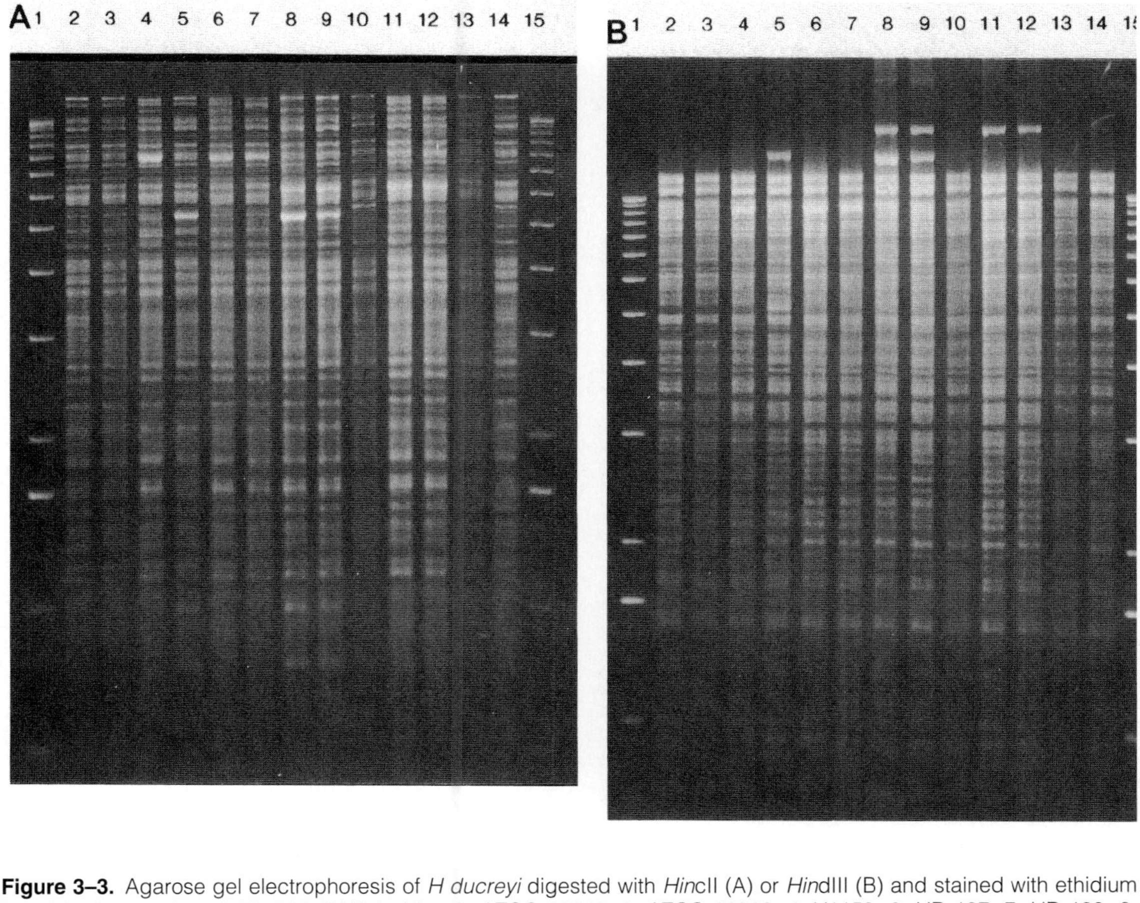

Figure 3–3. Agarose gel electrophoresis of *H ducreyi* digested with *Hinc*II (A) or *Hind*III (B) and stained with ethidium bromide. Lanes: 1 and 15: 1-kb DNA ladder; 2, ATCC 33940; 3, ATCC 33922; 4, V1159; 6, HD-187; 7, HD-188; 8, HD-181; 9, HD-182; 10, HD-179; 11, HD-185; 12, HD-186; 13, HD-174; 14, HD-189. (Reproduced, with permission, from Sarafian SK et al: Ribotyping of *H ducreyi*. J Clin Microbiol 1991;29:1949.)

Southern blot analysis, named after the investigator who developed the technique, has been used as a subtyping method to identify isolates associated with outbreaks. Following agarose gel electrophoresis, the separated restriction fragments are transferred to a nitrocellulose or nylon membrane. Using a labeled fragment of DNA as a probe, it is possible to identify the restriction or fragments containing sequences (loci) that are homologous to the probe. Variations in the number and size of these fragments are referred to as restriction fragment length polymorphisms (RFLPs) and reflect variations in both the number of loci that are homologous to the probe and the location of restriction sites that are within or flanking those loci. Ribotyping is a method which uses Southern blot analysis to detect polymorphisms of rRNA genes, which are present in all bacteria. Because ribosomal sequences are highly conserved, they can be detected with a common probe prepared from the 16S and 23S rRNA of *E coli.* Many organisms have multiple copies (five to seven) of these genes, resulting in patterns with a sufficient number of bands to provide good discriminatory power (Figure 3–4); however, ribotyping will be of limited value for some microorganisms like mycobacteria, which have only a single copy of these genes.

PCR has proved useful for the detection and identification of infectious agents without the need for culture. PCR has also been used in several subtyping methods. The most direct use of PCR involves the amplification of a specific gene, the subsequent digestion of the amplification product with restriction endonucleases, and the analysis of the resulting fragments by electrophoresis. An example of the way this method has been used is that the pattern of the restriction fragments from the major outer membrane protein (MOMP) gene of *Chlamydia trachomatis* can be correlated with results of a MOMP-based serotyping system. Thus, *C trachomatis,* an obligate intracellular pathogen, can be rapidly typed for epidemiologic or other purposes directly from clinical specimens without the need for culture.

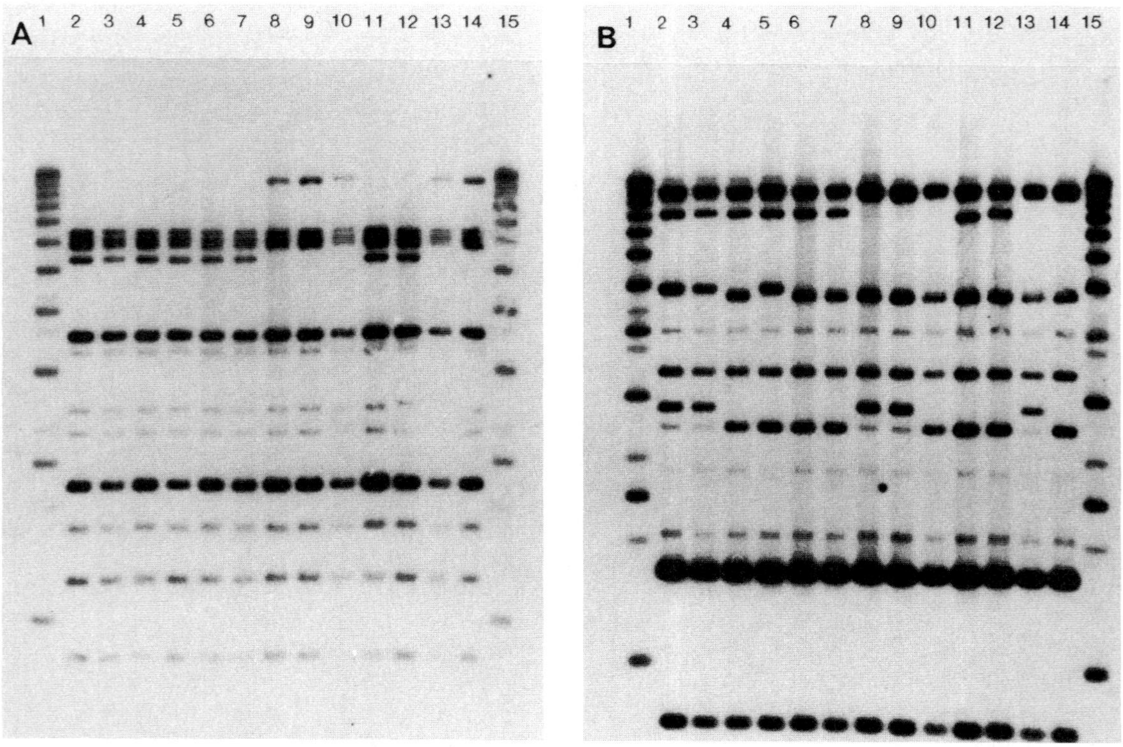

Figure 3–4. Southern blots of *H ducreyi* DNA, digested with *Hin*II (A) or *Hind*III (B), separated by agarose gel electrophoresis and hybridized with ^{32}P-labeled 16S and 23S *E coli* rRNA. Lanes: 1 and 15, 1-kb DNA ladder labeled with ^{32}P by nick translation; 2, ATCC 33940; 3, ATCC 33922; 4, V 1159; 5, C148; 6, HD-187; 7, HD-188; 8, HD-181; 9, HD-182; 10, HD-179; 11, HD-185; 12, HD-186; 13, HD-174; 14, HD-189. (Reproduced, with permission, from Sarafian SK et al: Ribotyping of *H ducreyi.* J Clin Microbiol 1991;29:1949.)

REFERENCES

Books

Balows A et al (editors): *The Prokaryotes,* 2nd ed. *A Handbook on the Biology of Bacteria: Ecophysiology, Isolation, Identification, Applications.* Springer, 1991.

Buchanan RE et al (editors): *Index Bergeyana. A Companion to Bergey's Manual of Determinative Bacteriology.* Williams & Wilkins, 1965.

Gibbons NE et al (editors): *Supplement to Index Bergeyana.* Williams & Wilkins, 1981.

Goodfellow M, Board RG (editors): *Microbiological Classification and Identification.* Academic Press, 1980.

Holt JG et al (editors): *Bergey's Manual of Determinative Bacteriology,* 9th ed. Williams & Wilkins, 1994.

Krieg NR (editor): *Bergey's Manual of Systematic Bacteriology,* 1st ed. Vol 1. Williams & Wilkins, 1984.

Persing DH et al (editors): *Diagnostic Molecular Microbiology. Principles and Applications.* American Society for Microbiology, 1993.

Sneath PHA et al (editors): *Bergey's Manual of Systematic Bacteriology,* 1st ed. Vol 2. Williams & Wilkins, 1986.

Sneath PHA (editor): *International Code of Nomenclature of Bacteria* (1990 Revision). American Society for Microbiology, 1992.

Sneath PHA, Sokal RR: *Numerical Taxonomy: The Principles and Practice of Numerical Classification.* Freeman, 1973.

Sokatch JR: *The Bacteria. A Treatise on Structure and Function.* Vol 10. Academic Press, 1986.

Staley JT et al (editors): *Bergey's Manual of Systematic Bacteriology,* 1st ed. Vol 3. Williams & Wilkins, 1989.

Stanier RY et al: *The Microbial World,* 5th ed. Prentice-Hall, 1979.

Williams ST et al (editors): *Bergey's Manual of Systematic Bacteriology,* 1st ed. Vol 4. Williams & Wilkins, 1989.

Articles & Reviews

Jones D, Sneath PHA: Genetic transfer and bacterial taxonomy. Bacteriol Rev 1970;34:40.

Maniloff J: Evolution of wall-less prokaryotes. Annu Rev Microbiol 1983;37:477.

Maslow JN, Mulligan ME, Arbeit RD: Molecular epidemiology: Application of contemporary techniques to the typing of microorganisms. Clin Infect Dis 1993;17:153.

Mayer LW: Use of plasmid profiles in epidemiologic surveillance of disease outbreaks in tracing the transmission of antibiotic resistance. Clin Microbiol Rev 1988;1:228.

Olsen GJ et al: Microbial ecology and evolution: A ribosomal RNA approach. Annu Rev Microbiol 1986;40:337.

Olsen GL, Woese CR, Overbeek R: The winds of (evolutionary) change: Breathing new life into microbiology. J Bacteriol 1994;176:1.

Razin S: The mycoplasmas. Microbiol Rev 1978;42:414.

Reeve JN: Molecular biology of methanogens. Ann Rev Microbiol 1992;46:165.

Roth RR, James WE: Microbial ecology of the skin. Annu Rev Microbiol 1989;43:441.

Sanderson KE: Genetic relatedness in the family Enterobacteriaceae. Annu Rev Microbiol 1976;30:327.

Schleifer KH, Stackebrandt E: Molecular systematics of prokaryotes. Annu Rev Microbiol 1983;37:143.

Skerman VBD, McGowan V, Sneath PHA (editors): Approved lists of bacterial names. Int J Systematic Bacteriol 1980;30:225.

Woese CR, Magrum LJ, Fox GE: Archaebacteria. J Mol Evol 1978;11:245.

4 The Growth, Survival, & Death of Microorganisms

SURVIVAL OF MICROORGANISMS IN THE NATURAL ENVIRONMENT

The population of microorganisms in the biosphere is roughly constant: growth is counterbalanced by death. The survival of any microbial group within its niche is determined in large part by successful competition for nutrients and by maintenance of a pool of living cells during nutritional deprivation. It is increasingly evident that many microorganisms exist in consortia formed by representatives of different genera. Other microorganisms, often characterized as single cells in the laboratory, form cohesive colonies in the natural environment.

Most of our understanding of microbial physiology has come from the study of isolated cell lines growing under optimal conditions, and this knowledge forms the basis for this section. Nevertheless, it should be remembered that many microorganisms compete in the natural environment while under nutritional stress, a circumstance that may lead to a physiologic state quite unlike that observed in the laboratory. Furthermore, it should be recognized that a vacant microbial niche in the environment will soon be filled. Public health procedures that eliminate pathogenic microorganisms by clearing their niche are likely to be less successful than methods that leave the niche occupied by successful nonpathogenic competitors.

THE MEANING OF GROWTH

Growth is the orderly increase in the sum of all the components of an organism. Thus, the increase in size that results when a cell takes up water or deposits lipid or polysaccharide is not true growth. Cell multiplication is a consequence of growth; in unicellular organisms, growth leads to an increase in the number of individuals making up a population or culture.

The Measurement of Microbial Concentrations

Microbial concentrations can be measured in terms of cell concentration (the number of viable cells per unit volume of culture) or of biomass concentration (dry weight of cells per unit volume of culture). These two parameters are not always equivalent, because the average dry weight of the cell varies at different stages in the history of a culture. Nor are they of equal significance: in studies of microbial genetics or the inactivation of cells, cell concentration is the significant quantity; in studies on microbial biochemistry or nutrition, biomass concentration is the significant quantity.

A. Cell Concentration: The viable cell count (Table 4–1) is usually considered the measure of cell concentration. However, for many purposes the turbidity of a culture, measured by photoelectric means, may be related to the viable count in the form of a **standard curve.** A rough visual estimate is sometimes possible: a barely turbid suspension of *Escherichia coli* contains about 10^7 cells per milliliter, and a fairly turbid suspension contains about 10^8 cells per milliliter. In using turbidimetric measurements, it must be remembered that the correlation between turbidity and viable count can vary during the growth and death of a culture; cells may lose viability without producing a loss in turbidity of the culture.

B. Biomass Density: In principle, biomass can be measured directly by determining the dry weight of a microbial culture after it has been washed with distilled water. In practice, this procedure is cumbersome, and the investigator customarily prepares a standard curve that correlates dry weight with turbidity. Alternatively, the concentration of biomass can be estimated indirectly by measuring an important cellular component such as protein or by determining the volume occupied by cells that have settled out of suspension.

EXPONENTIAL GROWTH

The Growth Rate Constant

The growth rate of cells unlimited by nutrient is first-order: the rate of growth (measured in grams of biomass produced per hour) is the product of the **growth rate constant,** *k,* and the biomass concentration, *B:*

$$\frac{dB}{dt} = kB \qquad (1)$$

Table 4–1. Example of a viable count.

Dilution	Plate Count[1]
Undiluted	Too crowded to count
10^{-1}	Too crowded to count
10^{-2}	510
10^{-3}	72
10^{-4}	6
10^{-5}	1

[1] Each count is the average of 3 replicate plates.

Rearrangement of equation (1) demonstrates that the growth rate constant is the rate at which cells are producing more cells:

$$k = \frac{Bdt}{dB} \tag{2}$$

A growth rate constant of 4.3 h^{-1}, one of the highest recorded, means that each gram of cells produces 4.3 g of cells per hour during this period of growth. Slowly growing organisms may have growth rate constants as low as 0.02 h^{-1}. With this growth rate constant, each gram of cells in the culture produces 0.02 g of cells per hour.

Integration of equation (1) yields

$$\ln \frac{B_1}{B_0} = 23 \log_{10} \frac{B_1}{B_0} = k(t_1 - t_0) \tag{3}$$

The natural logarithm of the ratio of B_1 (the biomass at time 1 [t_1]) to B_0 (the biomass at time zero [t_0]) is equal to the product of the growth rate constant *(k)* and the difference in time ($t_1 - t_0$). Growth obeying equation (3) is termed exponential because biomass increases exponentially with respect to time. Linear plots of exponential growth can be produced by plotting the logarithm of biomass concentration *(B)* as a function of time *(t)*.

Calculation of the Growth Rate Constant & Prediction of the Amount of Growth

Many bacteria reproduce by binary fission, and the average time required for the population, or the biomass, to double is known as the **generation time** or **doubling time** t_D. Usually the t_D is determined by plotting the amount of growth on a semilogarithmic scale as a function of time; the time required for doubling the biomass is t_D (Figure 4–1). The growth rate constant can be calculated from the doubling time by substituting the value 2 for B_1/B_0 and t_D for $t_1 - t_0$ in equation (3), which yields

$$\ln 2 = kt_D$$

$$k = \frac{\ln 2}{t_D} \tag{4}$$

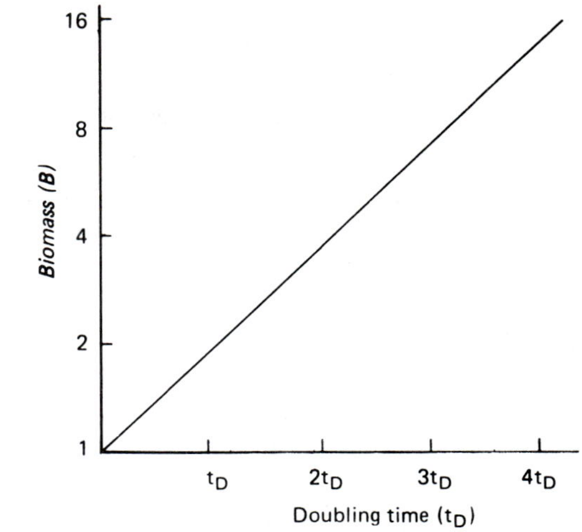

Figure 4–1. Exponential growth. The biomass (B) doubles with each doubling time (t_D).

A rapid doubling time corresponds to a high growth rate constant. For example, a doubling time of 10 min (0.17 h) corresponds to a growth rate constant of 4.1 h^{-1}. The relatively long doubling time of 35 hours corresponds to a growth rate constant of 0.02 h^{-1}.

The calculated growth rate constant can be used either to determine the amount of growth that will occur in a specified period of time or to calculate the amount of time required for a specified amount of growth.

The amount of growth within a specified period of time can be predicted on the basis of the following rearrangement of equation (3):

$$\log_{10} \frac{B_1}{B_0} = \frac{k(t_1 - t_0)}{2.3} \tag{5}$$

For example, it is possible to determine the amount of growth that would occur if a culture with a growth rate constant of 4.1 h^{-1} grew exponentially for 5 hours:

$$\log_{10} \frac{B_1}{B_0} = \frac{4.1\ h^{-1} \times 5\ h}{2.3} \tag{6}$$

In this example, the increase in biomass is 10^{-9}; a single bacterial cell with a dry weight of 2×10^{-13} g would give rise to 0.2 mg of biomass, a quantity that would densely populate a 5-mL culture. Clearly, this rate of growth cannot be sustained for a long period of time. Another 5 hours of growth at this rate would produce 200 kg dry weight of biomass, roughly a ton of cells.

Another rearrangement of equation (3) allows calculation of the amount of time required for a specified amount of growth to take place. In equation (7), shown below, *N*, cell concentration, is substituted for B, biomass concentration, to permit calculation of the time required for a specified increase in cell number.

$$t_1 - t_0 = \frac{2.3 \log_{10}(N_1/N_0)}{k} \qquad (7)$$

Using equation (7), it is possible, for example, to determine the time required for a slowly growing organism with a growth rate constant of 0.02 h^{-1} to grow from a single cell into a barely turbid cell suspension with a concentration of 10^7 cells/mL.

$$t_1 - t_0 = \frac{2.3 \times 7}{0.02\ h^{-1}} \qquad (8)$$

Solution of equation (8) reveals that about 800 hours—slightly more than a month—would be required for this amount of growth to occur. The survival of slowly growing organisms implies that the race for biologic survival is not always to the swift—those species flourish that compete successfully for nutrients and avoid annihilation by predators and other environmental hazards.

THE GROWTH CURVE

If a liquid medium is inoculated with microbial cells taken from a culture that has previously been grown to saturation and the number of viable cells per milliliter determined periodically and plotted, a curve of the type shown in Figure 4–2 is usually obtained. The curve may be discussed in terms of six phases, represented by the letters A–F (Table 4–2).

The Lag Phase (A)

The lag phase represents a period during which the cells, depleted of metabolites and enzymes as the result of the unfavorable conditions that obtained at the end of their previous culture history, adapt to their new environment. Enzymes and intermediates are formed and accumulate until they are present in concentrations that permit growth to resume.

If the cells are taken from an entirely different medium, it often happens that they are genetically incapable of growth in the new medium. In such cases a long lag may occur, representing the period necessary for a few mutants in the inoculum to multiply sufficiently for a net increase in cell number to be apparent.

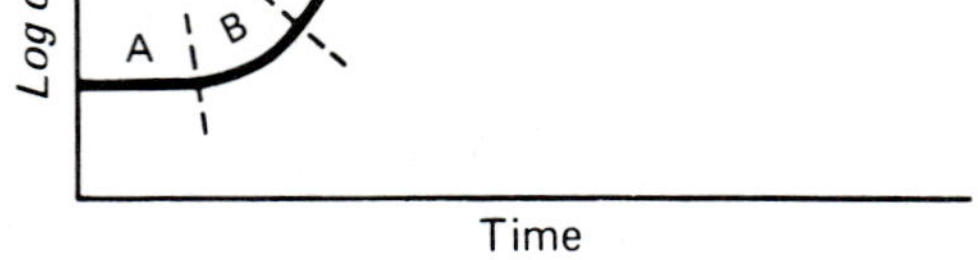

Figure 4–2. Cell concentration curve.

Table 4–2. Phases of microbial death curve.

Section of Curve	Phase	Growth Rate
A	Lag	Zero
B	Acceleration	Increasing
C	Exponential	Constant`
D	Retardation	Decreasing
E	Maximum stationary	Zero
F	Decline	Negative (death)

The Exponential Phase (C)

During the exponential phase, the mathematics of which has already been discussed, the cells are in a steady state. New cell material is being synthesized at a constant rate, but the new material is itself catalytic, and the mass increases in an exponential manner. This continues until one of two things happens: either one or more nutrients in the medium become exhausted, or toxic metabolic products accumulate and inhibit growth. For aerobic organisms, the nutrient that becomes limiting is usually oxygen. When the cell concentration exceeds about 1×10^7/mL (in the case of bacteria), the growth rate will decrease unless oxygen is forced into the medium by agitation or by bubbling in air. When the bacterial concentration reaches 4–5 $\times$ 10^9/mL, the rate of oxygen diffusion cannot meet the demand even in an aerated medium, and growth is progressively slowed.

The Maximum Stationary Phase (E)

Eventually, the exhaustion of nutrients or the accumulation of toxic products causes growth to cease completely. In most cases, however, cell turnover takes place in the stationary phase: there is a slow loss of cells through death, which is just balanced by the formation of new cells through growth and division. When this occurs, the total cell count slowly increases although the viable count stays constant.

The Phase of Decline (The Death Phase, F)

After a period of time in the stationary phase, which varies with the organism and with the culture conditions, the death rate increases until it reaches a steady level. The mathematics of steady-state death are discussed below. Frequently, after the majority of cells have died, the death rate decreases drastically, so that a small number of survivors may persist for months or even years. This persistence may in some cases reflect cell turnover, a few cells growing at the expense of nutrients released from cells that die and lyse.

MAINTENANCE OF CELLS IN THE EXPONENTIAL PHASE

Cells can be maintained in exponential phase by transferring them repeatedly into fresh medium of identical composition while they are still growing exponentially. Two devices have been invented for carrying out this process automatically: the chemostat and the turbidostat.

The Chemostat

This device consists of a culture vessel equipped with an overflow siphon and a mechanism for dripping in fresh medium from a reservoir at a regulated rate. The medium in the culture vessel is stirred by a stream of sterile air; each drop of fresh medium that enters causes a drop of culture to siphon out.

The medium is prepared so that one nutrient limits growth yield. The vessel is inoculated, and the cells grow until the limiting nutrient is exhausted; fresh medium from the reservoir is then allowed to flow in at such a rate that the cells use up the limiting nutrient as fast as it is supplied. Under these conditions, the cell concentration remains constant and the growth rate is directly proportionate to the flow rate of the medium.

DEFINITION & MEASUREMENT OF DEATH

The Meaning of Death

For a microbial cell, death means the irreversible loss of the ability to reproduce (grow and divide). The empirical test of death is the culture of cells on solid media: a cell is considered dead if it fails to give rise to a colony on any medium. Obviously, then, the reliability of the test depends upon choice of medium and conditions: a culture in which 99% of the cells appear "dead" in terms of ability to form colonies on one medium may prove to be 100% viable if tested on another medium. Furthermore, the detection of a few viable cells in a large clinical specimen may not be possible by directly plating a sample, as the sample fluid itself may be inhibitory to microbial growth. In such cases, the sample may have to be diluted first into liquid medium, permitting the outgrowth of viable cells before plating.

The conditions of incubation in the first hour following treatment are also critical in the determination of "killing." For example, if bacterial cells are irradiated with ultraviolet light and plated immediately on any medium, it may appear that 99.99% of the cells have been killed. If such irradiated cells are first incubated in a suitable buffer for 20 minutes, however, plating will indicate only 10% killing. In other words, irradiation determines that a cell will "die" if plated immediately but will live if allowed to repair radiation damage before plating.

A microbial cell that is not physically disrupted is thus "dead" only in terms of the conditions used to test viability.

The Measurement of Death

When dealing with microorganisms, one does not customarily measure the death of an individual cell, but the death of a population. This is a statistical problem: under any condition that may lead to cell death, the probability of a given cell's dying is constant per unit time. For example, if a condition is employed that causes 90% of the cells to die in the first 10 minutes, the probability of any one cell dying in a 10-minute interval is 0.9. Thus, it may be expected that 90% of the surviving cells will die in each succeeding 10-minute interval, and a death curve similar to those shown in Figure 4–3 will be obtained.

The number of cells dying in each time interval is thus a function of the number of survivors present, so

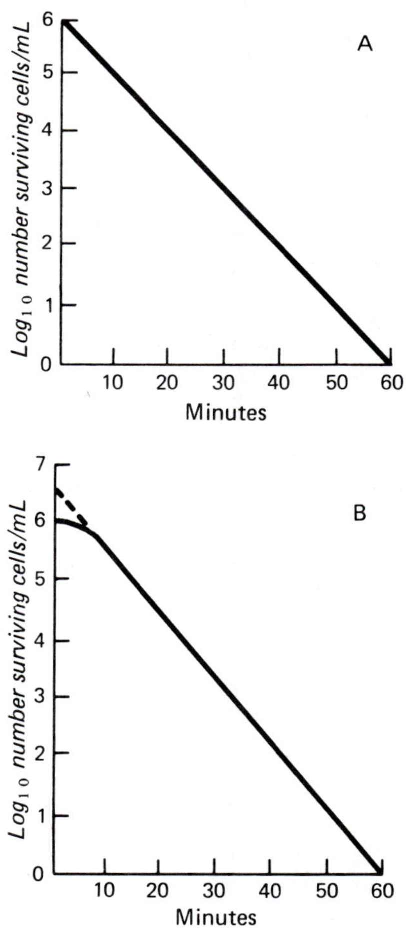

Figure 4–3. Death curve of microorganisms. ***A:*** Single-hit curve. ***B:*** Multi-hit curve. The straight-line portion extrapolates to 6.5, corresponding to 4×10^6 cells. The number of targets is thus 4×10^6, or four per cell.

that death of a population proceeds as an exponential process according to the general formula

$$S = S_0 e^{-kt} \quad (9)$$

where S_0 is the number of survivors at time zero, and S is the number of survivors at any later time t. As in the case of exponential growth, $-k$ represents the rate of exponential death when the fraction $ln\ (S/S_0)$ is plotted against time.

The one-hit curve shown in Figure 4–3A is typical of the kinetics of inactivation observed with many antimicrobial agents. The fact that it is a straight line from time zero (dose zero)—rather than exhibiting an initial shoulder—means that a single "hit" by the inactivating agent is sufficient to kill the cell, ie, only a single target must be damaged in order for the entire cell to be inactivated. Such a target might be the chromosome of a uninucleate bacterium or the cell membrane; conversely, it could not be an enzyme or other cell constituent that is present in multiple copies.

A cell that contains several copies of the target to be inactivated exhibits a multi-hit curve of the type shown in Figure 4–3B. Extrapolation of the straight-line portion of the curve to the ordinate permits an estimate of the number of targets (eg, 4 in Figure 4–3B).

Sterilization

In practice, we speak of "sterilization" as the process of killing all of the organisms in a preparation. From the above considerations, however, we see that no set of conditions is guaranteed to sterilize a preparation. Consider Figure 4–3, for example. At 60 minutes, there is one organism (10^0) left per milliliter. At 70 minutes there would be 10^{-1}, at 80 minutes 10^{-2}, etc. By 10^{-2} organisms per milliliter we mean that in a total volume of 100 mL, one organism would survive. How long, then, does it take to "sterilize" the culture? All we can say is that after any given time of treatment, the probability of having any surviving organisms in 1 mL is that given by the curve. After 2 hours, in the above example, the probability is 1×10^{-6}. This would usually be considered a safe sterilization time, but a 1000-liter lot might still contain one viable organism.

Note that such calculations depend upon the curve's remaining unchanged in slope over the entire time range. Unfortunately, it is very common for the curve to bend upward after a certain period, as a result of the population being heterogeneous with respect to sensitivity to the inactivation agent. Extrapolations are dangerous and can lead to errors such as those encountered in early preparations of sterile poliovaccine.

The Effect of Drug Concentration

When antimicrobial substances (drugs) are used to inactivate microbial cells, it is commonly observed that the concentration of drug employed is related to the time required to kill a given fraction of the population by the following expression:

$$C^n t = K \quad (10)$$

In this equation, C is the drug concentration, t is the time required to kill a given fraction of the cells, and n and K are constants.

This expression says that, for example, if $n = 5$ (as it is for phenol), then doubling the concentration of the drug will reduce the time required to achieve the same extent of inactivation 32-fold. That the effectiveness of a drug varies with the fifth power of the concentration suggests that five molecules of the drug are required to inactivate a cell, although there is no direct chemical evidence for this conclusion.

In order to determine the value of n for any drug, inactivation curves are obtained for each of several concentrations, and the time required at each concentration to inactivate a fixed fraction of the population is determined. For example, let the first concentration used be C_1 and the time required to inactivate 99% of the cells be t_1. Similarly, let C_2 and t_2 be the second concentration and time required to inactivate 99% of the cells. From equation (12), we see that

$$C_1^n t_1 = C_2^n t_2 \quad (11)$$

Solving for n gives

$$n = \frac{\log t_2 - \log t_1}{\log C_1 - \log C_2} \quad (12)$$

Thus, n can be determined by measuring the slope of the line that results when log t is plotted against log C (Figure 4–4). If n is experimentally determined in this manner, K can be determined by substituting observed values for C, t, and n in equation (12).

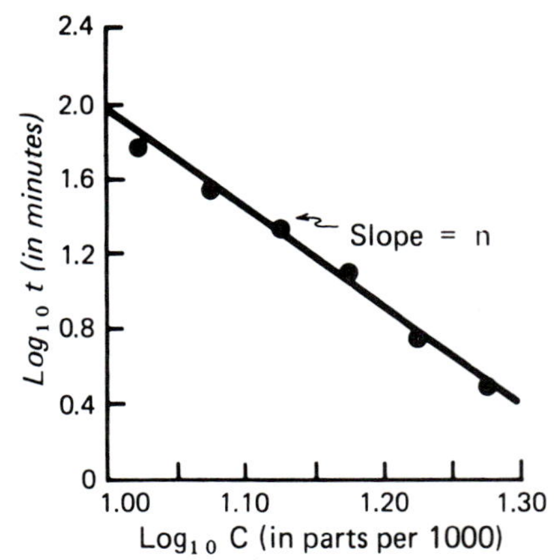

Figure 4–4. Relationship between drug concentration and time required to kill a given fraction of a cell population.

ANTIMICROBIAL AGENTS

Definitions

The following terms are commonly employed in connection with antimicrobial agents and their uses.

A. Bacteriostatic: Having the property of inhibiting bacterial multiplication; multiplication resumes upon removal of the agent.

B. Bactericidal: Having the property of killing bacteria. Bactericidal action differs from bacteriostasis only in being irreversible; ie, the "killed" organism can no longer reproduce, even after being removed from contact with the agent. In some cases the agent causes lysis (dissolving) of the cells; in other cases the cells remain intact and may even continue to be metabolically active.

C. Sterile: Free of life of every kind. Sterilization may be accomplished by filtration (in the case of liquids or air) or by treatment with microbicidal agents. Since the criterion of death for microorganisms is the inability to reproduce, sterile material may contain intact, metabolizing microbial cells.

D. Disinfectant: A chemical substance used to kill microorganisms on surfaces but too toxic to be applied directly to tissues.

E. Septic: Characterized by the presence of pathogenic microbes in living tissue.

F. Aseptic: Characterized by absence of pathogenic microbes.

Modes of Action

A. Damage to DNA: A number of antimicrobial agents act by damaging DNA; these include ionizing radiations, ultraviolet light, and DNA-reactive chemicals. Among the last category are alkylating agents and other compounds that react covalently with purine and pyrimidine bases to form DNA adducts or interstrand cross-links. Radiations damage DNA in several ways: ultraviolet light, for example, induces cross-linking between adjacent pyrimidines on one or the other of the two polynucleotide strands, forming pyrimidine dimers; ionizing radiations produce breaks in single and double strands. Radiation-induced and chemically induced DNA lesions kill the cell mainly by interfering with DNA replication. See Chapter 7 for a discussion of DNA repair systems.

B. Protein Denaturation: Proteins exist in a folded, 3-dimensional state determined by intramolecular covalent disulfide linkages and a number of noncovalent linkages such as ionic, hydrophobic, and hydrogen bonds. This state is called the tertiary structure of the protein; it is readily disrupted by a number of physical or chemical agents, causing the protein to become nonfunctional. The disruption of the tertiary structure of a protein is called protein denaturation.

C. Disruption of Cell Membrane or Wall: The cell membrane acts as a selective barrier, allowing some solutes to pass through and excluding others. Many compounds are actively transported through the membrane, becoming concentrated within the cell. The membrane is also the site of enzymes involved in the biosynthesis of components of the cell envelope. Substances that concentrate at the cell surface may alter the physical and chemical properties of the membrane, preventing its normal functions and therefore killing or inhibiting the cell.

The cell wall acts as a corseting structure, protecting the cell against osmotic lysis. Thus, agents that destroy the wall (eg, lysozyme) or prevent its normal synthesis (eg, penicillin) may bring about lysis of the cell.

D. Removal of Free Sulfhydryl Groups: Enzyme proteins containing cysteine have side chains terminating in sulfhydryl groups. In addition to these, coenzymes such as coenzyme A and dihydrolipoate contain free sulfhydryl groups. Such enzymes and coenzymes cannot function unless the sulfhydryl groups remain free and reduced. Oxidizing agents thus interfere with metabolism by tying neighboring sulfhydryls in disulfide linkages:

$$\text{R—SH} + \text{HS—R} \xrightarrow{-2\text{H}} \text{R—S—S—R}$$

Many metals such as mercuric ion likewise interfere by combining with sulfhydryls:

$$\begin{matrix}\text{R—SH} \\ \text{R—SH}\end{matrix} + \text{Cl—Hg—Cl} \longrightarrow \begin{matrix}\text{R—SH} \\ \text{R—SH}\end{matrix} \Big> \text{Hg} + 2\text{HCl}$$

There are many sulfhydryl enzymes in the cell; therefore, oxidizing agents and heavy metals do widespread damage.

E. Chemical Antagonism: The interference by a chemical agent with the normal reaction between a specific enzyme and its substrate is known as "chemical antagonism." The antagonist acts by combining with some part of the holoenzyme (either the protein apoenzyme, the mineral activator, or the coenzyme), thereby preventing attachment of the normal substrate. ("Substrate" is here used in the broad sense to include cases in which the inhibitor combines with the apoenzyme, thereby preventing attachment to it of coenzyme.)

An antagonist combines with an enzyme because of its chemical affinity for an essential site on that enzyme. Enzymes perform their catalytic function by virtue of their affinity for their natural substrates; hence any compound structurally resembling a substrate in essential aspects may also have an affinity for the enzyme. If this affinity is great enough, the "analogue" will displace the normal substrate and prevent the proper reaction from taking place.

Many holoenzymes include a mineral ion as a bridge either between enzyme and coenzyme or between enzyme and substrate. Chemicals that combine readily with these minerals will again prevent attachment of coenzyme or substrate; for example, carbon monoxide and cyanide (−C−N) combine with the iron atom in the porphyrin enzymes and prevent their function in respiration.

Chemical antagonists can be conveniently discussed under two headings: antagonists of energy-yielding processes, and antagonists of biosynthetic processes. The former include poisons of respiratory enzymes (carbon monoxide, cyanide) and of oxidative phosphorylation (dinitrophenol); the latter include analogues of the building blocks of proteins (amino acids) and of nucleic acids (nucleotides). In some cases the analogue simply prevents incorporation of the normal metabolite (eg, 5-methyltryptophan prevents incorporation of tryptophan into protein), and in other cases the analogue replaces the normal metabolite in the macromolecule, causing it to be nonfunctional. The incorporation of *p*-fluorophenylalanine in place of phenylalanine in proteins is an example of the latter type of antagonism.

Reversal of Antibacterial Action

In the section on definitions, the point was made that bacteriostatic action is, by definition, reversible. Reversal can be brought about in several ways.

A. Removal of Agent: When cells that are inhibited by the presence of a bacteriostatic agent are removed by centrifugation, washed thoroughly in the centrifuge, and resuspended in fresh growth medium, they will resume normal multiplication.

B. Reversal by Substrate: When a chemical antagonist of the analogue type forms a dissociating complex with the enzyme, it is possible to displace it by adding a high concentration of the normal substrate. Such cases are termed "competitive inhibition." The ratio of inhibitor concentration to concentration of substrate reversing the inhibition is called the **antimicrobial index;** it is usually very high (100–10,000), indicating a much greater affinity of enzyme for its normal substrate.

C. Inactivation of Agent: An agent can often be inactivated by adding to the medium a substance that combines with it, preventing its combination with cellular constituents. For example, mercuric ion can be inactivated by addition to the medium of sulfhydryl compounds such as thioglycolic acid.

D. Protection Against Lysis: Osmotic lysis can be prevented by making the medium isotonic for naked bacterial protoplasts. Concentrations of 10–20% sucrose are required. Under such conditions penicillin-induced protoplasts remain viable and continue to grow as L forms.

Resistance to Antibacterial Agents

The ability of bacteria to become resistant to antibacterial agents is an important factor in their control. The mechanisms by which resistance is acquired are discussed in Chapters 7 and 10.

Physical Agents

A. Heat: Application of heat is the simplest means of sterilizing materials, provided the material is itself resistant to heat damage. A temperature of 100 °C will kill all but spore forms of bacteria within 2–3 minutes in laboratory-scale cultures; a temperature of 121 °C for 15 minutes is utilized to kill spores. Steam is generally used, both because bacteria are more quickly killed when moist and because steam provides a means for distributing heat to all parts of the sterilizing vessel. Steam must be kept at a pressure of 15 lb/sq in above atmospheric pressure to obtain a temperature of 121 °C; autoclaves or pressure cookers are used for this purpose. For sterilizing materials that must remain dry, circulating hot air electric ovens are available; since heat is less effective on dry material, it is customary to apply a temperature of 160–170 °C for 1 hour or more.

Under the conditions described above (ie, excessive temperatures applied for long periods of time), heat acts by denaturing cell proteins and nucleic acids and by disrupting cell membranes.

B. Radiation: Ultraviolet light and ionizing radiations have various applications as sterilizing agents. Their modes of action are discussed on p 49.

Chemical Agents

Because antibacterial agents must be safe for the host organism under the conditions employed (selective toxicity), the number of commonly used antibacterial agents is much lower than the number of cell poisons and inhibitors available. Thus cyanide, arsenic, and other poisons are not included below because of the limitations on their practical usefulness.

A. Alcohols: Compounds with the structure $R-CH_2OH$ (where R means "alkyl group") are toxic to cells at relatively high concentrations. Ethyl alcohol (CH_3CH_2OH) and isopropyl alcohol ($[CH_3]_2CHOH$) are commonly used. At the concentrations generally employed (70% aqueous solutions), they act as protein denaturants.

B. Phenol: Phenol and many phenolic compounds are strong antibacterial agents. At the high concentrations generally employed (1–2% aqueous solutions), they denature proteins.

C. Heavy Metal Ions: Mercury, copper, and silver salts are all protein denaturants at high concentrations but are too injurious to human tissues to be used in this manner. They are commonly used at very low concentrations, under which conditions they act by combining with sulfhydryl groups. Mercury can be made safer for external use by combining it with organic compounds (eg, Mercurochrome, Merthiolate). Except when used on clean skin surfaces, these organic mercurials are of doubtful practical value, since they are readily inactivated by extraneous organic matter.

D. Oxidizing Agents: Strong oxidizing agents inactivate cells by oxidizing free sulfhydryl groups. Use-

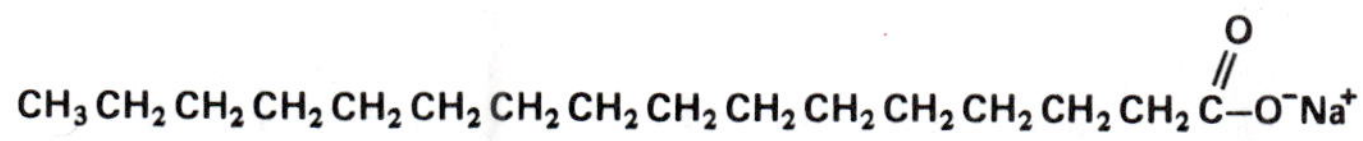

Figure 4–5. Sodium salt of palmitic acid (a soap).

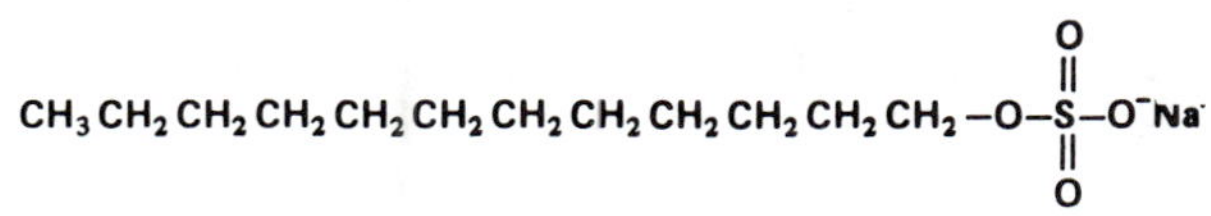

Figure 4–6. Sodium lauryl sulfate (a synthetic anionic detergent, Duponol WA).

ful agents include hydrogen peroxide, iodine, hypochlorite, chlorine, and compounds slowly liberating chlorine (chloride of lime).

E. Alkylating Agents: A number of agents react with compounds in the cell to substitute alkyl groups for labile hydrogen atoms. The two agents of this type that are commonly used for disinfection purposes are formaldehyde (sold as the 37% aqueous solution **formalin**) and **ethylene oxide.** Ethylene oxide gas, rendered inexplosive by mixture with 90% CO_2 or a fluorocarbon, is the most reliable disinfectant available for dry surfaces. It is extensively used for the disinfection of surgical instruments and materials, which must be placed in special vacuum chambers for the purpose.

F. Detergents: Compounds that have the property of concentrating at interfaces are called "surface-active agents," or "detergents." The interface between the lipid-containing membrane of a bacterial cell and the surrounding aqueous medium attracts a particular class of surface-active compounds, namely those possessing both a fat-soluble group and a water-soluble group. Long-chain hydrocarbons are very fat-soluble, while charged ions are very water-soluble; a compound possessing both structures will thus concentrate at the surface of the bacterial cell.

Two general types of such surface-active agents, or detergents, are known: anionic and cationic.

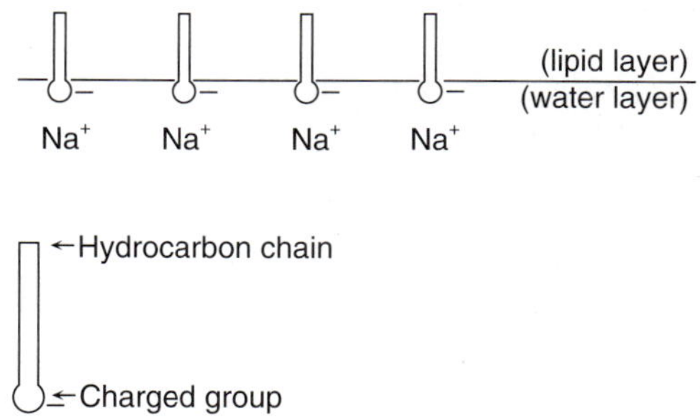

1. Anionic detergents–Detergents in which the long-chain hydrocarbon has a negative charge are called "anionic." These include soaps (sodium salts of long-chain carboxylic acids); synthetic products resembling soaps (except that the carboxyl group is replaced by a sulfonic acid group); and bile salts, in which the fat-soluble portion has a steroid structure. Some examples are shown in Figures 4–5, 4–6, and 4–7.

The synthetic detergents have advantages in solubility and cost over the natural soaps (obtained by saponification of animal fat). Bile salts are notable in that they completely dissolve pneumococcal cells, thus providing an aid in identification.

2. Cationic detergents–The fat-soluble moiety can be made to have a positive charge by combining it

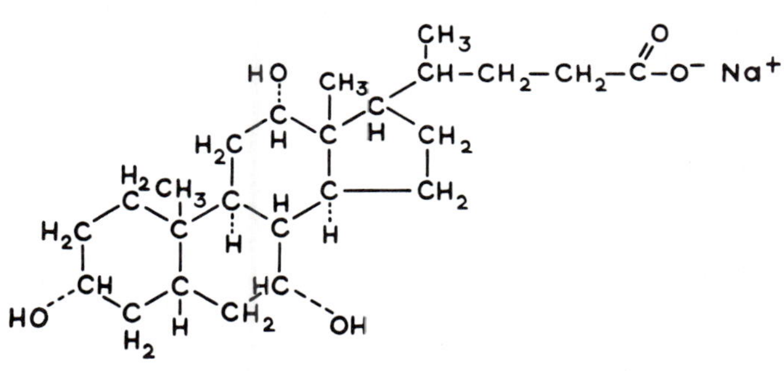

Figure 4–7. Sodium salt of cholic acid (a bile salt).

with a quaternary (valence = +5) nitrogen atom (Figure 4–8).

Since the detergents concentrate at the cell membrane, and since the latter is a delicate, essential cell component, the inference is drawn that detergents act by disrupting the normal function of the cell membrane. Support for this view comes from experiments showing that cells exposed to detergents leak soluble nitrogen and phosphorus compounds into the medium.

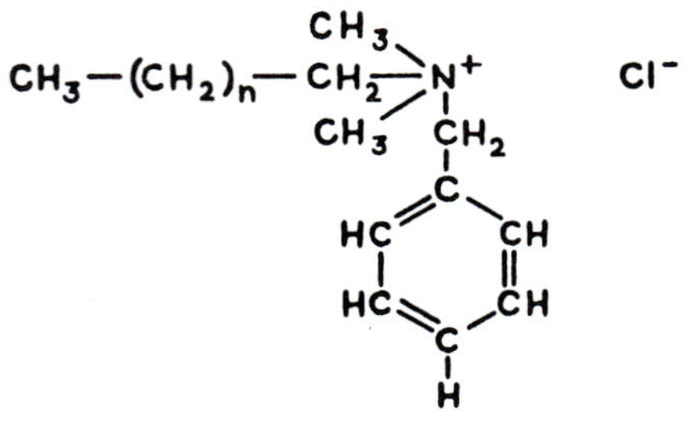

Figure 4–8. Alkyldimethylbenzylammonium chloride.

Chemotherapeutic Agents

To be a useful chemotherapeutic agent, a compound must be either bacteriostatic or bactericidal in vivo (action not reversed by substances in host tissues or fluids) and at the same time remain noninjurious to the host. These requirements for in vivo effectiveness and selective toxicity narrow the list of important chemotherapeutic agents to a very few compounds, including the sulfonamides, the antibiotics, and the antituberculosis agents.

The natures and modes of action of these drugs are discussed in Chapter 10.

REFERENCES

Books

Block SS (editor): *Disinfection, Sterilization, and Preservation,* 2nd ed. Lea & Febiger, 1977.

Gerhardt P et al (editors): *Manual of Methods for General Bacteriology.* American Society for Microbiology, 1981.

Hanawalt PC et al (editors): *DNA Repair Mechanisms.* Academic Press, 1978.

Hugo WB (editor): *Inhibition and Destruction of the Microbial Cell.* Academic Press, 1971.

Ingraham JL, Maaløe O, Neidhardt FC: *Growth of the Bacterial Cell.* Sinauer, 1983.

Kjelleberg S (editor): *Starvation in Bacteria.* Plenum Press, 1993.

Mandelstam J, McQuillen K, Dawes I: *Biochemistry of Bacterial Growth,* 3rd ed. Halsted, 1982.

Rehm HJ, Reed G (editors): *Biotechnology.* Vol 1: *Microbial Fundamentals.* Verlag Chemie, 1981.

Russell AD: *The Destruction of Bacterial Spores.* Academic Press, 1982.

Articles & Reviews

Donohue WD: The cell cycle of *Escherichia coli.* Annu Rev Microbiol 1993;47:199.

Franklin WA, Haseltine WA: Removal of UV light-induced pyrimidine-pyrimidone(6–4) products from *Escherichia coli* DNA requires the uvrB, and uvrC gene products. Proc Natl Acad Sci USA 1984;81: 3821.

Howard-Flanders P: Inducible repair of DNA. Sci Am (Nov) 1981;245:72.

Kjelleberg S et al: The transient phase between growth and nongrowth of heterotrophic bacteria. Annu Rev Microbiol 1987;41:25.

Kolter R, Siegels DA, Tormo A: The stationary phase of the bacterial life cycle. J Bacteriol 1992;174:345.

Lambert PA: Membrane-active antimicrobial agents. Prog Med Chem 1978;15:87.

Matin A et al: Genetic basis of starvation-survival in nondifferentiating bacteria. Annu Rev Microbiol 1989;43: 293.

Meyer HP, Käppeli O, Fiechter A: Growth control in microbial cultures. Annu Rev Microbiol 1985;39:299.

Sancar A, Sancar GB: DNA repair enzymes. Annu Rev Biochem 1988;57:29.

Siegels DA, Kolter R: Life after log. J Bacteriol 1992;174: 345.

Tempest DW, Niejssel OM: The status of YAPT and maintenance energy as biologically interpretable phenomena. Annu Rev Microbiol 1984;38:459.

Cultivation of Microorganisms 5

Cultivation is the process of propagating organisms by providing the proper environmental conditions. Growing microorganisms are making replicas of themselves, and they require the elements present in their chemical composition. Nutrients must provide these elements in metabolically accessible form. In addition, the organisms require metabolic energy in order to synthesize macromolecules and maintain essential chemical gradients across their membranes. Factors that must be controlled during growth include the nutrients, pH, temperature, aeration, salt concentration, and ionic strength of the medium.

REQUIREMENTS FOR GROWTH

Most of the dry weight of microorganisms is organic matter containing the elements carbon, hydrogen, nitrogen, oxygen, phosphorus, and sulfur. In addition, inorganic ions such as potassium, sodium, iron, magnesium, calcium, and chloride are required to facilitate enzymatic catalysis and to maintain chemical gradients across the cell membrane.

For the most part, the organic matter is in macromolecules formed by **anhydride bonds** between building blocks. Synthesis of the anhydride bonds requires chemical energy, which is provided by the two phosphodiester bonds in ATP (adenosine triphosphate; see Chapter 6). Additional energy required to maintain a relatively constant cytoplasmic composition during growth in a range of extracellular chemical environments is derived from the **proton motive force.** The proton motive force is the potential energy that can be derived by passage of a proton across a membrane. In eukaryotes, the membrane may be part of the mitochondrion or the chloroplast. In prokaryotes, the membrane is the cytoplasmic membrane of the cell.

The proton motive force is an electrochemical gradient with two components: a difference in pH (hydrogen ion concentration) and a difference in ionic charge. The charge on the outside of the bacterial membrane is more positive than the charge on the inside, and the difference in charge contributes to the free energy released when a proton enters the cytoplasm from outside the membrane. Metabolic processes that generate the proton motive force are discussed in Chapter 6. The free energy may be used to move the cell, to maintain ionic or molecular gradients across the membrane, to synthesize anhydride bonds in ATP, or for a combination of these purposes. Alternatively, cells given a source of ATP may use its anhydride bond energy to create a proton motive force that in turn may be used to move the cell and to maintain chemical gradients.

In order to grow, an organism requires all of the elements in its organic matter and the full complement of ions required for energetics and catalysis. In addition, there must be a source of energy to establish the proton motive force and to allow macromolecular synthesis. Microorganisms vary widely in their nutritional demands and their sources of metabolic energy.

SOURCES OF METABOLIC ENERGY

The three major mechanisms for generating metabolic energy are fermentation, respiration, and photosynthesis. At least one of these mechanisms must be employed if an organism is to grow.

Fermentation

The formation of ATP in fermentation is not coupled to the transfer of electrons. Fermentation is characterized by **substrate phosphorylation,** an enzymatic process in which a pyrophosphate bond is donated directly to ADP (adenosine diphosphate) by a phosphorylated metabolic intermediate. The phosphorylated intermediates are formed by metabolic rearrangement of a fermentable substrate such as glucose, lactose, or arginine. Because fermentations are not accompanied by a change in the overall oxidation-reduction state of the fermentable substrate, the elemental composition of the products of fermentation must be identical to those of the substrates. For example, fermentation of a molecule of glucose ($C_6H_{12}O_6$) by the Embden-Meyerhof pathway (see Chapter 6) yields a net gain of two pyrophosphate bonds in ATP and produces two molecules of lactic acid ($C_3H_6O_3$).

Respiration

Respiration is analogous to the coupling of an energy-dependent process to the discharge of a battery. Chemical reduction of an oxidant (electron acceptor) through a specific series of electron carriers in the membrane establishes the proton motive force across the bacterial membrane. The reductant (electron donor) may be organic or inorganic: for example, lactic acid serves as a reductant for some organisms, and hydrogen gas is a reductant for other organisms. Gaseous oxygen (O_2) often is employed as an oxidant, but alternative oxidants that are employed by some organisms include carbon dioxide (CO_2), sulfate (SO_4^{2-}), and nitrate (NO_3^-).

Photosynthesis

Photosynthesis is similar to respiration in that the reduction of an oxidant via a specific series of electron carriers establishes the proton motive force. The difference in the two processes is that in photosynthesis the reductant and oxidant are created photochemically by light energy absorbed by pigments in the membrane; thus, photosynthesis can continue only as long as there is a source of light energy. Plants and some bacteria are able to invest a substantial amount of light energy in making water a reductant for carbon dioxide. Oxygen is evolved in this process, and organic matter is produced. Respiration, the energetically favorable oxidation of organic matter by an electronic acceptor such as oxygen, can provide photosynthetic organisms with energy in the absence of light.

NUTRITION

Nutrients in growth media must contain all the elements necessary for the biologic synthesis of new organisms. In the following discussion, nutrients are classified according to the elements they supply.

Carbon Source

As mentioned above, plants and some bacteria are able to use photosynthetic energy to reduce carbon dioxide at the expense of water. These organisms belong to the group of **autotrophs,** creatures that do not require organic nutrients for growth. Other autotrophs are the **chemolithotrophs,** organisms that use an inorganic substrate such as hydrogen or thiosulfate as a reductant and carbon dioxide as a carbon source.

Heterotrophs require organic carbon for growth, and the organic carbon must be in a form that can be assimilated. Naphthalene, for example, can provide all the carbon and energy required for respiratory heterotrophic growth, but very few organisms possess the metabolic pathway necessary for naphthalene assimilation. Glucose, on the other hand, can support the fermentative or respiratory growth of many organisms. It is important that growth substrates be supplied at levels appropriate for the microbial strain that is being grown: levels that will support the growth of one organism may inhibit the growth of another organism.

Carbon dioxide is required for a number of biosynthetic reactions. Many respiratory organisms produce more than enough carbon dioxide to meet this requirement, but others require a source of carbon dioxide in their growth medium.

Nitrogen Source

Nitrogen is a major component of proteins and nucleic acids, accounting for about 10% of the dry weight of a typical bacterial cell. Nitrogen may be supplied in a number of different forms (Table 5–1), and microorganisms vary in their abilities to assimilate nitrogen. The end product of all pathways for nitrogen assimilation is the most reduced form of the element, ammonium ion (NH_4^+).

Many microorganisms possess the ability to assimilate nitrate (NO_3^-) and nitrite NO_2^-) reductively by conversion of these ions to ammonia (NH_3). These pathways for **assimilation** differ from pathways used for **dissimilation** of nitrate and nitrite. The dissimilatory pathways are used by organisms that employ the ions as terminal electron acceptors in respiration; this process is known as **denitrification,** and its product is nitrogen gas (N_2), which is evolved into the atmosphere.

The ability to assimilate N_2 reductively via NH_3, which is called **nitrogen fixation,** is a property unique to prokaryotes, and relatively few bacteria possess this metabolic capacity. The process requires a large amount of metabolic energy and is readily inactivated by oxygen. The capacity for nitrogen fixation is found in widely divergent bacteria that have evolved quite different biochemical strategies to protect their nitrogen-fixing enzymes from oxygen.

Most microorganisms can use NH_4^+ as a sole nitrogen source, and many organisms possess the ability to produce NH_4^+ from amines ($R-NH_2$). Ammonia is introduced into organic matter by biochemical pathways involving glutamate and glutamine. These pathways are discussed in Chapter 6.

Sulfur Source

Like nitrogen, sulfur is a component of many organic cell substances. It forms part of the structure of several coenzymes and is found in the cysteinyl and methionyl side chains of proteins. Most microorganisms can use sulfate (SO_4^{2-}) as a sulfur source, reducing the sulfate to the level of hydrogen sulfide (H_2).

Table 5–1. Sources of nitrogen in microbial nutrition.

Compound	Valence of N
No_3^-	+5
NO_2^-	+3
N_2	0
NH_4^+	−3
$R-NH_2$[1]	−3

[1] R = Organic radical.

Some microorganisms can assimilate H_2 directly from the growth medium, but this compound can be toxic to many organisms.

Phosphorus Source

Phosphate (PO_4^{3-}) is required as a component of ATP, nucleic acids, and such coenzymes as NAD, NADP, and flavins. In addition, many metabolites and some proteins are phosphorylated. Phosphate is always assimilated as free inorganic phosphate (P_i).

Mineral Sources

Numerous minerals are required for enzyme function. Magnesium ion (Mg^{2+}) and ferrous ion (Fe^{2+}) are also found in porphyrin derivatives: magnesium in the chlorophyll molecule, and iron as part of the coenzymes of the cytochromes and peroxidases. Mg^{2+} and K^+ are both essential for the function and integrity of ribosomes. Ca^{2+} is required as a constituent of gram-positive cell walls, though it is dispensable for gram-negative bacteria. Many marine organisms require Na^+ for growth. In formulating a medium for the cultivation of most microorganisms, it is necessary to provide sources of potassium, magnesium, calcium, and iron, usually as their ions (K^+, Mg^{2+}, Ca^{2+}, and Fe^{2+}). Many other minerals (eg, Mn^{2+}, Mo^{2+}, Co^{2+}, Cu^{2+}, and Zn^{2+}) are required; these frequently can be provided in tap water or as contaminants of other medium ingredients.

The uptake of iron, which forms insoluble hydroxides at neutral pH, is facilitated in many bacteria and fungi by their production of **siderophores**—compounds that chelate iron and promote its transport as a soluble complex. These include hydroxamates ($-CONH_2OH$) called sideramines, and derivatives of catechol (eg, 2,3-dihydroxybenzoylserine). Plasmid-determined siderophores play a major role in the invasiveness of some bacterial pathogens (see Chapter 7).

Growth Factors

A growth factor is an organic compound which a cell must contain in order to grow but which it is unable to synthesize. Many microorganisms, when provided with the nutrients listed above, are able to synthesize all of the building blocks for macromolecules (Figure 5–1): amino acids; purines, pyrimidines, and pentoses (the metabolic precursors of nucleic acids); additional carbohydrates (precursors of polysaccharides); and fatty acids and isoprenoid compounds. In addition, free-living organisms must be able to synthesize the complex vitamins that serve as precursors of coenzymes.

Each of these essential compounds is synthesized by a discrete sequence of enzymatic reactions; each enzyme is produced under the control of a specific gene. When an organism undergoes a gene mutation resulting in failure of one of these enzymes to function, the chain is broken and the end product is no longer produced. The organism must then obtain that compound from the environment: the compound has become a **growth factor** for the organism. This type of mutation can be readily induced in the laboratory.

Different microbial species vary widely in their growth factor requirements. The compounds involved are found in and are essential to all organisms; the differences in requirements reflect differences in synthetic abilities. Some species require no growth factors, while others—like some of the lactobacilli—have lost, during evolution, the ability to synthesize as many as 30–40 essential compounds and hence require them in the medium.

ENVIRONMENTAL FACTORS AFFECTING GROWTH

A suitable growth medium must contain all the nutrients required by the organism to be cultivated, and such factors as pH, temperature, and aeration must be carefully controlled. A liquid medium is used; the medium can be gelled for special purposes by adding agar or silica gel. Agar, a polysaccharide extract of a marine alga, is uniquely suitable for microbial cultivation because it is resistant to microbial action and because it dissolves at 100 °C but does not gel until cooled below 45 °C; cells can be suspended in the medium at 45 °C and the medium quickly cooled to a gel without harming them.

Nutrients

On the previous pages, the function of each type of nutrient is described and a list of suitable substances presented. In general, the following must be provided: (1) Hydrogen donors and acceptors: about 2 g/L. (2) Carbon source: about 1 g/L. (3) Nitrogen source: about 1 g/L. (4) Minerals: sulfur and phosphorus, about 50 mg/L of each; trace elements, 0.1–1 mg/L of each. (5) Growth factors: amino acids, purines, pyrimidines, about 50 mg/L of each; vitamins, 0.1–1 mg/L of each.

For studies of microbial metabolism, it is usually necessary to prepare a completely synthetic medium in which the exact characteristics and concentration of every ingredient are known. Otherwise, it is much cheaper and simpler to use natural materials such as yeast extract, protein digest, or similar substances. Most free-living microbes will grow well on yeast extract; parasitic forms may require special substances found only in blood or in extracts of animal tissues.

For many organisms, a single compound (such as an amino acid) may serve as energy source, carbon source, and nitrogen source; others require a separate compound for each. If natural materials for nonsynthetic media are deficient in any particular nutrient, they must be supplemented.

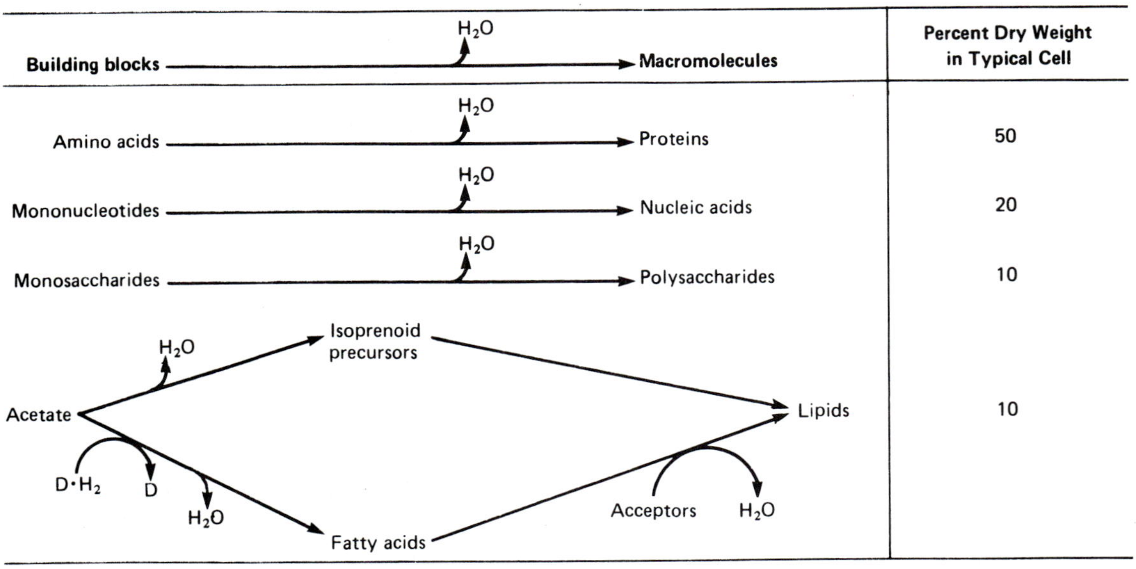

Figure 5–1. Macromolecular synthesis. Polymerization of building blocks into macromolecules is achieved largely by the introduction of anhydride bonds. Formation of fatty acids from acetate requires several steps of biochemical reduction using organic hydrogen donors (D · H_2).

Hydrogen Ion Concentration (pH)

Most organisms have a fairly narrow optimal pH range. The optimal pH must be empirically determined for each species. Most organisms (neutrophils) grow best at a pH of 6.0–8.0, although some forms (acidophils) have optima as low as pH 3.0 and others (alkalophils) have optima as high as pH 10.5.

Microorganisms regulate their internal pH over a wide range of external pH values. Acidophils maintain an internal pH of about 6.5 over an external range of 1.0–5.0; neutrophils maintain an internal pH of about 7.5 over an external range of 5.5–8.5; and alkalophils maintain an internal pH of about 9.5 over an external range of 9.0–11.0. Internal pH is regulated by a set of proton transport systems in the cytoplasmic membrane, including a primary, ATP-driven proton pump and a Na^+/H^+ exchanger. A K^+/H^+ exchange system has also been proposed to contribute to internal pH regulation in neutrophils.

Temperature

Different microbial species vary widely in their optimal temperature ranges for growth: psychrophilic forms grow best at low temperatures (15–20 °C); mesophilic forms grow best at 30–37 °C; and most thermophilic forms grow best at 50–60 °C. Most organisms are mesophilic; 30 °C is optimal for many free-living forms, and the body temperature of the host is optimal for symbionts of warm-blooded animals.

The upper end of the temperature range tolerated by any given species correlates well with the general thermal stability of that species' proteins as measured in cell extracts. Microorganisms share with plants and animals the **heat-shock response,** a transient synthesis of a set of "heat-shock proteins" when exposed to a sudden rise in temperature above the growth optimum. These proteins appear to be unusually heat-resistant and to stabilize the heat-sensitive proteins of the cell.

The relationship of growth rate to temperature for any given microorganism is seen in a typical Arrhenius plot (Figure 5–2). Arrhenius showed that the logarithm of the velocity of any chemical reaction (log k) is a linear function of the reciprocal of the temperature (1/T); since cell growth is the result of a set of chemical reactions, it might be expected to show this relationship. Figure 5–2 shows this to be the case over the normal range of temperatures for a given species: log k decreases linearly with 1/T. Above and below the normal range, however, log k drops rapidly, so that maximum temperature values are defined.

Beyond their effects on growth rate, extremes of temperature kill microorganisms. Extreme heat is used to sterilize preparations (see Chapter 4); extreme cold also kills microbial cells, although it cannot be used safely for sterilization. Bacteria also exhibit a phenomenon called **cold shock:** the killing of cells by rapid—as opposed to slow—cooling. For example, the rapid cooling of *Escherichia coli* from 37 °C to 5 °C can kill 90% of the cells. A number of compounds protect cells from either freezing or cold shock; glycerol and dimethysulfoxide are most commonly used.

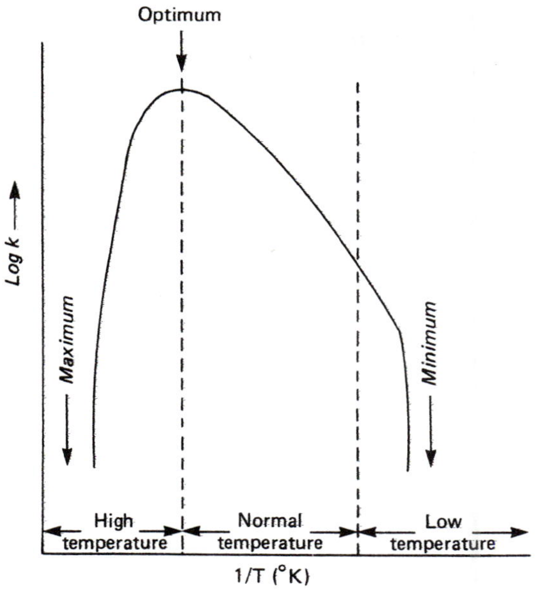

Figure 5–2. General form of an Arrhenius plot of bacterial growth. (After Ingraham JL, Maaløe O, Neidhardt FC: *Growth of the Bacterial Cell.* Sinauer Associates, 1983.)

Aeration

The role of oxygen as hydrogen acceptor is discussed in Chapter 6. Many organisms are obligate aerobes, specifically requiring oxygen as hydrogen acceptor; some are facultative, able to live aerobically or anaerobically; and others are obligate anaerobes, requiring a substance other than oxygen as hydrogen acceptor and being sensitive to oxygen inhibition.

The toxicity of O_2 results from its reduction by enzymes in the cell (such as flavoproteins) to hydrogen peroxide (H_2O_2) and by ferrous ion to the even more toxic free radical, superoxide (O_2^-). Aerobes and aerotolerant anaerobes are protected from these products by the presence of superoxide dismutase, an enzyme that catalyzes the reaction

$$2O_2^- + 2H^+ \rightarrow O_2 + H_2O_2$$

and by the presence of catalase, an enzyme that catalyzes the reaction

$$2H_2O_2 \rightarrow 2H_2O + O_2$$

One exception to this rule is the lactic acid bacteria, aerotolerant anaerobes that do not contain catalase. This group relies instead on peroxidases, which reduce H_2O_2 to $2H_2O$ at the expense of oxidizable organic substrates. All strict anaerobes lack both superoxide dismutase and catalase; the former enzyme is indispensable for survival in the presence of O_2.

Hydrogen peroxide owes much of its toxicity to the damage it causes to DNA. DNA repair-deficient mutants are exceptionally sensitive to hydrogen peroxide; the *recA* gene product, which functions in both genetic recombination and repair, has been shown to be more important than either catalase or superoxide dismutase in protecting *E coli* cells against hydrogen peroxide toxicity.

The supply of air to cultures of aerobes is a major technical problem. Vessels are usually shaken mechanically to introduce oxygen into the medium, or air is forced through the medium by pressure. The diffusion of oxygen often becomes the limiting factor in growing aerobic bacteria; when a cell concentration of $4–5 \times 10^9$/mL is reached, the rate of diffusion of oxygen to the cells sharply limits the rate of further growth.

Obligate anaerobes, on the other hand, present the problem of oxygen exclusion. Many methods are available for this: reducing agents such as sodium thioglycolate can be added to liquid cultures; tubes of agar can be sealed with a layer of petrolatum and paraffin; the culture vessel can be placed in a container from which the oxygen is removed by evacuation or by chemical means; or the organism can be handled within an anaerobic glove-box.

Ionic Strength & Osmotic Pressure

To a lesser extent, such factors as osmotic pressure and salt concentration may have to be controlled. For most organisms, the properties of ordinary media are satisfactory; but for marine forms and organisms adapted to growth in strong sugar solutions, for example, these factors must be considered. Organisms requiring high salt concentrations are called **halophilic;** those requiring high osmotic pressures are called **osmophilic.**

Most bacteria are able to tolerate a wide range of external osmotic pressures and ionic strengths because of their ability to regulate internal osmolality and ion concentration. Osmolality is regulated by the active transport of K^+ ions into the cell; internal ionic strength is kept constant by a compensating excretion of the positively charged organic polyamine putrescine. Since putrescine carries several positive charges per molecule, a large drop in ionic strength is effected at only a small cost in osmotic strength.

CULTIVATION METHODS

Two problems will be considered: the choice of a suitable medium and the isolation of a bacterial organism in pure culture.

The Medium

The technique used and the type of medium selected depend upon the nature of the investigation. In general, three situations may be encountered: (1) one may need to raise a crop of cells of a particular species that is on hand; (2) one may need to determine the numbers and types of organisms present in a given material; or (3) one may wish to isolate a particular type of microorganism from a natural source.

A. Growing Cells of a Given Species: Microorganisms observed microscopically to be growing in a natural environment may prove exceedingly difficult to grow in pure culture in an artificial medium. Certain parasitic forms, for example, have never been cultivated outside the host. In general, however, a suitable medium can be devised by carefully reproducing the conditions found in the organism's natural environment. The pH, temperature, and aeration are simple to duplicate; the nutrients present the major problem. The contribution made by the living environment is important and difficult to analyze; a parasite may require an extract of the host tissue, and a free-living form may require a substance excreted by a microorganism with which it is associated in nature. Considerable experimentation may be necessary in order to determine the requirements of the organism, and success depends upon providing a suitable source of each category of nutrient listed at the beginning of this chapter. The cultivation of obligate parasites such as rickettsiae is discussed in Chapter 47.

B. Microbiologic Examination of Natural Materials: A given natural material may contain many different microenvironments, each providing a niche for a different species. Plating a sample of the material under one set of conditions will allow a selected group of forms to produce colonies but will cause many other types to be overlooked. For this reason, it is customary to plate out samples of the material using as many different media and conditions of incubation as is practicable. Six to eight different culture conditions are not an unreasonable number if most of the forms present are to be discovered.

Since every type of organism present must have a chance to grow, solid media are used and crowding of colonies is avoided. Otherwise, competition will prevent some types from forming colonies.

C. Isolation of a Particular Type of Microorganism: A small sample of soil, if handled properly, will yield a different type of organism for every microenvironment present. For fertile soil (moist, aerated, rich in minerals and organic matter) this means that hundreds or even thousands of types can be isolated. This is done by selecting for the desired type. One gram of soil, for example, is inoculated into a flask of liquid medium that has been made up for the purpose of favoring one type of organism, eg, aerobic nitrogen fixers *(Azotobacter)*. In this case, the medium contains no combined nitrogen and is incubated aerobically. If cells of *Azotobacter* are present in the soil, they will grow well in this medium; forms unable to fix nitrogen will grow only to the extent that the soil has introduced contaminating fixed nitrogen into the medium. When the culture is fully grown, therefore, the percentage of *Azotobacter* in the total population will have increased greatly; the method is thus called "enrichment culture." Transfer of a sample of this culture to fresh medium will result in further enrichment of *Azotobacter*; after several serial transfers, the culture can be plated out on a solidified enrichment medium and colonies of *Azotobacter* isolated.

Liquid medium is used to permit competition and hence optimal selection, even when the desired type is represented in the soil as only a few cells in a population of millions. Advantage can be taken of "natural enrichment." For example, in looking for kerosene oxidizers, oil-laden soil is chosen, since it is already an enrichment environment for such forms.

Enrichment culture, then, is a procedure whereby the medium is prepared so as to duplicate the natural environment ("niche") of the desired microorganism, thereby selecting for it. An important principle involved in such selection is the following: The organism selected for will be the type whose nutritional requirements are barely satisfied. *Azotobacter*, for example, grows best in a medium containing organic nitrogen, but its minimum requirement is the presence of N_2; hence it is selected for in a medium containing N_2 as the sole nitrogen source. If organic nitrogen is added to the medium, the conditions no longer select for *Azotobacter* but rather for a form for which organic nitrogen is the minimum requirement.

When searching for a particular type of organism in a natural material, it is advantageous to plate the organisms obtained on a differential medium if available. A differential medium is one that will cause the colonies of a particular type of organism to have a distinctive appearance. For example, colonies of *E coli* have a characteristic iridescent sheen on agar containing the dyes eosin and methylene blue (EMB agar). EMB agar containing a high concentration of one sugar will also cause organisms which ferment that sugar to form reddish colonies. Differential media are used for such purposes as recognizing the presence of enteric bacteria in water or milk and the presence of certain pathogens in clinical specimens.

Table 5–2 presents examples of enrichment culture conditions and the types of bacteria they will select.

Isolation of Microorganisms in Pure Culture

In order to study the properties of a given organism, it is necessary to handle it in pure culture free of all other types of organisms. To do this, a single cell must be isolated from all other cells and cultivated in such a manner that its collective progeny also remain isolated. Several methods are available.

A. Plating: Unlike cells in a liquid medium, cells in or on a gelled medium are immobilized. Therefore, if few enough cells are placed in or on a gelled medium, each cell will grow into an isolated colony. The ideal gelling agent for most microbiologic media

Table 5–2. Some enrichment cultures.
Constituents of all media: $MgSO_4$, K_2HPO_4, $FeCl_3$, $CaCl_2$, $CaCO_3$, trace elements.

Nitrogen Source	Carbon Source	Atmosphere	Illumination	Predominant Organism Initially Enriched
N_2	Cl_2	Aerobic or anaerobic	Dark	None
			Light	Cyanobacteria
	Alcohol, fatty acids, etc	Anaerobic	Dark	None
		Air	Dark	*Azotobacter*
	Glucose	Anaerobic	Dark	*Clostridium pasteurianum*
		Air	Dark	*Azotobacter*
$NaNO_3$	CO_2	Aerobic or anaerobic	Dark	None
			Light	Green algae and cyanobacteria
	Alcohol, fatty acids, etc	Anaerobic	Dark	Denitrifiers
		Air	Dark	Aerobes
	Glucose	Anaerobic	Dark	Fermenters
		Air	Dark	Aerobes
NH_4Cl	CO_2	Anaerobic	Dark	None
		Aerobic	Dark	*Nitrosomonas*
		Aerobic or anaerobic	Light	Green algae and cyanobacteria
	Alcohol, fatty acids, etc	Anaerobic	Dark	Sulfate or carbonate reducers
		Aerobic	Dark	Aerobes
	Glucose	Anaerobic	Dark	Fermenters
		Aerobic	Dark	Aerobes

is **agar,** an acidic polysaccharide extracted from certain red algae. A 1.5–2% suspension in water dissolves at 100 °C, forming a clear solution that gels at 45 °C. Thus, a sterile agar solution can be cooled to 50 °C, bacteria or other microbial cells added, and then the solution quickly cooled below 45 °C to form a gel. (Although most microbial cells are killed at 50 °C, the time-course of the killing process is sufficiently slow at this temperature to permit this procedure; see Figure 4–3.) Once gelled, agar will not again liquefy until it is heated above 80 °C, so that any temperature suitable for the incubation of a microbial culture can subsequently be used. In the pour-plate method, a suspension of cells is mixed with melted agar at 50 °C and poured into a Petri dish. When the agar solidifies, the cells are immobilized in the agar and grow into colonies. If the cell suspension was sufficiently dilute, the colonies will be well separated, so that each has a high probability of being derived from a single cell. To make certain of this, however, it is necessary to pick a colony of the desired type, suspend it in water, and replate. Repeating this procedure several times ensures that a pure culture will be obtained.

Alternatively, the original suspension can be streaked on an agar plate with a wire loop. As the streaking continues, fewer and fewer cells are left on the loop, and finally the loop may deposit single cells on the agar. The plate is incubated, and any well-isolated colony is then removed, resuspended in water, and again streaked on agar. If a suspension (and not just a bit of growth from a colony or slant) is streaked, this method is just as reliable as and much faster than the pour-plate method.

B. Dilution: A much less reliable method is that of extinction dilution. The suspension is serially diluted, and samples of each dilution are plated. If only a few samples of a particular dilution exhibit growth, it is presumed that some of these cultures started from single cells. This method is not used unless plating is for some reason impossible. An undesirable feature of this method is that it can only be used to isolate the predominant type of organism in a mixed population.

REFERENCES

Books

Alexander M: *Microbial Ecology.* Wiley, 1971.

Cohen G, Greenwald RA (editors): *Oxy Radicals and Their Scavenger Systems.* Vol 1: *Molecular Aspects.* Vol 2: *Cellular and Medical Aspects.* Elsevier, 1983.

Gerhardt P et al (editors): *Manual of Methods for General Bacteriology.* American Society for Microbiology, 1981.

Lichstin HC (editor): *Bacterial Nutrition.* Van Nostrand Reinhold, 1983.

Oberley LW (editor): *Superoxide Dismutase.* CRC Press, 1982.

Pirt SJ: *Principles of Microbe and Cell Cultivation.* Wiley, 1975.

Precht H et al (editors): *Temperature and Life.* Springer-Verlag, 1973.

Schlegel HG (editor): *Enrichment Culture and Mutant Selection.* Fischer, 1965.

Stanier RY et al: *The Microbial World,* 5th ed. Prentice-Hall, 1979.

Articles & Reviews

Adams MWW: Enzymes and proteins from organisms that grow near or above 100 °C. Annu Rev Microbiol 1993;37:627.

Alexander M: Why microbial predators and parasites do not eliminate their prey and hosts. Annu Rev Microbiol 1981;35:113.

Baross JA, Deming JW: Growth of "black smoker" bacteria at temperatures of at least 250 °C. Nature 1983; 303:423.

Fridovich I: Oxygen: Boon and bane. Am Sci 1975;63:54.

Harder W, Dijkhuizen L: Physiological responses to nutrient limitation. Annu Rev Microbiol 1983;37:1.

Hutner SH: Inorganic nutrition. Annu Rev Microbiol 1972;26:313.

Krulevitch TA, Guffanti AA: Alkalophilic bacteria. Annu Rev Microbiol 1989;43:435.

Marzlut GA: Regulation of sulfur and nitrogen metabolism in filamentary fungi. Annu Rev Microbiol 1993; 42:89.

Minton KW et al: Nonspecific stabilization of stress susceptible proteins by stress-resistant proteins: A model for the biological role of heat shock proteins. Proc Natl Acad Sci USA 1982;79:7107.

Morris JG: The physiology of obligate anaerobiosis. Adv Microb Physiol 1975;12:169.

Nielands JB: Hydroxamic acids in nature. Science 1967;156:1443.

Padan E, Zilberstein D, Schuldiner S: pH homeostasis in bacteria. Biochim Biophys Acta 1981;650:151.

Microbial Metabolism 6

ROLE OF METABOLISM IN BIOSYNTHESIS & GROWTH

Microbial growth requires the polymerization of biochemical building blocks into proteins, nucleic acids, polysaccharides, and lipids. The building blocks must come preformed in the growth medium or must be synthesized by the growing cells. Additional biosynthetic demands are placed by the requirement for coenzymes that participate in enzymatic catalysis. Biosynthetic polymerization reactions demand the transfer of anhydride bonds from ATP. Growth demands a source of metabolic energy for the synthesis of anhydride bonds and for the maintenance of transmembrane gradients of ions and metabolites.

The biosynthetic origins of building blocks and coenzymes can be traced to relatively few precursors, called **focal metabolites.** Figures 6–1, 6–2, 6–3, and 6–4 illustrate how the respective focal metabolites glucose 6-phosphate, phosphoenolpyruvate, oxaloacetate, and α-ketoglutarate give rise to most biosynthetic end products. Microbial metabolism can be divided into four general categories: (1) pathways for the interconversion of focal metabolites, (2) assimilatory pathways for the formation of focal metabolites, (3) biosynthetic sequences for the conversion of focal metabolites to end products, and (4) pathways that yield metabolic energy for growth and maintenance.

When provided with building blocks and a source of metabolic energy, a cell synthesizes macromolecules. The sequence of building blocks within a macromolecule is determined in one of two ways. In nucleic acids and proteins, it is **template-directed:** DNA serves as the template for its own synthesis and for the synthesis of the various types of RNA; messenger RNA serves as the template for the synthesis of proteins. In carbohydrates and lipids, on the other hand, the arrangement of building blocks is determined entirely by enzyme specificities. Once the macromolecules have been synthesized, they self-assemble to form the supramolecular structures of the cell, eg, ribosomes, membranes, cell wall, flagella, pili.

The rate of macromolecular synthesis and the activity of metabolic pathways must be regulated so that biosynthesis is balanced. All of the components required for macromolecular synthesis must be present for orderly growth, and control must be exerted so that the resources of the cell are not expended on products that do not contribute to growth or survival.

This chapter contains a review of microbial metabolism and its regulation. Microorganisms represent extremes of evolutionary divergence, and a vast array of metabolic pathways are found within the group. For example, any of more than half a dozen different metabolic pathways may be used for assimilation of a relatively simple compound, benzoate, and a single pathway for benzoate assimilation may be regulated by any of more than half a dozen control mechanisms. Our goal will be to illustrate the principles that underlie metabolic pathways and their regulation. The primary principle that determines metabolic pathways is that they are achieved by organizing relatively few biochemical type reactions in a specific order. Many biosynthetic pathways can be deduced by examining the chemical structures of the starting material, the end product, and, perhaps, one or two metabolic intermediates. The primary principle underlying metabolic regulation is that enzymes tend to be called into play only when their catalytic activity is demanded. The activity of an enzyme may be changed by varying either the amount of enzyme or the amount of substrate. In some cases, the activity of enzymes may be altered by the binding of specific **effectors,** metabolites that modulate enzyme activity.

FOCAL METABOLITES & THEIR INTERCONVERSION

Glucose 6-Phosphate & Carbohydrate Interconversions

Figure 6–1 illustrates how glucose 6-phosphate is converted to a range of biosynthetic end products via phosphate esters of carbohydrates with different chain lengths. Carbohydrates possess the empirical formula $(CH_2O)_n$, and the primary objective of carbohydrate metabolism is to change *n*, the length of the carbon chain. Mechanisms by which the chain lengths of carbohydrate phosphates are interconverted are summarized in Figure 6–5. In one case, oxidative reactions are used to remove a single carbon from glucose 6-phosphate, producing the pentose derivative ribu-

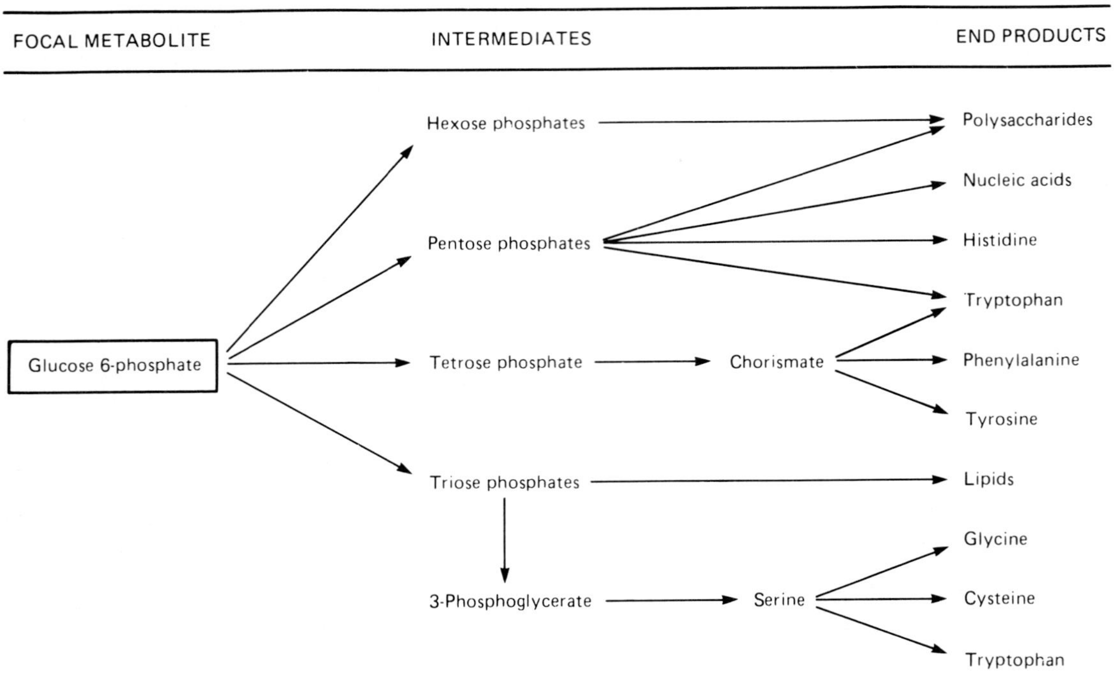

Figure 6–1. Biosynthetic end products formed from glucose 6-phosphate. Carbohydrate phosphate esters of varying chain length serve as intermediates in the biosynthetic pathways.

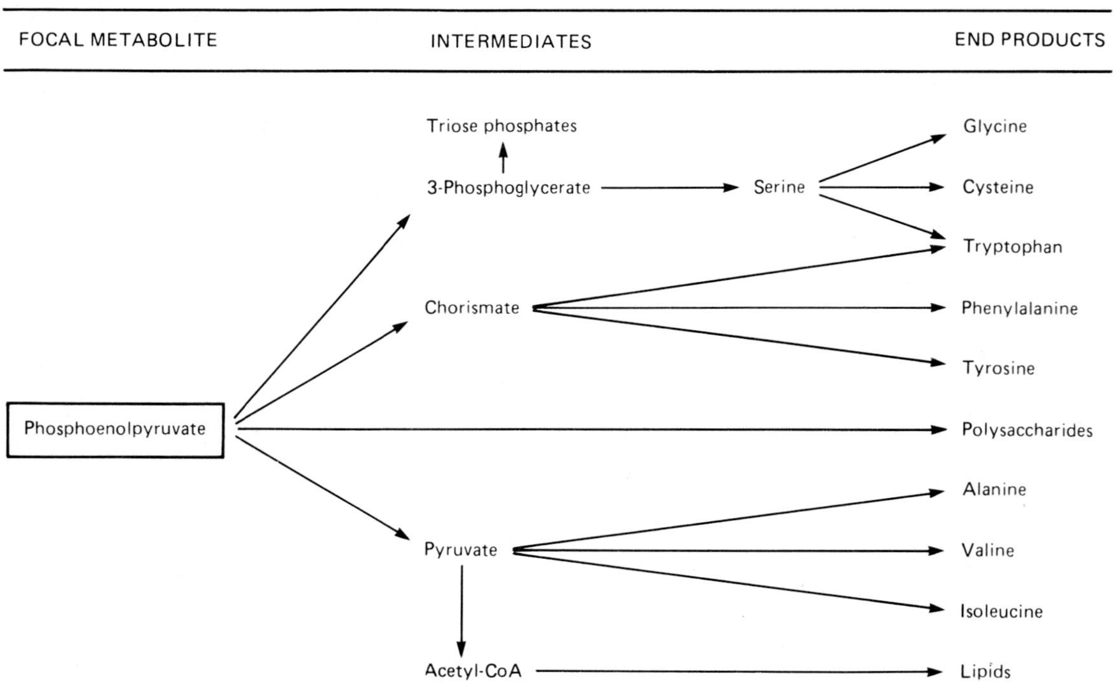

Figure 6–2. Biosynthetic end products formed from phosphoenolpyruvate.

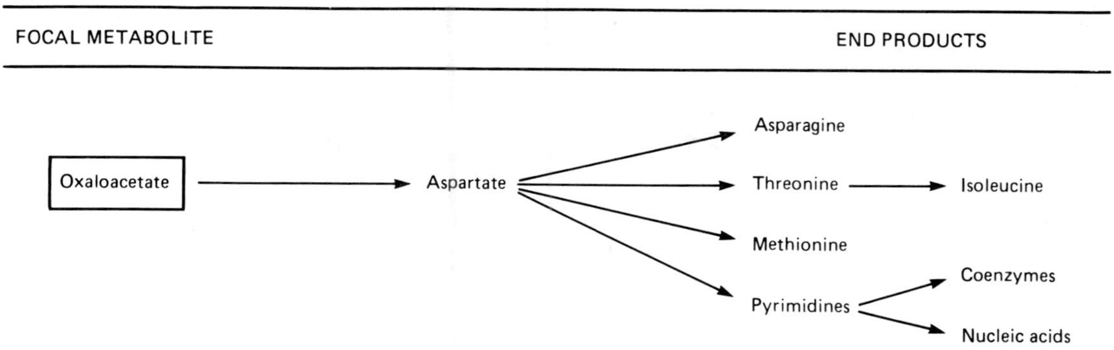

Figure 6–3. Biosynthetic end products formed from oxaloacetate. The end products threonine and pyrimidines serve as intermediates in the synthesis of additional compounds.

lose 5-phosphate. Isomerase and epimerase reactions interconvert the most common biochemical forms of the pentoses: ribulose 5-phosphate, ribose 5-phosphate, and xylulose 5-phosphate. Transketolases transfer a two-carbon fragment from a donor to an acceptor molecule. These reactions allow pentoses to form or to be formed from carbohydrates of varying chain lengths. As shown in Figure 6–5, two pentose 5-phosphates ($n = 5$) are interconvertible with triose 3-phosphate ($n = 3$) and heptose 7-phosphate ($n = 7$); pentose 5-phosphate ($n = 5$) and tetrose 4-phosphate ($n = 4$) are interconvertible with triose 3-phosphate ($n = 3$) and hexose 6-phosphate ($n = 6$).

The six-carbon hexose chain of fructose 6-phosphate can be converted to two three-carbon triose derivatives by the consecutive action of a kinase and an aldolase on fructose 6-phosphate. Alternatively, aldolases, acting in conjunction with phosphatases, can be used to lengthen carbohydrate molecules: triose phosphates give rise to fructose 6-phosphate; a triose phosphate and tetrose 4-phosphate form heptose 7-phosphate. The final form of carbohydrate chain length interconversion is the transaldolase reaction, which interconverts heptose 7-phosphate and triose 3-phosphate with tetrose 4-phosphate and hexose 6-phosphate.

The coordination of different carbohydrate rearrangement reactions to achieve an overall metabolic goal is illustrated by the hexose monophosphate shunt (Figure 6–6). This metabolic cycle is used by blue-green bacteria for the reduction of NAD^+ to NADH, which serves as a reductant for respiration in the dark. Many organisms use the hexose monophosphate shunt to reduce $NADP^+$ to NADPH, which is used for biosynthetic reduction reactions. The first steps in the hexose monophosphate shunt are the oxidative reactions that shorten six hexose 6-phosphates (abbreviated as six C_6 in Figure 6–6) to six pentose 5-phosphates (abbreviated six C_5). Carbohydrate rearrangement reactions convert the six C_5 molecules to five C_6 molecules so that the oxidative cycle may continue.

Clearly, all reactions for interconversion of carbohydrate chain lengths are not called into play at the same time. Selection of specific sets of enzymes, essentially the determination of the metabolic pathway taken, is dictated by the source of carbon and the biosynthetic demands of the cell. For example, a cell given triose phosphate as a source of carbohydrate will use the aldolase-phosphatase combination to form fructose 6-phosphate; the kinase that acts on fructose 6-phosphate in its conversion to triose phosphate

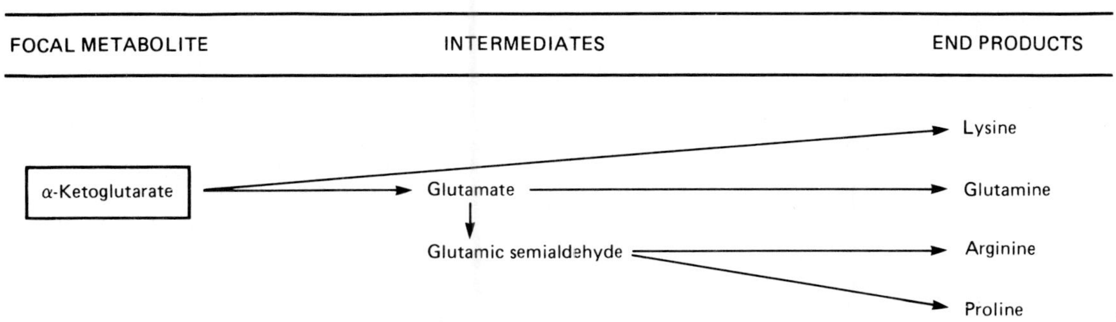

Figure 6–4. Biosynthetic end products formed from α-ketoglutarate.

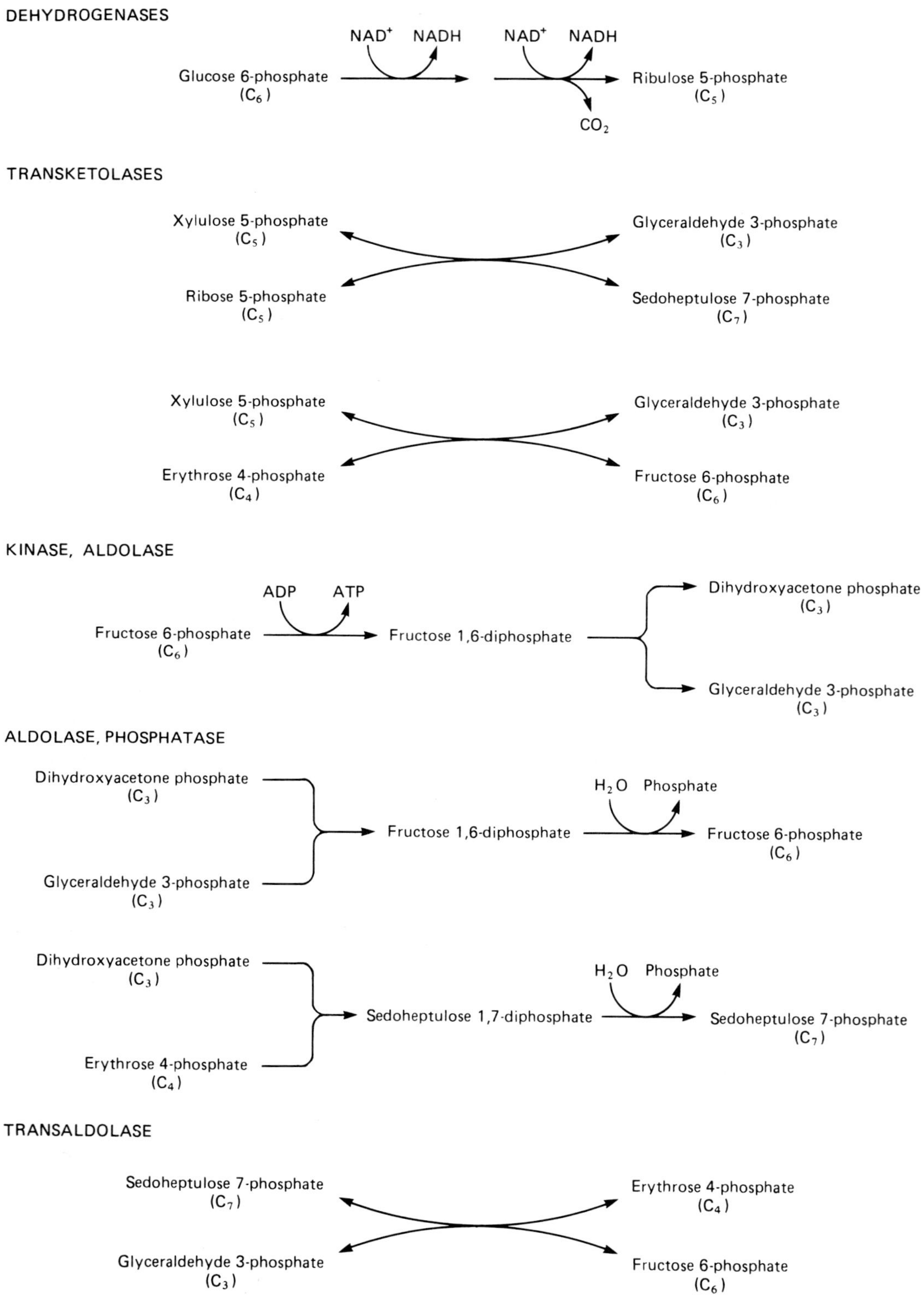

Figure 6–5. Biochemical mechanisms for changing the length of carbohydrate molecules. The general empirical formula for carbohydrate phosphate esters, $(C_nH_{2n}O_n)$-N-phosphate, is abbreviated (C_n) in order to emphasize changes in chain length.

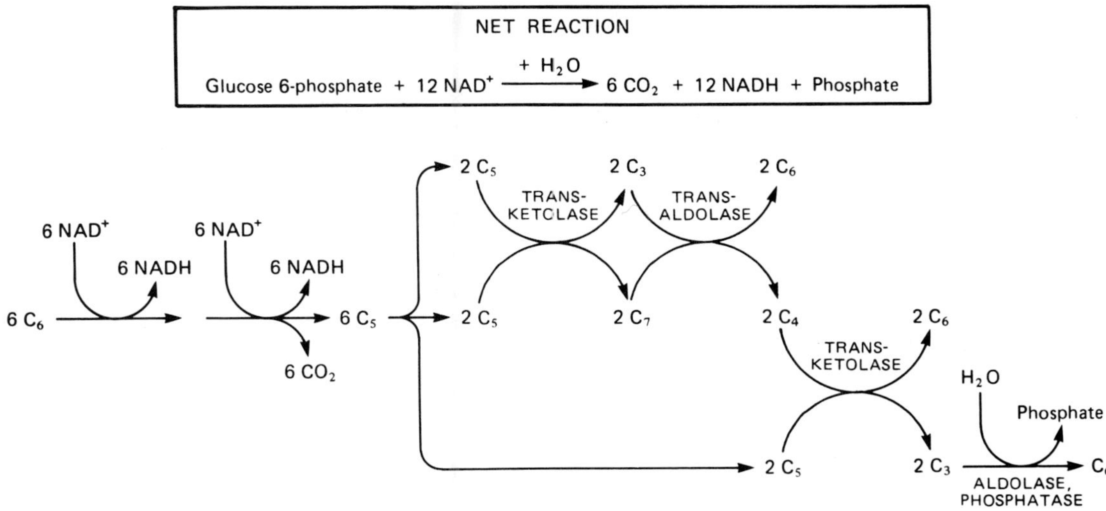

Figure 6–6. The hexose monophosphate shunt. Oxidative reactions (Figure 6–5) reduce NAD^+ and produce CO_2, resulting in the shortening of the six hexose phosphates (abbreviated C_6) to six pentose phosphates (abbreviated C_5). Carbohydrate rearrangements (Figure 6–5) convert the pentose phosphates to hexose phosphates so that the oxidative cycle may continue.

would not be expected to be active under these circumstances. If demands for pentose 5-phosphate are high, as in the case of photosynthetic carbon dioxide assimilation, transketolases that can give rise to pentose 5-phosphates are very active.

In sum, glucose 6-phosphate can be regarded as a focal metabolite because it serves both as a direct precursor for metabolic building blocks and as a source of carbohydrates of varying length that are used for biosynthetic purposes. Glucose 6-phosphate itself may be generated from other phosphorylated carbohydrates by selection of pathways from a set of reactions for chain length interconversion. The reactions chosen are determined by the genetic potential of the cell, the primary carbon source, and the biosynthetic demands of the organism. Metabolic regulation is required to ensure that reactions which meet the requirements of the organism are selected.

Formation & Utilization of Phosphoenolpyruvate

Triose phosphates, formed by the interconversion of carbohydrate phosphoesters, are converted to phosphoenolpyruvate by the series of reactions shown in Figure 6–7. Oxidation of glyceraldehyde 3-phosphate by NAD^+ is accompanied by the formation of the acid anhydride bond on the one-carbon of 1,3-diphosphoglycerate. This phosphate anhydride is transferred in a **substrate phosphorylation** to ADP, yielding an energy-rich bond in ATP. Another energy-rich phosphate bond is formed by dehydration of 2-phosphoglycerate to phosphoenolpyruvate; and via another substrate phosphorylation, phosphoenolpyruvate can donate the energy-rich bond to ADP, yielding ATP and pyruvate. Thus, two energy-rich bonds in ATP can be obtained by the metabolic conversion of triose phosphate to pyruvate. This is an oxidative process, and in the absence of an exogenous electron acceptor, the NADH generated by oxidation of glyceraldehyde 3-phosphate must be oxidized to NAD^+ by pyruvate or by metabolites derived from pyruvate. The products formed as a result of this process vary and, as described later in this chapter, can be used in the identification of clinically significant bacteria.

Formation of phosphoenolpyruvate from pyruvate (Figure 6–8) requires a substantial amount of metabolic energy, and two anhydride ATP bonds invariably are invested in the process. Some organisms—*Escherichia coli,* for example—directly phosphorylate pyruvate with ATP, yielding AMP and inorganic phosphate (P_i). Other organisms use two metabolic steps: one ATP pyrophosphate bond is invested in the carboxylation of pyruvate to oxaloacetate, and a second pyrophosphate bond (often carried to GTP rather than ATP) is used to generate phosphoenolpyruvate from oxaloacetate.

Formation & Utilization of Oxaloacetate (Figure 6–9)

As described above, many organisms form oxaloacetate by the ATP-dependent carboxylation of pyruvate (Figure 6–8). Other organisms, such as *E coli,* which form phosphoenolpyruvate directly from pyruvate, synthesize oxaloacetate by carboxylation of phosphoenolpyruvate (Figure 6–9).

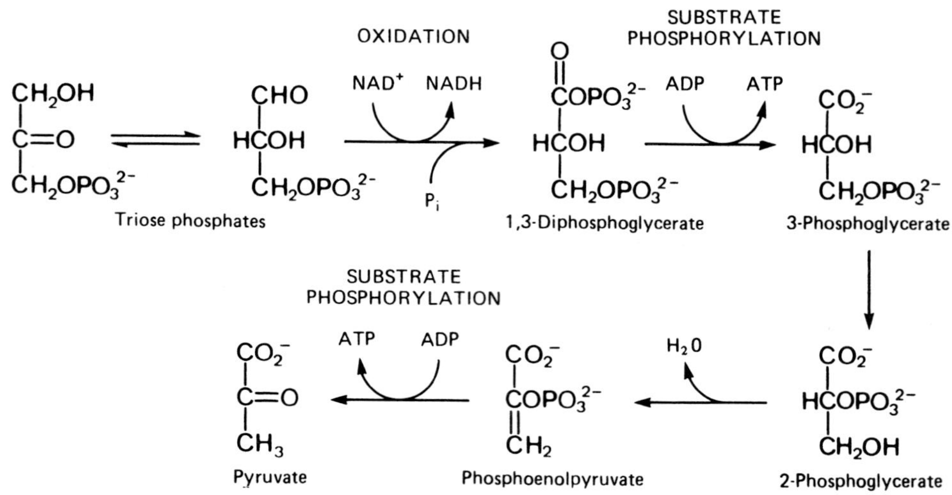

Figure 6–7. Formation of phosphoenolpyruvate and pyruvate from triose phosphate. The figure draws attention to two sites of substrate phosphorylation and to the oxidative step that results in the reduction of NAD^+ to NADH. Repetition of this energy-yielding pathway demands a mechanism for oxidizing NADH to NAD^+. Fermentative organisms achieve this goal by using pyruvate or metabolites derived from pyruvate as oxidants.

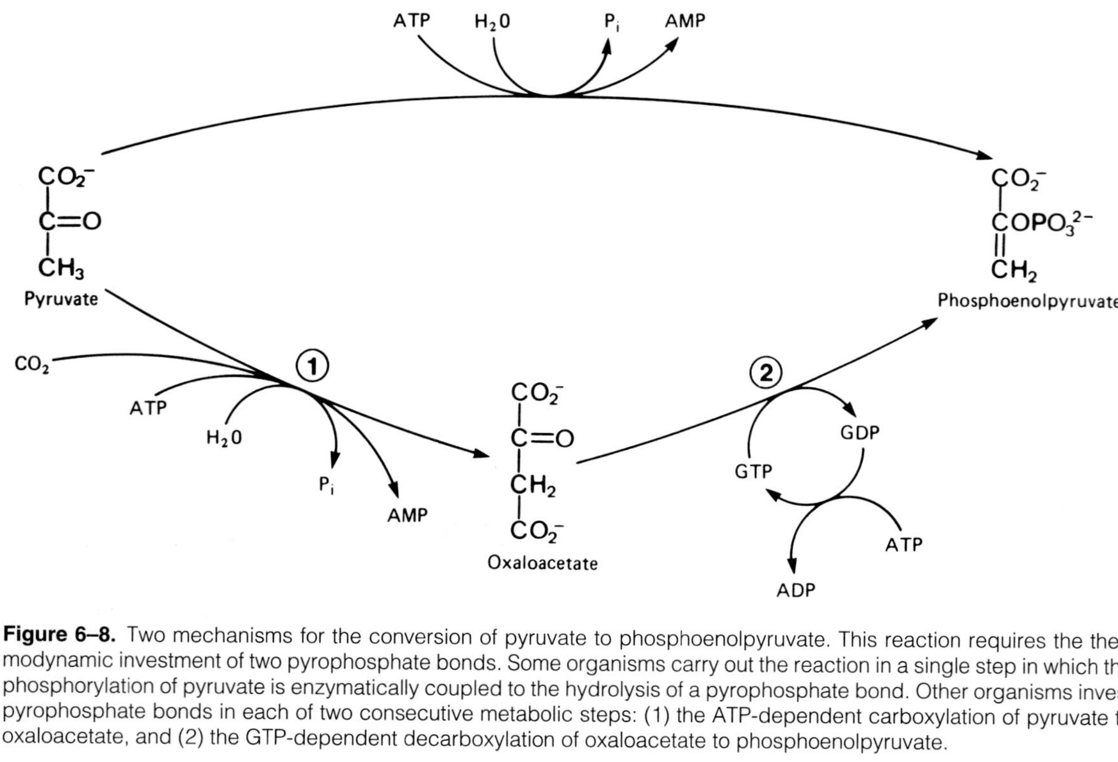

Figure 6–8. Two mechanisms for the conversion of pyruvate to phosphoenolpyruvate. This reaction requires the thermodynamic investment of two pyrophosphate bonds. Some organisms carry out the reaction in a single step in which the phosphorylation of pyruvate is enzymatically coupled to the hydrolysis of a pyrophosphate bond. Other organisms invest pyrophosphate bonds in each of two consecutive metabolic steps: (1) the ATP-dependent carboxylation of pyruvate to oxaloacetate, and (2) the GTP-dependent decarboxylation of oxaloacetate to phosphoenolpyruvate.

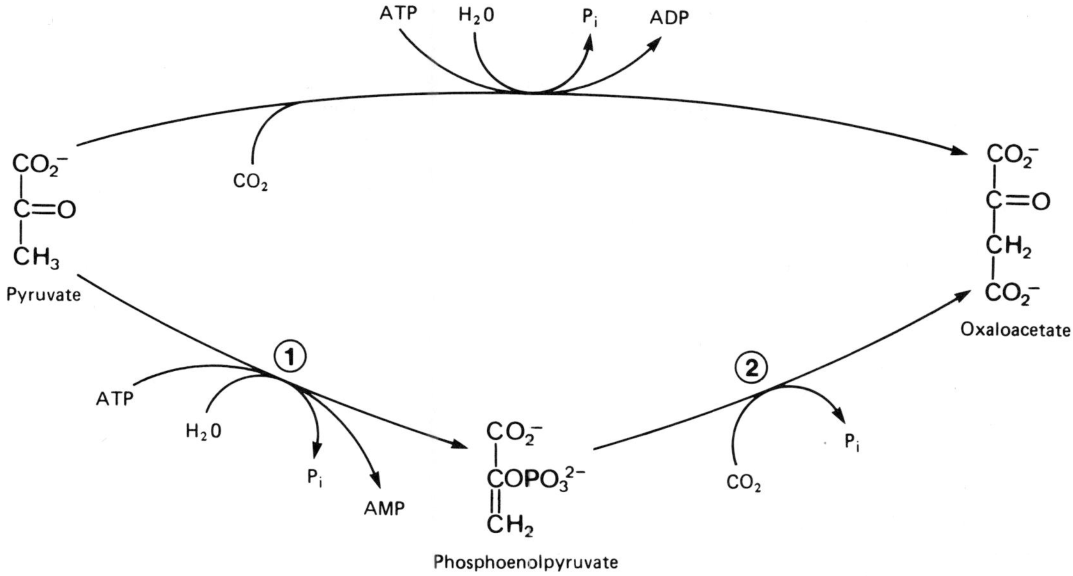

Figure 6–9. Formation of oxaloacetate from pyruvate. As described in Figure 6–8, some organisms carboxylate pyruvate directly to oxaloacetate in an ATP-dependent reaction. The organisms that convert pyruvate directly to phosphoenolpyruvate (Figure 6–8) carboxylate phosphoenolpyruvate to oxaloacetate.

Succinyl-CoA is a required biosynthetic precursor for the synthesis of porphyrins and other essential compounds. Some organisms form succinyl-CoA by reduction of oxaloacetate via malate and fumarate (Figure 6–10). These reactions represent a reversal of the metabolic flow observed in the conventional tricarboxylic acid cycle (Figure 6–13).

Formation of α-Ketoglutarate From Pyruvate (Figure 6–11)

Conversion of pyruvate to α-ketoglutarate requires a metabolic pathway that diverges and then converges (Figure 6–11). In one branch, oxaloacetate is formed by carboxylation of pyruvate or phosphoenolpyruvate. In the other branch, pyruvate is oxidized to acetyl-CoA. It is noteworthy that, regardless of the enzymatic mechanism used for the formation of oxaloacetate, acetyl-CoA is required as a positive metabolic effector for this process. Thus, the synthesis of oxaloacetate is balanced with the production of acetyl-CoA. Condensation of oxaloacetate with acetyl-CoA yields citrate. Isomerization of the citrate molecule produces isocitrate, which is oxidatively decarboxylated to α-ketoglutarate.

Growth With Acetate

Acetate is metabolized via acetyl-CoA, and many organisms possess the ability to form acetyl-CoA (Fig-

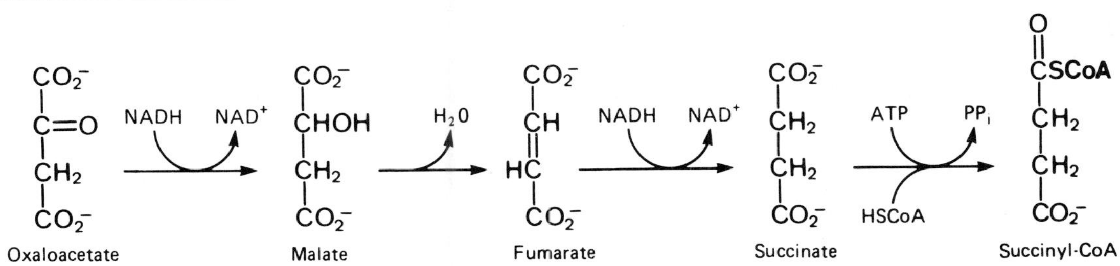

Figure 6–10. Reductive conversion of oxaloacetate to succinyl-CoA. This reductive series of reactions is used as a biosynthetic route in organisms that do not employ a conventional tricarboxylic acid cycle (Figure 6–13), and the direction of metabolic flow is the reverse of that found in the tricarboxylic acid cycle. The reactions that result in the oxidation of NADH are used by some fermentative organisms to generate NAD^+ so that the energy-yielding metabolism of triose phosphates (Figure 6–7) can continue.

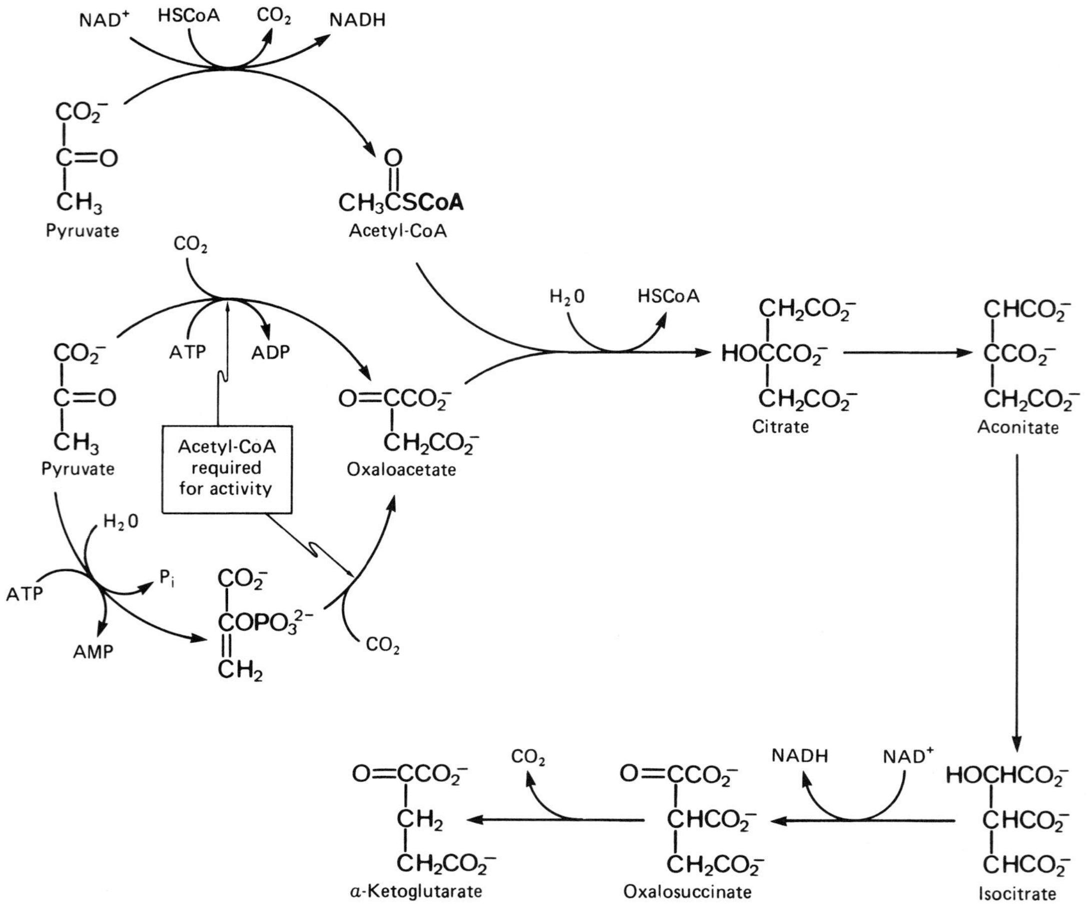

Figure 6–11. Conversion of pyruvate to α-ketoglutarate. Pyruvate is converted to α-ketoglutarate by a branched biosynthetic pathway. In one branch, pyruvate is oxidized to acetyl-CoA; in the other, pyruvate is carboxylated to oxaloacetate. As noted in Figure 6–9, the latter can proceed through either of two mechanisms.

ure 6–12). Acetyl-CoA is used in the biosynthesis of α-ketoglutarate, and in most respiratory organisms, the acetyl fragment in acetyl-CoA is oxidized completely to carbon dioxide via the tricarboxylic acid cycle (Figure 6–13). The ability to utilize acetate as a net source of carbon, however, is limited to relatively few microorganisms and plants. Net synthesis of biosynthetic precursors from acetate is achieved by coupling reactions of the tricarboxylic acid cycle with two additional reactions catalyzed by isocitrate lyase and malate synthase. As shown in Figure 6–14, these reactions allow the *net* oxidative conversion of two acetyl moieties from acetyl-CoA to one molecule of succinate. Succinate may be used for biosynthetic purposes after its conversion to oxaloacetate, α-ketoglutarate, phosphoenolpyruvate, or glucose 6-phosphate.

Growth With Carbon Dioxide: The Calvin Cycle

Like plants and algae, a number of microbial species can use carbon dioxide as a sole source of carbon. In almost all of these organisms, the primary route of carbon assimilation is via the Calvin cycle, in which carbon dioxide and ribulose diphosphate combine to form two molecules of 3-phosphoglycerate (Figure 6–15A). 3-Phosphoglycerate is phosphorylated to 1,3-diphosphoglycerate, and this compound is reduced to the triose derivative, glyceraldehyde 3-phosphate. Carbohydrate rearrangement reactions (Figure 6–5) allow triose phosphate to be converted to the pentose derivative ribulose 5-phosphate, which is phosphorylated to regenerate the acceptor molecule, ribulose 1,5-diphosphate (Figure 6–15B). Additional reduced carbon, formed by the reductive assimilation of carbon dioxide, is converted to focal metabolites for biosynthetic pathways.

Cells that can use carbon dioxide as a sole source of carbon are termed **autotrophic,** and the demands for this pattern of carbon assimilation can be summarized briefly as follows: In addition to the primary assimilatory reaction giving rise to 3-phosphoglycerate, there must be a mechanism for regenerating the acceptor

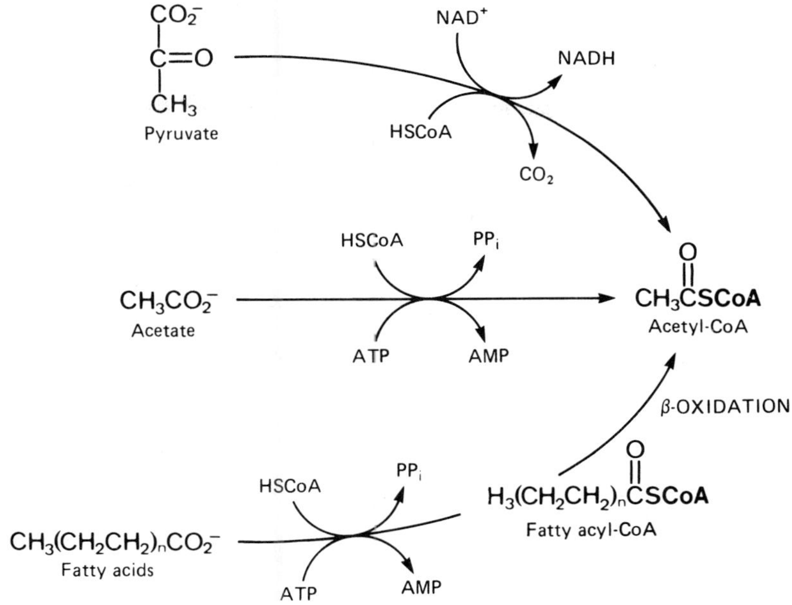

Figure 6–12. Biochemical sources of acetyl-CoA.

molecule, ribulose 1,5-diphosphate. This process demands the energy-dependent reduction of 3-phosphoglycerate to the level of carbohydrate. Thus, autotrophy requires carbon dioxide, ATP, NADPH, and a specific set of enzymes.

Depolymerases

Many potential growth substrates occur as building blocks within the structure of biologic polymers. These large molecules are not readily transported across the cell membrane and often are affixed to even larger cellular structures. Many microorganisms elaborate extracellular depolymerases that hydrolyze proteins, nucleic acids, polysaccharides, and lipids. The pattern of depolymerase production can be useful in the identification of microorganisms.

Oxygenases

Many compounds in the environment are relatively resistant to enzymatic modification, and utilization of these compounds as growth substrates demands a special class of enzymes, oxygenases. These enzymes directly employ the potent oxidant molecular oxygen as a substrate in reactions that convert a relatively intractable compound to a form in which it can be assimilated by thermodynamically favored reactions. The action of oxygenases is illustrated in Figure 6–16, which shows the role of two different oxygenases in the utilization of benzoate.

Reductive Pathways

Some microorganisms live in extremely reducing environments that favor chemical reactions which would not occur in organisms using oxygen as an electron acceptor. In these organisms, powerful reductants can be used to drive reactions that allow the assimilation of relatively intractable compounds. An example is the reductive assimilation of benzoate (Figure 6–17), a process in which the aromatic ring is reduced and opened to form the dicarboxylic acid pimelate. Further metabolic reactions convert pimelate to focal metabolites.

Nitrogen Assimilation

The reductive assimilation of molecular nitrogen (Figure 6–18) is required for continuation of life on our planet. Nitrogenase, the enzyme catalyzing the reaction, is found only in bacteria and demands a substantial amount of metabolic energy: 12–15 molecules of ATP are hydrolyzed as a single N_2 molecule is reduced to two molecules of NH_3 by three molecules of NADPH.

Additional physiologic demands are placed by the fact that nitrogenase is readily inactivated by oxygen. Aerobic organisms that employ nitrogenase have developed elaborate mechanisms to protect the enzyme against inactivation. Some form specialized cells in which nitrogen fixation takes place, and others have developed elaborate electron transport chains to protect nitrogenase against inactivation by oxygen. The most significant of these bacteria in agriculture are the Rhizobiaceae, organisms that fix nitrogen symbiotically in the root nodules of leguminous plants.

The capacity to use ammonia as a nitrogen source is widely distributed among organisms. The primary portal of entry of nitrogen into carbon metabolism is gluta-

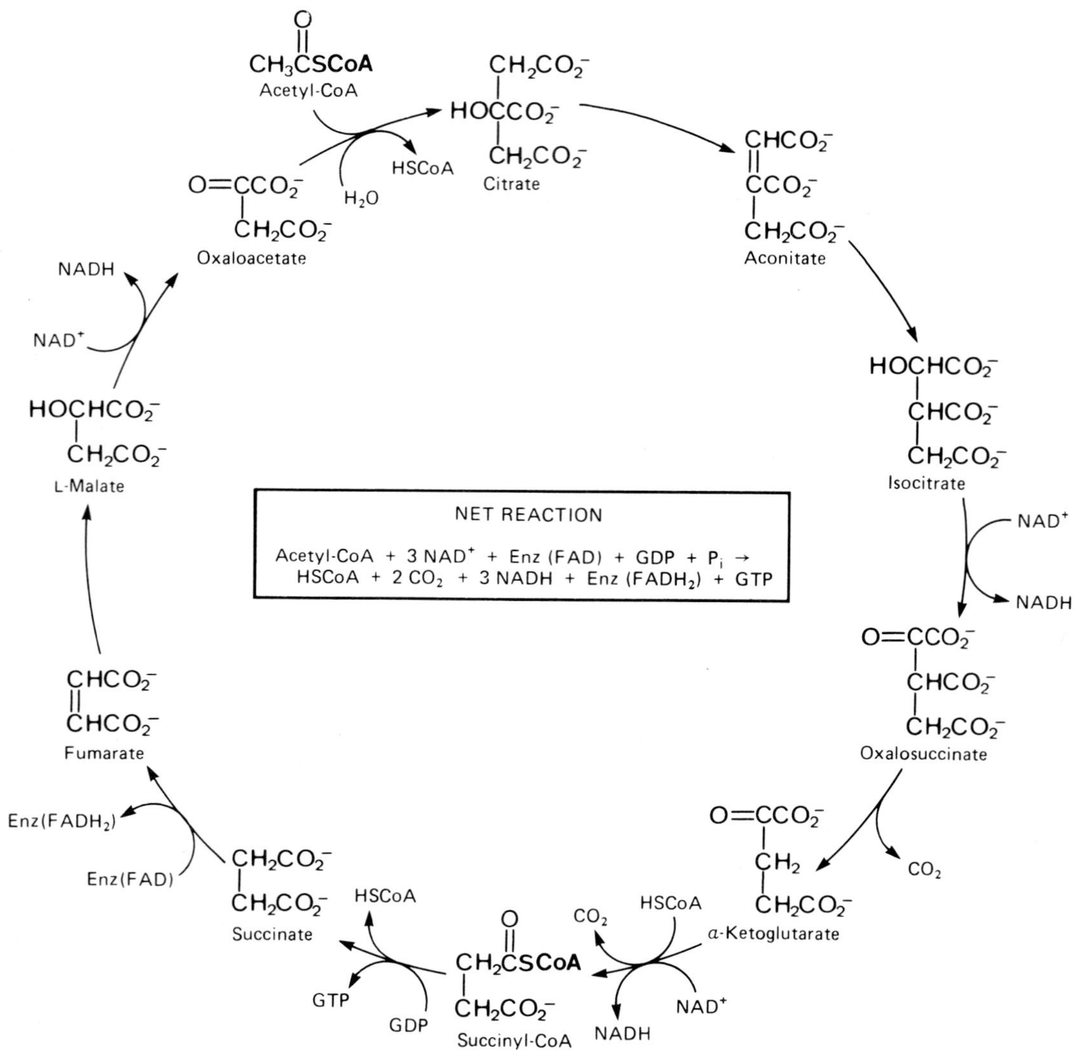

Figure 6–13. The tricarboxylic acid cycle. There are four oxidative steps, three giving rise to NADH and one giving rise to a reduced flavoprotein, Enz($FADH_2$). The cycle can continue only if electron acceptors are available to oxidize the NADH and reduced flavoprotein.

mate, which is formed by reductive amination of α-ketoglutarate. As shown in Figure 6–19, there are two biochemical mechanisms by which this can be achieved. One, the single-step reduction catalyzed by glutamate dehydrogenase (Figure 6–19A), is effective in environments in which there is an ample supply of ammonia. The other, a two-step process in which glutamine is an intermediate (Figure 6–19B), is employed in environments in which ammonia is in short supply. The latter mechanism allows cells to invest the free energy formed by hydrolysis of a pyrophosphate bond in ATP into the assimilation of ammonia from the environment.

The amide nitrogen of glutamine, an intermediate in the two-step assimilation of ammonia into glutamate (Figure 6–19B), is also transferred directly into organic nitrogen appearing in the structures of purines, pyrimidines, arginine, tryptophan, and glucosamine. The activity and synthesis of glutamine synthase are regulated by the ammonia supply and by the availability of metabolites containing nitrogen derived directly from the amide nitrogen of glutamine.

Most of the organic nitrogen in cells is derived from the α-amino group of glutamate, and the primary mechanism by which the nitrogen is transferred is **transamination,** illustrated in Figure 6–20. The usual acceptor in these reactions is an α-keto acid, which is transformed to the corresponding α-amino acid. α-Ketoglutarate, the other product of the transamination reaction, may be converted to glutamate by reductive amination (Figure 6–19).

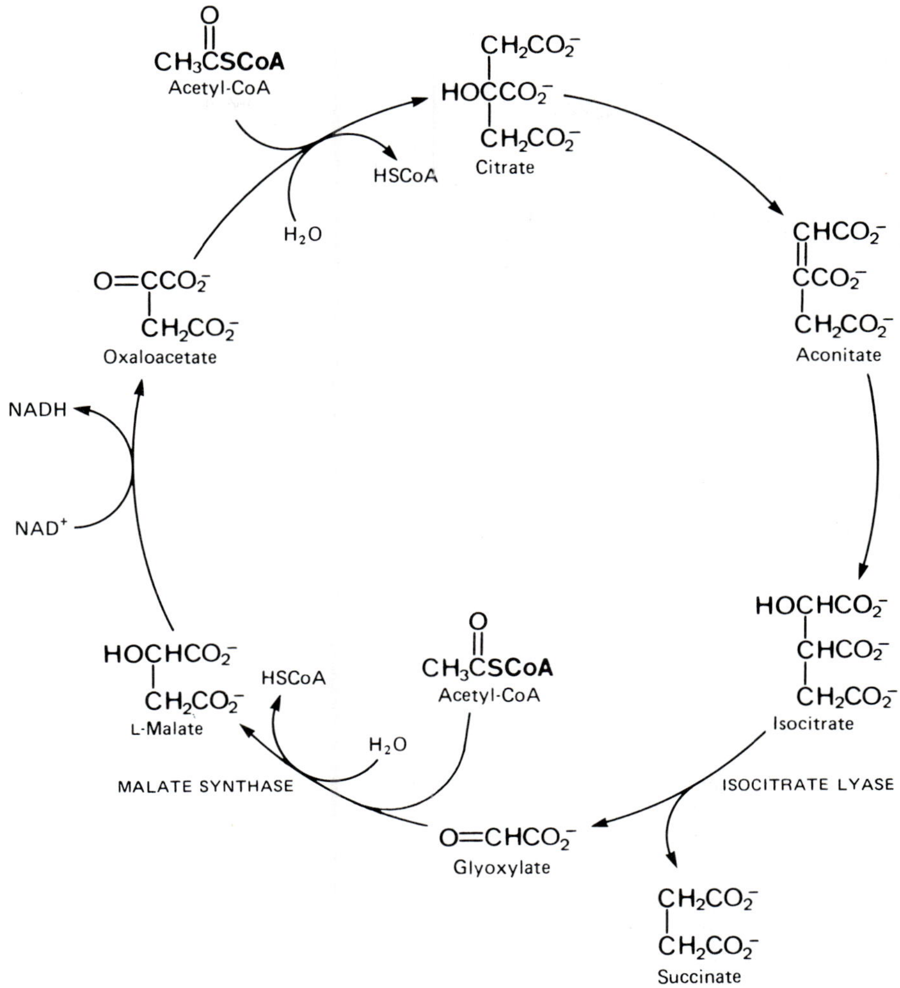

Figure 6–14. The glyoxylate cycle. Note that the reactions which convert malate to isocitrate are shared with the tricarboxylic acid cycle (Figure 6–13). Metabolic divergence at the level of isocitrate and the action of two enzymes, isocitrate lyase and malate synthase, modify the tricarboxylic acid cycle so that it reductively converts two molecules of acetyl-CoA to succinate.

BIOSYNTHETIC PATHWAYS

Tracing the Structures of Biosynthetic Precursors: Glutamate & Aspartate

In many cases, the carbon skeleton of a metabolic end product may be traced to its biosynthetic origins. Glutamine, an obvious example, clearly is derived from glutamate (Figure 6–21). The glutamate skeleton in the structures of arginine and proline (Figure 6–21) is less obvious but readily discernible. Similarly, the carbon skeleton of aspartate, directly derived from the focal metabolite oxaloacetate, is evident in the structures of asparagine, threonine, methionine, and pyrimidines (Figure 6–22). In some cases, different carbon skeletons combine in a biosynthetic pathway. For example, aspartate semialdehyde and pyruvate combine to form the metabolic precursor of lysine, diaminopimelic acid, and dipicolinic acid (Figure 6–23). The latter two compounds are found only in prokaryotes. Diaminopimelic acid is a component of peptidoglycan in the cell wall, and dipicolinic acid represents a major portion of endospores.

Synthesis of Cell Wall Peptidoglycan

The structure of peptidoglycan is shown in Figure 2–14; the pathway by which it is synthesized is shown in simplified form in Figure 6–24. The synthesis of peptidoglycan begins with the stepwise synthesis in the cytoplasm of UDP-N-acetylmuramic acid-pentapeptide. N-Acetylglucosamine is first attached to

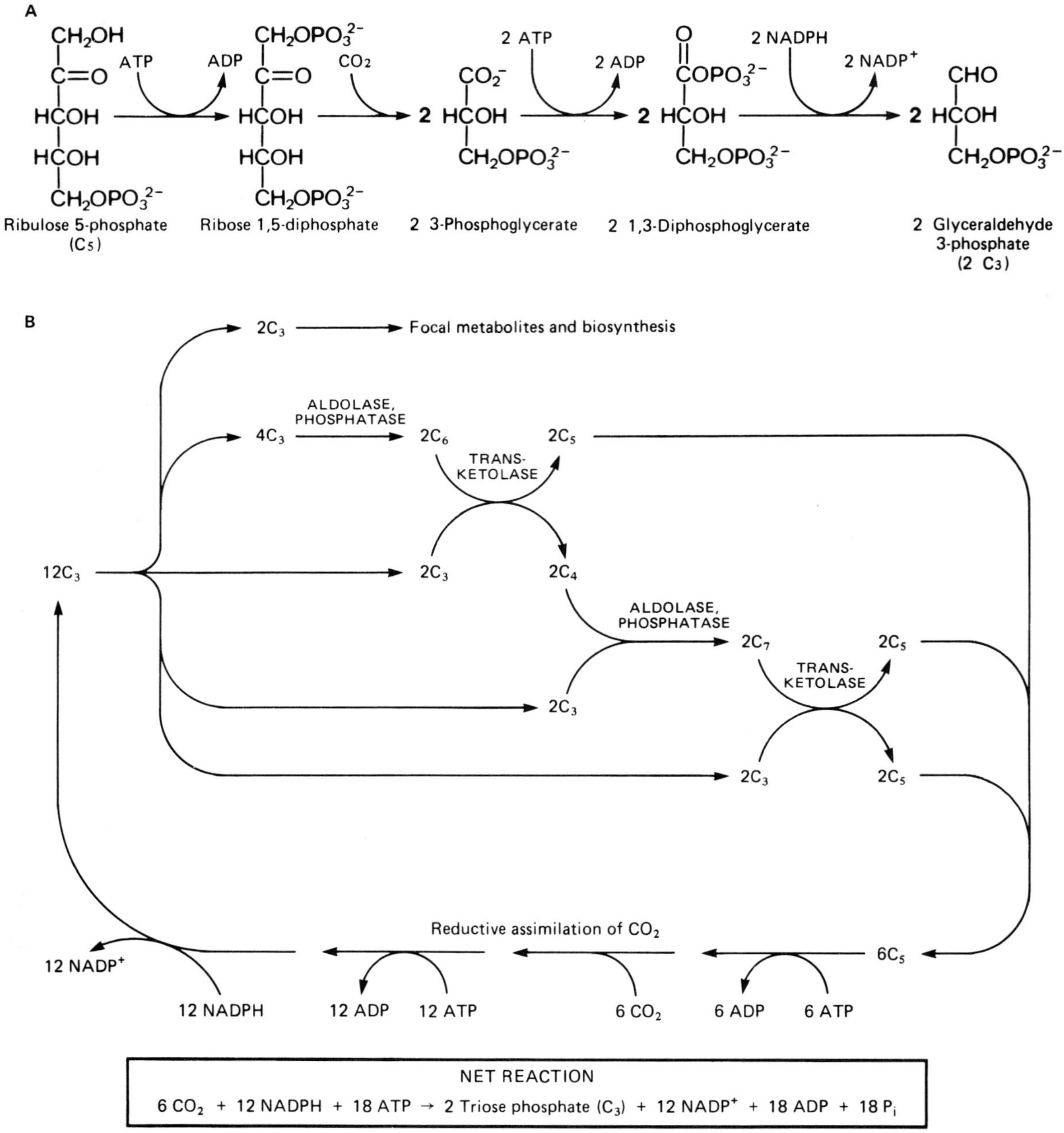

Figure 6–15. The Calvin cycle. ***A:*** Reductive assimilation of CO_2. ATP and NADPH are used to reductively convert pentose 5-phosphate (C_5) to two molecules of triose phosphate (C_3). ***B:*** The Calvin cycle is completed by carbohydrate rearrangement reactions (Figure 6–5) that allow the net synthesis of carbohydrate and the regeneration of pentose phosphate so that the cycle may continue.

UDP and then converted to UDP-N-acetylmuramic acid by condensation with phosphoenolpyruvate and reduction. The amino acids of the pentapeptide are sequentially added, each addition catalyzed by a different enzyme and each involving the split of ATP to ADP + P_i.

The UDP-N-acetylmuramic acid-pentapeptide is attached to bactoprenol (a lipid of the cell membrane) and receives a molecule of N-acetylglucosamine from UDP. The pentaglycine derivative is next formed in a series of reactions using glycyl-tRNA as the donor; the completed disaccharide is polymerized to an oligo-

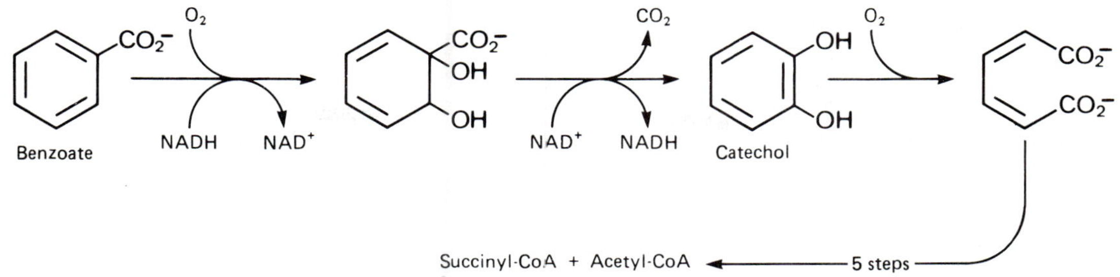

Figure 6–16. The role of oxygenases in aerobic utilization of benzoate as a carbon source. Molecular oxygen participates directly in the reactions that disrupt the aromaticity of benzoate and catechol.

meric intermediate before being transferred to the growing end of a glycopeptide polymer in the cell wall.

Final cross-linking is accomplished by a transpeptidation reaction in which the free amino group of a pentaglycine residue displaces the terminal d-alanine residue of a neighboring pentapeptide. Transpeptidation is catalyzed by one of a set of enzymes called penicillin-binding proteins (PBPs). PBPs bind penicillin and other β-lactam antibiotics covalently; they have both transpeptidase and carboxypeptidase activities, their relative rates perhaps controlling the degree of cross-linking in peptidoglycan (a factor important in cell septation).

The biosynthetic pathway is of particular importance in medicine, as it provides a basis for the selective antibacterial action of several chemotherapeutic agents. Unlike their host cells, bacteria are not isotonic with the body fluids. Their contents are under high osmotic pressure, and their viability depends on the integrity of the peptidoglycan lattice in the cell wall being maintained throughout the growth cycle. Any compound that inhibits any step in the biosynthesis of peptidoglycan causes the wall of the growing bacterial cell to be weakened and the cell to lyse. The sites of action of several antibiotics are shown in Figure 6–24.

Synthesis of Cell Wall Lipopolysaccharide

The general structure of the antigenic lipopolysaccharide of gram-negative cell walls is shown in Figure 2–17. The biosynthesis of the repeating end-group, which gives the cell wall its antigenic specificity, is shown in Figure 6–25. Note the resemblance to peptidoglycan synthesis: in both cases, a series of subunits is assembled on a lipid carrier in the membrane and then transferred to open ends of the growing polymer fabric of the cell wall.

Synthesis of Extracellular Capsular Polymers

The capsular polymers, a few examples of which are listed in Table 2–1, are enzymatically synthesized

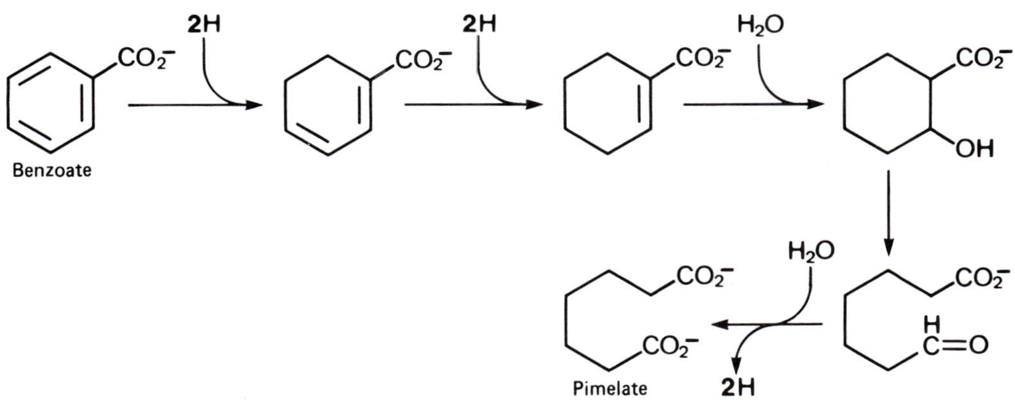

Figure 6–17. Reductive reactions in anaerobic utilization of benzoate as a carbon source. Individual steps in the pathway are somewhat speculative; for example, benzoate may be metabolized as its CoA thioester. The metabolic sequence illustrates that, in a strongly reducing environment, the aromatic ring of benzoate can be reduced, with the result that the dicarboxylate pimelate is produced as a source of carbon.

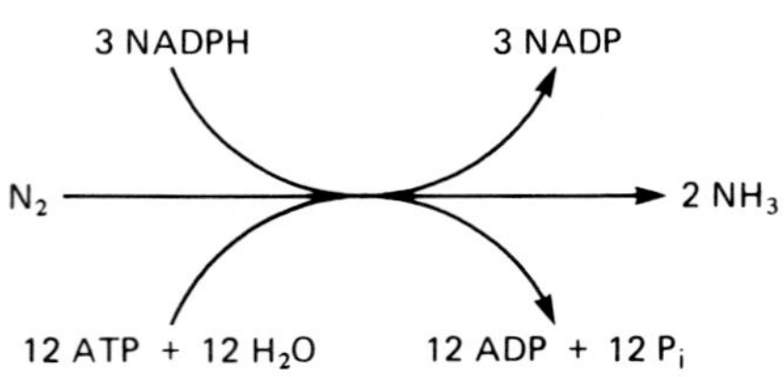

Figure 6–18. Reduction of N_2 to two molecules of NH_3. In addition to reductant, the nitrogenase reaction requires a substantial amount of metabolic energy. The number of ATP molecules required for reduction of a single nitrogen molecule to ammonia is uncertain; the value appears to lie between 12 and 15.

from activated subunits. No membrane-bound lipid carriers have been implicated in this process. The presence of a capsule is often environmentally determined: dextrans and levans, for example, can only be synthesized using the disaccharide sucrose (fructose-glucose) as the source of the appropriate subunit, and their synthesis thus depends on the presence of sucrose in the medium.

Synthesis of Reserve Food Granules

When nutrients are present in excess of the requirements for growth, bacteria convert certain of them to intracellular reserve food granules. The principal ones are starch, glycogen, poly-β-hydroxybutyrate (PBHB), and volutin, which consists mainly of inorganic polyphosphate. The type of granule formed is

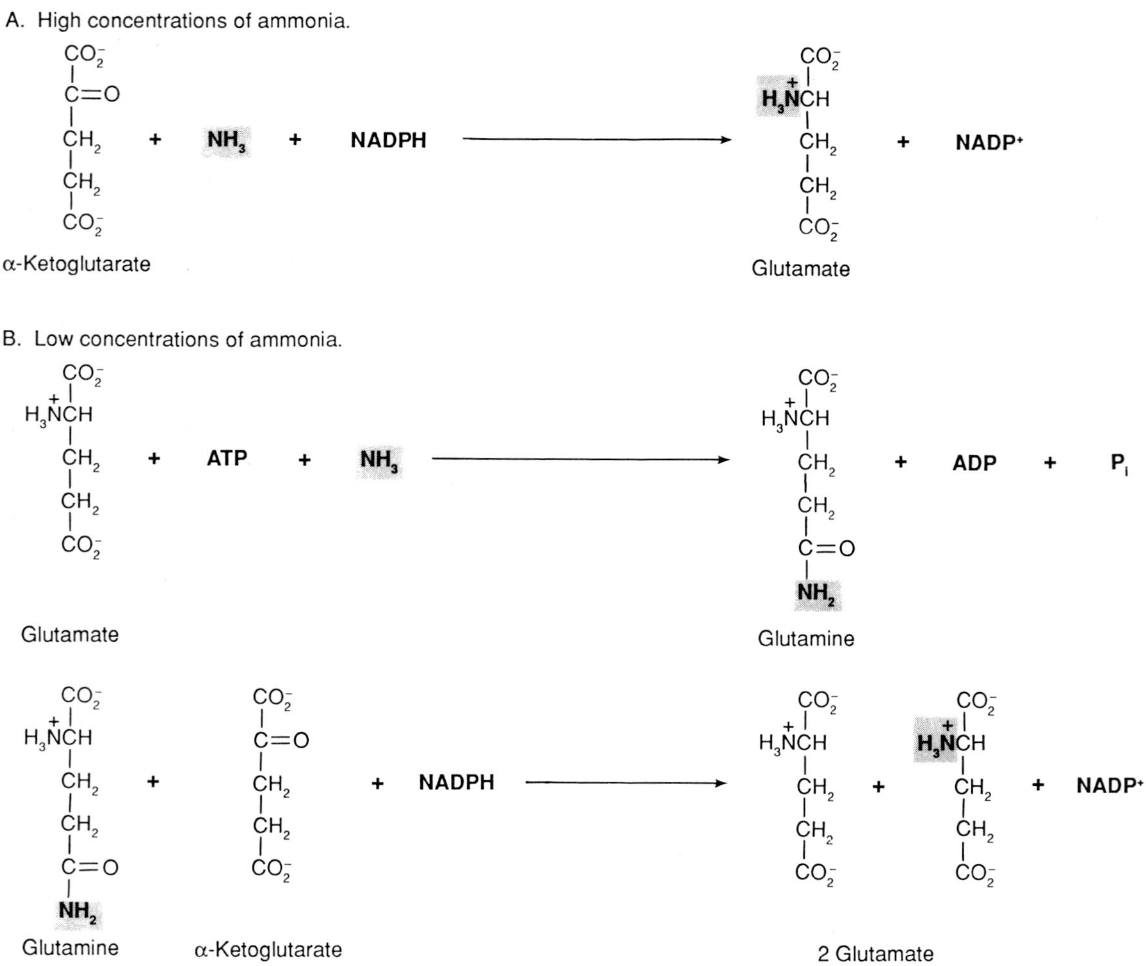

Figure 6–19. Mechanisms for the assimilation of NH_3. ***A:*** When the NH_3 concentration is high, cells are able to assimilate the compound via the glutamate dehydrogenase reaction. ***B:*** When, as most often is the case, the NH_3 concentration is low, cells couple the glutamine synthase and glutamate synthase reactions in order to invest the energy produced by hydrolysis of a pyrophosphate bond into ammonia assimilation.

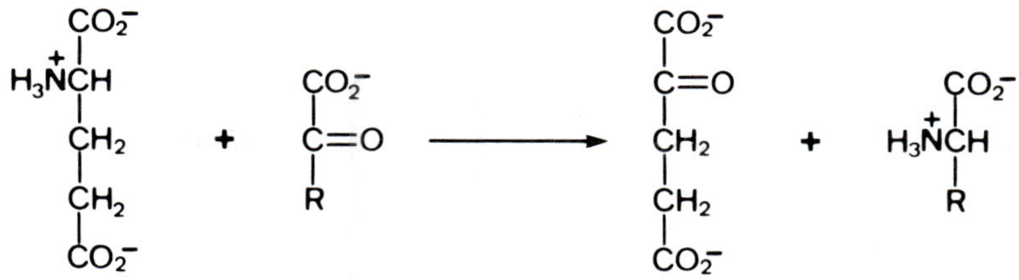

Glutamate Acceptor α-Ketoglutarate Amino acid

Figure 6–20. Transamination, the major mechanism for forming the α-amino group of amino acids. R, organic radical.

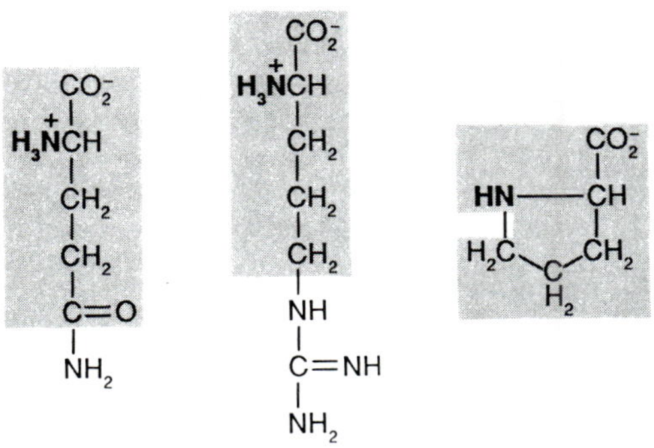

Glutamine Arginine Proline

Figure 6–21. Amino acids formed from glutamate.

species-specific. The granules are degraded when exogenous nutrients are depleted.

PATTERNS OF MICROBIAL ENERGY-YIELDING METABOLISM

As described in Chapter 5, there are two major metabolic mechanisms for generating the energy-rich acid pyrophosphate bonds in ATP: **substrate phosphorylation** (the direct transfer of a phosphate anhydride bond from an organic donor to ADP) and phosphorylation of ADP by inorganic phosphate. The latter reaction is energetically unfavorable and must be driven by a transmembrane electrochemical gradient, the **proton motive force.** In respiration, the electrochemical gradient is created from externally supplied reductant and oxidant. Energy released by transfer of electrons from the reductant to the oxidant through membrane-bound carriers is coupled to the formation of the transmembrane electrochemical gradient. In photosynthesis, light energy generates membrane-associated reductants and oxidants; the proton motive force is generated as these electron carriers return to the ground state. These processes are discussed below.

Pathways of Fermentation

A. Strategies for Substrate Phosphorylation: In the absence of respiration or photosynthesis, cells are entirely dependent upon substrate phosphorylation for their energy: generation of ATP must be coupled to chemical rearrangement of organic compounds. Many compounds can serve as fermentable growth substrates, and many pathways for their fermentation have evolved. These pathways have the following three general stages: (1) Conversion of the fermentable compound to the phosphate donor for substrate phosphorylation. This stage often contains metabolic reactions in which NAD^+ is reduced to NADH. (2) Phosphorylation of ADP by the energy-rich phosphate donor. (3) Metabolic steps that bring the products of the fermentation into chemical balance with the starting materials. The most frequent requirement in the last stage is a mechanism for oxidation of NADH, gen-

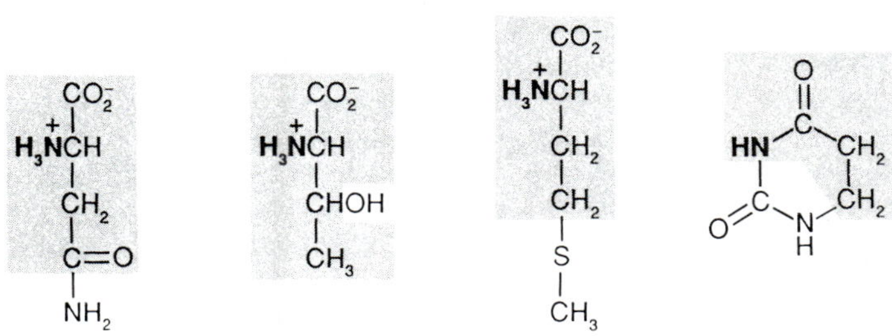

Asparagine Threonine Methionine Uracil

Figure 6–22. Biosynthetic end products formed from aspartate.

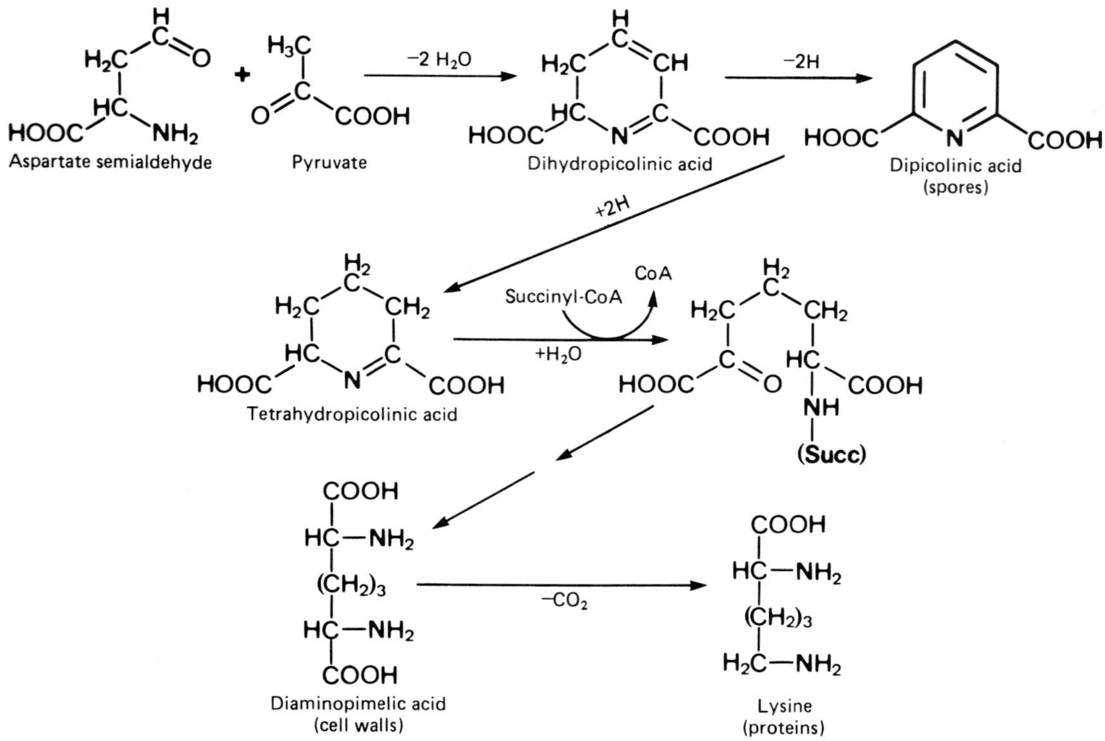

Figure 6–23. Biosynthetic end products formed from aspartate semialdehyde and pyruvate.

erated in the first stage of fermentation, to NAD^+ so that the fermentation may proceed. In the following sections, examples of each of the three stages of fermentation are considered.

B. Fermentation of Glucose: The diversity of fermentative pathways is illustrated by consideration of some of the mechanisms used by microorganisms to achieve substrate phosphorylation at the expense of glucose. In principle, the phosphorylation of ADP to ATP can be coupled to either of two chemically balanced transformations:

$$\underset{(C_6H_{12}O_6)}{\text{Glucose}} \longrightarrow \underset{(C_3H_6O_3)}{\text{2 Lactic acid}}$$

or

$$\underset{(C_6H_{12}O_6)}{\text{Glucose}} \longrightarrow \underset{(C_2H_6O)}{\text{2 Ethanol}} + \underset{(CO_2)}{\text{2 Carbon dioxide}}$$

The biochemical mechanisms by which these transformations are achieved vary considerably.

In general, the fermentation of glucose is initiated by its phosphorylation to glucose 6-phosphate. There are two mechanisms by which this can be achieved: (1) Extracellular glucose may be transported across the cytoplasmic membrane into the cell and then phosphorylated by ATP to yield glucose 6-phosphate and ADP (Figure 6–26A). (2) In many microorganisms, extracellular glucose is phosphorylated as it is being transported across the cytoplasmic membrane by an enzyme system in the cytoplasmic membrane that phosphorylates extracellular glucose at the expense of phosphoenolpyruvate, producing intracellular glucose 6-phosphate and pyruvate (Figure 6–26B). The latter process is an example of **vectorial metabolism,** a set of biochemical reactions in which both the structure and the location of a substrate are altered. It should be noted that the choice of ATP or phosphoenolpyruvate as a phosphorylating agent does not alter the ATP yield of fermentation, because phosphoenolpyruvate is used as a source of ATP in the later stages of fermentation (Figure 6–7).

C. The Embden-Meyerhof Pathway: This pathway (Figure 6–27), a commonly encountered mechanism for the fermentation of glucose, uses a kinase and an aldolase (Figure 6–5) to transform the hexose (C_6) phosphate to two molecules of triose (C_3) phosphate. Four substrate phosphorylation reactions accompany the conversion of the triose phosphate to two molecules of pyruvate. Thus, taking into account the two ATP pyrophosphate bonds required to form triose phosphate from glucose, the Embden-Meyerhof pathway produces a net yield of two ATP pyrophosphate bonds. Formation of pyruvate from triose phosphate is an oxidative process, and the NADH formed in the

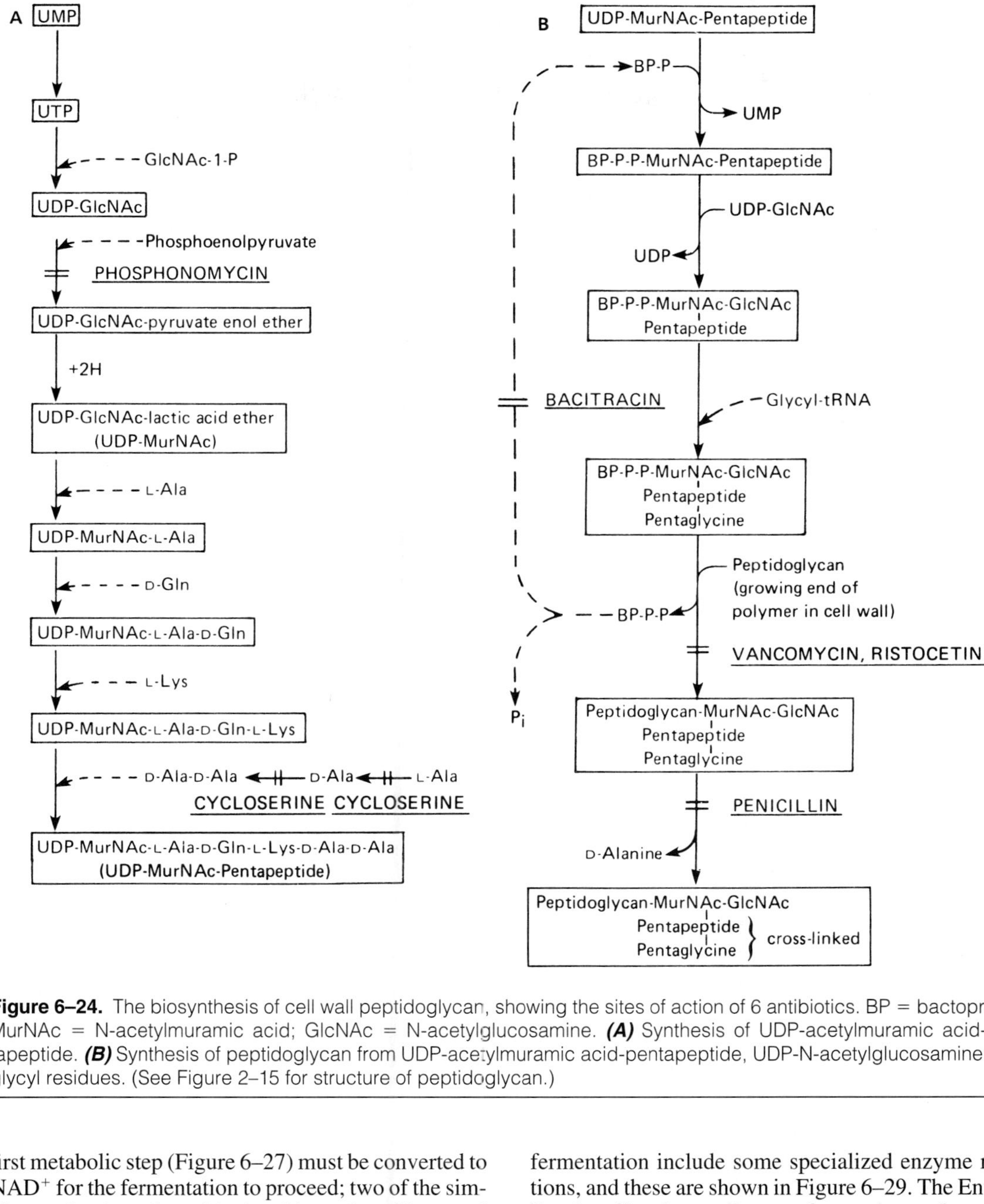

Figure 6–24. The biosynthesis of cell wall peptidoglycan, showing the sites of action of 6 antibiotics. BP = bactoprenol; MurNAc = N-acetylmuramic acid; GlcNAc = N-acetylglucosamine. ***(A)*** Synthesis of UDP-acetylmuramic acid-pentapeptide. ***(B)*** Synthesis of peptidoglycan from UDP-acetylmuramic acid-pentapeptide, UDP-N-acetylglucosamine, and glycyl residues. (See Figure 2–15 for structure of peptidoglycan.)

first metabolic step (Figure 6–27) must be converted to NAD^+ for the fermentation to proceed; two of the simpler mechanisms for achieving this goal are illustrated in Figure 6–28. Direct reduction of pyruvate by NADH produces lactate as the end product of fermentation and thus results in acidification of the medium. Alternatively, pyruvate may be decarboxylated to acetaldehyde, which is then used to oxidize NADH, resulting in production of the neutral product ethanol. The pathway taken is determined by the evolutionary history of the organism and, in some microorganisms, by the growth conditions.

D. The Entner-Doudoroff and Heterolactate Fermentations: Alternative pathways for glucose fermentation include some specialized enzyme reactions, and these are shown in Figure 6–29. The Entner-Doudoroff pathway diverges from other pathways of carbohydrate metabolism by a dehydration of 6-phosphogluconate followed by an aldolase reaction that produces pyruvate and triose phosphate (Figure 6–29A). The heterolactate fermentation and some other fermentative pathways depend upon a phosphoketolase reaction (Figure 6–29B) that phosphorolytically cleaves a ketose-phosphate to produce acetyl phosphate and triose phosphate. The acid anhydride acetyl phosphate may be used to synthesize ATP or may allow the oxidation of two NADH molecules to NAD^+ as it is reduced to ethanol.

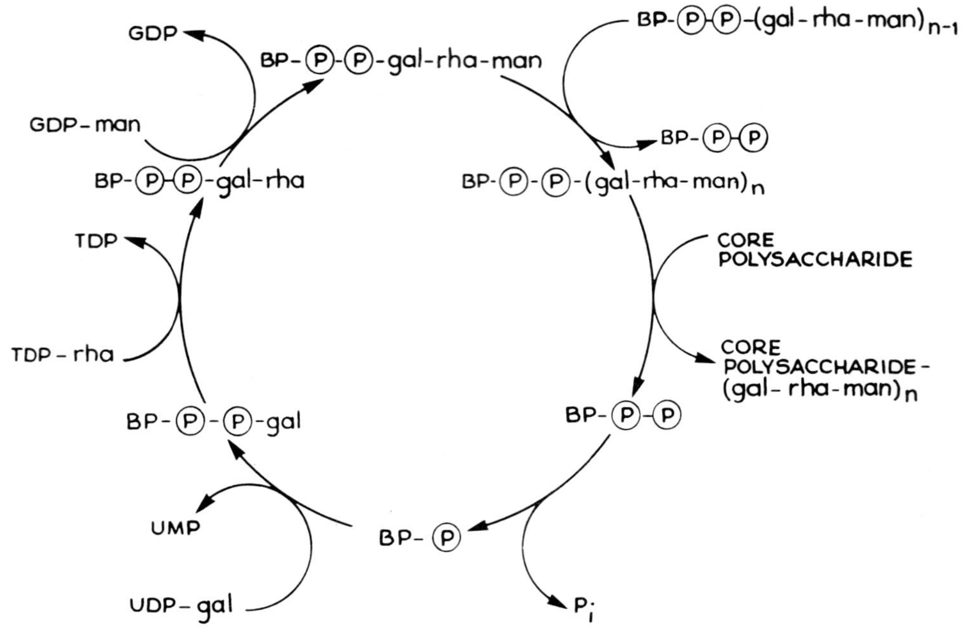

Figure 6–25. Synthesis of the repeating unit of the polysaccharide side chain of *Salmonella newington* and its transfer to the lipopolysaccharide core. BP = bactoprenol.

The overall outlines of the respective Entner-Doudoroff and heterolactate pathways are shown in Figures 6–30 and 6–31. The pathways yield only a single molecule of triose phosphate from glucose, and the energy yield is correspondingly low: unlike the Embden-Meyerhof pathway, the Entner-Doudoroff and heterolactate pathways yield only a single net substrate phosphorylation of ADP per molecule of glucose fermented. Why have the alternative pathways for glucose fermentation been selected in the natural environment? In answering this question, two facts should be kept in mind. First, in direct growth competition between two microbial species, the rate of substrate utilization can be more important than the amount of growth. Second, glucose is but one of many carbohydrates encountered by microorganisms in their natural environment. Pentoses, for example, can be fermented quite efficiently by the heterolactate pathway.

E. Additional Variations in Carbohydrate Fermentations: Pathways for carbohydrate fermentation can accommodate many more substrates than described here, and the end products may be far more diverse than suggested thus far. For example, there are numerous mechanisms for oxidation of NADH at the expense of pyruvate. One such pathway is the reductive formation of succinate (Figure 6–10). Many clinically significant bacteria form pyruvate from glucose via the Embden-Meyerhof pathway, and they may be distinguished on the basis of reduction products formed from pyruvate, reflecting the enzymatic constitution of different species. The major products of fermentation, listed in Table 6–1, form the basis for many diagnostic tests.

F. Fermentation of Other Substrates: Carbohydrates are by no means the only fermentable substrates. Metabolism of amino acids, purines, and pyrimidines may allow substrate phosphorylations to occur. For example, arginine may serve as an energy source by giving rise to carbamoyl phosphate, which can be used to phosphorylate ADP to ATP. Some organisms ferment pairs of amino acids, using one as an electron donor and the other as an electron acceptor:

$$\underset{\text{Alanine}}{CH_3CHNH_2COOH} \longrightarrow \underset{\text{Acetate}}{CH_3COOH} \quad (4H)$$

$$\underset{\text{Glycine}}{2\ CH_2NH_2COOH} \xrightarrow{4H} \underset{\text{Acetate}}{2\ CH_3COOH} + \underset{\text{Ammonia}}{2\ NH_3}$$

Patterns of Respiration

Respiration requires a closed membrane. In bacteria, the membrane is the cell membrane. Electrons are passed from a chemical reductant to a chemical oxidant through a specific set of electron carriers within the membrane, and as a result, the proton motive force is established (Figure 6–32); return of protons across the membrane is coupled to the synthesis of ATP. As suggested in Figure 6–32, the biologic reductant for respiration frequently is NADH, and the oxidant often is oxygen.

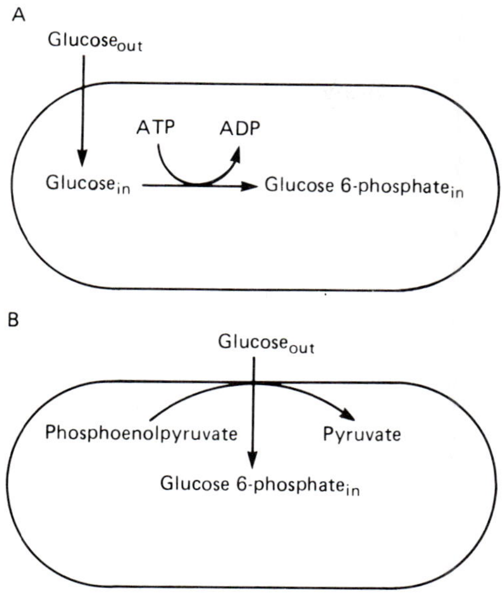

Figure 6–26. Phosphorylation of glucose to form glucose 6-phosphate. ***A:*** After transport across the cell membrane, glucose is phosphorylated by a kinase. ***B:*** Glucose is phosphorylated by phosphoenolpyruvate as it crosses the cell membrane.

Tremendous microbial diversity is exhibited in the sources of reductant used to generate NADH, and many microorganisms can use electron acceptors other than oxygen. Organic growth substrates are converted to focal metabolites that may reduce NAD^+ to NADH either by the hexose monophosphate shunt (Figure 6–6) or by the tricarboxylic acid cycle (Figure 6–13). Additional reductant may be generated during the breakdown of some growth substrates, eg, fatty acids (Figure 6–12).

Some bacteria, called **chemolithotrophs,** are able to use inorganic reductants for respiration. These energy sources include hydrogen, ferrous iron, and several reduced forms of sulfur and nitrogen. ATP derived from respiration and NADPH generated from the reductants can be used to drive the Calvin cycle (Figure 6–15).

Compounds and ions other than O_2 may be used as terminal oxidants in respiration. This ability, the capacity for **anaerobic respiration,** is a widespread microbial trait. Suitable electron acceptors include nitrate, sulfate, and carbon dioxide. Respiratory metabolism dependent upon carbon dioxide as an electron acceptor is a property found among representatives of a large and recently defined microbial group, the **archaebacteria.** Representatives of this group possess, for example, the ability to reduce carbon dioxide to acetate as a mechanism for generating metabolic energy.

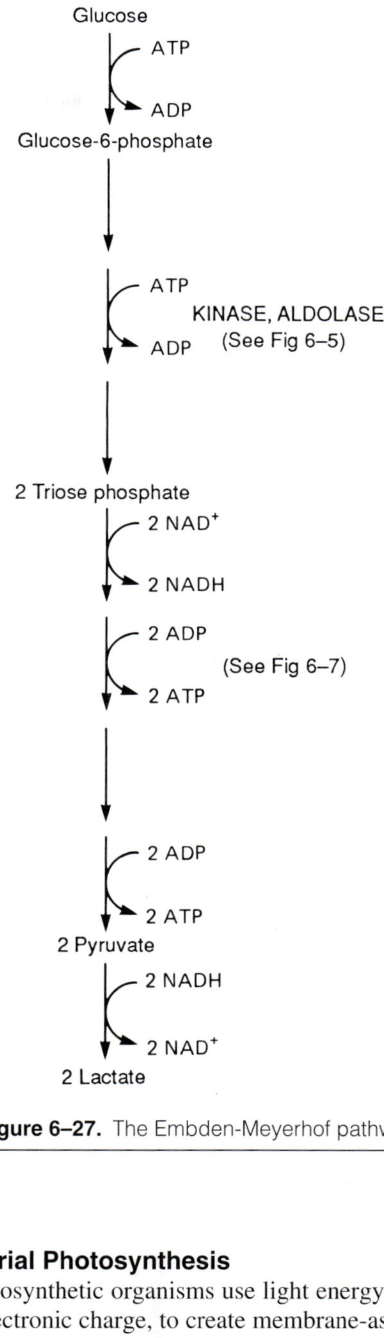

Figure 6–27. The Embden-Meyerhof pathway.

Bacterial Photosynthesis

Photosynthetic organisms use light energy to separate electronic charge, to create membrane-associated reductants and oxidants as a result of a photochemical event. Transfer of electrons from the reductant to the oxidant creates a proton motive force. Many bacteria carry out a photosynthetic metabolism that is entirely independent of oxygen. Light is used as a source of metabolic energy, and carbon for growth is derived either from organic compounds or from a combination of an inorganic reductant (eg, thiosulfate) and carbon dioxide. These bacteria possess a single photosystem that, although sufficient to provide energy for the synthesis of ATP and for the generation of essential trans-

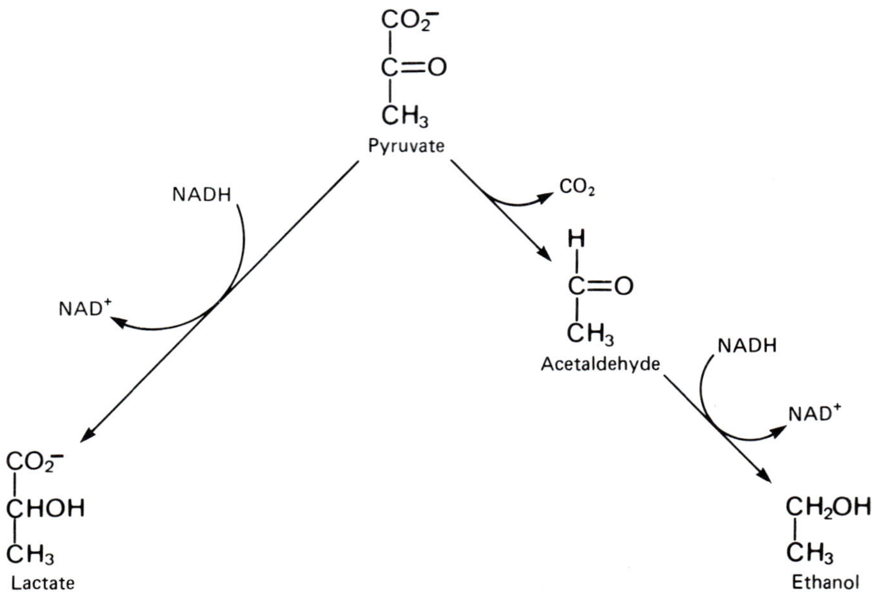

Figure 6–28. Two biochemical mechanisms by which pyruvate can oxidize NADH. ***Left:*** Direct formation of lactate, which results in net production of lactic acid from glucose. ***Right:*** Formation of the neutral products carbon dioxide and ethanol.

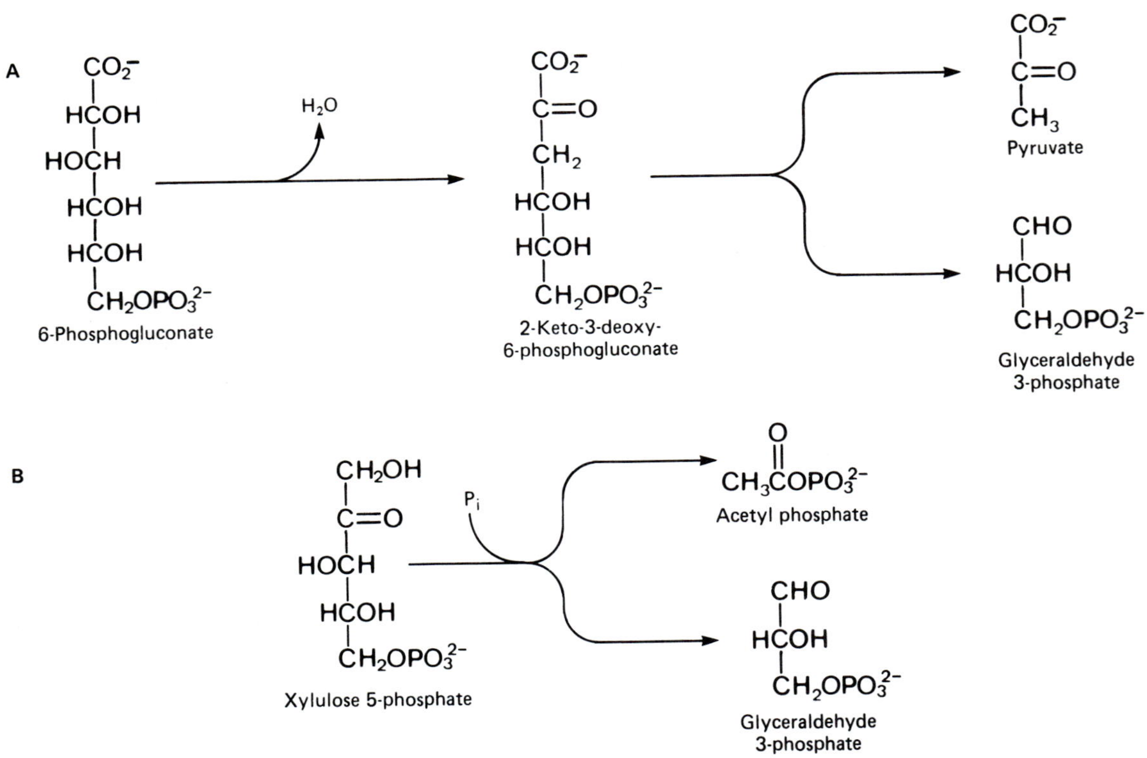

Figure 6–29. Reactions associated with specific pathways of carbohydrate fermentation: ***A:*** Dehydratase and aldolase reactions used in the Entner-Doudoroff pathway. ***B:*** The phosphoketolase reaction. This reaction, found in several pathways for fermentation of carbohydrates, generates the mixed acid anhydride acetyi phosphate, which can be used for substrate phosphorylation of ADP.

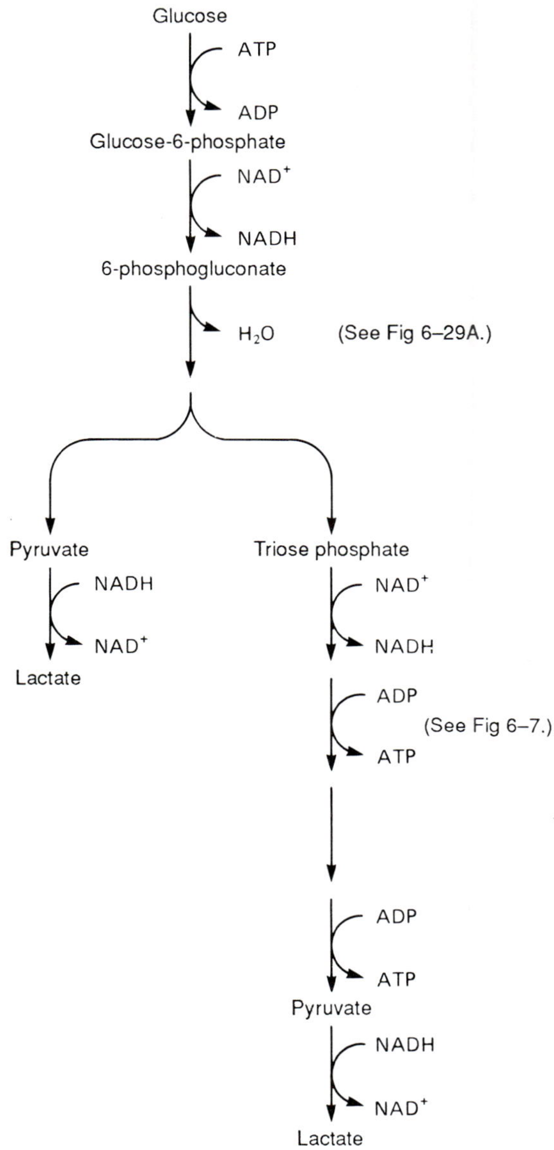

Figure 6–30. The Entner-Doudoroff pathway.

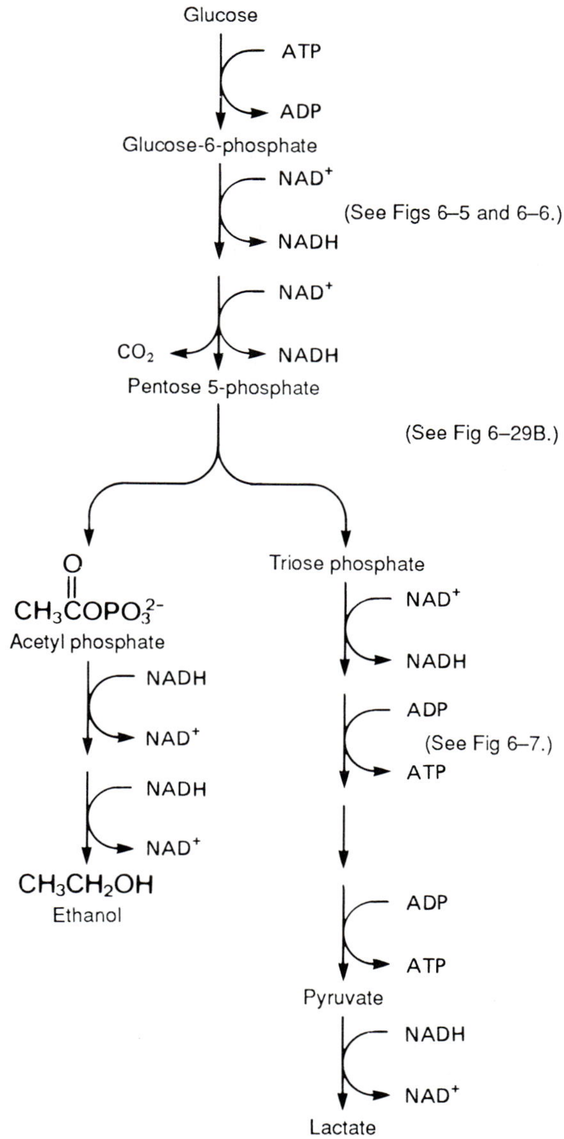

Figure 6–31. The heterolactic fermentation of glucose.

membrane ionic gradients, does not allow the highly exergonic reduction of $NADP^+$ at the expense of water. This process, essential for oxygen-evolving photosynthesis, rests upon additive energy derived from the coupling of two different photochemical events, driven by two independent photochemical systems. Among prokaryotes, this trait is found solely in the cyanobacteria (blue-green bacteria). Among eukaryotic organisms, the trait is shared by algae and plants in which the essential energy-providing organelle is the chloroplast.

REGULATION OF METABOLIC PATHWAYS

In their normal environment, microbial cells generally regulate their metabolic pathways so that no intermediate is made in excess. Each metabolic reaction is regulated not only with respect to all others in the cell but also with respect to the concentrations of nutrients in the environment. Thus, when a sporadically available carbon source suddenly becomes abundant, the enzymes required for its catabolism increase in

Table 6–1. Microbial fermentations based on the Embden-Meyerhof pathway.

Fermentation	Organisms	Products
Ethanol	Some fungi (notably some yeasts)	Ethanol, CO_2.
Lactate (homofermentation)	*Streptococcus* Some species of *Lactobacillus*	Lactate (accounting for at least 90% of the energy source carbon).
	Enterobacter *Aeromonas* *Bacillus polymyxa*	Ethanol, acetoin, 2,3-butylene glycol, CO_2, lactate, acetate, formate. (Total acids = 21 mol[1])
Propionate	*Clostridium propionicum* *Propionibacterium* *Corynebacterium diphtheriae* Some species of: *Neisseria* *Veillonella* *Micromonospora*	Propionate, acetate, succinate, CO_2.
Mixed acid	*Escherichia* *Salmonella* *Shigella* *Proteus*	Lactate, acetate, formate, succinate, H_2, CO_2, ethanol. (Total acids = 159 mol[1])
Butanol-butyrate	*Butyribacterium* *Zymosarcina maxima* Some species of: *Clostridium* *Neisseria*	Butanol, butyrate, acetone, isopropanol, acetate, ethanol, H_2, CO_2.

[1]Per 100 mol of glucose fermented.

both amount and activity; conversely, when a building block (such as an amino acid) suddenly becomes abundant, the enzymes required for its biosynthesis decrease in both amount and activity.

The regulation of enzyme activity as well as enzyme synthesis provides both fine control and coarse control of metabolic pathways. For example, the inhibition of enzyme activity by the end product of a pathway constitutes a mechanism of fine control, since the flow of carbon through that pathway is instantly and precisely regulated. The inhibition of enzyme synthesis by the same end product, on the other hand, constitutes a mechanism of coarse control. The preexisting enzyme molecules continue to function until they are diluted out by further cell growth, although unnecessary protein synthesis ceases immediately.

The mechanisms by which the cell regulates enzyme activity are discussed in the following section. The regulation of enzyme synthesis is discussed in Chapter 7.

The Regulation of Enzyme Activity

A. Enzymes as Allosteric Proteins: In many cases, the activity of an enzyme catalyzing an early step in a metabolic pathway is inhibited by the end product of that pathway. Such inhibition cannot depend on competition for the enzyme's substrate binding site, however, because the structures of the end product and the early intermediate (substrate) are usually quite different. Instead, inhibition depends on the fact that regulated enzymes are **allosteric:** each enzyme possesses not only a catalytic site, which binds substrate, but also one or more other sites that bind small regulatory molecules, or **effectors.** The binding of an effector to its site causes a conformational

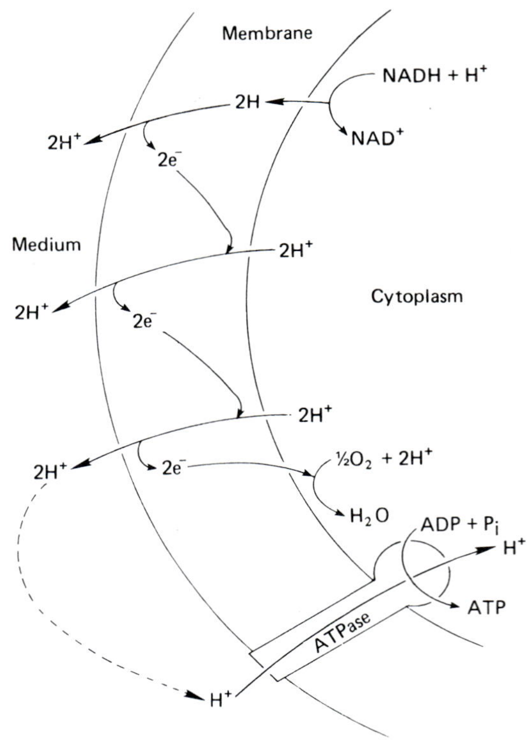

Figure 6–32. The coupling of electron transport in respiration to the generation of ATP. The indicated movements of protons and electrons are mediated by carriers (flavoprotein, quinone, cytochromes) associated with the membrane. The flow of protons down their electrochemical gradient, via the membrane ATPase, furnishes the energy for the generation of ATP from ADP and P_i. See text for explanation. (After Harold FM: Chemiosmotic interpretation of active transport in bacteria. Ann NY Acad Sci 1974;227:297.)

change in the enzyme such that the affinity of the catalytic site for the substrate is reduced (allosteric inhibition) or increased (allosteric activation).

Allosteric proteins are usually oligomeric. In some cases, the subunits are identical, each subunit possessing both a catalytic site and an effector site; in other cases, the subunits are different, one type possessing only a catalytic site and the other only an effector site.

B. Feedback Inhibition: The general mechanism which has evolved in microorganisms for regulating the flow of carbon through biosynthetic pathways is the most efficient that one can imagine. The end product in each case allosterically inhibits the activity of the first—and only the first—enzyme in the pathway. For example, the first step in the biosynthesis of isoleucine not involving any other pathway is the conversion of L-threonine to α-ketobutyric acid, catalyzed by threonine deaminase. Threonine deaminase is allosterically and specifically inhibited by L-isoleucine and by no other compound (Figure 6–33); the other four enzymes of the pathway are not affected (although their synthesis is repressed).

C. Allosteric Activation: In some cases, it is advantageous to the cell for an end product or an intermediate to activate rather than inhibit a particular enzyme. In the breakdown of glucose by *E coli,* for example, overproduction of the intermediates glucose 6-phosphate and phosphoenolpyruvate signals the diversion of some glucose to the pathway of glycogen synthesis; this is accomplished by the allosteric activation of the enzyme converting glucose 1-phosphate to ADP-glucose (Figure 6–34).

D. Cooperativity: Many oligomeric enzymes, possessing more than one substrate binding site, show cooperative interactions of substrate molecules. The binding of substrate by one catalytic site increases the affinity of the other sites for additional substrate molecules. The net effect of this interaction is to produce an exponential increase in catalytic activity in response to an arithmetic increase in substrate concentration.

E. Covalent Modification of Enzymes: The regulatory properties of some enzymes are altered by covalent modification of the protein. For example, the response of glutamine synthetase to metabolic effectors is altered by adenylation, the covalent attachment of ADP to a specific tyrosyl side chain within each enzyme subunit. The enzymes controlling adenylation also are controlled by covalent modification. The activity of other enzymes is altered by their phosphorylation.

F. Enzyme Inactivation: The activity of some enzymes is removed by their hydrolysis. This process can be regulated and sometimes is signaled by covalent modification of the enzyme targeted for removal.

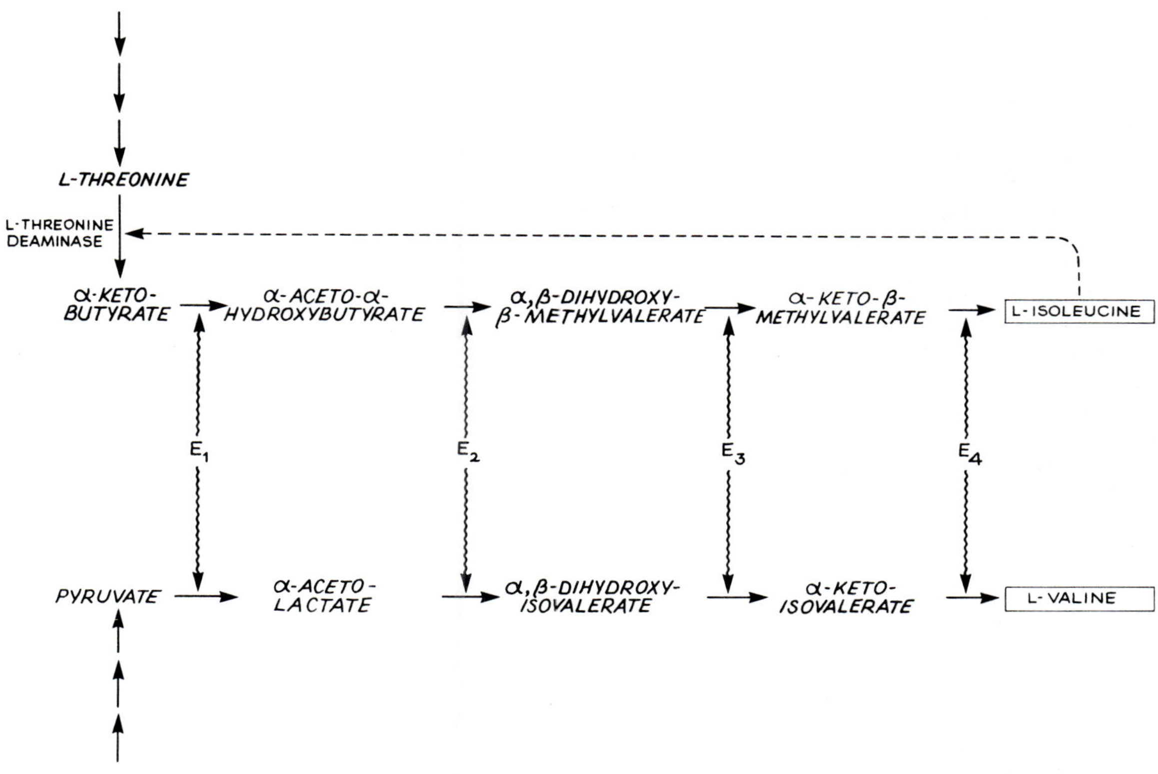

Figure 6–33. Feedback inhibition of L-threonine deaminase by L-isoleucine (dashed line). The pathways for the biosynthesis of isoleucine and valine are mediated by a common set of 4 enzymes, as shown.

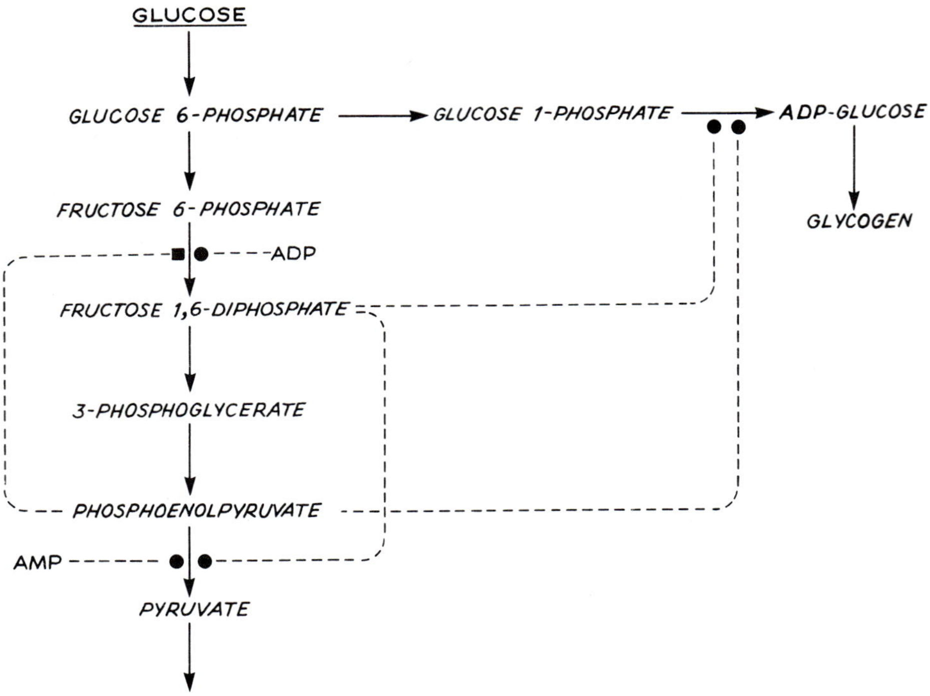

Figure 6–34. Regulation of glucose utilization by a combination of allosteric activation (●) and allosteric inhibition (■). (After Stanier RY, Adelberg EA, Ingraham JL: *The Microbial World,* 4th ed. Prentice-Hall, 1976.)

REFERENCES

Books

Chakrabarty AM (editor): *Biodegradation and Detoxification of Environmental Pollutants.* CRC Press, 1982.

Cohen GN: *Biosynthesis of Small Molecules.* Harper, 1967.

Gottschalk G: *Bacterial Metabolism.* Springer-Verlag, 1986.

Gunsalus IC, Stanier RY (editors): *The Bacteria: A Treatise on Structure and Function. Vol 2: Metabolism,* 1961; Vol 3: *Biosynthesis,* 1961. Academic Press.

Ingraham JL, Maaløe O, Neidhardt FC: *Growth of the Bacterial Cell.* Sinauer Associates, 1983.

Kornberg A: *Supplement to DNA Replication.* Freeman, 1980.

Kulaev JS, Tempest DW, Dawes EA (editors): *Environmental Regulation of Microbial Metabolism.* Academic Press, 1985.

Laskin AI, Lechevalier H (editors): *CRC Handbook of Microbiology,* 2nd ed. Vol 3: *Microbial Composition: Amino Acids, Proteins, and Nucleic Acids;* Vol 4: *Microbial Composition: Carbohydrates, Lipids, and Minerals.* CRC Press, 1981.

Mandelstam J, McQuillen K, Dawes I: *Biochemistry of Bacterial Growth,* 3rd ed. Halsted, 1982.

Nicholls DG: Bioenergetics: *An Introduction to the Chemiosmotic Theory.* Academic Press, 1983.

Ornston LN, Sokatch JR (editors): *Bacterial Diversity.* Vol. 6 of: *The Bacteria: A Treatise on Structure and Function.* Gunsalus IC, Stanier RY (editors). Academic Press, 1978.

Postgate JR: *Fundamentals of Nitrogen Fixation.* Cambridge Univ Press, 1983.

Rosen BP: *Bacterial Transport.* Dekker, 1978.

Sokatch JR, Ornston LN (editors): *Mechanisms of Adaptation.* Vol 7 of: *The Bacteria: A Treatise on Structure and Function.* Gunsalus IC, Stanier RY (editors). Academic Press, 1979.

Stryer L: *Biochemistry,* 2nd ed. Freeman, 1981.

Watson JD et al: *Molecular Biology of the Gene,* 4th ed. Benjamin Cummings, 1987.

Woese CR, Wolfe RS (editors): *Archaebacteria.* Vol 8 of: *The Bacteria: A Treatise on Structure and Function.* Gunsalus IC, Stanier RY (editors). Academic Press, 1985.

Articles & Reviews

Cundliffe E: How antibiotic producing organisms avoid suicide. Annu Rev Microbiol 1989;43:207.

Dagley S: A biochemical approach to some problems of environmental pollution. Pages 81–138 in: *Essays in Biochemistry.* Vol 11. Campbell PN, Aldridge WN (editors). Academic Press, 1975.

Felix CR, Ljungdahl LG: The cellulosome: The exocellular organelle of *Clostridium.* Annu Rev Microbiol 1993;49:791.

Finnety WR: Physiology and biochemistry of bacterial phospholipid metabolism. Adv Microb Physiol 1978; 18:177.

Goldin BR: In situ bacterial metabolism and colon mutagens. Annu Rev Microbiol 1986;40:367.

Harold FM: Membranes and energy transduction in bacteria. Curr Top Bioenerg 1977;6:83.

Ingledew WJ, Poole RK: The respiratory chains of *Escherichia coli.* Microbiol Rev 1984;48:222.

Kinoshita N, Unemoto T, Kobayashi H: Sodium-stimulated ATPase in *Streptococcus faecalis.* J Bacteriol 1984;158:844.

Lamond AI: The control of stable RNA synthesis in bacteria. Trends Biochem Sci 1985;10:271.

Ljungdahl LG: The autotrophic pathway of acetate synthesis in acetogenic bacteria. Annu Rev Microbiol 1986;40:415.

Lovely DR: Dissimulatory metal reduction. Annu Rev Microbiol 1993;47:263.

Mitchell P: Vectorial chemiosmotic processes. Annu Rev Biochem 1977;46:996.

Morris JG: The physiology of obligate anaerobiosis. Adv Microb Physiol 1975;12:169.

Nierlich DP: Regulation of bacterial growth, RNA and protein synthesis. Annu Rev Microbiol 1978;32: 393.

Priest FG: Extracellular enzyme synthesis in the genus *Bacillus.* Bacteriol Rev 1977;41:711.

Tabor CW, Tabor H: Polyamines in microorganisms. Microbiol Rev 1985;49:81.

Umbarger HE: Amino acid biosynthesis and its regulation. Annu Rev Biochem 1978;47:532.

Vanden Boom T, Croner JE Jr: Genetics and regulation of bacterial lipid metabolism. Annu Rev Microbiol 1989;43:317.

Waxman DJ, Strominger JL: Penicillin-binding proteins and the mechanism of action of β-lactam antibiotics. Annu Rev Biochem 1983;53:825.

7 Microbial Genetics

The science of **genetics** defines and analyzes **heredity,** or constancy and change in the vast array of physiologic functions that form the properties of organisms. The unit of heredity is the **gene,** a segment of DNA that carries in its nucleotide sequence information for a specific biochemical or physiologic property. The traditional approach to genetics has been to identify genes on the basis of their contribution to **phenotype,** or the collective structural and physiologic properties of a cell or an organism. A phenotypic property, be it eye color in a human or resistance to an antibiotic in a bacterium, is generally observed at the level of the organism. The chemical basis for variation in phenotype is change in **genotype,** or alteration in the sequence of DNA within a gene or in the organization of genes.

Traditional microbial genetics is based largely upon observation of growth. Phenotypic variation has been observed on the basis of a gene's capacity to permit growth under conditions of **selection;** eg, a bacterium containing a gene that confers resistance to ampicillin can be distinguished from a bacterium lacking the gene by its growth in the presence of the antibiotic, which serves as the agent of selection. Note that selection of the gene requires its **expression,** which under appropriate conditions can be observed at the level of phenotype.

Microbial genetics has revealed that genes consist of DNA, an observation that laid the foundation for molecular biology. Subsequent investigations of bacteria revealed the presence of **restriction enzymes** that cleave DNA at specific sites, giving rise to DNA **restriction fragments. Plasmids** were identified as small genetic elements capable of independent replication in bacteria and yeasts. The introduction of a DNA restriction fragment into a plasmid allows the fragment to be amplified many times. Amplification of specific regions of DNA also can be achieved with bacterial enzymes through **polymerase chain reaction (PCR)** testing. DNA within such regions can be placed under control of high-expression bacterial **promoters** that allow encoded proteins to be expressed at high levels. Thus, bacterial genetics fostered development of **genetic engineering,** a technology that has introduced tremendous advances into the field of medicine.

ORGANIZATION OF GENES

The Structure of DNA & RNA

Genetic information is stored as a sequence of bases in **deoxyribonucleic acid (DNA).** Most DNA molecules are double-stranded, with **complementary bases** (A-T; G-C) paired by hydrogen bonding in the center of the molecule (Figure 7–1). The complementarity of the bases enables one strand to provide the information for copying or expression of information in the other strand (Figure 7–2). The base pairs are stacked within the center of the DNA double helix (Figure 7–2), and they determine its genetic information. Each of the four bases is bonded to phospho-2′-deoxyribose to form a **nucleotide.** The negatively charged phosphodiester backbone of DNA faces the solvent, and charge repulsion contributes to the roughly linear structure assumed over long stretches of the molecule. The length of a DNA molecule is usually expressed in thousands of base pairs, or **kilobase pairs (kbp).** A small virus may contain a single DNA molecule of 5 kbp, whereas the single DNA molecule that forms the *Escherichia coli* chromosome is about 4000 kbp. Each base pair is separated from the next by about 0.34 nm, or 3.4×10^{-7} mm, so that the total length of the *E coli* chromosome is roughly 1 mm. Since the overall dimensions of the bacterial cell are roughly 1000-fold smaller than this length, it is evident that a substantial amount of folding, or **supercoiling,** contributes to the physical structure of the molecule in vivo.

Ribonucleic acid (RNA) most frequently occurs in single-stranded form. The base uracil (U) serves in RNA the hybridization function that thymine (T) serves in DNA, so the complementary bases that determine the structure of RNA are A-U and C-G. The overall structure of single-stranded RNA molecules is determined by hybridization between base sequences that form loops, with the result that single-stranded RNA molecules assume a compact structure capable of expressing genetic information contained in DNA.

A few RNA molecules have been shown to function as enzymes. The most general function of RNA is communication of DNA gene sequences in the form of **messenger RNA (mRNA)** to **ribosomes.** Within ri-

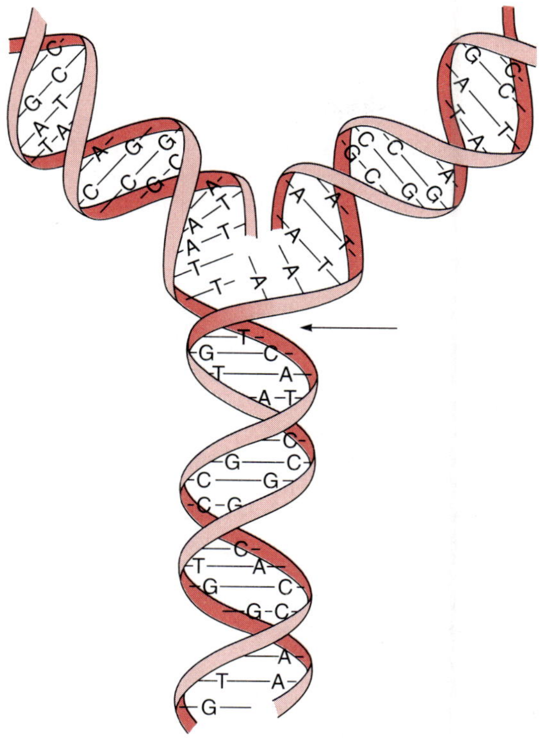

Figure 7–1. Structure and replication of DNA according to the Watson and Crick model. The vertical double strand is unwinding at the point indicated by the arrow, and the two arms have acted as templates for the synthesis of complementary strands. Synthesis is proceeding downward along the vertical double strand.

bosomes, which contain **ribosomal RNA (rRNA),** messages are translated into the amino acid structure of proteins via **transfer RNA (tRNA).** RNA molecules range in size from the small tRNAs, which contain fewer than 100 bases, to mRNAs, which may carry genetic messages extending to several thousand bases. Bacterial ribosomes contain three kinds of rRNA with respective sizes of 120, 1500, and 2900 bases. Corresponding rRNA molecules in eukaryotic ribosomes are somewhat larger. The need for expression of individual genes changes in response to physiologic demand, and requirements for flexible gene expression are reflected in the rapid metabolic turnover of most mRNAs. On the other hand, tRNAs and rRNAs—which are associated with the universally required function of protein synthesis—tend to be stable.

The Eukaryotic Genome

The **genome** is the totality of genetic information in an organism. Almost all of the eukaryotic genome is carried on two or more linear chromosomes separated from the cytoplasm within the membrane of the nucleus. **Diploid** eukaryotic cells contain two **homologues** (divergent evolutionary copies) of each chromosome. **Mutations,** or genetic changes, frequently cannot be detected in diploid cells because the contribution of one gene copy compensates for changes in the function of its homologue. A gene that does not achieve phenotypic expression in the presence of its homologue is **recessive,** whereas a gene that overrides the effect of its homologue is **dominant.** The effects of mutations can be most readily discerned in **haploid** cells, which carry only a single copy of most genes. Yeast cells (which are eukaryotic) are frequently investigated because they can be maintained and analyzed in the haploid state.

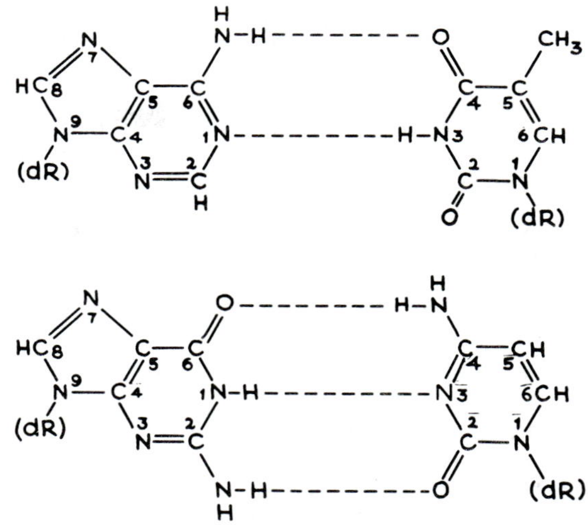

Figure 7–2. Normal base-pairing in DNA. Hydrogen bonds are indicated by dotted lines. (dR, deoxyribose of the sugar-phosphate backbone of DNA.) ***Top:*** Adenine-thymine pair. ***Bottom:*** Guanine-cytosine pair.

Eukaryotic cells contain mitochondria and, in some cases, chloroplasts. Within each of these organelles is a circular molecule of DNA that contains a few genes whose function relates to that particular organelle. Most genes associated with organelle function, however, are carried on eukaryotic chromosomes. Many yeasts contain an additional genetic element, an independently replicating 2-μm circle containing about 6.3 kbp of DNA. Such small circles of DNA, termed **plasmids,** are frequently encountered in the genetics of prokaryotes. The small size of plasmids renders them amenable to genetic manipulation and, after their alteration, may allow their introduction into cells. Therefore, plasmids are frequently called upon in genetic engineering.

Unlike prokaryotic DNA, eukaryotic DNA carries large amounts of repetitive DNA that does not code for any known function. In addition, many eukaryotic genes are interrupted by **introns,** intervening sequences of DNA that are not translated into gene products. Introns have been observed in archaeobacterial genes but have not been found in bacterial genes.

The Prokaryotic Genome

Most prokaryotic genes are carried on the bacterial chromosome, a single circle containing about 4000 kbp of DNA. Many bacteria contain additional genes on plasmids that range in size from several to 100 kbp. DNA circles (chromosome and plasmid), which contain genetic information necessary for their own replication, are called **replicons.** Membranes do not separate bacterial genes from cytoplasm as in eukaryotes. With few exceptions, bacterial genes are haploid.

Genes essential for bacterial growth are carried on the chromosome, and plasmids carry genes associated with specialized functions (Table 7–1). Many plasmids carry genes that mediate their transfer from one organism to another as well as other genes associated with acquisition or rearrangement of DNA. Therefore, genes with independent evolutionary origins may be assimilated by plasmids that are widely disseminated among bacterial populations. A consequence of such genetic events has been observed in the swift spread among bacterial populations of plasmid-borne resistance to antibiotics after their liberal use in hospitals.

Transposons are genetic elements that contain several kbp of DNA, including the information necessary for their migration from one genetic locus to another. Simple transposons, **insertion sequences,** carry only this genetic information. Complex transposons carry genes for specialized functions such as antibiotic resistance and are flanked by insertion sequences. Unlike plasmids, transposons do not contain genetic information necessary for their own replication. Selection of transposons depends upon their replication as part of a replicon. Detection or genetic exploitation of transposons is achieved by selection of the specialized genetic information (normally, resistance to an antibiotic) that they carry.

Table 7–1. Examples of metabolic activities determined by plasmids.

Organism	Activity
Pseudomonas spp	Degradation of camphor, toluene, octane, salicylic acid.
Bacillus stearothermophilus	α-Amylase.
Alcaligenes eutrophus	Utilization of H_2 as oxidizable energy source.
Escherichia coli	Sucrose uptake and metabolism, citrate uptake.
Klebsiella spp	Nitrogen fixation.
Streptococcus (group N)	Lactose utilization, galactose phosphotransferase system, citrate metabolism.
Rhodospirillum rubrum	Synthesis of photosynthetic pigment.
Flavobacterium spp	Nylon degradation.

The Viral Genome

Viruses are capable of survival, but not growth, in the absence of a cell host. Replication of the viral genome depends upon the metabolic energy and the macromolecular synthetic machinery of the host. Frequently, this form of genetic parasitism results in debilitation or death of the host cell. Therefore, successful propagation of the virus requires (1) a stable form that allows the virus to survive in the absence of its host, (2) a mechanism for invasion of a host cell, (3) genetic information required for replication of the viral components within the cell, and (4) additional information that may be required for packaging the viral components and liberating the resulting virus from the host cell.

Distinctions are frequently made between viruses associated with eukaryotes and viruses associated with prokaryotes, the latter being termed **bacteriophage.** It is appropriate to focus attention upon viral subgroups, but one should never forget the dictum of André Lwoff: "Viruses are viruses." Much of our understanding of viruses—indeed, many fundamental concepts of molecular biology—has emerged from investigation of the bacteriophage, and it is this group of viruses that is discussed in this chapter.

The nucleic acid molecule of bacteriophage is surrounded by a protein coat. Some phages also contain lipid, but these are exceptional. Considerable variability is found in the nucleic acid of phage. Many phages contain double-stranded DNA, others contain single-stranded RNA, and some contain single-stranded DNA. Unusual bases such as hydroxymethylcytosine are sometimes found in the phage nucleic acid. Many phages contain specialized syringe-like structures that bind to receptors on the cell surface and inject the phage nucleic acid into a host cell (Figure 7–3).

Phages can be distinguished on the basis of their mode of propagation. **Lytic phages** produce many

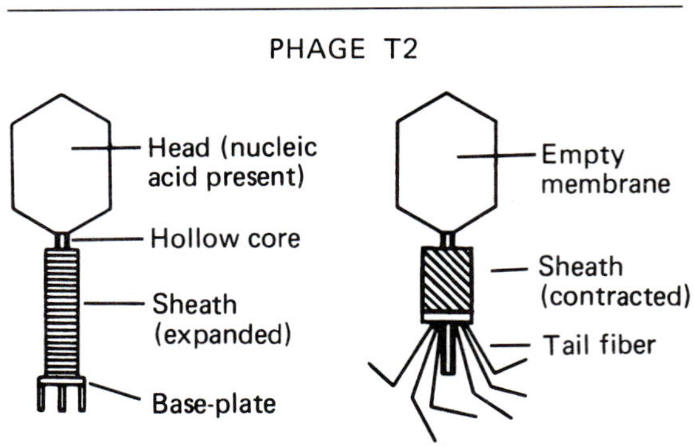

Figure 7–3. Diagrams of phage T2 based on electron micrographic observation.

copies of themselves as they kill their host cell. The most thoroughly studied lytic phages, the T-even phages of *Escherichia coli,* have demonstrated the need for precisely timed expression of viral genes in order to coordinate events associated with phage formation. Detailed analysis of these phages revealed the only introns that have been discovered among prokaryotes or their infective agents. **Temperate phages** are able to enter a nonlytic **prophage** state in which replication of their nucleic acid is linked to replication of host cell DNA. Bacteria carrying prophage are termed **lysogenic** because a physiologic signal can trigger a lytic cycle resulting in death of the host cell and liberation of many copies of the phage. The best characterized temperate phage is the *E coli* phage λ (lambda). Genes that determine the lytic or lysogenic response to λ infection have been identified and their complex interactions explored in detail.

Filamentous phages, exemplified by the well-studied *E coli* phage M13, are exceptional in several respects. Their filaments contain single-stranded DNA complexed with protein and are extruded from their hosts, which are debilitated but not killed by the phage infection. Engineering of DNA into phage M13 has provided single strands that are valuable sources for DNA analysis and manipulation.

REPLICATION

Double-stranded DNA is synthesized by **semiconservative replication.** As the parental duplex unwinds, each strand serves as a template (ie, the source of sequence information) for DNA replication. New strands are synthesized with their bases in an order complementary to that in the preexisting strands (Figure 7–2). When synthesis is complete, each daughter molecule contains one parental strand and one newly synthesized strand.

Eukaryotic DNA

Replication of eukaryotic DNA begins at several growing points along the linear chromosome. Accurate replication of the ends of linear chromosomes requires enzymatic activities different from the normal functions associated with DNA replication. These activities may involve **telomeres,** specialized DNA sequences (carried on the ends of eukaryotic chromosomes) that seem to be associated with accurate replication of chromosome ends. Eukaryotes have evolved specialized machinery, called a **spindle,** that pulls daughter chromosomes into separate nuclei newly formed by the process of **mitosis.** More extensive division of nuclei by **meiosis** halves the chromosomal number of diploid cells to form haploid cells. Accurate segregation of chromosomes during the reductive divisions of meiosis is an important factor in maintaining chromosomal structure within a species. Frequently, the haploid cells are **gametes.** Formation of gametes followed by their fusion to form diploid **zygotes** is the primary source of genetic variability via recombination in eukaryotes.

Bacterial DNA

Bacteria lack anything resembling the complex structures associated with the segregation of eukaryotic chromosomes into different daughter nuclei. Prokaryotic replicons are believed to be linked to the cell membrane, and segregation of daughter chromosomes and plasmids is thought to be coupled to elongation and septation of the membrane (Figure 7–4). Replication of the bacterial chromosome is tightly controlled, and the number of chromosomes per growing cell falls between one and four. Some bacterial plasmids may have as many as 30 copies in one bacterial cell, and mutations causing relaxed control of plasmid replication can result in even higher copy numbers.

Replication of circular double-stranded bacterial DNA begins at the *ori* locus, a region of DNA believed to be associated with the cell membrane. Replication of chromosomal DNA proceeds in two directions from the point of origin, and completion of the process at a distant site yields two daughter chromosomes that undergo segregation. Similar processes lead to the replication of plasmid DNA, except that in some cases replication is unidirectional.

Transposons

Transposons do not carry the genetic information required to couple their own replication to cell division, and their propagation therefore depends on their physical integration with a bacterial replicon. This association is fostered by the ability of transposons to form copies of themselves, which may be inserted within the same replicon or may be integrated into another replicon. The specificity of sequence at the insertion site is generally low, so that transposons often seem to insert in a random pattern. Since many of these insertions disrupt genes, transposons frequently cause mutations. Many plasmids are transferred among bacterial cells, and insertion of a transposon into such a plasmid can lead to its dissemination throughout a population.

Phage

Bacteriophages exhibit considerable diversity in the nature of their nucleic acid, and this diversity is reflected in different modes of replication. Fundamentally different propagation strategies are exhibited by lytic and temperate phages. Lytic phages produce many copies of themselves in a single burst of growth. Temperate phages establish themselves as prophages either by becoming part of an established replicon or by forming an independent replicon.

The double-stranded DNA of many lytic phages is linear, and the first stage in their replication is the formation of circular DNA. This process depends upon **cohesive ends,** complementary single-stranded tails of

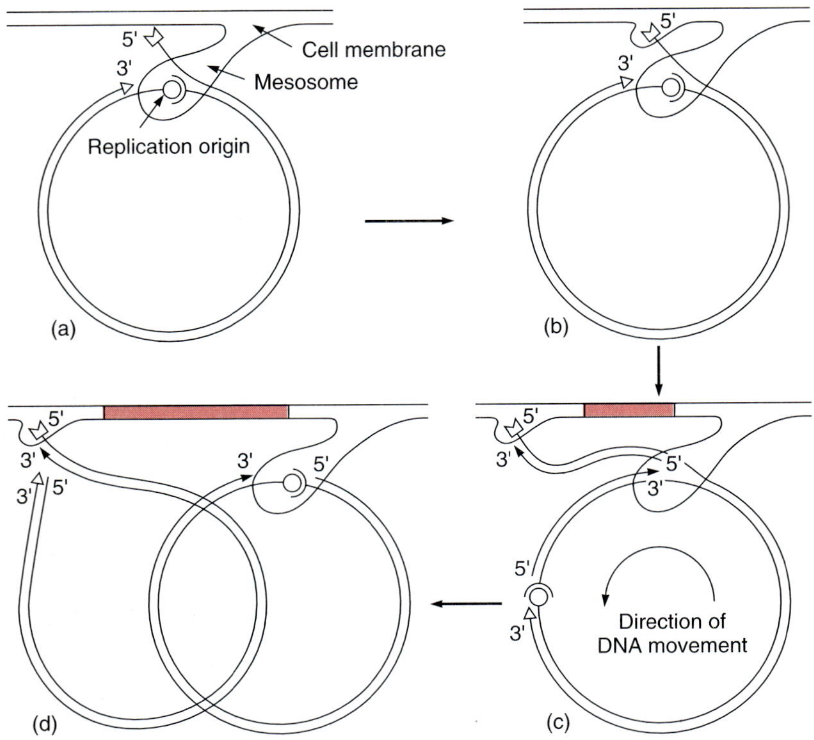

Figure 7–4. Replication of the bacterial chromosome, according to the model of Jacob and Brenner. ***(a)*** The chromosome is attached to a mesosome at the replication origin site, which serves as a swivel. One of the strands is broken. ***(b)*** The 5′ end of the broken strand attaches to a new site in the membrane. ***(c)*** The chromosome rotates counterclockwise past the mesosomal attachment site, at which is fixed the replicating enzyme system. Newly synthesized strands are shown as dashed lines. The attachment sites are separated by localized membrane synthesis (shown by shaded area). (d) The cycle of replication has been completed. The final step will be the joining of the free ends of one strand of the new chromosome (solid line). (From Stanier RY, Doudoroff M, Adelberg EA: *The Microbial World,* 3rd ed. Copyright © 1970. By permission of Prentice-Hall, Inc., Englewood Cliffs, NJ.)

DNA that hybridize. **Ligation,** formation of a phosphodiester bond between the tails, gives rise to covalently bonded circular DNA that may undergo replication in a manner similar to that used for other replicons. Cleavage of the circles produces linear DNA that is packaged inside protein coats to form daughter phages.

The single-stranded DNA of filamentous phages is converted to a circular double-stranded replicative form. One strand of the replicative form is used as a template in a continuous process that produces single-stranded DNA. The template is a rolling circle, and the single-stranded DNA it produces is cleaved and packaged with protein for extracellular extrusion.

Represented among the single-stranded RNA phages are the smallest extracellular particles containing information that allows for their own replication. The RNA of phage MS2, for example, contains (in fewer than 4000 nucleotides) three genes that can act as mRNA following infection. One gene encodes the coat protein, and another encodes an RNA polymerase that forms a double-stranded RNA replicative form. Single-stranded RNA produced from the replicative form is the core of new infective particles. The mechanism of propagation of RNA bacteriophage via RNA intermediates contrasts strongly with propagation of **retroviruses,** animal RNA viruses that use RNA as a template for DNA synthesis.

Some temperate bacteriophages, exemplified by *E coli* phage P1, can be established in the prophage state as plasmids. The double-stranded DNA of other temperate bacteriophages is established as prophage by its insertion into the host chromosome. The site of insertion may be quite specific, as exemplified by integration of *E coli* phage λ at a single *int* locus on the bacterial chromosome. The specificity of integration is determined by identity of the shared DNA sequence by the *int* locus and a corresponding region of the phage genome. Other temperate phages, such as *E coli* phage Mu, integrate in any of a wide range of chromosomal sites and in this respect resemble transposons.

Prophages contain genes required for lytic replication (also called vegetative replication), and expression of these genes is repressed during maintenance of the prophage state. A manifestation of repression is that established prophage frequently confers cellular immunity against lytic infection by similar phage. A cascade of molecular interactions triggers **derepression** (release from repression), so that a prophage undergoes vegetative replication, leading to formation of a burst of infectious particles. Artificial stimuli such as ultraviolet light may cause depression of prophage. The switch between lysogeny—propagation of the phage genome with the host—and vegetative phage growth at the expense of the cell may be determined in part by the cell's physiologic state. A nongrowing cell will not support vegetative growth of phage, whereas a vigorously growing cell contains sufficient energy and building blocks to support rapid phage replication.

TRANSFER OF DNA

Interstrain transfer of DNA among prokaryotes is widespread and makes a major contribution to the remarkable genetic diversity of bacteria. Genetic recombination among bacteria is quite unlike the fusion of zygotes observed with eukaryotes. Bacterial genetic exchange is typified by transfer of a relatively small fragment of a donor genome to a recipient cell. Successful genetic recombination demands that this donor DNA be replicated in the recombinant organism. Replication can be achieved either by integration of the donor DNA into the recipient's replicon or by establishment of donor DNA as an independent replicon.

Restriction & Other Constraints on Gene Transfer

Restriction enzymes (restriction endonucleases) provide bacteria with a mechanism to distinguish between their own DNA and DNA from other biologic sources. These enzymes hydrolyze DNA at restriction sites determined by specific DNA sequences ranging from four to 13 bases. In this specificity of sequence recognition lies the selectivity of DNA fragment preparation that is the foundation of much genetic engineering. Many restriction enzymes contain a modification function that methylates bases within restriction sites, thus providing a chemical signal that protects the sites in host DNA against cleavage. A direct biologic consequence of restriction can be cleavage of donor DNA before it has an opportunity to become established as part of a recombinant replicon. Therefore, many recipients used in genetic engineering are dysfunctional in the *res* genes associated with restriction.

Some plasmids exhibit a narrow host range and are able to replicate only in a closely related set of bacteria. Other plasmids, exemplified by some drug resistance plasmids, replicate in a wide range of bacterial recombinants. However, there are only a limited number of plasmid **compatibility groups,** and plasmids from the same compatibility group cannot replicate in the same bacterium. Plasmids that can replicate in a single cell line are called **compatible plasmids.**

Mechanisms of Recombination

Donor DNA that does not carry information necessary for its own replication must recombine with recipient DNA in order to become established in a recipient strain. The recombination may be **legitimate,** a consequence of close similarity in the sequences of donor and recipient DNA, or **illegitimate,** the result of enzyme-catalyzed recombination between dissimilar DNA sequences. Legitimate recombination almost always involves exchange between genes that share common ancestry and is therefore frequently called **homologous** recombination. The process requires a set of genes designated *rec,* and dysfunctions in these genes give rise to bacteria that can maintain closely homologous genes in the absence of recombination. Illegitimate **(nonhomologous)** recombination depends on enzymes encoded by the integrated DNA and is most clearly exemplified by the insertion of DNA into a recipient to form a copy of a donor transposon.

The mechanism of recombination mediated by *rec* gene products is reciprocal: introduction of a donor sequence into a recipient is mirrored by transfer of the homologous recipient sequence into the donor DNA. Increasing scientific attention is being paid to the role of **gene conversion**—the nonreciprocal transfer of DNA sequences from donor to recipient—in the acquisition of genetic diversity.

Mechanisms of Gene Transfer

The three major forms of prokaryotic genetic exchange are distinguished by the form of the donor DNA. In **conjugation,** the donor cell contributes energy and building blocks to the synthesis of a new strand of DNA, which is physically transferred to the recipient cell. The recipient completes the structure of double-stranded DNA by synthesizing the strand that complements the strand acquired from the donor. In **transduction,** donor DNA is carried in a phage coat and is transferred into the recipient by the mechanism used for phage infection. **Transformation,** the direct uptake of donor DNA by the recipient cell, may be natural or forced. Relatively few bacterial strains are naturally competent for transformation; these strains assimilate donor DNA in linear form. Forced transformation is induced in the laboratory, where, after treatment with high salt and temperature shock, many bacteria are rendered competent for the assimilation of extracellular plasmids. The capacity to force bacteria to incorporate extracellular plasmids by transformation is fundamental to genetic engineering.

A. Conjugation: Plasmids are the genetic elements most frequently transferred by conjugation. Genetic functions required for transfer are carried by the *tra* genes, which are carried by self-transmissible **plasmids.** Some self-transmissible plasmids can mobilize other plasmids or portions of the chromosome for transfer. In some cases mobilization is achieved because the *tra* genes provide functions necessary for transfer of an otherwise nontransmissible plasmid. In other cases, the self-transmissible plasmid integrates with the DNA of another replicon and, as an extension of itself, carries a strand of this DNA into a recipient cell.

Genetic analysis of *E coli* was greatly advanced by elucidation of fertility factors carried on a plasmid designated F^+. This plasmid confers certain donor characteristics upon cells; these characteristics include a sex pilus, an extracellular protein extrusion that attaches donor cells to recipient organisms lacking the fertility factor. A bridge between the cells allows a strand of the F^+ plasmid, synthesized by the donor, to pass into the recipient, where the complementary strand of DNA is formed (Figure 7–5). The F^+ fertility factor can integrate into numerous loci in the chromosome of donor cells. The integrated fertility factor creates **Hfr (high-frequency recombination)** donors from which chromosomal DNA is transferred (from the site of insertion) in a direction determined by the orientation of insertion.

The rate of chromosomal transfer from Hfr cells is constant, and compilation of results from many conjugation experiments has allowed preparation of an *E coli* **genetic map** in which distances between loci are measured in number of minutes required for transfer in conjugation. A similar map has been constructed for the related coliform bacterium *Salmonella typhimurium,* and comparison of the two maps shows related patterns of gene organization, although several major chromosomal rearrangements have accompanied divergence of the two bacterial species.

Analogous procedures with other plasmids have enabled researchers to map the circular chromosomes of members of distant bacterial genera; eg, drug resistance plasmids, termed **R factors,** can promote chromosomal transfer from diverse bacteria, including *Pseudomonas* species. Comparison of chromosomal maps of *Pseudomonas aeruginosa* and *Pseudomonas putida* shows that few, albeit significant, genetic rearrangements accompanied divergence of these two closely related species. *Pseudomonas* maps have little in common with those of the biologically distant coliform bacteria.

Integration of chromosomal DNA into a conjugal plasmid can produce a recombinant replicon—a **prime, F** (fertility)′ or **R** (resistance)′, depending on the plasmid—in which the integrated chromosomal DNA can be replicated on the plasmid independently of the chromosome. Bacteria carrying gene copies, a full set on the chromosome and a partial set on a prime, are partial diploids, or **merodiploids.** A wild-type gene frequently complements its mutant homologue, and selection for the wild-type phenotype can allow maintenance of merodiploids in the laboratory. Such strains can allow analysis of interactions between different **alleles,** genetic variants of the same gene. Merodiploids frequently are genetically unstable because recombination between the plasmid and the homologous chromosome can result in loss or exchange of mutant or wild-type alleles. This problem can frequently be circumvented by maintenance of merodiploids in a genetic background in which *recA,* a gene required for recombination between homologous segments of DNA, has been inactivated by mutation.

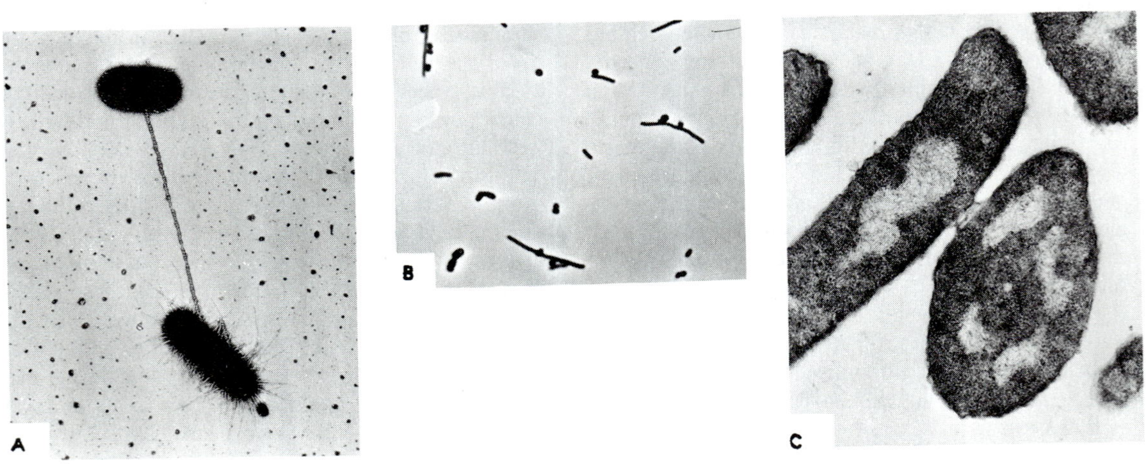

Figure 7–5. ***A:*** A male and a female cell joined by an F pilus (sex pilus). The F pilus has been "stained" with male-specific RNA phage particles. The male cell also possesses ordinary F pili, which do not adsorb male-specific phages and are not involved in mating. ***B:*** Mating pairs of *E coli* cells. Hfr cells are elongated. ***C:*** Electron micrograph of a thin section of a mating pair. The cell walls of the mating partners are in intimate contact in the "bridge" area. (Electron micrograph [A] by Carnahan J and Brinton C. From Stanier RY, Doudoroff M, Adelberg EA: *The Microbial World,* 3rd ed. Copyright © 1970. By permission of Prentice-Hall, Inc., Englewood Cliffs, NJ. Photographs [B] and [C] from Gross JD and Caro LG: DNA transfer in bacterial conjugation. J Mol Biol 1966;16:269.)

Homologous genes from different organisms may have diverged to an extent that prevents recombination between them but does not alter the capacity of one gene to complement the missing activity of another. For example, the genetic origin of an enzyme required for amino acid biosynthesis is unlikely to influence catalytic activity in the cytoplasm of a biologically distant host. A merodiploid carrying a gene for such an enzyme would also carry flanking genes derived from the donor organism. Therefore, conventional microbial genetics, based on selection of prime plasmids, can be used to isolate genes from fastidious organisms in *E coli* or *P aeruginosa.* The significance of this technology lies in its ability to simplify or to circumvent the relatively expensive procedures demanded by genetic engineering.

B. Transduction: Transduction is phage-mediated genetic recombination in bacteria. In simplest terms, a transducing particle might be regarded as bacterial DNA in a phage coat. Even a lytic phage population may contain some particles in which the phage coat surrounds DNA derived from the bacterium rather than from the phage. Such populations have been used to transfer genes from one bacterium to another. Temperate phages are preferred vehicles for gene transfer because infection of recipient bacteria under conditions that favor lysogeny minimizes cell lysis and thus favors survival of recombinant strains. Indeed a recipient bacterium carrying an appropriate prophage may form a repressor that renders the cell immune to lytic infection; such cells may still take up bacterial DNA from transducing particles. Transducing mixtures carrying donor DNA can be prepared under conditions that favor the lytic phage cycle.

The size of DNA in transducing particles is usually no more than several percent of the bacterial chromosome, and therefore **cotransduction**—transfer of more than one gene at a time—is limited to linked bacterial genes. The process is of particular value in mapping genes that lie too close together to be placed in map order on the basis of conjugal transfer. Mutant phages can be identified on the basis of the morphology of the **plaque** they form by lysis of a lawn of bacteria growing on solidified agar medium. Genetic maps for phages have been constructed by analysis of plaques arising from bacteria that have been simultaneously infected with two different phages.

The speed with which phages recombine and replicate has made them central subjects for study of these processes, and many generalizations concerning the underlying mechanisms have emerged from phage genetics. The capacity of phages to make rapid replicas of their DNA makes them valuable to genetic engineering. Of particular value are recombinant phages engineered so that they contain DNA inserts from another biologic source. Inserted DNA can be replicated with the swiftness that characterizes phage DNA and regained in a form useful for manipulation. Single-stranded DNA, produced by phage M13 and its derivatives, serves as a template for sequencing and site-directed mutagenesis.

C. Transformation: Direct uptake of donor DNA by recipient cells depends on their competence for transformation. Natural occurrence of this property is unusual among bacteria, and some of these strains are transformable only in the presence of **competence factors,** produced only at a specific point in the growth cycle. Other strains readily undergo natural transformation, and these organisms offer promise for genetic engineering because of the ease with which they incorporate modified DNA into their chromosomes. DNA fragments containing genes from such organisms can be readily identified on the basis of their ability to transform mutant cells to the wild type. These techniques represent a substantial advance over the laborious procedures used by Avery and his associates to demonstrate that the pneumococcus transforming principle was DNA.

Natural transformation is an active process demanding specific enzymes produced by the recipient cell. Many bacteria, unable to undergo natural transformation, can be forced to incorporate plasmids by treatment with calcium chloride and temperature shock. Transformation with engineered recombinant plasmids by this procedure is a cornerstone of modern molecular biology because it enables DNA from diverse biologic sources to be established as part of well-characterized bacterial replicons.

MUTATION & GENE REARRANGEMENT

Spontaneous Mutations

Mutations are changes in DNA sequence. Spontaneous mutations for a given gene generally occur with a frequency of 10^{-8}–10^{-6} in a population derived from a single bacterium. The mutations include **base substitutions, deletions, insertions,** and **rearrangements.** Base substitutions can arise as a consequence of mispairing between complementary bases during replication. Establishment of such mutations is minimized by enzymes associated with **mismatch repair,** a process that essentially proofreads a newly synthesized strand to ensure that it perfectly complements its template. The enzymes distinguish the newly synthesized strand from the preexisting strand on the basis of methylation of adenine in GATC sequences of the preexisting strand. A special DNA repair system, the **SOS response,** is called into play in cells in which DNA has been damaged.

Many base substitutions escape detection at the phenotypic level because they do not significantly disrupt the function of the gene product. For example, **missense mutations,** which result in substitution of one amino acid for another, may be without discernible phenotypic effect. **Nonsense mutations** terminate synthesis of proteins and thus result in a protein truncated at the site of mutation. The gene products of nonsense mutations are usually inactive.

The consequences of deletion or insertion mutations also are severe because they can drastically alter the amino acid sequence of gene products. As described below, accurate expression of DNA sequences depends on translation of nucleotide triplet codons in perfect phase. Insertion or deletion of a single nucleotide disrupts the phase of translation and thus introduces an entirely different protein sequence distal to the amino acid codon altered by the mutation.

A substantial fraction of spontaneous mutations are deletions that remove large portions of genes or even sets of genes. Other spontaneous mutations cause duplication, frequently in tandem, of comparable lengths of DNA. Such mutations usually are unstable and revert readily. Other mutations can invert lengthy DNA sequences or transpose such sequences to new loci. Comparative gene maps of related bacterial strains have shown that such rearrangements can be fixed in natural populations. These observations point to the fact that linear separation of DNA fragments does not completely disrupt possibilities for physical and chemical interaction among them.

Mutagens

The frequency of mutation is greatly enhanced by exposure of cells to mutagens. Ultraviolet (UV) light is a **physical mutagen** that damages DNA by linking neighboring thymine bases to form dimers. Sequence errors can be introduced during enzymatic repair of this genetic damage. **Chemical mutagens** may act by altering either the chemical or the physical structure of DNA. Reactive chemicals alter the structure of bases in DNA. For example, nitrous acid (HNO_2) substitutes hydroxyl groups for amino groups. The resulting DNA has altered template activity during subsequent rounds of replication. **Frameshift mutations**—introduction or removal of a single base pair from DNA—are caused by slight slippage of DNA strands. This slippage is favored by acridine dyes, which can intercalate between bases.

In general, the direct effect of chemical or physical mutagens is damage to DNA. The resulting mutations are introduced by enzymes associated with replication or repair. Mutations that change the properties of these enzymes can make them biologic mutagens, the products of mutator genes. Other forms of biologic mutagenesis are insertions into repair genes caused by transposons such as the phage Mu.

Reversion & Suppression

Regaining an activity lost as a consequence of mutation, termed **phenotypic reversion,** may or may not result from restoration of the original DNA sequence, as would be demanded by **genotypic reversion.** Frequently, a mutation at a second locus, called a **suppressor mutation,** restores the lost activity. In **intragenic suppression,** after a primary mutation has changed an enzyme's structure so that its activity has been lost, a second mutation, at a different site in the enzyme's gene, restores the structure required for activity. **Extragenic suppression** is caused by a second mutation lying outside the originally affected gene. Well-characterized examples are **nonsense suppressors,** which allow introduction of amino acids at sites where nonsense mutations cause the termination of the synthesis of a protein. Nonsense suppressors can exert their effect on nonsense mutations in many different genes.

GENE EXPRESSION

The tremendous evolutionary separation of eukaryotic and prokaryotic genomes is illustrated by comparing their mechanisms of gene expression, which share certain properties. In both groups, genetic information is encoded in DNA, transcribed into mRNA, and translated on ribosomes through tRNA into the structure of proteins (Figure 7–6). The triplet nucleotide codons used in translation are generally shared, and many enzymes associated with macromolecular synthesis in the two biologic groups have similar properties. Beyond these generalizations, there are striking differences between eukaryotes and prokaryotes at each step in gene expression. The mechanism by which the sequence of nucleotides in a gene determines the sequence of amino acids in a protein is as follows:

(1) RNA polymerase forms a single polyribonucleotide strand, called "messenger RNA" (mRNA), using DNA as a template; this process is called **transcription.** The mRNA has a nucleotide sequence complementary to one of the strands in the DNA double helix.

(2) Amino acids are enzymatically activated and transferred to specific adapter molecules of RNA, called "transfer RNA" (tRNA). Each adapter molecule has at one end a triplet of bases complementary to a triplet of bases on mRNA, and at the other end its specific amino acid. The triplet of bases on mRNA is called the **codon** for that amino acid.

(3) mRNA and tRNA come together on the surface of the ribosome. As each tRNA finds its complementary nucleotide triplet on mRNA, the amino acid that it carries is put into peptide linkage with the amino acid of the preceding (neighboring) tRNA molecule. The ribosome moves along the mRNA, the polypeptide growing sequentially until the entire mRNA molecule has been translated into a corresponding sequence of amino acids. This process, called **translation,** is diagrammed in Figure 7–6.

Genes associated with related functions are frequently clustered in prokaryotes, whereas such clustering among eukaryotic genes is unusual. **Enhancer sequences** are regions of eukaryotic DNA that increase transcription and may lie distantly upstream

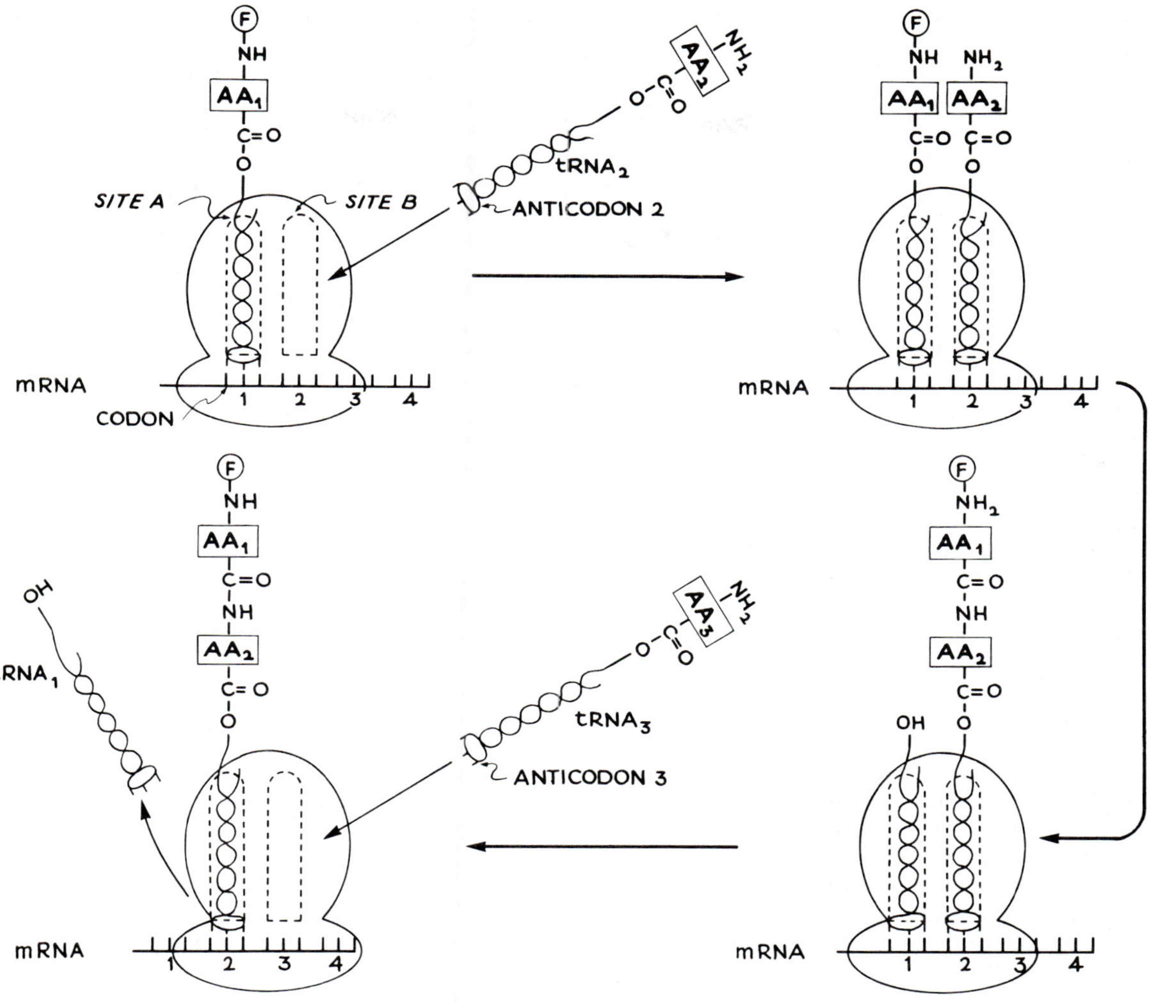

Figure 7–6. Four stages in the lengthening of a polypeptide chain on the surface of a 70S ribosome. ***Top left:*** A tRNA molecule bearing the anticodon complementary to codon 1 at one end and $AA_1$1 at the other, binds to site A. AA_1 is attached to the tRNA through its carboxyl group; its amino nitrogen bears a formyl group (F). ***Top right:*** A tRNA molecule bearing AA_2 binds to site B; its anticodon is complementary to codon 2. ***Bottom right:*** An enzyme complex catalyzes the transfer of AA_1 to the amino group of AA_2, forming a peptide bond. (Note that transfer in the opposite direction is blocked by the prior formylation of the amino group of AA_1.) ***Bottom left:*** The ribosome moves to the right, so that sites A and B are now opposite codons 2 and 3; in the process, $tRNA_1$ is displaced and $tRNA_2$ moves to site A. Site B is again vacant and is ready to accept $tRNA_3$ bearing AA_3. (When the polypeptide is completed and released, the formyl group is enzymatically removed.) (Redrawn and reproduced by permission of Stanier RY, Doudoroff M, Adelberg EA: *The Microbial World,* 3rd ed. Copyright © 1970. Prentice-Hall, Inc., Englewood Cliffs, NJ.)

from the transcribed gene. Eukaryotic genes carry **introns,** DNA insertions that generally are not found in prokaryotic genes. Introns separate **exons,** the coding regions of eukaryotic genes. Transcribed introns are removed from eukaryotic transcripts during RNA processing, a series of enzymatic reactions that take place in the nucleus. As far as is known, prokaryotic mRNA is turned over rapidly, whereas some eukaryotic mRNA molecules, exemplified by the hemoglobin RNA of erythrocytes, are quite stable.

Eukaryotic and prokaryotic ribosomes differ in many respects. Eukaryotic ribosomes are larger and have a sedimentation coefficient of 80S compared with the 70S sedimentation coefficient of prokaryotic ribosomes. The 40S and 60S eukaryotic ribosomal subunits are larger than the corresponding 30S and 50S ribosomes of prokaryotes, and the eukaryotic ribosomes are relatively rich in protein. Significant differences are inherent in the sensitivity of the ribosomal activities to antibiotics, many of which selectively inhibit protein synthesis in prokaryotic but not in eukaryotic cytoplasm (see Chapter 9). It should be remembered, however, that mitochondrial ribosomes in eukaryotes resemble those from prokaryotes.

Regulation of Gene Expression

Eukaryotic mRNA is transported from the nucleus to the cytoplasm, where translation occurs. In contrast, the translation of prokaryotic mRNA is coupled to its synthesis, and in this coupling lie opportunities for regulation that may be uniquely prokaryotic. For example, **attenuation**—the premature termination of mRNA transcribed from biosynthetic genes—is effected by the cellular capacity to synthesize a leader peptide. Blockage of the leader peptide's synthesis, favored by deprivation of an amino acid component, causes the mRNA to assume a structure that masks the termination signal and allows transcription to proceed into structural genes. Thus, in the absence of the amino acids required for synthesis of the peptide, the biosynthetic end product reduces attenuation and leads to increased levels of biosynthetic enzymes.

Specific proteins, the products of regulatory genes, govern expression of structural genes that encode enzymes. Transcription of DNA into mRNA begins at the **promoter,** the DNA sequence that binds RNA polymerase. The level of gene expression is determined in part by the ability of a promoter to bind the polymerase, and the intrinsic effectiveness of promoters differs widely. Further controls over gene expression are exerted by regulatory proteins that can bind to regions of DNA near promoters.

Some prokaryotic structural genes that encode a series of metabolic reactions are clustered in an **operon.** Such genes are expressed as a single mRNA transcript, and expression of the transcript may be governed by a single regulatory gene. For example, five genes associated with tryptophan biosynthesis are clustered in the *trp* operon of *E coli.* Gene expression is governed by attenuation, as described above, and is also controlled by repression: binding of tryptophan by a **repressor protein** gives it a conformation that allows it to attach to the *trp* **operator,** a short DNA sequence that helps to regulate gene expression. Binding of the repressor protein to the operator prevents transcription of the *trp* genes. This form of control is independent of attenuation, which also is used to govern *trp* gene expression.

Prevention of transcription by a repressor protein is called **negative control.** The opposite form of transcriptional regulation—initiation of transcription in response to binding of an **activator protein**—is termed **positive control.** Both forms of control are exerted over expression of the *lac* operon, genes associated with fermentation of lactose in *E coli.* The operon contains three structural genes. Transport of lactose into the cell is mediated by the product of the *lacY* gene. Beta-galactosidase, the enzyme that hydrolyzes lactose to galactose and glucose, is encoded by the *lacZ* gene. The product of the third gene *(lacA)* is a transacetylase; the physiologic function of this enzyme has not been clearly elucidated.

As a by-product of its normal function, β-galactosidase produces allolactose, a structural isomer of lactose. Lactose itself does not influence regulation of transcription. This function is served by allolactose, which is the **inducer** of the *lac* operon because it is the metabolite that most directly elicits gene expression. In the absence of allolactose, the *lac* repressor, a product of the independently controlled *lacI* gene, exerts negative control over transcription of the *lac* operon by binding to the *lac* operator. In the presence of the inducer, the repressor is released from the operator, and transcription takes place.

Expression of the *lac* operon and many other operons for enzymes associated with fermentation is enhanced by the binding of **cyclic AMP binding protein (CAP)** to a specific DNA sequence near the promoter for the regulated operon. The protein exerts positive control by enhancing RNA polymerase activity. The metabolite that triggers the positive control by binding to CAP is 3′,5′-cyclic AMP (cAMP). This compound, formed in energy-deprived cells, acts through CAP to enhance expression of catabolic enzymes that give rise to metabolic energy.

Cyclic AMP is not alone in its ability to exert control over unlinked genes in *E coli.* A number of different genes respond to the nucleotide ppGpp (in which "p" denotes phosphodiester and "G" denotes guanine) as a signal of amino acid starvation, and unlinked genes are expressed as part of the SOS response to DNA damage. Yet another set of unlinked genes is called into play in response to heat shock. This response is found in both prokaryotes and eukaryotes.

Elucidation of prokaryotic systems of transcriptional control has proved to have both conceptual and technical value. The *lac* operon has provided a useful model for comparative studies of gene expression. For example, the phenomenon of repression, first clearly described for the *lac* operon, accounts for the lysogenic response to infection by temperature phage such as λ. Thorough study of the *E coli lac* system has provided many genetic derivatives that are useful in genetic engineering. Insertion of foreign DNA into plasmids to form **recombinant vectors** is frequently monitored phenotypically by use of a color test to monitor insertional inactivation of the *lacY* gene, and the *lac* promoter is often used to achieve controlled expression of inserted genes.

GENETIC ENGINEERING

Engineering is the application of science to social needs. In recent years, engineering based on bacterial genetics has transformed biology. Specified DNA fragments can be isolated and amplified, and their genes can be expressed at high levels. The nucleotide specificity required for cleavage by restriction enzymes allows fragments containing genes or parts of genes to be covalently bound to plasmids ("vectors") that can then be inserted into bacterial hosts. Bacterial colonies or **clones** carrying specified genes can be identified by **hybridization** of DNA or RNA with chemical or radiochemical **probes.** Alternatively, protein products encoded by the genes can be recognized either by enzyme activity or by immunologic techniques. The latter procedures have been greatly enhanced by the remarkable selectivity with which **monoclonal antibodies** (see Chapter 8) bind to specific antigenic determinants in proteins. Thus, genetic engineering techniques can be used to isolate virtually any gene with a biochemically recognizable property.

Isolated genes can be used for a variety of purposes. **Site-directed mutagenesis** can identify and alter the DNA sequence of a gene. Nucleotide residues essential for gene function can thus be determined and, if desired, altered. With hybridization techniques, DNA can be used as a probe that recognizes nucleic acids corresponding to the sequence of its own DNA. For example, a latent virus in animal tissue can be detected with a DNA probe even in the absence of viral activity. The protein products of isolated viral genes offer great promise as vaccines because they can be prepared without genes that encode the replication of viral nucleic acid. Moreover, proteins such as insulin that have useful functions can be prepared in large quantities from bacteria that express cloned genes.

PREPARATION OF DNA FRAGMENTS WITH RESTRICTION ENZYMES

The genetic diversity of bacteria is reflected in their remarkable range of **restriction enzymes,** which possess remarkable selectivity that allows them to recognize specific regions of DNA for cleavage. DNA sequences recognized by restriction enzymes are predominantly palindromes (inverted sequence repetitions). A typical sequence palindrome, recognized by the frequently used restriction enzyme *Eco*R1, is GAATTC; the inverted repetition, inherent in the complementarity of the G-C and A-T base pairs, results in the 5′ sequence TTC being reflected as AAG in the 3′ strand.

The length of DNA fragments produced by restriction enzymes varies tremendously because of the individuality of DNA sequences. The average length of the DNA fragment is determined in large part by the number of specific bases recognized by an enzyme. In general, restriction enzymes recognize four, six, or eight base sequences. Recognition of four bases yields fragments with an average length of 250 base pairs and therefore is generally useful for analysis or manipulation of gene fragments. Complete genes are frequently encompassed by restriction enzymes that recognize six bases and produce fragments with an average size of about 4000 base pairs. Restriction enzymes that recognize eight bases produce fragments with a typical size of 64,000 base pairs and are useful for analysis of large genetic regions.

PHYSICAL SEPARATION OF DIFFERENTLY SIZED DNA FRAGMENTS

Much of the simplicity underlying genetic engineering techniques lies in the fact that **gel electrophoresis** permits DNA fragments to be separated on the basis of size (Figure 7–7A): the smaller the fragment, the more rapid the rate of migration. Overall rate of migration and optimal range of size for separation are determined by the chemical nature of the gel and by the degree of its cross-linking. Highly cross-linked gels optimize the separation of small DNA fragments. The dye **ethidium bromide** forms a brightly fluorescent adduct as it binds to DNA, so that small amounts of separated DNA fragments can be photographed on gels (Figure 7–7). Specific DNA fragments can be recognized by probes containing complementary sequences (Figures 7–7B and C).

Pulsed gel electrophoresis allows the separation of DNA fragments containing up to 100,000 base pairs (100 kilobase pairs [kbp]). Characterization of such large fragments has allowed construction of a physical map for the chromosomes from several bacterial species. In one instance, the bacterial genes have been shown to be organized in two separate chromosomes.

CLONING OF DNA RESTRICTION FRAGMENTS

Overview

Many restriction enzymes cleave asymmetrically and produce DNA fragments with **cohesive (sticky) ends** that may hybridize with one another. This DNA can be used as a donor with plasmid recipients to form genetically engineered recombinant plasmids. For example, cleavage of DNA with *Eco*R1 produces DNA containing the 5′ tail sequence AATT and the complementary 3′ tail sequence TTAA (Figure 7–8). Cleavage of a plasmid (a circular piece of DNA) with the same restriction enzyme produces a linear fragment with cohesive ends that are identical to one another. Enzymatic removal of the free phosphate groups from these ends ensures that they will not be ligated to form the original circular plasmid (Figure 7–8). Ligation in the presence of other DNA fragments containing free phosphate groups produces **recombinant plasmids,** or **chimeric plasmids,** which contain DNA fragments as inserts in covalently closed circular DNA

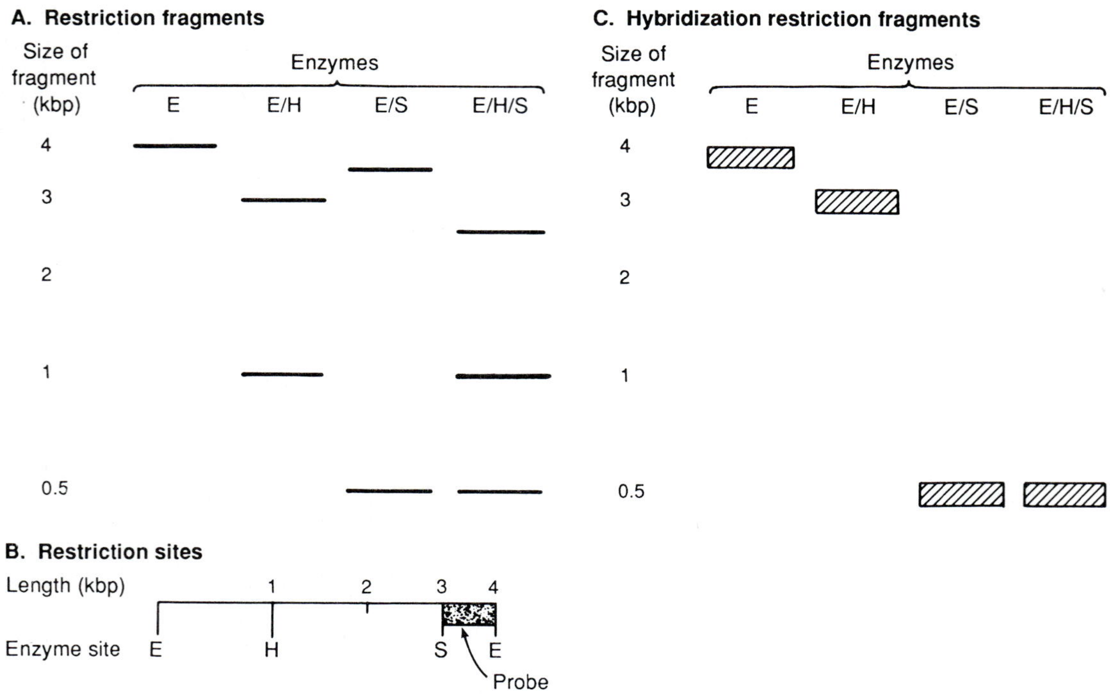

Figure 7–7. ***A:*** Separation of DNA fragments on the basis of size by electrophoresis through a gel. Smaller fragments migrate more rapidly than large fragments, and, over a range determined by the properties of the gel, the distance migrated is roughly proportionate to the logarithm of the size of the fragment. DNA fragments can be visualized on the basis of their fluorescence after staining with a dye. ***B:*** The size of restriction fragments is determined by the location of restriction sites within the DNA. In this example, a 4.0-kbp (kilobase pair) fragment formed by restriction enzyme *Eco*R1 (E) contains respective sites for restriction enzymes *HinD*III (H) and *Sal*I (S) at positions corresponding to 1.0 and 3.5 kbp. The electrophoretic pattern in ***A*** reveals that restriction enzyme E does not cut the 4.0-kbp fragment (first lane); cleavage with restriction enzyme H produces fragments of 3.0 and 1.0 kbp (second lane); cleavage with restriction enzyme S yields fragments of 3.5 and 0.5 kbp (third lane); cleavage with both H and S forms fragments of 2.5, 1.0 and 0.5 kbp (fourth lane). The 0.5-kbp fragment lying between the S and E sites was selected as a probe to determine DNA with hybridizing sequences as shown in ***C. C:*** Identification of hybridizing fragments. Restriction fragments were separated as in ***A.*** The hybridization procedure reveals those fragments that hybridized with the 0.5-kbp probe. These are the 4.0-kbp fragment formed by restriction enzyme E, the 3.0-kbp fragment lying between the E and H sites, and the 0.5-kbp fragment lying between the S and H sites.

(Figure 7–8). Plasmids must be in circular form in order to replicate in a bacterial host.

Recombinant plasmids may be introduced into a bacterial host, frequently *Escherichia coli,* by transformation. Transformed cells may be selected on the basis of one or more drug resistance factors encoded by plasmid genes (Figure 7–8). The resulting bacterial population contains a **library** of recombinant plasmids carrying various cloned inserted restriction fragments derived from the donor DNA. Hybridization techniques may be used to identify bacterial colonies carrying specific DNA fragments or, if the plasmid expresses the inserted gene, colonies can be screened for the gene product (Figure 7–9).

Electroporation is a recently developed procedure for introduction of DNA into bacteria. The procedure gives rise to the possibility that diverse bacteria may be used as hosts for engineered genes.

CHARACTERIZATION OF CLONED DNA

Restriction Mapping

Manipulation of cloned DNA requires an understanding of its structure. Preparation of a **restriction map** is the first step in gaining this understanding. A restriction map is constructed much like a jigsaw puzzle from fragment sizes produced by **single digests,** which are prepared with individual restriction enzymes, and by **double digests,** which are formed with pairs of restriction enzymes (Figure 7–7). Restriction maps are also the initial step toward DNA sequencing, because they identify fragments that will provide **subclones** (relatively small fragments of DNA) that may be subjected to more rigorous analysis, which may involve DNA sequencing. In addition, restriction maps provide a highly specific information base that allows

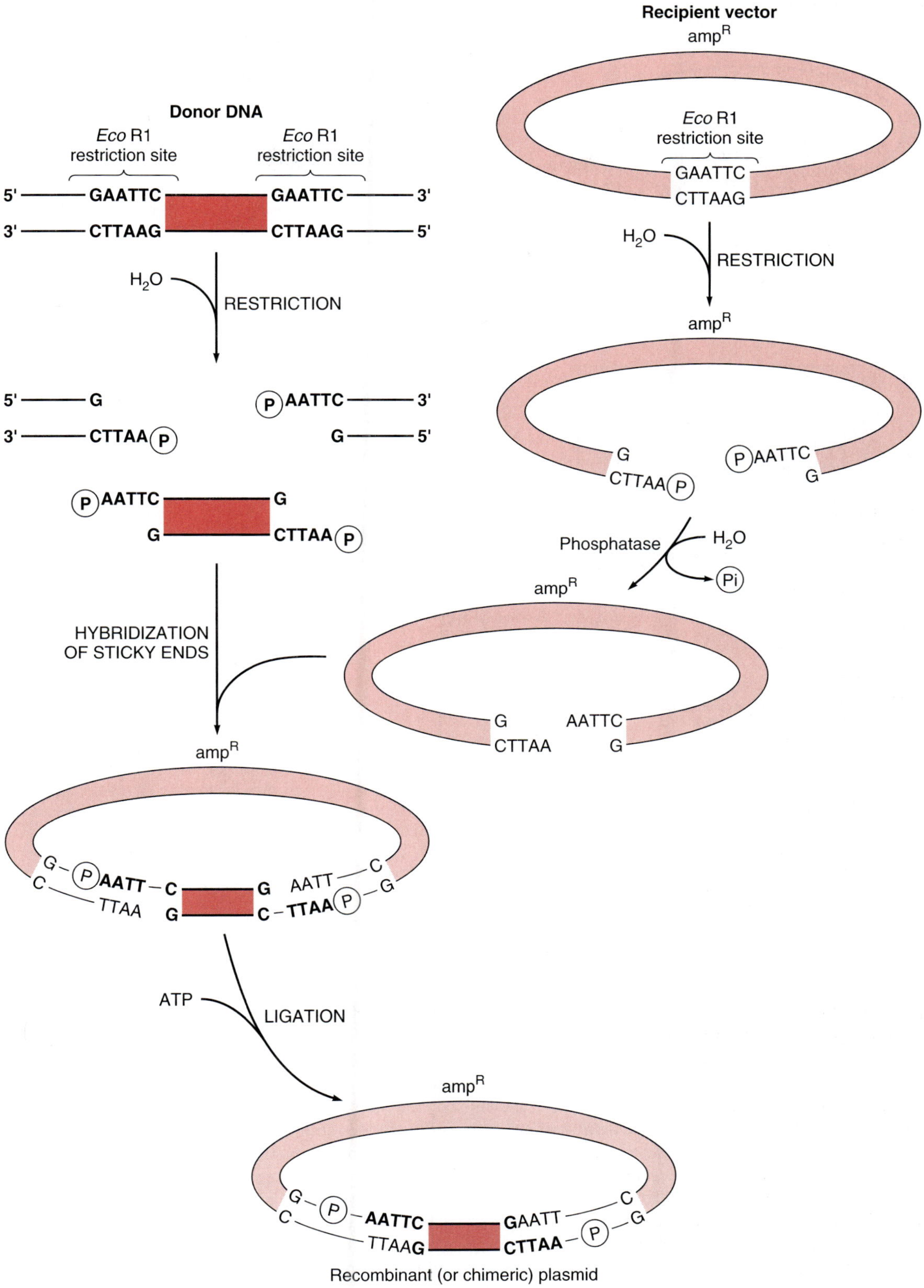

Figure 7–8. Formation of a recombinant, or chimeric, plasmid from donor DNA and a recipient vector. The vector, a plasmid which carries an *Eco*R1 restriction site, is cleaved by the enzyme and prepared for ligation by removal of the terminal phosphate groups. This step prevents the sticky ends of the plasmid from being ligated in the absence of an insert. The donor DNA is treated with the same restriction enzyme and covalently bound circles are formed by ligation. A drug resistance marker, shown as amp^R on the plasmid, can be used to select the recombinant plasmids after their transformation into *E coli*. Enzymes of the host bacterium complete covalent bonding of the circular DNA and mediate its replication.

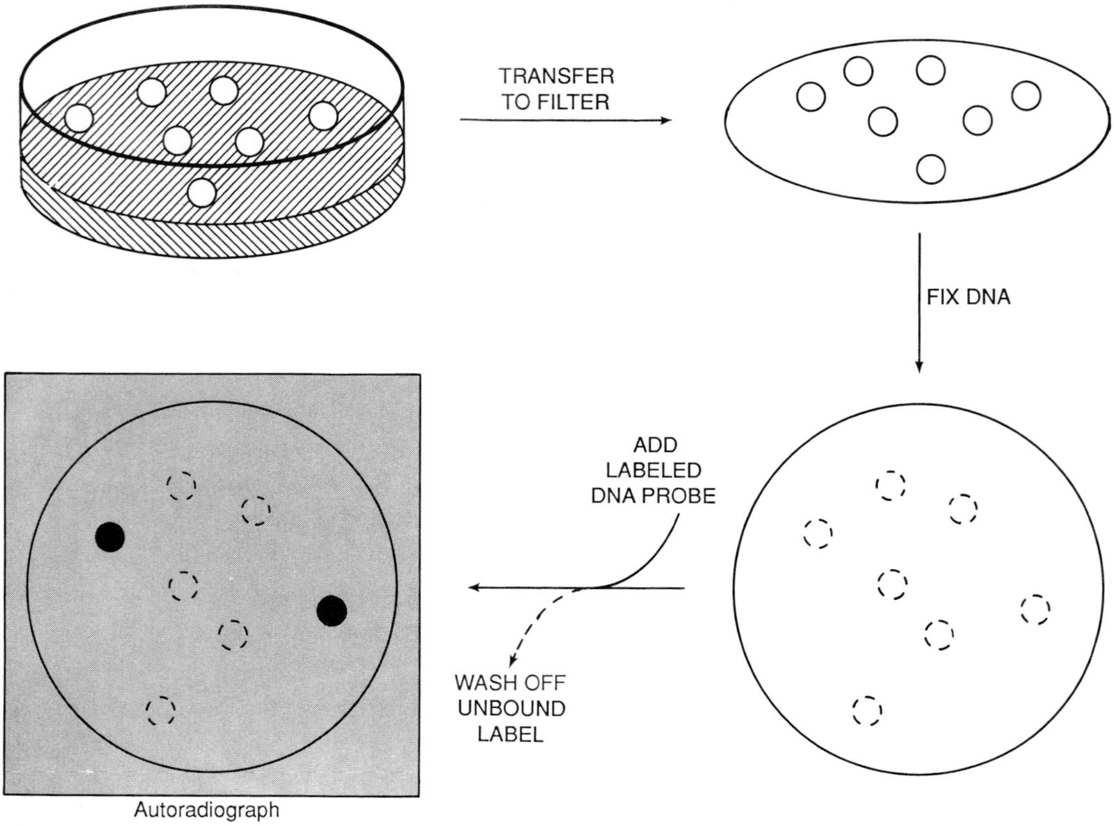

Figure 7–9. Use of probes to identify clones containing a specific fragment of DNA. Colonies may be transferred to a filter and baked so that the cells lyse and the DNA adheres to the filter. The filter can then be treated with a solution containing a suitably labeled DNA probe, which specifically hybridizes to the desired clones. Subsequent autoradiography of the filter identifies these clones (dark circles). Alternatively, the clones may be probed with antibodies to determine if they have synthesized a specific protein product.

DNA fragments, identified on the basis of size, to be associated with specific gene functions.

Sequencing

DNA sequencing displays gene structure and enables researchers to deduce the structure of gene products. In turn, this information makes it possible to manipulate genes in order to understand or alter their function. In addition, DNA sequence analysis reveals regulatory regions that control gene expression and genetic "hot spots" particularly susceptible to mutation. Comparison of DNA sequences reveals evolutionary relationships that provide a framework for unambiguous classification of organisms and viruses. Such comparisons may facilitate identification of conserved regions that may prove particularly useful as specific hybridization probes to detect the organisms or viruses in clinical samples.

The two generally employed methods of DNA sequence determination are the **Maxam-Gilbert technique,** which relies on the relative chemical liability of different nucleotide bonds, and the **Sanger (dideoxy termination) method,** which interrupts elongation of DNA sequences by incorporating dideoxynucleotides into the sequences.

Both techniques produce a nested set of oligonucleotides starting from a single origin and entail separation on a sequencing gel of DNA strands that differ by the increment of a single nucleotide. A sequencing gel separates strands that differ in length from one to several hundred nucleotides and reveals DNA sequences of varying lengths. A sequence is displayed by running similar reaction mixes in four parallel lanes, each of which exposes a specified nucleotide in the overall sequence (Figure 7–10). For example, terminating elongation by incorporating 2′,3′-deoxyadenine-5′-phosphate reveals the relative length of a strand containing adenine at the terminated position. A series of such strands, each terminated at a different position, is created by including some of the dideoxynucleotide in a DNA polymerase reaction mixture.

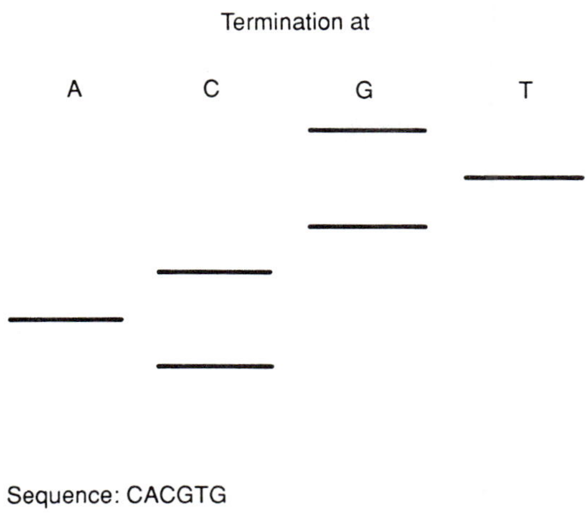

Figure 7–10. Determination of a DNA sequence by the Sanger (dideoxy termination) method. Enzymatic elongation of DNA is interrupted by inclusion of dideoxy analogues of the trinucleotides corresponding to A, C, G, and T separately in parallel reaction mixes. The resulting sets of interrupted elongated strands are separated on a sequencing gel, and the sequence can be deduced by noting the base corresponding to each increment of chain length.

Four parallel lanes on the same gel reveal the relative length of strands undergoing dideoxy termination at adenine, cytidine, guanidine, and thymidine. Comparison of four lanes containing reaction mixes that differ solely in the method of chain termination makes it possible to determine DNA sequence by the Sanger method (Figure 7–10).

The relative simplicity of the Sanger method has led to its more general use, but the Maxam-Gilbert technique is widely employed because it can expose regions of DNA that are protected by specific binding proteins against chemical modification.

DNA sequencing is greatly facilitated by genetic manipulation of *E coli* bacteriophage M13, which contains single-stranded DNA. The replicative form of the phage DNA is a covalently closed circle of double-stranded DNA that has been engineered so that it contains a multiple cloning site that permits integration of specific DNA fragments that have been previously identified by restriction mapping. Bacteria infected with the replicative form secrete modified phages containing, within their protein coat, single-stranded DNA that includes the inserted sequence. This DNA serves as the **template** for elongation reactions. The origin for elongation is determined by a DNA **primer,** which can be synthesized by highly automated machines for **chemical oligonucleotide synthesis.** Such machines, which can produce DNA strands containing 75 or more oligonucleotides in a predetermined sequence, are extremely useful in sequencing and in the modification of DNA by site-directed mutagenesis.

Chemically synthesized oligonucleotides can serve as primers for the **polymerase chain reaction (PCR),** a procedure that allows amplification and sequencing of DNA lying between the primers. Thus, in many instances, DNA need not be cloned in order to be sequenced or to be made available for engineering.

SITE-DIRECTED MUTAGENESIS

Chemical synthesis of oligonucleotides enables researchers to perform controlled introduction of base substitutions into a DNA sequence. The specified substitution may be used to explore the effect of a predesigned mutation on gene expression, to examine the contribution of a substituted amino acid to protein function, or—on the basis of prior information about residues essential for function—to inactivate a gene. Single-stranded oligonucleotides containing the specified mutation are synthesized chemically and hybridized to single-stranded bacteriophage DNA, which carries the wild-type sequence as an insert (Figure 7–11). The resulting partially double-stranded DNA is enzymatically converted to the fully double-stranded replicative form. This DNA, which contains the wild-type sequence on one strand and the mutant sequence on the other, is used to infect a bacterial host by transformation. Replication results in segregation of wild-type and mutant DNA, and the double-stranded mutant gene can be isolated and subsequently cloned from the replicative form of the phage.

Chemical oligonucleotide synthesis permits formation of synthetic genes containing widely distributed restriction sites that allow modular substitution of DNA sequences that encode for mutant proteins. Multiple mutations can thus be readily introduced. In principle, a desired property (such as antigenicity) can be retained, while an undesirable property (such as toxicity) can be eliminated.

ANALYSIS WITH CLONED DNA: HYBRIDIZATION PROBES

Hybridization probes are used routinely in the cloning of DNA. The amino acid sequence of a protein can be used to deduce the DNA sequence from which a probe may be constructed and employed to detect a bacterial colony containing the cloned gene. **Complementary DNA,** or **cDNA,** encoded by mRNA, can be used to detect the gene that encoded that mRNA. Hybridization of DNA to RNA by **Northern blots** can provide quantitative information about RNA synthesis. Specific DNA sequences in restriction fragments separated on gels can be revealed by **Southern blots,** a method that uses hybridization of DNA to DNA. These blots can be used to detect overlapping restriction fragments. Cloning of these fragments makes it possible to isolate flanking regions of DNA by a tech-

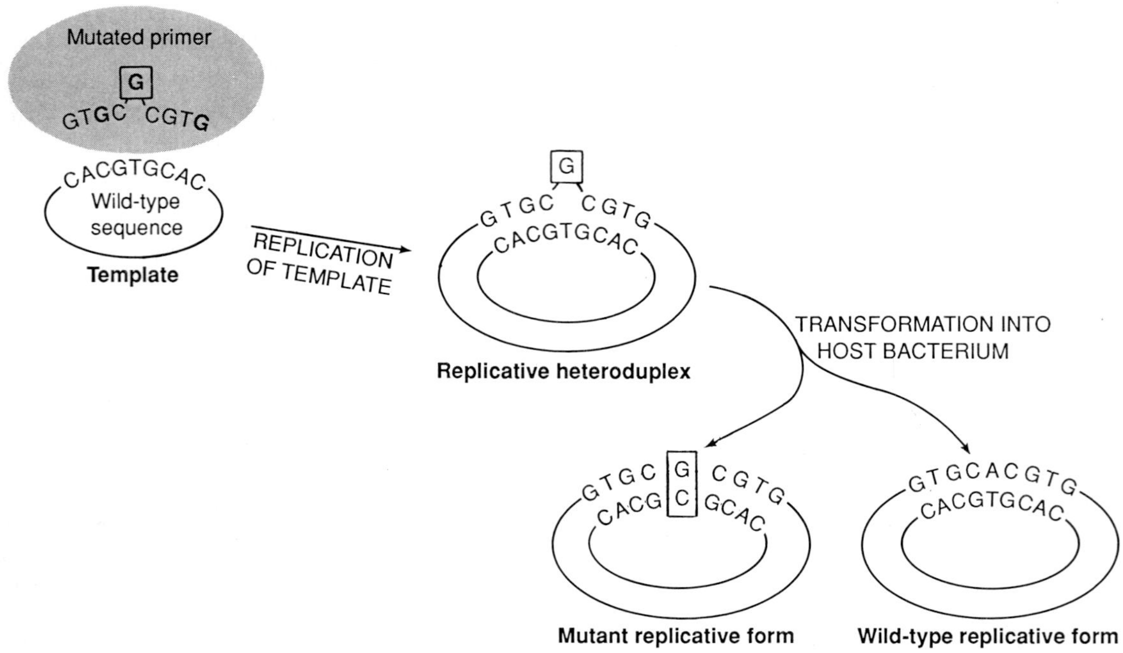

Figure 7–11. Site-directed mutagenesis. A chemically synthesized primer containing mutation G (in box) is hybridized to a wild-type sequence inserted in DNA from a single-stranded phage. Polymerization reactions are used to form the double-stranded heteroduplex carrying the mutation on one strand. Introduction of the heteroduplex into a host bacterium followed by segregation produces derivation strains carrying replicative forms with either the wild-type insert or an insert that has acquired the chemically designed mutation.

nique known as **chromosomal walking** (Figure 7–12). With **Western blots,** another frequently employed detection technique, antibodies are used to detect cloned genes by binding to their protein products.

Probes can be used in a broad range of analytic procedures. Some regions of human DNA exhibit substantial variability in the distribution of restriction sites. This variability is termed **restriction fragment length polymorphism,** or **RFLP.** Oligonucleotide probes that hybridize with RFLP DNA fragments can be used to trace DNA from a small sample to its human donor. Thus, the technique promises to be valuable to forensic science. Applications of RFLP to medicine include identification of genetic regions that are closely linked to human genes with dysfunctions coupled to genetic disease. This information will be a valuable aid in **genetic counseling.**

DNA probes offer the promise of techniques for rapidly identifying fastidious organisms in clinical specimens that are difficult to grow in a microbiology laboratory. Furthermore, extensions of the technique afford opportunities to identify pathogenic agents rapidly and directly in infected tissue. Kits for identification of some specific pathogens have been developed, and rapid advances in this field can be anticipated.

Application of diagnostic DNA probes requires an appreciation of (1) the probes themselves, (2) systems used to detect the probes, (3) targets (the DNA to which the probes hybridize), and (4) the conditions of hybridization. Probes may be relatively large restriction fragments derived from cloned DNA or oligonucleotides corresponding to a specific region of DNA. Larger probes may provide greater accuracy because they are less sensitive to single base changes in target DNA. On the other hand, hybridization reactions occur more rapidly with small probes, and they can be designed against conserved regions of DNA in which base substitutions are unlikely to have occurred.

Radiochemical techniques traditionally have been used to detect probes in research laboratories. Most frequently DNA has been labeled with ^{32}P phosphate by **nick translation,** a process in which breaks or "nicks" are introduced into DNA strands. Radioactive nucleotides are introduced into the DNA by a polymerase that replaces nucleotides at positions starting at the break sites. Unfortunately, the half-life of radioactive phosphate is only 2 weeks, and the radioactivity poses possible hazards in the laboratory. These problems can be circumvented by use of a **reporter molecule** that is covalently bonded to the probe. The reporter may be an enzyme that generates a colored product or a relatively small molecule to which a protein specifically binds after hybridization has taken place. Linkage of the protein to an enzyme that yields a colored product reveals the hybridized probe.

Preparation of target DNA for hybridization includes procedures that ensure lysis of cells containing the DNA, thereby exposing the DNA for hybridization.

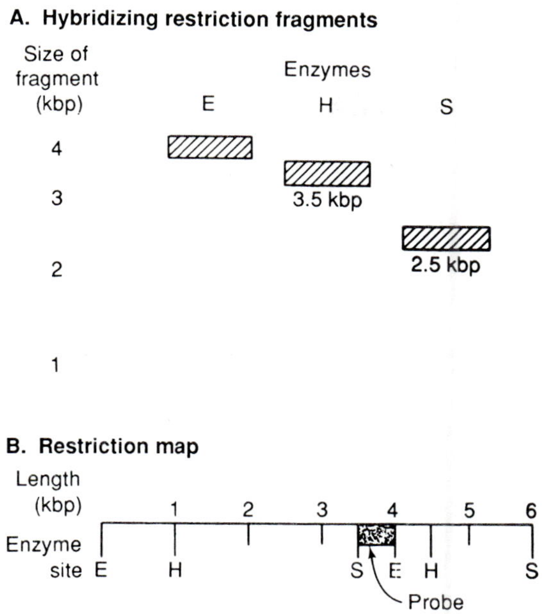

Figure 7–12. Use of hybridization to identify DNA flanking a probe from a cloned fragment of DNA. The DNA fragment and the 0.5-kbp (kilobase pair) probe produced by restriction enzymes S and E were described in Figure 7–7. Here we note respective sites for H at 4.5 kbp and S at 6.0 kbp in the restriction map ***(B).*** The presence of these sites can be deduced from the appearance of a 3.5-kbp hybridizing H fragment and a 2.5-kbp hybridizing S fragment after electrophoresis of restricted chromosomal DNA ***(A).*** Purification of fragments of this size, followed by cloning and screening with the probe, should yield a flanking region ranging from 4 kbp to 6 kbp on the restriction map.

Possibilities for hybridization are determined by the **stringency** of the procedure. Stringency, determined by physical and chemical conditions, establishes the degree of hybridization. Probes containing relatively few nucleotides are most sensitive to changes in stringency conditions. In some cases changes in stringency can be used to control the range of organisms revealed by hybridization: a broad biologic group containing a number of nucleotide substitutions may be revealed under conditions of low stringency, whereas the same probe may detect only closely related organisms under highly stringent conditions.

MANIPULATION OF CLONED DNA

Genetic engineering techniques permit separation and entirely independent expression of genes associated with pathogens. Vaccines prepared with engineered genes afford previously unattainable measures of safety. For example, a vaccine might be prepared against a viral coat protein that was produced in the absence of any genes associated with replicative viral functions; inoculation with such a vaccine would therefore entail no risk of introducing functional virus. Potential difficulties in the development of such vaccines stem from the ease with which viral mutations may produce genetic variants that are not recognized by the immune defense system of a vaccinated individual. Ultimately, vaccines may contain a range of proteins that anticipate the genetic response of pathogens.

RECOMBINANT STRAINS IN THE ENVIRONMENT

Major scientific advances have sometimes elicited adverse public reactions, so it is prudent to consider the potential consequences of genetic engineering. Of most immediate concern are known pathogens that have undergone relatively slight genetic modification. These have been and should be investigated in laboratories specially designed to contain them. The need for containment diminishes after genes for specific functions, such as protein coats, are separated from genes associated with replication or toxicity of a pathogen. For the most part, standard precautions associated with microbiology laboratories should be observed, if for no other reason than that they foster habits which are valuable if a potential pathogen enters the laboratory.

Interesting exceptions to this general rule are engineered organisms that may provide a social benefit if introduced into the environment. Many such organisms derive from nonpathogenic bacteria that occur naturally with a frequency as high as 10^5/g of soil. The available evidence suggests that predation and competition rapidly eliminate engineered bacterial strains after they are introduced into the environment. The primary challenge would thus seem to be to maintain engineered organisms in the environment rather than to eliminate them.

The best known example of engineered organisms are *Pseudomonas* strains that produce a protein that favors formation of ice crystals. The value of these wild-type organisms is appreciated by ski slope owners, who have deliberately introduced the bacteria into the environment without arousing any public concern. An unfortunate side effect of the introduction of these organisms is that the ice crystals they promote can injure sensitive crops such as lettuce during seasons in which light frost is likely. Mutant bacteria that do not form ice crystals were designed by microbiologists who hoped that the mutant organisms might protect lettuce crops by temporarily occupying the niche normally inhabited by the ice-forming strains; however, attempts to use the mutant organisms in field studies were met with substantial protest, and studies were conducted only after lengthy and expensive legal delays. Perhaps legal precedents emerging from this and related cases will establish guidelines for the progressive and beneficial use of genetic engineering techniques and facilitate determination of situations in which extreme caution is justified.

REFERENCES

Books

Ausubel FM et al: *Current Protocols in Molecular Biology.* Wiley, 1987.

Bainbridge BW: *Genetics of Microbes,* 2nd ed. Chapman & Hall, 1987.

Freifelder D: *Molecular Biology: A Comprehensive Introduction to Prokaryotes and Eukaryotes.* Science Books International, 1983.

Ganesan AT, Chang S, Hoch JA (editors): *Molecular Cloning and Gene Regulation in Bacilli.* Academic Press, 1982.

Hardy K: *Bacterial Plasmids.* American Society for Microbiology, 1981.

Hofschneider PH, Goebel W (editors): *Gene Cloning in Organisms Other Than* Escherichia coli. Springer-Verlag, 1982.

Hood LE et al: *Immunology,* 2nd ed. Benjamin/Cummings, 1984.

Inouye M (editor): *Experimental Manipulation of Gene Expression.* Academic Press, 1983.

Kornberg A: *DNA Replication.* Freeman, 1980.

Lewin B: *Genes,* 3rd ed. Wiley, 1987.

Maniatis T, Fitsch EF, Sambrook J: *Molecular Cloning: A Laboratory Manual.* Cold Spring Harbor Laboratory, 1982.

Miller JH, Reznikoff WS: *The Operon,* 2nd ed. Cold Spring Harbor Laboratory, 1980.

Oliver SG, Brown TA: *Microbial Extrachromosomal Genetics.* American Society for Microbiology, 1985.

Ptashne M: *A Genetic Switch: Gene Control and Phage Lambda.* Blackwell, 1987.

Razin AM, Cedar H, Riggs AD (editors): *DNA Methylation: Biochemistry and Biological Significance.* Springer-Verlag, 1984.

Riley M, Drlica K (editors): *The Bacterial Chromosome.* American Society for Microbiology, 1990.

Scaife J, Leach D, Galizzi A (editors): *Genetics of Bacteria.* Academic Press, 1985.

Shapiro JA (editor): *Mobile Genetic Elements.* Academic Press, 1983.

Simon M, Herskowitz I (editors): *Genome Rearrangement.* Alan R. Liss, 1985.

Singleton P: *A Dictionary of Microbiology and Molecular Biology,* 2nd ed. Wiley, 1987.

Suzuki DT et al: *An Introduction to Genetic Analysis,* 3rd ed. Freeman, 1985.

Trautner TA (editor): *Methylation of DNA.* Springer-Verlag, 1984.

Watson JD et al: *Molecular Biology of the Gene,* 4th ed. 2 vols. Benjamin/Cummings, 1987.

Watson JD, Tooze J, Kurtz DT: *Recombinant DNA: A Short Course.* Scientific American, 1983.

Williamson R (editor): *Genetic Engineering.* Vols 1 and 2, 1981; Vols 3 and 4, 1982. Academic Press.

Wu R, Grossman L, Moldave K (editors): *Recombinant DNA.* Parts B and C. Vols 100 and 101 of: *Methods in Enzymology.* Academic Press, 1983.

Articles & Reviews

Bachmann BJ: Linkage map of *Escherichia coli* K-12, edition 8. Microbial Rev 1990;54:130.

Blake LW: DNA packaging in dsDNA bacteriophage. Annu Rev Microbiol 1989;43:267.

Campbell A: Evolutionary significance of accessory DNA elements in bacteria. Annu Rev Microbiol 1981;35:55.

Clark AJ, Warren GJ: Conjugal transmission of plasmids. Annu Rev Genet 1979;13:99.

Cohen SN, Shapiro JA: Transposable genetic elements. Sci Am (Feb) 1980;242:40.

Dressler D, Potter H: Molecular mechanisms in genetic recombination. Annu Rev Biochem 1982;51:727.

Firshein WD: Role of the DNA/membrane complex in prokaryotic DNA replication. Annu Rev Microbiol 1989;43:89.

Holloway BW: Genetics for all bacteria. Annu Rev Microbiol 1993;47:659.

Miller JH: Mutational specificity in bacteria. Annu Rev Genet 1983;17:215.

Miller LK: Baculoviruses as gene expression vectors. Annu Rev Microbiol 1988;42:177.

Miller RV: Potential for transfer and establishment of engineered genetic sequences. Trends Eco Evol 1988; 3:S23.

Platt T: Transcription termination and the regulation of gene expression. Annu Rev Biochem 1986;55:339.

Radding CM: Homologous pairing and strand exchange in genetic recombination. Annu Rev Genet 1982;16: 405.

Radding CM: Recombination activities of *Escherichia coli recA* protein. Cell 1981;25:3.

Reznikoff WS et al: The regulation of transcription initiation in bacteria. Annu Rev Genet 1985;19:355.

Riggs AD et al: Synthesis, cloning, and expression of hormone genes in *Escherichia coli.* Recent Prog Horm Res 1980;36:261.

Ripley LS: The specificity of infidelity of DNA polymerase. Base Life Sci 1983;23:83.

Sancar A, Sancar GB: DNA repair enzymes. Annu Rev Biochem 1988;57:29.

Shapiro JA: Changes in gene order and gene expression. Natl Cancer Inst Monogr 1982;60:87.

Singer B: Mutagenic effects of nucleic acid modification and repair assessed by in vitro transcription. Basic Life Sci 1983;23:1.

Singer GR, Kusmierek JT: Chemical mutagenesis. Annu Rev Biochem 1982;52:655.

Smith GR: Chi hotspots of generalized recombination. Cell 1983;34:709.

Walker GC: Mutagenesis and inducible responses to deoxyribonucleic acid damage in *Escherichia coli.* Microbiol Rev 1984;48:60.

Willets N, Skurray R: The conjugation system of F-like plasmids. Annu Rev Genet 1980;14:41.

Williamson VM: Transposable elements in yeast. Int Rev Cytol 1983;83:1.

Wilson M, Lindow SE: Release of recombinant organisms. Annu Rev Microbiol 1993;47:913.

Zoller MJ, Smith M: Oligonucleotide-directed mutagenesis of DNA fragments cloned into M13 vectors. Methods Enzymol 1983;100:468.

Immunology 8

*Roderick Nairn, PhD**

The study of immunology, a broad field encompassing basic research and clinical application, deals with antigens, antibodies, and cell-mediated host defense functions, especially as they relate to immunity to disease, hypersensitive biologic reactions, allergies, and rejection of foreign tissues. This chapter presents the basic principles of immunology, particularly as they are oriented toward infection. The reader is referred to texts on immunology for more detailed discussions.

Terms commonly used in immunology are defined in the glossary included with this chapter.

IMMUNITY & THE IMMUNE RESPONSE

Immunity can be natural (innate) or acquired (adaptive).

Natural Immunity

Natural immunity is resistance that is not acquired through contact with an antigen. It is nonspecific and includes barriers to infectious agents—eg, skin and mucous membranes, natural killer (NK) cells, phagocytosis, inflammation, interferon, and a variety of other nonspecific factors. It may vary with age and with hormonal or metabolic activity.

Acquired Immunity

Acquired immunity, which occurs after exposure to an antigen, eg, an infectious agent, is specific and is mediated by either antibody or lymphoid cells. It can be passive or active.

A. Passive Immunity: Passive immunity is transmitted by antibodies or lymphocytes preformed in another host. The passive administration of antibody (in antisera) against bacteria (eg, diphtheria, tetanus, botulism) makes immediately available excess antitoxin to neutralize the toxins. Likewise, preformed antibodies to certain viruses (eg, rabies, hepatitis A and B) can be injected during the incubation period to limit viral multiplication. The main advantage of passive immunization with preformed antibodies is the prompt availability of large amounts of antibody; disadvantages are the short life span of these antibodies and possible hypersensitivity reactions if antibodies (immunoglobulins) from another species are administered.

B. Active Immunity: Active immunity is induced after contact with foreign antigens (eg, microorganisms or their products). This contact may consist of clinical or subclinical infection, immunization with live or killed infectious agents or their antigens, exposure to microbial products (eg, toxins, toxoids), or transplantation of foreign cells. In all these instances the host actively produces antibodies, and lymphoid cells acquire the ability to respond to the antigens. Advantages of active immunity include long-term resistance (based on memory of prior contact with antigen and the capacity to respond faster and to a greater extent on subsequent contact with the same antigen); disadvantages include the slow onset of resistance and the need for prolonged or repeated contact with the antigen.

MECHANISMS OF NONSPECIFIC HOST DEFENSE

Physiologic Barriers at the Portal of Entry

A. The Skin: Few microorganisms are capable of penetrating intact skin, but many can enter sweat or sebaceous glands and hair follicles and establish themselves there. Sweat and sebaceous secretions—by virtue of their acid pH and certain chemical substances (especially fatty acids)—have antimicrobial properties that tend to eliminate pathogenic organisms. Lysozyme, an enzyme that dissolves some bacterial cell walls, and perhaps other enzymes are also present on the skin. Lysozyme is also present in tears and in respiratory and cervical secretions.

Skin resistance may vary with age. For example, children are highly susceptible to ringworm infection. After puberty, resistance to such fungi increases markedly with the increased content of saturated fatty acids in sebaceous secretions.

*Associate Professor of Microbiology and Immunology, Department of Microbiology and Immunology, and Director, Medical Scientist Training Program, University of Michigan Medical School, Ann Arbor.

GLOSSARY*

Anaphylatoxin: A substance produced by complement activation (especially C3a, C5a) that results in increased vascular permeability through release of pharmacologically active mediators from mast cells.

Antibody (Ab): A protein that is produced as a result of the introduction of an antigen and has the ability to combine with the antigen that stimulated its production.

Antigen (Ag): A subtance that can induce a detectable immune response when introduced into an animal.

B cell (also B lymphocyte): Strictly, a bursa-derived cell in avian species and, by analogy, a cell derived from the equivalent of the bursa in non-avian species. B cells are the precursors of plasma cells that produce antibody.

Cell-mediated (cellular) immunity: Immunity in which the participation of lymphocytes and macrophages is predominant. Cell-mediated immunity is a term generally applied to the type IV hypersensitivity reaction (see below).

Chemotaxis: A process whereby phagocytic cells are attracted to the vicinity of invading pathogens.

Complement: A system of serum proteins that is the primary mediator of antigen-antibody reactions.

Cytokine: A factor such as a lymphokine or monokine produced by cells that affect other cells (eg, lymphocytes and macrophages) and have multiple immunomodulating functions. Cytokines include interleukins and interferons.

Cytolysis: The lysis of bacteria or of cells such as tumor or red blood cells by insertion of the membrane attack complex derived from complement activation.

Hapten: A molecule that is not immunogenic by itself but can react with specific antibody.

Histocompatible: Sharing transplantation antigens.

Humoral immunity: Pertaining to immunity in a body fluid and used to denote immunity mediated by antibody and complement.

Hypersensitivity reactions: These occur in 4 types:

(1) Antibody-mediated hypersensitivity:

Type I. Anaphylactic ("immediate"): IgE antibody is induced by allergen and binds via its Fc receptor to mast cells and basophils. After encountering the antigen again, the fixed IgE becomes cross-linked, inducing degranulation and release of mediators, especially histamine.

Type II. Cytotoxic: Antigens on a cell surface combine with antibody, which leads to complement-mediated lysis (eg, transfusion or Rh reactions) or other cytotoxic membrane damage (eg, autoimmune hemolytic anemia).

Type III. Immune complex: Antigen-antibody immune complexes are deposited in tissues, complement is activated, and polymorphonuclear cells are attracted to the site, causing tissue damage.

(2) Cell-mediated hypersensitivity:

Type IV. Delayed: T lymphocytes, sensitized by an antigen, release lymphokines upon second contact with the same antigen. The lymphokines induce inflammation and activate macrophages.

Immunity:

(1) Natural immunity: Nonspecific resistance not acquired through contact with an antigen. It includes skin and mucous membrane barriers to infectious agents and a variety of non-specific immunologic factors, and it may vary with age and hormonal or metabolic activity.

(2) Acquired immunity: Protection acquired by deliberate introduction of an antigen into a responsive host. Active immunity is specific and is mediated by either antibody or lymphoid cells (or both).

Immune response: Development of resistance (immunity) to a foreign substance (eg, infectious agent). It can be antibody-mediated (humoral), cell-mediated (cellular), or both.

Immunoglobulin: A glycoprotein, composed of H and L chains, that functions as antibody. All antibodies are immunoglobulins, but not all immunoglobulins have antibody function.

Immunoglobulin class: A subdivision of immunoglobulin molecules based on unique antigenic determinants in the Fc region of the H chains. In humans there are 5 immunoglobulin classes: IgG, IgM, IgA, IgE, and IgD.

Immunoglobulin subclass: A subdivision of the classes of immunoglobulins based on structural and antigenic differences in the H chains. For human IgG there are 4 subclasses: IgG1, IgG2, IgG3, and IgG4.

Interferon: One of a heterogeneous group of low-molecular-weight proteins elaborated by infected host cells that protect noninfected cells from viral infection. Interferons, which are cytokines, also have immunomodulating functions.

*Modified and reproduced with permission, from Stites DP, Stobo JD, Wells JV (editors): *Basic & Clinical Immunology,* 6th ed. Appleton & Lange, 1987.

Interleukin: A cytokine that stimulates or otherwise affects the function of lymphocytes and some other cells.

(1) Interleukin-1: A macrophage-derived factor that promotes short-term proliferation of T cells.

(2) Interleukin-2: A lymphocyte-derived factor that promotes long-term proliferation of T cell lines in tissue culture.

(3) Interleukin-3: A T cell product that induces proliferation and differentiation in other lymphocytes and some hematopoietic cells.

Lymphocyte: A mononuclear cell 7–12 μm in diameter containing a nucleus with densely packed chromatin and a small rim of cytoplasm. Lymphocytes include the T cells and B cells, which have primary roles in immunity.

Lymphokine: A cytokine that is a soluble product of a lymphocyte. Lymphokines are responsible for multiple effects in a cellular immune reaction.

Macrophage: A phagocytic mononuclear cell derived from bone marrow monocytes and found in tissues and at the site of inflammation. Macrophages serve accessory roles in cellular immunity.

Major histocompatibility complex (MHC): A cluster of genes located in close proximity that determine histocompatibility antigens of members of a species.

Membrane attack complex: The end product of activation of the complement cascade, which contains C5, C6, C7, and C8 (and C9). The membrane attack complex makes holes in the membranes of gram-negative bacteria, killing them and, in red blood or other cells, resulting in lysis.

Monocyte: A circulating phagocytic blood cell that develops into tissue macrophages.

Opsonin: A substance capable of enhancing phagocytosis. Antibodies and complement are the 2 main opsonins.

Opsonization: The coating of an antigen or particle (eg, infectious agent) by substances such as antibodies, complement components, fibronectin, and so forth, that facilitate uptake of the foreign particle into a phagocytic cell.

Polymorphonuclear cell (PMN): Also known as a neutrophil or granulocyte, a PMN is derived from a hematopoietic cell of bone marrow and is characterized by a multilobed nucleus. PMNs migrate from the circulation to a site of inflammation by chemotaxis and are phagocytic for bacteria and other particles.

T cell (also T lymphocyte): A thymus-derived cell that participates in a variety of cell-mediated immune reactions.

B. Mucous Membranes: In the respiratory tract, a film of mucus covers the surface and is constantly being driven upward by ciliated cells toward the natural orifices. Bacteria tend to stick to this film. In addition, mucus and tears contain lysozyme and other substances with antimicrobial properties. For some microorganisms, the first step in infection is their attachment to surface epithelial cells by means of adhesive bacterial surface proteins, eg, the pili of gonococci and *Escherichia coli.* If such cells have IgA antibody on their surfaces—a host resistance mechanism—attachment may be prevented. (The organism can overcome this resistance mechanism by breaking down the antibody with a protease.)

When organisms enter the body via mucous membranes, they tend to be taken up by phagocytes and are transported into regional lymphatic channels that carry them to lymph nodes. These act as barriers to further spread of large numbers of bacteria. The mucociliary apparatus for removal of bacteria in the respiratory tract is aided by pulmonary macrophages. This entire defense system can be suppressed by alcohol, narcotics, cigarette smoke, hypoxia, acidosis, and other harmful influences. Special protective mechanisms in the respiratory tract include the hairs at the nares and the cough reflex, which prevents aspiration.

In the gastrointestinal tract, several systems function to inactivate bacteria: saliva contains numerous hydrolytic enzymes; the acidity of the stomach kills many ingested bacteria (eg, *V. cholerae*); the small intestine contains many proteolytic enzymes and active macrophages.

It must be remembered that most mucous membranes of the body carry a constant normal microbial flora that itself opposes establishment of pathogenic microorganisms ("bacterial interference") and has important physiologic functions. For example, in the adult vagina, an acid pH is maintained by normal lactobacilli, inhibiting establishment of yeasts, anaerobes, and gram-negative bacteria.

Nonspecific Immunologic Mechanisms

A. Phagocytosis: During bacterial infection the number of circulating phagocytic cells often increases. The main functions of phagocytic cells include migration, chemotaxis, ingestion, and microbial killing. Microorganisms (and other particles) that enter the lymphatics, lung, bone marrow, or bloodstream are engulfed by any of a variety of phagocytic cells. Among them are polymorphonuclear leukocytes (granulocytes), phagocytic monocytes (macrophages), and fixed macrophages of the reticuloendothelial system (see below). Many microorganisms elaborate chemotactic factors that attract phagocytic cells. Defects in chemotaxis may account for hypersusceptibility to certain infections; the defects may be acquired or inherited. Phagocytosis can occur in the absence of serum antibodies, particularly if aided by the architecture of tissue. Thus, phagocytic cells are inefficient in large, smooth, open spaces like the pleura, pericardium, or joints but may be more effective in ingesting microorganisms trapped in small tissue spaces (eg, alveoli) or on rough surfaces. Such "surface phagocytosis" occurs early in the infectious process before antibodies are available.

1. Factors affecting phagocytosis–Phagocytosis is made more efficient by the presence of antibodies (opsonins) that coat the surface of bacteria and facilitate their ingestion by phagocytes. Opsonization can occur by three mechanisms: (1) antibody alone can act as opsonin; (2) antibody plus antigen can activate complement via the classic pathway to yield opsonin; (3) opsonin may be produced by a heat-labile system in which immunoglobulin or other factors activate C3 via the alternative pathway. Macrophages have receptors on their membranes for the Fc portion of antibody and for the C3 component of complement. These receptors aid the phagocytosis of antibody-coated particles.

Hyperosmolality (eg, in the renal medulla) inhibits phagocytosis. Hypophosphatemia depletes ATP in granulocytes and reduces the efficiency of phagocytosis. Neutrophils from patients with diabetes (and perhaps other metabolic disorders) ingest bacteria normally but then are deficient in their killing ability. In contrast, during acute infections the killing power of neutrophils may be increased.

Ingestion of foreign particles, eg, microorganisms, has the following effects on phagocytic granulocytes: (1) oxygen consumption increases, and there is increased generation of superoxide anion (O_2^-) and increased release of H_2O_2; (2) glycolysis increases via the hexose monophosphate shunt; (3) lysosomes rupture, and their hydrolytic enzymes are discharged into the phagocytic vacuole to form a digestive vacuole, or "phagolysosome." Morphologically, this process appears as "degranulation" of granulocytes. Inhibition of these processes is an important part of the infectious process, or pathogenesis, of *Legionella pneumophila.*

2. Granulocytes (polymorphonuclear leukocytes)–Granulocytes contain at least two types of granules: (1) the azurophil or primary granules that contain lysozyme, other hydrolytic enzymes, and several cationic proteins, the defensins, that are antimicrobial; and (2) the secondary, or specific granules, that contain lactoferrin and collagenase, etc.

The functional mechanisms of intracellular killing of microorganisms in phagocytic granulocytes are not fully known. They include nonoxidative mechanisms (eg, activation of hydrolytic enzymes in contact with microorganisms, action of basic proteins) and oxidative mechanisms. Among the latter, the following have been implicated:

a. Increased oxidative activity results in accumulation of H_2O_2. In the presence of oxidizable cofactors (halides such as iodine, bromine, chlorine), an acid pH, and the enzyme myeloperoxidase, intensive oxidation results in microbial death.

Children suffering from chronic granulomatous disease have granulocytes that ingest microbes normally but lack the cytochrome b enzyme required to produce the superoxide anion so important in the antimicrobial activity of phagocytes. In Chédiak-Higashi syndrome, most microorganisms are phagocytosed normally but intracellular killing is impaired, perhaps because there is uncontrolled fusion of cytoplasmic granules.

b. In normal granulocytes, superoxide anion (O_2^-) is generated when particles are phagocytosed, and it is destroyed by superoxide dismutase. The superoxide radical may be directly lethal for many microorganisms. Granulocytes associated with chronic granulomatous disease have a greatly reduced capacity for generating superoxide radicals after ingestion of microorganisms. This defect may be responsible for the impaired killing ability of granulocytes associated with this disease and explains the susceptibility of patients to infections, especially those due to staphylococci. Another important toxic product generated after phagocytosis is nitric oxide (NO).

When the bone marrow of patients is suppressed by disease, drugs, or radiation, the number of functional granulocytes falls. If the granulocyte level drops below 500 polymorphonuclear neutrophils per microliter, the patient is highly susceptible to opportunistic infection by bacteria. The antibacterial defenses of such patients may be boosted by the provision of certain cytokines important in hematopoiesis, such as the colony stimulating-factors described later.

3. Macrophages (circulating phagocytic monocytes)–Macrophages are derived from monocyte stem cells in bone marrow, have a longer life span than circulating granulocytic phagocytes, and continue their activity at a lower pH.

Macrophages in blood can be activated by various stimulants, or "activators," including microbes and their products, antigen-antibody complexes, inflammation, sensitized T lymphocytes, lymphokines (see below), and injury. Activated macrophages have an increased number of lysosomes and produce and release interleukin-1, which has a wide range of activity in inflammation. Interleukin-1 participates in fever production and in activation of other phagocytic cells as well as T and B cells to produce their resulting effects.

Intracellular killing in macrophages probably includes mechanisms similar to those described above for granulocytes; however, the role of superoxide anion is less well defined. Activated macrophages also make nitric oxide (NO), a nitrogn metabolite with antimicrobial activity.

4. Outcome of phagocytosis–All types of phagocytic cells (granulocytes, macrophages in blood, and fixed macrophages of the reticuloendothelial system) may kill ingested microorganisms or may permit their prolonged survival or even their intracellular multiplication. The outcome of phagocytosis is determined by a complex set of factors, including the specific nature of the microorganism as well as the genetic and functional makeup and the preconditioning of phagocytic cells.

B. Reticuloendothelial System: This system involves mononuclear phagocytic cells present in blood, lymphoid tissue, liver, spleen, bone marrow, lung, and other tissues that are efficient in uptake and removal of particulate matter from lymph and bloodstream. It includes cells lining blood and lymph sinuses (Kupffer cells in the liver) and histiocytes of tissues (macrophages). An important function of the spleen, bone marrow, and other reticuloendothelial organs is filtering microorganisms from the bloodstream. Patients whose spleens have been removed or are nonfunctional (eg, in sickle cell disease) often suffer from bacterial sepsis, particularly with pneumococci and salmonellae. Phagocytosis by reticuloendothelial cells is greatly enhanced by opsonins.

C. Inflammatory Response: Any injury to tissue, such as that following establishment and multiplication of microorganisms, elicits an inflammatory response. This begins with dilation of local arterioles and capillaries, from which plasma escapes. Edema fluid accumulates in the area of injury, and fibrin forms a network and occludes the lymphatic channels, limiting the spread of organisms. Polymorphonuclear leukocytes in the capillaries stick to the walls and then migrate out of the capillaries toward the irritant. This migration (chemotaxis) is stimulated by substances in the inflammatory exudate. Phagocytes engulf the microorganisms, and intracellular digestion begins. Soon the pH of the inflamed area becomes more acid, and cellular proteases induce lysis of the leukocytes. Large mononuclear macrophages arrive on the site and, in turn, engulf leukocytic debris as well as microorganisms and pave the way for resolution of the local inflammatory process.

Cytokines and derivatives of arachidonic acid, including prostaglandins, leukotrienes, and thromboxanes, are mediators of the inflammatory response. Drugs that inhibit synthesis of prostaglandins (by blocking the enzyme cyclooxygenase) act as anti-inflammatory agents.

At different stages in the inflammatory sequence, different microorganisms may predominate as the inciting cause. Early edema fluid may actually promote bacterial growth. Localization of the process depends on the nature of the organism. For instance, spread of staphylococci is limited by the extensive lymphatic thrombus formation, fibrin walls, etc, precipitated by coagulase; conversely, hemolytic streptococci tend to spread rapidly through tissues as a result of the activity of streptokinase (fibrinolysin) and hyaluronidase. Phagocytosis and intracellular existence are destructive to some bacteria (eg, some pyogenic cocci), whereas for others (eg, tubercle bacilli) these factors constitute a means of transport, protection, and even multiplication.

D. Fever: Fever is the most common systemic manifestation of the inflammatory response and a cardinal symptom of infectious diseases.

1. Possible mechanisms of fever production–The ultimate regulator of body temperature is the thermoregulatory center in the hypothalamus, which is subject to physical and chemical stimuli. Direct mechanical injury or application of chemical substances to these centers results in fever. Neither of these obvious forms of stimulation is present in the many types of fever associated with infection, neoplasms, hypersensitivity, and other causes of inflammation, however.

Among the substances capable of inducing fever (pyrogens) are endotoxins of gram-negative bacteria and cytokines released from lymphoid cells, such as interleukin-1. These two substances differ as follows:

a. Endotoxins–Endotoxins are heat-stable lipopolysaccharides (discussed in Chapter 9). After intravenous injection, there is a 60- to 90-minute latent period until onset of fever. Repeated intravenous injection of endotoxin makes the recipient tolerant: no response occurs to repetitive injections of endotoxin.

b. Interleukin-1–Interleukin-1 was also called endogenous pyrogen, lymphocyte-activating factor, and many other terms depending on its effect. It is heat-labile (destroyed by heating at 90 °C for 30 minutes or more). After intravenous injection, fever begins in a few minutes, even in endotoxin-tolerant recipients. Repeated injection of interleukin-1 does not induce unresponsiveness.

Various activators can act upon mononuclear phagocytes and other cells and induce them to release interleukin-1. Among these activators (Figure 8–1) are microbes and their products; toxins, including endotoxins; antigen-antibody complexes; inflammatory processes; and many others. Interleukin-1 is carried by the bloodstream to the thermoregulatory center in the hypothalamus, where physiologic responses are initiated that result in fever (eg, increased heat production, reduced heat loss). Other effects of interleukin-1 are mentioned below.

Lymphokines are protein hormones that are produced by certain cells and influence other cells. Cytokines produced by lymphocytes are known as lymphokines; those produced in nonspecific immunity by phagocytes are sometimes known as monokines. Interleukin-1 promotes lymphocyte proliferation in addition to inducing fever. Interleukin-2 is produced by T cells. Gamma interferon, also produced by T cells, has numerous immunomodulating functions.

2. Beneficial effects of fever–It is possible to demonstrate some beneficial effects of fever on the control of infection in a few instances. For example, antibody production and T cell proliferation are more efficient at higher body temperatures than at normal

Activating agent	Activated cells	Substance released	Biologic effects and targets: Low IL-1 concentration	Biologic effects and targets: High IL-1 concentration
Bacterial products such as LPS Macrophage-derived cytokines such as TNF CD4 T cells	→ Mononuclear phagocytes and others, eg, epithelial and endothelial cells	→ IL-1	Local inflammation IL-1 synthesis by phagocytes increased Causes release of other cytokines by various cells	Systemic effects, eg, fever, synthesis of acute-phase plasma proteins by the liver and initiation of metabolic wasting (cachexia)

Figure 8–1. Scheme of interleukin-1 production and some of its effects.

levels. Poikilothermic lizards can resist bacterial infection at elevated environmental temperatures but will die of the same infection in a cool environment. However, in humans, no consistent benefits for the control of infection can be attributed to fever. Suppression of fever by drugs (eg, aspirin) is not harmful during infections and often makes febrile patients more comfortable.

MECHANISMS OF SPECIFIC HOST DEFENSE

Immune Response

The immune response can be antibody-mediated (humoral), cell-mediated (cellular), or both. An encounter with a microbial or viral agent usually elicits a complex variety of responses. An overview of these is given here, and details are presented later in this chapter.

Upon entry of a potential pathogen into the host, it or its major antigens are taken up by antigen-presenting cells (APCs), eg, macrophages. Such antigens reappear on the macrophage surface complexed with proteins encoded by the major histocompatibility complex (MHC) and are presented to T lymphocytes. The MHC-antigen complexes are recognized by specific receptors on the surface of T cells, and these cells then produce a variety of lymphokines that induce clonal proliferation. The two arms of the immune response—cell-mediated and antibody-mediated—develop concurrently.

In the **antibody-mediated** arm, helper (CD4) T lymphocytes recognize the pathogen's antigen complexed with class II MHC proteins on the surface of an antigen-presenting cell (macrophage or B cell) and produce lymphokines that activate B cells expressing antibodies that match the antigen. These B cells proliferate and differentiate to form plasma cells which then produce specific immunoglobulins (antibodies). Major host defense functions of antibodies include neutralization of toxins and viruses and opsonization (coating) of the pathogen, which aids its uptake by phagocytic cells. Antibody-mediated defense is important against pathogens that produce toxins (eg, *Clostridium tetani*) or have polysaccharide capsules that interfere with phagocytosis (eg, the pneumococcus). It applies mainly to extracellular pathogens.

In the **cell-mediated** arm, the antigen-MHC class II complex is recognized by helper (CD4) T lymphocytes, while the antigen-MHC I complex is recognized by cytotoxic (CD8) T lymphocytes. Each class of T cells produces lymphokines, becomes activated, and expands by clonal proliferation.

Helper T cell activity promotes the development of delayed hypersensitivity and serves in the defense against intracellular agents, including intracellular bacteria (eg, mycobacteria), fungi, protozoa, and some viruses. **Cytotoxic** T cell activity is aimed mainly at the destruction of cells in tissue grafts, tumor cells, or cells infected by some viruses. In addition to unaided killing by cytotoxic T lymphocytes, such cells may be killed by the combined action of cytotoxic T lymphocytes with antibody.

Figure 8–2 summarizes the specific and nonspecific host defense mechanisms used to combat microorganisms. The net result of effective immunity is the host's resistance to microbial and other pathogens and foreign cells. By contrast, impaired immunity manifests itself as excessive susceptibility to such pathogens or tumors. Specific examples are presented below.

Antigens

The features of antigens that determine immunogenicity in the immune response are as follows:

A. Foreignness: In general, molecules recognized as "self" are not immunogenic; for immunogenicity, molecules must be recognized as "nonself."

B. Molecular Size: The most potent immunogens are usually large proteins. Generally, molecules with a molecular weight less than 10,000 are weakly immunogenic, and very small ones (eg, amino acids) are nonimmunogenic. Certain small molecules (eg, haptens) become immunogenic only when linked to a carrier protein.

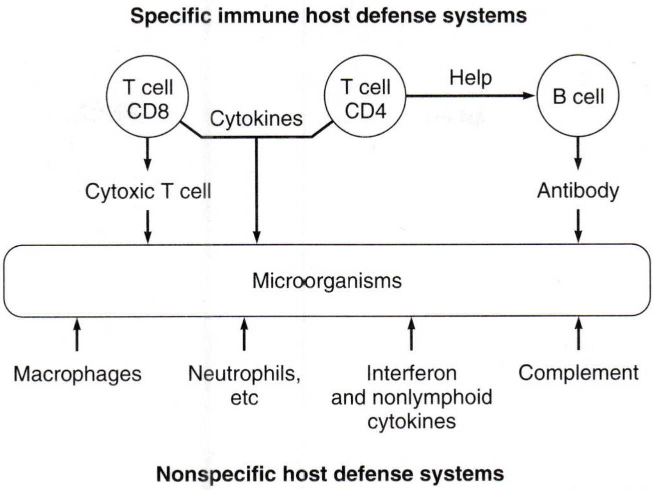

Figure 8–2. Host defense mechanisms against microbes.

C. Chemical and Structural Complexity: A certain amount of chemical complexity is required, eg, amino acid homopolymers are less immunogenic than heteropolymers containing two or three different amino acids.

D. Antigenic Determinants (Epitopes): The smallest unit of a complex antigen that is capable of binding to an antibody is known as an antigenic determinant, or epitope. An antigen can have one or more determinants. In general, a determinant is roughly five amino acids or sugars in size.

E. Genetic Constitution of the Host: Two strains of the same species of animal may respond differently to the same antigen because of a different composition of immune response genes.

F. Dosage, Route, and Timing of Antigen Administration: Since the degree of the immune response depends on the amount of antigen given, the immune response can be optimized by carefully defining the dosage (including number of doses), route of administration, and timing of administration (including intervals between doses).

Cellular Basis of the Immune Response

The capacity to respond to immunologic stimuli resides mainly in lymphoid cells. During embryonic development, blood cell precursors are found in fetal liver and other tissues; in postnatal life the stem cells reside in bone marrow. They can differentiate in several ways. In liver and bone marrow, stem cells may differentiate into cells of the red cell series or into cells of the lymphoid series. Lymphoid stem cells evolve into two main lymphocyte populations, B cells and T cells.

A. B Cells: B cells are lymphocytes that develop in gut lymphoid tissue and other equivalents of the avian bursa of Fabricius, a gut appendage in birds. They are the source of antibody development and humoral immunity. Antibodies are immunoglobulins. B cells do not require the thymus for maturation.

B. T Cells: T cells are lymphocytes that require maturation in the thymus and form many subclasses with specific functions. They are the source of cell-mediated immunity, discussed below.

Some lymphocytic cells (eg, natural killer cells; see below) lack features of B or T cells but have significant immunologic roles. Figure 8–3 presents an overview of immunologically active lymphocytes and their interactions.

ANTIGEN RECOGNITION MOLECULES

In order for the immune system to respond to nonself, ie, foreign antigen, a recognition system capable of precisely distinguishing self from nonself had to evolve. The next section of this chapter deals with the molecules used to recognize foreign antigens. First, we will review the structure and function of **antibodies,** the soluble recognition products of B lymphocytes. Then we will review some membrane-bound receptors for antigen, the **T cell antigen specific receptor,** and the products of the **major histocompatibility complex.**

ANTIBODIES (IMMUNOGLOBULINS)

Antibodies are formed by **clonal selection.** Each person has a large pool of B lymphocytes (about 10^9) that have a life span of days or weeks and are formed

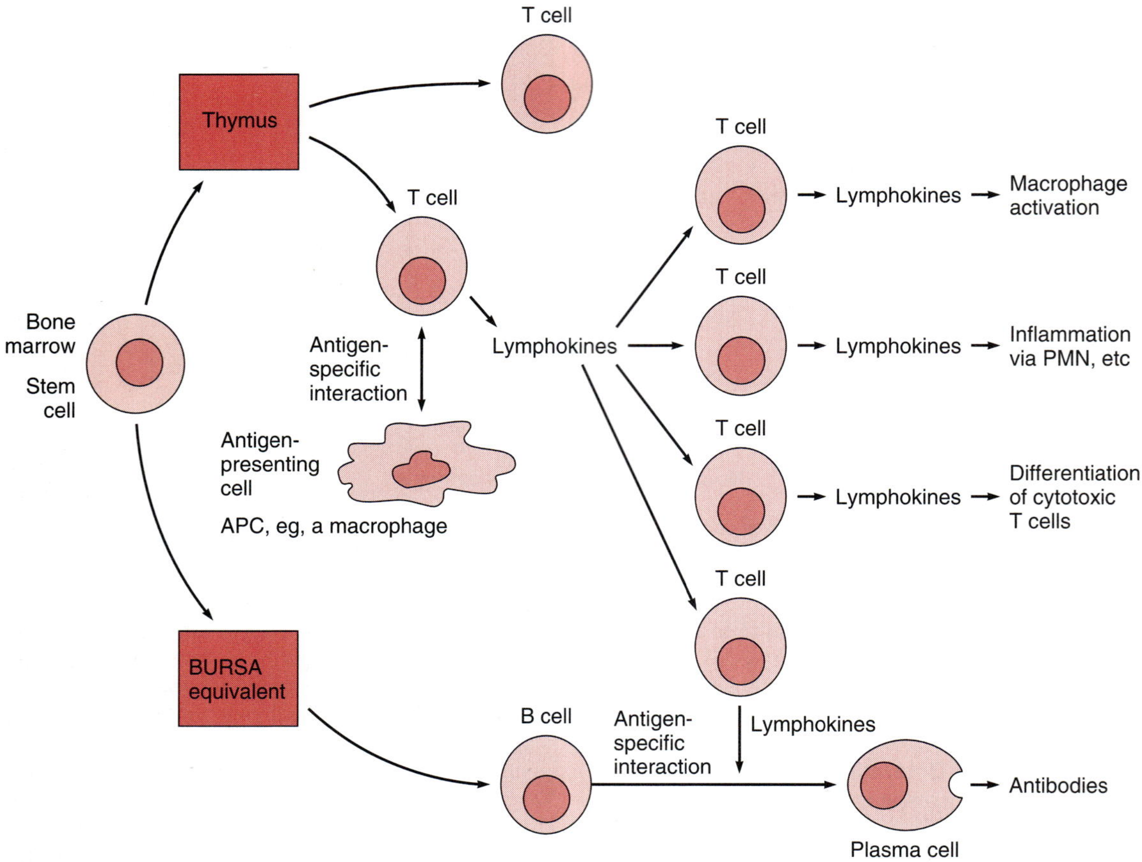

Figure 8–3. Schematic diagram of the cellular interactions in the specific immune response.

in the lymph nodes and gut-associated lymphoid tissues (eg, tonsils or appendix).

B cells display immunoglobulin molecules (10^5/cell) on their surface. These immunoglobulins serve as receptors for a specific antigen, so that each B cell can respond to only one antigen or a closely related group of antigens. All immature B cells carry IgM immunoglobulins on their surface, and most also carry IgD. B cells also have surface receptors for the Fc portion of immunoglobulins and for several complement components.

An antigen interacts with the B lymphocyte that shows the best "fit" by virtue of its immunoglobulin surface receptor. The antigen binds to this receptor, and the B cell is stimulated to divide and form a clone. Such selected B cells soon become plasma cells and secrete antibody. Since each person can make about 10^9 different antibody molecules, there is an antigen-binding site on a B cell to fit almost any antigenic determinant.

The initial step in antibody formation is phagocytosis of the antigen, usually by macrophages that process and present the antigen to T cells. These activated T cells then interact with B cells. B cells that carry the surface immunoglobulin that best fits the antigen are stimulated to proliferate and differentiate into plasma cells (see above), which form the specific antibody proteins. The plasma cells synthesize the same class of immunoglobulins (ie, same class H chain, same class L chain—except for isotype switch; see below) carried by the B precursor cells. Plasma cells can revert to small lymphocytes with a long life span, which serve as B memory cells.

Antibody Structure & Function

Antibodies are immunoglobulins that react specifically with the antigen that stimulated their production. They make up about 20% of plasma proteins.

Antibodies that arise in an animal in response to a single complex antigen are heterogeneous because they are formed by several different clones of cells, each expressing an antibody capable of reacting with a different antigenic determinant on the complex antigen. These antibodies are said to be **polyclonal.** Antibodies that arise from a single clone of cells, eg, in a plasma cell tumor (myeloma), are homogeneous—ie, they are **monoclonal.** Monoclonal antibodies can be made by fusing a myeloma cell with an antibody-producing lymphocyte. Such **hybridomas** produce virtually unlimited quantities of monoclonal antibodies *in vitro*. Important information about the structure and function of antibodies has been derived from the study of monoclonal antibodies.

All immunoglobulin molecules are made up of light and heavy polypeptide chains. The terms light and heavy refer to molecular weight—ie, light chains have a molecular weight of 25,000, whereas heavy chains have a molecular weight of 50,000–70,000. **Light (L) chains** belong to one of two types, κ (kappa) or λ (lambda); classification is made based on amino acid differences in their constant regions. Both types occur in all classes of immunoglobulin (IgG, IgM, IgA, IgE, and IgD), but any one immunoglobulin molecule contains only one type of L chain. The amino terminal portion of each L chain contains part of the antigen-binding site. **Heavy (H) chains** are distinct for each of the five immunoglobulin classes and are designated γ (gamma), μ (mu), α (alpha), δ (delta), and ϵ (epsilon) (Table 8–1). The amino terminal portion of each H chain participates in the antigen-binding site; the other (carboxy) terminal forms the Fc fragment, which has various biologic activities (eg, complement activation and binding to cell surface receptors).

An individual antibody molecule always consists of identical H chains and identical L chains. The simplest antibody molecule has a Y shape (Figure 8–4) and consists of four polypeptide chains: two H chains and two L chains. The four chains are covalently linked by disulfide bonds.

If such an antibody molecule is treated with a proteolytic enzyme (eg, papain), peptide bonds in the **hinge region** are broken. This breakage produces two identical Fab fragments, which carry the antigen-binding sites, and one Fc fragment, which is involved in placental transfer, complement fixation, attachment for various cells, and other biologic activities.

L and H chains are subdivided into **variable regions** and **constant regions.** The regions are composed of 3-dimensionally folded, repeating segments called domains. An L chain consists of one variable domain (VL) and one constant domain (CL). Most H chains consist of one variable domain (VH) and three or more constant domains (CH). Each domain is approximately 110 amino acids long. Variable regions are responsible for antigen binding; constant regions are responsible for the biologic functions described below.

In the variable regions of both L and H chains are three extremely variable **(hypervariable)** amino acid sequences that form the antigen-binding site. The hypervariable regions form the region complementary in structure to the antigenic determinant or epitope and are therefore also known as complementarity-determining regions (CDRs). Only five to ten amino acids in each hypervariable region constitute the antigen-binding site. Antigen binding is noncovalent, involving van der Waals, electrostatic, and other weak forces as well as hydrogen and other bonds.

Isotypes, Allotypes, & Idiotypes

Because immunoglobulins are proteins, they are antigenic. **Isotypes** are the antigenic features of a class of immunoglobulin H or L chain (eg, μH chain is isotypically different from γH chain). All normal humans share certain isotypes, because all produce the various H and L chains.

Allotypes are additional antigenic features of immunoglobulins that vary among individuals and are under genetic control. Thus, the γH chain contains an allotype called Gm; the κL chain contains an allotype called Km. Allotypes can be shared by some members of a species.

An **idiotype** is a unique antigenic determinant of the hypervariable region, produced by a specific clone of antibody-producing cells. An anti-idiotypic antibody reacts only with the V domain of the specific immunoglobulin molecule that induced it. Such an antibody may exert regulatory functions with respect to down-modulating an antibody response.

Immunoglobulin Classes

A. IgG: Each IgG molecule consists of two L chains and two H chains linked by disulfide bonds (molecular formula H_2L_2). Because it has two identical antigen-binding sites, it is said to be divalent. There are four subclasses (IgG1 to IgG4), based on antigenic differences in the H chains and on the number and location of disulfide bonds. IgG1 is 65% of the total IgG. IgG2 is directed against polysaccharide antigens and

Table 8–1. Properties of human immunoglobulins.

	IgG	IgA	IgM	IgE	IgD
Heavy chain symbol	γ	α	μ	ε	δ
Molecular weight (× 1000)	150	170 or 400[1]	900	190	150
Serum concentration (mg/mL)	0.5–10	0.5–3	1.5	0.003	0.03
Serum half-life (days)	23	6	5	1–5	2–8
Fixes complement	+	−	+	−	−
Percentage of total immunoglobulin in serum	80	13	6	<1	<1

[1]In secretions, eg, saliva, milk, and tears and in respiratory, intestinal, and genital tract secretion.

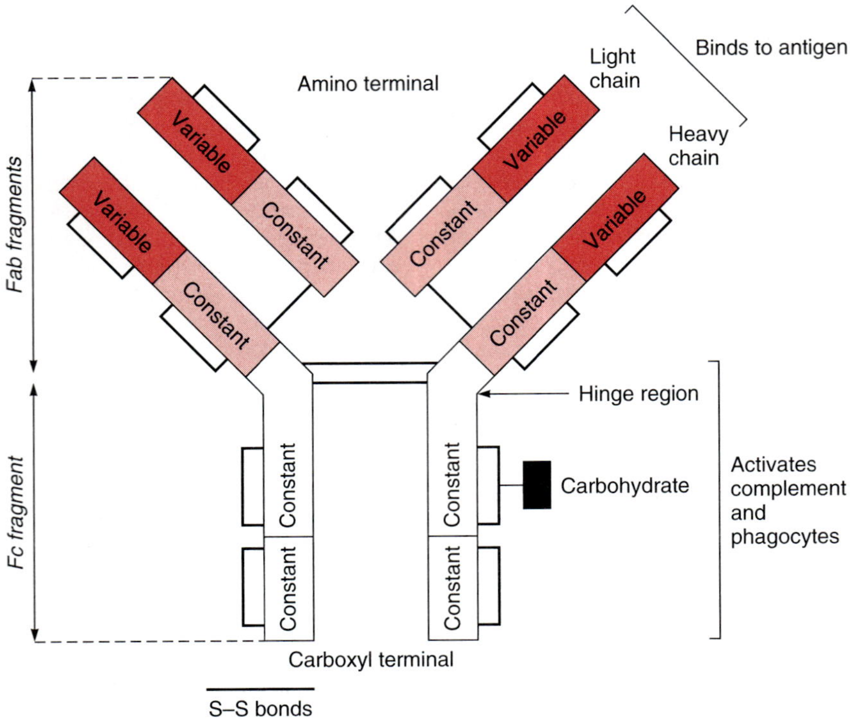

Figure 8–4. Schematic representation of an IgG molecule, indicating the location of the constant and the variable regions on the light and the heavy chains.

may be an important host defense against encapsulated bacteria.

IgG is the predominant antibody in secondary responses and constitutes an important defense against bacteria and viruses. It is the only antibody to pass the placenta and is therefore the most abundant immunoglobulin in newborns.

B. IgM: IgM is the main immunoglobulin produced early in the *primary* immune response. IgM is present on the surface of virtually all uncommitted B cells. It is composed of five H_2L_2 units (each similar to one IgG unit) and one molecule of J (joining) chain (Figure 8–5). The pentamer (MW 900,000) has a total of ten identical antigen-binding sites and thus a valence of 10. It is the most efficient immunoglobulin in agglutination, complement fixation, and other antigen-antibody reactions and is important also in defense against bacteria and viruses. It can be produced by a fetus with an infection. Since its interaction with antigen can involve all ten binding sites, it has the highest avidity of all immunoglobulins.

C. IgA: IgA is the main immunoglobulin in secretions such as milk, saliva, and tears and in secretions of the respiratory, intestinal, and genital tracts. It protects mucous membranes from attack by bacteria and viruses.

Each secretory IgA molecule (MW 400,000) consists of two H_2L_2 units and one molecule each of J chain and secretory component. The latter is a protein derived from cleavage of the poly Ig receptor. This receptor binds IgA dimers and facilitates their transport across mucosal epithelial cells. Some IgA exists in serum as a monomer H_2L_2 (MW 170,000). There are

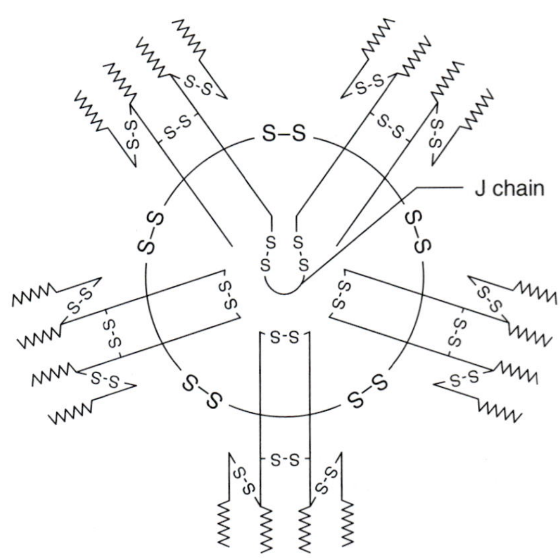

Figure 8–5. Schematic diagram of the pentameric structure of human IgM.

at least two subclasses, IgA1 and IgA2. Some bacteria (eg, *Neisseria*) can destroy IgA1 by producing a protease and can thus overcome antibody-mediated resistance on mucosal surfaces.

D. IgE: The Fc region of IgE binds to a receptor on the surface of mast cells and basophils. This bound IgE acts as a receptor for the antigen that stimulated its production, and the resulting antigen-antibody complex triggers allergic responses of the immediate (anaphylactic) type through the release of mediators. In persons with such antibody-mediated allergic hypersensitivity, IgE concentration is greatly increased, and IgE may appear in external secretions. Serum IgE is also typically increased during helminth (worm) infections.

E. IgD: IgD acts as an antigen receptor when present on the surface of certain B lymphocytes. It also occurs on cells of some lymphatic leukemias. In serum it is present only in trace amounts.

Immunoglobulin Genes/ Generation of Diversity

Special genetic mechanisms have evolved to produce the very large number of immunoglobulin molecules (about 10^9) that develop in the host in response to antigen stimulation without requiring excessive numbers of genes.

Each immunoglobulin chain consists of a variable (V) and a constant (C) region. For each type of immunoglobulin chain—ie, kappa light chain (κ), lambda light chain (λ), and the five heavy chains (γH, μH, αH, ϵH, and δH)—there is a separate pool of gene segments located on different chromosomes. Each of the three gene loci contains a set of different V gene segments widely separated from C gene segments. During B cell differentiation, the DNA is rearranged to bring the selected gene segments adjacent to each other in the genome. A family of enzymes known as **recombinases** is responsible for this gene rearrangement process.

The V region of each L chain is encoded by two gene segments, V and J. The V region of each H chain is encoded by three gene segments, V, D, and J. The segments are united into one functional V gene by DNA rearrangement. Each assembled V gene is then transcribed with the appropriate C-constant gene to produce a messenger RNA (mRNA) that codes for the complete peptide chain. L and H chains are synthesized separately on polysomes and finally assembled in the cytoplasm to form H_2L_2 units by means of disulfide bonds. The carbohydrate moiety is then added, and the immunoglobulin molecule is released from the cell.

This gene rearrangement mechanism permits the assembly of an enormous variety of immunoglobulin molecules. Antibody diversity depends on (1) multiple V, D, and J gene segments; (2) combinatorial association, ie, the association of any V gene segment with any D or J segment; (3) the random combining of different L and H chains; (4) somatic mutations; (5) junctional diversity, created by imprecise joining during rearrangement and leading to changes or deletions in amino acids in the hypervariable regions; and (6) insertional diversity, where the enzyme terminal deoxynucleotidyl transferase inserts small groups of nucleotides at V–D and D–J junctions (N region diversity.)

Immunoglobulin Class (Isotype) Switching

Initially, all B cells matched to an antigen carry IgM specific for that antigen and produce IgM in response to this exposure to antigen. Later, gene rearrangement permits elaboration of antibodies of the same antigenic specificity but of different immunoglobulin classes. In **class switching,** the same assembled VH gene can sequentially associate with different CH genes, so that the immunoglobulin produced later (either IgG, IgA, or IgE) has the same specificity as the original IgM but different biologic characteristics. Class switching is dependent on lymphokines released from T cells and also happens after antigenic stimulation.

CELL SURFACE RECEPTORS FOR ANTIGEN

1. B CELL RECEPTOR FOR ANTIGEN

B cells express a cell surface-located form of IgM. Cell surface IgM has the same antigen specificity as the secreted IgM antibody molecule. This is achieved by a differential RNA splicing mechanism. The μ-chain RNA transcript can include a sequence that encodes about 25 hydrophobic amino acids which enables the IgM molecule to sit in the cell membrane as a transmembrane receptor. Later in development of the B cell, the same process allows expression of a membrane-bound form of IgD, again with the same antigen-binding specificity. Throughout this process, the same V region segment is being expressed with different C region segments.

As a membrane-bound receptor, IgM or IgD interacts with other cell surface molecules that can transduce signals subsequent to antigen binding. These signals result in biochemical events involving intracellular tyrosine kinases, GTP-binding proteins, etc, that lead to cell activation.

2. THE ANTIGEN-SPECIFIC T CELL RECEPTOR

The T cell receptor is a transmembrane heterodimeric protein composed of two disulfide-linked chains. There are two different classes of T cell receptor. In one, the two chains are known as α and β, and in the other as γ and δ. γδ-expressing T cells are relatively infrequent in humans and seem to be predisposed toward recognition of bacterial antigens, eg, the highly conserved heat shock proteins of certain mycobacteria. αβ T cells make up the predominant T cell phenotype and are subdivided by their expression of other cell surface markers, the proteins known as CD4 and CD8, into helper and cytotoxic functional classes respectively.

The T cell receptor proteins have variable and constant regions similar to antibodies. The variable regions are located at the amino terminals of the polypeptide chain farthest away from the cell membrane. Both chains contribute to the variable domain that has been shown to interact with antigen.

Generation of diversity in the T cell receptor is accomplished in a fashion largely analogous to that described earlier for immunoglobulins. Thus, there are multiple variable region exons contributing a repertoire of different antigen specificities; multiple V, D, and J segments that can combine in different ways just as for antibodies; and random combination of a large number of α and β chains. There are two differences from the situation described earlier for antibodies: (1) no evidence for somatic mutation in T cell receptors has been obtained, and (2) the potential for increasing the repertoire of potential antigen specificities by junctional diversity is much greater for T cell receptors than for antibodies. In essence however, the encoding of T cell receptors is very much like that described for immunoglobulins. For example, the variable-regions of the α and γ chains of the T cell receptor are like the variable regions of immunoglobulin light-chains in having V and J segments, whereas the β and δ chains are like immunoglobulin heavy chains in being encoded by V, D, and J segments.

In all functional antigen-specific T cells, the T cell receptor chains are noncovalently associated with the five proteins of the CD3 complex. The CD3 complex is responsible for transducing the signal received by the T cell receptor on recognition of antigen to the inside of the cell. All five proteins of the CD3 complex are transmembrane proteins and interact with tyrosine kinases on the inside of the membrane. It is this interaction that begins the biochemical events of signal transduction leading to gene transcription, cell activation, and initiation of the functional activities of T cells.

3. THE MAJOR HISTOCOMPATIBILITY COMPLEX

The major histocompatibility complex (MHC) was first detected as the genetic locus encoding the molecules (transplantation antigens) responsible for the rapid rejection of tissue grafts transplanted between genetically nonidentical individuals. It is now known that MHC molecules bind peptide antigens and present them to T cells. Thus, these transplantation antigens are responsible for antigen recognition by the T cell receptor. In this respect, the T cell receptor is different from antibody. Antibody molecules interact with antigen directly; the T cell receptor only recognizes antigen presented by MHC molecules on another cell, the antigen presenting cell. The T cell receptor is specific for antigen, but the antigen must be presented on a self-MHC molecule. The T cell receptor is also specific for the MHC molecule. If the antigen is presented by another allelic form of the MHC molecule (normally only in an experimental situation), there is no recognition by the T cell receptor. This phenomenon is known as MHC restriction.

In humans, the MHC is a cluster of very extensively studied genes located on chromosome 6. Much is known about this important locus, and the reader is referred to more advanced texts for additional information. The most important genes in the human MHC, also known as HLA (for human leukocyte antigens), are those which encode the class I and class II MHC proteins. As outlined in Table 8–2, the class I proteins are encoded by the HLA-A, -B, and -C genes. These proteins are made up of two chains. A transmembrane glycoprotein of MW 45,000, noncovalently associated with a non-MHC-encoded polypeptide of MW 12,000 that is known as β_2-microglobulin. Class I molecules are to be found on virtually all nucleated cells in the body.

The class II proteins are encoded by the HLA-D region. As shown in Table 8–2, there are three main sets: the DP-, DQ-, and DR-encoded molecules. This locus retains control of immune responsiveness, and different allelic forms of these genes confer striking differences in the ability to mount an immune response against a given antigen.

The class II proteins are made up of two noncovalently associated transmembrane glycoproteins of about MW 33,000 and MW 29,000. Unlike class I proteins, they have a restricted tissue distribution and are chiefly found on macrophages, B cells, and other antigen-presenting cells. Their expression on other cells—eg, epithelial cells—can be induced by interferon, however.

Table 8–2. Important features of human MHC gene products.

	Class I	Class II
Genetic loci	HLA-A, -B, and -C	HLA-DP, -DQ, and -DR
Polypeptide composition	MW 45,000 + β_2M (MW 12,000)	α chain (MW 33,000) β chain (MW 29,000) Ii chain (MW 30,000)
Cell distribution	All nucleated somatic cells	Antigen-presenting cells (macrophages, B cells, etc), activated human T cells
Present peptide antigens to	Cytotoxic Tcells	Helper T cells

The genes of the MHC exhibit a remarkable **polymorphism.** Thus, a large number of alleles exist in the population. Each individual inherits a restricted set of alleles from the parents. Sets of MHC genes tend to be inherited as a block or **haplotype,** as there are relatively infrequent cross-over events at this locus.

Much is known about the organization and sequence of MHC genes and proteins. Perhaps the most important information, however, has come from the x-ray analysis of crystals of MHC proteins. It was these studies that clearly explained the function of the MHC proteins. The x-ray analysis (Figure 8–6) shows that the domains of the molecule farthest away from the membrane are composed of two parallel α-helices above a platform created by a β-pleated sheet. The whole structure undoubtedly looks like a **cleft** whose sides are formed by the α-helices and floored by the β-sheets. The x-ray analysis also showed that the cleft was occupied by a peptide. In essence, then, the T cell receptor sees the peptide antigen bound in a cleft provided by the MHC protein. A simplified diagram of this interaction is provided in Figure 8–7A.

MHC proteins show a broad specificity for peptide antigens, and many different peptides can be presented by any given MHC allele (albeit one peptide is bound at a time). The α-helices that form the binding cleft are the location of the amino acid residues that are polymorphic in MHC proteins (ie, those that vary between alleles). This means that different alleles can bind and present different peptide antigens.

Analysis of the function of T cells with respect to interaction with MHC molecules reveals that peptide antigens associated with class I MHC molecules are recognized by CD8-positive cytotoxic T lymphocytes, whereas class II-associated peptide antigens are recognized by CD4-positive helper T cells.

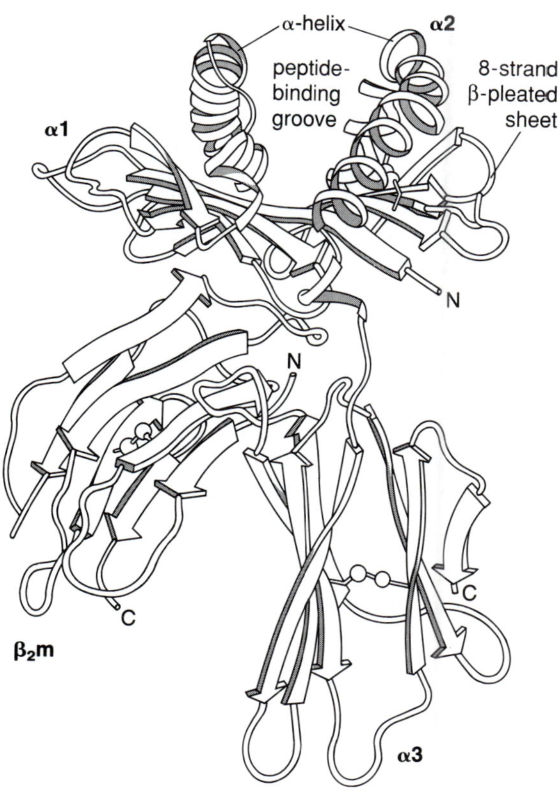

Figure 8–6. Diagrammatic structure of a class I HLA molecule.

4. THE IMMUNOGLOBULIN SUPERGENE FAMILY

It is important to note that all the molecules discussed—antibodies, the T cell receptor, and MHC proteins—have structural features in common. All of these molecules—and a long list of other immunologically relevant molecules, including the T cell subpopulation markers CD4 and CD8—have a domain structure built on the three-dimensional feature known as the **immunoglobulin fold.** Undoubtedly, the members of this family evolved to supply a common function to the organism. One part of this function is to act as a recognition unit or receptor at the cell surface.

5. ANTIGEN PROCESSING & PRESENTATION

Proteins from exogenous antigens, such as bacteria, are internalized via endocytic vesicles into antigen-presenting cells such as macrophages. Then, as illustrated in Figure 8–8, they are exposed to cellular proteases in intracellular vesicles. Peptides, approximately 10–30 amino acid residues in length, are generated in endosomal vesicles. The endosomic vesicles can then fuse with exocytics vesicle containing class II MHC molecules.

The class II MHC molecules are synthesized, as for other membrane glycoproteins, in the rough endoplasmic reticulum and then proceed out through the Golgi apparatus. A third polypeptide, **the invariant chain (Ii),** protects the binding site of the class II αβ dimer until the lowered pH of the compartment created after fusion with an endosomal vesicle causes a dissociation of the Ii chain. The MHC class II-peptide antigen complex is then transported to the cell surface for display and recognition by a T cell receptor.

Endogenous antigens, eg, cytosolic viral proteins synthesized in an infected cell, are processed for presentation by class I MHC molecules. Some of the steps involved are diagrammed in Figure 8–8. In brief, cytosolic proteins are broken down by a peptidase complex known as the **proteasome.** The cytosolic peptides gain access to nascent MHC class I molecules in the rough endoplasmic reticulum via peptide transporter systems (transporters associated with antigen process-

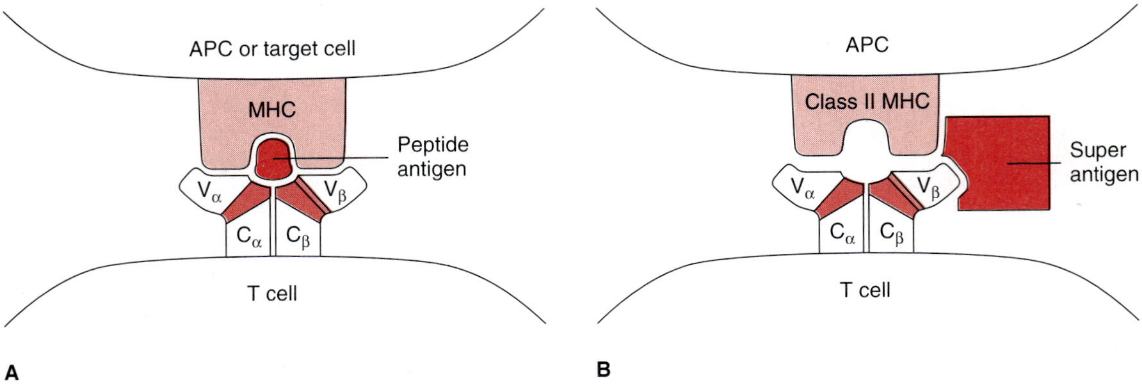

Figure 8–7. Binding of antigen by MHC and T cell receptor. In Panel A, a model of the interaction between peptide antigen, MHC, and the T cell receptor is shown. The V_α and V_β regions of the TCR are shown interacting with the α-helices that form the peptide binding groove of MHC. The J_α and J_β regions (cross-hatched) and the D_β region (stippled) are shown interacting with the peptide antigen. In Panel B, a model of the interaction between a superantigen, MHC, and the T cell receptor is shown. The superantigen interacts with the V_β region of the TCR and with Class II MHC outside the peptide binding groove. Modified and reproduced with permission from Stites et al. Basic and Clinical Immunology 8th ed. Appleton & Lange, 1994.

ing; TAP). Within the lumen of the endoplasmic reticulum, peptide antigens approximately 9–11 residues in length complex with nascent MHC class I proteins and cooperate with β_2-microglobulin to create a stable fully-folded MHC class I-peptide antigen complex that is then transported to the cell surface for display and recognition by cytotoxic T cells.

The binding groove of the class I molecule is more constrained than that of the class II molecule, and for that reason shorter peptides are found in class I than in class II MMC molecules.

It is important to note that an understanding of the details of antigen processing has greatly clarified thinking about T cell function. Thus, it is now clear why T cells do not respond to carbohydrate antigens (they would not fit in the groove) and why T cells only recognize linear antigenic determinants (they only respond to proteolytically processed antigen). It should also be pointed out that whether an antigen is destined for class I or class II presentation depends only on the intracellular compartments that it traverses.

Some antigens, known as **superantigens,** are able to bind to MHC molecules outside of the peptide-binding cleft. One consequence of this is that whereas an individual peptide complexed to an MHC molecule will normally stimulate only a small percentage of the T cells in an individual, superantigens cause large percentages of T cells to be nonspecifically activated. Examples of superantigens include certain bacterial toxins, including the staphylococcal enterotoxins, toxic shock syndrome toxin, group A streptococcal pyrogenic exotoxin A, and others. These antigens bind to the "outside" of the MHC protein and to the T cell receptor (Figure 8–7B). They are active at very low concentrations (10^{-9} mol/L) and cause T cells expressing particular Vβ sequences to be stimulated and release large amounts of cytokines, including IL-1 and tumor necrosis factor (TNF). It is the release of large amounts of cytokines from stimulation of a high percentage of the pool of T lymphocytes that explains to a large extent the pathogenesis of diseases caused by organisms with superantigens.

ANTIBODY-MEDIATED (HUMORAL) IMMUNITY

The Primary Response

When an individual encounters an antigen for the first time, antibody to that antigen is detectable in the serum within days or weeks, depending on the nature and dose of the antigen and the route of administration (eg, oral, parenteral). The serum antibody concentration continues to rise for several weeks and then declines; it may drop to very low levels (Figure 8–9). The first antibodies formed are IgM, followed by IgG, IgA, or both. IgM levels tend to decline sooner than IgG levels.

The Secondary Response

In the event of a second encounter with the same antigen (or a closely related, "cross-reacting" one) months or years after the primary response, the antibody response is more rapid and rises to higher levels than during the primary response. This change in response is attributed to the persistence of antigen-sensitive "memory cells" following the first immune response. In the secondary response, the amount of IgM produced is similar to that after the first contact with antigen; however, much more IgG is produced, and the level of IgG tends to persist much longer than in the primary response. Furthermore, such antibody tends to bind antigen more firmly (ie, to have higher affinity) and thus to dissociate less easily.

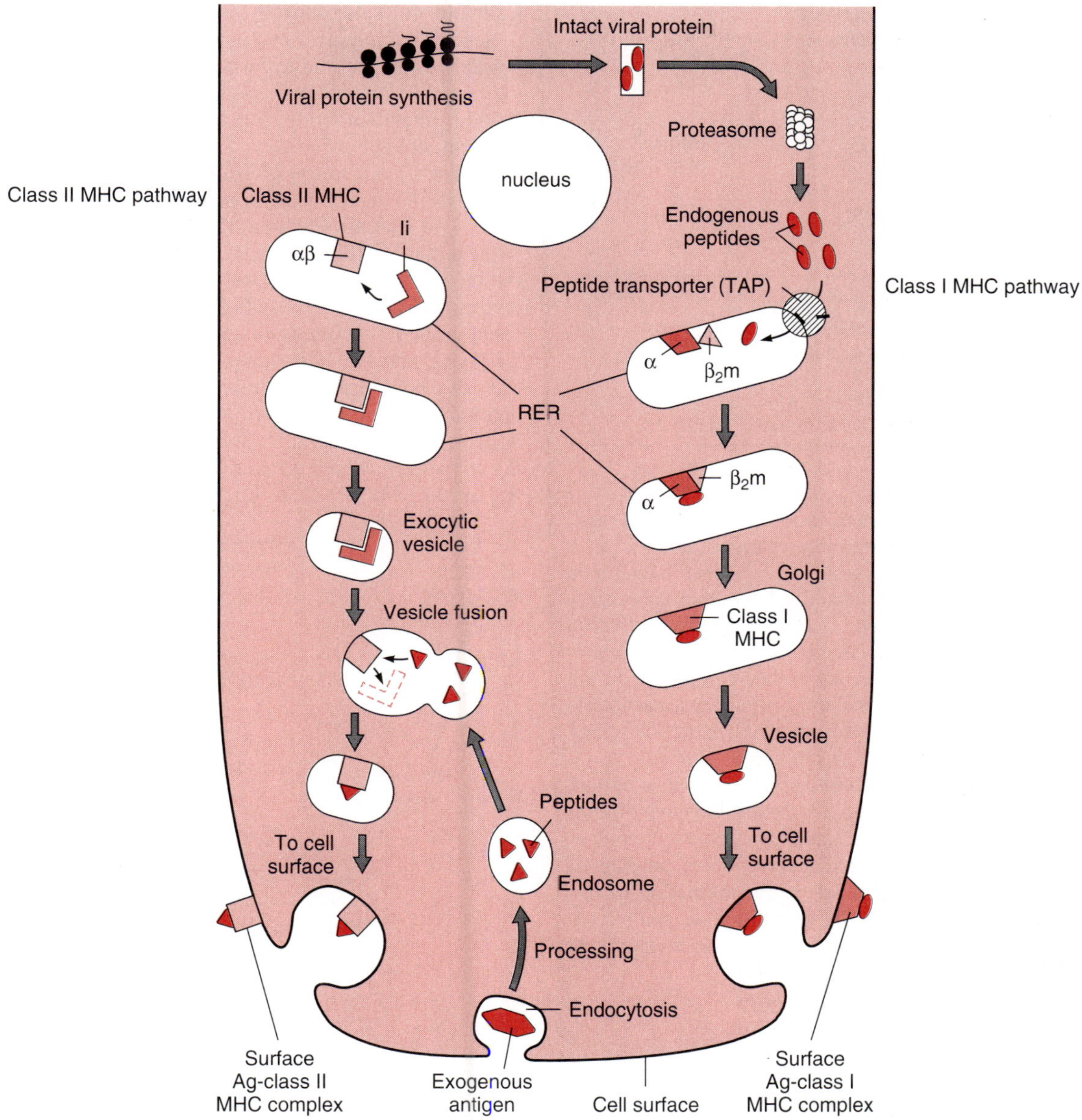

Figure 8–8. Antigen-processing pathways.

Protective Functions of Antibodies

Because of the close structural complementarity between antibodies and the antigen that elicited them, the two tend to bind to each other whenever they meet, in vitro and in vivo. This binding is noncovalent and involves electrostatic, van der Waals, and other weak forces as well as hydrogen and other bonds. Antibodies can produce resistance to infection by opsonizing (coating) organisms, which makes them more readily ingested by phagocytes; antibodies can bind to viruses and reduce their ability to invade host cells; most importantly, antibodies can neutralize toxins of microorganisms (eg, diphtheria, tetanus, and botulism) and inactivate their harmful effects.

Antibodies can be induced actively in the host by administering appropriate antigens or preparations containing them (toxoids of diphtheria, tetanus), but results are delayed until the antibodies reach helpful concentrations. In contrast, antibodies can be administered passively (ie, preformed in another host), which makes them immediately available for preventive or therapeutic purposes. The latter approach is used in the management of clinical diphtheria, tetanus, and botulism. It is important in the prevention of some viral infections, including rabies, hepatitis A, hepatitis B, varicella-

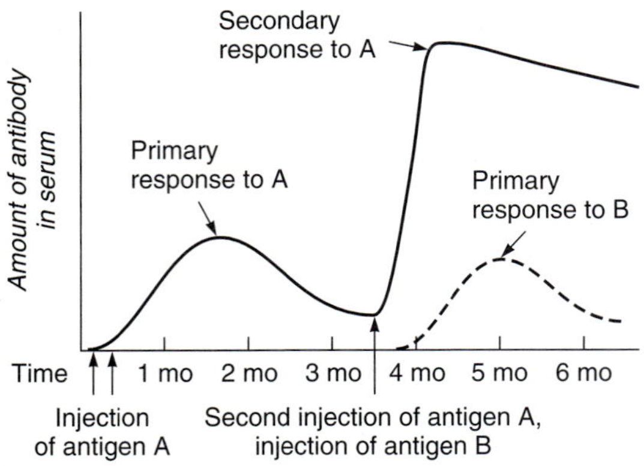

Figure 8–9. Rate of antibody production following initial antigen administration and a "booster" injection.

zoster in immunodeficient children, perhaps cytomegalovirus infections in transplant patients, and others.

Antibody-mediated immunity against bacteria is most effective when directed against microbial infections in which virulence is related to polysaccharide capsules (eg, pneumococcus, *Haemophilus, Neisseria*). In such infections, antibodies complex with the capsular antigens and make the organisms susceptible to ingestion by phagocytic cells and destruction within the cells.

Many cell-mediated immune responses also require the cooperation of antibodies directed against offending antigens before the latter can be inactivated or eliminated (see below). Conversely, the binding of antibodies to antigens leads to the formation of immune complexes, and the deposition of such complexes may be an important feature in the development of organ dysfunction.

THE COMPLEMENT SYSTEM

The complement system includes serum and membrane-bound proteins that function in both the acquired and constitutive (natural) host defense systems. These proteins are highly regulated and interact via a series of proteolytic cascades. The term "complement" refers to the ability of these proteins to complement (ie, augment) the effects of other components of the immune system (eg, antibody). Complement has several main effects: (1) lysis of cells (eg, bacteria and tumor cells), (2) production of mediators that participate in inflammation and attract phagocytes, (3) opsonization of organisms and immune complexes for clearance by phagocytosis, and (4) enhancement of antibody-mediated immune responses. Complement proteins are synthesized mainly by the liver and by phagocytic cells. Complement, being **heat-labile,** is inactivated at 56 °C for 30 minutes; immunoglobulins are not inactivated at this temperature.

Complement Activation

Several complement components are proenzymes, which must be cleaved to form active enzymes. Activation of the complement system can be initiated either by antigen-antibody complexes or by a variety of nonimmunologic molecules.

Sequential activation of complement components (Figure 8–10) occurs via two pathways:

A. The Classic Pathway: Only IgM and IgG activate or fix complement via the "classic" pathway. Of the IgGs, only IgG subclasses 1, 2, and 3 fix complement; IgG4 does not. C1, which is bound to a site located in the Fc region, is composed of three proteins, C1q, C1r, and C1s. C1q is an aggregate of polypeptides that bind to the Fc portion of IgG and IgM. The antibody-antigen, complexed with C1, activates C1s, which cleaves C4 and C2 to form C4b2b. The latter is C3 convertase, which cleaves C3 molecules into two fragments, C3a and C3b. C3a, an anaphylatoxin, is

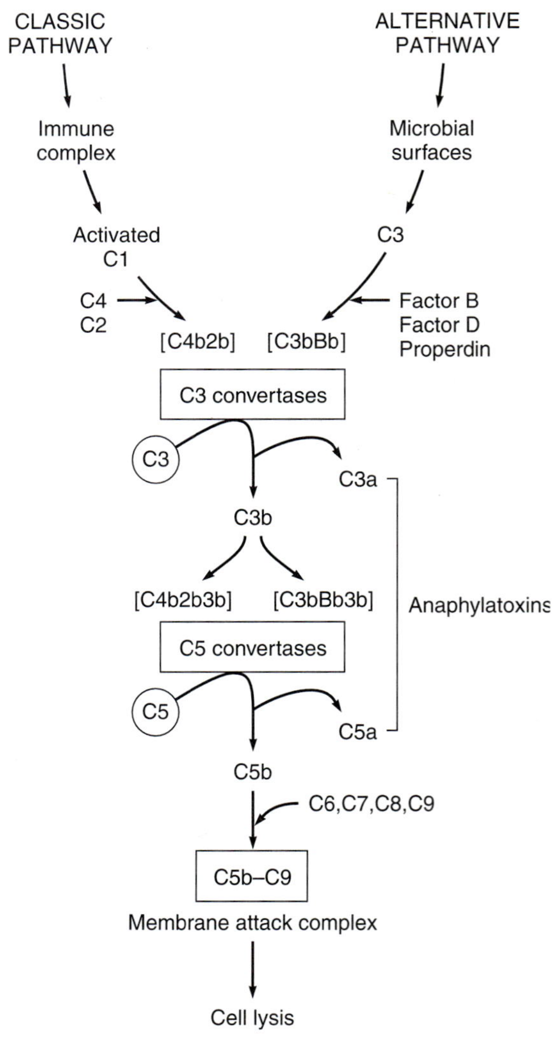

Figure 8–10. Complement reaction sequence.

discussed below. C3b forms a complex with C4b2b, producing a new enzyme, C5 convertase, which cleaves C5 to form C5a and C5b. C5a is an anaphylatoxin and a chemotactic factor (see below). C5b binds to C6 and C7 to form a complex that inserts into the membrane bilayer. C8 then binds to the C5b/C6/C7 complex, followed by the polymerization of up to 16 C9 molecules to produce the membrane attack complex that causes cytolysis.

B. The Alternative Pathway: Many unrelated substances, from complex chemicals (eg, endotoxin) to infectious agents (eg, parasites), activate a different alternative pathway. C3 is cleaved, and a C3 convertase is generated via the action of factors B, D, and properdin. The alternative C3 convertase (C3bBb) generates more C3b. The additional C3b binds to the C3 convertase to form C3bBbC3b, which is the alternative pathway C5 convertase that generates C5b, leading to production of the membrane attack complex described above.

Regulation of the Complement System

Several serum proteins regulate the complement system at different stages: (1) C1 inhibitor (C1 INH) binds to and inactivates the serine protease activity of C1r and C1s; (2) factor I cleaves C3b and C4b, thereby reducing the amount of C5 convertase available; (3) factor H enhances the effect of factor I on C3b; (4) factor P (properdin) protects C3b and stabilizes the C3 convertase of the alternative pathway; (5) regulation is also provided by proteins that have the ability to accelerate the decay of the complement proteins, eg, DAF (decay-accelerating factor), a membrane-bound protein found on most blood cell surfaces that can act to accelerate dissociation of the C3 convertases of both pathways.

Major Biologic Effects of Complement

A. Opsonization: Cells, antigen-antibody complexes, and other particles are phagocytosed much more efficiently in the presence of C3b because of the presence of C3b receptors on the surface of many phagocytes.

B. Chemotaxis: C5a stimulates movement of neutrophils.

C. Anaphylatoxins: C3a, C4a, and C5a can produce degranulation of mast cells with release of mediators, leading to increased vascular permeability and smooth muscle contraction.

D. Cytolysis: Insertion of the C5b6789 complex into the cell surface leads to killing or lysis of many types of cells, including erythrocytes, bacteria, and tumor cells.

Clinical Consequences of Complement Deficiencies

Many genetic deficiencies of complement proteins have been described, and these generally lead to enhanced susceptibility to infectious disease, eg, C2 deficiency frequently leads to serious pyogenic bacterial infections. Deficiency in components of the membrane attack complex greatly enhances susceptibility to *Neisseria* infections. Deficiencies in components of the alternative pathway are also known, eg, properdin deficiency makes people more susceptible to meningococcal disease.

PHAGOCYTOSIS

Particles, including microorganisms, and some soluble molecular complexes in blood lymph and tissues are often engulfed by specialized cells in a process called phagocytosis. The principal phagocytic cells are **macrophages (mononuclear phagocytes)** and **granulocytes (polymorphonuclear leukocytes).** These two types are sometimes called "professional phagocytes" to distinguish them from other cells that occasionally ingest particles (eg, fibroblasts and epithelial cells). Phagocytosis is an essential host defense mechanism both in normal tissues and in the inflammatory response. A detailed discussion of the events involved is provided earlier in this chapter.

CELL-MEDIATED IMMUNITY

As described earlier, antibody-mediated immunity is most important in toxin-induced disorders, in microbial infections in which polysaccharide capsules determine virulence, and in the prevention of some viral infections. However, in most microbial infections, it is cell-mediated immunity that imparts resistance and aids in recovery, although the cooperation of antibodies may be required. Furthermore, cell-mediated immunity is central in the defense against parasites, tumors, and foreign (grafted) cells. The important role of cell-mediated immunity is underlined in clinical situations in which its suppression (eg, AIDS) results in overwhelming infections or tumors.

The cell-mediated immune system includes several cell types and their products. Macrophages present antigen to T lymphocytes via their cell surface-located MHC proteins. T cell receptors recognize the antigen, and a specific T cell clone becomes activated and begins to proliferate. Because the number of T cell subpopulations is large and because their interactions (either directly or through the production of soluble lymphokines) result in a very complex response system, selected aspects of the system are discussed separately below. Natural killer (NK) cells are briefly described because of their distinctive features and functions.

Development of T Cells

Within the thymus, T cell progenitor cells undergo differentiation (under the influence of thymic hormones) into T cell subpopulations. Much has been learned about this process in recent years, and this remains an area of active investigation. T cells differentiate in the thymus into committed cells expressing a specific T cell receptor and become either CD4- or CD8-positive. CD4 and CD8 are cell surface proteins that define the major subpopulations of T cells, the helper (CD4) T cells and cytotoxic (CD8) T cells. After differentiation in the thymus, T cells undergo a selection process that results in the retention of only those cells with the most useful receptors, ie, those that are foreign antigen-specific and self-MHC restricted. Those clones that are potentially anti-self are deleted or functionally inactivated (made *anergic*). A consequence of the selection processes is that about 95% of thymocytes die in the thymus. Only a minority of developing T cells express the appropriate receptors.

T Cell Activation

T cell proliferation depends on a variety of events. Resting T cells must receive two signals for activation to occur. One signal comes from the T cell receptor interacting with an MHC-antigen complex presented on another cell. Recognition of antigen triggers a set of biochemical pathways in the cell that result eventually in DNA synthesis and mitosis. Critical to the signaling event are the proteins of the CD3 complex associated with the T cell receptor chains. CD3 transduces the signal to the cytoplasm that results in biochemical events such as increased cytoplasmic Ca^{2+} levels, increased protein kinase C activity, protein phosphorylation to activate transcription factors, and eventually transcription of, for example, IL-2 and IL-2 receptor genes. Release of IL-2 results in activation of other T cells bearing IL-2 receptors. Another separate signal is required for T cell activation, and that comes from an interaction between a molecule known as B7 which is found on B cells and macrophages and its receptor partner, CD28, on the T cell. Without this second signal, exposure of T cells to antigen may lead to their functional inactivation or death.

Main Categories of T Cells

T cells fall into two broad categories: CD4 cells and CD8 cells. CD4 cells predominate in human thymic medulla, tonsils, and blood, whereas CD8 cells predominate in human bone marrow and gut lymphoid tissue. The number of T cells specific for a single antigen is only about 1 in 10^5. To achieve immune reactivity, these few cells secrete soluble lymphokines, which activate large numbers of additional lymphocytes.

T cells constitute 65–80% of the recirculating pool of small lymphocytes. Their life span is relatively long—months or years.

A. CD4 Lymphocytes: These include the following main subpopulations:

1. Helper cells for B cells to develop into antibody-producing plasma cells.

2. Helper cells for CD8 T cells to become functionally mature and capable of cytolytic activity.

3. Cells that activate macrophages containing intracellular bacteria, thereby allowing them to destroy the bacteria.

4. Effector cells for delayed hypersensitivity reactions.

B. CD8 Lymphocytes: These include the following main subpopulations:

1. Cytotoxic cells that can kill virus-infected, tumor, and allograft cells.

2. Suppressor cells, which may inhibit antibody production and reactions of delayed hypersensitivity.

T Cell Functions

T cells have both effector and regulatory functions.

A. Effector Functions: Cell-mediated immunity and delayed hypersensitivity reactions are produced particularly against antigens of intracellular parasites, including viruses, fungi, some protozoa, and bacteria (eg, mycobacteria). A deficiency in cell-mediated immunity manifests itself mainly as marked susceptibility to infection by such parasites and to certain tumors.

In the response to allografts or tumors, CD4-positive cells recognize class II MHC molecules in addition to specific antigens and are activated. Then CD8-positive cytotoxic T cells respond to the production of interleukin-2 (and other soluble factors) by CD4 cells, recognize class I MHC molecules on the "foreign" cells, and proceed to destroy these cells. In the case of virus-infected cells, the CD8 lymphocytes must recognize both virus-determined antigens and class I MHC molecules on infected cells.

B. Regulatory Functions: T cells play a central role in regulating both humoral (antibody-mediated) and cellular (cell-mediated) immunity. Antibody production by B cells usually requires the participation of T helper cells (T cell-dependent response), but antibodies to some antigens (eg, polymerized macromolecules such as bacterial capsular polysaccharide) are the result of a T cell-independent response.

In the T cell-dependent B cell response to antigen, both B and T cells must have the same class II MHC specificity. In such T cell-dependent responses, the antigen interacts with IgM on the B cell surface. It is then internalized and modified. Fragments of the antigen are returned to the B cell surface in association with class II MHC molecules. These interact with the T cell receptor on the T helper cell, which produces lymphokines that enhance division of the B cells and make them differentiate into antibody-producing plasma cells.

In cell-mediated responses, the antigen is processed by macrophages, and fragments are presented in conjunction with class II MHC molecules on the macrophage surface. These interact with the T cell receptor on T helper cells, which produce lymphokines to stimulate growth of appropriate CD4 (T helper) cells. Important lymphokines are briefly described below.

When an imbalance exists in the number of active CD4 and CD8 cells, cellular immune mechanisms are grossly impaired. Thus, in AIDS, the normal ratio of CD4 to CD8 cells (>1.5) is lost. Some CD4 cells are destroyed by HIV. This results in a CD4:CD8 ratio of less than 1, leading to extreme susceptibility to development of many opportunistic infections and certain tumors.

NATURAL KILLER (NK) CELLS

Natural killer cells appear to represent a distinct functional population of lymphocytes. They resemble large, granular lymphocytes morphologically related to T cells and are capable of spontaneous cytotoxic activity against a variety of target cells without a need for antibody and independent of major histocompatibility antigens. Their target specificity is unknown, and they do not express T cell receptor-like proteins. They can lyse target cells that have undergone malignant transformation and may play a role in immune surveillance against tumor establishment. They can kill virus-infected cells. The lytic activity of NK cells is enhanced by high levels of alpha and beta interferons.

CYTOKINES

These molecules are the soluble mediators of host defense responses, both specific and nonspecific. As such they have a critically important role in the effector mechanisms involved in eliminating foreign antigens such as microorganisms. Table 8–3 lists a small number of important cytokines.

New cytokines are still being discovered, and much remains to be learned about their structure and function as well as how to make the best use of these **biologic response modifiers.** Many different cytokines are produced during immune responses. The same cytokine can be produced by multiple cell types and can have multiple effects on the same cell and also act on many different cell types. This has created considerable difficulty in fully understanding these important molecules. Their effects are mediated by binding to specific receptors on target cells. Thus, cytokines are like other hormones in that their effects are mediated through receptors that signal target cells to respond. As can be appreciated from Table 8–3, cytokines (like other hormones) frequently act as growth factors.

HYPERSENSITIVITY

"Hypersensitivity," or "allergy," denotes a condition in which an immune response results in exaggerated or inappropriate reactions that are harmful to the host. Such reactions typically occur in a given individual after the second contact with a specific antigen (allergen). The first contact (occurring earlier in the individual's life) is a necessary preliminary event and induces sensitization to that allergen.

There are four main types of hypersensitivity reactions. Types I, II, and III are antibody-mediated; type IV is cell-mediated.

Type I: Immediate (Anaphylactic) Hypersensitivity

This type of hypersensitivity manifests itself in tissue reactions occurring within minutes after the antigen combines with the matching antibody. If such a reaction can occur in any member of a species, it is called **anaphylaxis.** If it occurs only in certain predisposed members of a species, it is termed **atopy.**

The general mechanism of immediate hypersensitivity involves the following steps. An antigen induces the formation of IgE antibody, which binds firmly by its Fc portion to a receptor on basophils and mast cells. Some weeks later, a second contact of the individual with the same antigen results in the antigen's fixation

Table 8–3. Selected important cytokines.

Name	Major Cellular Source	Selected Biological Effects
IFN-α, -β	Phagocytes	Antiviral, pyrogenic
IFN-γ (interferon)	T cells	Activates mononuclear phagocytes
TNF (tumor necrosis factor)	Phagocytes, T cells	Cell activation, fever, cachexia, antitumor
LT (lymphotoxin)	T cells	Activates leukocytes, antitumor
TGF-β (transforming growth factor)	T cells, macrophages	Leukocyte growth regulation, angiogenesis
IL-1 (interleukin-1)	Phagocytes	Cell activation, fever, cachexia
IL-2 (interleukin-2)	T cells	T cell growth and activation
IL-3 (interleukin-3)	T cells	Hematopoiesis
IL-4 (interleukin-4)	Helper T cells	Isotype (class) switching to IgE
IL-10 (interleukin-10)	Helper T cells	Activates B cells, inhibits T cells
GM-CSF (granulocyte-macrophage colony-stimulating factor)	T cells, phagocytes, etc	Hematopoiesis of granulocyte, monocyte lineage
M-CSF	Macrophages, etc	Differentiation to monocytes
G-CSF (granulocyte colony-stimulating factor)	T cells, phagocytes, etc	Differentiation to granulocytes

to cell-bound IgE, cross-linking of IgE molecules, and release of pharmacologically active mediators from cells within minutes. Cyclic nucleotides and calcium are essential in the release of mediators. The reactivity can be transferred by serum but not by lymphoid cells.

A. Mediators of Anaphylactic Hypersensitivity: Some important mediators and their main effects are listed below.

1. Histamine–Histamine exists in a preformed state in platelets and in granules of tissue mast cells and basophils. Its release causes vasodilation, increased capillary permeability, and smooth muscle contraction (eg, bronchospasm). Antihistamine drugs can block histamine receptor sites and are relatively effective in allergic rhinitis but not in asthma (see below).

2. Prostaglandins and thromboxanes–Related to leukotrienes, prostaglandins and thromboxanes are derived from arachidonic acid via the cyclooxygenase pathway. Prostaglandins produce bronchoconstriction and dilatation and increased permeability of capillaries. Thromboxanes aggregate platelets.

The mediators listed above are active only for some minutes after release: they are enzymatically inactivated and resynthesized at a slow rate.

B. Treatment and Prevention of Anaphylactic Reactions: Treatment aims to counteract the action of mediators by maintaining the airway, ventilation, and cardiac function. One or more of the following may be given: epinephrine, antihistamines, corticosteroids, or cromolyn sodium. The last prevents release of mediators (eg, histamine) from mast cell granules. Prevention relies on identification of the allergen (often by skin test) and subsequent avoidance of that antigen.

Type II: Cytotoxic Hypersensitivity

Antibody directed at cell surface antigens activates complement (or other effectors) to damage the cells. The antibody (IgG or IgM) attaches to the antigen via the Fab region and acts as a bridge to complement via the Fc region. As a result, there may be complement-mediated lysis, as occurs in hemolytic anemias, ABO transfusion reactions, or Rh hemolytic disease.

Drugs such as penicillin, phenacetin, and quinidine can attach to surface proteins on red blood cells and initiate antibody formation. Such autoimmune antibodies (IgGs) may then combine with the cell surface, with resulting hemolysis. Certain infections (eg, *Mycoplasma pneumoniae*) can induce antibodies that cross-react with red cell antigens, resulting in hemolytic anemia. In rheumatic fever, antibodies against group A streptococci cross-react with cardiac tissue. In Goodpasture's syndrome, antibody to basement membranes of kidney and lung forms, resulting in severe damage to the membranes through activity of complement-attracted leukocytes.

Type III: Immune Complex Hypersensitivity

When antibody combines with its specific antigen, immune complexes are formed. Normally, they are promptly removed by the reticuloendothelial system, but occasionally they persist and are deposited in tissues, resulting in several disorders. In persistent microbial or viral infections, immune complexes may be deposited in organs (eg, the kidneys), resulting in dysfunction. In autoimmune disorders, "self" antigens may elicit antibodies that bind to organ antigens or are deposited in organs as complexes, especially in joints (arthritis), kidneys (nephritis), or blood vessels (vasculitis).

Wherever immune complexes are deposited, they activate the complement system, and polymorphonuclear cells are attracted to the site, where they cause inflammation and tissue injury. A typical type III hypersensitivity reaction is serum sickness.

A. Serum Sickness: Following the injection of foreign serum (or certain drugs), the antigen is slowly cleared from the circulation and antibody production begins. Simultaneous presence of antigen and antibody leads to production of immune complexes, which may circulate or may be deposited at various sites. Typical serum sickness results in fever, urticaria, arthralgia, lymphadenopathy, and splenomegaly a few days to 2 weeks after injection of the foreign serum. Symptoms improve as the immune elimination of antigen continues and subside when it is complete. Today, serum sickness less frequently follows the injection of foreign sera than the administration of drugs (eg, penicillin). Although it takes several days for symptoms to appear, serum sickness is classed as an immediate reaction, since symptoms occur promptly after immune complexes form.

B. Immune Complex Disease: Many clinical disorders associated with immune complexes have been described, though the antigen often cannot be identified. A representative example is glomerulonephritis. Acute poststreptococcal glomerulonephritis is a well-known immune complex disease. Its onset occurs several weeks after a group A β-hemolytic streptococcal infection, particularly of the skin, and often occurs in infection due to nephritogenic types of streptococci. The complement level is typically low, suggesting an antigen-antibody reaction. Lumpy deposits of immunoglobulin and C3 are seen along glomerular basement membranes stained by immunofluorescence, suggesting antigen-antibody complexes; streptococcal antigens have been rarely demonstrated, however. It is assumed that streptococcal antigen-antibody complexes are filtered out by glomeruli and that they fix complement, attract polymorphs, and start the inflammatory process.

C. Atopy: Atopic hypersensitivity disorders exhibit a strong familial predisposition and are associated with elevated IgE levels. Predisposition to atopy is clearly genetic, but symptoms are induced by exposure to specific allergens. These antigens are typically environmental allergens (eg, respiratory allergy to pollens, ragweed, or house dust) or foods (eg, intestinal allergy to shellfish or nuts). Common clinical manifestations include hay fever, asthma, eczema, and urticaria. Many sufferers give immediate type reactions to skin tests (injection, patch, scratch, etc) using the offending antigen.

Type IV: Cell-Mediated (Delayed) Hypersensitivity

Cell-mediated hypersensitivity is a function of T lymphocytes, not of antibody. It can be transferred by immunologically committed T cells but not by serum. The response is **delayed**—ie, it starts hours (or days) after contact with the antigen and often lasts for days. It consists mainly of mononuclear cell infiltration and tissue induration, as typified by the tuberculin skin test. Delayed hypersensitivity and cell-mediated immunity are closely related.

A. Contact Hypersensitivity: This manifestation of cell-mediated hypersensitivity occurs after sensitization with simple chemicals (eg, nickel, formaldehyde), plant materials (poison ivy, poison oak), topically applied drugs (eg, sulfonamides, neomycin), some cosmetics, soaps, and other substances. In all cases, small molecules enter the skin and then—acting as haptens—attach to body proteins to serve as complete antigen. Cell-mediated hypersensitivity is induced, particularly in skin. When the skin again comes in contact with the offending agent, the sensitized person develops erythema, itching, vesication, eczema, or necrosis of skin within 12–48 hours. Patch testing on a small area of skin can sometimes identify the offending antigen. Subsequent avoidance of the material will prevent recurrences. The antigen-presenting cell in contact sensitivity is probably the Langerhans cell in the epidermis.

B. Tuberculin-Type Hypersensitivity: Delayed hypersensitivity to antigens of microorganisms occurs in many infectious diseases and has been used as an aid in diagnosis. It is typified by the tuberculin reaction. When a small amount of tuberculin is injected into the epidermis of a patient previously exposed to *Mycobacterium tuberculosis,* there is little immediate reaction; gradually, however, induration and redness develop and reach a peak in 48–72 hours. A positive skin test indicates that the person has been infected with the agent, but it implies no current disease. However, a skin test that changes from negative to positive suggests recent infection and possible current activity.

A positive skin test response assists in diagnosis and provides support for chemoprophylaxis or chemotherapy. In leprosy, a positive lepromin test indicates tuberculoid leprosy—with active cell-mediated immunity, whereas a negative lepromin test suggests lepromatous leprosy—with impaired cell-mediated immunity. In systemic mycotic infections (eg, coccidioidomycosis, histoplasmosis, blastomycosis), a positive delayed-type skin test with the specific antigen helps to determine exposure to the organism. Cell-mediated hypersensitivity develops in many viral infections (eg, herpes simplex, mumps). However, serologic tests are more specific both for diagnosis and for assessment of immunity. In protozoan and helminthic infections, skin tests may be positive but they are generally not as useful as specific serologic tests.

IMMUNOLOGICAL TECHNIQUES: IN VITRO ANTIGEN-ANTIBODY REACTIONS

Reactions of antigens and antibodies are highly specific. An antigen will react only with antibody elicited by its own kind or by a closely related antigen. Because of this high specificity, reactions between an antigen and an antibody can be used to identify one by means of the other. This specificity is the basis of serologic reactions. Possible cross-reactions between related antigens can limit the test's specificity.

Antigen-antibody reactions are used to identify specific components in mixtures of either one. Microorganisms and other cells possess a variety of antigens and may thus react with many different antibodies. Monoclonal antibodies are excellent tools for identification of antigens because heterogeneity of antibodies is absent.

Radioimmunoassay (RIA)

This method is used to quantitate antigens or haptens that can be radioactively labeled. It is based on the competition for specific antibody between the labeled (known) and the unlabeled (unknown) concentration of material. The complexes that form between antigen and antibody can then be separated and the amount of radioactivity measured. The concentration of the unknown (unlabeled) antigen or hapten is determined by comparing the results with those obtained using several concentrations of a predetermined standard antigen. RIA is a highly sensitive method applied to the assay of hormones or drugs in serum. A specialized RIA, the radioallergosorbent test (RAST), is used to measure the amount of serum IgE antibody that reacts with a known allergen (antigen).

Enzyme Immunoassay (EIA)

This method, which has many variations, depends on the conjugation of an enzyme to either an antigen or an antibody. The enzyme is detected by assaying for enzyme activity with its substrate. Although the method is nearly as sensitive as RIA, it requires no special equipment or radioactive labels.

To measure antibody, known antigens are fixed to a solid phase (eg, plastic microdilution plate), incubated with test serum dilutions, washed, and reincubated with an anti-immunoglobulin labeled with an enzyme (eg, horseradish peroxidase). Enzyme activity, measured by adding the specific substrate and estimating the color reaction, is a direct function of the amount of antibody bound.

Immunofluorescence

Fluorescent dyes (eg, fluorescein, rhodamine) can be covalently attached to antibody molecules and made visible by ultraviolet light in the fluorescence microscope. Such labeled antibody can be used to identify antigens (eg, on the surface of bacteria such as streptococci or treponemes) or in cells in histologic section or other specimens. A **direct immunofluorescence** reaction occurs when known labeled antibody interacts directly with unknown antigen. An **indirect immunofluorescence** reaction occurs when a 2-stage process is used—eg, known antigen is attached to a slide, unknown serum is added, and the preparation is washed. If the unknown serum antibody matches the antigen, it will remain fixed to it on the slide and can be detected by adding a fluorescent-labeled antiglobulin antibody or other antibody-specific reagent such as *Staphylococcus* protein A and examining the slide by ultraviolet microscopy. The indirect test is often more sensitive than the direct test, because more labeled antibody adheres per antigenic site. Furthermore, the labeled antiglobulin becomes a "universal reagent" (independent of the nature of the antigen used) reactive with all IgG of that species.

Another use of fluorescent-tagged antibody molecules is, by virtue of the process of **flow cytometry** and a complex machine known as a **fluorescence-activated cell sorter (FACS)** to enumerate and classify cells.

Flow cytometry analyses a single-cell suspension flowing through a set of laser beams to measure the relative amount of light scattered by microscopic particles (thereby gaining information on relative size and granularity) and the relative fluorescence of those particles. For a mixture of white blood cells then, it is relatively easy to separate the cells in this mixture into major classes, eg, small lymphocytes separated from granulocytes which are larger and contain more granules (scatter more light). With the availability of panels of monoclonal antibodies (that can be detected by fluorescent anti-globulins) to cell surface proteins, it is also possible to enumerate subpopulations of cells, eg, CD4 expressing helper T cells from CD8 expressing cytolytic T cells, or antibody expressing B cells from T cells etc. This technology is widely used in clinical medicine and biomedical research.

Immunoblotting

Immunoblotting (sometimes called "Western blotting") is a method for identifying a particular antigen in a complex mixture of proteins. The complex mixture of proteins is subjected to sodium dodecyl sulfate (SDS)–polyacrylamide gel electrophoresis (PAGE). This separates the proteins according to molecular size. The gel is then covered with a membrane (usually a sheet of nitrocellulose), and the proteins are "transferred" by electrophoresis to the membrane. The nitrocellulose membrane (blot) acquires a replica of the proteins separated by SDS-PAGE. During the transfer, the SDS is largely removed from the proteins and, at least for some proteins, there is refolding into a conformation such that antibodies can react with the proteins on the membrane.

The nitrocellulose membrane is then incubated with either a radioactive or enzyme-labeled antibody in a direct test or in an indirect test with antibody followed by a labeled antiglobulin. The protein antigen then becomes visible as a band on the membrane. None of the other proteins in the mixture are detected.

REFERENCES

Abbas AK, Lichtman AH, Pober JS: *Cellular and Molecular Immunology,* 2nd ed. Saunders, 1994.

Janeway CA Jr, Travers P: *Immunobiology.* Current Biology/Garland, 1994.

Klein J: *Immunology.* Blackwell, 1990.

"Life, Death and the Immune System." Scientific American, September, 1993.

Paul WE (editor): *Fundamental Immunology,* 2nd ed. Raven Press, 1989.

Roitt I: *Essential Immunology,* 8th ed. Blackwell, 1994.

Stites DP, Terr AI, Parslow TG (editors): *Basic and Clinical Immunology,* 8th ed. Appleton & Lange, 1994.

Pathogenesis of Bacterial Infection

9

The pathogenesis of bacterial infection includes the initiation of the infectious process and the mechanisms that lead to the development of signs and symptoms of disease. Characteristics of bacteria that are pathogens include transmissibility, adherence to host cells, invasion of host cells and tissues, toxigenicity, and ability to evade the host's immune system. Many infections caused by bacteria that are commonly considered to be pathogens are inapparent or asymptomatic. Disease occurs if the bacteria or immunologic reactions to their presence cause sufficient harm to the person.

Terms frequently used in describing aspects of pathogenesis are defined in the Glossary (see at right). Refer to the Glossary in Chapter 8 for definitions of terms used in immunology and in describing aspects of the host's response to infection.

IDENTIFYING BACTERIA THAT CAUSE DISEASE

Humans and animals have abundant normal flora that usually do not produce disease (see Chapter 11) but achieve a balance that ensures the survival, growth, and propagation of both the bacteria and the host. Some bacteria that are important causes of disease are cultured commonly with the normal flora (eg, *Streptococcus pneumoniae, Staphylococcus aureus*). Sometimes bacteria that are clearly pathogens (eg, *Salmonella typhi*) are present, but infection remains latent or subclinical and the host is a "carrier" of the bacteria.

It can be difficult to show that a specific bacterial species is the cause of a particular disease. In 1884, Robert Koch proposed a series of postulates that have been applied broadly to link many specific bacterial species with particular diseases. **Koch's postulates** are summarized as follows:

(1) The microorganism should be found in all cases of the disease in question, and its distribution in the body should be in accordance with the lesions observed.

(2) The microorganism should be grown in pure culture in vitro (or outside the body of the host) for several generations.

(3) When such a pure culture is inoculated into susceptible animal species, the typical disease must result.

GLOSSARY

Adherence (adhesion, attachment): The process by which bacteria stick to the surface of host cells. Once bacteria have entered the body, adherence is a major initial step in the infection process. The terms adherence, adhesion, and attachment are often used interchangeably.

Carrier: A person or animal with asymptomatic infection that can be transmitted to another susceptible person or animal.

Infection: Multiplication of an infectious agent within the body. Multiplication of the bacteria that are part of the normal flora of the gastrointestinal tract, skin, etc, is generally not considered an infection; on the other hand, multiplication of pathogenic bacteria (eg, *Salmonella* species)—even if the person is asymptomatic—is deemed an infection.

Invasion: The process whereby bacteria, animal parasites, fungi, and viruses enter host cells or tissues and spread in the body.

Nonpathogen: A microorganism that does not cause disease; may be part of the normal flora.

Opportunistic pathogen: An agent capable of causing disease only when the host's resistance is impaired (eg, the patient is "immunocompromised").

Pathogen: A microorganism capable of causing disease.

Pathogenicity: The ability of an infectious agent to cause disease. (Also see virulence).

Toxigenicity: The ability of a microorganism to produce a toxin that contributes to the development of disease.

Virulence: The quantitative ability of an agent to cause disease. Virulent agents cause disease when introduced into the host in small numbers. Virulence involves invasiveness and toxigenicity (see above).

(4) The microorganism must again be isolated from the lesions of such experimentally produced disease.

Koch's postulates have remained a mainstay of microbiology; however, since the late 19th century, many microorganisms that do not meet the criteria of the postulates have been shown to cause disease. For example, *Treponema pallidum* (syphilis) and *Mycobacterium leprae* (leprosy) cannot be grown in vitro; however, there are animal models of infection with these agents. In another example, *Neisseria gonorrhoeae* (gonorrhea), there is no animal model of infection even though the bacteria can readily be cultured in vitro; experimental infection in humans has been produced, which substitutes for an animal model.

In other instances, Koch's postulates have been at least partially satisfied by showing bacterial pathogenicity in an in vitro model of infection rather than in an animal model. For example, some forms of *E coli*-induced diarrhea (Chapter 16) have been defined by the interaction of the *E coli* with host cells in culture.

The host's immune responses also should be considered when an organism is being investigated as the possible cause of a disease. Thus, development of a rise in specific antibody during recovery from disease is an important adjunct to Koch's postulates.

Modern-day microbial genetics has opened new frontiers to study pathogenic bacteria and differentiate them from nonpathogens. Molecular cloning has allowed investigators to isolate and modify specific virulence genes and study them with models of infection. The ability to study genes associated with virulence has led to a proposed form of **molecular Koch's postulates.** These postulates are paraphrased as follows:

(1) The phenotype, or property, under investigation should be significantly associated with pathogenic strains of a species and not with nonpathogenic strains.

(2) Specific inactivation of the gene or genes associated with the suspected virulence trait should lead to a measurable decrease in pathogenicity or virulence.

(3) Reversion or replacement of the mutated gene with the "wild type" gene should lead to restoration of pathogenicity or virulence.

Analysis of infection and disease through the application of principles such as Koch's postulates leads to classification of bacteria as pathogens, opportunistic pathogens, or nonpathogens. Some bacterial species are always considered to be pathogens, and their presence is abnormal; examples include *Mycobacterium tuberculosis* (tuberculosis) and *Yersinia pestis* (plague). Such bacteria readily meet the criteria of Koch's postulates. Other species are commonly part of the normal flora of humans (and animals) but also can frequently cause disease. For example, *Escherichia coli* is part of the gastrointestinal flora of normal humans but is also a common cause of urinary tract infections, traveler's diarrhea, and other diseases. Strains of *E coli* that cause disease are differentiated from those that do not by determining (1) whether they are virulent in animals or in vitro models of infection and (2) whether they have a genetic makeup that is significantly associated with production of disease. Other bacteria (eg, *Pseudomonas* species, *Xanthomonas maltophilia*, and many yeasts and molds) only cause disease in immunosuppressed and debilitated persons and are **opportunistic pathogens.**

TRANSMISSION OF INFECTION

Bacteria (and other microorganisms) adapt to the environment, including animals and humans, where they normally reside and subsist. In doing so the bacteria ensure their survival and enhance the possibility of transmission. By producing asymptomatic infection or mild disease, rather than death of the host, microorganisms that normally live in people enhance the possibility of transmission from one person to another.

Some bacteria that commonly cause disease in humans exist primarily in animals and incidentally infect humans. For example, *Salmonella* and *Campylobacter* species typically infect animals and are transmitted in food products to humans. Other bacteria produce infection of humans that is inadvertent, a mistake in the normal life cycle of the organism; the organisms have not adapted to humans, and the disease they produce may be severe. For example, *Yersinia pestis* (plague) has a well-established life cycle in rodents and rodent fleas, and transmission by the fleas to humans is inadvertent; *Bacillus anthracis* (anthrax) lives in the environment, occasionally infects animals, and is transmitted to humans by products such as raw hair from infected animals. The *Clostridium* species are ubiquitous in the environment and are transmitted to humans by ingestion (eg, *C perfringens* gastroenteritis and *C botulinum* [botulism]) or when wounds are contaminated by soil (eg, *C perfringens* gas gangrene and *C tetani* [tetanus]).

The clinical manifestations of diseases (eg, diarrhea, cough, genital discharge) produced by microorganisms often promote transmission of the agents. Examples of clinical syndromes and how they enhance transmission of the causative bacteria are as follows: *Vibrio cholerae* can cause voluminous diarrhea which may contaminate salt and fresh water; drinking water or seafood such as oysters and crabs may be contaminated; ingestion of contaminated water or seafood can produce infection and disease. Similarly, contamination of food products with sewage containing *E coli* that cause diarrhea results in transmission of the bacteria. *Mycobacterium tuberculosis* (tuberculosis) naturally infects only humans; it produces respiratory disease with cough and production of aerosols, resulting in transmission of the bacteria from one person to another.

Many bacteria are transmitted from one person to another on hands. A person with *S aureus* carriage in the anterior nares may rub his nose, pick up the staphylococci on the hands, and spread the bacteria to other parts of the body or to another person, where infection results. Many opportunistic pathogens that cause nosocomial infections are transmitted from one patient to another on the hands of hospital personnel. Hand washing is thus an important component of infection control.

The most frequent **portals of entry of pathogenic bacteria** into the body are the sites where mucus membranes meet with the skin: respiratory (upper and lower airways), gastrointestinal (primarily mouth), genital, and urinary tracts. Abnormal areas of mucous membranes and skin (eg, cuts, burns, and other injuries) are also frequent sites of entry. Normal skin and mucus membranes provide the primary defense against infection. The normal physiologic barriers to infection are discussed in Chapter 8. To cause disease, pathogens must overcome these barriers.

THE INFECTIOUS PROCESS

Once in the body, bacteria must attach or adhere to host cells, usually epithelial cells (see below). After the bacteria have established a primary site of infection, they multiply and spread directly through tissues or via the lymphatic system to the bloodstream. This infection (bacteremia) can be transient or persistent. Bacteremia allows bacteria to spread widely in the body and permits them to reach tissues particularly suitable for their multiplication.

Pneumococcal pneumonia is an example of the infectious process. *S pneumoniae* can be cultured from the nasopharynx of 5–40% of healthy people. Occasionally, pneumococci from the nasopharynx are aspirated into the lungs; aspiration occurs most commonly in debilitated people and in settings such as coma when normal gag and cough reflexes are diminished. Infection develops in the terminal air spaces of the lungs in persons who do not have protective antibodies against that capsular polysaccharide type of pneumococci. Multiplication of the pneumococci and resultant inflammation lead to pneumonia. The pneumococci enter the lymphatics of the lung and move to the bloodstream. Between 10% and 20% of persons with pneumococcal pneumonia have bacteremia at the time the diagnosis of pneumonia is made. Once bacteremia occurs, the pneumococci can spread to secondary sites of infection (eg, cerebrospinal fluid, heart valves, joint spaces). The major complications of pneumococcal pneumonia are meningitis, endocarditis, and septic arthritis.

The infectious process in cholera involves ingestion of *Vibrio cholerae,* chemotactic attraction of the bacteria to the gut epithelium, motility of the bacteria by a single polar flagellum, and penetration of the mucus layer on the intestinal surface. The *V cholerae* adherence to the epithelial cell surface is mediated by pili and possibly other adhesins. Production of cholera toxin results in flow of chloride and water into the lumen of the gut, causing diarrhea and electrolyte imbalance.

THE CLONAL NATURE OF BACTERIAL PATHOGENS

Bacteria are haploid (Chapter 7) and limit genetic interactions that might change their chromosomes and potentially disrupt their adaptation and survival in specific environmental niches. The primary mechanism for exchange of genetic information between bacteria is transfer of extrachromosomal mobile genetic elements, plasmids or phages. The genes that code for many bacterial virulence factors commonly are on plasmids or are carried by phages. Transfer of these mobile genetic elements between members of one species or, less commonly, between species can result in transfer of virulence factors. Sometimes the genetic elements are part of highly mobile DNA (transposons; Chapter 7) and there is recombination between the extrachromosomal DNA and the chromosome (illegitimate or nonhomologous recombination; Chapter 7). If this recombination occurs, the genes coding for virulence factors may become chromosomal.

One important result of the conservation of chromosomal genes in bacteria is that the organisms are clonal. For most pathogens there are only one or a few clonal types that are spread in the world during a period of time. For example, epidemic serogroup A meningococcal meningitis occurs in Asia, the Middle East, and Africa, and occasionally spreads into Northern Europe and the Americas. On several occasions, over a period of decades, single clonal types of serogroup A *Neisseria meningitidis* have been observed to appear in one geographic area and subsequently spread to others with resultant epidemic disease. There are over 100 clonal types of *H influenzae* but only a small number of types are commonly associated with disease. There are two clonal types of *Bordetella pertussis,* both associated with disease. Similarly, *Salmonella typhi* (typhoid fever) from patients is of two clonal types.

REGULATION OF BACTERIAL VIRULENCE FACTORS

Pathogenic bacteria (and other pathogens) have adapted both to saprophytic or free-living states, possibly environments outside of the body, and to the human host. In the adaptive process, pathogens husband their metabolic needs and products. They have evolved complex signal transduction systems to regulate the genes important for virulence. Environmental signals often control the expression of the virulence genes. Common signals include temperature, iron availability, osmolality, growth phase, pH, and specific ions (eg, Ca^{2+}) or nutrient factors. A few examples are presented in the following paragraphs.

The gene for diphtheria toxin from *Corynebacterium diphtheriae* is carried on temperate bacteriophages.

Toxin is produced only by strains lysogenized by the phages. Toxin production is greatly enhanced when *C diphtheriae* are grown in medium with low iron.

Expression of virulence genes of *Bordetella pertussis* is enhanced when the bacteria are grown at 37 °C and suppressed when they are grown at lower temperatures or in the presence of high concentrations of magnesium sulfate or nicotinic acid.

The virulence factors of *Vibrio cholerae* are regulated on multiple levels and by many environmental factors. Expression of the cholera toxin is higher at pH 6.0 than at pH 8.5 and higher also at 30 °C than at 37 °C. Osmolality and amino acid composition also are important. As many as 20 other genes of *V cholerae* are similarly regulated.

Yops are a series of *Yersinia* virulence plasmid-encoded proteins that result in antiphagocytic function. Yops are expressed maximally at 37 °C in the absence of calcium. When calcium is present, the production of Yops still is higher than at 25 °C. Thus, production of the antiphagocytic virulence factors is highest at the body temperatures of animals and humans rather than at the ambient temperature of rodent fleas, where antiphagocytic factors are not important to the bacteria. The regulation of other virulence factors in *Yersinia* species also is influenced by environmental factors.

Motility of bacteria enables them to spread and multiply in their environmental niches or in patients. *Yersinia enterocolitica* and *Listeria monocytogenes* are ubiquitous in the environment where motility is important to them. Presumably, motility is not important in the pathogenesis of the diseases caused by these bacteria. *Y enterocolitica* is motile when grown at 25 °C but not when grown at 37 °C. Similarly, *Listeria* is motile when grown at 25 °C and not motile or minimally motile when grown at 37 °C.

BACTERIAL VIRULENCE FACTORS

Many factors determine bacterial virulence, or ability to cause infection and disease.

Adherence Factors

Once bacteria enter the body of the host, they must adhere to cells of a tissue surface. If they did not adhere, they would be swept away by mucus and other fluids that bathe the tissue surface. Adherence, which is only one step in the infectious process, is followed by development of microcolonies and subsequent steps in the pathogenesis of infection.

The interactions between bacteria and tissue cell surfaces in the adhesion process are complex. Several factors play important roles: surface hydrophobicity and net surface charge; binding molecules on bacteria (ligands) and host cell receptor interactions. Bacteria and host cells commonly have net negative surface charges and, therefore, repulsive electrostatic forces. These forces are overcome by hydrophobic and other more specific interactions between bacteria and host cells. In general, the more hydrophobic the bacterial cell surface, the greater the adherence to the host cell. Different strains of bacteria within a species may vary widely in their hydrophobic surface properties and ability to adhere to host cells.

Bacteria also have specific surface molecules that interact with host cells. Many bacteria have **pili,** hair-like appendages that extend from the bacterial cell surface and help mediate adherence of the bacteria to host cell surfaces. For example, some *E coli* strains have type 1 pili, which adhere to epithelial cell receptors containing D-mannose; adherence can be blocked in vitro by addition of D-mannose to the medium. *E coli* organisms that cause urinary tract infections commonly do not have D-mannose-mediated adherence but have P-pili, which attach to a portion of the P blood group antigen; the minimal recognition structure is the disaccharide α-D-galactopyranosyl-(1–4)-β-D-ga-lactopyranoside (GAL-GAL binding adhesion). The *E coli* that cause diarrheal diseases (see Chapter 16) have pilus-mediated adherence to intestinal epithelial cells, though the pili and specific molecular mechanisms of adherence appear to be different depending upon the form of the *E coli* that induce the diarrhea.

Other specific ligand-receptor mechanisms have evolved to promote bacterial adherence to host cells, illustrating the diverse mechanisms employed by bacteria. Group A streptococci and *Streptococcus pyogenes* (see Chapter 15) also have hair-like appendages, termed fimbriae, that extend from the cell surface. **Lipoteichoic acid** and M protein are found on the fimbriae. The lipoteichoic acid causes adherence of the streptococci to buccal epithelial cells; this adherence is mediated by the lipid portion of the lipoteichoic acid, which acts as the ligand, and by fibronectin, which acts as the host cell receptor molecule. M protein acts as an antiphagocytic molecule.

Antibodies that act against the specific bacterial ligands that promote adherence (eg, pili and lipoteichoic acid) can block adherence to host cells and protect the host from infection.

Invasion of Host Cells & Tissues

For many disease-causing bacteria, invasion of the host's epithelium is central to the infectious process. Some bacteria (eg, *Salmonella* species) invade tissues through the junctions between epithelial cells. Other bacteria (eg, *Yersinia* species, *N gonorrhoeae, Chlamydia trachomatis*) invade specific types of the host's epithelial cells and may subsequently enter the tissue. Once inside the host cell, bacteria may remain enclosed in a vacuole composed of the host cell membrane, or the vacuole membrane may be dissolved and bacteria may be dispersed in the cytoplasm. Some bacteria (eg, *Shigella* species) multiply within host cells, whereas other bacteria do not.

"Invasion" is the term commonly used to describe the entry of bacteria into host cells, implying an active role for the organisms and a passive role for the host cells. In many infections, the bacteria produce virulence factors that influence the host cells, causing them to engulf (ingest) the bacteria. The host cells play a very active role in the process.

Toxin production and other virulence properties are generally independent of the ability of bacteria to invade cells and tissues. For example, *Corynebacterium diphtheriae* is able to invade the epithelium of the nasopharynx and cause symptomatic sore throat even when the *C diphtheriae* strains are nontoxigenic.

In vitro studies with cells in tissue culture have helped characterize the mechanisms of invasion for some pathogens; however, the in vitro models have not necessarily provided a complete picture of the invasion process. Full understanding of the invasion process, as it occurs in naturally acquired infection, has required study of genetically engineered mutants and their ability to infect susceptible animals and humans. Thus, understanding of eukaryotic cell invasion by bacteria requires satisfying much of Koch's postulates and the molecular Koch's postulates. The following paragraphs contain examples of bacterial invasion of host cells as part of the infectious process.

Shigella species adhere to host cells in vitro. Commonly, HeLa cells are used; these undifferentiated unpolarized cells were derived from a cervical carcinoma. The adherence causes actin polymerization in the nearby portion of the HeLa cell, which induces the formation of pseudopods by the HeLa cells and engulfment of the bacteria. Adherence and invasion are mediated at least in part by products of genes located on a large plasmid common to many *Shigella.* At least three proteins (*i*nvasion *p*lasmid *a*ntigens, Ipa), IpaB, IpaC, and IpaD contribute to the process. Once inside the HeLa cells, the *Shigella* either are released or escape from the phagocytic vesicle, where they multiply in the cytoplasm. Actin polymerization propels the *Shigella* within an HeLa cell and from one cell into another. The pathogenesis of *Shigella* adherence and invasion in vivo appears to be somewhat different and less well understood at the molecular level. The *Shigella* adhere to integrins on the surface of M cells in Peyer's patches and not to the polarized absorptive cells of the mucosa. M cells normally sample antigens and present them to macrophages in the submucosa. *Shigella* are phagocytosed by the M cells, pass through the M cells, and escape killing by macrophages. The *Shigella* are thought to adhere to integrins on the basal surfaces of nearby mucosal cells followed by engulfment by the mucosal cells and spread to adjacent cells in a manner similar to the in vitro cell invasion model.

From studies using cells in vitro, it appears that the adherence/invasion process with *Y enterocolitica* is similar to that of *Shigella.* The *Yersinia* adhere to the host cell membrane and cause it to extrude protoplasmic projections. The bacteria are then engulfed by the host cell with vacuole formation. Invasion is enhanced when the bacteria are grown at 22 °C rather than at 37 °C. Once *Yersinia* has entered the cell, the vacuolar membrane dissolves and the bacteria are released into the cytoplasm. In vivo, the *Yersinia* are thought to adhere to and invade the M cells of Peyer's patches rather than the polarized absorptive mucosal cells, much like *Shigella.*

L monocytogenes from the environment are ingested in food. Presumably, the bacteria adhere to and invade the intestinal mucosa, reach the bloodstream, and disseminate. The pathogenesis of this process has been studied in vitro. *L monocytogenes* adhere to and readily invade macrophages and cultured undifferentiated intestinal cells. The *Listeria* induce engulfment by the host cells. An 80,000 MW protein, **internalin,** appears have a primary role in this process. The engulfment process, movement within a cell, and movement between cells, requires actin polymerization to propel the bacteria, as with *Shigella.*

Legionella pneumophila infects pulmonary macrophages and causes pneumonia. Adherence of the *Legionella* to the macrophage induces formation of a long, thin pseudopod which then coils around the bacteria, forming a vesicle **(coiling phagocytosis).** The vesicle remains intact, phagolysosome fusion is inhibited, and the bacteria multiply within the vesicle.

Neisseria gonorrhoeae use pili as primary adhesins and **opacity associated proteins (Opa)** as secondary adhesins to host cells. Certain Opa proteins mediate adherence to polymorphonuclear cells. Some gonococci survive after phagocytosis by these cells. Pili and Opa together enhance the invasion of cells cultured in vitro. In uterine (fallopian) tube organ cultures, the gonococci adhere to the microvilli of nonciliated cells and appear to induce engulfment by these cells. The gonococci multiply intracellularly and migrate to the subepithelial space by an unknown mechanism.

Toxins

Toxins produced by bacteria are generally classified into two groups: exotoxins and endotoxins. The primary features of the two groups are listed in Table 9–1.

A. Exotoxins: Many gram-positive and gram-negative bacteria produce exotoxins of considerable medical importance. Some of these toxins have had major roles in world history. For example, tetanus caused by the toxin of *C tetani* killed as many as 50,000 soldiers of the Axis powers in World War II; the Allied forces, however, immunized military personnel against tetanus, and very few died of that disease. Vaccines have been developed for some of the exotoxin-mediated diseases and continue to be important in the prevention of disease. These vaccines—called **toxoids**—are made from exotoxins, which are modified so that they are no longer toxic. Many exotoxins consist of A and B subunits: The B subunit generally mediates adherence of the toxin complex to a host cell and aids en-

Table 9–1. Characteristics of exotoxins and endotoxins (lipopolysaccharides).

Exotoxins	Endotoxins
Excreted by living cell; high concentrations in liquid medium.	Integral part of the cell wall of gram-negative bacteria. Released on bacterial death and in part during growth. May not need to be released to have biologic activity.
Produced by both gram-positive and gram-negative bacteria.	Found only in gram-negative bacteria.
Polypeptides with a molecular weight of 10,000–900,000.	Lipopolysaccharide complexes. Lipid A portion probably responsible for toxicity.
Relatively unstable; toxicity often destroyed rapidly by heating at temperatures above 60 °C.	Relatively stable; withstand heating at temperatures above 60 °C for hours without loss of toxicity.
Highy antigenic; stimulate formation of high-titer antitoxin. Antitoxin neutralizes toxin.	Weakly immunogenic; antibodies are antitoxic and protective. Relationship between antibody titers and protection from disease is less clear than with exotoxins.
Converted to antigenic, nontoxic toxoids by formalin, acid, heat, etc. Toxoids are used to immunize (eg, tetanus toxoid).	Not converted to toxoids.
Highly toxic; fatal to animals in microgram quantities or less.	Moderately toxic; fatal for animals in tens to hundreds of micrograms.
Usually bind to specific receptors on cells.	Specific receptors not found on cells.
Usually do not produce fever in the host.	Usually produce fever in the host by release of interleukin-1 and other mediators.
Frequently controlled by extrachromosomal genes (eg, . plasmids).	Synthesis directed by chromosomal genes.

trance of the exotoxin into the host cell. The A subunit provides the toxic activity. Examples of some pathogenetic mechanisms associated with exotoxins are given below. Toxins of specific bacteria are discussed in the chapters covering those bacteria.

C diphtheriae is a gram-positive rod that can grow on the mucous membranes of the upper respiratory tract or in minor skin wounds (Chapter 13). Strains of *C diphtheriae* that carry a temperate bacteriophage with the structural gene for the toxin are toxigenic and produce **diphtheria toxin** and cause **diphtheria.** Many factors regulate toxin production; when the availability of inorganic iron is the factor limiting the growth rate, then maximal toxin production occurs. The toxin molecule is secreted as a single polypeptide molecule (MW 62,000). This native toxin is enzymatically degraded into two fragments, A and B, linked together by a disulfide bond. Fragment B (MW 40,700) binds to specific host cell receptors and facilitates the entry of fragment A (MW 21,150) into the cytoplasm. Fragment A inhibits peptide chain elongation factor EF-2 by catalyzing a reaction that yields free nicotinamide plus an inactive adenosine diphosphate-ribose-EF-2 complex. Arrest of protein synthesis disrupts normal cellular physiologic functions. Diphtheria toxin can be lethal in a dose of 0.1 mg/kg.

C tetani is an anaerobic gram-positive rod that causes tetanus (Chapter 12). *C tetani* from the environment contaminate wounds, and the spores germinate in the anaerobic environment of the devitalized tissue. Infection often is minor and not clinically apparent. The vegetative forms of *C tetani* produce the toxin **tetanospasmin** (MW 150,000). The released toxin has two peptides (MW 50,000 and 100,000) linked by disulfide bonds. The large peptide binds to gangliosides, whereas the small peptide appears to have the toxic activity. Toxin reaches the central nervous system by retrograde transport along axons and through the systemic circulation. The toxin acts by blocking release of an inhibitory mediator in motor neuron synapses. The result is initially localized, then generalized, muscle spasms. Extremely small amounts of toxin can be lethal for humans. Tetanus is totally preventable in immunologically normal people by immunization with tetanus toxoid.

C botulinum causes **botulism.** *C botulinum* is found in soil or water and may grow in foods (canned, vacuum-packed, etc) if the environment is appropriately anaerobic. An exceedingly potent toxin (the most potent toxin known) is produced. It is heat-labile and is destroyed by sufficient heating. There are multiple distinct serologic types of toxin. Types A, B, and E are most commonly associated with human disease. The toxin is absorbed from the gut and carried to motor nerves, where it blocks the release of acetylcholine at synapses and neuromuscular junctions. Muscle contraction does not occur, and paralysis results.

Spores of *C perfringens* are introduced into wounds by contamination with soil or feces. In the presence of necrotic tissue (an anaerobic environment), spores germinate and vegetative cells can produce several different toxins. Many of these are necrotizing and hemolytic and—together with distention of tissue by gas formed from carbohydrates and interference with blood supply—favor the spread of **gas gangrene.** The **alpha toxin** of *C perfringens* is a **lecithinase** that damages cell membranes by splitting lecithin to phosphorylcholine and diglyceride. Theta toxin also has a necrotizing effect. Collagenases and DNAses are produced by clostridia as well.

Some *S aureus* strains growing on mucous membranes (eg, the vagina in association with menstruation), or in wounds, elaborate **toxic shock syndrome toxin-1 (TSST-1),** which causes **toxic shock syndrome** (Chapter 14). The illness is characterized by shock, high fever, and a diffuse red rash that later desquamates; multiple other organ systems are involved as well. TSST-1 is a super antigen and stimulates lymphocytes to produce large amounts of IL-1 and TNF (Chapter 8). The major clinical manifestations of the disease appear to be secondary to the effects of the cytokines. TSST-1 may act synergistically with low levels of lipopolysaccharide to yield the toxic effect. Many of the systemic effects of TSST-1 are similar to those of toxicity due to lipopolysaccharide (below).

Some strains of group A beta-hemolytic streptococci produce **pyrogenic exotoxin A** that is similar to or the same as streptococcal erythrogenic toxin, which results in scarlet fever. Rapidly progressive soft tissue infection by streptococci that produce the pyrogenic exotoxin A has many clinical manifestations similar to those of staphylococcal toxic shock syndrome. The pyrogenic exotoxin A also is a super antigen that acts in a manner similar to TSST-1.

B. Exotoxins Associated With Diarrheal Diseases and Food Poisoning: Exotoxins associated with diarrheal diseases are frequently called enterotoxins. (See also Table 48–3.) Characteristics of some important enterotoxins are discussed below.

V cholerae has produced epidemic diarrheal disease **(cholera)** in many parts of the world (Chapter 18) and is another toxin-produced disease of historical and current importance. After entering the host via contaminated food or drink, *V cholerae* penetrates the intestinal mucosa and attaches to microvilli of the brush border of gut epithelial cells. *V cholerae,* usually of the serotype O1 (and O139), can produce an enterotoxin with a molecular weight of 84,000. The toxin consists of two subunits, A (two peptides) and B, linked by a disulfide bond. Subunit B has five identical peptides and rapidly binds the toxin to cell membrane ganglioside molecules. Subunit A enters the cell membrane and causes a large increase in adenylyl cyclase activity and in the concentration of cAMP. The net effect is rapid secretion of electrolytes into the small bowel lumen, with impairment of sodium and chloride absorption and loss of bicarbonate. Life-threatening massive diarrhea (eg, 20–30 L/d) can occur, and acidosis develops. The deleterious effects of cholera are due to fluid loss and acid-base imbalance; treatment, therefore, is by electrolyte and fluid replacement.

Some strains of *S aureus* produce enterotoxins while growing in meat, dairy products, or other foods. In typical cases, the food has been recently prepared but not properly refrigerated. There are at least six distinct types of the **staphylococcal enterotoxin.** After the preformed toxin is ingested, it is absorbed in the gut, where it stimulates neural receptors. The stimulus is transmitted to the vomiting center in the central nervous system. Vomiting, often projectile, results within hours. Diarrhea is less frequent. Staphylococcal food poisoning is the most common form of food poisoning. *S aureus* enterotoxins are super antigens.

Enterotoxins are also produced by some strains of *Y enterocolitica* (Chapter 20), *Vibrio parahaemolyticus* (Chapter 18), *Aeromonas* species (Chapter 18), and other bacteria, but the role of these toxins in pathogenesis is not defined. The enterotoxin produced by *C perfringens* is discussed in Chapter 12.

C. Lipopolysaccharides of Gram-Negative Bacteria: The lipopolysaccharides (LPS, endotoxin) of gram-negative bacteria are derived from cell walls and are often liberated when the bacteria lyse. The substances are heat-stable, have molecular weights between 3000 and 5000 **(lipooligosaccharides, LOS)** and several million **(lipopolysaccharides, LPS),** and can be extracted (eg, with phenol-water). They have three main regions (Table 9–2; Figure 2–18).

The **pathophysiologic effects of LPS** are similar regardless of their bacterial origin except for those of *Bacteroides* species, which have a different structure and are less toxic (Chapter 11). LPS in the bloodstream is initially bound to circulating proteins which then interact with receptors on macrophages and monocytes and other cells of the reticuloendothelial system. IL-1, TNF, and other cytokines are released, and the complement and coagulation cascades are activated. The following can be observed clinically or experimentally: fever, leukopenia, and hypoglycemia; hypotension and shock resulting in impaired perfusion of essential organs (eg, brain, heart, kidney); intravascular coagulation; and death from massive organ dysfunction.

Table 9–2. Composition of lipopolysaccharide "endotoxins" in the cell walls of gram-negative bacteria.

Chemistry	Common Name
(a) Repeating oligosaccharide (eg, man-rha-gal) combinations make up type-specific haptenic determinants (outermost in cell wall).	(a) O-specific polysaccharide. Induce specific immunity.
(b) (N-Acetylglucosamine, glucose, galactose, heptose.) Same in all gram-negative bacteria.	(b) Common core polysaccharide.
(c) Backbone of alternating heptose and phosphate groups linked through KDO (2-keto-3-deoxyoctonic acid) to lipid. Lipid is linked to peptidoglycan (by glycoside bonds). (See Fig 2–18.)	(c) Lipid A with KDO responsible for primary toxicity.

Injection of LPS produces **fever** after 60–90 minutes, the time needed for the body to release IL-1. Injection of IL-1 produces fever within 30 minutes. Repeated injection of IL-1 produces the same fever response each time, but repeated injection of LPS causes a steadily diminishing fever response because of tolerance due in part to reticuloendothelial blockade and in part to IgM antibodies to LPS.

Injection of LPS produces early **leukopenia,** as does bacteremia with gram-negative organisms. Secondary leukocytosis occurs later. The early leukopenia coincides with the onset of fever due to liberation of IL-1. LPS enhances glycolysis in many cell types and can lead to **hypoglycemia.**

Hypotension occurs early in gram-negative bacteremia or following injection of LPS. There may be widespread arteriolar and venular constriction followed by peripheral vascular dilatation, increased vascular permeability, decrease in venous return, lowered cardiac output, stagnation in the microcirculation, peripheral vasoconstriction, shock, and impaired organ perfusion and its consequences. Disseminated intravascular coagulation also contributes to these vascular changes.

LPS are among the many different agents that can activate the alternative pathway of the **complement cascade,** precipitating a variety of complement-mediated reactions (anaphylatoxins, chemotactic responses, membrane damage, etc) and a drop in serum levels of complement components (C3, C5–9).

Disseminated intravascular coagulation (DIC) is a frequent complication of gram-negative bacteremia and can also occur in other infections. LPS activates factor XII (Hageman factor)—the first step of the intrinsic clotting system—and sets into motion the coagulation cascade, which culminates in the conversion of fibrinogen to fibrin. At the same time, plasminogen can be activated by LPS to plasmin (a proteolytic enzyme), which can attack fibrin with the formation of fibrin split products. Reduction in platelet and fibrinogen levels and detection of fibrin split products are evidence of DIC. Heparin can sometimes prevent the lesions associated with DIC.

LPS causes platelets to adhere to vascular endothelium and occlusion of small blood vessels, causing ischemic or hemorrhagic necrosis in various organs.

Endotoxin levels can be assayed by the limulus test: a lysate of amebocytes from the horseshoe crab *(Limulus)* gels or coagulates in the presence of 0.0001 μg/mL of endotoxin.

D. Peptidoglycan of Gram-Positive Bacteria: The peptidoglycan of gram-positive bacteria are cross-linked macromolecules that surround the bacterial cells (Chapter 2 and Figure 2–15). Vascular changes leading to shock may also occur in infections due to gram-positive bacteria that contain no LPS. Gram-positive bacteria have considerably more cell wall-associated peptidoglycan than do gram-negative bacteria. Peptidoglycan released during infection may yield many of the same biologic activities as LPS, though peptidoglycan is invariably much less potent than LPS.

Enzymes

Many species of bacteria produce enzymes that are not intrinsically toxic but do play important roles in the infectious process. Some of these enzymes are discussed below.

A. Tissue-Degrading Enzymes: Many bacteria produce tissue-degrading enzymes. The best-characterized are enzymes from *C perfringens* (Chapter 12), *S aureus* (Chapter 14), group A streptococci (Chapter 15), and, to a lesser extent, anaerobic bacteria (Chapter 22). The roles of tissue-degrading enzymes in the pathogenesis of infections appear obvious but have been difficult to prove, especially those of individual enzymes. For example, antibodies against the tissue-degrading enzymes of streptococci do not modify the features of streptococcal disease.

In addition to **lecithinase, C perfringens** produces the proteolytic enzyme **collagenase,** which degrades collagen, the major protein of fibrous connective tissue, and promotes spread of infection in tissue.

S aureus produces **coagulase,** which works in conjunction with serum factors to coagulate plasma. Coagulase contributes to the formation of fibrin walls around staphylococcal lesions, which helps them persist in tissues. Coagulase also causes deposition of fibrin on the surfaces of individual staphylococci, which may help protect them from phagocytosis or from destruction within phagocytic cells.

Hyaluronidases are enzymes that hydrolyze hyaluronic acid, a constituent of the ground substance of connective tissue. They are produced by many bacteria (eg, staphylococci, streptococci, and anaerobes) and aid in their spread through tissues.

Many hemolytic streptococci produce **streptokinase (fibrinolysin),** a substance that activates a proteolytic enzyme of plasma. This enzyme is then able to dissolve coagulated plasma and probably aids in the rapid spread of streptococci through tissues. Streptokinase is used in treatment of acute myocardial infarction to dissolve fibrin clots.

Many bacteria produce substances that are **cytolysins**—ie, they dissolve red blood cells **(hemolysins)** or kill tissue cells or leukocytes **(leukocidins). Streptolysin O,** for example, is produced by group A streptococci and is lethal for mice and hemolytic for red blood cells from many animals. Streptolysin O is oxygen-labile and can therefore be oxidized and inactivated, but it is reactivated by reducing agents. It is antigenic. The same streptococci also produce oxygen-stable **streptolysin S,** which is not antigenic. Clostridia produce various hemolysins, including the lecithinase described above. Hemolysins are produced by most strains of *S aureus*; staphylococci also produce leukocidins. Most gram-negative rods isolated from sites of disease produce hemolysins. For example, *E coli* strains that cause urinary tract infections typically produce hemolysins, whereas those strains that are part of the normal gastrointestinal flora may or may not produce hemolysins.

B. IgA1 Proteases: Immunoglobulin A is the secretory antibody on mucosal surfaces. It has two primary forms, IgA1 and IgA2, that differ near the center, or hinge, region of the heavy chains of the molecules (Chapter 8). IgA1 has a series of amino acids in the hinge region that are not present in IgA2. Some bacteria that cause disease produce enzymes, **IgA1 proteases,** that split IgA1 at specific proline-threonine or proline-serine bonds in the hinge region and inactivate its antibody activity. IgA1 protease is an important virulence factor of the pathogens *N gonorrhoeae, N meningitidis, H influenzae,* and *S pneumoniae.* The enzymes are also produced by some strains of *Prevotella melaninogenica,* some streptococci associated with dental disease, and a few strains of other species that occasionally cause disease. Nonpathogenic species of the same genera do not have genes coding for the enzyme and do not produce it. Production of IgA1 protease allows pathogens to inactivate the primary antibody found on mucosal surfaces and thereby eliminate protection of the host by the antibody.

Antiphagocytic Factors

Many bacterial pathogens are rapidly killed once they are ingested by polymorphonuclear cells or macrophages. Some pathogens evade phagocytosis or leukocyte microbicidal mechanisms by adsorbing normal host components to their surfaces. For example, *S aureus* has surface protein A, which binds to the Fc portion of IgG. Other pathogens have surface factors that impede phagocytosis—eg, *S pneumoniae, N meningitidis;* and many other bacteria have polysaccharide capsules. *S pyogenes* (group A streptococci) have M protein. *N gonorrhoeae* (gonococci) have pili. Most of these antiphagocytic surface structures show much antigenic heterogeneity. For example, there are more than 80 pneumococcal capsular polysaccharide types and more than 80 M protein types of group A streptococci. Antibodies against one type of the antiphagocytic factor (eg, capsular polysaccharide, M protein) protect the host from disease caused by bacteria of that type but not from those with other types of the same factor.

A few bacteria (eg, *Capnocytophaga* and *Bordetella*) produce soluble factors or toxins that inhibit chemotaxis by leukocytes and thus evade phagocytosis by a different mechanism.

Intracellular Pathogenicity

Some bacteria (eg, *M tuberculosis, Brucella* species, and *Legionella* species) live and grow in the hostile environment within polymorphonuclear cells, macrophages, or monocytes. The bacteria accomplish this feat by several mechanisms: they may avoid entry into phagolysosomes and live within the cytosol of the phagocyte; they may prevent phagosome-lysosome fusion and live within the phagosome; or they may be resistant to lysosomal enzymes and survive within the phagolysosome.

Many bacteria can live within nonphagocytic cells (see Invasion of Host Cells and Tissues, above).

Antigenic Heterogeneity

The surface structures of bacteria (and of many other microorganisms) have considerable antigenic heterogeneity. Often these antigens are used as part of a serologic classification system for the bacteria. The classification of the 2000 or so different *Salmonella* species is based principally on the types of the O (lipopolysaccharide side chain) and H (flagellar) antigens. Similarly, there are more than 100 *E coli* O types and more than 100 *E coli* K (capsule) types. The antigenic type of the bacteria may be a marker for virulence, related to the clonal nature of pathogens, though it may not actually be the virulence factor (or factors). *V cholerae* O antigen type 1 and some O antigen type 139 typically produce cholera toxin, whereas very few of the many other O types produce the toxin. Only some of the 70 or more group A streptococcal M protein types are associated with a high incidence of poststreptococcal glomerulonephritis. *N meningitidis* capsular polysaccharide types A and C are associated with epidemic meningitis. In the examples cited above and in other typing systems that use surface antigens in serologic classification, antigenic types for a given isolate of the species remain constant during infection and on subculture of the bacteria.

Some bacteria and other microorganisms have the ability to make frequent shifts in the antigenic form of their surface structures in vitro and presumably in vivo. One well-known example is *Borrelia recurrentis,* which causes relapsing fever. A second widely studied example is *N gonorrhoeae* (see Chapter 21). The gonococcus has three surface-exposed antigens that switch forms at very high rates of about one in every 1000: lipooligosaccharide, 6–8 types; pili, innumerable types; and Opa (protein II), 8–12 types for each strain. The number of antigenic forms is so large that each strain of *N gonorrhoeae* appears to be antigenically distinct from every other strain. Switching of forms for each of the three antigens appears to be under the control of different genetic mechanisms. It is presumed that frequent switching of antigenic forms allows gonococci to evade the host's immune system; gonococci that are not attacked by the immune system survive and cause disease.

The Requirement for Iron

Pathogenic bacteria must be able to compete successfully for nutrients with nonpathogenic bacteria and with host cells, or they must alter the environment to suit their needs. Iron is the most thoroughly studied nutrient essential to the infectious process. Iron has a wide oxidation-reduction potential which makes it important in a variety of metabolic functions.

Like other cells, bacteria require 0.4–4 μmol/L of iron in order to grow. Humans and animals have an abundant amount of iron; however, most of it is located intracellularly (ie, in hemoglobin and myoglobin) and is not accessible to bacteria. Free iron in its ferric form (Fe^{3+}) occurs primarily as highly insoluble hydroxides, carbonates, and phosphates. The concentration of free ionic iron in blood, lymph, extracellular tissue fluid, and external secretions is very low, on the order of 10^{-18} mol/L Fe^{3+}. This low concentration of free ionic iron is due to the host's iron-binding and transport proteins, transferrin in blood and lymph, and lactoferrin in external secretions. Transferrin and lactoferrin have high association constants for Fe^{3+} and are only partially saturated under conditions of normal iron metabolism. Thus, the host's iron metabolism denies pathogenic bacteria an adequate source of iron for growth.

Bacteria have developed several methods to obtain sufficient iron for essential metabolism. Most bacteria have a low-affinity iron assimilation system, which permits them to use the polymeric forms of iron in spite of the low solubility of the ferric compounds. Some bacteria have evolved high-affinity iron assimilation systems. Part of these high-affinity systems involves **siderophores,** which are small (MW 500–1000) ligands that are specific for ferric iron and thus supply iron to the bacterial cell. Much variation exists among the siderophores that have been characterized, but most fall into two categories: catechols (phenolates), of which enterobactin is the best-characterized; and hydroxamates, of which ferrichrome is the best-characterized. Enterobactin is produced by *E coli* and some other Enterobacteriaceae. Hydroxamates are commonly found in fungi. Siderophore production is genetically responsive to the concentration of iron in the medium. For example, enterobactin is produced only under low-iron conditions. Siderophores function to capture iron; enterobactin can remove iron from transferrin. Once the siderophore captures the iron, it is internalized into the cell through the action of specific outer membrane protein receptors, which also are synthesized under conditions of low iron.

Some bacteria do not have demonstrable siderophores. *Y pestis* can utilize iron from hemin and may be able to initiate infection using iron from hemin in the gut of the biting flea. *N gonorrhoeae* makes a series of iron-regulated outer membrane proteins, but the mechanism by which these proteins function to capture and internalize iron is not well understood. Other bacteria (eg, *Legionella pneumophila, Listeria,* and *Salmonella* species and other bacteria) can obtain iron from the hosts' intracellular iron pools.

The availability of iron affects the virulence of pathogens. For example, the virulence of *N meningitidis* for mice is increased 1000-fold or more when the bacteria are grown under iron-limited conditions. Similar effects of iron on virulence have been shown for other species of bacteria. Some plasmids that have genes for virulence also encode for iron-sequestering systems.

REFERENCES

Brunham RC, Plummer FA, Stepehens RS: Bacterial antigenic variation, host immune response, and pathogen-host coevolution. Infect Immun 1993;61:2273.

Falkow S: Molecular Koch's postulates applied to microbial pathogenicity. Rev Infect Dis 1988;10(Suppl 3):S274.

Relman DA, Falkow S: A molecular perspective of microbial pathogenicity. In: *Principles and Practice of Infectious Diseases*, 4th ed. Mandell GL, Dolin R, Bennett JE, Dolan R (editors). Churchill Livingstone, 1995.

Salyers AA, Whitt DD: *Bacterial Pathogenesis: A Molecular Approach.* American Society for Microbiology Press, 1994.

Antimicrobial Chemotherapy 10

Chemicals have been used for the treatment of infectious diseases since the 17th century (eg, quinine for malaria and emetine for amebiasis); however, the science of chemotherapy began with Paul Ehrlich in the first decade of the 20th century. Ehrlich formulated the principles of selective toxicity and recognized the specific chemical relationships between parasites and drugs, the development of drug-fastness in parasites, and the role of combined therapy in combating this development. Ehrlich's experiments led to the arsphenamines, the first major triumph of planned chemotherapy.

The current era of antimicrobial chemotherapy began in 1935, with the discovery of the sulfonamides. In 1940, it was demonstrated that penicillin, which was discovered in 1929, could be made into an effective therapeutic substance. During the next 25 years, research on chemotherapeutic agents largely centered around substances of microbial origin called antibiotics. The isolation, concentration, purification, and mass production of penicillin were followed by the development of streptomycin, tetracyclines, chloramphenicol, and many other agents. These substances were originally isolated from filtrates of media in which their respective molds had grown. Subsequently, others have been synthesized, and in recent years biosynthetic modification of molecules has been a prominent method in the development of new antimicrobial agents.

Summaries of antimicrobial agents commonly employed in medical treatment of bacterial infections are presented in this chapter. The chemotherapy of viruses, fungi, and parasites are discussed in Chapters 30, 45, and 46, respectively. Additional comments on antimicrobial susceptibility testing for bacteria are offered in Chapter 47.

MECHANISMS OF ACTION OF CLINICALLY USED ANTIMICROBIAL DRUGS

Selective Toxicity

An ideal antimicrobial agent exhibits selective toxicity. This term implies that a drug is harmful to a parasite without being harmful to the host. Often, selective toxicity is relative rather than absolute; this implies that a drug in a concentration tolerated by the host may damage a parasite.

Selective toxicity may be a function of a specific receptor required for drug attachment, or it may depend on the inhibition of biochemical events essential to the parasite but not to the host. The mechanism of action of most antimicrobial drugs is not completely understood. However, these mechanisms of action can be placed under four headings:

(1) Inhibition of cell wall synthesis.

(2) Inhibition of cell membrane function.

(3) Inhibition of protein synthesis (ie, inhibition of translation and transcription of genetic material).

(4) Inhibition of nucleic acid synthesis.

Antimicrobial Action Through Inhibition of Cell Wall Synthesis (*Examples:* Bacitracin, Cephalosporins, Cycloserine, Penicillins, Vancomycin)

Bacteria possess a rigid outer layer, the cell wall. It maintains the shape of the microorganism and "corsets" the bacterial cell, which has a high internal osmotic pressure. The internal pressure is three to five times greater in gram-positive than in gram-negative bacteria. Injury to the cell wall (eg, by lysozyme) or inhibition of its formation may lead to lysis of the cell. In a hypertonic environment (eg, 20% sucrose), damaged cell wall formation leads to formation of spherical bacterial "protoplasts" from gram-positive organisms or "spheroplasts" from gram-negative organisms; these forms are limited by the fragile cytoplasmic membrane. If such **protoplasts** or **spheroplasts** are placed in an environment of ordinary tonicity, they take up fluid rapidly, swell, and may explode.

The cell wall contains a chemically distinct complex polymer "mucopeptide" ("murein," "peptidoglycan") consisting of polysaccharides and a highly cross-linked polypeptide. The polysaccharides regularly contain the amino sugars N-acetylglucosamine and acetylmuramic acid. The latter is found only in bacteria. To the amino sugars are attached short peptide chains. The final rigidity of the cell wall is imparted by cross-linking of the peptide chains (eg, through pentaglycine bonds) as a result of transpeptidation reactions carried out by several enzymes. The peptidoglycan layer is much thicker in the cell wall of gram-positive than of gram-negative bacteria.

All β-lactam drugs are selective inhibitors of bacterial cell wall synthesis and, thus, active against growing bacteria. This inhibition is only one of several different activities of these drugs, but it is the best understood. The initial step in drug action consists of binding of the drug to cell receptors ("penicillin-binding proteins," PBPs). There are 3–6 PBPs (MW 4–12 $\times 10^5$), some of which are transpeptidation enzymes. Different receptors have different affinities for a drug, and each may mediate a different effect. For example, attachment of penicillin to one PBP may result chiefly in abnormal elongation of the cell, whereas attachment to another PBP may lead to a defect in the periphery of the cell wall, with resulting cell lysis. PBPs are under chromosomal control, and mutations may alter their number or their affinity for β-lactam drugs.

After a β-lactam drug has attached to one or more receptors, the transpeptidation reaction is inhibited and peptidoglycan synthesis is blocked. The next step probably involves the removal or inactivation of an inhibitor of autolytic enzymes in the cell wall. This activates the lytic enzyme and results in lysis if the environment is isotonic. In a markedly hypertonic environment, the microbes change to protoplasts or spheroplasts, covered only by the fragile cell membrane. In such cells, synthesis of proteins and nucleic acids may continue for some time.

The inhibition of the transpeptidation enzymes by penicillins and cephalosporins may be due to a structural similarity of these drugs to acyl-D-alanyl-D-alanine. The transpeptidation reaction involves loss of a D-alanine from the pentapeptide.

The remarkable lack of toxicity of β-lactam drugs to mammalian cells must be attributed to the absence of a bacterial type cell wall, with its peptidoglycan, in animal cells. The difference in susceptibility of gram-positive and gram-negative bacteria to various penicillins or cephalosporins probably depends on structural differences in their cell walls (eg, amount of peptidoglycan, presence of receptors and lipids, nature of cross-linking, activity of autolytic enzymes) that determine penetration, binding, and activity of the drugs.

Resistance to penicillins may be determined by the organism's production of penicillin-destroying enzymes (β-lactamases). **Beta-lactamases** open the β-lactam ring of penicillins and cephalosporins and abolish their antimicrobial activity. Beta-lactamases have been described for many species of gram-positive and gram-negative bacteria. Some β-lactamases are plasmid-mediated (eg, penicillinase of *Staphylococcus aureus*). while others are chromosomally mediated (eg, many species gram-negative bacteria). All of the more than 30 plasmid-mediated β-lactamases are produced constitutively; many are encoded by genes on plasmids and have a high propensity to move from one species of bacteria to another (eg, β-lactamase-producing *Neisseria gonorrhoeae, Haemophilus influenzae,* and, most recently, enterococci). Chromosomally mediated β-lactamases may be constitutively produced (eg, *Bacteroides, Acinetobacter*), or they may be inducible (eg, *Enterobacter, Citrobacter, Pseudomonas*).

The classification of β-lactamases is complex, based upon the genetics, biochemical properties, and substrate affinity for a β-lactamase inhibitor (clavulanic acid). Clavulanic acid, sulbactam, and tazobactam are β-lactamase inhibitors that have a high affinity for and irreversibly bind some β-lactamases (eg, penicillinase of *Staphylococcus aureus*) but are not hydrolyzed by the β-lactamase. These inhibitors protect simultaneously present hydrolyzable penicillins (eg, ampicillin, amoxicillin, and ticarcillin) from destruction. Certain penicillins (eg, cloxacillin) also have a high affinity for β-lactamases.

There are two other types of resistance mechanisms. One is due to the absence of some penicillin receptors (PBPs) and occurs as a result of chromosomal mutation; the other results from failure of the β-lactam drug to activate the autolytic enzymes in the cell wall. As a result, the organism is inhibited but not killed. Such **tolerance** has been observed especially with staphylococci and certain streptococci.

Several other drugs, including bacitracin, teichoplanin, vancomycin, ristocetin, and novobiocin, inhibit early steps in the biosynthesis of the peptidoglycan. Since the early stages of synthesis take place inside the cytoplasmic membrane, these drugs must penetrate the membrane to be effective. For these drugs, inhibition of peptidoglycan synthesis is not the sole mode of antibacterial action.

Antimicrobial Action Through Inhibition of Cell Membrane Function (*Examples:* Amphotericin B, Colistin, Imidazoles, Polyenes, Polymyxins)

The cytoplasm of all living cells is bounded by the cytoplasmic membrane, which serves as a selective permeability barrier, carries out active transport functions, and thus controls the internal composition of the cell. If the functional integrity of the cytoplasmic membrane is disrupted, macromolecules and ions escape from the cell, and cell damage or death ensues. The cytoplasmic membrane of bacteria and fungi has a structure different from that of animal cells and can be more readily disrupted by certain agents. Consequently, selective chemotherapy is possible.

Examples of this mechanism are the polymyxins acting on gram-negative bacteria and polyenes acting on fungi. Polyenes require binding to a sterol which is present in the fungal cell membrane but lacking in the bacterial cell membrane. Conversely, polymyxins are inactive against fungi and polyenes are inactive against bacteria—a striking example of selective toxicity.

Antimicrobial Action Through Inhibition of Protein Synthesis (*Examples:* Chloramphenicol, Erythromycins, Lincomycins, Tetracyclines; Aminoglycosides)

It is established that chloramphenicol, tetracyclines, aminoglycosides, erythromycins, and lincomycins can inhibit protein synthesis in bacteria. The precise mechanisms of action are not fully established for these drugs.

Bacteria have 70S ribosomes, whereas mammalian cells have 80S ribosomes. The subunits of each type of ribosome, their chemical composition, and their functional specificities are sufficiently different to explain why antimicrobial drugs can inhibit protein synthesis in bacterial ribosomes without having a major effect on mammalian ribosomes.

In normal microbial protein synthesis, the mRNA message is simultaneously "read" by several ribosomes that are strung out along the mRNA strand. These are called **polysomes**.

A. Aminoglycosides: The mode of action of streptomycin has been studied far more than that of other aminoglycosides (kanamycin, neomycin, gentamicin, tobramycin, amikacin, etc), but probably all act similarly. The first step is the attachment of the aminoglycoside to a specific receptor protein (P 12 in the case of streptomycin) on the 30S subunit of the microbial ribosome. Second, the aminoglycoside blocks the normal activity of the "initiation complex" of peptide formation (mRNA + formyl methionine + tRNA). Third, the mRNA message is misread on the "recognition region" of the ribosome; consequently the wrong amino acid is inserted into the peptide, resulting in a nonfunctional protein. Fourth, aminoglycoside attachment results in the breakup of polysomes and their separation into **monosomes** incapable of protein synthesis. These activities occur more or less simultaneously, and the overall effect is usually an irreversible event—killing of the bacterium.

Chromosomal resistance of microbes to aminoglycosides principally depends on the lack of a specific protein receptor on the 30S subunit of the ribosome. Plasmid-dependent resistance to aminoglycosides depends on the production by the microorganism of adenylylating, phosphorylating, or acetylating enzymes that destroy the drugs. A third type of resistance consists of a "permeability defect," an outer membrane change that reduces active transport of the aminoglycoside into the cell so that the drug cannot reach the ribosome. Often this is plasmid-mediated.

B. Tetracyclines: Tetracyclines bind to the 30S subunit of microbial ribosomes. They inhibit protein synthesis by blocking the attachment of charged aminoacyl-tRNA. Thus, they prevent introduction of new amino acids to the nascent peptide chain. The action is usually inhibitory and reversible upon withdrawal of the drug. Resistance to tetracyclines results from changes in permeability of the microbial cell envelope. In susceptible cells, the drug is concentrated from the environment and does not readily leave the cell. In resistant cells, the drug is not actively transported into the cell or leaves it so rapidly that inhibitory concentrations are not maintained. This is often plasmid-controlled. Mammalian cells do not actively concentrate tetracyclines.

C. Chloramphenicol: Chloramphenicol binds to the 50S subunit of the ribosome. It interferes with the binding of new amino acids to the nascent peptide chain, largely because chloramphenicol inhibits peptidyl transferase. Chloramphenicol is mainly bacteriostatic, and growth of microorganisms resumes (ie, drug action is reversible) when the drug is withdrawn. Microorganisms resistant to chloramphenicol produce the enzyme chloramphenicol acetyltransferase, which destroys drug activity. The production of this enzyme is usually under control of a plasmid.

D. Macrolides (Erythromycins, Azithromycin, Clarithromycin): These drugs bind to the 50S subunit of the ribosome, and the binding site is a 23S rRNA. They may interfere with formation of initiation complexes for peptide chain synthesis or may interfere with aminoacyl translocation reactions. Some macrolide-resistant bacteria lack the proper receptor on the ribosome (through methylation of the rRNA). This may be under plasmid or chromosomal control.

E. Lincomycins (Lincomycin, Clindamycin): Lincomycins bind to the 50S subunit of the microbial ribosome and resemble macrolides in binding site, antibacterial activity, and mode of action. There may be mutual interference between these drugs. Chromosomal mutants are resistant because they lack the proper binding site on the 50S subunit.

Antimicrobial Action Through Inhibition of Nucleic Acid Synthesis (*Examples:* Quinolones, Pyrimethamine, Rifampin, Sulfonamides, Trimethoprim)

Rifampin inhibits bacterial growth by binding strongly to the DNA-dependent RNA polymerase of bacteria. Thus, it inhibits bacterial RNA synthesis. Rifampin resistance results from a change in RNA polymerase due to a chromosomal mutation that occurs with high frequency. The mechanism of rifampin action on viruses is different. It blocks a late stage in the assembly of poxviruses.

All quinolones and fluoroquinolones inhibit microbial DNA synthesis by blocking DNA gyrase.

For many microorganisms, p-aminobenzoic acid (PABA) is an essential metabolite. The specific mode of action of PABA involves an adenosine triphosphate (ATP)-dependent condensation of a pteridine with PABA to yield dihydropteroic acid, which is subsequently converted to folic acid. PABA is involved in the synthesis of folic acid, an important precursor to the synthesis of nucleic acids. Sulfonamides are structural analogues of PABA and inhibit dihydropteroate synthetase.

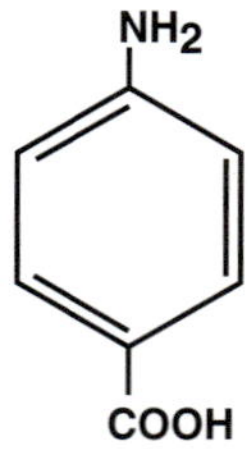

p–Aminobenzoic acid (PABA)

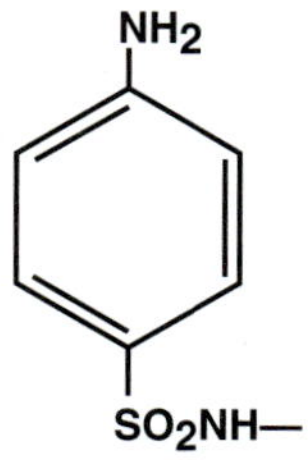

Basic ring structure of sulfonamides

Sulfonamides can enter into the reaction in place of PABA and compete for the active center of the enzyme. As a result, nonfunctional analogues of folic acid are formed, preventing further growth of the bacterial cell. The inhibiting action of sulfonamides on bacterial growth can be counteracted by an excess of PABA in the environment (competitive inhibition). Animal cells cannot synthesize folic acid and must depend upon exogenous sources. Some bacteria, like animal cells, are not inhibited by sulfonamides. Many other bacteria, however, synthesize folic acid as mentioned above and consequently are susceptible to action by sulfonamides.

Trimethoprim (3,4,5-trimethoxybenzyl pyrimidine) inhibits dihydrofolic acid reductase 50,000 times more efficiently in bacteria than in mammalian cells. This enzyme reduces dihydrofolic to tetrahydrofolic acid, a stage in the sequence leading to the synthesis of purines and ultimately of DNA. Sulfonamides and trimethoprim each can be used alone to inhibit bacterial growth. If used together, they produce sequential blocking, resulting in a marked enhancement (synergism) of activity. Such mixtures of sulfonamide (5 parts) + trimethoprim (1 part) have been used in the treatment of *Pneumocystis* pneumonia, malaria, *Shigella* enteritis, systemic *Salmonella* infections, urinary tract infections, and many others.

Pyrimethamine also inhibits dihydrofolate reductase, but it is more active against the enzyme in mammalian cells and therefore is more toxic than trimethoprim. Pyrimethamine plus sulfonamide or clindamycin is the current treatment of choice in toxoplasmosis and some other protozoal infections. A number of inhibitors of nucleic acid synthesis are sufficiently selective to serve as antiviral drugs (see Chapter 30).

RESISTANCE TO ANTIMICROBIAL DRUGS

There are many different mechanisms by which microorganisms might exhibit resistance to drugs. The following are fairly well supported.

(1) Microorganisms produce enzymes that destroy the active drug. ***Examples:*** Staphylococci resistant to penicillin G produce a β-lactamase that destroys the drug. Other β-lactamases are produced by gram-negative rods. Gram-negative bacteria resistant to aminoglycosides (by virtue of a plasmid) produce adenylylating, phosphorylating, or acetylating enzymes that destroy the drug. Gram-negative bacteria may be resistant to chloramphenicol if they produce a chloramphenicol acetyltransferase.

(2) Microorganisms change their permeability to the drug. ***Examples:*** Tetracyclines accumulate in susceptible bacteria but not in resistant bacteria. Resistance to polymyxins is also associated with a change in permeability to the drugs. Streptococci have a natural permeability barrier to aminoglycosides. This can be partly overcome by the simultaneous presence of a cell wall-active drug, eg, a penicillin. Resistance to amikacin and to some other aminoglycosides may depend on a lack of permeability to the drugs, apparently due to an outer membrane change that impairs active transport into the cell.

(3) Microorganisms develop an altered structural target for the drug. ***Examples:*** Chromosomal resistance to aminoglycosides is associated with the loss or alteration of a specific protein in the 30S subunit of the bacterial ribosome that serves as a binding site in susceptible organisms. Erythromycin-resistant organisms have an altered receptor on the 50S subunit of the ribosome, resulting from methylation of a 23S ribosomal RNA. Resistance to some penicillins and cephalosporins may be a function of the loss or alteration of PBPs.

(4) Microorganisms develop an altered metabolic pathway that bypasses the reaction inhibited by the drug. Example: Some sulfonamide-resistant bacteria do not require extracellular PABA but, like mammalian cells, can utilize preformed folic acid.

(5) Microorganisms develop an altered enzyme that can still perform its metabolic function but is much less affected by the drug than the enzyme in the susceptible organism. ***Example:*** In trimethoprim-resistant bacteria, the dihydrofolic acid reductase is inhibited far less efficiently than in trimethoprim-susceptible bacteria.

ORIGIN OF DRUG RESISTANCE

The origin of drug resistance may be genetic or nongenetic.

Nongenetic Origin

Active replication of bacteria is usually required for most antibacterial drug actions. Consequently, microorganisms that are metabolically inactive (nonmultiplying) may be phenotypically resistant to drugs. However, their offspring are fully susceptible. ***Example:*** Mycobacteria often survive in tissues for many years after infection yet are restrained by the host's defenses and do not multiply. Such "persisting" organisms are resistant to treatment and cannot be eradicated by drugs. Yet if they start to multiply (eg, following suppression of cellular immunity in the patient), they are fully susceptible to the same drugs.

Microorganisms may lose the specific target structure for a drug for several generations and thus be resistant. ***Example:*** Penicillin-susceptible organisms may change to cell wall-deficient L forms during penicillin administration. Lacking cell walls, they are resistant to cell wall-inhibitor drugs (penicillins, cephalosporins) and may remain so for several generations. When these organisms revert to their bacterial parent forms by resuming cell wall production, they are again susceptible to penicillin.

Genetic Origin

Most drug-resistant microbes emerge as a result of genetic change and subsequent selection processes by antimicrobial drugs.

A. Chromosomal Resistance: This develops as a result of spontaneous mutation in a locus that controls susceptibility to a given antimicrobial drug. The presence of the antimicrobial drug serves as a selecting mechanism to suppress susceptible organisms and favor the growth of drug-resistant mutants. Spontaneous mutation occurs with a frequency of 10^{-12} to 10^{-7} and thus is an infrequent cause of the emergence of clinical drug resistance in a given patient. However, chromosomal mutants resistant to rifampin occur with high frequency (about 10^{-7} to 10^{-5}). Consequently, treatment of bacterial infections with rifampin as the sole drug often fails. Chromosomal mutants are most commonly resistant by virtue of a change in a structural receptor for a drug. Thus, the P 12 protein on the 30S subunit of the bacterial ribosome serves as a receptor for streptomycin attachment. Mutation in the gene controlling that structural protein results in streptomycin resistance. A narrow region of the bacterial chromosome contains structural genes that code for a number of drug receptors, including those for erythromycin, lincomycin, and aminoglycosides. Mutation can also result in the loss of PBPs, making such mutants resistant to β-lactam drugs.

B. Extrachromosomal Resistance: Bacteria often contain extrachromosomal genetic elements called plasmids. Their features are described in Chapter 7.

R factors are a class of plasmids that carry genes for resistance to one—and often several—antimicrobial drugs and heavy metals. Plasmid genes for antimicrobial resistance often control the formation of enzymes capable of destroying the antimicrobial drugs. Thus, plasmids determine resistance to penicillins and cephalosporins by carrying genes for the formation of β-lactamases. Plasmids code for enzymes that destroy chloramphenicol (acetyltransferase); for enzymes that acetylate, adenylylate, or phosphorylate various aminoglycosides; for enzymes that determine the active transport of tetracyclines across the cell membrane; and for others.

Genetic material and plasmids can be transferred by the following mechanisms:

1. Transduction–Plasmid DNA is enclosed in a bacterial virus and transferred by the virus to another bacterium of the same species. ***Example:*** The plasmid carrying the gene for β-lactamase production can be transferred from a penicillin-resistant to a susceptible *Staphylococcus* if carried by a suitable bacteriophage. Similar transduction occurs in salmonellae.

2. Transformation–Naked DNA passes from one cell of a species to another cell, thus altering its genotype. This can occur through laboratory manipulation.

3. Conjugation–A unilateral transfer of genetic material between bacteria of the same or different genera occurs during a mating (conjugation) process. This is mediated by a fertility (F) factor that results in the extension of sex pili from the donor (F^+) cell to the recipient. Plasmid or other DNA is transferred through these protein tubules from the donor to the recipient cell. A series of closely linked genes, each determining resistance to one drug, may thus be transferred from a resistant to a susceptible bacterium. This is the commonest method by which multidrug resistance spreads among different genera of gram-negative bacteria. Transfer of resistance plasmids also occurs among some gram-positive cocci.

4. Transposition–A transfer of short DNA sequences (transposons, transposable elements) occurs between one plasmid and another or between a plasmid and a portion of the bacterial chromosome within a bacterial cell.

Cross-Resistance

Microorganisms resistant to a certain drug may also be resistant to other drugs that share a mechanism of action. Such relationships exist mainly between agents that are closely related chemically (eg, different aminoglycosides) or that have a similar mode of binding or action (eg, macrolides-lincomycins). In certain classes of drugs, the active nucleus of the chemical is so similar among many congeners (eg, tetracyclines) that extensive cross-resistance is to be expected.

Limitation of Drug Resistance

Emergence of drug resistance in infections may be minimized in the following ways: (1) maintain sufficiently high levels of the drug in the tissues to inhibit both the original population and first-step mutants; (2) simultaneously administer two drugs that do not give cross-resistance, each of which delays the emergence of mutants resistant to the other drug (eg, rifampin and isoniazid in the treatment of tuberculosis); and (3) avoid exposure of microorganisms to a particularly valuable drug by limiting its use, especially in hospitals and in animal feeds.

Clinical Implications of Drug Resistance

A few examples will illustrate the impact of the emergence of drug-resistant organisms and their selection by the widespread use of antimicrobial drugs.

(1) Gonococci: When sulfonamides were first employed in the late 1930s for the treatment of gonorrhea, virtually all isolates of gonococci were susceptible and most infections were cured. A few years later, most strains had become resistant to sulfonamides, and gonorrhea was rarely curable by these drugs. Most gonococci were still highly susceptible to penicillin. Over the next decades, there was a gradual increase in resistance to penicillin, but large doses of that drug were still curative. In the 1970s, β-lactamase-producing gonococci appeared, first in the Philippines and in West Africa, and then spread to form endemic foci worldwide. Such infections could not be treated effectively by penicillin but were treated with spectinomycin. Resistance to spectinomycin has appeared. Second- and third-generation cephalosporins or quinolones are recommended to treat gonorrhea.

(2) Meningococci: Until 1962, meningococci were uniformly susceptible to sulfonamides, and these drugs were effective for both prophylaxis and therapy. Subsequently, sulfonamide-resistant meningococci spread widely, and the sulfonamides have now lost most of their usefulness against meningococcal infections. Penicillins remain effective for therapy, and rifampin is employed for prophylaxis. However, rifampin-resistant meningococci persist in about 1% of individuals who have received rifampin for prophylaxis.

(3) Staphylococci: In 1944, most staphylococci were susceptible to penicillin, although a few resistant strains had been observed. After massive use of penicillin, 65–85% of staphylococci isolated from hospitals in 1948 were β-lactamase producers and thus resistant to penicillin G. The advent of β-lactamase-resistant penicillins (eg, methicillin) provided a temporary respite, but outbreaks of infections due to methicillin-resistant staphylococci now occur intermittently. In 1986, penicillin-resistant staphylococci included not only those acquired in hospital but also 80–90% of those isolated in the community. These organisms also tend to be resistant to other drugs, eg, tetracyclines. Methicillin-resistant staphylococci produce intermittent hospital outbreaks but are fortunately still susceptible to vancomycin.

(4) Pneumococci: Until 1963, pneumococci were uniformly susceptible to penicillin G; in that year, some relatively penicillin-resistant pneumococci were found in New Guinea. Such organisms have been encountered since 1977 in hospital outbreaks, first in South Africa and then elsewhere. While they do not produce β-lactamase, they are resistant or relatively resistant to penicillin G, probably because of altered PBPs.

(5) Gram-negative enteric bacteria: Most drug resistance in enteric bacteria is attributable to the widespread transmission of resistance plasmids among different genera. About half the strains of *Shigella* species in many parts of the world are now resistant to multiple drugs.

Salmonellae carried by animals have developed resistance also, particularly to drugs (especially tetracyclines) incorporated in animal feeds. The practice of incorporating drugs into animal feeds causes farm animals to grow more rapidly but is associated with an increase in drug-resistant enteric organisms in the fecal flora of farm workers. A concomitant rise in drug-resistant *Salmonella* infections in Britain led to a restriction on antibiotic supplements in animal feeds. Continued use of tetracycline supplements in animal feeds in the USA may contribute to the spread of resistance plasmids and of drug-resistant salmonellae.

Plasmids carrying drug resistance genes occur in many gram-negative bacteria of the normal gut flora. The abundant use of antimicrobial drugs—particularly in hospitalized patients—leads to the suppression of drug-susceptible organisms in the gut flora and favors the persistence and growth of drug-resistant bacteria, including *Enterobacter, Klebsiella, Proteus, Pseudomonas, Serratia,* and fungi. Such organisms present particularly difficult problems in granulopenic and immunocompromised patients. The closed environment of hospitals favors transmission of such resistant organisms through personnel and fomites as well as by direct contact.

(6) Tubercle bacilli: Drug-resistant mutants have arisen in tuberculosis, especially in patients infected with HIV. Resistant tubercle bacilli may complicate the treatment of individual patients in whom they arise and may be transmitted to contacts, giving rise to primary drug-resistant infections.

ANTIMICROBIAL ACTIVITY IN VITRO

Antimicrobial activity is measured in vitro in order to determine (1) the potency of an antibacterial agent in solution, (2) its concentration in body fluids or tissues, and (3) the sensitivity of a given microorganism to known concentrations of the drug.

Measurement of Antimicrobial Activity

Determination of these quantities may be undertaken by one of two principal methods: dilution or diffusion.

Using an appropriate standard test organism and a known sample of drug for comparison, these methods can be employed to estimate either the potency of antibiotic in the sample or the sensitivity of the microorganism.

A. Dilution Method: Graded amounts of antimicrobial substances are incorporated into liquid or solid bacteriologic media. The media are subsequently inoculated with test bacteria and incubated. The end point is taken as that amount of antimicrobial substance required to inhibit the growth of, or to kill, the test bacteria. Agar-dilution susceptibility tests are time-consuming, and their use is limited to special circumstances. Broth-dilution tests were cumbersome and little used when dilutions had to be made in test tubes; however, the advent of prepared broth-dilution series for many different drugs in microdilution plates has greatly enhanced and simplified the method. The advantage of microdilution broth-dilution tests is that they permit a quantitative result to be reported, indicating the amount of a given drug necessary to inhibit (or kill) the microorganisms tested.

B. Diffusion Method: A filter paper disk, a porous cup, or a bottomless cylinder containing measured quantities of drug is placed on a solid medium that has been heavily seeded with the test organisms. After incubation, the diameter of the clear zone of inhibition surrounding the deposit of drug is taken as a measure of the inhibitory power of the drug against the particular test organism. This method is subject to many physical and chemical factors in addition to the simple interaction of drug and organisms (eg, nature of medium and diffusibility, molecular size, and stability of drug). Nevertheless, standardization of conditions permits quantitative assay of drug potency or sensitivity of the organism.

When determining bacterial sensitivity by the diffusion method, most laboratories use disks of antibiotic-impregnated filter paper. A concentration gradient of antibiotic is produced in the medium by diffusion from the disk. As the diffusion is a continuous process, the concentration gradient is never stable for long; but some stabilization can be achieved by allowing diffusion to start before bacterial growth begins. The greatest difficulties arise from the varying growth rates of different microorganisms.

Interpretation of the results of diffusion tests must be based on comparisons between dilution and diffusion methods. Such comparisons have led to the establishment of reference standards. Linear regression lines can express the relationship between log of minimum inhibitory concentration in dilution tests and diameter of inhibition zones in diffusion tests.

Use of a single disk for each antibiotic with careful standardization of the test conditions permits the report of susceptible or resistant for a microorganism by comparing the size of the inhibition zone against a standard of the same drug (Kirby-Bauer method).

Inhibition around a disk containing a certain amount of antimicrobial drug does not imply susceptibility to that same concentration of drug per milliliter of medium, blood, or urine.

Factors Affecting Antimicrobial Activity

Among the many factors that affect antimicrobial activity in vitro, the following must be considered, because they significantly influence the results of tests.

A. pH of Environment: Some drugs are more active at acid pH (eg, nitrofurantoin); others, at alkaline pH (eg, aminoglycosides, sulfonamides).

B. Components of Medium: Sodium polyanethol sulfonate and other anionic detergents inhibit aminoglycosides. PABA in tissue extracts antagonizes sulfonamides. Serum proteins bind penicillins in varying degrees, ranging from 40% for methicillin to 98% for dicloxacillin. Addition of NaCl to the medium enhances the detection of methicillin resistance in *S aureus*.

C. Stability of Drug: At incubator temperature, several antimicrobial agents lose their activity. Chlortetracycline is inactivated rapidly and penicillins more slowly, whereas aminoglycosides, chloramphenicol, and ciprofloxacin are quite stable for long periods.

D. Size of Inoculum: In general, the larger the bacterial inoculum, the lower the apparent "sensitivity" of the organism. Large bacterial populations are less promptly and completely inhibited than small ones. In addition, a resistant mutant is much more likely to emerge in large populations.

E. Length of Incubation: In many instances, microorganisms are not killed but only inhibited upon short exposure to antimicrobial agents. The longer incubation continues, the greater the chance for resistant mutants to emerge or for the least susceptible members of the antimicrobial population to begin multiplying as the drug deteriorates.

F. Metabolic Activity of Microorganisms: In general, actively and rapidly growing organisms are more susceptible to drug action than those in the resting phase. Metabolically inactive organisms that survive long exposure to a drug may have offspring that are fully susceptible to the same drug.

ANTIMICROBIAL ACTIVITY IN VIVO

The problem of the activity of antimicrobial agents is much more complex in vivo than in vitro. It involves not only drug and parasite but also a third factor, the host. The interrelationships of host, drug, and parasite are diagrammed in Figure 10–1. Drug-parasite and host-parasite relationships are discussed in the following paragraphs. Host-drug relationships (absorption, excretion, distribution, metabolism, and toxicity) are dealt with mainly in pharmacology texts.

DRUG-PARASITE RELATIONSHIPS

Several important interactions between drug and parasite have been discussed in the preceding pages. The following are additional important in vivo factors.

Environment

The environment in the test tube is constant for all members of a microbial population. In the host, how-

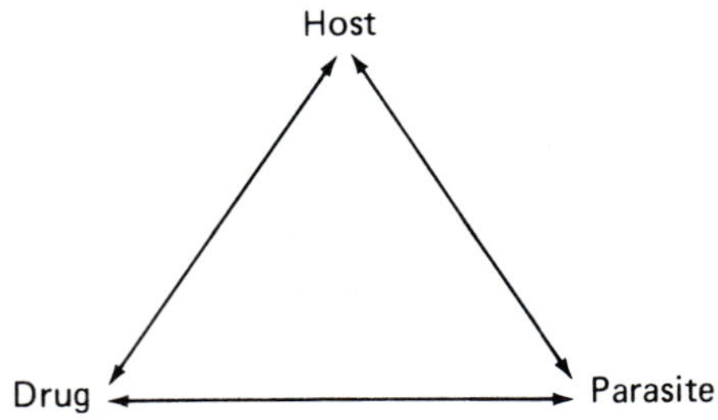

Figure 10–1. Interrelationships of host, drug, and parasite.

ever, varying environment influences affect microorganisms located in different tissues and in different parts of the body. Therefore, the response of the microbial population is much less uniform within the host than in the test tube.

A. State of Metabolic Activity: In the test tube, the state of metabolic activity is relatively uniform for the majority of microorganisms. In the body, it is diverse; undoubtedly, many organisms are at a low level of biosynthetic activity and are thus relatively insusceptible to drug action. These "dormant" microorganisms often survive exposure to high concentrations of drugs and subsequently may produce a clinical relapse of the infection. Alternatively, cell wall-deficient forms may be insusceptible to drugs that inhibit cell wall formation.

B. Distribution of Drug: In the test tube, all microorganisms are equally exposed to the drug. In the body, the antimicrobial agent is unequally distributed in tissues and fluids. Many drugs do not reach the central nervous system effectively. The concentration in urine is often much greater than the concentration in blood or tissue. The tissue response induced by the microorganism may protect it from the drug. Necrotic tissue or pus may adsorb the drug and thus prevent its contact with bacteria.

C. Location of Organisms: In the test tube, the microorganisms come into direct contact with the drug. In the body, they may often be located within tissue cells. Drugs enter tissue cells at different rates. Some (eg, tetracyclines) reach about the same concentration inside monocytes as in the extracellular fluid. With others (eg, streptomycin), the intracellular concentration is only a small fraction (perhaps 5–10%) of the extracellular concentration.

D. Interfering Substances: In the test tube, drug activity may be impaired by binding of the drug to protein or to lipids or by interaction with salts. The biochemical environment of microorganisms in the body is very complex and results in significant interference with drug action. The drug may be bound by blood and tissue proteins or phospholipids; it may also react with nucleic acids in pus and may be physically adsorbed onto exudates, cells, and necrotic debris. In necrotic tissue, the pH may be highly acid and thus unfavorable for drug action (eg, aminoglycosides).

Concentration

In the test tube, microorganisms are exposed to an essentially constant concentration of drug. In the body, this is not so.

A. Absorption: The absorption of drugs from the intestinal tract (if taken by mouth) or from tissues (if injected) is irregular. There is also a continuous excretion as well as inactivation of the drug. Consequently, the levels of drug in body compartments fluctuate continually, and the microorganisms are exposed to varying concentrations of the antimicrobial agent.

B. Distribution: The distribution of drugs varies greatly with different tissues. Some drugs penetrate certain tissues poorly (eg, central nervous system, prostate). Drug concentrations following systemic administration may therefore be inadequate for effective treatment. In such situations, the drug may be administered locally (eg, injection of drugs into the central nervous system). On surface wounds or mucous membranes, local (topical) application of poorly absorbed drugs permits highly effective local concentrations without toxic side effects. Alternatively, some drugs applied topically on surface wounds are well absorbed. Drug concentrations in urine are often much higher than in blood.

C. Variability of Concentration: It is critical to maintain an effective concentration of a drug where the infecting microorganisms proliferate for a sufficient length of time to eradicate them. Because the drug is administered intermittently and is absorbed and excreted irregularly, the levels constantly fluctuate at the site of infection. In order to maintain sufficient drug concentrations for a sufficient time, the time-dose relationship has to be considered. The larger each individual drug dose, the longer the permissible interval between doses. The smaller the individual dose, the shorter the interval that will ensure adequate drug levels. A good general rule in antimicrobial therapy is as follows: Give a sufficiently large amount of an effective drug as early as possible and continue treatment long enough to ensure eradication of infection, but give an antimicrobial drug only when it is indicated by rational choice.

HOST-PARASITE RELATIONSHIPS

Host-parasite relationships may be altered by antimicrobial drugs in several ways.

Alteration of Tissue Response

The inflammatory response of the tissue to infections may be altered if the drug suppresses the multiplication of microorganisms but does not eliminate them from the body, and an acute process may in this way be transformed into a chronic one. Conversely, the suppression of inflammatory reactions in tissues by impairment of cell-mediated immunity in recipients of tissue transplants, antineoplastic therapy, or immunocompromise by disease (eg, AIDS) causes enhanced susceptibility to infection and diminished response to antimicrobial drugs.

Alteration of Immune Response

If an infection is modified by an antimicrobial drug, the immune response of the host may also be altered. An example will suffice to illustrate this phenomenon.

Infection with β-hemolytic group A streptococci is followed frequently by the development of antistreptococcal antibodies and occasionally by rheumatic fever. If the infective process can be interrupted early and completely with antimicrobial drugs, the development of an immune response and of rheumatic fever can be prevented (presumably by rapid elimination of the antigen). Drugs and doses that rapidly eradicate the infecting streptococci (eg, penicillin) are more effective in preventing rheumatic fever than those that merely suppress the microorganisms temporarily (eg, tetracycline).

Alteration of Microbial Flora

Antimicrobial drugs affect not only the infecting microorganisms but also susceptible members of the normal microbial flora of the body. An imbalance is thus created that in itself may lead to disease. A few examples will serve:

(1) In hospitalized patients who receive antimicrobials, the normal microbial flora is suppressed. This creates a partial void that is filled by the organisms most prevalent in the environment, particularly drug-resistant gram-negative aerobic bacteria (eg, *Pseudomonas*), staphylococci, fungi, etc. Such superinfecting organisms subsequently may produce serious drug-resistant infections.

(2) In women taking antibiotics by mouth, the normal vaginal flora may be suppressed, permitting marked overgrowth of *Candida.* This leads to unpleasant local inflammation (vaginitis) and itching that is difficult to control.

(3) In the presence of urinary tract obstruction, the tendency to bladder infection is great. When such urinary tract infection due to a sensitive microorganism (eg, *Escherichia coli*) is treated with an appropriate drug, the organism may be eradicated. However, very often a reinfection due to drug-resistant *Proteus, Pseudomonas,* or *Enterobacter* occurs after the drug-sensitive microorganisms are eliminated. A similar process accounts for respiratory tract superinfections in patients given antimicrobials for chronic bronchitis.

(4) In persons receiving antimicrobial drugs by mouth for several days, parts of the normal intestinal flora may be suppressed. Drug-resistant organisms may establish themselves in the bowel in great numbers and may precipitate serious enterocolitis (*Clostridium difficile,* staphylococci, etc).

CLINICAL USE OF ANTIBIOTICS

Selection of Antibiotics

The rational selection of antimicrobial drugs depends upon the following:

A. Diagnosis: A specific etiologic diagnosis must be formulated. This can often be done on the basis of a clinical impression. Thus, in typical lobar pneumonia or acute urinary tract infection, the relationship between clinical picture and causative agent is sufficiently constant to permit selection of the antibiotic of choice on the basis of clinical impression alone. Even in these cases, however, as a safeguard against diagnostic error, it is preferable to obtain a representative specimen for bacteriologic study before giving antimicrobial drugs.

In most infections, the relationship between causative agent and clinical picture is not constant. It is therefore important to obtain proper specimens for bacteriologic identification of the causative agent. As soon as such specimens have been secured, chemotherapy can be started on the basis of the "best guess." Once the causative agent has been identified by laboratory procedures, empirical chemotherapy can be modified as necessary.

The "best guess" of a causative organism is based on the following considerations, among others: (1) the site of infection (eg, pneumonia, urinary tract infection); (2) the age of the patient (eg, meningitis: neonatal, young child, adult); (3) the place where the infection was acquired (hospital versus community); (4) mechanical predisposing factors (intravenous drip, urinary catheter, respirator, exposure to vector); and (5) predisposing host factors (immunodeficiency, corticosteroids, transplant, cancer chemotherapy, etc).

When the causative agent of a clinical infection is known, the drug of choice can often be selected on the basis of current clinical experience. At other times, laboratory tests for antibiotic susceptibility (see below) are necessary to determine the drug of choice.

B. Susceptibility Tests: Laboratory tests for antibiotic susceptibility are indicated in the following circumstances: (1) when the microorganism recovered is of a type that is often resistant to antimicrobial drugs (eg, gram-negative enteric bacteria); (2) when an infectious process is likely to be fatal unless treated specifically (eg, meningitis, septicemia); (3) in certain infections where eradication of the infectious organisms requires the use of drugs that are rapidly bactericidal, not merely bacteriostatic (eg, infective endocarditis). The laboratory aspects of antibiotic sensitivity testing are discussed in Chapter 47.

Dangers of Indiscriminate Use

(1) Widespread sensitization of the population, with resulting hypersensitivity, anaphylaxis, rashes, fever, blood disorders, cholestatic hepatitis, and perhaps collagen-vascular diseases.

(2) Changes in the normal flora of the body, with disease resulting from "superinfection" due to overgrowth of drug-resistant organisms.

(3) Masking serious infection without eradicating it. For example, the clinical manifestations of an abscess may be suppressed while the infectious process continues.

(4) Direct drug toxicity (eg, granulopenia or thrombocytopenia with cephalosporins and penicillins and renal damage or auditory nerve damage due to aminoglycosides).

(5) Development of drug resistance in microbial populations, chiefly through the elimination of drug-sensitive microorganisms from antibiotic-saturated environments (eg, hospitals) and their replacement by drug-resistant microorganisms.

ANTIMICROBIAL DRUGS USED IN COMBINATION

Indications

Possible reasons for employing two or more antimicrobials simultaneously instead of a single drug are as follows:

(1) To give prompt treatment in desperately ill patients suspected of having a serious microbial infection. A good guess about the most probable two or three pathogens is made, and drugs are aimed at those organisms. Before such treatment is started, it is essential that adequate specimens be obtained for identifying the etiologic agent in the laboratory. Suspected gram-negative or staphylococcal sepsis in immunocompromised patients and bacterial meningitis in children are foremost indications in this category.

(2) To delay the emergence of microbial mutants resistant to one drug in chronic infections by the use of a second or third non-cross-reacting drug. The most prominent example is active tuberculosis of an organ, with large microbial populations.

(3) To treat mixed infections, particularly those following massive trauma or those involving vascular structures. Each drug is aimed at an important pathogenic microorganism. However, many drugs can be used as monotherapy.

(4) To achieve bactericidal synergism or to provide bactericidal action (see below). In a few infections, eg, enterococcal sepsis, a combination of drugs is more likely to eradicate the infection than either drug used alone. Such synergism is only partially predictable, and a given drug pair may be synergistic for only a single microbial strain. Occasionally, simultaneous use of two drugs permits significant reduction in dose and thus avoids toxicity but still provides satisfactory antimicrobial action.

Disadvantages

The following disadvantages of using antimicrobial drugs in combinations must always be considered:

(1) The physician may feel that since several drugs are already being given, everything possible has been done for the patient, leading to relaxation of the effort to establish a specific diagnosis. It may also give a false sense of security.

(2) The more drugs that are administered, the greater the chance for drug reactions to occur or for the patient to become sensitized to drugs.

(3) The cost is unnecessarily high.

(4) Antimicrobial combinations usually accomplish no more than an effective single drug.

(5) Very rarely, one drug may antagonize a second drug given simultaneously (see below).

Mechanisms

When two antimicrobial agents act simultaneously on a homogeneous microbial population, the effect may be one of the following: (1) indifference, ie, the combined action is no greater than that of the more effective agent when used alone; (2) addition, ie, the combined action is equivalent to the sum of the actions of each drug when used alone; (3) synergism, ie, the combined action is significantly greater than the sum of both effects; (4) antagonism, ie, the combined action is less than that of the more effective agent when used alone. All these effects may be observed in vitro (particularly in terms of bactericidal rate) and in vivo.

Antagonism is sharply limited by time-dose relationships and is therefore a rare event in clinical antimicrobial therapy. Antagonism resulting in higher morbidity and mortality rates has been most clearly demonstrated in bacterial meningitis. It occurred when a bacteriostatic drug (which inhibited protein synthesis in bacteria) such as chloramphenicol or tetracycline was given with a bactericidal drug such as a penicillin or an aminoglycoside. Antagonism occurred mainly if the bacteriostatic drug reached the site of infection before the bactericidal drug; if the killing of bacteria was essential for cure; and if only minimal effective doses of either drug in the pair were present. Another example is combining β-lactam drugs in treatment of *Pseudomonas aeruginosa* infections (eg, imipenem and piperacillin, where imipenem is a potent β-lactamase inducer and the β-lactamase breaks down the less stable piperacillin). Antagonism can be overcome by large excess amounts of one or both drugs in the pair—a common event clinically—and very rarely affects the outcome of clinical therapy.

Synergism

Antimicrobial synergism can occur in several types of situations. Synergistic drug combinations must be selected by complex laboratory procedures.

(1) Two drugs may sequentially block a microbial metabolic pathway. Sulfonamides inhibit the use of extracellular *p*-aminobenzoic acid by some microbes for the synthesis of folic acid. Trimethoprim or pyrimethamine inhibits the next metabolic step, the reduction of dihydro- to tetrahydrofolic acid. The simulta-

neous use of a sulfonamide plus trimethoprim is effective in some bacterial *(Shigella, Salmonella, Serratia)* and some parasitic (*Pneumocystis carinii*, malaria) infections. Pyrimethamine plus a sulfonamide or clindamycin is used in toxoplasmosis.

(2) A drug such as a cell wall inhibitor (a penicillin or cephalosporin) may enhance the entry of an aminoglycoside into bacteria and thus produce synergistic effects. Penicillins enhance the uptake of gentamicin or streptomycin by enterococci. Thus, ampicillin plus gentamicin may be essential for the eradication of *Enterococcus faecalis*, particularly in endocarditis. Similarly, piperacillin plus tobramycin may be synergistic against some strains of *Pseudomonas.*

(3) One drug may affect the cell membrane and facilitate the entry of the second drug. The combined effect may then be greater than the sum of its parts. For example, amphotericin has been synergistic with flucytosine against certain fungi, eg, *Cryptococcus, Candida.*

(4) One drug may prevent the inactivation of a second drug by microbial enzymes. Thus, inhibitors of β-lactamase (eg, clavulanic acid, sulbactam, tazobactam) can protect amoxicillin, ticarcillin, or piperacillin from inactivation by β-lactamases. In such circumstances, a form of synergism takes place.

The effects that can be achieved with combinations of antimicrobial drugs vary with different combinations and are specific for each strain of microorganism. Thus, no combination is uniformly synergistic. Combined effects cannot be predicted from the behavior of the microorganism toward single drugs.

Combined therapy should not be used indiscriminately; every effort should be made to employ the single antibiotic of choice. In resistant infections, detailed laboratory study can at times define synergistic drug combinations that may be essential to eradicate the microorganisms.

ANTIMICROBIAL CHEMOPROPHYLAXIS

Anti-infective chemoprophylaxis implies the administration of antimicrobial drugs to prevent infection. In a broader sense, it also includes the use of antimicrobial drugs soon after the acquisition of pathogenic microorganisms (eg, after compound fracture) but before the development of signs of infection.

Useful chemoprophylaxis is limited to the action of a specific drug on a specific organism. An effort to prevent all types of microorganisms in the environment from establishing themselves only selects the most drug-resistant organisms as the cause of a subsequent infection. In all proposed uses of prophylactic antimicrobials, the risk of the patient's acquiring an infection must be weighed against the toxicity, cost, inconvenience, and enhanced risk of superinfection resulting from the prophylactic drug.

Prophylaxis in Persons of Normal Susceptibility Exposed to a Specific Pathogen

In this category, a specific drug is administered to prevent one specific infection. Outstanding examples are the injection of benzathine penicillin G intramuscularly once every 3–4 weeks to prevent reinfection with group A hemolytic streptococci in rheumatic patients; prevention of meningitis by eradicating the meningococcal carrier state with rifampin; prevention of syphilis by the injection of benzathine penicillin G; prevention of plague pneumonia in those exposed to infectious droplets by oral administration of tetracycline; prevention of clinical rickettsial disease (but not of infection) by the daily ingestion of tetracycline during exposure; and prevention of leptospirosis with oral administration of doxycycline in a hyperendemic environment.

Early treatment of an asymptomatic infection is sometimes called prophylaxis. Thus, administration of isoniazid, orally for 6–12 months, to an asymptomatic person who converts from a negative to a positive tuberculin skin test may prevent later clinically active tuberculosis.

Prophylaxis in Persons of Increased Susceptibility

Certain anatomic or functional abnormalities predispose to serious infections. It may be feasible to prevent or abort such infections by giving a specific drug for short periods. Some important examples are listed below:

A. Heart Disease: Persons with heart valve abnormalities or with prosthetic heart valves are unusually susceptible to implantation of microorganisms circulating in the bloodstream. This bacterial endocarditis can sometimes be prevented if the proper drug can be used during periods of bacteremia. Large numbers of viridans streptococci are pushed into the circulation during dental procedures and operations on the mouth or throat. At such times, the increased risk warrants the use of a prophylactic antimicrobial drug aimed at viridans streptococci. For example, amoxicillin taken orally before the procedure and 2 hours later can be effective. Persons allergic to penicillin can take erythromycin orally. Other oral and parenteral dosage schedules can be effective.

Enterococci cause 5–15% of cases of infective endocarditis. They reach the bloodstream from the urinary, gastrointestinal, or female genital tract. During procedures in these areas, persons with prostheses or heart valve abnormalities can be given ampicillin combined with an aminoglycoside, eg, gentamicin, both administered intramuscularly or intravenously 30 minutes before the procedure.

During and after cardiac catheterization, blood cultures may be positive in 10–20% of patients. Many of these persons also have fever, but very few acquire endocarditis. Prophylactic antimicrobials do not appear to influence these events.

B. Respiratory Tract Disease: Persons with functional and anatomic abnormalities of the respiratory tract—eg, emphysema or bronchiectasis—are subject to attacks of chronic bronchitis. This is a recurrent bacterial infection, often precipitated by acute viral infections and resulting in respiratory decompensation. The most common organisms are pneumococci and *H influenzae.* Chemoprophylaxis consists of giving tetracycline or ampicillin orally, during the "respiratory disease season." This is successful only in patients who are not hospitalized; otherwise, superinfection with *Pseudomonas, Proteus,* or yeasts is common. Simple prophylaxis of bacterial infection has been applied to children with cystic fibrosis who are not hospitalized. In spite of this, such children contract complicating infections caused by *Pseudomonas* and staphylococci. Trimethoprim-sulfamethoxazole orally or pentamidine aerosol are used for prophylaxis for *P carinii* pneumonia in AIDS patients.

C. Recurrent Urinary Tract Infection: For certain women who are subject to frequently recurring urinary tract infections, the oral intake either daily or three times weekly of nitrofurantoin or trimethoprim-sulfamethoxazole can markedly reduce the frequency of symptomatic recurrences over long periods.

Certain women tend to develop symptoms of cystitis after sexual intercourse. The ingestion of a single dose of antimicrobial drug (nitrofurantoin, trimethoprim-sulfamethoxazole, etc) can prevent this postcoital cystitis by early inhibition of growth of bacteria moved into the proximal urethra or bladder from the introitus during intercourse.

D. Opportunistic Infections in Severe Granulocytopenia: Immunocompromised patients receiving organ transplants or antineoplastic chemotherapy often develop profound leukopenia. When the neutrophil count falls below 1000/μL, they become unusually susceptible to opportunistic infections, most often gram-negative sepsis. Such persons are sometimes given a fluoroquinolone or a drug combination (eg, vancomycin, gentamicin, cephalosporin) directed at the most prevalent opportunists at the earliest sign—or even without clinical evidence—of infection. This is continued for several days until the granulocyte count rises again. Retrospective studies suggest that there is some benefit to this procedure.

In other centers, such patients are given oral insoluble antimicrobials (neomycin + polymyxin + nystatin) during the period of granulopenia to reduce the incidence of gram-negative sepsis. Some benefit has been reported from this approach.

Prophylaxis in Surgery

A major portion of all antimicrobial drugs used in hospitals is employed on surgical services with the stated intent of prophylaxis. The administration of antimicrobials before and after surgical procedures is sometimes viewed as "banning the microbial world" both from the site of the operation and from other organ systems that suffer postoperative complications. The provable benefit of antimicrobial prophylaxis in surgery is much more limited.

Several general features of surgical prophylaxis merit consideration:

(1) In clean elective surgical procedures (ie, procedures during which no tissue bearing normal flora is traversed, other than the prepared skin), the disadvantages of "routine" antibiotic prophylaxis (allergy, toxicity, superinfection) generally outweigh the possible benefits. However, even in "clean" herniorrhaphy, a single preoperative dose of cefonicid resulted in measurable benefit.

(2) Prophylactic administration of antibiotics should generally be considered only if the expected rate of infectious complications is 3–5%. An exception to this rule is the elective insertion of prostheses (cardiovascular, orthopedic), where a possible infection would have a catastrophic effect.

(3) If prophylactic antimicrobials are to be effective, a sufficient concentration of a drug must be present at the site and time of the operative procedure to inhibit or kill bacteria that might settle there. Thus, it is essential that drug administration begin 1–3 hours before operation.

(4) Prolonged administration of antimicrobial drugs tends to alter the normal flora of organ systems, suppressing the susceptible microorganisms and favoring the implantation of drug-resistant ones. Thus, antimicrobial prophylaxis should usually continue only 1 day after the procedure to prevent superinfection.

(5) Systemic levels of antimicrobial drugs usually do not prevent wound infection, pneumonia, or urinary tract infection if physiologic abnormalities or foreign bodies are present.

In major surgical procedures, the administration of a broad-spectrum bactericidal drug from just before until 1 day after the procedure has been found effective. Thus, cefazolin given intravenously 2 hours before gastrointestinal, pelvic, or orthopedic procedures and again at 2, 10, and 18 hours after the operation results in a demonstrable lowering of the risk of deep infection at the operative site. A single preoperative dose of cefonicid significantly reduced the risk of infection with breast operations. In cardiovascular surgery, antimicrobials directed at the most common organisms producing infection are begun just prior to the procedure and continued for 2 or 3 days thereafter. While this prevents drug-susceptible organisms from producing endocarditis, pericarditis, or similar complications, it may favor the implantation of drug-resistant bacteria or fungi.

Other forms of surgical prophylaxis attempt to reduce normal flora or existing bacterial contamination at the site. Thus, the colon is routinely prepared not only by mechanical cleansing through cathartics and enemas but also by the oral administration of insoluble drugs (eg, neomycin plus erythromycin every 6 hours) for 1 day before operation. In the case of a perforated viscus resulting in peritoneal contamination, immediate treatment with an aminoglycoside, a penicillin, or clindamycin reduces the impact of seeded infection. Similarly, grossly infected compound fractures or war wounds benefit from a penicillin or cephalosporin plus an aminoglycoside. In all these instances, the antimicrobials tend to reduce the likelihood of rapid and early invasion of the bloodstream and tend to help localize the infectious process—although they generally are incapable of preventing it altogether. The surgeon must be watchful for the selection of the most resistant members of the flora, which tend to manifest themselves 2 or 3 days after the beginning of prophylaxis. Such prophylaxis is really an attempt at very early treatment.

Whenever antimicrobials are administered for prophylactic purposes, the risk from these same drugs (allergy, toxicity, selection of superinfecting microorganisms) must be evaluated daily, and the course of prophylaxis must be kept as brief as possible.

Topical antimicrobials (intravenous tube site, catheter, closed urinary drainage, within a surgical wound, acrylic bone cement, etc) may have limited usefulness but must always be viewed with suspicion.

DISINFECTANTS

Disinfectants and antiseptics differ from systemically active antimicrobials in that they possess little selective toxicity: they are toxic not only for microbial parasites but for host cells as well. Therefore, they can be used only to inactivate microorganisms in the inanimate environment or, to a limited extent, on skin surfaces. They cannot be administered systemically.

The antimicrobial action of disinfectants is determined by concentration, time, and temperature; and the evaluation of their effect may be complex. A few examples of disinfectants that are used in medicine or public health are listed in Table 10–1.

Table 10–1. Practical chemical disinfectants.

Disinfection of inanimate environment	
Table tops, instruments	5% Lysol or other phenolic compound 1–10% Formaldehyde 2% Aqueous glutaraldehyde Quaternary ammonium compounds (0.1%)
Excreta, bandages, bedpans	1% Sodium hypochlorite 5% Lysol or other phenolic compound
Air	Propylene glycol mist or aerosol Formaldehyde vapor
Heat-sensitive instruments	Ethylene oxide gas (alkylates nucleic acids; residual gas must be removed by aeration)
Disinfection of skin or wounds	
	Washing with soap and water Soaps or detergents containing 2% hexachlorophene or 1.5% trichlorocarbanilide or chlorhexidine 2% Tincture of iodine 70% Ethyl alcohol; 70–90% isopropyl alcohol Povidone-iodine (water-soluble) Nitrofurazone, 0.2% jelly or solution
Topical drugs to skin or mucous membranes	
In candidiasis	Nystatin cream, 100,000 units/g Candicidin ointment, 0.6 mg/g Miconazole, 2% cream
In burns	Mafenide acetate cream Silver sulfadiazine
In dermatophytosis	Undecylenic acid powder or 5–10% cream Tolnaftate cream, 1%
In pyoderma	Bacitracin-neomycin-polymyxin ointment Potassium permanganate, 0.01%
In pediculosis	Lindane, malathion, or permethrin, 0.5–1% lotion
Topical application of drugs to eyes	
For gonorrhea prophylaxis	Erythromycin or tetracycline ointment
For bacterial conjunctivitis	Sulfacetamide ointment Chloramphenicol ointment

ANTIMICROBIAL DRUGS FOR SYSTEMIC ADMINISTRATION

Refer to Table 10–2 for a list of infecting organisms and their respective primary and alternative drug choices.

PENICILLINS

The penicillins are derived from molds of the genus *Penicillium* (eg, *Penicillium notatum*) and obtained by extraction of submerged cultures grown in special media. The most widely used natural penicillin is penicillin G. From fermentation brews of *Penicillium*, 6-aminopenicillanic acid has been isolated on a large scale. This makes it possible to synthesize an almost unlimited variety of penicillin compounds by coupling the free amino group of the penicillanic acid to free carboxyl groups of different radicals.

All penicillins share the same basic structure (see 6-aminopenicillanic acid in Figure 10–2). A thiazolidine ring (a) is attached to a β-lactam ring (b) that carries a free amino group (c). The acidic radicals attached to the amino group can be split off by bacterial and other amidases. The structural integrity of the 6-aminopenicillanic acid nucleus is essential to the biologic activity of the compounds. If the β-lactam ring is enzymatically cleaved by β-lactamases (penicilli-

Table 10–2. Drugs of choice for suspected or proved microbial pathogens, 1994. (± = alone or combined with)

Suspected or Proved Etiologic Agent	Drug(s) of First Choice	Alternative Drug(s)
Gram-negative cocci		
Moraxella catarrhalis	TMP-SMZ[1]	Newer cephalosporins,[2] erythromycin,[3] tetracycline,[4] azithromycin, amoxicillin-clavulanic acid
Niesseria gonorrhoeae (gonococcus)	Ceftriaxone	Cefixime, ciprofloxacin, spectinomycin, ofloxacin, cefpodoxime proxetil
Neisseria meningitidis	Penicillin[5]	Newer cephalosporins,[2] ampicillin, chloramphenicol
Gram-positive cocci		
Pneumococcus *(Streptococcus pneumoniae)*	Penicillin[5]	Erythromycin,[3] cephalosporin,[6] vancomycin
Streptococcus hemolytic, groups A, B, C, G	Penicillin[5]	Erythromycin,[3] cephalosporin,[6] vancomycin, clindamycin, azithromycin, clarithromycin
Streptococcus viridans	Penicillin[5] ± aminoglycosides[7]	Cephalosporin,[6] vancomycin
Staphylococcus, methicillin-resistant	Vancomycin ± gentamicin or rifampin (or both)	TMP-SMZ
Staphylococcus, non-penicillinase-producing	Penicillin	Cephalosporin,[6] vancomycin
Staphylococcus, penicillinase-producing	Penicillinase-resistant penicillin[8]	Vancomycin, cephalosporin,[6] clindamycin, amoxicillin-clavulanic acid, ticarcillin-clavulanic acid, ampicillin-sulbactam
Streptococcus faecalis (enterococcus)	Ampicillin + gentamicin	Vancomycin + gentamicin
Gram-negative rods		
Acinetobacter	Imipenem	Minocycline, TMP-SMZ,[1] doxycycline, aminoglycosides,[7] pipericillin
Bacteroides, oropharyngeal strains	Penicillin,[5] clindamycin	Metronidazole, cefoxitin, cefotetan
Bacteroides, gastrointestinal strains	Metronidazole	Cefoxitin, chloramphenicol, clindamycin, cefotetan, cefmetazole, imipenem, ticarcillin-clavulanic acid, ampicillin-sulbactam
Brucella	Tetracycline[4] + gentamicin	TMP-SMZ[1]
Campylobacter	Erythromycin[3]	Tetracycline,[4] ciprofloxacin, ofloxacin
Enterobacter	TMP-SMZ,[1] imipenem	Newer cephalosporins,[2] aminoglycoside,[7] ciprofloxacin, ofloxacin
Escherichia coli (sepsis)	Newer cephalosporins[2]	Ampicillin, TMP-SMZ,[1] ciprofloxacin, imipenem, aminoglycosides
Escherichia coli (first urinary infection)	Sulfonamide,[9] TMP-SMZ[1]	Ampicillin, cephalosporin,[6] ciprofloxacin, ofloxacin
Haemophilus (meningitis, respiratory infections)	Newer cephalosporins[2]	Ampicillin and chloramphenicol[1]
Klebsiella	Newer cephalosporins[2]	TMP-SMZ,[1] aminoglycoside,[7] imipenem, ciprofloxacin, ofloxacin
Legionella sp (pneumonia)	Erythromycin[3] + rifampin	TMP-SMZ,[1] clarithromycin, azithromycin, ciprofloxacin
Pasteurella (Yersinia) (plaque, tularemia)	Streptomycin	Chloramphenicol, a tetracycline,[4] gentamicin
Proteus mirabilis	Ampicillin	Newer cephalosporins,[2] aminoglycoside,[7] TMP-SMZ,[1] ciprofloxacin, ofloxacin
Proteus vulgaris and other species	Newer cephalosporins[2]	Aminoglycoside,[7] imipenem. TMP-SMZ,[1] ciprofloxacin, ofloxacin
Pseudomonas aeruginosa	Aminoglycoside[7] + antipseudomonal penicillin[10]	Ceftazidime ± aminoglycoside; imipenem ± aminoglycoside; aztreonam ± aminoglycoside; ciprofloxacin
Pseudomonas pseudomallei (melioidosis)	Ceftazidime	Chloramphenicol, tetracycline,[4] TMP-SMZ,[1] amoxicillin-clavulanic acid
Pseudomonas mallei (glanders)	Streptomycin + tetracycline[4]	Chloramphenicol + streptomycin
Salmonella	Ceftriaxone	TMP-SMZ,[1] ciprofloxacin, ampicillin, ofloxacin, chloramphenicol
Serratia, Providencia	Newer cephalosporins,[2] ciprofloxacin ofloxacin	TMP-SMZ,[1] aminoglycosides,[7] ciprofloxacin, ofloxacin
Shigella	Ciprofloxacin, ofloxacin	Ampicillin, TMP-SMZ[1]
Vibrio (cholera, sepsis)	Tetracycline[4]	TMP-SMZ,[1] ciprofloxacin

(continued)

Table 10–2. Drugs of choice for suspected or proved microbial pathogens, 1994. (continued)

Suspected or Proved Etiologic Agent	Drug(s) of First Choice	Alternative Drug(s)
Gram-positive rods		
Actinomyces	Penicillin[5]	Tetracycline[4]
Bacillus (eg, anthrax)	Penicillin[5]	Erythromycin,[3] tetracycline[4]
Clostridium (eg, gas gangrene, tetanus)	Penicillin[5]	Metronidazole, chloramphenicol, clindamycin
Corynebacterium diphtheriae	Erythromycin[3]	Penicillin[5]
Corynebacterium jeikeium	Vancomycin	Ciprofloxacin, penicillin and gentamicin
Listeria	TMP-SMZ[1]	Ampicillin ± aminoglycoside[7]
Acid-fast rods		
Mycobacterium tuberculosis	INH + rifampin + pyrazinamide + ethambutol	Other antituberculous drugs
Mycobacterium teprae	Dapsone + rifampin ± clofazimine	Minocycline, ofloxacin
Mycobacterium kansasii	INH + rifampin ± ethambutol	Ethionamide, cycloserine
Mycobacterium avium-intracellulare	Clarithromycin + ethambutol + rifampin+ clofazimine ± ciprofloxacin ± amikacin	Other antituberculous drugs
Mycobacterium fortuitum-chelonei	Amikacin 1 doxycycline	Cefoxitin, erythromycin, sulfonamide
Nocardia	TMP-SMZ[1]	Minocycline, imipenem, sulfonamide[9]
Spirochetes		
Borrelia burgdorferi (Lyme disease)	Tetracycline[4]	Amoxicillin, ceftriaxone, erythromycin, cefuroxime axetil, azithromycin
Borrelia recurrentis (relapsing fever)	Tetracycline[4]	Penicillin
Leptospira	Penicillin[5]	Tetracycline[4]
Treponema pallidum (syphilis)	Penicillin[5]	Tetracycline,[4] ceftriaxone
Treponema pertenue (yaws)	Penicillin[5]	Tetracycline[4]
Mycoplasmas	Erythromycin[3] or tetracycline[4]	Clarithromycin
Chlamydiae		
C psittaci	Tetracycline[4]	Chloramphenicol
C trachomatis (urethritis or pelvic inflammatory disease)	Doxycycline or erythromycin[3]	Ofloxacin or axithromycin
C pneumoniae	Tetracycline[4]	Erythromcyin,[3] clarithromycin
Rickettsiae	Tetracycline[4]	Chloramphenicol

[1] TMP-SMZ is a mixture of 1 part trimethoprim and 5 parts sulfamethoxazole.

[2] Newer cephalosporins (1994) include cefotaxime, cefuroxime, ceftriaxone, ceftazidime, ceftizoxime, cefuroxime axetil, cefixime, and others.

[3] Erythromycin estolate is best absorbed orally but carries the highest risk of hepatitis; erythromycin stearate and erythromycin ethylsuccinate are also available.

[4] All tetracyclines have similar activity against microorganisms. Dosage is determined by rates of absorption and excretion of various preparations.

[5] Penicillin G is preferred for parenteral injection; penicillin V for oral administration—to be used only in treating infections due to highly sensitive organisms.

[6] Older cephalosporins are cephalothin, cefazolin, cephapirin, and cefoxitin for parenteral injection; cephalexin and cephradine can be given orally.

[7] Aminoglycosides—gentamicin, tobramycin, amikacin, netilmicin—should be chosen on the basis of local patterns of susceptibility.

[8] Parenteral nafcillin or oxacillin; oral dicloxacillin, cloxacillin, or oxacillin.

[9] Oral sulfisoxazole and trisulfapyrimidines are highly soluble in urine; parenteral sodium sulfadiazine can be injected intravenously in treating severely ill patients.

[10] Antipseudomonal penicillins; ticarcillin, carbenicillin, mezlocillin, azlocillin, pipericillin.

[11] First choice for previously untreated urinary tract infection is a highly soluble sulfonamide (see Not e 9). TMP-SMZ (see Note 1) is acceptable.

nases), the resulting product, penicilloic acid, is devoid of antibacterial activity. However, it carries an antigenic determinant of the penicillins and acts as a sensitizing hapten when attached to carrier proteins.

The different radicals (R) attached to the aminopenicillanic acid determine the essential pharmacologic properties of the resulting drugs. The clinically important penicillins fall into four principal groups: (1) Highest activity against gram-positive organisms, spirochetes, and some others but susceptible to hydrolysis by β-lactamases and acid-labile (eg, penicillin G). (2) Relative resistance to β-lactamases but lower activity against gram-positive organisms and inactivity against gram-negatives (eg, nafcillin). (3) Rela-

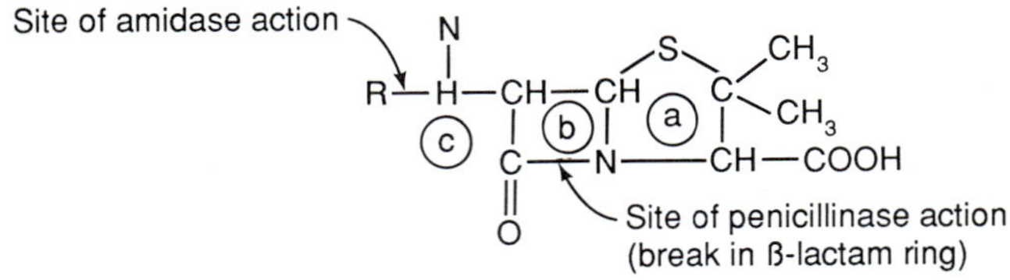

6-Aminopenicillanic acid

The following structures can each be substituted at the R to produce a new penicillin.

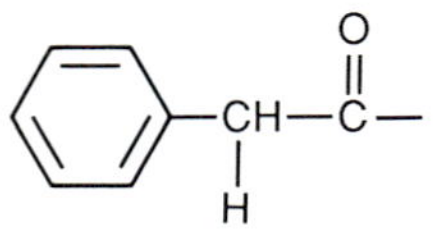

Penicillin G (benzylpenicillin):
High activity against gram-positive bacteria. Low activity against gram-negative bacteria. Acid-labile. Destroyed by ß-lactamase. 60% protein-bound.

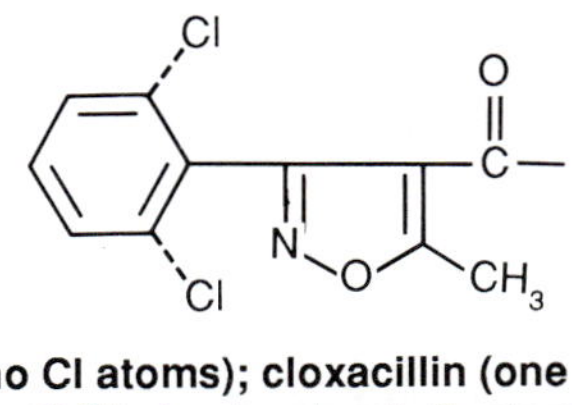

Oxacillin (no Cl atoms); cloxacillin (one Cl in structure) dicloxacillin (2 Cls in structure); flucloxacillin (one Cl and one F in structure) (isoxazolyl penicillins):
Similar to methicillin in ß-lactamase resistance, but acid-stable. Can be taken orally. Highly protein-bound (95–98%).

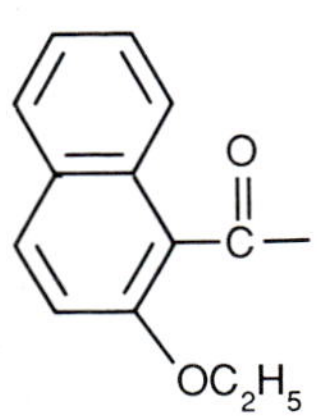

Nafcillin (ethoxynaphthamidopenicillin):
Similar to isoxazolyl penicillins. Less strongly protein-bound (90%). Can be given by mouth or by vein. Resistant to staphylococcal ß-lactamase.

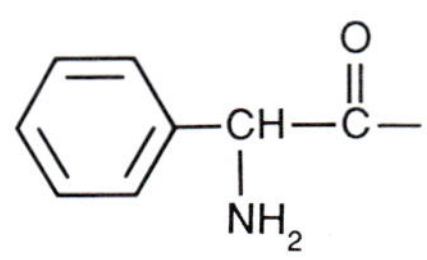

Ampicillin (alpha-aminobenzylpenicillin):
Similar to penicillin G (destroyed by ß-lactamase) but acid-stable and more active against gram-negative bacteria. Carbenicillin has –COONa instead of $-NH_2$ group.

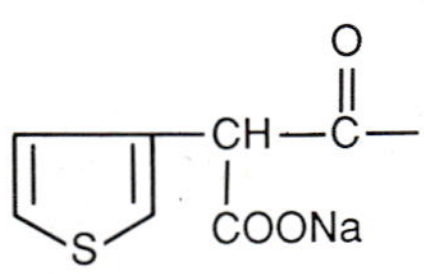

Ticarcillin:
Similar to carbenicillin but gives higher blood levels. Piperacillin, azlocillin, and mezlocillin resemble ticarcillin in action against gram-negative aerobes.

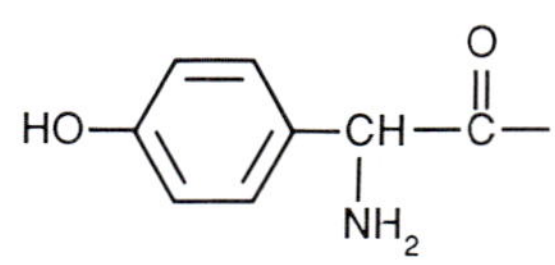

Amoxicillin:
Similar to ampicillin but better absorbed, gives higher blood levels.

Figure 11–2. Structures of some penicillins.

tively high activity against both gram-positive and gram-negative organisms but destroyed by β-lactamases (eg, ampicillin, pipericillin). (4) Relative stability to gastric acid and suitable for oral administration (eg, penicillin V, cloxacillin, amoxicillin). Some representatives are shown in Figure 10–2. Most penicillins are dispensed as sodium or potassium salts of the free acid. Potassium penicillin G contains about 1.7 meq of K^+ per million units (2.8 meq/g). Procaine salts and benzathine salts of penicillin provide repository forms for intramuscular injection. In dry form, penicillins are stable, but solutions rapidly lose their activity and must be prepared fresh for administration.

Antimicrobial Activity

The initial step in penicillin action is binding of the drug to cell receptors. These receptors are PBPs, at least some of which are enzymes involved in transpeptidation reactions. From three to six (or more) PBPs per cell can be present. After penicillin molecules have attached to the receptors, peptidoglycan synthesis is inhibited as final transpeptidation is blocked. A final bactericidal event is the removal or inactivation of an inhibitor of autolytic enzymes in the cell wall. This activates the autolytic enzymes and results in cell lysis. Organisms with defective autolysin function are inhibited but not killed by β-lactam drugs, and they are said to be "tolerant."

Since active cell wall synthesis is required for penicillin action, metabolically inactive microorganisms, L forms, or mycoplasmas are insusceptible to such drugs.

Penicillin G and penicillin V are often measured in units (1 million = 0.6 g), but the semisynthetic penicillins are measured in grams. Whereas 0.002–1 μg/mL of penicillin G is lethal for a majority of susceptible gram-positive organisms, 10–100 times more is required to kill gram-negative bacteria (except neisseriae).

Resistance

Resistance to penicillins falls into several categories: (1) Production of β-lactamases by staphylococci, gram-negative bacteria, *Haemophilus,* gonococci, and others. More than 50 different β-lactamases are known, most of them produced under the control of bacterial plasmids. Some β-lactamases are inducible by the newer cephalosporins. (2) Lack of penicillin receptors (PBPs) or inaccessibility of receptors because of permeability barriers of bacterial outer membranes. These are often under chromosomal control. (3) Failure of activation of autolytic enzymes in the cell wall, which can result in inhibition without killing bacteria (eg, tolerance of some staphylococci). (4) Failure to synthesize peptidoglycans, eg, in mycoplasmas, L forms, or metabolically inactive bacteria.

Absorption, Distribution, & Excretion

After intramuscular or intravenous administration, absorption of most penicillins is rapid and complete. After oral administration, only 5–30% of the dose for most penicillins is absorbed, depending on acid stability, binding to foods, pres...
cillin is well absorbed. Af...
widely distributed in tiss...

Special dosage forms ...
layed absorption to yield ...
After a single intramuscu...
cillin, 1.5 g (2.4 million ...
unit/mL are maintained fo...
unit/mL for 3 weeks. Pro...
muscularly yields therape...

In many tissues, penici...
lar to those in serum. Lo...
prostate, and the central ...
in meningitis, penetratio...
0.2 μg/mL occur in the ...
daily parenteral dose of ...
and pneumococcal meni...
temic penicillin, and int...
abandoned.

Most of the penicillins are rapidly excreted by the kidneys. About 10% of renal excretion is by glomerular filtration and 90% by tubular secretion. The latter can be partially blocked by probenecid to achieve higher systemic and cerebrospinal fluid levels. In the newborn and in persons with renal failure, penicillin excretion is reduced and systemic levels remain elevated longer. Some penicillins (eg, nafcillin) are eliminated mainly by nonrenal mechanisms.

Clinical Uses

Penicillins are the most widely used antibiotics, particularly in the following areas.

Penicillin G is the drug of choice in most infections caused by streptococci, pneumococci, meningococci, spirochetes, clostridia, aerobic gram-positive rods, non-penicillinase-producing staphylococci and gonococci and *Actinomyces.*

Penicillin G is inhibitory for enterococci (*E faecalis*), but for bactericidal effects (eg, in enterococcal endocarditis), an aminoglycoside must be added. Penicillin G in ordinary doses is excreted into the urine in sufficiently high concentrations to inhibit some gram-negative organisms, unless they produce a large amount of β-lactamases.

Benzathine penicillin G is a salt of very low solubility given intramuscularly for low but prolonged drug levels. A single injection of 1.2 million units (0.7 g) is satisfactory treatment for group A streptococcal pharyngitis and primary syphilis. The same injection once every 3–4 weeks is satisfactory prophylaxis against group A streptococcal reinfection in rheumatic patients. A dose of 2.4 million units one to three times at weekly intervals is effective in early syphilis.

Infection with β-lactamase-producing staphylococci is the only indication for the use of lactamase-resistant penicillins, eg, nafcillin or oxacillin. Cloxacillin or dicloxacillin by mouth can be given for milder staphylococcal infections. Staphylococci resistant to methicillin and nafcillin probably lack drug receptors

...ly for treatment of
...ith coliforms. Oral
...han ampicillin and
...given together with
...ase-producing *H in-*
...npicillin but is more
...It is usually given in
...ion with an amino-
...acillin, mezlocillin,
...tive against aerobic
...*eudomonas.*

...oxicity than most of
...t serious side effects

...nay produce central
...at are irritating. In

patients with renal failure, smaller doses may produce encephalopathy, delirium, and convulsions. With such doses, direct cation toxicity (K^+) may also occur. Nafcillin occasionally causes granulocytopenia. Oral penicillins can cause diarrhea. High doses of penicillins may cause a bleeding tendency.

B. Allergy: All penicillins are cross-sensitizing and cross-reacting. Any material (including milk, cosmetics) containing penicillin may induce sensitization. The responsible antigens are degradation products, eg, penicilloic acid, bound to host protein. Skin tests with penicilloyl-polylysine, with alkaline hydrolysis products, and with undegraded penicillin identify many hypersensitive persons. Among positive reactors to skin tests, the incidence of major immediate allergic reactions is high. Such reactions are associated with cell-bound IgE antibodies. IgG antibodies to penicillin are common and are not associated with allergic reactions except rare hemolytic anemia. A history of a penicillin reaction in the past is not reliable, but the drug must be administered with caution to such persons, or a substitute drug should be chosen.

Allergic reactions may occur as typical anaphylactic shock, typical serum sickness type reactions (urticaria, joint swelling, angioneurotic edema, pruritus, respiratory embarrassment within 7–12 days of penicillin dosage), and a variety of skin rashes, fever, nephritis, eosinophilia, vasculitis, etc. The incidence of hypersensitivity to penicillin is negligible in children but may be 1–5% among adults in the USA. Acute anaphylactic life-threatening reactions are very rare (0.5%). Corticosteroids can sometimes suppress allergic manifestations to penicillins.

CEPHALOSPORINS

Some *Cephalosporium* fungi yield antimicrobial substances called cephalosporins. These are β-lactam compounds with a nucleus of 7-aminocephalosporanic acid, instead of the penicillins' 6-aminopenicillanic acid (Figure 10–3). Natural cephalosporins have low antibacterial activity, but the attachment of various R side-groups has resulted in the proliferation of an enormous array of drugs with varying pharmacologic properties and antimicrobial spectra and activity. Cephamycins are similar to cephalosporins but are derived from actinomycetes.

The mechanism of action of cephalosporins is analogous to that of penicillins: (1) binding to specific PBPs that serve as drug receptors on bacteria; (2) inhibiting cell wall synthesis by blocking the transpeptidation of peptidoglycan; and (3) activating autolytic enzymes in the cell wall that can produce lesions resulting in bacterial death. Resistance to cephalosporins can be attributed to (1) poor permeation of bacteria by the drug; (2) lack of PBP for a specific drug; and (3) degradation of drug by β-lactamases, many of which exist. Certain third-generation cephalosporins can induce special β-lactamases in gram-negative bacteria. In general, however, cephalosporins tend to be resistant to the β-lactamases produced by staphylococci and common gram-negative bacteria that hydrolyze and inactivate many penicillins.

For easy reference, cephalosporins have been arranged into three major groups, or "generations," discussed below (Table 10–3). Many cephalosporins are mainly excreted by the kidney and may accumulate and induce toxicity in renal insufficiency.

First-Generation Cephalosporins

First-generation cephalosporins are very active against gram-positive cocci—except enterococci and methicillin-resistant staphylococci—and moderately active against some gram-negative rods—primarily E coli, Proteus, and *Klebsiella.* Anaerobic cocci are often sensitive, but *Bacteroides fragilis* is not.

Cephalexin, cephradine, and cefadroxil are absorbed from the gut to a variable extent and can be used to treat urinary and respiratory tract infections. Other first-generation cephalosporins must be injected to give adequate levels in blood and tissues. Cefazolin is a choice for surgical prophylaxis because it gives the highest (90–120 μg/mL) levels. Cephalothin and cephapirin in the same dose give lower levels. None of the first-generation drugs penetrate the central nervous system, and they are not drugs of first choice for any infection.

Second-Generation Cephalosporins

The second-generation cephalosporins are a heterogeneous group. All are active against organisms covered by first-generation drugs but have extended coverage against gram-negative rods—including *Klebsiella, Enterobacter,* and *Proteus* but not *Pseudomonas aeruginosa.*

Oral second-generation cephalosporins can be used to treat sinusitis and otitis caused by *Haemophilus influenzae,* including β-lactamase-producing strains.

Cefoxitin and cefotetan are particularly active against B fragilis and thus are used in mixed anaerobic infections, including peritonitis or pelvic inflammatory disease. Cefamandole, cefuroxime, cefonicid, and ceforanide are injected intravenously at intervals in the treatment of gram-negative bacterial pneumonias or other community-acquired infections. The dosage must be reduced in renal failure.

Third-Generation Cephalosporins

Third-generation cephalosporins have little activity against gram-positive cocci; staphylococci and especially enterococci often produce superinfections during their use. A major advantage of third-generation drugs is their enhanced activity against gram-negative rods. Whereas second-generation drugs tend to fail against *P aeruginosa,* ceftazidime or cefoperazone may succeed. Thus, third-generation drugs are very

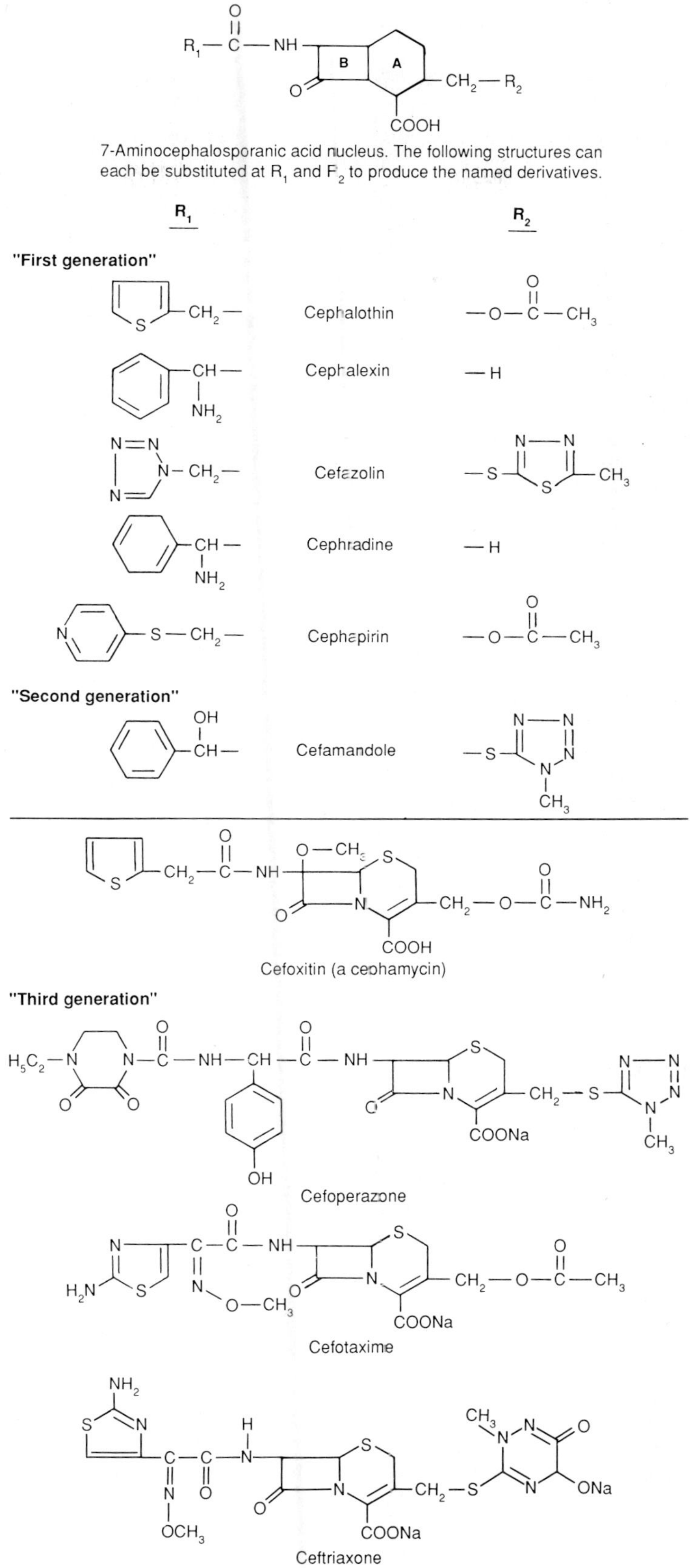

Figure 10–3. Structures of some cephalosporins.

Table 10–3. Major groups of cephalosporins.

First-Generation	Second-Generation	Third-Generation	Fourth-Generation
Parenteral	**Parenteral**	**Parenteral**	**Parenteral**
Cefazolin	Cefamandole	Cefoperazone	Cefepime
Cephalothin	Cefmetazole	Cefotaxime	
Cephapirin	Cefonicid	Ceftazidime	
Oral	Ceforanide	Ceftizoxime	
Cephradine[1]	Cefotetan	Ceftriaxone	
Cephalexin	Cefoxitin	**Oral**	
Cefadroxil	Cefuroxime	Cefixime	
	Oral		
	Cefaclor		
	Cefpodoxime proxetil		
	Cefprozil		
	Cefuroxime axetil		
	Loracarbef[2]		

[1]Parenteral and oral agent.
[2]Carbacephem analogue of cefaclor.

useful in the management of hospital-acquired gram-negative bacteremia. In immunocompromised patients, these drugs are often combined with an aminoglycoside. Ceftazidime may also be lifesaving in severe melioidosis (*P pseudomallei* infection).

Another important distinguishing feature of several third-generation drugs—except cefoperazone—is the ability to reach the central nervous system and to appear in the spinal fluid in sufficient concentrations to treat meningitis caused by gram-negative rods. Cefotaxime, ceftriaxone, or ceftizoxime given intravenously is the choice for management of gram-negative bacterial sepsis and meningitis.

Fourth-Generation Cephalosporins

Some new cephalosporins are being classified as fourth-generation drugs. The new agents have comparable or slightly enhanced activity against some Enterobacteriaceae that are resistant to third-generation cephalosporins. They are not active against *P aeruginosa* that are resistant to the third-generation drugs. The activity against streptococci and nafcillin-susceptible staphylococci is comparable to that of the third-generation compounds.

Adverse Effects of Cephalosporins

A. Allergy: Cephalosporins are sensitizing and can elicit a variety of hypersensitivity reactions, including anaphylaxis, fever, skin rashes, nephritis, granulocytopenia, and hemolytic anemia. The frequency of cross-allergy between cephalosporins and penicillins is approximately 5%. Patients with minor penicillin allergy can often tolerate cephalosporins, but those with a history of anaphylaxis cannot.

B. Toxicity: Thrombophlebitis can occur after intravenous injection. Hypoprothrombinemia is frequent with cephalosporins that have a methylthiotetrazole group (eg, cefamandole, cefmetazole, cefotetan, cefoperazone). Oral administration of vitamin K (10 mg) twice weekly can prevent this complication. These same drugs can also cause severe disulfiram reactions, and use of alcohol must be avoided.

C. Superinfection: Since many second-, third-, and fourth-generation cephalosporins have little activity against gram-positive organisms, particularly staphylococci and enterococci, superinfection with these organisms and with fungi may occur.

OTHER BETA-LACTAM DRUGS

Monobactams

Monobactams have a monocyclic β-lactam ring and are resistant to β-lactamases. They are active against gram-negative rods but not against gram-positive bacteria or anaerobes. The first such drug to become available was aztreonam, which resembles aminoglycosides in activity and is given intravenously or intramuscularly every 8 or 12 hours in a dose of 1–2 g. Penicillin-allergic patients can apparently tolerate it without reaction, and—apart from skin rashes and minor transaminase disturbances—no major toxicity has been reported. Superinfections with staphylococci and enterococci can occur. The clinical usefulness of aztreonam has not yet been well defined.

Carbapenems

These drugs are structurally related to β-lactam antibiotics. Imipenem, the first such agent to become available, has good activity against many gram-negative rods, gram-positive organisms, and anaerobes. It is resistant to β-lactamases but is inactivated by dihydropeptidases in renal tubules. Consequently, it is administered together with a peptidase inhibitor, cilastatin.

Imipenem penetrates body tissues and fluids well, including cerebrospinal fluid. The drug is given intravenously every 6 hours and in reduced dosage in renal insufficiency. Imipenem may be indicated for infections due to organisms that are resistant to other drugs. *Pseudomonas* species rapidly develop resistance, and therefore the concomitant use of an aminoglycoside is required. Such a combination may be effective treatment for febrile neutropenic patients.

Adverse effects of imipenem include vomiting, diarrhea, skin rashes, and reactions at the infusion sites. Excessive levels in patients with renal failure may lead to seizures. Patients allergic to penicillins may be allergic to imipenem as well.

TETRACYCLINES

The tetracyclines have virtually identical antimicrobial properties and give complete cross-resistance. However, they differ in physical and pharmacologic characteristics. All tetracyclines are readily absorbed from the intestinal tract and distributed widely in tissues but penetrate into the cerebrospinal fluid poorly. Some can also be administered intramuscularly or intravenously. They are excreted in stool and into bile and urine at varying rates. With doses of tetracycline hydrochloride, 2 g/d orally, blood levels reach 8 μg/mL. Demeclocycline, minocycline, and doxycycline are excreted more slowly and therefore are administered at longer intervals.

The tetracyclines have the basic structure shown below. The following radicals occur in the different forms:

	R	R_1	R_2	Renal Clearance (mL/min)
Tetracycline	—H	$—CH_3$	—H	65
Oxytetracycline	—H	$—CH_3$	—OH	90
Demeclocycline	—Cl	—H	—H	35
Doxycycline	—H	$—CH_3$	—OH	16
Minocycline	$—N(CH_3)_2$	—H	—H	<10

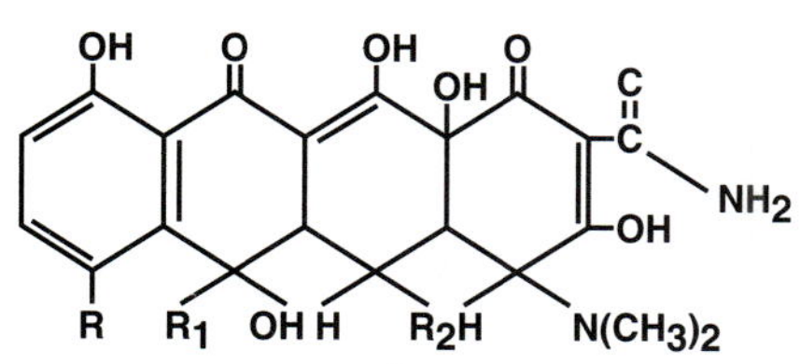

Antimicrobial Activity

Tetracyclines are concentrated by susceptible bacteria and inhibit protein synthesis by inhibiting the binding of aminoacyl-tRNA to the 30S unit of bacterial ribosomes. Resistant bacteria fail to concentrate the drug. This resistance is under the control of transmissible plasmids.

The tetracyclines are principally bacteriostatic agents. They inhibit the growth of susceptible gram-positive and gram-negative bacteria (inhibited by 0.1–10 μg/mL) and are drugs of choice in infections caused by rickettsiae, chlamydiae, and *Mycoplasma pneumoniae*. Tetracyclines are used in cholera to shorten excretion of vibrios, and in shigellosis. Tetracycline hydrochloride or doxycycline orally for 7 days is effective against chlamydial genital infection. Tetracyclines are sometimes employed in combination with streptomycin to treat *Brucella, Yersinia,* and *Francisella* infections. Minocycline is often active against *Nocardia* and can eradicate the meningococcal carrier state. Low doses of tetracycline for many months are given for acne to suppress both skin bacteria and their lipases, which promote inflammatory changes.

Tetracyclines do not inhibit fungi. They temporarily suppress parts of the normal bowel flora, but superinfections may occur, particularly with tetracycline-resistant *Pseudomonas, Proteus,* staphylococci, and yeasts.

Side Effects

The tetracyclines produce varying degrees of gastrointestinal upset (nausea, vomiting, diarrhea), skin rashes, mucous membrane lesions, and fever in many patients, particularly when administration is prolonged and dosage high. It is not definitely known what part is played by allergy and what part by direct toxicity. Replacement of bacterial flora (see above) occurs commonly. Overgrowth of yeasts on anal and vaginal mucous membranes during tetracycline administration leads to inflammation and pruritus. Overgrowth of organisms in the intestine may lead to enterocolitis.

Tetracyclines are deposited in bony structures and teeth, particularly in the fetus and during the first 6 years of life. Discoloration and fluorescence of the teeth occur in newborns if tetracyclines are taken for prolonged periods by pregnant women. Hepatic damage may occur. Outdated tetracycline can produce renal damage. Demeclocycline causes photosensitization. Minocycline can cause marked vestibular disturbances.

Bacteriologic Examination

Antimicrobial efficacy of the tetracyclines is virtually identical, so that only one stable tetracycline need be included in antibiotic sensitivity tests. Cross-resistance of microorganisms to tetracyclines is extensive; an organism resistant to one of the drugs may be assumed to be resistant to the others also.

CHLORAMPHENICOL

Chloramphenicol is a substance produced originally from cultures of *Streptomyces venezuelae* but now manufactured synthetically.

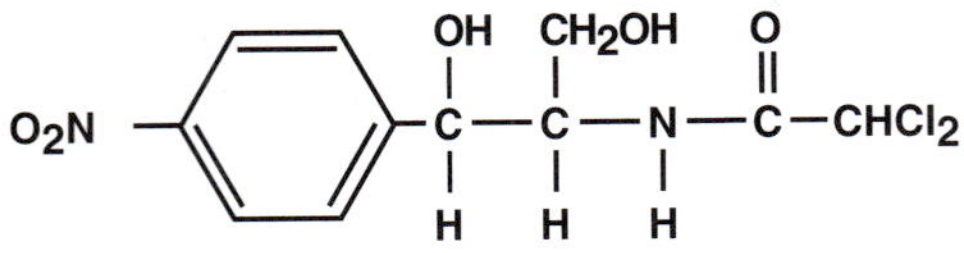

Chloramphenicol

Crystalline chloramphenicol is a stable compound that is rapidly absorbed from the gastrointestinal tract and widely distributed into tissues and body fluids, including the central nervous system and cerebrospinal fluid; it penetrates cells well. Most of the drug is inactivated in the liver by conjugation with glucuronic acid or by reduction to inactive arylamines. Excretion is mainly in the urine, 90% in inactive form. Although chloramphenicol is usually administered orally, the succinate can be injected intravenously in similar dosage.

Antimicrobial Activity

Chloramphenicol is a potent inhibitor of protein synthesis in microorganisms. It blocks the attachment of amino acids to the nascent peptide chain on the 50S unit of ribosomes by interfering with the action of peptidyl transferase. Chloramphenicol is principally bacteriostatic, and its spectrum, dosage, and blood levels are similar to those of the tetracyclines. Chloramphenicol is a drug of possible first choice in (1) symptomatic *Salmonella* infections, eg, typhoid fever (although resistant strains are increasing); (2) *H influenzae* infections due to β-lactamase-producing strains; (3) meningococcal infections in patients hypersensitive to penicillin; (4) anaerobic or mixed infections in the central nervous system, eg, brain abscess; (5) severe rickettsial infections, as a substitute for tetracyclines; and (6) occasional topical use in eye infections.

Chloramphenicol resistance is due to destruction of the drug by an enzyme (chloramphenicol acetyltransferase) that is under plasmid control.

Side Effects

Chloramphenicol infrequently causes gastrointestinal upsets. However, administration of more than 3 g/d regularly induces disturbances in red cell maturation, elevation of serum iron, and anemia. These changes are reversible upon discontinuance of the drug. Very rarely, individuals exhibit an apparent idiosyncrasy to chloramphenicol and develop severe or fatal depression of bone marrow function. The mechanism of this aplastic anemia is not understood, but it is distinct from the dose-related reversible effect described above. For these reasons, the use of chloramphenicol is generally restricted to those infections where it is clearly the most effective drug by laboratory test or experience.

In premature and newborn infants, chloramphenicol can induce collapse ("gray syndrome") because the normal mechanism of detoxification (glucuronide conjugation in the liver) is not yet developed.

Bacteriologic Examination

Chloramphenicol is very stable and diffuses well in agar media. For these reasons, it tends to give large zones of growth inhibition by the "disk test." An enzymatic assay (using acetyltransferase) permits estimation of chloramphenicol concentration in body fluids.

ERYTHROMYCINS (Macrolides)

Erythromycin is obtained from *Streptomyces erythreus* and has the chemical formula $C_{37}H_{67}NO_{13}$. Drugs related to erythromycin are clarithromycin, azithromycin, and others. Erythromycins attach to a receptor (a 23S rRNA) on the 50S subunit of the bacterial ribosome. They inhibit protein synthesis by interfering with translocation reactions and the formation of initiation complexes. Resistance to erythromycins results from an alteration (methylation) of the rRNA receptor. This is under control of a transmissible plasmid. The activity of erythromycins is greatly enhanced at alkaline pH.

Erythromycins in concentrations of 0.1–2 μg/mL are active against gram-positive bacteria, including pneumococci, streptococci, and corynebacteria. *Mycoplasma, Chlamydia trachomatis, Legionella pneumophila,* and *Campylobacter jejuni* are also susceptible. Resistant variants occur in susceptible microbial populations and tend to emerge during treatment, especially in staphylococcal infections.

Erythromycins may be drugs of choice in infections caused by the organisms listed above and are substitutes for penicillins in persons hypersensitive to the latter. Erythromycin stearate, succinate, or estolate orally four times a day yields serum levels of 0.5–2 μg/mL. Special forms (erythromycin gluceptate or lactobionate) are given intravenously.

Undesirable side effects are drug fever, mild gastrointestinal upsets, and cholestatic hepatitis as a hypersensitivity reaction, especially to the estolate. Hepatotoxicity may be increased during pregnancy. Erythromycin tends to increase levels of simultaneously administered anticoagulants, cyclosporine, and other drugs by depressing microsomal enzymes.

Clarithromycin and azithromycin are macrolides chemically related to erythromycin. Like erythromycin, both clarithromycin and azithromycin are active against staphylococci and streptococci. Clarithromycin has enhanced activity against *Legionella pneumophila, Helicobacter pylori, Moraxella catarrhalis, Chlamydia trachomatis,* and *Borrelia burgdorferi.* Azithromycin has enhanced activity against *Campylobacter jejuni, Haemophilus influenzae, Mycoplasma pneumoniae, Moraxella catarrhalis, Neisseria gonorrhoeae,* and *Borrelia burgdorferi.* Clarithromycin is active against *Mycobacterium avium,* and both drugs inhibit *Mycobacterium chelonei* and *Mycobacterium fortuitum.* Bacteria resistant to erythromycin are also resistant to clarithromycin and azithromycin. The chemical modifications prevent the metabolism of clarithromycin and azithromycin to inactive forms, and the drugs are given twice daily (clarithromycin) or once daily (azithromycin). Both drugs are associated with a much lower incidence of gastrointestinal side effects than erythromycin.

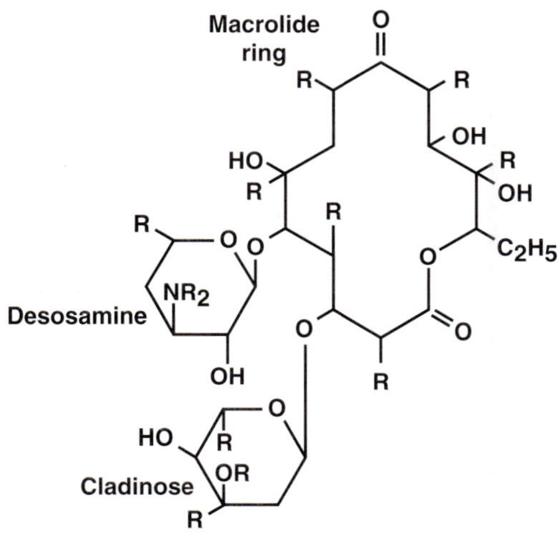

Erythromycin (R = CH_3)

CLINDAMYCIN & LINCOMYCIN

Lincomycin (derived from *Streptomyces lincolnensis*) and clindamycin (a chlorine-substituted derivative) resemble erythromycins in mode of action, antibacterial spectrum, and ribosomal receptor site but are chemically distinct. Clindamycin is very active against *Bacteroides* and other anaerobes.

The drugs are acid-stable and can be given by mouth or intravenously. They are widely distributed in tissues, except the central nervous system. Excretion is mainly through liver, bile, and urine.

Probably the most important indication for intravenous clindamycin is the treatment of severe anaerobic infections, including those caused by *B fragilis.* Successful treatment of staphylococcal infections of bone with lincomycins has been recorded. Lincomycins should not be used in meningitis. Clindamycin has been prominent in antibiotic-associated colitis caused by *C difficile.* This organism is generally clindamycin-resistant and gains prominence in bowel flora during treatment with this—or occasionally other—drugs. It produces a necrotizing toxin and results in pseudomembranous colitis, which may be fatal. Early diagnosis and treatment with oral vancomycin or metronidazole are necessary.

VANCOMYCIN

Vancomycin is a glycopeptide (MW 1450) produced by *Streptomyces orientalis.* It is poorly absorbed from the intestine.

Vancomycin is markedly bactericidal for staphylococci, some clostridia, and some bacilli. The drug inhibits early stages in cell wall peptidoglycan synthesis. Drug-resistant strains do not emerge rapidly. Vancomycin is given intravenously for serious systemic staphylococcal infections, including endocarditis, especially if resistant to nafcillin. For enterococcal sepsis or endocarditis, vancomycin can be effective if combined with a penicillin. Oral vancomycin is indicated in antibiotic-associated pseudomembranous colitis (see Clindamycin).

Undesirable side effects are thrombophlebitis, skin rashes, nerve deafness, and perhaps kidney damage when used in combination with an aminoglycoside.

TEICHOPLANIN

Teichoplanin is a glycopeptide with a structure similar to that of vancomycin. It is active against staphylococci (including nafcillin-resistant strains), streptococci, enterococci, and many other gram-positive bacteria. The drug has a long half-life and is administered once a day. Adverse effects include localized irritation at injection sites, hypersensitivity, and the potential for ototoxicity and nephrotoxicity.

BACITRACIN

Bacitracin is a polypeptide obtained from a strain of *Bacillus subtilis* (Tracy strain). It is stable and poorly absorbed from the intestinal tract. Its only use is for topical application to skin, wounds, or mucous membranes.

Bacitracin is mainly bactericidal for gram-positive bacteria, including penicillin-resistant staphylococci. For topical use, concentrations of 500–2000 units per milliliter of solution or gram of ointment are used. In combination with polymyxin B or neomycin, bacitracin is useful for the suppression of mixed bacterial flora in surface lesions.

Bacitracin is toxic for the kidney, causing proteinuria, hematuria, and nitrogen retention. For this reason, it has no place in systemic therapy. Bacitracin is said not to induce hypersensitivity readily.

POLYMYXINS

Polymyxins are basic, cationic polypeptides that are nephrotoxic and neurotoxic. Polymyxins can be bactericidal for many gram-negative aerobic rods—including *Pseudomonas* and *Serratia*—by binding to cell membranes rich in phosphatidylethanolamine and destroying membrane functions of active transport and permeability barrier. Because of their toxicity and poor distribution to tissues, polymyxins are used primarily topically and rarely for systemic infections. Solutions of polymyxin B sulfate (1 mg/mL) can be applied to infected surfaces or injected subconjunctivally or into the pleural cavity or joint spaces. Ointments of 0.5 mg/g polymyxin B sulfate in mixture with neomycin or bacitracin are often applied to superficial infected skin lesions. Rarely, polymyxin E (colistin) is given orally to suppress aerobic gram-negative bowel flora in immunocompromised patients. Polymyxin E is not significantly absorbed from the bowel, is said not to induce hypersensitivity, and is rapidly bound by purulent exudates.

AMINOGLYCOSIDES

Aminoglycosides are a group of drugs sharing chemical, antimicrobial, pharmacologic, and toxic characteristics. At present, the group includes streptomycin, neomycin, kanamycin, amikacin, gentamicin, tobramycin, sisomicin, netilmicin, and others. All inhibit protein synthesis of bacteria by attaching to and inhibiting the function of the 30S subunit of the bacterial ribosome. Resistance is based on (1) a deficiency of the ribosomal receptor (chromosomal mutant), (2) enzymatic destruction of the drug (plasmid-mediated transmissible resistance of clinical importance), or (3) lack of permeability to the drug molecule and lack of active transport into the cell. The last can be chromosomal (eg, streptococci are relatively impermeable to aminoglycosides), or it can be plasmid-mediated (eg, in gram-negative enteric bacteria). Anaerobic bacteria are often resistant to aminoglycosides because transport through the cell membrane is an energy-requiring process that is oxygen-dependent.

All aminoglycosides are more active at alkaline pH than at acid pH. All are potentially ototoxic and nephrotoxic, though to different degrees. All can accumulate in renal failure; therefore, marked dosage adjustments must be made when nitrogen retention occurs. Aminoglycosides are used most widely against gram-negative enteric bacteria or when there is suspicion of sepsis. In the treatment of bacteremia or endocarditis caused by fecal streptococci or some gram-negative bacteria, the aminoglycoside is given together with a penicillin that facilitates the entry of the aminoglycoside. Aminoglycosides are selected according to recent susceptibility patterns in a given area or hospital until susceptibility tests become available on a specific isolate. The clinical usefulness of aminoglycosides has declined with the advent of cephalosporins and quinolones, but they continue to be used in combinations (eg, with cephalosporins for multiresistant gram-negative bacteremias). All positively charged aminoglycosides are inhibited in blood cultures by sodium polyanethol sulfonate and other polyanionic detergents. Some aminoglycosides (especially streptomycin) are useful as antimycobacterial drugs.

1. NEOMYCIN & KANAMYCIN

Kanamycin is a close relative of neomycin, with similar activity and complete cross-resistance. Paromomycin is also closely related and is used in amebiasis. These drugs are stable and poorly absorbed from the intestinal tract and other surfaces. Neither drug is used systemically because of ototoxicity and neurotoxicity. Oral doses of both neomycin and kanamycin are used for reduction of intestinal flora before large bowel surgery, often in combination with erythromycin. Otherwise, these drugs are mainly limited to topical application on infected surfaces (skin and wounds).

2. AMIKACIN

Amikacin is a semisynthetic derivative of kanamycin. It is relatively resistant to several of the enzymes that inactivate gentamicin and tobramycin and therefore can be employed against some microorganisms resistant to the latter drugs. However, bacterial resistance due to impermeability to amikacin is slowly increasing. Many gram-negative enteric bacteria are inhibited by amikacin in concentrations obtained after injection. Central nervous system infections require intrathecal or intraventricular injection.

Like all aminoglycosides, amikacin is nephrotoxic and ototoxic (particularly for the auditory portion of the eighth nerve). Its level should be monitored in patients with renal failure.

3. GENTAMICIN

In concentrations of 0.5–5 μg/mL, gentamicin is bactericidal for many gram-positive and gram-negative bacteria, including many strains of *Proteus, Serratia,* and *Pseudomonas.* Gentamicin is ineffective against streptococci and *Bacteroides.*

Gentamicin has been used in serious infections caused by gram-negative bacteria insusceptible to other drugs. Penicillins may precipitate gentamicin in vitro (and thus must not be mixed), but in vivo they may facilitate the aminoglycoside entrance into streptococci and gram-negative rods and result in bactericidal synergism, beneficial in sepsis and endocarditis.

Gentamicin is toxic, particularly in the presence of impaired renal function. Gentamicin sulfate, 0.1%, has been used topically in creams or solutions for infected burns or skin lesions. Such creams tend to select gentamicin-resistant bacteria, and patients receiving them must remain in strict isolation.

4. TOBRAMYCIN

This aminoglycoside closely resembles gentamicin, and there is some cross-resistance between them. Separate susceptibility tests are desirable.

The pharmacologic properties of tobramycin are virtually identical to those of gentamicin. Most of the drug is excreted by glomerular filtration. In renal failure, the drug dosage must be reduced, and monitoring of blood levels is desirable.

Like other aminoglycosides, tobramycin is ototoxic but perhaps less nephrotoxic than gentamicin. It should not be used concurrently with other drugs having similar adverse effects or with diuretics, which tend to enhance aminoglycoside tissue concentrations.

5. NETILMICIN

Netilmicin shares many characteristics with gentamicin and tobramycin, but it is not inactivated by some bacteria that are resistant to the other drugs.

The principal indication for netilmicin may be iatrogenic infections in immunocompromised and severely ill patients at very high risk for gram-negative bacterial sepsis in the hospital setting.

Netilmicin may be somewhat less ototoxic and nephrotoxic than the other aminoglycosides.

6. STREPTOMYCIN

Streptomycin was the first aminoglycoside—it was discovered in the 1940s as a product of *Streptomyces griseus.* It was studied in great detail and became the prototype of this class of drugs. For this reason, its properties are listed here, although widespread resistance among microorganisms has greatly reduced its clinical usefulness. Dihydrostreptomycin has been abandoned because of excessive ototoxicity.

After intramuscular injection, streptomycin is rapidly absorbed and widely distributed in tissues except the central nervous system. Only 5% of the extracellular concentration of streptomycin reaches the interior of the cell. Absorbed streptomycin is excreted by glomerular filtration into the urine. After oral administration, it is poorly absorbed from the gut; most of it is excreted in feces.

Streptomycin inhibits protein synthesis in bacteria and is bactericidal for susceptible microorganisms.

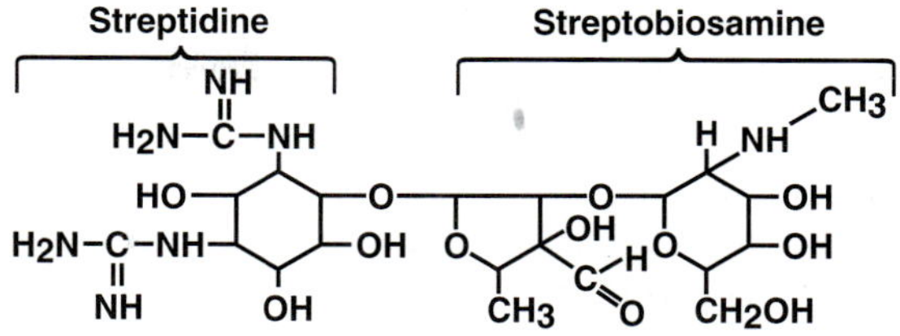

Streptomycin

Streptomycin may be bactericidal for enterococci (eg, in endocarditis) when combined with a penicillin. In tularemia and plague, it may be given with a tetracycline. In tuberculosis, it is used in combination with other antituberculosis drugs (isoniazid, rifampin).

The therapeutic effectiveness of streptomycin is limited by the rapid emergence of resistant mutants. All microbial strains produce streptomycin-resistant chromosomal mutants with relatively high frequency. Chromosomal mutants have an alteration in the P 12 receptor on the 30S ribosomal subunit. Plasmid-mediated resistance results in enzymatic destruction of the drug. Enterococci resistant to high levels of streptomycin (2000 μg/mL; or gentamicin, 500 μg/mL) are resistant to the synergistic actions of these drugs with penicillin. In tuberculosis, combination of streptomycin with other antituberculosis drugs results in a marked delay in the emergence of resistance.

Fever, skin rashes, and other allergic manifestations may result from hypersensitivity to streptomycin. This occurs most frequently upon prolonged contact with the drug, in patients receiving a protracted course of treatment (eg, for tuberculosis), or in personnel preparing and handling the drug. (Those preparing solutions should wear gloves.)

Streptomycin is markedly toxic for the vestibular portion of the eighth cranial nerve, causing tinnitus, vertigo, and ataxia, which are often irreversible. It is moderately nephrotoxic.

SPECTINOMYCIN

This is an aminocyclitol antibiotic (related to aminoglycosides) for intramuscular administration. Its sole application is in the single-dose treatment of gonorrhea caused by β-lactamase-producing gonococci or occurring in individuals hypersensitive to penicillin. About 5–10% of gonococci are probably resistant. There is usually pain at the injection site, and there may be nausea and fever.

ISONIAZID (Isonicotinic Acid Hydrazide, INH)

Isoniazid has little effect on most bacteria but is strikingly active against mycobacteria, especially *Mycobacterium tuberculosis.* Most tubercle bacilli are inhibited and killed in vitro by isoniazid, 0.1–1 μg/mL, but large populations of tubercle bacilli usually contain some isoniazid-resistant organisms. For this reason, the drug is employed in combination with other antimycobacterial agents (especially ethambutol or rifampin) to reduce the emergence of resistant tubercle bacilli. Isoniazid acts on mycobacteria by inhibiting the synthesis of mycolic acids. Isoniazid and pyridoxine are structural analogues. Patients receiving isoniazid excrete pyridoxine in excessive amounts, which results in peripheral neuritis. This can be prevented by the administration of pyridoxine, which does not interfere with the antituberculosis action of isoniazid.

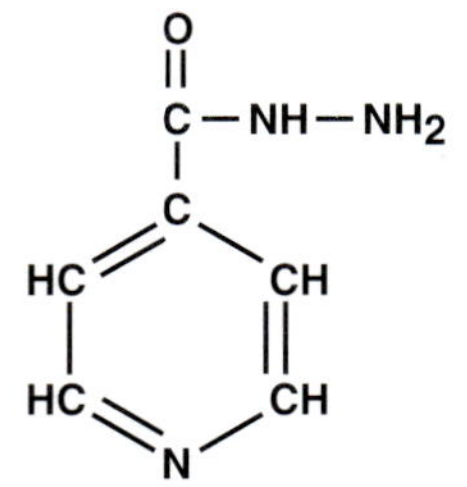

Isoniazid

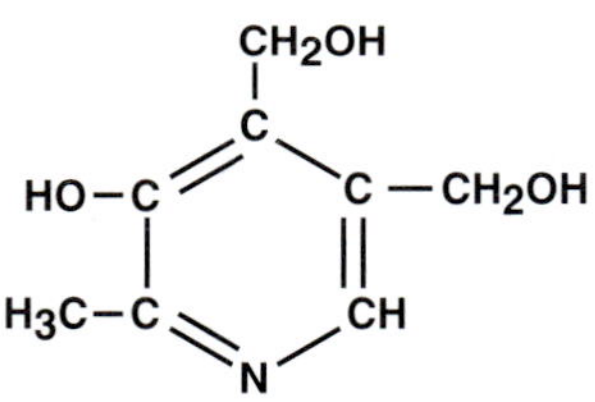

Pyridoxine

Isoniazid is rapidly and completely absorbed from the gastrointestinal tract and is in part acetylated and in part excreted in the urine. With usual doses, toxic manifestations, eg, hepatitis, are infrequent. Isoniazid freely diffuses into tissue fluids, including the cerebrospinal fluid.

In converters from negative to positive tuberculin skin tests who have no evidence of disease, isoniazid may be used as prophylaxis.

ETHAMBUTOL

Ethambutol is a synthetic, water-soluble, heat-stable D-isomer of the structure shown below.

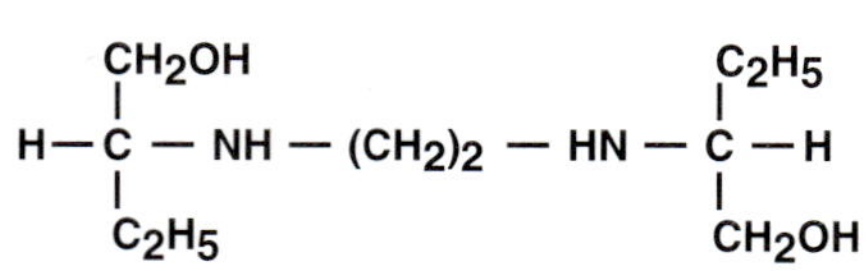

Ethambutol

Many strains of M tuberculosis and of "atypical" mycobacteria are inhibited in vitro by ethambutol, 1–5 μg/mL. The mechanism of action is not known.

Ethambutol is well absorbed from the gut. About 20% of the drug is excreted in feces and 50% in urine, in unchanged form. Excretion is delayed in renal failure. In meningitis, ethambutol appears in the cerebrospinal fluid.

Resistance to ethambutol emerges fairly rapidly among mycobacteria when the drug is used alone. Therefore, ethambutol is always given in combination with other antituberculosis drugs.

Ethambutol is usually given as a single oral daily dose. Hypersensitivity to ethambutol occurs infrequently. The commonest side effects are visual disturbances: reduction in visual acuity, optic neuritis, and perhaps retinal damage occur in some patients given high doses for several months. Most of these changes apparently regress when ethambutol is discontinued. However, periodic visual acuity testing is mandatory during treatment. With low doses, visual disturbances are very rare.

RIFAMPIN

Rifampin is a semisynthetic derivative of rifamycin, an antibiotic produced by *Streptomyces mediterranei*. It is active in vitro against some gram-positive and gram-negative cocci, some enteric bacteria, mycobacteria, chlamydiae, and poxviruses. Although many meningococci and mycobacteria are inhibited by less than 1 μg/mL, highly resistant mutants occur in all microbial populations in a frequency of 10^{-6} to 10^{-5}. The prolonged administration of rifampin as a single drug permits the emergence of these highly resistant mutants. There is no cross-resistance to other antimicrobial drugs.

Rifampin binds strongly to DNA-dependent RNA polymerase and thus inhibits RNA synthesis in bacteria. It blocks a late stage in the assembly of poxviruses. Rifampin penetrates phagocytic cells well and can kill intracellular organisms. Rifampin-resistant mutants exhibit an altered RNA polymerase.

Rifampin is well absorbed after oral administration, widely distributed in tissues, and excreted mainly through the liver and to a lesser extent into the urine.

In tuberculosis, a single oral dose is administered together with ethambutol, isoniazid, or another antituberculosis drug in order to delay the emergence of rifampin-resistant mycobacteria. A similar regimen may apply to atypical mycobacteria. In short-term treatment schedules for tuberculosis, rifampin is given orally, first daily (together with isoniazid) and then two or three times weekly for 6–9 months. However, no less than two doses weekly should be given to avoid a "flu syndrome" and anemia. Rifampin used in conjunction with a sulfone is effective in leprosy.

Oral rifampin can eliminate a majority of meningococci from carriers. Unfortunately, some highly resistant meningococcal strains are selected out by this procedure. Close contacts of children with *H influenzae* infections (eg, in the family or in day care centers) can receive rifampin as prophylaxis. In urinary tract infections and in chronic bronchitis, rifampin is not useful because resistance emerges promptly.

Rifampin imparts an orange color to urine, sweat, and contact lenses, which is harmless. Occasional adverse effects include rashes, thrombocytopenia, light chain proteinuria, and impairment of liver function. Rifampin induces microsomal enzymes (eg, cytochrome P450).

Rifabutin is a related new antimycobacterial drug, active in the prevention of infection due to *M avium-intracellulare.*

AMINOSALICYLIC ACID

Aminosalicylic acid (*p*-aminosalicylic acid; PAS) closely resembles *p*-aminobenzoic acid and sulfonamides. Most bacteria are not inhibited by PAS, but tubercle bacilli are usually inhibited by drug levels of 1–5 μg/mL. Atypical mycobacteria are resistant. In susceptible mycobacterial populations, PAS-resistant mutants tend to emerge. The simultaneous use of a second antituberculosis drug inhibits this development. Full oral doses of PAS often caused with severe gastrointestinal side effects. Therefore, the use of PAS has been largely abandoned.

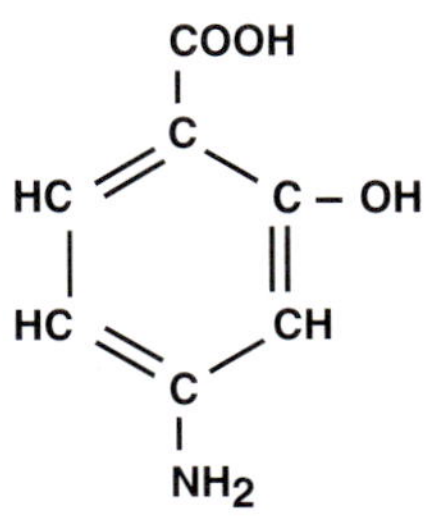

Aminosalicylic acid

PYRAZINAMIDE

Pyrazinamide is related to nicotinamide. It is readily absorbed from the gastrointestinal tract and widely distributed in tissues. *Mycobacterium tuberculosis* readily develops resistance to pyrazinamide, but there is no cross-resistance with isoniazid or other antituberculosis drugs. The major adverse effects of pyrazinamide are hepatotoxicity (1–5%), nausea, vomiting, hypersensitivity, and hyperuricemia.

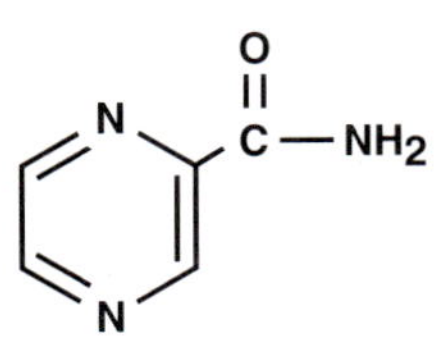

Pyrazinamide (PZA)

CYCLOSERINE

Cycloserine is an antibiotic active against many types of microorganisms, including coliform bacteria, Proteus, and tubercle bacilli. It acts by inhibiting the incorporation of D-alanine into peptidoglycan of bacterial cell walls by blocking alanine racemase. It can be used in urinary tract infections but often causes neurotoxic side effects or shock and is therefore rarely used.

QUINOLONES

Quinolones are synthetic analogues of nalidixic acid. They are active against many gram-positive and gram-negative bacteria. The mode of action of all quinolones involves inhibition of bacterial DNA synthesis by blocking of the DNA gyrase.

The earlier quinolones (nalidixic acid, oxolinic acid, cinoxacin) did not achieve systemic antibacterial levels after oral intake and thus were useful only as urinary antiseptics (see below). The newer fluorinated derivatives (eg, norfloxacin, ciprofloxacin, enoxacin, pefloxacin, and others; see Figure 10–4 for structures) have greater antibacterial activity and low toxicity and achieve clinically useful levels in blood and tissues.

Antimicrobial Activity & Resistance

The fluoroquinolones inhibit many types of gram-negative bacteria—including Enterobacteriaceae, neisseriae, chlamydiae, and others—in concentrations of 0.1–5 μg/mL. Gram-negative organisms and legionellae are inhibited by somewhat larger amounts of these drugs, and anaerobes are even less susceptible. During fluoroquinolone therapy, the emergence of resistance of *Pseudomonas, Staphylococcus,* and other pathogens has been observed.

Chromosomal resistance develops by mutation and involves one of two mechanisms: either an alteration in the A subunit of the target enzyme, DNA gyrase; or a change in outer membrane permeability, resulting in decreased drug accumulation in the bacterium.

Absorption & Excretion

After oral administration, representative fluoroquinolones are well absorbed and widely distributed in body fluids and tissues to varying degrees, but they do not reach the central nervous system to a significant extent. The serum half-life is variable (3–8 hours) and is greatly prolonged in renal failure depending upon the specific drug used.

The fluoroquinolones are mainly excreted into the urine via the kidney, but some of the dose may be metabolized in the liver.

Clinical Uses

Fluoroquinolones are generally effective in urinary tract infections, and several of them benefit prostatitis.

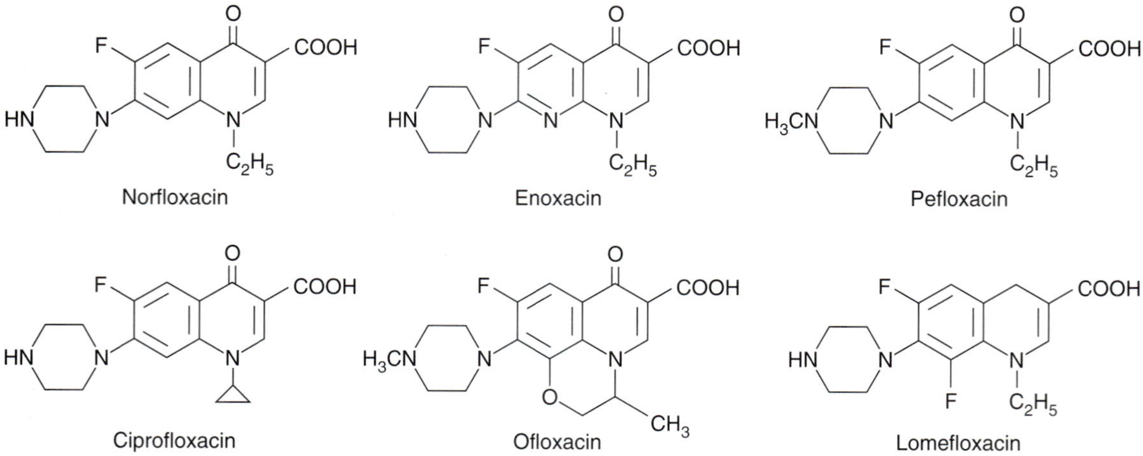

Figure 10–4. Structures of some fluoroquinolones.

Some fluoroquinolones (eg, ofloxacin) are valuable in the treatment of sexually transmitted diseases caused by *N gonorrhoeae* and *C trachomatis* but have no effect on *T pallidum.* These drugs can control lower respiratory infections due to *H influenzae* (but may not be drugs of choice) and enteritis caused by salmonellae, shigellae, or campylobacters. Fluoroquinolones may be suitable for the treatment of major gynecologic and soft tissue bacterial infections and for osteomyelitis of gram-negative or polymicrobic origin. Perhaps they can be used for antimicrobial prophylaxis in neutropenic patients. While they can benefit some exacerbations of cystic fibrosis caused by *Pseudomonas*, about one-third of such mucoid organisms are drug-resistant.

Adverse Effects

Most prominent are nausea, insomnia, headache, and dizziness. Occasionally, there are other gastrointestinal disturbances, impaired liver function, skin rashes, and superinfections, particularly with enterococci and staphylococci. In animals, prolonged administration of fluoroquinolones produces joint damage, and for that reason fluoroquinolones are seldom prescribed for children.

SULFONAMIDES & TRIMETHOPRIM

The sulfonamides are a large group of compounds with the basic formula shown on p 140. By substituting various R-radicals, a series of compounds is obtained with somewhat varying physical, pharmacologic, and antibacterial properties. The basic mechanism of action of all of these compounds is the competitive inhibition of *p*-aminobenzoic acid (PABA) utilization. The simultaneous use of sulfonamides with trimethoprim results in the inhibition of sequential metabolic steps and possible antibacterial synergism.

The sulfonamides are bacteriostatic for some gram-negative and gram-positive bacteria, chlamydiae, nocardiae, and protozoa.

The "soluble" sulfonamides (eg, trisulfapyrimidines, sulfisoxazole) are readily absorbed from the intestinal tract after oral administration of 4–8 g/d and are distributed in all tissues and body fluids (required blood levels: 8–12 mg/dL). Most sulfonamides are excreted rapidly in the urine. Some (eg, sulfamethoxypyridazine) are excreted very slowly and thus tend to be toxic. At present, sulfonamides are particularly useful in the treatment of nocardiosis and first attacks of urinary tract infections due to coliform bacteria. By contrast, many meningococci, shigellae, group A streptococci, and organisms causing recurrent urinary tract infections are now resistant. A mixture of five parts sulfamethoxazole plus one part trimethoprim is widely used in urinary tract infections, shigellosis, and salmonellosis and in infections with other gram-negative bacterial infections and *P carinii* pneumonia.

Trimethoprim alone can be effective treatment for uncomplicated urinary tract infections. Its extensive use in Finland has led to widespread bacterial resistance there.

Resistance

Microorganisms that do not use extracellular PABA but, like mammalian cells, can use preformed folic acid are resistant to sulfonamides. In some sulfonamide-resistant mutants, the tetrahydropteroic acid synthetase has a much higher affinity for PABA than for sulfonamides. The opposite is true for sulfonamide-susceptible organisms.

Side Effects

The soluble sulfonamides may produce side effects that fall into two categories:

A. Allergic Reactions: Many individuals develop hypersensitivity to sulfonamides after initial contact with these drugs and, on reexposure, may develop fever, hives, skin rashes, and chronic vascular diseases such as polyarteritis nodosa.

B. Direct Toxic Effects: There may be fever, skin rashes, gastrointestinal disturbances, depression of the bone marrow leading to anemia or agranulocytosis, hemolytic anemia, and toxic effects on the liver and kidney. Toxicity is especially frequent in patients with AIDS.

Bacteriologic Examination

When culturing specimens from patients receiving sulfonamides, the incorporation of PABA (5 mg/dL) into the medium overcomes sulfonamide inhibition.

DAPSONE

Dapsone is a sulfone, closely related to the sulfonamides. Combined therapy with dapsone and rifampin is often given in the initial therapy of leprosy. Dapsone also may be used to treat *Pneumocystis carinii* pneumonia in AIDS patients. Dapsone is well absorbed from the gastrointestinal tract and is widely distributed in tissues. Side effects are common, including hemolytic anemia, gastrointestinal intolerance, fever, itching, and rashes.

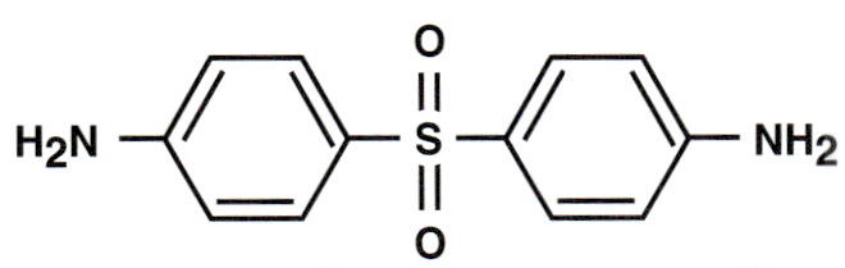

Dapsone

METRONIDAZOLE

Metronidazole is an antiprotozoal drug used in treating *Trichomonas, Giardia,* and amebic infections. It also has striking effects in anaerobic bacterial infections, eg, those due to *Bacteroides* species, and in bacterial vaginosis. It appears to be effective for the preoperative preparation of the colon and in antibiotic-associated diarrhea caused by toxigenic *Clostridium difficile.* Adverse effects include stomatitis, diarrhea, and nausea.

URINARY ANTISEPTICS

These are drugs with antibacterial effects limited to the urine. They fail to produce significant levels in tissues and thus have no effect on systemic infections. However, they effectively lower bacterial counts in the urine and thus greatly diminish the symptoms of lower urinary tract infection. They are used only in the management of urinary tract infections.

The following are commonly used urinary antiseptics: nitrofurantoin, nalidixic acid, methenamine mandelate, and methenamine hippurate. Nitrofurantoin is active against many bacteria but may cause gastrointestinal distress. Nalidixic acid, a quinolone, is effective only in urine, but resistant bacteria may rapidly emerge in the urine. Both methenamine mandelate and methenamine hippurate acidify the urine and liberate formaldehyde there. Other substances that acidify urine (eg, methionine, cranberry juice) may result in bacteriostasis in urine.

Systemically absorbed oral drugs that are excreted in high concentrations in urine are usually preferred in acute urinary tract infections. These include ampicillin, amoxicillin, sulfonamides, quinolones, and others.

REFERENCES

Bahal N, Nahata MC: The new macrolide antibiotics: Azithromycin, clarithromycin, dirithromycin, and roxithromycin. Ann Pharmacother 1992;26:46.

Brewer NS, Hellinger WC: The monobactams. Mayo Clin Proc 1991;66:1152.

Campoli-Richards DM, Brogden RN, Faulds D: Teicoplanin: A review of its antibacterial activity, pharmacokinetic properties and therapeutic potential. Drugs 1990; 40:449.

Donowitz GR, Mandell GL: Drug therapy: Beta-lactam antibiotics. (Two parts.) N Engl J Med 1988;318:419, 490.

Edson RS, Terrell CL: The aminoglycosides. Mayo Clin Proc 1991;66:1158.

Goldman P: Metronidazole. N Engl J Med 1980;303:1212.

Gustaferro CA, Steckelberg JM: Cephalosporin antimicrobial agents and related compounds. Mayo Clin Proc 1991;66:1073.

Handwerger S, Tomasz A: Antibiotic tolerance among clinical isolates of bacteria. Rev Infect Dis 1985;7:368.

Hellinger WC, Brewer NS: Imipenem. Mayo Clin Proc 1991;66:1081.

Ho JL (editor): β-Lactamase inhibition: Therapeutic implications in infectious diseases. Rev Infect Dis 1991;13 (Suppl 9):S573.

Hooper DC, Wolfson JS: Fluoroquinolone antimicrobial agents. N Engl J Med 1991;324:384.

Katzung BG (editor): *Basic & Clinical Pharmacology,* 6th ed. Appleton & Lange, 1994.

Livermore DM: Determinants of the activity of β-lactamase inhibitor combinations. J Antimicrob Chemother 1993;31 (Suppl A):9.

Moellering RC Jr: Meeting the challenges of β-lactamases. J Antimicrob Chemother 1993;31(Suppl A):1.

Nathwani D, Wood MJ: Penicillins: A current review of their clinical pharmacology and therapeutic use. Drugs 1993; 45:866.

Neu HC: New macrolide antibiotics: Azithromycin and clarithromycin. Ann Intern Med 1992;116:517.

Neu HC: Relation of structural properties of beta-lactam antibiotics to antibacterial activity. Am J Med 1985;79 (No. 2A):2.

O'Brien TF et al: Resistance of bacteria to antibacterial agents. Rev Infect Dis 1987;9(Suppl 3):S244.

Petz LD: Immunologic cross-reactivity between penicillins and cephalosporins: A review. J Infect Dis 1978;137 (Suppl):S74.

Rubin RH, Swartz MN: Trimethoprim-sulfamethoxazole. N Engl J Med 1980;303:426.

Russell AD, Hugo WB, Ayliffe GA (editors): *Principles and Practice of Disinfection, Preservation and Sterilization.* Blackwell, 1982.

Siegel D: Tetracyclines: New look at an old antibiotic. 1. Clinical pharmacology, mechanism of action, and untoward effects. N Y State J Med 1978;78:950.

Snider DE Jr et al: Standard therapy for tuberculosis 1985. Chest 1985;87(2 Suppl):117S.

Wilhelm MP: Vancomycin. Mayo Clin Proc 1991;66:1165.

Wright AJ, Wilkowske CJ: The penicillins. Mayo Clin Proc 1991;66:1047.

Normal Microbial Flora of the Human Body

11

The term "normal microbial flora" denotes the population of microorganisms that inhabit the skin and mucous membranes of healthy normal persons. It is doubtful whether a normal viral flora exists in humans.

The skin and mucous membranes always harbor a variety of microorganisms that can be arranged into two groups: (1) The resident flora consists of relatively fixed types of microorganisms regularly found in a given area at a given age; if disturbed, it promptly reestablishes itself. (2) The transient flora consists of nonpathogenic or potentially pathogenic microorganisms that inhabit the skin or mucous membranes for hours, days, or weeks; it is derived from the environment and does not establish itself permanently on the surface. Members of the transient flora are generally of little significance so long as the normal resident flora remains intact. However, if the resident flora is disturbed, transient microorganisms may colonize, proliferate, and produce disease.

Organisms frequently encountered in specimens obtained from various areas of the human body—and considered normal flora—are listed in Table 11–1. The classification of anaerobic normal bacterial flora is discussed in Chapter 22.

ROLE OF THE RESIDENT FLORA

The microorganisms that are constantly present on body surfaces are commensals. Their flourishing in a given area depends upon physiologic factors of temperature, moisture, and the presence of certain nutrients and inhibitory substances. Their presence is not essential to life, because "germ-free" animals can be reared in the complete absence of a normal microbial flora. Yet the resident flora of certain areas plays a definite role in maintaining health and normal function. Members of the resident flora in the intestinal tract synthesize vitamin K and aid in the absorption of nutrients. On mucous membranes and skin, the resident flora may prevent colonization by pathogens and possible disease through "bacterial interference." The mechanism of bacterial interference is not clear. It may involve competition for receptors or binding sites on host cells, competition for nutrients, mutual inhibition by metabolic or toxic products, mutual inhibition by antibiotic materials or bacteriocins, or other mechanisms. Suppression of the normal flora clearly creates a partial local void that tends to be filled by organisms from the environment or from other parts of the body. Such organisms behave as opportunists and may become pathogens.

On the other hand, members of the normal flora may themselves produce disease under certain circumstances. These organisms are adapted to the noninvasive mode of life defined by the limitations of the environment. If forcefully removed from the restrictions of that environment and introduced into the bloodstream or tissues, these organisms may become pathogenic. For example, streptococci of the viridans group are the most common resident organisms of the upper respiratory tract. If large numbers of them are introduced into the bloodstream (eg, following tooth extraction or tonsillectomy), they may settle on deformed or prosthetic heart valves and produce infective endocarditis. Small numbers occur transiently in the bloodstream with minor trauma (eg, dental scaling or vigorous brushing). *Bacteroides* are the commonest resident bacteria of the large intestine and are quite harmless in that location. If introduced into the free peritoneal cavity or into pelvic tissues along with other bacteria as a result of trauma, they cause suppuration and bacteremia. There are many other examples, but the important point is that microbes of the normal resident flora are harmless and may be beneficial in their normal location in the host and in the absence of coincident abnormalities. They may produce disease if introduced into foreign locations in large numbers and if predisposing factors are present.

NORMAL FLORA OF THE SKIN

Because of its constant exposure to and contact with the environment, the skin is particularly apt to contain transient microorganisms. Nevertheless, there is a constant and well-defined resident flora, modified in different anatomic areas by secretions, habitual wearing of clothing, or proximity to mucous membranes (mouth, nose, and perineal areas).

The predominant resident microorganisms of the skin are aerobic and anaerobic diphtheroid bacilli (eg,

Table 11–1. Normal bacteria flora.

Skin

1. *Staphylococcus epidermidis.*
2. *Staphylococcus aureus* (in small numbers).
3. *Micrococcus* species.
4. Nonpathogenic *Neisseria* species.
5. Alpha-hemolytic and nonhemolytic streptococci.
6. Diphtheroids
7. *Propionibacterium* species.
8. *Peptostreptococcus* species.
9. Small numbers of other organisms (*Candida* species, *Acinetobacter* species, etc).

Nasopharynx

1. Any amount of the following: Diphtheroids, nonpathogenic *Neisseria* species, α-hemolytic streptococci; *S epidermidis,* nonhemolytic streptococci, anaerobes (too many species to list; varying amounts of *Prevotella* species, anaerobic cocci, diphtheroids, *Fusobacterium* species, etc).
2. Lesser amounts of the following when accompanied by organisms listed above: yeasts, *Haemophilus* species, pneumococci, *S aureus,* gram-negative rods, *Neisseria meningitidis.*

Gastrointestinal tract and rectum

1. Various Enterobacteriaceae except *Salmonella, Shigella, Yersinia, Vibrio,* and *Campylobacter* species.
2. Non-dextrose-fermenting gram-negative rods.
3. Enterococci.
4. *S epidermidis.*
5. Alpha-hemolytic and nonhemolytic streptococci.
6. Diphtheroids.
7. *S aureus* in small numbers.
8. Yeasts in small numbers.
9. Anaerobes in large numbers (too many species to list).

Genitalia

1. Any amount of the following: *Corynebacterium* species, *Lactobacillus* species, α-hemolytic and nonhemolytic streptococci, nonpathogenic *Neisseria* species.
2. The following when mixed and not predominant; enterococci, Enterobacteriaceae and other gram-negative rods, *S epidermidis, Candida albicans* and other yeasts.
3. Anaerobes (too many species to list); the following may be important when in pure growth or clearly predominant: *Prevotella, Clostridium,* and *Peptostreptococcus* species.

Corynebacterium, Propionibacterium); nonhemolytic aerobic and anaerobic staphylococci (*Staphylococcus epidermidis,* occasionally *Staphylococcus aureus,* and *Peptostreptococcus* species); gram-positive, aerobic, spore-forming bacilli that are ubiquitous in air, water, and soil; alpha-hemolytic streptococci *(viridans streptococci)* and enterococci (*Enterococcus* species); and gram-negative coliform bacilli and *Acinetobacter.* Fungi and yeasts are often present in skin folds; acid-fast, nonpathogenic mycobacteria occur in areas rich in sebaceous secretions (genitalia, external ear).

Among the factors that may be important in eliminating nonresident microorganisms from the skin are the low pH, the fatty acids in sebaceous secretions, and the presence of lysozyme. Neither profuse sweating nor washing and bathing can eliminate or significantly modify the normal resident flora. The number of superficial microorganisms may be diminished by vigorous daily scrubbing with soap containing hexachlorophene or other disinfectants, but the flora is rapidly replenished from sebaceous and sweat glands even when contact with other skin areas or with the environment is completely excluded. Placement of an occlusive dressing on skin tends to result in a large increase in the total microbial population and may also produce qualitative alterations in the flora.

Anaerobes and aerobic bacteria often join to form synergistic infections (gangrene, necrotizing fasciitis, cellulitis) of skin and soft tissues. The bacteria are frequently part of the normal microbial flora. It is usually difficult to pinpoint one specific organism as being responsible for the progressive lesion, since mixtures of organisms are usually involved.

NORMAL FLORA OF THE MOUTH & UPPER RESPIRATORY TRACT

The flora of the nose consists of prominent corynebacteria, staphylococci *(S epidermidis, S aureus),* and streptococci.

The mucous membranes of the mouth and pharynx are often sterile at birth but may be contaminated by passage through the birth canal. Within 4–12 hours after birth, viridans streptococci become established as the most prominent members of the resident flora and remain so for life. They probably originate in the respiratory tracts of the mother and attendants. Early in life, aerobic and anaerobic staphylococci, gram-negative diplococci (neisseriae, *Moraxella catarrhalis*), diphtheroids, and occasional lactobacilli are added. When teeth begin to erupt, the anaerobic spirochetes, *Prevotella* (especially *P melaninogenica*), *Fusobacterium* species, *Rothia* and *Capnocytophaga* species (see below), and some anaerobic vibrios and lactobacilli establish themselves. *Actinomyces* species are normally present in tonsillar tissue and on the gingivae in adults, and various protozoa may also be present. Yeasts (*Candida* species) occur in the mouth.

In the pharynx and trachea, a similar flora establishes itself, whereas few bacteria are found in normal bronchi. Small bronchi and alveoli are normally sterile. The predominant organisms in the upper respiratory tract, particularly the pharynx, are nonhemolytic and alpha-hemolytic streptococci and neisseriae. Staphylococci, diphtheroids, *Haemophilus, pneumococci, Mycoplasma,* and *Prevotella* are also encountered.

Infections of the mouth and respiratory tract often include anaerobes. Periodontal infections, perioral abscesses, sinusitis, and mastoiditis may involve predominantly *Prevotella melaninogenica, Fusobacterium,* and peptostreptococci. Aspiration of saliva (containing up to 10^2 of these organisms and aerobes) may result in necrotizing pneumonia, lung abscess, and empyema.

The Role of the Normal Mouth Flora in Dental Caries

Caries is a disintegration of the teeth beginning at the surface and progressing inward. First the surface enamel, which is entirely noncellular, is demineralized. This has been attributed to the effect of acid products of bacterial fermentation. Subsequent decomposition of the dentin and cement involves bacterial digestion of the protein matrix.

An essential first step in caries production appears to be the formation of plaque on the hard, smooth enamel surface. The plaque consists mainly of gelatinous deposits of high-molecular-weight glucans in which acid-producing bacteria adhere to the enamel. The carbohydrate polymers (glucans) are produced mainly by streptococci (*Streptococcus mutans*, peptostreptococci), perhaps in association with actinomycetes. There appears to be a strong correlation between the presence of *S mutans* and caries on specific enamel areas. The essential second step in caries production appears to be the formation of large amounts of acid (pH < 5.0) from carbohydrates by streptococci and lactobacilli in the plaque. High concentrations of acid demineralize the adjoining enamel and initiate caries.

In experimental "germ-free" animals, cariogenic streptococci can induce the formation of plaque and caries. Adherence to smooth surfaces requires both the synthesis of water-insoluble glucan polymers by glucosyltransferases and the participation of binding sites on the surface of microbial cells. (Perhaps carbohydrate polymers also aid the attachment of some streptococci to endocardial surfaces.) Other members of the oral microflora, eg, *Veillonella*, may complex with glucosyltransferase of *Streptococcus salivarius* in saliva and then synthesize water-insoluble carbohydrate polymers to adhere to tooth surfaces. Adherence may be initiated by salivary IgA antibody to *S mutans*. Certain diphtheroids and streptococci that produce levans can induce specific soft tissue damage and bone resorption typical of periodontal disease. Proteolytic organisms, including actinomycetes and bacilli, play a role in the microbial action on dentin that follows damage to the enamel. The development of caries also depends on genetic, hormonal, nutritional, and many other factors. Control of caries involves physical removal of plaque, limitation of sucrose intake, good nutrition with adequate protein intake, and reduction of acid production in the mouth by limitation of available carbohydrates and frequent cleansing. The application of fluoride to teeth or its ingestion in water results in enhancement of acid resistance of the enamel. Control of periodontal disease requires removal of calculus (calcified deposit) and good mouth hygiene.

Periodontal pockets in the gingiva are particularly rich sources of organisms, including anaerobes, that are rarely encountered elsewhere. While they may participate in periodontal disease and tissue destruction, attention is drawn to them when they are implanted elsewhere, eg, producing infective endocarditis or bacteremia in a granulopenic host. Examples are *Capnocytophaga* species and *Rothia dentocariosa*. *Capnocytophaga* species are fusiform, gram-negative, gliding anaerobes; *Rothia* species are pleomorphic, aerobic, gram-positive rods. Both probably participate in the complex microbial flora of periodontal disease with prominent bone destruction. In granulopenic immunodeficient patients, they can lead to serious opportunistic lesions in other organs.

NORMAL FLORA OF THE INTESTINAL TRACT

At birth the intestine is sterile, but organisms are soon introduced with food. In breast-fed children, the intestine contains large numbers of lactic acid streptococci and lactobacilli. These aerobic and anaerobic, gram-positive, nonmotile organisms (eg, *Bifidobacterium*) produce acid from carbohydrates and tolerate pH 5.0. In bottle-fed children, a more mixed flora exists in the bowel, and lactobacilli are less prominent. As food habits develop toward the adult pattern, the bowel flora changes. Diet has a marked influence on the relative composition of the intestinal and fecal flora. Bowels of newborns in intensive care nurseries tend to be colonized by Enterobacteriaceae, eg, *Klebsiella, Citrobacter, Enterobacter*.

In the normal adult, the esophagus contains microorganisms arriving with saliva and food. The stomach's acidity keeps the number of microorganisms at a minimum (10^3–10^5/g of contents) unless obstruction at the pylorus favors the proliferation of gram-positive cocci and bacilli. The normal acid pH of the stomach markedly protects against infection with some enteric pathogens, eg, cholera. Administration of cimetidine for peptic ulcer leads to a great increase in microbial flora of the stomach, including many organisms usually prevalent in feces. As the pH of intestinal contents becomes alkaline, the resident flora gradually increases. In the adult duodenum, there are 10^3–10^6 bacteria per gram of contents; in the jejunum and ileum, 10^5–10^8 bacteria per gram; and in the cecum and transverse colon, 10^8–10^{10} bacteria per gram. In the upper intestine, lactobacilli and enterococci predominate, but in the lower ileum and cecum, the flora is fecal. In the sigmoid colon and rectum, there are about 10^{11} bacteria per gram of contents, constituting 10–30% of the fecal mass. In diarrhea, the bacterial content may diminish greatly, whereas in intestinal stasis the count rises.

In the normal adult colon, 96–99% of the resident bacterial flora consists of anaerobes: *Bacteroides*, especially *Bacteroides fragilis; Fusobacterium* species; anaerobic lactobacilli, eg, *Bifidobacterium;* clostridia (*Clostridium perfringens*, 10^3–10^5/g); and anaerobic gram-positive cocci (*Peptostreptococcus* species). Only 1–4% are facultative aerobes (gram-negative coliform bacteria, enterococci, and small numbers of *Proteus, Pseudomonas,* lactobacilli, *Candida,* and other organisms). More than 100 distinct types of organisms occur regularly in normal fecal flora. Minor trauma (eg, sigmoidoscopy, barium enema) may induce transient bacteremia in about 10% of procedures.

Intestinal bacteria are important in synthesis of vitamin K, conversion of bile pigments and bile acids, absorption of nutrients and breakdown products, and antagonism to microbial pathogens. The intestinal flora produces ammonia and other breakdown products that are absorbed and can contribute to hepatic coma. Among aerobic coliform bacteria, only a few serotypes persist in the colon for prolonged periods, and most serotypes of *Escherichia coli* are present only over a period of a few days.

Antimicrobial drugs taken orally can, in humans, temporarily suppress the drug-susceptible components of the fecal flora. This is commonly done by the preoperative oral administration of insoluble drugs. For example, neomycin plus erythromycin can in 1–2 days suppress part of the bowel flora, especially aerobes. Metronidazole accomplishes that for anaerobes. If lower bowel surgery is performed when the counts are at their lowest, some protection against infection by accidental spill can be achieved. However, soon thereafter the counts of fecal flora rise again to normal or higher than normal levels, principally of organisms selected out because of relative resistance to the drugs employed. The drug-susceptible microorganisms are replaced by drug-resistant ones, particularly staphylococci, *Enterobacter,* enterococci, *Proteus, Pseudomonas, Clostridium difficile,* and yeasts.

The feeding of large quantities of *Lactobacillus acidophilus* may result in the temporary establishment of this organism in the gut and the concomitant partial suppression of other gut microflora.

The anaerobic flora of the colon including *B fragilis,* clostridia, and peptostreptococci, plays a main role in abscess formation originating in perforation of the bowel. *Prevotella bivia* and *Prevotella disiens* are important in abscesses of the pelvis originating in the female genital organs. Like *B fragilis,* these species are relatively penicillin-resistant; therefore, another effective agent should be used.

NORMAL FLORA OF THE URETHRA

The anterior urethra of both sexes contains small numbers of the same types of organisms found on the skin and perineum. These organisms regularly appear in normal voided urine in numbers of 10^2–10^4/mL.

NORMAL FLORA OF THE VAGINA

Soon after birth, aerobic lactobacilli appear in the vagina and persist as long as the pH remains acid (several weeks). When the pH becomes neutral (remaining so until puberty), a mixed flora of cocci and bacilli is present. At puberty, aerobic and anaerobic lactobacilli reappear in large numbers and contribute to the maintenance of acid pH through the production of acid from carbohydrates, particularly glycogen. This appears to be an important mechanism in preventing the establishment of other, possibly harmful microorganisms in the vagina. If lactobacilli are suppressed by the administration of antimicrobial drugs, yeasts or various bacteria increase in numbers and cause irritation and inflammation. After menopause, lactobacilli again diminish in number and a mixed flora returns. The normal vaginal flora often includes also group B hemolytic streptococci, anaerobic streptococci (peptostreptococci), *Prevotella* species, clostridia, *Gardnerella vaginalis, Ureaplasma urealyticum,* and sometimes *Listeria* or *Mobiluncus* species. The cervical mucus has antibacterial activity and contains lysozyme. In some women, the vaginal introitus contains a heavy flora resembling that of the perineum and perianal area. This may be a predisposing factor in recurrent urinary tract infections. Vaginal organisms present at time of delivery may infect the newborn (eg, group B streptococci).

NORMAL FLORA OF THE EYE (Conjunctiva)

The predominant organisms of the conjunctiva are diphtheroids *(Corynebacterium xerosis), S epidermidis,* and nonhemolytic streptococci. Neisseriae and gram-negative bacilli resembling *Haemophilus* (*Moraxella* species) are also frequently present. The conjunctival flora is normally held in check by the flow of tears, which contain antibacterial lysozyme.

REFERENCES

Aly R et al: Correlation of human in vivo and in vitro cutaneous antimicrobial factors. J Infect Dis 1975;131:579.

Bartlett JB, Polk BF: Bacterial flora of the vagina: Quantitative study. Rev Infect Dis 1984;6(Suppl 1):S67.

Bentley DW et al: The microflora of the human ileum and colon. J Lab Clin Med 1972;79:421.

Drude RB Jr, Hines C Jr: The pathophysiology of intestinal bacterial overgrowth syndromes. Arch Intern Med 1980; 140:1349.

Fainstein V et al: Patterns of oropharyngeal and fecal flora in patients with acute leukemia. J Infect Dis 1981;144: 10.

Finegold SM, George WL (editors): *Anaerobic Infections in Humans.* Academic Press, 1989.

Glickman I: Periodontal disease. N Engl J Med 1971; 284:1071.

Goldmann DA et al: Bacterial colonization of neonates admitted to an intensive care environment. J Pediatr 1978; 93:288.

Hentges DJ: The anaerobic microflora of the human body. Clin Infect Dis 1993;16(Suppl 4):S175.

Leyden JJ et al: Age-related changes in the resident bacterial flora of the human face. J Invest Dermatol 1975;65:379.

Macowiak PA: The normal microbial flora. N Engl J Med 1982;307:83.

McCormack WM et al: Sexually transmitted conditions among women college students. Am J Obstet Gynecol 1981;139:130.

Onderdonk AB et al: Normal vaginal microflora during use of various forms of catamenial protection. Rev Infect Dis 1989;11(Suppl 1):S61.

Redondo-Lopez V, Cook RL, Sobel JD: Emerging role of lactobacilli in the control and maintenance of the vaginal bacterial microflora. Rev Infect Dis 1990;12:856.

Scherp HW: Dental caries. Science 1971;173:1199.

Shooter RA et al: *E coli* serotypes in the faeces of healthy adults over a period of several months. J Hyg 1977;78:95.

Simon GL, Gorbach SL: Intestinal microflora. Med Clin North Am 1982;66:557.

Sutter VL: Anaerobes as normal oral flora. Rev Infect Dis 1984;6(Suppl 1):S62.

12 Spore-Forming Gram-Positive Bacilli: *Bacillus* & *Clostridium* Species

The gram-positive spore-forming bacilli are the *Bacillus* and *Clostridium* species. These bacilli are ubiquitous, and because they form spores, they can survive in the environment for many years. *Bacillus* species are aerobes, whereas clostridia are obligate anaerobes.

Of the many species of both *Bacillus* and *Clostridium* genera, most do not cause disease and are not well characterized in medical microbiology. Several species, however, cause important disease in humans. Anthrax, a prototype disease in the history of microbiology, is caused by *Bacillus anthracis.* Anthrax remains an important disease of animals and occasionally of humans, and *B anthracis* could be a major agent of biological warfare. *Bacillus cereus* causes food poisoning and occasionally eye or other localized infections. Clostridia cause several important toxin-mediated diseases: *Clostridium tetani,* tetanus; *Clostridium botulinum,* botulism; *Clostridium perfringens,* gas gangrene; and *Clostridium difficile,* pseudomembranous colitis. Other clostridia are also found in mixed anaerobic infections in humans (see Chapter 22).

BACILLUS SPECIES

The genus *Bacillus* includes large aerobic, gram-positive rods occurring in chains. Most members of this genus are saprophytic organisms prevalent in soil, water, and air and on vegetation, such as *Bacillus cereus* and *Bacillus subtilis*. Some are insect pathogens. *B cereus* can grow in foods and produce an enterotoxin or an emetic toxin and cause food poisoning. Such organisms may occasionally produce disease in immunocompromised humans (eg, meningitis, endocarditis, endophthalmitis, conjunctivitis, or acute gastroenteritis). *B anthracis,* which causes **anthrax,** is the principal pathogen of the genus.

Morphology & Identification

A. Typical Organisms: The typical cells, measuring 1 × 3–4 μm, have square ends and are arranged in long chains; spores are located in the center of the nonmotile bacilli.

B. Culture: Colonies of *B anthracis* are round and have a "cut glass" appearance in transmitted light. Hemolysis is uncommon with *B anthracis* but common with the saprophytic bacilli. Gelatin is liquefied, and growth in gelatin stabs resembles an inverted fir tree.

C. Growth Characteristics: The saprophytic bacilli utilize simple sources of nitrogen and carbon for energy and growth. The spores are resistant to environmental changes, withstand dry heat and certain chemical disinfectants for moderate periods, and persist for years in dry earth. Animal products contaminated with anthrax spores (eg, hides, bristles, hair, wool, bone) can be sterilized only by autoclaving.

1. *BACILLUS ANTHRACIS* (Figure 12–1)

Antigenic Structure

The capsular substance of *B anthracis,* which consists of a polypeptide of high molecular weight composed of D-glutamic acid, is a hapten. The bacterial bodies contain protein and a somatic polysaccharide, both of which are antigenic.

Pathogenesis

Anthrax is primarily a disease of sheep, cattle, horses, and many other animals; humans are affected only rarely. The infection is usually acquired by the entry of spores through injured skin or mucous membranes, rarely by inhalation of spores into the lung. In animals, the portal of entry is the mouth and the gastrointestinal tract. Spores from contaminated soil find easy access when ingested with spiny or irritating vegetation. In humans, scratches in the skin or inhalation (see below) leads to infection.

The spores germinate in the tissue at the site of entry, and growth of the vegetative organisms results in formation of a gelatinous edema and congestion. Bacilli spread via lymphatics to the bloodstream, and they multiply freely in the blood and tissues shortly before and after the animal's death. In the plasma of animals dying from anthrax, a toxic factor has been demonstrated. This material kills mice or guinea pigs upon inoculation and is specifically neutralized by anthrax antiserum.

The exudate in anthrax contains a polypeptide, identical with that in the capsule of the *Bacillus*, which can

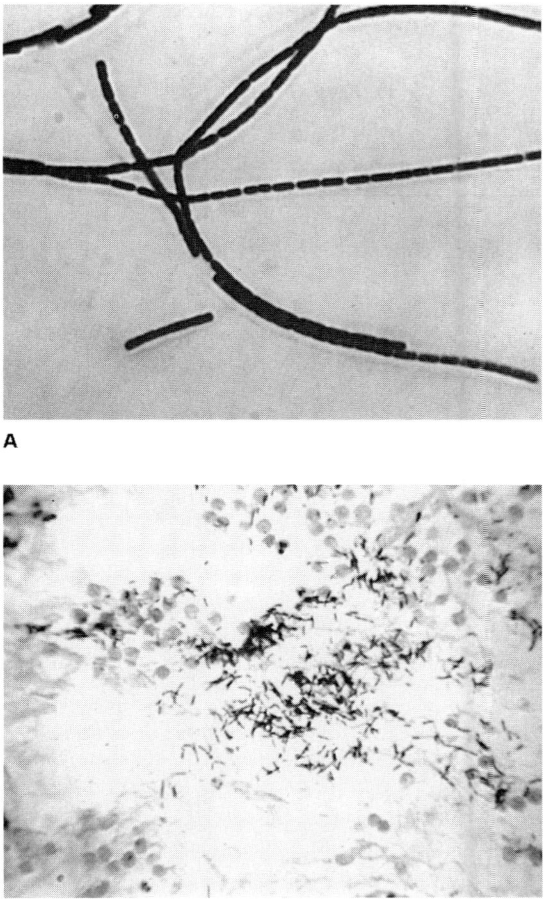

Figure 12–1. *Bacillus anthracis* in culture ***(A)*** and in tissue ***(B).*** (Photos courtesy of Dr Philip S. Brachman, Emory University School of Public Health and Center for International Health.)

evoke histologic reactions similar to those of anthrax infection. Other proteins isolated from exudate stimulate solid immunity to anthrax upon injection into animals. From culture filtrates ("anthrax toxin"), three substances have been separated by glass filtration and chromatography: (1) protective antigen, (2) edema factor, and (3) lethal factor. Mixtures of (1), (2), and (3) are more toxic in animals and more immunogenic than single substances. Toxin production is under genetic control of a plasmid, loss of which results in loss of toxin production.

Another type of anthrax is inhalation anthrax ("woolsorter's disease"). The inhalation of anthrax spores from the dust of wool, hair, or hides results in germination of the spores in the lungs or in tracheobronchial lymph nodes and the production of hemorrhagic mediastinitis, pneumonia, meningitis, and sepsis, which are usually rapidly fatal. In anthrax sepsis, the number of organisms in the blood exceeds 10^7/mL just prior to death.

Pathology

In susceptible animals, the organisms proliferate at the site of entry. The capsules remain intact, and the organisms are surrounded by a large amount of proteinaceous fluid containing few leukocytes from which they rapidly disseminate and reach the bloodstream.

In resistant animals, the organisms proliferate for a few hours, by which time there is massive accumulation of leukocytes. The capsules gradually disintegrate and disappear. The organisms remain localized.

Clinical Findings

In humans, anthrax gives rise to an infection of the skin (malignant pustule). A papule first develops within 12–36 hours after entry of the organisms or spores through a scratch. This papule rapidly changes into a vesicle, then a pustule, and finally a necrotic ulcer from which the infection may disseminate, giving rise to septicemia.

In inhalation anthrax, early manifestations may be mediastinitis, sepsis, meningitis, or hemorrhagic pulmonary edema. Hemorrhagic pneumonia with shock is a terminal event.

Whereas animals often acquire anthrax through ingestion of spores and spread of the organisms from the intestinal tract, this is exceedingly rare in humans. Thus, abdominal pain, vomiting, and bloody diarrhea are rare clinical signs.

Diagnostic Laboratory Tests

A. Specimens: Fluid or pus from local lesion; blood, sputum.

B. Stained Smears: From the local lesion or blood of dead animals; chains of large gram-positive rods are often seen. Anthrax can be identified in dried smears by immunofluorescence staining techniques.

C. Culture: When grown on blood agar plates, the organisms produce nonhemolytic gray colonies with typical microscopic morphology. Carbohydrate fermentation is not useful. In semisolid medium, anthrax bacilli are always nonmotile, whereas related nonpathogenic organisms (eg, *B cereus*) exhibit motility by "swarming." Virulent anthrax cultures kill mice or guinea pigs upon intraperitoneal injection.

D. Serologic Tests: Precipitating or hemagglutinating antibodies can be demonstrated in the serum of vaccinated or infected persons or animals.

Resistance & Immunity

Some animals (guinea pig) are highly susceptible, whereas others (rat) are very resistant to anthrax infection. This fact has been attributed to a variety of defense mechanisms: leukocytic activity, body temperature, and the bactericidal action of the blood. Certain basic polypeptides that kill anthrax bacilli have been isolated from animal tissues. A synthetic polylysine has a similar action.

Active immunity to anthrax can be induced in susceptible animals by vaccination with live attenuated bacilli, with spore suspensions, or with protective antigens from culture filtrates (see above). Immune serum is sometimes injected together with live bacilli into animals. Anthrax immunization is based on the classic experiments of Louis Pasteur, who in 1881 proved that cultures that had been grown in broth at 42–52 °C for several months lost much of their virulence and could be injected live into sheep and cattle without causing disease; subsequently, such animals proved to be immune. There are great variations in the efficacy of various vaccines.

Treatment

Many antibiotics are effective against anthrax in humans, but treatment must be started early. Penicillin is satisfactory treatment except in inhalation anthrax, in which the mortality rate remains high. Some other gram-positive bacilli may be resistant to penicillin by virtue of β-lactamase production. Tetracyclines, erythromycin, or clindamycin may be effective.

Epidemiology, Prevention, & Control

Soil is contaminated with anthrax spores from the carcasses of dead animals. These spores remain viable for decades. Perhaps spores can germinate in soil at pH 6.5 at proper temperature. Grazing animals infected through injured mucous membranes serve to perpetuate the chain of infection. Contact with infected animals or with their hides, hair, and bristles is the source of infection in humans. Control measures include (1) disposal of animal carcasses by burning or by deep burial in lime pits, (2) decontamination (usually by autoclaving) of animal products, (3) protective clothing and gloves for handling potentially infected materials, and (4) active immunization of domestic animals with live attenuated vaccines. Persons with high occupational risk should be immunized with a cell-free vaccine obtainable from the Centers for Disease Control and Prevention, Atlanta, GA 30333.

2. *BACILLUS CEREUS*

Food poisoning caused by *Bacillus cereus* has two distinct forms, the emetic type and the diarrheal type associated with meat dishes and sauces. *B cereus* produces toxins that cause disease which is more an intoxication than a food-borne infection. The emetic form is manifested by nausea, vomiting, abdominal cramps, and occasionally diarrhea and is self-limiting, with recovery occurring within 24 hours. It begins 1–5 hours after ingestion of rice and occasionally pasta dishes. *B cereus* is a soil organism that commonly contaminates rice. When large amounts of rice are cooked and allowed to cool slowly, the *B cereus* spores germinate and the vegetative cells produce the toxin during log-phase growth or during sporulation. The diarrheal form has an incubation period of 1–24 hours and is manifested by profuse diarrhea with abdominal pain and cramps; fever and vomiting are uncommon. The enterotoxin may be preformed in the food or produced in the intestine. The presence of *B cereus* in a patient's stool is not sufficient to make a diagnosis of *B cereus* disease, since the bacteria may be present in normal stool specimens; a concentration of 10^5 bacteria or more per gram of food is considered diagnostic.

B cereus is an important cause of eye infections, severe keratitis, endophthalmitis, and panophthalmitis. Typically, the organisms are introduced into the eye by foreign bodies associated with trauma. *B cereus* has also been associated with localized infections and with systemic infections, including endocarditis, meningitis, osteomyelitis, and pneumonia; the presence of a medical device or intravenous drug use predisposes to these infections.

Other *Bacillus* species are rarely associated with human disease. It is difficult to differentiate superficial contamination with *Bacillus* from genuine disease caused by the organism. Five *Bacillus* species (*B thuringiensis, B popilliae, B sphaericus,* B larvae, and *B lentimorbus*) are pathogens for insects, and some have been used as commercial insecticides.

CLOSTRIDIUM SPECIES

The clostridia are large anaerobic, gram-positive, motile rods. Many decompose proteins or form toxins, and some do both. Their natural habitat is the soil or the intestinal tract of animals and humans, where they live as saprophytes. Among the pathogens are the organisms causing **botulism, tetanus, gas gangrene,** and **pseudomembranous colitis.**

Morphology & Identification

A. Typical Organisms: Spores of clostridia are usually wider than the diameter of the rods in which they are formed (Figure 12-2). In the various species, the spore is placed centrally, subterminally, or terminally. Most species of clostridia are motile and possess peritrichous flagella.

B. Culture: Clostridia grow only under anaerobic conditions, established by one of the following means (see Chapter 22):

1. Agar plates or culture tubes are placed in an airtight jar from which air is removed and replaced by nitrogen with 10% CO_2, or oxygen may be removed by other means (Gaspack).

2. Fluid media are put in deep tubes containing either fresh animal tissue (eg, chopped cooked meat) or 0.1% agar and a reducing agent such as thioglycolate. Such tubes can be handled like aerobic media, and growth will occur from the bottom up to within 15 mm of the surface exposed to air.

C. Colony Forms: Some organisms produce large raised colonies with entire margins (eg, *C perfringens*); others produce smaller colonies that extend in a meshwork of the fine filaments (eg, *C tetani*). Many clostridia produce a zone of hemolysis on blood agar. *C perfringens* typically produces multiple zones of hemolysis around colonies.

D. Growth Characteristics: The outstanding characteristic of anaerobic microorganisms is their inability to utilize oxygen as the final hydrogen acceptor. They lack cytochrome and cytochrome oxidase and are unable to break down hydrogen peroxide because they lack catalase and peroxidase. Therefore, H_2O_2 tends to accumulate to toxic concentrations in the presence of oxygen. Clostridia and other obligate anaerobes probably also lack superoxide dismutase and consequently permit the accumulation of the toxic free radical superoxide anion. Such anaerobes can carry out their metabolic reactions only at a negative oxidation-reduction potential (E_h), ie, in an environment that is strongly reducing.

Clostridia can ferment a variety of sugars; many can digest proteins. Milk is turned acid by some and digested by others and undergoes "stormy fermentation" (ie, clot torn by gas) with a third group (eg, *C perfringens*). Various enzymes are produced by different species (see below).

E. Antigenic Characteristics: Clostridia share some antigens but also possess specific soluble antigens that permit grouping by precipitin tests.

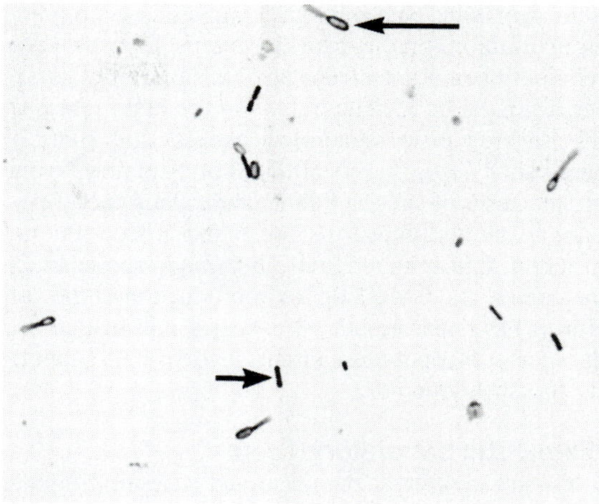

Figure 12–2. *Clostridium* Gram stain. Individual gram-positive bacilli are present (short arrow). Some bacilli have terminal spores (long arrow).

1. *CLOSTRIDIUM BOTULINUM*

Clostridium botulinum, which causes **botulism,** is worldwide in distribution; it is found in soil and occasionally in animal feces.

Types of *C botulinum* are distinguished by the antigenic type of toxin they produce. Spores of the organism are highly resistant to heat, withstanding 100 °C for at least 3–5 hours. Heat resistance is diminished at acid pH or high salt concentration.

Toxin

During the growth of *C botulinum* and during autolysis of the bacteria, toxin is liberated into the environment. Seven antigenic varieties of toxin (A–G) are known. Types A, B, and E (and occasionally F) are the principal causes of human illness. Types A and B have been associated with a variety of foods, and type E predominantly with fish products. Type C produces limberneck in birds; type D, botulism in mammals. The toxins are neurotoxic proteins (MW 150,000) of similar structure and action. They are made up of heavy and light chains linked by a disulfide bond. The heavy chain is thought to specifically and avidly bind the toxin to the motor nerve endplates and with the internalization of the toxin. The light chain blocks the calcium-mediated release of acetylcholine. *C botulinum* toxins are among the most highly toxic substances known: the lethal dose for a human is probably about 1–2 μg. The toxins are destroyed by heating for 20 minutes at 100 °C. Toxin production is under control of a viral gene. Some toxigenic *C botulinum* strains yield bacteriophages that may infect nontoxigenic strains and convert them to toxigenicity.

Pathogenesis

Although *C botulinum* types A and B have been implicated in rare cases of wound infection and botulism, the illness is not an infection. Botulism is an intoxication resulting from the ingestion of food in which *C botulinum* has grown and produced toxin. The most common offenders are spiced, smoked, vacuum-packed, or canned alkaline foods that are eaten without cooking. In such foods, spores of *C botulinum* germinate; under anaerobic conditions, vegetative forms grow and produce toxin.

The toxin acts by blocking release of acetylcholine at synapses and neuromuscular junctions. Flaccid paralysis results. The electromyogram and edrophonium (Tensilon) strength tests are typical.

Clinical Findings

Symptoms begin 18–24 hours after ingestion of the toxic food, with visual disturbances (incoordination of eye muscles, double vision), inability to swallow, and speech difficulty; signs of bulbar paralysis are progressive, and death occurs from respiratory paralysis or cardiac arrest. Gastrointestinal symptoms are not regularly prominent. There is no fever. The patient remains fully conscious until shortly before death. The mortality rate is high. Patients who recover do not develop antitoxin in the blood.

In the United States, infant botulism is as common as or more common than the classic form of paralytic botulism associated with the ingestion of toxin-contaminated food. The infants in the first months of life develop poor feeding, weakness, and signs of paralysis ("floppy baby"). Infant botulism may be one of the causes of sudden infant death syndrome. *C botulinum* and botulinus toxin are found in feces but not in serum. It is assumed that *C botulinum* spores are in the babies' food, yielding toxin production in the gut. Honey has been implicated as a possible vehicle for the spores. Most of these infants recover with supportive therapy alone.

Diagnostic Laboratory Tests

Toxin can often be demonstrated in serum from the patient, and toxin may be found in leftover food. Mice injected intraperitoneally die rapidly. The antigenic type of toxin is identified by neutralization with specific antitoxin in mice. *C botulinum* may be grown from food remains and tested for toxin production, but this is rarely done and is of questionable significance. In infant botulism, *C botulinum* and toxin can be demonstrated in bowel contents but not in serum. Toxin may be demonstrated by passive hemagglutination or radioimmunoassay.

Treatment

Potent antitoxins to three types of botulinus toxins have been prepared in animals. Since the type responsible for an individual case is usually not known, trivalent (A, B, E) antitoxin (available from the Centers for Disease Control, Atlanta, GA 30333; central telephone number 404-639-3311) must be promptly administered intravenously with customary precautions. Adequate ventilation must be maintained by mechanical respirator, if necessary. These measures have reduced the mortality rate from 65% to below 25%.

Epidemiology, Prevention, & Control

Since spores of *C botulinum* are widely distributed in soil, they often contaminate vegetables, fruits, and other materials. A large restaurant-based outbreak was associated with sautéed onions. When such foods are canned or otherwise preserved, they either must be sufficiently heated to ensure destruction of spores or must be boiled for 20 minutes before consumption. Strict regulation of commercial canning has largely overcome the danger of widespread outbreaks, but commercially canned mushrooms and vichyssoise have caused deaths. At present, the chief danger lies in home-canned foods, particularly string beans, corn, peppers, olives, peas, and smoked fish or vacuum-packed fresh fish in plastic bags. Toxic foods may be spoiled and rancid, and cans may "swell"; or the appearance may be innocuous. The risk from home-canned foods can be reduced if the food is boiled for more than 20 minutes before consumption. Toxoids are used for active immunization of cattle in South Africa.

2. *CLOSTRIDIUM* TETANI

Clostridium tetani, which causes **tetanus,** is worldwide in distribution in the soil and in the feces of horses and other animals. Several types of *C tetani* can be distinguished by specific flagellar antigens. All share a common O (somatic) antigen, which may be masked, and all produce the same antigenic type of neurotoxin, tetanospasmin.

Toxin

Vegetative cells of *C tetani* produce tetanospasmin and release it mainly when they lyse. Toxin production appears to be under control of a plasmid gene. The intracellular toxin is a polypeptide (MW 160,000) that proteolytic enzymes split into two fragments of increased toxicity. Purified toxin contains more than 2×10^7 mouse lethal doses per milligram. Tetanospasmin acts in several ways upon the central nervous system. It inhibits release of acetylcholine, thus interfering with neuromuscular transmission. The most important action, however, is the inhibition of postsynaptic spinal neurons by blocking the release of an inhibitory mediator. This results in generalized muscular spasms, hyperreflexia, and seizures.

Pathogenesis

C tetani is not an invasive organism. The infection remains strictly localized in the area of devitalized tissue (wound, burn, injury, umbilical stump, surgical suture) into which the spores have been introduced. The volume of infected tissue is small, and the disease is almost entirely a toxemia. Germination of the spore and development of vegetative organisms that produce toxin are aided by (1) necrotic tissue, (2) calcium salts, and (3) associated pyogenic infections, all of which aid establishment of low oxidation-reduction potential.

The toxin released from vegetative cells may reach the central nervous system by retrograde axonal transport or via the bloodstream. In the central nervous system, the toxin rapidly becomes fixed to gangliosides in spinal cord and brain stem and exerts the actions described above.

Clinical Findings

The incubation period may range from 4–5 days to as many weeks. The disease is characterized by convulsive tonic contraction of voluntary muscles. Muscular spasms often involve first the area of injury and infection and then the muscles of the jaw (trismus, lockjaw), which contract so that the mouth cannot be opened. Gradually, other voluntary muscles become involved, resulting in tonic spasms. Any external stimulus may precipitate a tetanic seizure. The patient is fully conscious, and pain may be intense. Death usually results from interference with the mechanics of respiration. The mortality rate in generalized tetanus is very high.

Diagnosis

The diagnosis rests on the clinical picture and a history of injury, although only 50% of patients with tetanus have an injury for which they seek medical attention. The primary differential diagnosis of tetanus is strychnine poisoning. Anaerobic culture of tissues from contaminated wounds may yield *C tetani,* but neither preventive nor therapeutic use of antitoxin should ever be withheld pending such demonstration. Proof of isolation of *C tetani* must rest on production of toxin and its neutralization by specific antitoxin.

Prevention & Treatment

The results of treatment of tetanus are not satisfactory. Therefore, prevention is all-important. Prevention of tetanus depends upon (1) active immunization with toxoids; (2) proper care of wounds contaminated with soil, etc; (3) prophylactic use of antitoxin; and (4) administration of penicillin.

A. Antitoxin: Tetanus antitoxin, prepared in animals or humans, can neutralize the toxin, but only before it becomes fixed onto nervous tissue. Because of the frequency of hypersensitivity reactions to foreign serum and because of the rapidity with which foreign serum is eliminated, the administration of human antitoxin is preferable. The intramuscular administration of 250–500 units of human antitoxin (tetanus immune globulin) gives adequate systemic protection (0.01 unit or more per milliliter of serum) for 2–4 weeks. Active immunization with tetanus toxoid should accompany antitoxin prophylaxis.

Patients who develop symptoms of tetanus should receive muscle relaxants, sedation, and assisted ventilation. Sometimes they are given very large doses of antitoxin (3000–10,000 units of tetanus immune globulin) intravenously in an effort to neutralize toxin that has not yet been bound to nervous tissue. However, the efficacy of antitoxin for treatment is doubtful except in neonatal tetanus, where it may be lifesaving.

B. Surgical Measures: Surgical debridement is vitally important because it removes the necrotic tissue that is essential for proliferation of the organisms. Hyperbaric oxygen has no proved effect.

C. Antibiotics: Penicillin strongly inhibits the growth of *C tetani* and stops further toxin production. Antibiotics may also control associated pyogenic infection.

D. Tetanus Toxoid: When a previously immunized individual sustains a potentially dangerous wound, an additional dose of toxoid should be injected to restimulate antitoxin production. This "recall" injection of toxoid may be accompanied by a dose of antitoxin if the patient has not had current immunization or boosters or if the history of immunization is unknown.

Control

Tetanus is a totally preventable disease. Universal active immunization with tetanus toxoid should be mandatory. Tetanus toxoid is produced by detoxifying the toxin with formalin and then concentrating it. Aluminum-salt-adsorbed toxoids are employed. Three injections comprise the initial course of immunization, followed by another dose about 1 year later. Initial immunization should be carried out in all children during the first year of life. A "booster" injection of toxoid is given upon entry into school. Thereafter, "boosters" can be spaced 10 years apart to maintain serum levels of more than 0.01 unit antitoxin per milliliter. In young children, tetanus toxoid is often combined with diphtheria toxoid and pertussis vaccine.

Control measures are not possible because of the wide dissemination of the organism in the soil and the long survival of its spores. Narcotics addicts who inject drugs subcutaneously are a high-risk group.

3. CLOSTRIDIA THAT PRODUCE INVASIVE INFECTIONS (*Clostridium perfringens* & Related Clostridia) (Figure 12–3)

Many different toxin-producing clostridia can produce invasive infection (including **myonecrosis** and **gas gangrene**) if introduced into damaged tissue.

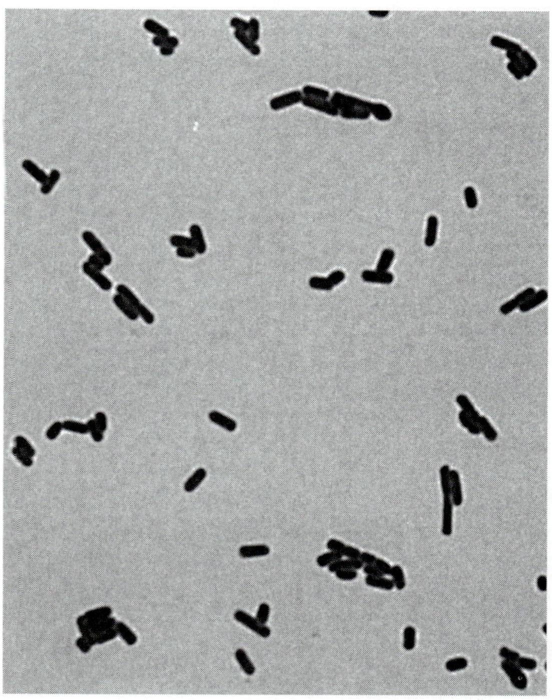

Figure 12–3. Gas gangrene bacilli. *C perfringens* typically does not form spores when grown on laboratory media.

About 30 species of clostridia may produce such an effect, but the most common in invasive disease is *Clostridium perfringens* (90%). An enterotoxin of *C perfringens* is a common cause of food poisoning.

Toxins

The clostridia produce a large variety of toxins and enzymes that result in a spreading infection. Many of these toxins have lethal, necrotizing, and hemolytic properties. In some cases, these are different properties of a single substance; in other instances, they are due to different chemical entities. The alpha toxin of *C perfringens* type A is a lecithinase, and its lethal action is proportionate to the rate at which it splits lecithin (an important constituent of cell membranes) to phosphorylcholine and diglyceride. The theta toxin has similar hemolytic and necrotizing effects but is not a lecithinase. DNase and hyaluronidase, a collagenase that digests collagen of subcutaneous tissue and muscle, are also produced.

Some strains of *C perfringens* produce a powerful enterotoxin, especially when growing in meat dishes. The action of *C perfringens* enterotoxin involves marked hypersecretion in the jejunum and ileum, with loss of fluids and electrolytes in diarrhea. The precise mechanism is not established, but it may not involve stimulation of adenylyl cyclase or guanylyl cyclase. When more than 10^8 vegetative cells are ingested and sporulate in the gut, enterotoxin is formed. The enterotoxin is a protein (MW 35,000) that appears identical with a component of the spore coat, is distinct from other clostridial toxins, and induces intense diarrhea in 6–18 hours. This illness is similar to that produced by *B cereus* and tends to be self-limited.

Pathogenesis

Clostridial spores reach tissue either by contamination of traumatized areas (soil, feces) or from the intestinal tract. The spores germinate at low oxidation-reduction potential; vegetative cells multiply, ferment carbohydrates present in tissue, and produce gas. The distention of tissue and interference with blood supply, together with the secretion of necrotizing toxin and hyaluronidase, favor the spread of infection. Tissue necrosis extends, providing an opportunity for increased bacterial growth, hemolytic anemia, and, ultimately, severe toxemia and death.

In gas gangrene (clostridial myonecrosis), a mixed infection is the rule. In addition to the toxigenic clostridia, proteolytic clostridia and various cocci and gram-negative organisms are also usually present. *C perfringens* occurs in the genital tract of 5% of women. Before legalization of abortion in the United States, clostridial uterine infections followed instrumental abortions. Clostridial bacteremia is a frequent occurrence in patients with neoplasms. In New Guinea, *C perfringens* type C produces a necrotizing enteritis (pigbel) that can be highly fatal in children. Immunization with type C toxoid appears to have preventive value.

Clinical Findings

From a contaminated wound (eg, a compound fracture, postpartum uterus), the infection spreads in 1–3 days to produce crepitation in the subcutaneous tissue and muscle, foul-smelling discharge, rapidly progressing necrosis, fever, hemolysis, toxemia, shock, and death. Treatment is with early surgery (amputation) and antitoxin administration. Until the advent of specific therapy, early amputation was the only treatment. At times, the infection results only in anaerobic fasciitis or cellulitis.

C perfringens food poisoning usually follows the ingestion of large numbers of clostridia that have grown in warmed meat dishes. The toxin forms when the organisms sporulate in the gut, with the onset of diarrhea—usually without vomiting or fever—in 6–18 hours. The illness lasts only 1–2 days.

Diagnostic Laboratory Tests

A. Specimens: Material from wounds, pus, tissue.

B. Smears: The presence of large gram-positive rods in Gram-stained smears suggests gas gangrene clostridia; spores are not regularly present.

C. Culture: Material is inoculated into chopped meat-glucose medium and thioglycolate medium and onto blood agar plates incubated anaerobically. The growth from one of the media is transferred into milk. A clot torn by gas in 24 hours is suggestive of *C perfringens*. Once pure cultures have been obtained by selecting colonies from anaerobically incubated blood plates, they are identified by biochemical reactions (various sugars in thioglycolate, action on milk), hemolysis, and colony form. Lecithinase activity is evaluated by the precipitate formed around colonies on egg yolk media. Final identification rests on toxin production and neutralization by specific antitoxin. *C perfringens* rarely produces spores when cultured on agar in the laboratory.

Treatment

The most important aspect of treatment is prompt and extensive surgical debridement of the involved area and excision of all devitalized tissue, in which the organisms are prone to grow. Administration of antimicrobial drugs, particularly penicillin, is begun at the same time. Hyperbaric oxygen may be of help in the medical management of clostridial tissue infections. It is said to "detoxify" patients rapidly.

Antitoxins are available against the toxins of *C perfringens, Clostridium novyi, Clostridium histolyticum,* and *Clostridium septicum,* usually in the form of concentrated immune globulins. Polyvalent antitoxin (containing antibodies to several toxins) has been used. Although such antitoxin is sometimes administered to individuals with contaminated wounds containing much devitalized tissue, there is no evidence for its efficacy. Food poisoning due to *C perfringens* enterotoxin usually requires only symptomatic care.

Prevention & Control

Early and adequate cleansing of contaminated wounds and surgical debridement, together with the administration of antimicrobial drugs directed against clostridia (eg, penicillin), are the best available preventive measures. Antitoxins should not be relied on. Although toxoids for active immunization have been prepared, they have not come into practical use.

4. *CLOSTRIDIUM DIFFICILE* & DIARRHEAL DISEASE

Pseudomembranous Colitis

Pseudomembranous colitis is diagnosed by detection of one or both *C difficile* toxins in stool and by endoscopic observation of pseudomembranes or microabscesses in patients who have diarrhea and have been given antibiotics. Plaques and microabscesses may be localized to one area of the bowel. The diarrhea may be watery or bloody, and the patient frequently has associated abdominal cramps, leukocytosis, and fever. Although many antibiotics have been associated with pseudomembranous colitis, the most common are ampicillin and clindamycin. The disease is treated by discontinuing administration of the offending antibiotic and orally giving either metronidazole or vancomycin.

Administration of antibiotics results in proliferation of drug-resistant *C difficile* that produce two toxins. Toxin A (MW 440,000–500,000), a potent enterotoxin that also has some cytotoxic activity, binds to the brush border membranes of the gut at receptor sites. Toxin B (MW 360,000–470,000) is a potent cytotoxin. Both toxins are found in the stools of patients with pseudomembranous colitis. Not all strains of *C difficile* produce the toxins, and though the *tox* genes apparently are not carried on plasmids or phage, the genetic regulation of toxin production is unknown.

Antibiotic-Associated Diarrhea

The administration of antibiotics frequently leads to a mild to moderate form of diarrhea, termed antibiotic-associated diarrhea. This disease is generally less severe than the classic form of pseudomembranous colitis. As many as 25% of cases of antibiotic-associated diarrhea may be associated with *C difficile.*

REFERENCES

Abramova et al: Pathology of inhalation anthrax in 42 cases from the Sverdlovsk outbreak in 1979. Proc Nat Acad Sci (USA) 1993;90:2291.

Arnon SS et al: Intestinal infection and toxin production by *Clostridium botulinum* as one cause of sudden infant death syndrome. Lancet 1978;1:1273.

Bartlett JG: Antibiotic-associated diarrhea. Clin Infect Dis 1992;15:573.

Brachman PS: Inhalation anthrax. Ann NY Acad Sci 1980; 353:83.

Caplan ES, Kluge RM: Gas gangrene: Review of 34 cases. Arch Intern Med 1976;136:788.

Davey RT Jr, Tauber WB: Posttraumatic endophthalmitis: The emerging role of *Bacillus cereus* infection. Rev Infect Dis 1987;9:110.

Drobniewski FA: *Bacillus cereus* and related species. Clin Microbiol Rev 1993;6:324.

Edmondson RS, Flowers MW: Intensive care in tetanus: Management, complications and mortality in 100 cases. Br Med J 1979;1:1401.

Hambleton P: *Clostridium botulinum* toxins: A general review of involvement in disease, structure, mode of action and preparation for clinical use. J Neurol 1992;239:16.

Hatheway CL: Toxigenic clostridia. Clin Microbiol Rev 1990;3:66.

Laird WJ et al: Plasmid-associated toxigenicity in *Clostridium tetani.* J Infect Dis 1980;142:623.

Lyerly DM et al: *Clostridium difficile:* Its disease and toxins. Clin Microbiol Rev 1988;1:1.

Midura TF et al: Isolation of *Clostridium botulinum* from honey. J Clin Microbiol 1979;9:282.

Simpson LL: The action of botulinal toxin. Rev Infect Dis 1979;1:656.

Stark RL: Biological characteristics of *C perfringens.* Infect Immun 1971;4:89.

Stevens DL et al: Lethal effects and cardiovascular effects of purified α- and θ-toxins from *Clostridium perfringens.* J Infect Dis 1988;157:272.

Sugiyama H: *Clostridium botulinum* neurotoxicity. Microbiol Rev 1980;44:419.

Thomas M et al: Hospital outbreak of *Clostridium perfringens* food poisoning. Lancet 1977;1:1046.

Weinstein L: Tetanus. N Engl J Med 1973;289:1293.

Wilson KH: The microecology of *Clostridium difficile.* Clin Infect Dis 1993;16(Suppl 4):S214.

13 Non-Spore-Forming Gram-Positive Bacilli: *Corynebacterium, Propionibacterium, Listeria, Erysipelothrix,* & Related Species

The non-spore-forming gram-positive bacilli are a diverse group of bacteria. Many members of the genus *Corynebacterium* and their anaerobic equivalents, *Propionibacterium* species, are members of the normal flora of skin and mucous membranes of humans. Other corynebacteria are found in animals and plants. *Corynebacterium diphtheriae* is the most important member of the group, as it can produce a powerful exotoxin that causes diphtheria in humans. *Listeria monocytogenes* and *Erysipelothrix rhusiopathiae* are primarily found in animals and occasionally cause severe disease in humans.

CORYNEBACTERIUM DIPHTHERIAE

Morphology & Identification

A. Typical Organisms: Corynebacteria are 0.5–1 μm in diameter and several micrometers long. Characteristically, they possess irregular swellings at one end that give them a "club-shaped" appearance (Figure 13–1). Irregularly distributed within the rod (often near the poles) are granules staining deeply with aniline dyes (metachromatic granules) that give the rod a beaded appearance. Individual corynebacteria in stained smears tend to lie parallel or at acute angles to one another. True branching is rarely observed in cultures.

B. Culture: On blood agar, the *C diphtheriae* colonies are small, granular, and gray, with irregular edges, and may have small zones of hemolysis. On agar containing potassium tellurite, the colonies are brown to black because the tellurite is reduced intracellularly (staphylococci and streptococci can also produce black colonies). Three biovars of *C diphtheriae* have been widely recognized: *gravis, mitis,* and *intermedius.* These variants have been classified on the basis of growth characteristics such as colony morphology, biochemical reactions, and, severity of disease produced by infection. Very few reference laboratories provide the biovar characterization; the incidence of diphtheria has greatly decreased and the association of severity of disease with biovar is not important to clinical or public health management of cases or outbreaks. If necessary in the setting of an outbreak, immunochemical and molecular methods can be used to type the *C diphtheriae* isolates.

C. Growth Characteristics: *C diphtheriae* and other corynebacteria grow aerobically on most ordinary laboratory media. *Propionibacterium* is an anaerobe. On Loeffler's serum medium, corynebacteria grow much more readily than other respiratory pathogens, and the morphology of organisms is typical in smears. Acid, but not gas, is formed from some carbohydrates, as illustrated in Table 13–1.

D. Variation and Conversion: Corynebacteria tend to pleomorphism in microscopic and colonial morphology. When some nontoxigenic diphtheria organisms are infected with bacteriophage from certain toxigenic diphtheria bacilli, the offspring of the exposed bacteria are lysogenic and toxigenic, and this trait is subsequently hereditary. When toxigenic diphtheria bacilli are serially subcultured in specific antiserum against the temperate phage that they carry, they tend to become nontoxigenic. Thus, acquisition of phage leads to toxigenicity (lysogenic conversion). The actual production of toxin occurs perhaps only when the prophage of the lysogenic *C diphtheriae* becomes induced and lyses the cell. Whereas toxigenicity is under control of the phage gene, invasiveness is under control of bacterial genes.

Antigenic Structure

Serologic differences have been observed between types and within each type of *C diphtheriae,* but no satisfactory serologic classification exists. Serologic tests are not usually employed in identification.

Pathogenesis

The principal human pathogen of the group is *C diphtheriae.* In nature, *C diphtheriae* occurs in the respiratory tract, in wounds, or on the skin of infected persons or normal carriers. It is spread by droplets or by contact to susceptible individuals; the bacilli then grow on mucous membranes or in skin abrasions, and those that are toxigenic start producing toxin.

All toxigenic *C diphtheriae* are capable of elaborating the same disease-producing exotoxin. In vitro production of this toxin depends largely on the con-

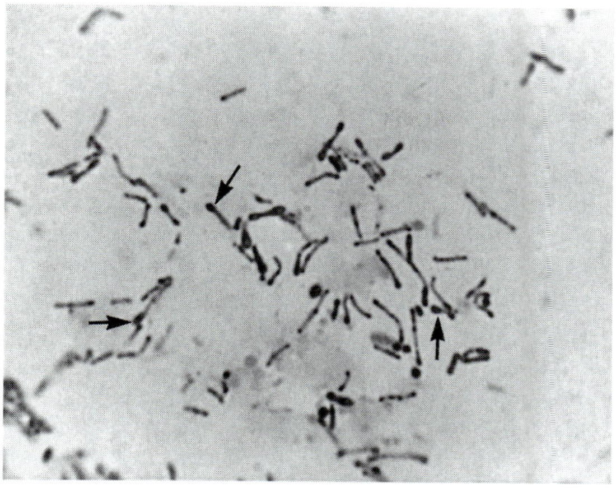

Figure 13–1. *C diphtheriae* from Pai medium and stained with methylene blue.

centration of iron. Toxin production is optimal at 0.14 μg of iron per milliliter of medium but is virtually suppressed at 0.5 μg/mL. Other factors influencing the yield of toxin in vitro are osmotic pressure, amino acid concentration, pH, and availability of suitable carbon and nitrogen sources. The factors that control toxin production in vivo are not well understood.

Diphtheria toxin is a heat-labile polypeptide (MW 62,000) that can be lethal in a dose of 0.1 μg/kg. If disulfide bonds are broken, the molecule can be split into two fragments. Fragment B (MW ≈ 38,000) has no independent activity but is required for the transport of fragment A into the cell. Fragment A inhibits polypeptide chain elongation—provided nicotinamide adenine dinucleotide (NAD) is present—by inactivating the elongation factor EF-2. This factor is required for translocation of polypeptidyl-transfer RNA from the acceptor to the donor site on the eukaryotic ribosome. Toxin fragment A inactivates EF-2 by catalyzing a reaction that yields free nicotinamide plus an inactive adenosine diphosphate-ribose-EF-2 complex. It is assumed that the abrupt arrest of protein synthesis is responsible for the necrotizing and neurotoxic effects of diphtheria toxin. An exotoxin with a similar mode of action can be produced by strains of *Pseudomonas aeruginosa.*

Table 13–1. Examples of metabolic reactions.

	Glucose[1]	Maltose[1]	Sucrose[1]	Urease[1]
C diphtheriae	+	+	–	–
C xerosis	+	+	+	–
C pseudodiphtheriticum[2]	–	–	–	+
C pyogenes (C haemolyticum)	+	+	+	–

[1]Acid but no gas formed.
[2]Also called *C hofmannii.*

Pathology

Diphtheria toxin is absorbed into the mucous membranes and causes destruction of epithelium and a superficial inflammatory response. The necrotic epithelium becomes embedded in exuding fibrin and red and white cells, so that a grayish "pseudomembrane" is formed—commonly over the tonsils, pharynx, or larynx. Any attempt to remove the pseudomembrane exposes and tears the capillaries and thus results in bleeding. The regional lymph nodes in the neck enlarge, and there may be marked edema of the entire neck. The diphtheria bacilli within the membrane continue to produce toxin actively. This is absorbed and results in distant toxic damage, particularly parenchymatous degeneration, fatty infiltration, and necrosis in heart muscle, liver, kidneys, and adrenals, sometimes accompanied by gross hemorrhage. The toxin also produces nerve damage, resulting often in paralysis of the soft palate, eye muscles, or extremities.

Wound or skin diphtheria occurs chiefly in the tropics. A membrane may form on an infected wound that fails to heal. However, absorption of toxin is usually slight and the systemic effects negligible. The "virulence" of diphtheria bacilli is due to their capacity for establishing infection, growing rapidly, and then quickly elaborating toxin that is effectively absorbed. *C diphtheriae* does not need to be toxigenic to establish localized infection—in the nasopharynx or skin, for example—but nontoxigenic strains do not yield the localized or systemic toxic effects. *C diphtheriae* does not actively invade deep tissues and practically never enters the bloodstream.

Clinical Findings

When diphtheritic inflammation begins in the respiratory tract, sore throat and fever usually develop. Prostration and dyspnea soon follow because of the obstruction caused by the membrane. This obstruction may even cause suffocation if not promptly relieved by intubation or tracheostomy. Irregularities of cardiac rhythm indicate damage to the heart. Later, there may be difficulties with vision, speech, swallowing, or movement of the arms or legs. All of these manifestations tend to subside spontaneously.

In general, var *gravis* tends to produce more severe disease than var *mitis,* but similar illness can be produced by all types.

Diagnostic Laboratory Tests

These serve to confirm the clinical impression and are of epidemiologic significance. ***Note:*** Specific treatment must never be delayed for laboratory reports if the clinical picture is strongly suggestive of diphtheria.

A. Specimens: Swabs from the nose, throat, or other suspected lesions must be obtained before antimicrobial drugs are administered.

B. Smears: Smears stained with alkaline methylene blue or Gram's stain show beaded rods in typical arrangement.

C. Culture: Inoculate a blood agar plate (to rule out hemolytic streptococci), a Loeffler slant, and a tellurite plate (eg, cystine-tellurite agar or modified Tinsdale medium) and incubate all three at 37 °C. Unless the swab can be inoculated promptly, it should be kept moistened with sterile horse serum so the bacilli will remain viable. In 12–18 hours, the Loeffler slant may yield organisms of typical "diphtheria-like" morphology. In 36–48 hours, the colonies on tellurite medium are sufficiently definite for recognition of *C diphtheriae.*

Any diphtheria-like organism cultured must be submitted to a "virulence" test before the bacteriologic diagnosis of diphtheria is definite. Such tests are really tests for toxigenicity of an isolated diphtheria-like organism. They can be done in one of three ways as follows:

1. In vivo test–A culture from a Loeffler slant is emulsified in water and 4 mL is injected subcutaneously into each of two guinea pigs, one of which has received 1000–2000 units of diphtheria antitoxin intraperitoneally 2 hours previously. The unprotected animal should die in 2–3 days, whereas the protected animal survives.

2. In vitro test–A strip of filter paper saturated with antitoxin is placed on an agar plate containing 20% horse serum. The cultures to be tested for toxigenicity are streaked across the plate at right angles to the filter paper. After 48 hours' incubation, the antitoxin diffusing from the paper strip has precipitated the toxin diffusing from toxigenic cultures and resulted in lines radiating from the intersection of the strip and the bacterial growth.

3. Tissue culture test–The toxigenicity of *C diphtheriae* can be shown by incorporation of bacteria into an agar overlay of cell culture monolayers. Toxin produced diffuses into cells below and kills them.

Resistance & Immunity

Since diphtheria is principally the result of the action of the toxin formed by the organism rather than invasion by the organism, resistance to the disease depends largely on the availability of specific neutralizing antitoxin in the bloodstream and tissues. It is generally true that diphtheria occurs only in persons who possess no antitoxin (or less than 0.01 Lf unit/mL).

The relative amount of antitoxin that a person possesses can be estimated, but the two tests used for this purpose are not readily available: titration of serum for antitoxin content is too complex for routine use; and the **Schick test,** based on the irritating action of and local reaction to the Schick antigen (diluted diphtheria toxin) with antitoxin-treated controls, is seldom if ever performed and the antigen is not generally available. These tests are of historical interest. Assessment of immunity to diphtheria toxin for individual patients can best be made by review of documented diphtheria toxoid immunizations and primary or booster immunization if needed.

Treatment

The treatment of diphtheria rests largely on rapid suppression of toxin-producing bacteria by antimicrobial drugs and the early administration of specific antitoxin against the toxin formed by the organisms at their site of entry and multiplication. Diphtheria antitoxin is produced in various animals (horses, sheep, goats, and rabbits) by the repeated injection of purified and concentrated toxoid. Treatment with antitoxin is mandatory when there is strong clinical suspicion of diphtheria. From 20,000 to 100,000 units are injected intramuscularly or intravenously after suitable precautions have been taken (skin or conjunctival test) to rule out hypersensitivity to the animal serum. The antitoxin should be given on the day the clinical diagnosis of diphtheria is made and need not be repeated. Intramuscular injection may be used in mild cases.

Antimicrobial drugs (penicillin, erythromycin) inhibit the growth of diphtheria bacilli. Although these drugs have virtually no effect on the disease process, they arrest toxin production. They also help to eliminate coexistent streptococci and *C diphtheriae* from the respiratory tracts of patients or carriers.

Epidemiology, Prevention, & Control

Before artificial immunization, diphtheria was mainly a disease of small children. The infection occurred either clinically or subclinically at an early age and resulted in the widespread production of antitoxin in the population. An asymptomatic infection during adolescence and adult life served as a stimulus for maintenance of high antitoxin levels. Thus, most members of the population, except children, were immune.

By age 6–8 years, approximately 75% of children in developing countries where skin infections with *C diphtheriae* are common have protective serum antitoxin levels. Absorption of small amounts of diphtheria toxin from the skin infection presumably provides the antigenic stimulus for the immune response; the amount of absorbed toxin does not produce disease.

Active immunization in childhood with diphtheria toxoid yields antitoxin levels that are generally adequate until adulthood. Young adults should be given boosters of toxoid, because toxigenic diphtheria bacilli are not sufficiently prevalent in the population of many developed countries to provide the stimulus of subclinical infection with stimulation of resistance. Levels of antitoxin decline with time, and many older persons have insufficient amounts of circulating antitoxin to protect them against diphtheria.

The principal aims of prevention are to limit the distribution of toxigenic diphtheria bacilli in the population and to maintain as high a level of active immunization as possible.

A. Isolation: To limit contact with diphtheria bacilli to a minimum, patients with diphtheria should be isolated. Without treatment, a large percentage of infected persons continue to shed diphtheria bacilli for weeks or months after recovery (convalescent carriers). This danger may be greatly reduced by active early treatment with antibiotics. However, there are some healthy carriers from whom diphtheria bacilli cannot be readily eradicated with penicillin or erythromycin.

B. Active Immunization: The following preparations have been employed:

1. Fluid toxoid–A filtrate of broth culture of a toxigenic strain is treated with 0.3% formalin and incubated at 37 °C until toxicity has disappeared. Toxoid is purified and standardized in flocculating units (Lf doses). Fluid toxoid itself is not often used for immunization now.

2. Toxoids for delayed absorption–Fluid toxoids prepared as above are adsorbed onto aluminum hydroxide or aluminum phosphate. This material remains longer in a depot after injection and is a better antigen. Such toxoids are commonly combined with tetanus toxoid and sometimes with pertussis vaccine as a single injection to be used in initial immunization of children. For booster injection of adults, only Td toxoids are used; these combine a full dose of tetanus toxoid with a tenfold smaller dose of diphtheria toxoid in order to diminish the likelihood of adverse reactions.

All children must receive an initial course of immunizations and boosters. Regular boosters with Td are particularly important for adults who travel to developing countries, where the incidence of clinical diphtheria may be 1000-fold higher than in developed countries, where immunization is universal.

OTHER CORYNEBACTERIA (DIPHTHEROIDS) & PROPIONIBACTERIA

Many other *Corynebacterium* and *Propionibacterium* species have been associated with disease in humans. *Corynebacterium jeikeium* (corynebacteria group JK) causes disease in immunocompromized patients and is important because it produces infections, including bacteremia, that have a high mortality rate and because it is resistant to many commonly used antimicrobial drugs. Other corynebacteria have been associated with disease in humans. For example, *Corynebacterium minutissimum* causes erythrasma, a superficial infection of axillary and pubic skin. The organism produces bright pink fluorescence under ultraviolet light in skin lesions and when cultured in Mueller-Hinton agar.

Other species that have been rarely associated with disease in humans include *C pseudodiphtheriticum, C hofmannii, C xerosis, C pyogenes,* and *C ulcerans*. They are normal inhabitants of the mucous membranes of the respiratory tract, urinary tract, and conjunctiva, and because they are part of the normal flora they are commonly called diphtheroids. A number of other diphtheroids cause infections in animals and, rarely, in humans.

Anaerobic diphtheroids (eg, *Propionibacterium* species) reside in normal skin. *Propionibacterium acnes*) participates in the pathogenesis of acne by producing lipases, which split free fatty acids off from skin lipids. These fatty acids can produce tissue inflammation and contribute to acne. Because *P acnes* is part of the normal skin flora, it occasionally appears in blood cultures and must be differentiated as a culture contaminant or a true cause of disease. *P acnes* occasionally causes infection of prosthetic heart valves and cerebrospinal fluid shunts.

Arcanobacterium haemolyticum (previously *Corynebacterium haemolyticum*) produces beta hemolysis on blood agar. It is occasionally associated with pharyngitis and can grow in selective media for streptococci. *A haemolyticum* is catalase-negative, like group A streptococci, and must be differentiated by Gram stain morphology (rods versus cocci) and biochemical characteristics.

LISTERIA MONOCYTOGENES

There are several species in the genus *Listeria*. Of these, *L monocytogenes* is important as a cause of a wide spectrum of disease in animals and humans.

Morphology & Identification

L monocytogenes is a short, gram-positive, non-spore-forming rod. It has a tumbling end-over-end motility at 22 °C but not at 37 °C; the motility test rapidly differentiates *Listeria* from diphtheroids that are members of the normal flora of the skin.

Culture & Growth Characteristics

Listeria grows on media such as Mueller-Hinton agar. Identification is enhanced if the primary cultures are done on agar containing sheep blood, because the characteristic small zone of hemolysis can be observed around and under colonies. Isolation can be enhanced if the tissue is kept at 4 °C for some days before inoculation into bacteriologic media. The organism is a facultative anaerobe and is catalase-positive and motile. *Listeria* produces acid but not gas in a variety of carbohydrates.

Antigenic Classification

Serologic classification requires typing of both O and H antigens, is done only in reference laboratories, and is primarily used for epidemiologic studies. Serotypes Ia, Ib, and IVb make up more than 90% of the isolates from humans. Serotype IVb was found to have caused an epidemic of listeriosis associated with cheese made from inadequately pasteurized milk.

Pathogenesis

The association of epidemics of listeriosis with contaminated food suggests that the natural route of infection with *Listeria* is the gastrointestinal tract. *Liste-*

ria can invade and multiply in nonphagocytic cells and may initially infect intestinal epithelial cells. *Listeria* also can survive and multiply within macrophages.

Listeria species that cause disease in humans produce hemolysis on sheep blood agar, implying that hemolysin is important for virulence. Studies of infection in mice with nonhemolytic mutants support this conclusion. Other studies have shown that the hemolysin is important in the ability of *Listeria* to survive within cells but is not the factor that induces uptake of the bacteria by cells.

Clinical Findings

Perinatal human listeriosis **(granulomatosis infantiseptica)** may be an intrauterine infection. The early-onset syndrome results in intrauterine sepsis and death before or after delivery. The late-onset syndrome causes the development of meningitis between birth and the third week of life; it is often caused by serotype IVb and has a significant mortality rate.

Adults can develop *Listeria* meningoencephalitis, bacteremia, and (rarely) focal infections. Meningoencephalitis and bacteremia occur most commonly in immunosuppressed patients, in whom *Listeria* is one of the more common causes of meningitis. Clinical presentation of *Listeria* meningitis in these patients varies from insidious to fulminant and is nonspecific. The route of infection for adults is uncertain. After ingestion of raw vegetables contaminated from soil or contaminated milk or cheese, the gut may be colonized by *Listeria.*

The diagnosis of listeriosis rests on isolation of the organism in cultures of blood and spinal fluid. *Listeria* infection leads to the production of cold agglutinins for human and sheep red cells as well as specific agglutinating antibodies.

Spontaneous infection occurs in many domestic and wild animals. In ruminants (eg, sheep) *Listeria* may cause meningoencephalitis with or without bacteremia. In smaller animals (eg, rabbits, chickens), there is septicemia with focal abscesses in the liver and heart muscle and marked monocytosis. A glyceride extracted from *Listeria* can likewise induce monocytosis in rabbits. This cellular reaction, however, is not related to human infectious mononucleosis.

Many antimicrobial drugs inhibit *Listeria* in vitro. Clinical cures have been obtained with ampicillin or penicillin plus an aminoglycoside; with erythromycin; and with intravenous trimethoprim-sulfamethoxazole.

ERYSIPELOTHRIX RHUSIOPATHIAE (Erysipelothrix insidiosa)

Erysipelothrix resembles *Listeria* but is nonmotile and produces an entirely different disease. In its smooth form, it grows as clear, minute colonies in which short, non-spore-forming rods are arranged in short chains; in its rough form, long filaments predominate. Growth is aided by blood and glucose in the medium. On blood agar, only slight hemolysis is produced. Carbohydrates are fermented irregularly, and catalase is not produced. Multiple serovars have been described.

Infection with *E rhusiopathiae* occurs worldwide in a variety of animals, especially swine. In swine, it causes swine erysipelas, which is different from erysipelas of humans; the latter is caused by group A β-hemolytic streptococci. *E rhusiopathiae* infection in humans occurs through skin abrasions and follows contact with contaminated fish, shellfish, meat, or poultry. The infection, called erysipeloid, is limited to the skin. There is pain, edema, and purplish erythema with sharp margins that extend peripherally but clear centrally. Relapses and extension of the lesions to distant areas are common, but there is usually no fever. Rarely, endocarditis occurs. There is no permanent immunity following an attack. The diagnosis rests on isolation of the organism in cultures from a skin biopsy. The fragments should be incubated in glucose broth for 24 hours and then subcultured on blood agar plates. Typical clinical appearance in a person with occupational exposure is highly suggestive of infection due to this organism.

Penicillin seems to be the antibiotic of choice.

ROTHIA

Rothia dentocariosa is a gram-positive rod that forms branching filaments. It has been associated with abscesses and endocarditis, presumably following entry into the blood from the mouth.

REFERENCES

Bach MC, Davis KM: *Listeria rhomboencephalitis* mimicking tuberculous meningitis. Rev Infect Dis 1987;9:130.

Bainton D et al: Immunity of children to diphtheria, tetanus and poliomyelitis. Br Med J 1979;1:854.

Barksdale L: Identifying *Rothia dentocariosa.* Ann Intern Med 1979;91:786.

Barresi JA: *Listeria monocytogenes:* A cause of premature labor and neonatal sepsis. Am J Obstet Gynecol 1980; 136:410.

Collier RJ: Diphtheria toxin: Mode of action and structure. Bacteriol Rev 1975;39:54.

Dan M et al: Cutaneous manifestations of infection with the *Corynebacterium* group JK. Rev Infect Dis 1988;10: 1204.

Farizo KM et al: Fatal respiratory disease due to *Corynebacterium diphtheriae*: Case report and review of guidelines for management, investigation, and control. Clin Infect Dis 1993;16:59.

Harnisch JP, et al: Diphtheria among alcoholic urban adults: A decade of experience in Seattle. Ann Intern Med 1989; 111:71.

Linnan MJ et al: Epidemic listeriosis associated with Mexican-style cheese. New Engl J Med 1988;319:823.

Rappuoli R, Perugini M, Falsen E: Molecular epidemiology of the 1984–1986 outbreak of diphtheria in Sweden. N Engl J Med 1988;318:12.

Reboli AC, Farrar WE: *Erysipelothrix rhusiopathiae:* An occupational pathogen. Clin Microbiol Rev 1989;2:354.

Rosenberg EW: Bacteriology of acne. Annu Rev Med 1969; 20:201.

Rozdzinski E et al: *Corynebacterium jeikeium* bacteremia in a tertiary care center. Infection 1991;19:201.

Schuster MG et al: Persistent bacteremia with *Erysipelothrix rhusiopathiae* in a hospitalized patient. Clin Infect Dis 1993;17:783.

Visintine AM, Oleske JM, Nahmias AJ: *Listeria monocytogenes* infection in infants and children. Am J Dis Child 1977;131:393.

Yocum RC et al: Septic arthritis caused by *Propionibacterium acnes.* JAMA 1982;248:1740.

14 The Staphylococci

The staphylococci are gram-positive spherical cells, usually arranged in grape-like irregular clusters. They grow readily on many types of media and are active metabolically, fermenting carbohydrates and producing pigments that vary from white to deep yellow. Some are members of the normal flora of the skin and mucous membranes of humans; others cause suppuration, abscess formation, a variety of pyogenic infections, and even fatal septicemia. The pathogenic staphylococci often hemolyze blood, coagulate plasma, and produce a variety of extracellular enzymes and toxins. The most common type of food poisoning is caused by a heat-stable staphylococcal enterotoxin. Staphylococci rapidly develop resistance to many antimicrobial agents and present difficult therapeutic problems.

The genus *Staphylococcus* has at least 30 species. The three main species of clinical importance are *Staphylococcus aureus, Staphylococcus epidermidis,* and *Staphylococcus saprophyticus. Staphylococcus aureus* is **coagulase-positive,** which differentiates it from the other species. *S aureus* is a major pathogen for humans. Almost every person will have some type of *S aureus* infection during a lifetime, ranging in severity from food poisoning or minor skin infections to severe life-threatening infections. The coagulase-negative staphylococci are normal human flora and sometimes cause infection, often associated with implanted appliances and devices, especially in very young, old, and immunocompromised patients. Approximately 75% of these infections caused by **coagulase-negative** staphylococci are due to *S epidermidis*; infections due to *Staphylococcus warneri*, *Staphylococcus hominis*, and other species are less common. *S saprophyticus* is a relatively common cause of urinary tract infections in young women. Other species are important in veterinary medicine.

Morphology & Identification

A. Typical Organisms: Staphylococci are spherical cells about 1 μm in diameter arranged in irregular clusters (Figure 14–1). Single cocci, pairs, tetrads, and chains are also seen in liquid cultures. Young cocci stain strongly gram-positive; on aging, many cells become gram-negative. Staphylococci are nonmotile and do not form spores. Under the influence of drugs like penicillin, staphylococci are lysed.

Micrococcus species often resemble staphylococci. They are found free-living in the environment and form regular packets of four or eight cocci. Their colonies can be yellow, red, or orange.

B. Culture: Staphylococci grow readily on most bacteriologic media under aerobic or microaerophilic conditions. They grow most rapidly at 37 °C but form pigment best at room temperature (20–25 °C). Colonies on solid media are round, smooth, raised, and glistening. *S aureus* usually forms gray to deep golden yellow colonies. *S epidermidis* colonies usually are gray to white on primary isolation; many colonies develop pigment only upon prolonged incubation. No pigment is produced anaerobically or in broth. Various degrees of hemolysis are produced by *S aureus* and occasionally by other species. *Peptostreptococcus* species, which are anaerobic cocci, often resemble staphylococci in morphology.

C. Growth Characteristics: The staphylococci produce catalase, which differentiates them from the streptococci. Staphylococci slowly ferment many carbohydrates, producing lactic acid but not gas. Proteolytic activity varies greatly from one strain to another. Pathogenic staphylococci produce many extracellular substances, which are discussed below.

Staphylococci are relatively resistant to drying, heat (they withstand 50 °C for 30 minutes), and 9% sodium chloride but are readily inhibited by certain chemicals, eg, 3% hexachlorophene.

Staphylococci are variably sensitive to many antimicrobial drugs. Resistance falls into several classes: (1) β-lactamase production is common, is under plasmid control, and makes the organisms resistant to many penicillins (penicillin G, ampicillin, ticarcillin, and similar drugs). The plasmids are transmitted by transduction and perhaps also by conjugation. (2) Resistance to nafcillin (and to methicillin and oxacillin) is independent of β-lactamase production. The genes for nafcillin resistance reside on the chromosome and are variably expressed. The mechanism of nafcillin resistance is related to the lack or inaccessibility of certain penicillin-binding proteins (PBPs) in the organisms. (3) "Tolerance" implies that staphylococci

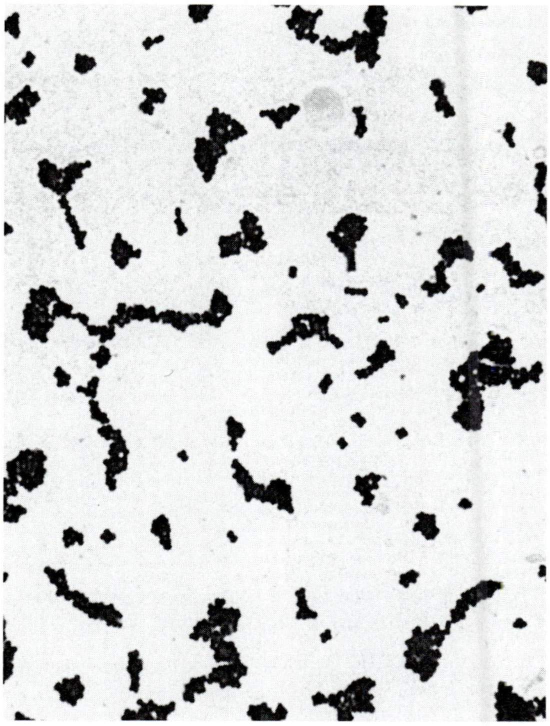

Figure 14–1. Gram stain of *Staphylococcus aureus* showing gram-positive cocci in pairs, tetrads, and clusters.

are inhibited by a drug but not killed by it, ie, there is a very large difference between minimal inhibitory and minimal lethal concentrations of an antimicrobial drug. Tolerance can at times be attributed to a lack of activation of autolytic enzymes in the cell wall. (4) Plasmids can also carry genes for resistance to tetracyclines, erythromycins, aminoglycosides, and other drugs. Staphylococci have remained susceptible to vancomycin.

D. Variation: A culture of staphylococci contains some bacteria that differ from the bulk of the population in expression of colony characteristics (colony size, pigment, hemolysis), in enzyme elaboration, in drug resistance, and in pathogenicity. In vitro, the expression of such characteristics is influenced by growth conditions: When nafcillin-resistant *S aureus* is incubated at 37 °C on blood agar, one in 10^7 organisms expresses nafcillin resistance; when it is incubated at 30 °C on agar containing 2–5% sodium chloride, one in 10^3 organisms expresses nafcillin resistance.

Antigenic Structure

Staphylococci contain antigenic polysaccharides and proteins as well as other substances important in cell wall structure (Figure 14–2). Peptidoglycan, a polysaccharide polymer containing linked subunits provides the rigid exoskeleton of the cell wall. Peptidoglycan is destroyed by strong acid or exposure to lysozyme. It is important in the pathogenesis of infection. It elicits production of interleukin-1 (endogenous pyrogen) and opsonic antibodies by monocytes. It can be a chemoattractant for polymorphonuclear leukocytes, have endotoxin-like activity, produce a localized Shwartzman phenomenon, and activate complement.

Teichoic acids, which are polymers of glycerol or ribitol phosphate, are linked to the peptidoglycan and can be antigenic. Antiteichoic antibodies detectable by gel diffusion may be found in patients with active endocarditis due to *S aureus*.

Protein A is a cell wall component of many *S aureus* strains that binds to the Fc portion of IgG molecules except IgG3. The Fab portion of IgG bound to protein A is free to combine with a specific antigen. Protein A has become an important reagent in immunology and diagnostic laboratory technology; for example, protein A with attached IgG molecules directed against a specific bacterial antigen will agglutinate bacteria that have that antigen ("coagglutination").

Some *S aureus* strains have capsules, which inhibit phagocytosis by polymorphonuclear leukocytes unless specific antibodies are present. Most strains of *S aureus* have coagulase, or clumping factor, on the cell wall surface; coagulase binds nonenzymatically to fibrinogen, yielding aggregation of the bacteria.

Serologic tests have limited usefulness in identifying staphylococci. Phage typing is based on the lysis of *S aureus* by one or a series of specific bacteriophages; it is done only in reference laboratories and has been used for epidemiologic studies.

Toxins & Enzymes

Staphylococci can produce disease both through their ability to multiply and spread widely in tissues and through their production of many extracellular substances. Some of these substances are enzymes; others are considered to be toxins, though they may function as enzymes. Many of the toxins are under the genetic control of plasmids; some may be under both chromosomal and extrachromosomal control; and for others the mechanism of genetic control is not well defined.

A. Catalase: Staphylococci produce catalase, which converts hydrogen peroxide into water and oxygen. The catalase test differentiates the staphylococci, which are positive, from the streptococci, which are negative.

B. Coagulase: *S aureus* produces coagulase, an enzyme-like protein that clots oxalated or citrated plasma in the presence of a factor contained in many sera. The serum factor reacts with coagulase to generate both esterase and clotting activities, in a manner similar to the activation of prothrombin to thrombin. The action of coagulase circumvents the normal

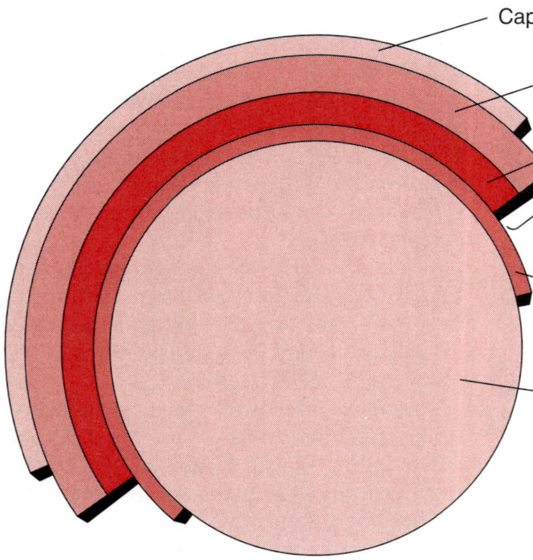

Figure 14–2. Antigenic structure of staphylococci. ***(a)*** Site of bacteriophage attachment. Species antigens present (antigenic determinant is N-acetylglucosamine linked to polyribitol phosphate). ***(b)*** Multiple antigens; several widely distributed.

plasma clotting cascade. Coagulase may deposit fibrin on the surface of staphylococci, perhaps altering their ingestion by phagocytic cells or their destruction within such cells. Coagulase production is considered synonymous with invasive pathogenic potential.

C. Other Enzymes: Other enzymes produced by staphylococci include a hyaluronidase, or spreading factor; a staphylokinase resulting in fibrinolysis but acting much more slowly than streptokinase; proteinases; lipases; and β-lactamase.

D. Exotoxins: These include several toxins that are lethal for animals on injection, cause necrosis in skin, and contain soluble hemolysins which can be separated by electrophoresis. The alpha toxin (hemolysin) is a heterogeneous protein that can lyse erythrocytes and damage platelets and is probably identical with the lethal and dermonecrotic factors of exotoxin. Alpha toxin also has a powerful action on vascular smooth muscle. Beta toxin degrades sphingomyelin and is toxic for many kinds of cells, including human red blood cells. These toxins and two others, the gamma and delta toxins, are antigenically distinct and bear no relationship to streptococcal lysins. Exotoxin treated with formalin gives a nonpoisonous but antigenic toxoid, but this is not clinically useful.

E. Leukocidin: This toxin of *S aureus* can kill exposed white blood cells of many animals. Its role in pathogenesis is uncertain, because pathogenic staphylococci may not kill white blood cells and may be phagocytosed as effectively as nonpathogenic varieties. However, they are capable of very active intracellular multiplication, whereas the nonpathogenic organisms tend to die inside the cell. Antibodies to leukocidin may play a role in resistance to recurrent staphylococcal infections.

F. Exfoliative Toxin: This toxin of *S aureus* includes at least two proteins that yield the generalized desquamation of the staphylococcal scalded skin syndrome. Specific antibodies protect against the exfoliative action of the toxin.

G. Toxic Shock Syndrome Toxin: Most *S aureus* strains isolated from patients with toxic shock syndrome produce a toxin called toxic shock syndrome toxin-1 (TSST-1), which is the same as enterotoxin F and pyrogenic exotoxin C. TSST-1 is the prototypical superantigen (see Chapter 8) which promotes the protean manifestations of the toxic shock syndrome. In humans, the toxin is associated with fever, shock, and multisystem involvement, including a desquamative skin rash. In rabbits, TSST-1 produces fever, enhanced susceptibility to the effects of bacterial lipopolysaccharides, and other biologic effects similar to toxic shock syndrome, but the skin rash and desquamation do not occur.

H. Enterotoxins: There are at least six (A–F) soluble toxins produced by nearly 50% of *S aureus* strains. Like TSST-1, the enterotoxins are superantigens that bind to MHC class II molecules, yielding T cell stimulation. The enterotoxins are heat-stable (they resist boiling for 30 minutes) and resistant to the action of gut enzymes. An important cause of food poisoning, enterotoxins are produced when *S aureus* grows in carbohydrate and protein foods. The gene for enterotoxin production may be on the chromosome, but a plasmid may carry a protein that regulates active toxin production. Ingestion of 25 μg of enterotoxin B by humans or monkeys results in vomiting and diarrhea. The emetic effect of enterotoxin is probably the result of central nervous system stimulation (vomiting center) after the toxin acts on neural receptors in the gut. Enterotoxins can be assayed by precipitin tests (gel diffusion).

Pathogenesis

Staphylococci, particularly *S epidermidis*, are members of the normal flora of the human skin and respiratory and gastrointestinal tracts. Nasal carriage of *S aureus* occurs in 40–50% of humans. Staphylococci are also found regularly on clothing, bed linens, and other fomites in human environments.

The pathogenic capacity of a given strain of *S aureus* is the combined effect of extracellular factors and toxins together with the invasive properties of the strain. At one end of the disease spectrum is staphylococcal food poisoning, attributable solely to the ingestion of preformed enterotoxin; at the other end are staphylococcal bacteremia and disseminated abscesses in all organs. The potential contribution of the various extracellular substances in pathogenesis is evident from the nature of their individual actions.

Pathogenic, invasive *S aureus* produces coagulase and tends to produce a yellow pigment and to be hemolytic. Nonpathogenic, noninvasive staphylococci such as *S epidermidis* are coagulase-negative and tend to be nonhemolytic. Such organisms rarely produce suppuration but may infect orthopedic or cardiovascular prostheses or cause disease in immunosuppressed persons. *S saprophyticus* is typically nonpigmented, novobiocin-resistant, and nonhemolytic; it causes urinary tract infections in young women.

Pathology

The prototype of a staphylococcal lesion is the furuncle or other localized abscess. Groups of *S aureus* established in a hair follicle lead to tissue necrosis (dermonecrotic factor). Coagulase is produced and coagulates fibrin around the lesion and within the lymphatics, resulting in formation of a wall that limits the process and is reinforced by the accumulation of inflammatory cells and, later, fibrous tissue. Within the center of the lesion, liquefaction of the necrotic tissue occurs (enhanced by delayed hypersensitivity), and the abscess "points" in the direction of least resistance. Drainage of the liquid center necrotic tissue is followed by slow filling of the cavity with granulation tissue and eventual healing.

Focal suppuration (abscess) is typical of staphylococcal infection. From any one focus, organisms may spread via the lymphatics and bloodstream to other parts of the body. Suppuration within veins, associated with thrombosis, is a common feature of such dissemination. In osteomyelitis, the primary focus of *S aureus* growth is typically in a terminal blood vessel of the metaphysis of a long bone, leading to necrosis of bone and chronic suppuration. *S aureus* may cause pneumonia, meningitis, empyema, endocarditis, or sepsis with suppuration in any organ. Staphylococci of low invasiveness are involved in many skin infections (eg, acne, pyoderma, or impetigo). Anaerobic cocci *(Peptostreptococcus)* participate in mixed anaerobic infections.

Staphylococci also cause disease through the elaboration of toxins, without apparent invasive infection. Bullous exfoliation, the scalded skin syndrome, is caused by the production of exfoliative toxin. Toxic shock syndrome is associated with toxic shock syndrome toxin-1 (TSST-1).

Clinical Findings

A localized staphylococcal infection appears as a "pimple," hair follicle infection, or abscess. There is usually an intense, localized, painful inflammatory reaction that undergoes central suppuration and heals quickly when the pus is drained. The wall of fibrin and cells around the core of the abscess tends to prevent spread of the organisms and should not be broken down by manipulation or trauma.

S aureus infection can also result from direct contamination of a wound, eg, postoperative staphylococcal wound infection or infection following trauma (chronic osteomyelitis subsequent to an open fracture, meningitis following skull fracture).

If *S aureus* disseminates and bacteremia ensues, endocarditis, acute hematogenous osteomyelitis, meningitis, or pulmonary infection can result. The clinical presentations resemble those seen with other bloodstream infections. Secondary localization within an organ or system is accompanied by the symptoms and signs of organ dysfunction and intense focal suppuration.

Food poisoning due to staphylococcal enterotoxin is characterized by a short incubation period (1–8 hours); violent nausea, vomiting, and diarrhea; and rapid convalescence. There is no fever.

Toxic shock syndrome is manifested by an abrupt onset of high fever, vomiting, diarrhea, myalgias, a scarlatiniform rash, and hypotension with cardiac and renal failure in the most severe cases. It often occurs within 5 days after the onset of menses in young women who use tampons, but it also occurs in children or in men with staphylococcal wound infections. The syndrome can recur. Toxic shock syndrome-associated *S aureus* can be found in the vagina, on tampons, in wounds or other localized infections, or in the throat but virtually never in the bloodstream.

Diagnostic Laboratory Tests

A. Specimens: Surface swab, pus, blood, tracheal aspirate, or spinal fluid for culture, depending upon the localization of the process. Antibody determinations in serum are of no value.

B. Smears: Typical staphylococci are seen in stained smears of pus or sputum. It is not possible to distinguish saprophytic *(S epidermidis)* from pathogenic *(S aureus)* organisms on smears.

C. Culture: Specimens planted on blood agar plates give rise to typical colonies in 18 hours at 37 °C, but hemolysis and pigment production may not occur until several days later and are optimal at room temperature. Specimens contaminated with a mixed flora can be cultured on media containing 7.5% NaCl; the salt inhibits most other normal flora but not *S aureus*.

D. Catalase Test: A drop of hydrogen peroxide solution is placed on a slide, and a small amount of the bacterial growth is placed in the solution. The formation of bubbles (the release of oxygen) indicates a positive test. The test can also be performed by pouring hydrogen peroxide solution over a heavy growth of the bacteria on an agar slant and observing for the appearance of bubbles.

E. Coagulase Test: Citrated rabbit (or human) plasma diluted 1:5 is mixed with an equal volume of broth culture or growth from colonies on agar and incubated at 37 °C. A tube of plasma mixed with sterile broth is included as a control. If clots form in 1–4 hours, the test is positive.

All coagulase-positive staphylococci are considered pathogenic for humans. Infections of prosthetic devices can be caused by organisms of the coagulase-negative *S epidermidis* group.

F. Susceptibility Testing: Broth microdilution or disk diffusion susceptibility testing should be done routinely on staphylococcal isolates from clinically significant infections. Resistance to penicillin G can be predicted by a positive test for β-lactamse; approximately 90% of *S aureus* produce β-lactamse. Resistance to nafcillin (and oxacillin and methicillin) occurs in 10–20% of *S aureus* and approximately 75% *S epidermidis* isolates. Nafcillin resistance correlates with the presence of *mec*A, the gene that codes for a penicillin-binding protein not affected by these drugs. The gene can be detected using the polymerase chain reaction, but this is not necessary because staphylococci that grow on Mueller-Hinton agar containing 4% NaCl and 6 μg/mL of oxacillin typically are *mec*A-positive and oxacillin-resistant.

G. Serologic and Typing Tests: Antibodies to teichoic acid can be detected in prolonged, deep infections (eg, staphylococcal endocarditis). These serologic tests have little practical value.

Antibiotic susceptibility patterns are helpful in tracing *S aureus* infections and in determining if multiple *S epidermidis* isolates from blood cultures represent bacteremia due to the same strain, seeded by a nidus of infection.

Phage typing is used for epidemiologic tracing of infection only in severe outbreaks of *S aureus* infections, as might occur in a hospital.

Treatment

Most persons harbor staphylococci on the skin and in the nose or throat. Even if the skin can be cleared of staphylococci (eg, in eczema), reinfection by droplets will occur almost immediately. Because pathogenic organisms are commonly spread from one lesion (eg, a furuncle) to other areas of the skin by fingers and clothing, scrupulous local antisepsis is important to control recurrent furunculosis.

Serious multiple skin infections (acne, furunculosis) occur most often in adolescents. Similar skin infections occur in patients receiving prolonged courses of corticosteroids. In acne, lipases of staphylococci and corynebacteria liberate fatty acids from lipids and thus cause tissue irritation. Tetracyclines are used for long-term treatment.

Abscesses and other closed suppurating lesions are treated by drainage, which is essential, and antimicrobial therapy. Many antimicrobial drugs have some effect against staphylococci in vitro. However, it is difficult to eradicate pathogenic staphylococci from infected persons, because the organisms rapidly develop resistance to many antimicrobial drugs and the drugs cannot act in the central necrotic part of a suppurative lesion. It is also difficult to eradicate the *S aureus* carrier state.

Acute hematogenous osteomyelitis responds well to antimicrobial drugs. In chronic and recurrent osteomyelitis, surgical drainage and removal of dead bone is accompanied by long-term administration of appropriate drugs, but eradication of the infecting staphylococci is difficult. Hyperbaric oxygen and the application of vascularized myocutaneous flaps have aided healing in chronic osteomyelitis.

Bacteremia, endocarditis, pneumonia, and other severe infections due to *S aureus* require prolonged intravenous therapy with a β-lactamase-resistant penicillin. Vancomycin is often reserved for use with nafcillin-resistant staphylococci. If the infection is found to be due to non-β-lactamase-producing *S aureus*, penicillin G is the drug of choice, but only a small percentage of *S aureus* strains are susceptible to penicillin G.

S epidermidis infections are difficult to cure because they occur in prosthetic devices where the bacteria can sequester themselves from the circulation and thus from antimicrobial drugs. *S epidermidis* is more often resistant to antimicrobial drugs than is *S aureus;* approximately 75% of *S epidermidis* strains are nafcillin-resistant.

Because of the frequency of drug-resistant strains, meaningful staphylococcal isolates should be tested for antimicrobial susceptibility to help in the choice of systemic drugs. Resistance to drugs of the erythromycin group tends to emerge so rapidly that these drugs should not be used singly for treatment of chronic infection. Drug resistance (to penicillins, tetracyclines, aminoglycosides, erythromycins, etc) determined by plasmids can be transmitted among staphylococci by transduction and perhaps by conjugation.

Penicillin G-resistant *S aureus* strains from clinical infections always produce penicillinase. They now constitute about 90% of *S aureus* isolates in communities in the USA. They are often susceptible to β-lactamase-resistant penicillins, cephalosporins, or vancomycin. Nafcillin resistance is independent of β-lactamase production, and its clinical incidence varies greatly in different countries and at different times. The selection pressure of β-lactamase-resistant antimicrobial drugs may not be the sole determinant for resistance to these drugs: For example, in Denmark, nafcillin-resistant *S aureus* comprised 40% of isolates in 1970 and only 10% in 1980, without notable changes in the use of nafcillin or similar drugs. In the USA, nafcillin-resistant *S aureus* accounted for only 0.1% of isolates in 1970 but in the 1990s constituted 10–30% of isolates from infections in some hospitals. Vancomycin remains the most widely effective drug against staphylococci.

Epidemiology & Control

Staphylococci are ubiquitous human parasites. The chief sources of infection are shedding human lesions, fomites contaminated from such lesions, and the human respiratory tract and skin. Contact spread of infection has assumed added importance in hospitals, where a large proportion of the staff and patients carry antibiotic-resistant staphylococci in the nose or on the skin. Although cleanliness, hygiene, and aseptic management of lesions can control the spread of staphylococci from lesions, few methods are available to prevent the wide dissemination of staphylococci from carriers. Aerosols (eg, glycols) and ultraviolet irradiation of air have little effect.

In hospitals, the areas at highest risk for severe staphylococcal infections are the newborn nursery, intensive care units, operating rooms, and cancer chemotherapy wards. Massive introduction of "epidemic" pathogenic *S aureus* into these areas may lead to serious clinical disease. Personnel with active *S aureus* lesions and carriers may have to be excluded from these areas. In such individuals, the application of topical antiseptics (eg, chlorhexidine or bacitracin cream) to nasal or perineal carriage sites may diminish shedding of dangerous organisms. Rifampin coupled with a second oral antistaphylococcal drug sometimes provides long-term suppression and possibly cure of nasal carriage; this form of therapy is usually reserved for major problems of staphylococcal carriage, because staphylococci can rapidly develop resistance to rifampin. Antiseptics such as hexachlorophene used on the skin of newborns diminish colonization by staphylococci, but toxicity prevents their widespread use.

REFERENCES

Chambers HF: Methicillin-resistant staphylococci. Clin Microbiol Rev 1988;1:173.

Hackbarth CJ, Chambers HF: Methicillin-resistant staphylococci: Genetics and mechanisms of resistance. Antimicrob Agents Chemother 1989;33:991.

Kim JH et al: *Staphylococcus aureus* meningitis: Review of 28 cases. Rev Infect Dis 1989;11:698.

Kloos WE, Bannerman TL: Update on clinical significance of coagulase-negative staphylococci. Clin Microbiol Rev 1994;7:117.

Labrecque N et al: Interactions between staphylococcal superantigens and MHC class II molecules. Semin Immunol 1993;5:23.

Micusan VV, Thibodeau J: Superantigens of microbial origin. Semin Immunol 1993;5:3.

Melish ME et al: The staphylococcal scalded skin syndrome: Isolation and partial characterization of the exfoliative toxin. J Infect Dis 1972;125:129.

Mulligan ME et al: Methicillin-resistant *Staphylococcus aureus*: A consensus review of the microbiology, pathogenesis, and epidemiology with implications for prevention and management. Am J Med 1993;94:313.

Pfaller MA, Herwald LA: Laboratory, clinical, and epidemiological aspects of coagulase-negative staphylococci. Clin Microbiol Rev 1988;1:281.

Sheagren JN: *Staphylococcus aureus:* The persistent pathogen. (Two parts.) N Engl J Med 1984;310:1368, 1437.

15 The Streptococci

The streptococci are gram-positive spherical bacteria that characteristically form pairs or chains during growth. They are widely distributed in nature. Some are members of the normal human flora; others are associated with important human diseases attributable in part to infection by streptococci, in part to sensitization to them. Streptococci elaborate a variety of extracellular substances and enzymes.

Streptococci are a heterogeneous group of bacteria, and no one system suffices to classify them. Twenty species, including *Streptococcus pyogenes* (group A), *Streptococcus agalactiae* (group B), and the enterococci (group D), are characterized by combinations of features: colony growth characteristics, hemolysis patterns on blood agar (α hemolysis, β hemolysis, or no hemolysis), antigenic composition of group-specific cell wall substances, and biochemical reactions. *Streptococcus pneumoniae* (pneumococcus) types are further classified by the antigenic composition of the capsular polysaccharides.

Morphology & Identification

A. Typical Organisms: Individual cocci are spherical or ovoid and are arranged in chains (Figure 15–1). The cocci divide in a plane perpendicular to the long axis of the chain. The members of the chain often have a striking diplococcal appearance, and rod-like forms are occasionally seen. The lengths of the chains vary widely and are conditioned by environmental factors. Streptococci are gram-positive. However, as a culture ages and the bacteria die, they lose their gram-positivity and appear to be gram-negative; this can occur after overnight incubation.

Some streptococci elaborate a capsular polysaccharide comparable to that of pneumococci. Most group A, B, and C strains (Table 15–1) produce capsules composed of hyaluronic acid. The capsules are most noticeable in very young cultures. They impede phagocytosis. The streptococcal cell wall contains proteins (M, T, R antigens), carbohydrates (group-specific), and peptidoglycans (Figure 15–2). Hair-like pili project through the capsule of group A streptococci. The pili consist partly of M protein and are covered with **lipoteichoic acid.** The latter is important in the attachment of streptococci to epithelial cells.

B. Culture: Most streptococci grow in solid media as discoid colonies, usually 1–2 mm in diameter. Strains that produce capsular material often give rise to mucoid colonies. Matt and glossy colonies of group A strains are discussed below. *Peptostreptococcus* is an obligate anaerobe.

C. Growth Characteristics: Energy is obtained principally from the utilization of sugars. Growth of streptococci tends to be poor on solid media or in broth unless enriched with blood or tissue fluids. Nutritive requirements vary widely among different species. The human pathogens are most exacting, requiring a variety of growth factors. Growth and hemolysis are aided by incubation in 10% CO_2.

Whereas most pathogenic hemolytic streptococci grow best at 37 °C, group D enterococci grow well at between 15 °C and 45 °C. Enterococci also grow in high (6.5%) sodium chloride concentrations, in 0.1% methylene blue, and in bile-esculin agar. Most streptococci are facultative anaerobes.

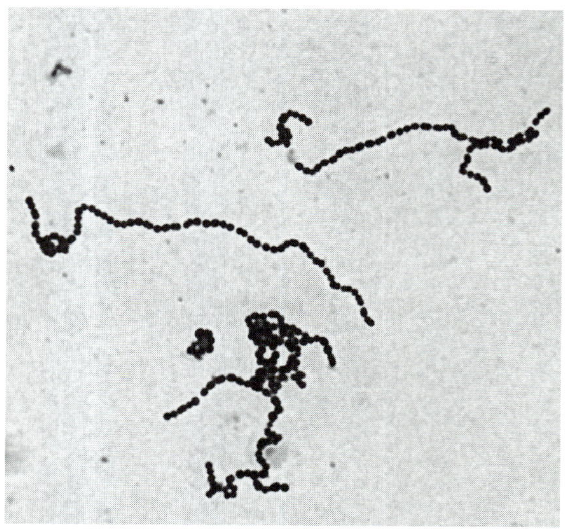

Figure 15–1. Streptococci grown in broth, showing gram-positive cocci in chains.

Table 15–1. Characteristics of medically important streptococci.

Name	Group-Specific Substance[1]	Hemolysis[2]	Habitat	Important Laboratory Criteria	Common and Important Diseases
Streptococcus pyogenes	A	Beta	Throat, skin	PYR[3] test positive, inhibited by bacitracin	Pharyngitis, impetigo, rheumatic fever, glomerulonephritis
Streptococcus agalactiae	B	Beta	Female genital tract	Hippurate hydrolysis, CAMP-positive[4]	Neonatal sepsis and meningitis
Enterococcus faecalis (and other enterococci)	D	None, alpha	Colon	Growth in presence of bile, hydrolyze esculin, growth in 6.5% NaCl, PYR-positive	Abdominal abscess, urinary tract infection, endocarditis
Streptococcus bovis (non-*enterococcus*)	D	None	Colon	Growth in presence of bile, hydrolyze esculin, no growth in 6.5% NaCl, degrades starch	Endocarditis, common blood isolate in colon cancer
Streptococcus anginosus	F(ACg) and untypable	Beta	Throat, colon, female genital tract	Small ("minute") colony variants of beta-hemolytic species. Group A are bacitracin-resistant and PYR-negative.	Pyogenic infections, including brain abscesses
	Usually not typed or untypable	Alpha, none	Throat, colon, female genital tract	Carbohydrate fermentation patterns	Not well defined
Viridans streptococci (multiple species)	Usually not typed or untypable	Alpha, none	Mouth, throat, colon, female genital tract	Optochin-resistant. Colonies not soluble in bile. Carbohydrate fermentation patterns	Dental caries *(S mutans)*, endocarditis, abscesses (with many other bacterial species)
Streptococcus pneumoniae	None	Alpha	Throat	Susceptible to optochin. Colonies soluble in bile, Quellung reaction-positive	Pneumonia, meningitis, endocarditis
Peptostreptococcus (many species)	None	None, alpha	Mouth, colon, female genital tract	Obligate anaerobes	Abscesses (with multiple other bacterial species)

[1]Lancefield classification.
[2]Hemolysis observed on 5% sheep blood agar after overnight incubation; alpha hemolysis screening of the agar; beta hemolysis is clearing of the agar.
[3]Hydrolysis of L-pyrrolidonyl-2-naphthylamide ("PYR").
[4]Christie, Atkins, Munch-Peterson test.

D. Variation: Variants of the same *Streptococcus* strain may show different colony forms. This is particularly marked among group A strains, giving rise to either matt or glossy colonies. Matt colonies consist of organisms that produce much M protein. Such organisms tend to be virulent and relatively insusceptible to phagocytosis by human leukocytes. Glossy colonies tend to produce little M protein and are often nonvirulent.

Antigenic Structure

Hemolytic streptococci can be divided into serologic groups (A–U), and certain groups can be subdivided into types. Several antigenic substances are found:

(1) Group-specific cell wall antigen: This carbohydrate is contained in the cell wall of many streptococci and forms the basis of serologic grouping **(Lancefield groups A–U).** Extracts of group-specific antigen for grouping streptococci may be prepared by extraction of centrifuged culture with hot hydrochloric acid, nitrous acid, or formamide; by enzymatic lysis of streptococcal cells (eg, with pepsin or trypsin); or by autoclaving of cell suspensions at 15 lb pressure for 15 minutes. The serologic specificity of the group-specific carbohydrate is determined by an amino sugar.

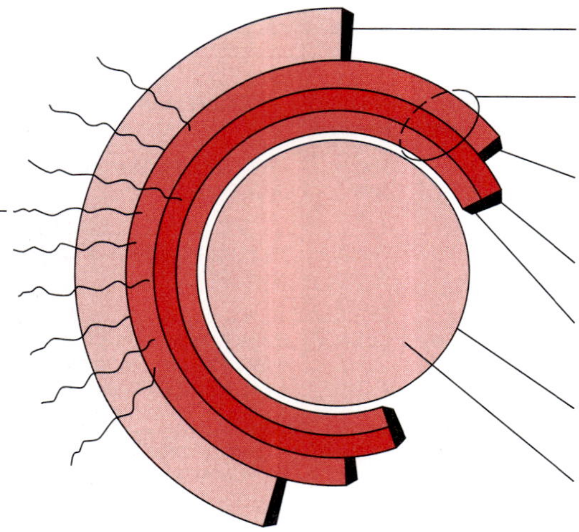

Figure 15–2. Antigenic structure of group A streptococcal cell. ***(a):*** Capsule is hyaluronic acid. ***(b):*** Cell wall protein antigens M, T, and R. ***(c):*** Group-specific carbohydrate of group A streptococci is rhamnose-N-acetylglucosamine.

For group A streptococci, this is rhamnose-N-acetylglucosamine; for group B, rhamnose-glucosamine polysaccharide; for group C, rhamnose-N-acetylgalactosamine; for group D, glycerol teichoic acid containing D-alanine and glucose; for group F, glucopyranosyl-N-acetylgalactosamine.

(2) M protein: This substance is a major virulence factor of group A *S pyogenes.* M protein appears as hair-like projections of the streptococcal cell wall. When M protein is present, the streptococci are virulent, and in the absence of M type-specific antibodies, they are able to resist phagocytosis by polymorphonuclear leukocytes. Group A streptococci that lack M protein are not virulent. Immunity to infection with group A streptococci is related to the presence of type-specific antibodies to M protein. Because there are more than 80 types of M protein, a person can have repeated infections with group A *S pyogenes* of different M types. Both group C and group G streptococci have genes homologous to the genes for M protein of group A, and M protein has been found on group G streptococci.

The structure and function characteristics of M protein have been studied extensively. The molecule has a rod-like coiled-coil structure that separates functional domains. The structure allows for a large number of sequence changes while maintaining function, and the M protein immunodeterminants thus can readily change. There are two major structural classes of M protein, classes I and II.

It appears that M protein and perhaps other streptococcal cell wall antigens have an important role in the pathogenesis of rheumatic fever. Purified streptococcal cell wall membranes induce antibodies that react with human cardiac sarcolemma; the characteristics of the cross-reactive antigens are not clear. A component of the cell wall of selected M types induces antibodies that react with cardiac muscle tissue. Conserved antigenic domains on the class I M protein cross-react with human cardiac muscle, and the class I M protein may be a virulence determinant for rheumatic fever.

(3) T substance: This antigen has no relationship to virulence of streptococci. Unlike M protein, T substance is acid-labile and heat-labile. It is obtained from streptococci by proteolytic digestion, which rapidly destroys M proteins. T substance permits differentiation of certain types of streptococci by agglutination with specific antisera, while other types share the same T substance. Yet another surface antigen has been called **R protein.**

(4) Nucleoproteins: Extraction of streptococci with weak alkali yields mixtures of proteins and other substances of little serologic specificity, called **P substances,** which probably make up most of the streptococcal cell body.

Toxins & Enzymes

More than 20 extracellular products that are antigenic are elaborated by group A streptococci, including the following:

(1) Streptokinase (fibrinolysin) is produced by many strains of group A β-hemolytic streptococci. It transforms the plasminogen of human plasma into plasmin, an active proteolytic enzyme that digests fibrin and other proteins. This process of digestion may be interfered with by nonspecific serum inhibitors and by a specific antibody, antistreptokinase. Streptokinase has been given intravenously for treatment of pulmonary emboli and of coronary artery and venous thromboses.

(2) Streptodornase (streptococcal deoxyribonuclease) depolymerizes DNA. The enzymatic activity can be measured by the decrease in viscosity of known DNA solutions. Purulent exudates owe their viscosity largely to deoxyribonucleoprotein. Mixtures of streptodornase and streptokinase are used in "enzymatic debridement." They help to liquefy exudates and facilitate removal of pus and necrotic tissue; antimicrobial drugs thus gain better access, and infected surfaces recover more quickly. An antibody to DNase develops after streptococcal infections (normal limit = 100 units), especially after skin infections with pyoderma.

(3) Hyaluronidase splits hyaluronic acid, an important component of the ground substance of connective tissue. Thus, hyaluronidase aids in spreading infecting microorganisms (spreading factor). Hyaluronidases are antigenic and specific for each bacterial or tissue source. Following infection with hyaluronidase-producing organisms, specific antibodies are found in the serum.

(4) Pyrogenic exotoxins A–C (erythrogenic toxin) is soluble and is destroyed by boiling for 1 hour. It causes the rash that occurs in scarlet fever. Only strains elaborating this toxin can cause scarlet fever. Pyrogenic exotoxin is elaborated only by lysogenic streptococci. Strains devoid of the temperate phage genome do not produce toxin. A nontoxigenic *Streptococcus,* after lysogenic conversion, will produce pyrogenic exotoxin.

(5) Diphosphopyridine nucleotidase is an enzyme elaborated into the environment by some streptococci. This substance may be related to the organism's ability to kill leukocytes. Proteinases and amylase are produced by some strains.

(6) Hemolysins: Many streptococci are able to hemolyze red blood cells in vitro in varying degrees. Complete disruption of erythrocytes with release of hemoglobin is called β hemolysis. Incomplete lysis of erythrocytes with the formation of green pigment is called **α hemolysis.**

β-Hemolytic group A *S pyogenes* elaborate two hemolysins (streptolysins):

Streptolysin O is a protein (MW 60,000) that is hemolytically active in the reduced state (available —SH groups) but rapidly inactivated in the presence of oxygen. Streptolysin O is responsible for some of the hemolysis seen when growth is in cuts deep into the medium in blood agar plates. It combines quantitatively with **antistreptolysin O,** an antibody that appears in humans following infection with any streptococci that produce streptolysin O. This antibody blocks hemolysis by streptolysin O. This phenomenon forms the basis of a quantitative test for the antibody. An antistreptolysin O (ASO) serum titer in excess of 160–200 units is considered abnormally high and suggests either recent infection with streptococci or persistently high antibody levels due to an exaggerated immune response to an earlier exposure in a hypersensitive person.

Streptolysin S is the agent responsible for the hemolytic zones around streptococcal colonies growing on the surface of blood agar plates. It is not antigenic, but it may be inhibited by a nonspecific inhibitor that is frequently present in the sera of humans and animals and is independent of past experience with streptococci.

Classification of Streptococci

Over many years, the classification of streptococci into major categories has been based on a series of observations: (1) colony morphology and hemolytic reactions on blood agar; (2) serologic specificity of the cell wall group-specific substance **(Lancefield classification)** and other cell wall or capsular antigens; (3) biochemical reactions and resistance to physical and chemical factors; and (4) ecologic features. Additional biochemical tests and molecular genetics also have been used to study the relationships of streptococcal species to each other. Combinations of the above methods have permitted the classification of streptococci for purposes of clinical and epidemiologic convenience, but new methods have been introduced as the classification has evolved, with the result that several classifications have been described. In some cases, different species names have been used to describe the same organisms; and in other instances, some members of the same species have been included in another species or classified separately. The genus *Enterococcus,* for example, now includes some species previously classified as group D streptococci.

The classification of streptococci described in the following paragraphs and summarized in Table 15–1 is one logical approach.

A. Hemolysis: The characteristics of β and α hemolysis (and nonhemolysis) are described in Table 15–1. In some classification systems, β-hemolytic strains include strains that show α hemolysis after overnight incubation on 5% sheep blood agar. In other classifications, only strains that show β hemolysis are considered to be hemolytic, and the α-hemolytic strains are included with the nonhemolytic strains. It is, however, most practical to consider the streptococci and enterococci as β-hemolytic, α-hemolytic, or nonhemolytic. The classification of hemolytic patterns is used primarily with the streptococci and not with other bacteria that cause disease and which typically produce a variety of hemolysins.

B. Group-Specific Substance (Lancefield Classification): Hot acid or enzyme extracts contain the carbohydrate group-specific substances. These give precipitin reactions with specific antisera that permit arrangement into groups A–H and K–U. Typing is generally done only for groups A–D, F, and G, which cause disease in humans and for which there are reagents that allow typing using simple agglutination or color reactions.

C. Capsular Polysaccharides: The antigenic specificity of the capsular polysaccharides is used to classify *S pneumoniae* into 84 types (American

System) and to type the group B streptococci *(S agalactiae).*

D. Biochemical Reactions: Biochemical tests include sugar fermentation reactions, tests for the presence of enzymes, and tests for susceptibility or resistance to certain chemical agents. Biochemical tests are most often used to classify streptococci after the colony growth and hemolytic characteristics have been observed. Biochemical tests are used for species that typically do not react with the commonly used antibody preparations for the group-specific substances, groups A, B, C, F, and G. For example, the viridans streptococci are α-hemolytic or nonhemolytic and do not react with the antibodies commonly used for the Lancefield classification. Speciation of the viridans streptococci requires a battery of biochemical tests.

Classification of Streptococci of Particular Medical Interest

The following streptococci and enterococci are of particular medical relevance. (Names of less common species are included to clarify the previous and current classifications.)

(1) *Streptococcus pyogenes:* Most streptococci that contain the group A antigen are *S pyogenes.* They are β-hemolytic. *S pyogenes* is the main human pathogen associated with local or systemic invasion and poststreptococcal immunologic disorders. *S pyogenes* typically produces large (1 cm in diameter) zones of β hemolysis around colonies greater than 0.5 mm in diameter. They are PYR-positive (hydrolysis of L-pyrrolidonyl-2-naphthylamide) and usually are susceptible to bacitracin.

(2) *Streptococcus agalactiae:* These are the **group B streptococci.** They are members of the normal flora of the female genital tract and an important cause of neonatal sepsis and meningitis. They typically are β-hemolytic and produce zones of hemolysis that are only slightly larger than the colonies (1–2 mm in diameter). The group B streptococci hydrolyze sodium hippurate and give a positive response in the so-called CAMP test (Christie, Atkins, Munch-Peterson; see Austr J Exp Biol Med 1944;22:197).

(3) Groups C and G: These streptococci occur sometimes in the nasopharynx and may cause sinusitis, bacteremia, or endocarditis. They often look like group A *S pyogenes* on blood agar medium and are β-hemolytic. They are identified by reactions with specific antisera for groups C or G.

(4) *Enterococcus faecalis (E faecium, E durans):* The enterococci react with group D antisera. Enterococci are part of the normal enteric flora. Because the group D antigen is a teichoic acid, it is not an antigenically good marker, and the enterococci are usually identified by other characteristics. They are usually nonhemolytic and occasionally α-hemolytic. They are PYR-positive. They grow in the presence of bile and hydrolyze esculin (bile esculin-positive). They grow in 6.5% NaCl. They are more resistant to penicillin G than the streptococci, and rare isolates have plasmids that encode for β-lactamase. Some strains are vancomycin-resistant.

(5) *Streptococcus bovis:* These are among the nonenterococcal group D streptococci. They are part of the enteric flora, occasionally cause endocarditis, and sometimes cause bacteremia in patients with colon carcinoma. They are nonhemolytic and PYR-negative. They grow in the presence of bile and hydrolyze esculin (bile esculin-positive) but do not grow in 6.5% NaCl. *S bovis* are often classified as viridans streptococci.

(6) *Streptococcus anginosus:* Other species names for *S anginosus* are *S milleri, S intermedius,* and *S constellatus.* These streptococci are part of the normal flora. They may be β-, α-, or nonhemolytic. *S anginosus* includes β-hemolytic streptococci that form minute colonies (< 0.5 mm in diameter) and react with groups A, C, or G antisera; and all β-hemolytic group F streptococci. Those that are group A are PYR-negative. *S anginosus* are Voges-Proskauer test-positive. They may be classified as viridans streptococci.

(7) Group N streptococci: They are rarely found in human disease states but produce normal coagulation ("souring") of milk.

(8) Groups E, F, G, H, and K–U streptococci: These streptococci occur primarily in animals other than humans with the exceptions noted.

(9) *Streptococcus pneumoniae:* Pneumococci are α-hemolytic. Their growth is inhibited by optochin (ethylhydrocupreine hydrochloride), and colonies are bile-soluble. Their role in disease is discussed separately below.

(10) Viridans streptococci include *S mitis, S mutans, S salivarius, S sanguis* (group H) and others. Typically they are α-hemolytic (hence the name viridans), but they may be nonhemolytic. Their growth is not inhibited by optochin, and colonies are not soluble in bile (deoxycholate). The viridans streptococci are the most prevalent members of the normal flora of the upper respiratory tract and are important for the healthy state of the mucous membranes there. They may reach the bloodstream as a result of trauma and are a principal cause of endocarditis on abnormal heart valves. Some viridans streptococci (eg, *S mutans*) synthesize large polysaccharides such as dextrans or levans from sucrose and contribute importantly to the genesis of dental caries.

(11) Nutritionally variant streptococci: The nutritionally variant streptococci (*Streptococcus defectivus* and *Streptococcus adjacens* have been known as "nutritionally deficient streptococci," "pyridoxal-dependent streptococci," and by other names. They require pyridoxal or cysteine for growth on blood agar or grow as satellite colonies around colonies of staphylococci and other bacteria. They are usually α-hemolytic but may be nonhemolytic. They are part of the normal flora and occasionally cause bacteremia or endocarditis and can be found in brain abscesses and other infections. Routinely supplementing blood agar medium with pyridoxyl allows recovery of these organisms.

(12) *Peptostreptococcus* (many species): These streptococci grow only under anaerobic or microaerophilic conditions and variably produce hemolysins. They are part of the normal flora of the mouth, upper respiratory tract, bowel, and female genital tract. They often participate with many other bacterial species in mixed anaerobic infections in the abdomen, pelvis, lung, or brain.

Pathogenesis & Clinical Findings

A variety of distinct disease processes are associated with streptococcal infections. The biologic properties of the infecting organisms, the nature of the host response, and the portal of entry of the infection all greatly influence the pathologic picture. Infections can be divided into several categories.

A. Diseases Attributable to Invasion by β-Hemolytic Group A Streptococci *(S pyogenes)*: The portal of entry determines the principal clinical picture. In each case, however, there is a diffuse and rapidly spreading infection that involves the tissues and extends along lymphatic pathways with only minimal local suppuration. From the lymphatics, the infection can extend to the bloodstream.

1. Erysipelas–If the portal of entry is the skin, erysipelas results, with massive brawny edema and a rapidly advancing margin of infection.

2. Puerperal fever–If the streptococci enter the uterus after delivery, puerperal fever develops, which is essentially a septicemia originating in the infected wound (endometritis).

3. Sepsis–Infection of traumatic or surgical wounds with streptococci results in sepsis or surgical scarlet fever.

B. Diseases Attributable to Local Infection With β-Hemolytic Group A *S pyogenes* and Their β Products:

1. Streptococcal sore throat–The most common infection due to β-hemolytic streptococci is streptococcal sore throat. Virulent group A streptococci adhere to the pharyngeal epithelium by means of lipoteichoic acid covering surface pili. The glycoprotein fibronectin (MW 440,000) on epithelial cells probably serves as lipoteichoic acid ligand. In infants and small children, the sore throat occurs as a subacute nasopharyngitis with a thin serous discharge and little fever but with a tendency of the infection to extend to the middle ear, the mastoid, and the meninges. The cervical lymph nodes are usually enlarged. The illness may persist for weeks. In older children and adults, the disease is more acute and is characterized by intense nasopharyngitis, tonsillitis, and intense redness and edema of the mucous membranes, with purulent exudate; enlarged, tender cervical lymph nodes; and (usually) a high fever. Twenty percent of infections are asymptomatic. A similar clinical picture can occur with infectious mononucleosis, diphtheria, gonococcal infection, and adenovirus infection.

If the infecting streptococci produce **erythrogenic toxin** and **pyrogenic exotoxins A–C** the patient has no antitoxic immunity, **scarlet fever rash** occurs. Antitoxin to the erythrogenic toxin prevents the rash but does not interfere with the streptococcal infection. With the most intense inflammation, tissues may break down and form peritonsillar abscesses (quinsy) or Ludwig's angina, where massive swelling of the floor of the mouth blocks air passages. Streptococcal toxic shock syndrome (see above) is associated with invasive group A streptococcal infection with strains that produce the pyrogenic exotoxin.

Streptococcal infection of the upper respiratory tract does not usually involve the lungs. Pneumonia due to β-hemolytic streptococci is rapidly progressive and severe and is most commonly a sequela to viral infections, eg, influenza or measles, which seem to enhance susceptibility greatly.

2. Streptococcal pyoderma–Local infection of superficial layers of skin, especially in children, is called **impetigo.** It consists of superficial blisters that break down and eroded areas whose denuded surface is covered with pus or crusts. It spreads by continuity and is highly communicable, especially in hot, humid climates. More widespread infection occurs in eczematous or wounded skin or in burns and may progress to cellulitis. Group A streptococcal skin infections are often attributable to M types 49, 57, and 59–61 and may precede glomerulonephritis but do not often lead to rheumatic fever.

C. Infective Endocarditis:

1. Acute endocarditis–In the course of bacteremia, β-hemolytic streptococci, pneumococci, or other bacteria may settle on normal or previously deformed heart valves, producing acute endocarditis. Rapid destruction of the valves frequently leads to fatal cardiac failure in days or weeks unless a prosthesis can be inserted during antimicrobial therapy. *S aureus* and gram-negative bacilli are encountered occasionally in this disease, particularly in narcotics users. Patients with prosthetic heart valves are at special risk.

2. Subacute endocarditis–Subacute endocarditis often involves abnormal valves (congenital deformities and rheumatic or atherosclerotic lesions). Although any organism reaching the bloodstream may establish itself on thrombotic lesions that develop on endothelium injured as a result of circulatory stresses, subacute endocarditis is most frequently due to members of the normal flora of the respiratory or intestinal tract that have accidentally reached the blood. After dental extraction, at least 30% of patients have viridans streptococcal bacteremia. These streptococci, ordinarily the most prevalent members of the upper respiratory flora, are also the most frequent cause of subacute bacterial endocarditis. The group D streptococci also are common causes of subacute endocarditis. About 5–10% of cases are due to enterococci originating in the gut or urinary tract. The lesion is slowly progressive, and a certain amount of healing accompanies the active inflammation; vegetations consist of fibrin, platelets, blood cells, and bacteria adherent to the valve leaflets. The clinical course is gradual, but the disease is invariably fatal in untreated cases. The typical clinical picture includes fever, anemia, weakness, a heart murmur, embolic phenomena, an enlarged spleen, and renal lesions.

D. Fulminant Group A Streptococcal Infections and Streptococcal Toxic Shock Syndrome: Fulminant, invasive group A streptococcal infections with streptococcal toxic shock syndrome are characterized by shock, bacteremia, respiratory failure, and multiorgan failure. Death occurs in about 30% of patients. The infections tend to follow minor trauma in otherwise healthy persons with several presentations of soft tissue infection. These include necrotizing fasciitis, a progressive infection of subcutaneous tissue with destruction of fascia and fat; myositis; and infections at other soft tissue sites, including tissues around the upper respiratory tract. Bacteremia occurs frequently in patients with these severe group A streptococcal infections. In some patients, particularly those infected with group A streptococci of M types 1 or 3, the disease presents with focal soft tissue infection accompanied by fever and rapidly progressive shock with multiorgan failure. Erythema and desquamation may occur. The group A streptococci of the M types 1 and 3 (and types 12 and 28) that make pyrogenic exotoxin A or B are associated with the severe infections. These toxins and the M proteins act as superantigens, which stimulate T cells by binding to the class II major histocompatibility complex in the V_β region of the T cell receptor. The activated T cells release cytokines that mediate shock and tissue injury. The mechanisms of action appear to be similar to those due to staphylococcal toxic syndrome toxin-1 and the staphylococcal enterotoxins.

E. Other Infections: Various streptococci, particularly enterococci, can cause urinary tract infections. Anaerobic streptococci *(Peptostreptococcus)* occur in the normal female genital tract, the mouth, and the intestine. They may give rise to suppurative lesions, sometimes alone but most often in association with other anaerobes, particularly *Bacteroides*. Such infections may occur in wounds, in the breast, in postpartum endometritis, following rupture of an abdominal viscus, or in chronic suppuration of the lung. The pus usually has a foul odor. A variety of other streptococci (groups C–L and O) that are usually found in animals may also occasionally produce infections in humans.

Group B streptococci are part of the normal vaginal flora in 5–25% of women. Group B streptococcal infection during the first month of life may present as fulminant sepsis, meningitis, or respiratory distress syndrome. Intrapartum intravenous ampicillin appears to prevent colonization of infants whose mothers carry group B streptococci.

F. Poststreptococcal Diseases (Rheumatic Fever, Glomerulonephritis): Following an acute group A streptococcal infection, there is a latent period of 1–4 weeks, after which nephritis or rheumatic fever occasionally develops. The latent period suggests that these poststreptococcal diseases are not attributable to the direct effect of disseminated bacteria but represent instead a hypersensitivity response. Nephritis is more commonly preceded by infection of the skin; rheumatic fever, by infection of the respiratory tract.

1. Acute glomerulonephritis–This sometimes develops 3 weeks after streptococcal skin infection, particularly with M types 12, 4, 2, and 49. Some strains are particularly nephritogenic. In one study, 23% of children with a skin infection with a type 49 strain developed nephritis or hematuria. Other nephritogenic M types are 59–61. After random streptococcal infections, the incidence of nephritis is less than 0.5%.

Glomerulonephritis may be initiated by antigen-antibody complexes on the glomerular basement membrane. The most important antigen is probably in the streptococcal protoplast membrane. In acute nephritis, there is blood and protein in the urine, edema, high blood pressure, and urea nitrogen retention; serum complement levels are low. A few patients die; some develop chronic glomerulonephritis with ultimate kidney failure; the majority recover completely.

2. Rheumatic fever–This is the most serious sequela of hemolytic streptococcal infection because it results in damage to heart muscle and valves. Certain strains of group A streptococci contain cell membrane antigens that cross-react with human heart tissue antigens. Sera from patients with rheumatic fever contain antibodies to these antigens.

The onset of rheumatic fever is often preceded by a group A *Streptococcus* infection 1–4 weeks earlier, although the infection may be mild and may not be detected. In general, however, patients with more severe streptococcal sore throats have a greater chance of developing rheumatic fever. Untreated streptococcal infections were followed by rheumatic fever in up to 3% of military personnel and 0.3% of civilian children in the 1950s. In the 1980s, rheumatic fever was relatively rare in the USA (< 0.05% of streptococcal infections), but it occurs up to 100 times more frequently in tropical countries, eg, Egypt.

Typical symptoms and signs of rheumatic fever include fever, malaise, a migratory nonsuppurative polyarthritis, and evidence of inflammation of all parts of the heart (endocardium, myocardium, pericardium). The carditis characteristically leads to thickened and deformed valves and to small perivascular granulomas in the myocardium (Aschoff bodies) that are finally replaced by scar tissue. Erythrocyte sedimentation rates, serum transaminase levels, electrocardiograms, and other tests are used to estimate rheumatic activity.

Rheumatic fever has a marked tendency to be reactivated by recurrent streptococcal infections, whereas nephritis does not. The first attack of rheumatic fever usually produces only slight cardiac damage, which, however, increases with each subsequent attack. It is therefore important to protect such patients from recurrent hemolytic group A streptococcal infections by prophylactic penicillin administration.

Diagnostic Laboratory Tests

A. Specimens: Specimens to be obtained depend upon the nature of the streptococcal infection. A throat swab, pus, or blood is obtained for culture. Serum is obtained for antibody determinations.

B. Smears: Smears from pus often show single cocci or pairs rather than definite chains. Cocci are sometimes gram-negative because the organisms are no longer viable and have lost their ability to retain blue dye (crystal violet) and be gram-positive. If smears of pus show streptococci but cultures fail to grow, anaerobic organisms must be suspected. Smears of throat swabs are rarely contributory, because streptococci (viridans) are always present and have the same appearance as group A streptococci on stained smears.

C. Culture: Specimens suspected of containing streptococci are cultured on blood agar plates. If anaerobes are suspected, suitable anaerobic media must also be inoculated. Incubation in 10% CO_2 often speeds hemolysis. Slicing the inoculum into the blood agar has a similar effect, because oxygen does not readily diffuse through the medium to the deeply embedded organisms, and it is oxygen that inactivates streptolysin O.

Blood cultures will grow hemolytic group A streptococci (eg, in sepsis) within hours or a few days. Certain α-hemolytic streptococci and enterococci may grow slowly, so blood cultures in cases of suspected endocarditis may not turn positive for 1 week or longer.

The degree and kind of hemolysis (and colonial appearance) may help place an organism in a definite group. Group A streptococci can be rapidly identified by a fluorescent antibody test, the PYR test, and by rapid tests specific for the presence of the group A-specific antigen. Serologic grouping and typing by means of precipitin tests or coagglutination should be performed when needed for definitive classification and for epidemiologic reasons. Streptococci belonging to group A may be presumptively identified by inhibition of growth by bacitracin, but this should be used only when more definitive tests are not available.

D. Antigen Detection Tests: Several commercial kits are available for rapid detection of group A streptococcal antigen from throat swabs. These kits use enzymatic or chemical methods to extract the antigen from the swab, then use EIA or agglutination tests to demonstrate the presence of the antigen. The tests can be completed minutes to hours after the specimen is obtained. They are 60–90% sensitive and 98–99% specific when compared to culture methods. Kit tests are more rapid than cultures.

E. Serologic Tests: A rise in the titer of antibodies to many group A streptococcal antigens can be estimated: such antibodies include antistreptolysin O (ASO), particularly in respiratory disease; anti-DNase and antihyaluronidase, particularly in skin infections; antistreptokinase; anti-M type-specific antibodies; and others. Of these, the anti-ASO titer is most widely used.

Immunity

Resistance against streptococcal diseases is type-specific. Thus, a host who has recovered from infection by one group A streptococcal M type is relatively insusceptible to reinfection by the same type but fully susceptible to infection by another M type. Anti-M type-specific antibodies can be demonstrated in a test that exploits the fact that streptococci are rapidly killed after phagocytosis. M protein interferes with phagocytosis, but in the presence of type-specific antibody to M protein, streptococci are killed by human leukocytes.

Immunity against erythrogenic toxin is due to antitoxin in the blood. This antitoxic immunity protects against the rash of scarlet fever but has no effect on infection with streptococci.

Antibody to streptolysin O (antistreptolysin O, ASO) develops following infection; it blocks hemolysis by streptolysin O but does not indicate immunity. High titers (> 250 units) indicate recent or repeated infections and are found more often in rheumatic individuals than in those with uncomplicated streptococcal infections.

Treatment

All β-hemolytic group A streptococci are sensitive to penicillin G, and most are sensitive to erythromycin. Some are resistant to tetracyclines. α-Hemolytic streptococci and enterococci vary in their susceptibility to antimicrobial agents. Particularly in bacterial endocarditis, antibiotic sensitivity tests are useful to determine which drugs may be used for optimal therapy. In these cases, laboratory tests should include determinations of both inhibitory and killing power of drugs or drug combinations. Aminoglycosides often enhance the rate of bactericidal action of penicillin on streptococci, particularly enterococci.

Antimicrobial drugs have no effect on established glomerulonephritis and rheumatic fever. However, in acute streptococcal infections, every effort must be made to rapidly eradicate streptococci from the patient, eliminate the antigenic stimulus (before day 8), and thus prevent poststreptococcal disease. Doses of penicillin or erythromycin that result in effective tissue levels for 10 days usually accomplish this. Antimicrobial drugs are also very useful in preventing reinfection with β-hemolytic group A streptococci in rheumatic fever patients.

Epidemiology, Prevention, & Control

Many streptococci (viridans streptococci, enterococci, etc) are members of the normal flora of the human body. They produce disease only when established in parts of the body where they do not normally occur (eg, heart valves). To prevent such accidents, particularly in the course of surgical procedures on the respiratory, gastrointestinal, and urinary tracts that result in temporary bacteremia, antimicrobial agents are often administered prophylactically to persons with known heart valve deformity and to those with prosthetic valves or joints.

The ultimate source of group A streptococci is a person harboring these organisms. The individual may have a clinical or subclinical infection or may be a carrier distributing streptococci directly to other persons via droplets from the respiratory tract or skin. The nasal discharges of a person harboring β-hemolytic streptococci are the most dangerous source for spread of these organisms. The role of contaminated bedding, utensils, or clothing is doubtful. The infected udder of a cow yields milk that may cause epidemic spread of hemolytic streptococci. Immunologic grouping and typing of streptococci are valuable tools for epidemiologic tracing of the transmission chain.

Control procedures are directed mainly at the human source: (1) Detection and early antimicrobial therapy of respiratory and skin infections with group A streptococci. This requires maintenance of adequate penicillin levels in tissues for 10 days (eg, benzathine penicillin G, 1.2 million units given once intramuscularly). Erythromycin is an alternative drug of choice. Prompt eradication of streptococci from early infections can effectively prevent the development of poststreptococcal disease. (2) Antistreptococcal chemoprophylaxis in persons who have suffered an attack of rheumatic fever. This involves giving one injection of benzathine penicillin G, 1.2 million units intramuscularly, every 3–4 weeks or daily oral penicillin or oral sulfonamide. The first attack of rheumatic fever infrequently causes major heart damage. However, such persons are particularly susceptible to reinfections with streptococci that precipitate relapses of rheumatic activity and give rise to cardiac damage. Chemoprophylaxis in such individuals, especially children, must be continued for years. Chemoprophylaxis is not used in glomerulonephritis because of the small number of nephritogenic types of streptococci. An exception may be family groups with a high rate of poststreptococcal nephritis. (3) Eradication of group A streptococci from carriers. This is especially important when carriers are in areas such as obstetric delivery rooms, operating rooms, classrooms, or nurseries. Unfortunately, it is often difficult to eradicate hemolytic streptococci from permanent carriers, and individuals may occasionally have to be shifted away from "sensitive" areas for some time. (4) Dust control, ventilation, air filtration, ultraviolet light, and aerosol mists are all of doubtful efficacy in the control of streptococcal transmission. Milk should always be pasteurized. (5) Group B streptococci account for most cases of neonatal sepsis at present. They are derived from the mother's genital tract, where carriage is asymptomatic. Neonatal illness may be favored by deficiency of maternal antibody. Group B streptococcal disease in the newborn can be prevented by drug prophylaxis in a mother with positive cultures in the setting of premature labor or prolonged rupture of the membranes.

STREPTOCOCCUS PNEUMONIAE (Pneumococcus)

The pneumococci *(S pneumoniae)* are gram-positive diplococci, often lancet-shaped or arranged in chains, possessing a capsule of polysaccharide that permits typing with specific antisera. Pneumococci are readily lysed by surface-active agents such as bile salts. Surface-active agents probably remove or inactivate the inhibitors of cell wall autolysins. Pneumococci are normal inhabitants of the upper respiratory tract of humans and can cause pneumonia, sinusitis, otitis, bronchitis, bacteremia, meningitis, and other infectious processes.

Morphology & Identification

A. Typical Organisms: The typical gram-positive, lancet-shaped diplococci (Figure 15–3) are often seen in specimens of young cultures. In sputum or pus, single cocci or chains are also seen. With age, the organisms rapidly become gram-negative and tend to lyse spontaneously.

Autolysis of pneumococci is greatly enhanced by surface-active agents. Lysis of pneumococci occurs in a few minutes when ox bile (10%) or sodium deoxycholate (2%) is added to a broth culture or suspension of organisms at neutral pH. Viridans streptococci do not lyse and are thus easily differentiated from pneumococci. On solid media, the growth of pneumococci is inhibited around a disk of optochin; viridans streptococci are not inhibited by optochin.

Other identifying points include almost uniform virulence for mice when injected intraperitoneally and the "capsule swelling test," or quellung reaction (see below).

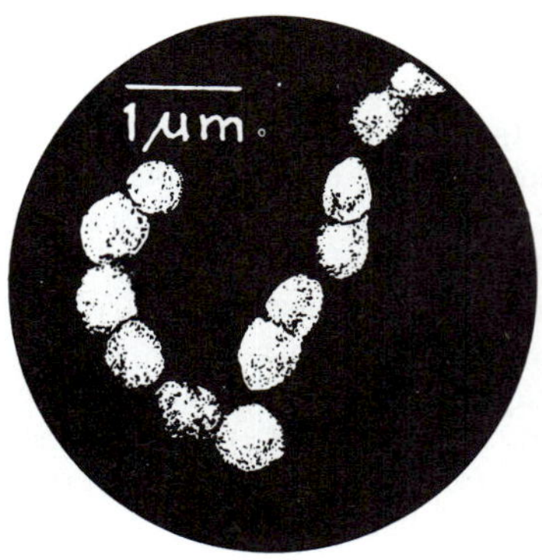

Figure 15–3. Drawing from electron micrograph of pneumococci.

B. Culture: Pneumococci form a small round colony, at first dome-shaped and later developing a central plateau with an elevated rim. Pneumococci are α-hemolytic on blood agar. Growth is enhanced by 5–10% CO_2.

C. Growth Characteristics: Most energy is obtained from fermentation of glucose; this is accompanied by the rapid production of lactic acid, which limits growth. Neutralization of broth cultures with alkali at intervals results in massive growth.

D. Variation: A culture of pneumococci contains a few organisms that are unable to produce capsular polysaccharide and thus give rise to rough colonies; most of the organisms are polysaccharide-producing and give rise to smooth colonies. Rough forms predominate if the culture is grown in type-specific antipolysaccharide serum.

E. Transformation: When pneumococci of a type that does not make polysaccharide capsules are grown in the presence of DNA extracted from a pneumococcus type that does produce capsular polysaccharide, encapsulated pneumococci of the latter type are formed. Similar transformation reactions have been performed that involve changes in drug resistance.

Antigenic Structure

A. Component Structures: The capsular polysaccharide is immunologically distinct for each of the 84 types. The polysaccharide is an antigen that primarily elicits a B cell response.

The somatic portion of the pneumococcus contains an M protein that is characteristic for each type and a group-specific carbohydrate that is common to all pneumococci. The carbohydrate can be precipitated by C-reactive protein, a substance found in the serum of certain patients.

B. Quellung Reaction: When pneumococci of a certain type are mixed with specific antipolysaccharide serum of the same type—or with polyvalent antiserum—on a microscope slide, the capsule swells markedly. This reaction is useful for rapid identification and for typing of the organisms, either in sputum or in cultures. The polyvalent antiserum, which contains antibody to more than 80 types ("omniserum"), is a good reagent for rapid microscopic determination of whether pneumococci are present in fresh sputum.

Pathogenesis

A. Types of Pneumococci: In adults, types 1–8 are responsible for about 75% of cases of pneumococcal pneumonia and for more than half of all fatalities in pneumococcal bacteremia; in children, types 6, 14, 19, and 23 are frequent causes.

B. Production of Disease: Pneumococci produce disease through their ability to multiply in the tissues. They produce no toxins of significance. The virulence of the organism is a function of its capsule, which prevents or delays ingestion of encapsulated cells by phagocytes. A serum that contains antibodies against the type-specific polysaccharide protects against infection. If such a serum is absorbed with the type-specific polysaccharide, it loses its protective power. Animals or humans immunized with a given type of pneumococcal polysaccharide are subsequently immune to that type of pneumococcus and possess precipitating and opsonizing antibodies for that type of polysaccharide.

C. Loss of Natural Resistance: Since 40–70% of humans are at some time carriers of virulent pneumococci, the normal respiratory mucosa must possess great natural resistance to the pneumococcus. Among the factors that probably lower this resistance and thus predispose to pneumococcal infection are the following:

1. Abnormalities of the respiratory tract– Viral and other infections that damage surface cells; abnormal accumulations of mucus (eg, allergy), which protect pneumococci from phagocytosis; bronchial obstruction (eg, atelectasis); and respiratory tract injury due to irritants disturbing its mucociliary function.

2. Alcohol or drug intoxication, which depresses phagocytic activity, depresses the cough reflex, and facilitates aspiration of foreign material.

3. Abnormal circulatory dynamics (eg, pulmonary congestion, heart failure).

4. Malnutrition, general debility, sickle cell anemia, hyposplenism, nephrosis, or complement deficiency.

Pathology

Pneumococcal infection causes an outpouring of fibrinous edema fluid into the alveoli, followed by red cells and leukocytes, which results in consolidation of portions of the lung. Many pneumococci are found throughout this exudate, and they may reach the bloodstream via the lymphatic drainage of the lungs. The alveolar walls remain normally intact during the infection. Later, mononuclear cells actively phagocytose the debris, and this liquid phase is gradually reabsorbed. The pneumococci are taken up by phagocytes and digested intracellularly.

Clinical Findings

The onset of pneumococcal pneumonia is usually sudden, with fever, chills, and sharp pleural pain. The sputum is similar to the alveolar exudate, being characteristically bloody or rusty colored. Early in the disease, when the fever is high, bacteremia is present in 10–20% of cases. Before the days of chemotherapy, recovery from the disease began between the fifth and tenth days and was associated with the development of type-specific antibodies. The mortality rate was as high as 30%, depending on age and underlying illness. Bacteremic pneumonia always has the highest mortality rate. With antimicrobial therapy, the illness is usually terminated promptly; if drugs are given early, the development of consolidation is interrupted.

Pneumococcal pneumonia must be differentiated from pulmonary infarction, atelectasis, neoplasm, congestive heart failure, and pneumonia caused by many other bacteria. Empyema (pus in the pleural space) is a significant complication and requires aspiration and drainage.

From the respiratory tract, pneumococci may reach other sites. The sinuses and middle ear are most frequently involved. Infection sometimes extends from the mastoid to the meninges. Bacteremia from pneumonia has a triad of severe complications: meningitis, endocarditis, and septic arthritis. With the early use of chemotherapy, acute pneumococcal endocarditis and arthritis have become rare.

Diagnostic Laboratory Tests

Blood is drawn for culture, and sputum is collected for demonstration of pneumococci by smear and culture. Serum antibody tests are impractical. Sputum may be examined in several ways.

(1) Stained smears: A Gram-stained film of rusty-red sputum shows typical organisms, many polymorphonuclear neutrophils, and many red cells.

(2) Capsule swelling tests: Fresh emulsified sputum mixed with antiserum gives capsule swelling (the quellung reaction) for identification of pneumococci and possible typing. Peritoneal exudate can also be used for capsule swelling tests.

(3) Culture: Sputum cultured on blood agar and incubated in CO_2 or a candle jar. Blood culture.

(4) Intraperitoneal injection of sputum into laboratory mice: Animals die in 18–48 hours; heart blood gives pure culture of pneumococci. This form of culture for pneumococci is very sensitive but seldom used because of the need to maintain a mouse colony.

(5) Pneumococcal meningitis should be diagnosed by prompt examination and culture of cerebrospinal fluid.

Immunity

Immunity to infection with pneumococci is type-specific and depends both on antibodies to capsular polysaccharide and on intact phagocytic function. Vaccines can induce production of antibodies to capsular polysaccharides (see below).

Treatment

Since pneumococci are sensitive to many antimicrobial drugs, early treatment usually results in rapid recovery, and antibody response seems to play a much diminished role. The penicillins are the drugs of choice. Recently, some drug resistance has appeared; pneumococci resistant to tetracyclines, erythromycin, and lincomycin have been isolated from patients. Pneumococci of increased resistance to penicillin (minimum inhibitory concentration, > 1 μg/mL) appear in New Guinea and South Africa. Similar penicillin-resistant pneumococci are found worldwide, including the United States. Some pneumococci that are moderately resistant to penicillin G (MICs 0.1–1 μg/mL) have been isolated in the USA and elsewhere. The penicillin G-resistant pneumococci from South Africa are resistant to multiple drugs, but no plasmids or β-lactamase production has been identified. Penicillin-resistant pneumococci present little difficulty in pneumonia, but in meningitis, where limited amounts of the drug reach the central nervous system, they are a severe management problem.

Epidemiology, Prevention, & Control

Pneumococcal pneumonia accounts for about 60% of all bacterial pneumonias. It is an endemic disease with a high incidence of carriers. In the development of illness, predisposing factors (see above) are more important than exposure to the infectious agent, and the healthy carrier is more important in disseminating pneumococci than the sick patient.

It is possible to immunize individuals with type-specific polysaccharides. Such vaccines can probably provide 90% protection against bacteremic pneumonia. Among workers in South African gold mines, vaccines containing 12 polysaccharide types gave good antibody response and good protection against disease. A vaccine containing 14 pneumococcal types was beneficial in patients with sickle cell disease or after splenectomy. In 1983, an expanded polysaccharide vaccine containing 23 types was licensed in the USA. Such vaccines are appropriate for children and for elderly, debilitated, or immunosuppressed individuals. Pneumococcal vaccines have greatly reduced immunogenicity in children under 2 years of age and in patients with lymphomas; in such high-risk patients, penicillin prophylaxis must accompany vaccination.

In addition, it is desirable to avoid predisposing factors, to establish the diagnosis promptly, and to begin adequate chemotherapy early. At present, most fatalities from pneumococcal pneumonia occur in persons over 50 years of age; persons with impaired natural resistance, eg, those with sickle cell disease or asplenia; and those with bacteremia.

ENTEROCOCCI

There are at least 12 species of enterococci. *Enterococcus faecalis* is the most common and causes 85–90% of enterococcal infections, while *Enterococcus faecium* causes 5–10%. The enterococci are among the most frequent causes of nosocomial infections, particularly in intensive care units, and are selected by therapy with cephalosporins and other antibiotics to which they are resistant. Enterococci are transmitted from one patient to another primarily on the hands of hospital personnel, some of whom may carry the enterococci in their gastrointestinal tracts. Enterococci occasionally are transmitted on medical devices. In patients, the most common sites of infection are the urinary tract, wounds, biliary tract, and blood. Enterococci may cause meningitis and bacteremia in neonates. In adults, enterococci can cause endocarditis. However, enterococci usually are cultured along with other species of bacteria, and it is difficult to define the pathogenic role of the enterococci.

Antibiotic Resistance

A major problem with the enterococci is that they can be very resistant to antibiotics. *E faecium* is usually much more antibiotic-resistant than *E faecalis.*

A. Intrinsic Resistance: Enterococci are intrinsically resistant to cephalosporins, penicillinase-resistant penicillins, and monobactams. They have intrinsic low-level resistance to many aminoglycosides, are of intermediate susceptibility or resistant to fluoroquinolones, and are less susceptible than streptococci (10- to 1000-fold) to penicillin and ampicillin. Enterococci are inhibited by β-lactams (eg, ampicillin) but generally are not killed by them.

B. Resistance to Aminoglycosides: Therapy with combinations of a cell wall-active antibiotic (a penicillin or vancomycin) plus an aminoglycoside (streptomycin or gentamicin) is essential for severe enterococcal infections, such as endocarditis. Although enterococci have intrinsic low-level resistance to aminoglycosides (MICs of 4–500 μg/mL), they have synergistic susceptibility when treated with a cell wall-active antibiotic plus an aminoglycoside. However, some enterococci have high-level resistance to aminoglycosides (MICs > 500 μg/mL) and are not susceptible to the synergism. This high-level aminoglycoside resistance is due to enterococcal aminoglycoside-modifying enzymes (Table 15–2). The genes that code for most of these enzymes are usually on conjugative plasmids or transposons. The enzymes have differential activity against the aminoglycosides. Resistance to gentamicin predicts resistance to the other aminoglycosides except streptomycin. (Susceptibility to gentamicin does not predict susceptibility to other aminoglycosides.) Resistance to streptomycin does not predict resistance to other aminoglycosides. The result is that only streptomycin or gentamicin (or both or neither) is likely to show synergistic activity with a cell wall-active antibiotic against enterococci. Enterococci from severe infections should have susceptibility tests (MICs > 500 μg/mL) for high-level resistance to gentamicin and streptomycin to predict therapeutic efficacy.

C. Vancomycin Resistance: Vancomycin is the primary alternative drug to a penicillin (plus an aminoglycoside) for treating enterococcal infections. In the United States, enterococci that are resistant to vancomycin have increased in frequency. These enterococci are not synergistically susceptible to vancomycin plus an aminoglycoside. Vancomycin resistance has been most common in *E faecium,* but vancomycin-resistant strains of *E faecalis* also occur.

There are three **vancomycin resistance phenotypes,** VanA, VanB, and VanC. VanA strains have inducible high-level resistance to vancomycin. The nine genes coding for the VanA phenotype are on a transposon and are self-transmissible to other enterococci by a conjugative plasmid. VanB strains have moderate to high level resistance to vancomycin. VanC strains have intermediate to moderate resistance to vancomycin. VanC is constitutive in the less commonly isolated species *Enterococcus gallinarum* and *Enterococcus casseliflavus.*

Teicoplanin is a glycopeptide drug with many similarities to vancomycin. Enterococci with the VanA phenotype are resistant to teicoplanin. Those with the VanB and VanC phenotypes usually are susceptible to teicoplanin.

D. β-Lactamase Production and Resistance to β-Lactams: β-Lactamase-producing *E faecalis* have been isolated from patients' specimens in the United States and other countries. There is great geographic variation. The isolates from the Northeastern and Southern United States appeared to be from dissemination of a single strain, suggesting there will be spread to additional geographical areas. The gene encoding for the enterococcal β-lactamase is the same

Table 15–2. Enterococcal aminoglycoside modifying enzymes that eliminate aminoglycoside-penicillin synergy.

Enzyme	Aminoglycoside			
	Streptomycin	Gentamicin	Tobramycin	Amikacin
6-Adenyltransferase	+	–	–	–
3'-Phosphotransferase	–	–	–	+
6'-Acetyltransferase	–	–	+	
4'-Adenyltransferase	–	–	+	±
2"-Phosphotransferase/6'-acetyltransferase	–	+	+	+

gene as found in *Staphylococcus aureus.* The gene is constitutively expressed in enterococci and inducible in staphylococci. Because enterococci may produce small amounts of the enzyme, they may appear to be susceptible to penicillin and ampicillin by routine susceptibility tests. The β-lactamase can be detected using a high inoculum and the chromogenic cephalosporin test or by other methods. High-level gentamicin resistance often accompanies the β-lactamase production. The genes coding for both of these properties reside on conjugative plasmids and can be transferred from one strain of enterococcus to another. Infections due to β-lactamase-producing enterococci can be treated with combination penicillin/β-lactamase inhibitors or vancomycin (and streptomycin), when in vitro susceptibility has been demonstrated.

E. Trimethoprim-Sulfamethoxazol Resistance: Enterococci often show susceptibility to this combination by in vitro testing, but the drugs are not effective in treating infections. This discrepancy is because enterococci are able to utilize exogenous folates available in vivo and thus escape inhibition by the drugs.

OTHER GRAM-POSITIVE VANCOMYCIN-RESISTANT & VANCOMYCIN-SUSCEPTIBLE COCCI & COCCOBACILLARY ORGANISMS

There are nonstreptococcal gram-positive cocci or coccobacilli that occasionally cause disease. These organisms have many growth and morphologic characteristics like viridans streptococci. They may be α-hemolytic or nonhemolytic. Most of them are catalase-negative; others may be weakly catalase-positive. *Pediococcus* and *Leuconostoc* are the genera whose members are **vancomycin-resistant.** Lactobacilli are anaerobes that can be microaerophilic and α-hemolytic, sometimes have coccobacillary forms similar to the viridans streptococci. Most (90%) **lactobacilli** are **vancomycin-resistant.** Other organisms that occasionally cause disease and should be differentiated from streptococci and enterococci include *Lactococcus, Aerococcus,* and *Gemella,* species that generally are **vancomycin-susceptible. Stomatococcus mucilaginosus** was previously considered a *Staphylococcus* species, but it is catalase-negative; colonies show a distinct adherence to agar.

REFERENCES

Group A Streptococci

Bisno AL: The resurgence of acute rheumatic fever in the United States. Ann Rev Med 1990;41:319.

Centor RM, Meier FA, Dalton HP: Throat cultures and rapid tests for diagnosis of group A streptococcal pharyngitis. Ann Intern Med 1986;105:892.

Charles D, Larsen B: Streptococcal puerperal sepsis and obstetric infections: A historical perspective. Rev Infect Dis 1986;8:411.

Dillon HC: Poststreptococcal glomerulonephritis following pyoderma. Rev Infect Dis 1979;1:935.

Fischetti VA: Streptococcal M protein: Molecular design and biological behavior. Clin Microbiol Rev 1989; 2:285.

Quinn RW: Comprehensive review of morbidity and mortality trends for rheumatic fever, streptococcal disease, and scarlet fever: The decline of rheumatic fever. Rev Infect Dis 1989;11:928.

Senitzer D, Freimer EH: Autoimmune mechanisms in the pathogenesis of rheumatic fever. Rev Infect Dis 1984; 6:832.

Stevens DL et al: Invasive group A streptococcus infections. Clin Infect Dis 1992;14:2.

Tomai MA et al: T cell receptor V gene usage by human T cells stimulated with the superantigen M protein. J Exp Med 1991;174:285.

Group B Streptococci

Baker CJ: Immunization to prevent group B streptococcal disease: Victories and vexations. J Infect Dis 1990; 161:917.

Boyer KM, Gotoff SP: Prevention of early-onset neonatal group B streptococcal disease with selective intrapartum chemoprophylaxis. N Engl J Med 1986;314:1 665.

Groups C, F, & G Streptococci

Jones KF, Fischetti VA: Biological and immunochemical identity of M protein on group G streptococci with M protein on group A streptococci. Infect Immun 1987;55:502.

Ruoff KL: *Streptococcus anginosus ("Streptococcus milleri"):* The unrecognized pathogen. Clin Microbiol Rev 1988;1:102.

Venezio FR et al: Group G streptococcal endocarditis and bacteremia. Am J Med 1986;81:29.

Viridans Streptococci; Nutritionally Variant Streptococci

Coykendall AL: Classification and identification of the viridans streptococci. Clin Microbiol Rev 1989;2:315.

Roberts RB et al: Viridans streptococcal endocarditis: The role of various species, including pyridoxal-dependent streptococci. Rev Infect Dis 1979;1:955.

Ruoff KL: Nutritionally variant streptococci. Clin Microbiol Rev 1991;4:184.

Sussman JI et al: Viridans streptococcal endocarditis: Clinical, microbiological, and echocardiographic correlations. J Infect Dis 1986;154:597.

Pneumococci

Bolan G et al: Pneumococcal vaccine efficacy in selected populations in the United States. Ann Intern Med 1986;104:1.

Burman LA, Norrby R, Trollfors B: Invasive pneumococcal infections: Incidence, predisposing factors, and prognosis. Rev Infect Dis 1985;7:133.

Hager HL, Woolley TW, Berk SL: Review of pneumococcal infections with attention to vaccine and nonvaccine serotypes. Rev Infect Dis 1990;12:267.

Jacobs MR: Treatment and diagnosis of infections caused by drug-resistant *Streptococcus pneumoniae.* Clin Infect Dis 1992;15:119.

Powderly WG, Stanley SL Jr, Medoff G: Pneumococcal endocarditis: Report of a series and review of the literature. Rev Infect Dis 1986;8:786.

Simberkoff MS et al: Efficacy of pneumococcal vaccine in high-risk patients: Results of a veterans administration cooperative study. N Engl J Med 1986;315:1318.

Enterococci

Gordon S et al: Antimicrobial susceptibility patterns of common and unusual species of enterococci causing infections in the United States. J Clin Microbiol 1992;30:2373.

Leclercq R et al: Resistance of enterococci to aminoglycosides and glycopeptides. Clin Infect Dis 1992;15:495.

Murray BE: The life and times of the enterococcus. Clin Microbiol Rev 1990;3:46.

Rhinehart E et al: Rapid dissemination of β-lactamase-producing, aminoglycoside-resistant *Enterococcus faecalis* among patients and staff on an infant-toddler surgical ward. N Engl J Med 1990;323:1814.

Nonstreptococcal Gram-Positive Cocci

Ascher DP et al: Infections due to *Stomatococcus mucilaginosus*: 10 cases and review. Rev Infect Dis 1991;13:1048.

Facklam R, Hollis, Collins MD: Identification of gram-positive coccal and coccobacillary vancomycin-resistant bacteria. J Clin Microbiol 1989;27:724.

Handwerger S et al: Infection due to *Leuconostoc* species: Six cases and review. Rev Infect Dis 1990;12:602.

Riebel WJ, Washington J: Clinical and microbiologic characteristics of pediococci. J Clin Microbiol 1990;28:1348.

16 Enteric Gram-Negative Rods (Enterobacteriaceae)

The Enterobacteriaceae are a large, heterogeneous group of gram-negative rods whose natural habitat is the intestinal tract of humans and animals. The family includes many genera (eg, *Escherichia, Shigella, Salmonella, Enterobacter, Klebsiella, Serratia, Proteus,*) and others. Some enteric organisms, eg, *Escherichia coli,* are part of the normal flora and incidentally cause disease, while others, the salmonellae and shigellae, are regularly pathogenic for humans. The Enterobacteriaceae are facultative anaerobes or aerobes, ferment a wide range of carbohydrates, possess a complex antigenic structure, and produce a variety of toxins and other virulence factors. Enterobacteriaceae, enteric gram-negative rods, and enteric bacteria are the terms used in this chapter, but these bacteria may also be called coliforms.

Classification

The taxonomy of the Enterobacteriaceae is complex and is rapidly changing as further DNA homology studies are performed. More than 20 genera and 100 species have been defined. In this chapter, taxonomy will be minimized and the names employed in the medical literature will generally be used. A comprehensive approach to the identification of Enterobacteriaceae is presented by Kelly and Farmer in *Manual of Clinical Microbiology,* 5th ed. Balows A et al (editor). American Society for Microbiology, 1991.

The family Enterobacteriaceae is characterized biochemically by the ability to reduce nitrates to nitrites and to ferment glucose with the production of acid or acid and gas. The Enterobacteriaceae do not require increased amounts of sodium chloride for growth and are oxidase-negative. Many biochemical tests are used to differentiate species of Enterobacteriaceae (Table 16–1); in laboratories in the USA, commercially prepared kits are used to a large extent for this purpose.

The major groups of Enterobacteriaceae are described and discussed briefly in the following paragraphs. Specific characteristics of salmonellae, shigellae, and the other medically important enteric gram-negative rods and the diseases they cause are discussed separately later in this chapter.

Morphology & Identification

A. Typical Organisms: The Enterobacteriaceae are short gram-negative rods that may form chains. Typical morphology is seen in growth on solid media in vitro, but morphology is highly variable in clinical specimens. Capsules are large and regular in *Klebsiella,* less so in *Enterobacter,* and uncommon in the other species.

B. Culture: *E coli* and most of the other enteric bacteria form circular, convex, smooth colonies with distinct edges. *Enterobacter* colonies are similar but somewhat more mucoid. *Klebsiella* colonies are large and very mucoid and tend to coalesce with prolonged incubation. The salmonellae and shigellae produce colonies similar to *E coli* but do not ferment lactose. Some strains of *E coli* produce hemolysis on blood agar.

C. Growth Characteristics: Carbohydrate fermentation patterns and the activity of amino acid decarboxylases and other enzymes are used in biochemical differentiation (Table 16–1). Some tests, eg, the production of indole from tryptophan, are commonly used in rapid identification systems, while others, eg, the Voges-Proskauer reaction (production of acetylmethylcarbinol from dextrose), are used less often. Culture on "differential" media that contain special dyes and carbohydrates (eg, eosin-methylene blue [EMB], MacConkey's, or deoxycholate medium) distinguishes lactose-fermenting (colored) from non-lactose-fermenting colonies (nonpigmented) and may allow rapid presumptive identification of enteric bacteria (Table 16–2).

Many complex media have been devised to help in identification of the enteric bacteria. One such medium is triple sugar iron (TSI) agar, which is often used to help differentiate salmonellae and shigellae from other enteric gram-negative rods in stool cultures. The medium contains 0.1% glucose, 1% sucrose, 1% lactose, ferrous sulfate (for detection of H_2S production), tissue extracts (protein growth substrate), and a pH indicator (phenol red). It is poured into a test tube to produce a slant with a deep butt and is inoculated by stabbing bacterial growth into the butt. If only glucose is fermented, the slant and the butt initially turn yellow from the small amount of acid produced; as the fermentation products are subsequently oxidized to CO_2 and H_2O and released from the slant and as oxidative decarboxylation of proteins continues with formation of amines, the slant turns alkaline (red). If lactose or

Table 16–1. Biochemical reaction patterns in primary tests for the common clinically significant Enterobacteriaceae.[1]

	Citrobacter	Enterobacter	Escherichia	Klebsiella	Morganella	Proteus	Providencia	Salmonella	Serratia	Shigella
Arginine	±	±	–	–	–	–	–	±	–	–
Citrate	+	+	–	+	–	±	+	±	+	–
DNase	–	–	–	–	–	–	–	–	+	–
Gas	+	+	+	±	±	±	±	±	±	–
Glucose	+	+	+	+	+	+	+	+	+	+
H_2S	±	–	–	–	–	+	–	±	–	–
Indole	±	–	+	±	+	±	+	–	–	±
Lysine	–	±	+	+	–	–	–	+	+	–
Motility	+	+	±	–	+	+	+	+	+	–
Ornithine	±	+	±	–	+	±	–	+	+	±
Phenylalanine	–	–	–	–	+	+	+	–	–	–
Sucrose	±	+	±	+	–	±	±	–	+	–
Urease	–	–	–	±	+	+	±	–	–	–
VP[2]	–	+	–	+	–	–	–	–	+	–
TSI[3] slant	Alk (A)	A	A (Alk)	A	Alk	Alk	Alk	Alk	Alk (A)	Alk
butt	AG	AG	AG	AG	AG	AG	AG	A; G±	A	A

[1]Results for common clinical isolates: ± = variable; + = most (usually ≥ 90%) of strains positive; – = few (usually ≤ 10%) of strains positive; A = acid (yellow); G = gas; Alk = alkaline. (Note: There are exceptions to nearly all of the results listed.)

[2]VP = Voges-Proskauer reaction.

[3]TSI = Triple sugar iron agar.

Table 16–2. Rapid, presumptive identification of gram-negative enteric bacteria.

Lactose Fermented Rapidly	Lactose Fermented Slowly	Lactose Not Fermented
Escherichia coli: Metallic sheen on differential media; motile; flat, nonviscous colonies. ***Enterobacter aerogenes:*** Raised colonies, no metallic sheen; often motile; more viscous growth. ***Klebsiella pneumoniae:*** Very viscous, mucoid growth; nonmotile.	*Edwardsiella, Serratia, Citrobacter, Arizona, Providencia, Erwinia*	Shigella *species:* Nonmotile; no gas from dextrose. Salmonella *species:* Motile; acid and usually gas from dextrose. Proteus *species:* "Swarming" on agar; urea rapidly hydrolyzed (smell of ammonia). Pseudomonas *species* (see Chapter 17): Soluble pigments, blue-green and fluorescing; sweetish smell.

sucrose is fermented, so much acid is produced that the slant and butt remain yellow (acid). Salmonellae and shigellae typically yield an alkaline slant and an acid butt (Table 16–1). Although *Proteus, Providencia,* and *Morganella* produce an alkaline slant, they can be identified by their rapid formation of red color in Christensen's urea medium or TSI agar. Organisms producing acid on the slant and acid and gas (bubbles) in the butt are other enteric bacteria.

1. *Escherichia*–*E coli* typically produces positive tests for indole, lysine decarboxylase, and mannitol fermentation and produces gas from glucose. An isolate from urine can be quickly identified as *E coli* by its hemolysis on blood agar, typical colonial morphology with an iridescent "sheen" on differential media such as EMB agar, and a positive spot indole test. Over 90% of *E coli* isolates are positive for β-glucuronidase using the substrate 4-methylumbelliferyl-β-glucuronide (MUG). Isolates from anatomic sites other than urine, with characteristic properties (above plus negative oxidase tests) often can be confirmed as *E coli* with a positive MUG test.

2. *Klebsiella-Enterobacter-Serratia* group– *Klebsiella* species exhibit mucoid growth, large polysaccharide capsules, and lack of motility, and they usually give positive tests for lysine decarboxylase and citrate. Most *Enterobacter* species give positive tests for motility, citrate, and ornithine decarboxylase and produce gas from glucose. *Enterobacter aerogenes* has small capsules. *Serratia* produces DNase, lipase, and gelatinase. *Klebsiella, Enterobacter,* and *Serratia* usually give positive Voges-Proskauer reactions.

3. *Proteus-Morganella-Providencia* group– The members of this group deaminate phenylalanine, are motile, grow on potassium cyanide medium (KCN), and ferment xylose. *Proteus* species move very actively by means of peritrichous flagella, resulting in "swarming" on solid media unless the swarming is inhibited by chemicals, eg, phenylethyl alcohol or CLED (*c*ystine-*l*actose-*e*lectrolyte-*d*eficient) medium. *Proteus* species and *Morganella morganii* are urease-positive, while *Providencia* species usually are urease-negative. The *Proteus-Providencia* group ferment lactose very slowly or not at all. *Proteus mirabilis* is more susceptible to antimicrobial drugs, including penicillins, than other members of the group.

4. *Citrobacter*–These bacteria typically are citrate-positive and differ from the salmonellae in that they do not decarboxylate lysine. They ferment lactose very slowly if at all.

5. The shigellae–(See p 212.) Shigellae are nonmotile and usually do not ferment lactose but do ferment other carbohydrates, producing acid but not gas. They do not produce H_2S. The four *Shigella* species are closely related to *E coli.* Many share common antigens with one another and with other enteric bacteria.

6. The salmonellae–(See p 214.) Salmonellae are motile rods that characteristically ferment glucose and mannose without producing gas but do not ferment lactose or sucrose. Most salmonellae produce H_2S. They are often pathogenic for humans or animals when ingested. *Arizona* is included in the *Salmonella* group.

7. Other Enterobacteriaceae–*Yersinia* species are discussed in Chapter 20. Other genera occasionally found in human infections include *Edwardsiella* and *Ewingella, Hafnia, Cedecea,* and *Kluyvera.*

Antigenic Structure

Enterobacteriaceae have a complex antigenic structure. They are classified by more than 150 different heat-stable somatic O (lipopolysaccharide) antigens, more than 100 heat-labile K (capsular) antigens, and more than 50 H (flagellar) antigens (Figure 16–1). In *Salmonella typhi* the capsular antigens are called Vi antigens.

O antigens are the most external part of the cell wall lipopolysaccharide and consist of repeating units of polysaccharide. Some O-specific polysaccharides contain unique sugars. O antigens are resistant to heat and alcohol and usually are detected by bacterial agglutination. Antibodies to O antigens are predominantly IgM.

While each genus of Enterobacteriaceae is associated with specific O groups, a single organism may carry several O antigens. Thus, most shigellae share one or more O antigens with *E coli. E coli* may cross-react with some *Providencia, Klebsiella,* and *Salmo-*

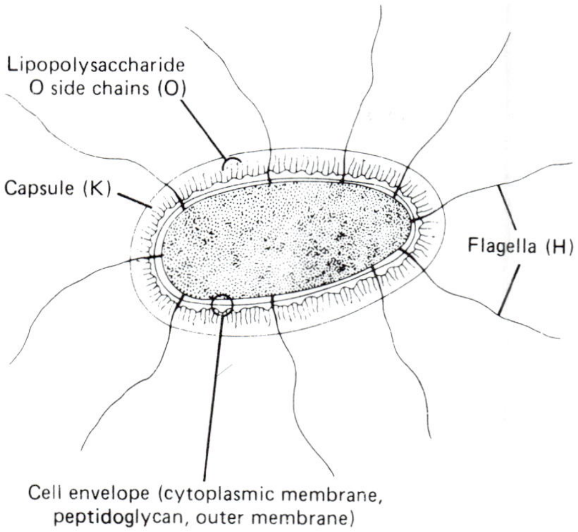

Figure 16–1. Antigenic structure of Enterobacteriaceae.

nella species. Occasionally, O antigens may be associated with specific human diseases, eg, specific O types of *E coli* are found in diarrhea and in urinary tract infections.

K antigens are external to O antigens on some but not all Enterobacteriaceae. Some are polysaccharides, including the K antigens of *E coli;* others are proteins. K antigens may interfere with agglutination by O antisera, and they may be associated with virulence (eg, *E coli* strains producing K1 antigen are prominent in neonatal meningitis, and K antigens of *E coli* cause attachment of the bacteria to epithelial cells prior to gastrointestinal or urinary tract invasion).

Klebsiellae form large capsules consisting of polysaccharides (K antigens) covering the somatic (O or H) antigens and can be identified by capsular swelling tests with specific antisera. Human infections of the respiratory tract are caused particularly by capsular types 1 and 2; those of the urinary tract, by types 8, 9, 10, and 24.

H antigens are located on flagella and are denatured or removed by heat or alcohol. They are preserved by treating motile bacterial variants with formalin. Such H antigens agglutinate with anti-H antibodies, mainly IgG. The determinants in H antigens are a function of the amino acid sequence in flagellar protein (flagellin). Within a single serotype, flagellar antigens may be present in either or both of two forms, called phase 1 (conventionally designated by lower-case letters) and phase 2 (conventionally designated by Arabic numerals). The organism tends to change from one phase to the other; this is called phase variation. H antigens on the bacterial surface may interfere with agglutination by anti-O antibody.

There are many examples of overlapping antigenic structures between Enterobacteriaceae and other bacteria. Most Enterobacteriaceae share the O14 antigen of *E coli.* The type 2 capsular polysaccharide of klebsiellae is very similar to the polysaccharide of type 2 pneumococci. Some K antigens cross-react with capsular polysaccharides of *Haemophilus influenzae* or *Neisseria meningitidis.* Thus, *E coli* O75:K100:H5 can induce antibodies that react with *H influenzae* type b.

The antigenic classification of Enterobacteriaceae often indicates the presence of each specific antigen. Thus, the antigenic formula of an *E coli* may be O55:K5:H21; that of *Salmonella schottmülleri* is O1,4,5,12:Hb:1,2.

Colicins (Bacteriocins)

Many gram-negative organisms produce bacteriocins. These virus-like bactericidal substances are produced by certain strains of bacteria active against some other strains of the same or closely related species. Their production is controlled by plasmids. Colicins are produced by *E coli,* marcescins by *Serratia,* and pyocins by *Pseudomonas.* Bacteriocin-producing strains are resistant to their own bacteriocin; thus, bacteriocins can be used for "typing" of organisms.

Toxins & Enzymes

Most gram-negative bacteria possess complex lipopolysaccharides in their cell walls. These substances, endotoxins, have a variety of pathophysiologic effects that are summarized in Chapter 9. Many gram-negative enteric bacteria also produce exotoxins of clinical importance. Some specific toxins are discussed in subsequent sections.

DISEASES CAUSED BY ENTEROBACTERIACEAE OTHER THAN *SALMONELLA* & *SHIGELLA*

Causative Organisms

E coli is a member of the normal intestinal flora (see Chapter 11). Other enteric bacteria (*Proteus, Enterobacter, Klebsiella, Morganella, Providencia, Citrobacter,* and *Serratia* species) are also found as members of the normal intestinal flora but are considerably less common than *E coli.* The enteric bacteria are sometimes found in small numbers as part of the normal flora of the upper respiratory and genital tracts. The enteric bacteria generally do not cause disease, and in the intestine they may even contribute to normal function and nutrition. When clinically important infections occur, they are usually caused by *E coli,* but the other enteric bacteria are causes of hospital-acquired infections and occasionally cause community-acquired infections. The bacteria become pathogenic only when they reach tissues outside of their normal intestinal or other less common normal flora sites. The most frequent sites of clinically important infection are the urinary tract, biliary tract, and other sites in the abdominal cavity, but any anatomic site (eg, bacteremia, prostate gland, lung, bone, meninges) can be the site of disease. Some of the enteric bacteria (eg, *Serratia marcescens, Enterobacter aerogenes*) are opportunistic pathogens. When normal host defenses are inadequate—particularly in infancy or old age, in the terminal stages of other diseases, after immunosuppression, or with indwelling venous or urethral catheters—localized clinically important infections can result, and the bacteria may reach the blood stream and cause sepsis.

Pathogenesis & Clinical Findings

The clinical manifestations of infections with *E coli* and the other enteric bacteria depend on the site of the infection and cannot be differentiated by symptoms or signs from processes caused by other bacteria.

A. *E coli*:

1. Urinary tract infection–*E coli* is the most common cause of urinary tract infection and accounts for approximately 90% of first urinary tract infections in young women (see Chapter 48). The symptoms and signs include urinary frequency, dysuria, hematuria, and pyuria. Flank pain is associated with upper tract infection. None of these symptoms or signs is specific for *E coli* infection. Urinary tract infection can result in bacteremia with clinical signs of sepsis.

Nephropathogenic *E coli* typically produce a hemolysin. Most of the infections are caused by *E coli* with a small number of O antigen types. K antigen appears to be important in the pathogenesis of upper tract infection. Pyelonephritis is associated with a specific type of pilus, P pilus, which binds to the P blood group substance.

2. *E coli*-associated diarrheal diseases–*E coli* that cause diarrhea are extremely common worldwide. These *E coli* are classified by the characteristics of their virulence properties (see below), and each group causes disease by a different mechanism. The small or large bowel epithelial cell adherence properties are encoded by genes on plasmids. Similarly, the toxins often are plasmid- or phage-mediated. Some clinical aspects of diarrheal diseases are discussed in Chapter 48.

Enteropathogenic *E coli* (EPEC) is an important cause of diarrhea in infants, especially in developing countries. EPEC previously was associated with outbreaks of diarrhea in nurseries in developed countries. EPEC adhere to the mucosal cells of the small bowel. Chromosomally mediated factors promote tight adherence. There is loss of microvilli (effacement), formation of filamentous actin pedestals or cup-like structures, and occasionally, entry of the EPEC into the mucosal cells. Characteristic lesions can be seen on electron micrographs of small bowel biopsy lesions. The result of EPEC infection is watery diarrhea, which is usually self-limited but can be chronic. EPEC diarrhea has been associated with multiple specific serotypes of *E coli;* strains are identified by O antigen and occasionally by H antigen typing. A two-stage infection model using HEp-2 cells also can be performed. Tests to identify EPEC are performed in reference laboratories. The duration of the EPEC diarrhea can be shortened and the chronic diarrhea cured by antibiotic treatment.

Enterotoxigenic *E coli* (ETEC) is a common cause of "traveler's diarrhea" and a very important cause of diarrhea in infants in developing countries. ETEC colonization factors specific for humans promote adherence of ETEC to epithelial cells of the small bowel. Some strains of ETEC produce a **heat-labile exotoxin** (LT)(MW 80,000) that is under the genetic control of a plasmid. Its subunit B attaches to the G_{M1} ganglioside at the brush border of epithelial cells of the small intestine and facilitates the entry of subunit A (MW 26,000) into the cell, where the latter activates adenylyl cyclase. This markedly increases the local concentration of cyclic adenosine monophosphate (cAMP), which results in intense and prolonged hypersecretion of water and chlorides and inhibits the reabsorption of sodium. The gut lumen is distended with fluid, and hypermotility and diarrhea ensue, lasting for several days. LT is antigenic and cross-reacts with the enterotoxin of *Vibrio cholerae.* LT stimulates the production of neutralizing antibodies in the serum (and perhaps on the gut surface) of persons previously infected with enterotoxigenic *E coli.* Persons residing in areas where such organisms are highly prevalent (eg, in some developing countries) are likely to possess antibodies and are less prone to develop diarrhea on reexposure to the LT-producing *E coli.* Assays for LT include the following: (1) fluid accumulation in the intestine of laboratory animals; (2) typical cytologic changes in cultured Chinese hamster ovary cells or other cell lines; (3) stimulation of steroid production in cultured adrenal tumor cells; and (4) binding and immunologic assays with standardized antisera to LT. These assays are done only in reference laboratories.

Some strains of ETEC produce the **heat-stable enterotoxin** ST_a (MW 1500–4000), which is under the genetic control of a heterogeneous group of plasmids. ST_a activates guanylyl cyclase in enteric epithelial cells and stimulates fluid secretion. A second heat-stable enterotoxin, ST_b, stimulates cyclic nucleotide-independent secretion with a short onset of action in vivo. Many ST_a-positive strains also produce LT. The strains with both toxins produce a more severe diarrhea.

The plasmids carrying the genes for enterotoxins (LT, ST) also may carry genes for the **colonization factors** that facilitate the attachment of *E coli* strains to intestinal epithelium. Recognized colonization factors occur with particular frequency in some serotypes. Certain serotypes of ETEC occur worldwide; others have a limited recognized distribution. It is possible that virtually any *E coli* may acquire a plasmid encoding for enterotoxins. There is no definite association of ETEC with the EPEC strains causing diarrhea in children. Likewise, there is no association between enterotoxigenic strains and those able to invade intestinal epithelial cells.

Care in the selection and consumption of foods potentially contaminated with ETEC is highly recommended to help prevent traveler's diarrhea. Antimicrobial prophylaxis can be effective but may result in increased antibiotic resistance in the bacteria and probably should not be uniformly recommended. Once diarrhea develops, antibiotic treatment effectively shortens the duration of disease.

Enterohemorrhagic *E coli* (EHEC) produce **verotoxin,** named for its cytotoxic effect on Vero cells, a line of African green monkey kidney cells. There are at least two antigenic forms of the toxin. EHEC has been associated with hemorrhagic colitis, a severe form of diarrhea, and with hemolytic uremic syndrome, a disease resulting in acute renal failure, microangiopathic hemolytic anemia, and thrombocytopenia. Verotoxin has many properties that are similar to the Shiga toxin produced by some strains of *Shigella dysenteriae* type 1; however, the two toxins are antigenically and genetically distinct. Of the *E coli* serotypes that produce verotoxin, O157:H7 is the most common and is the one that can be identified in clinical specimens. ETEC O157:H7 does not use sorbitol, unlike most other *E coli,* and is negative on sorbitol MacConkey agar (sorbitol is used instead of lactose; O157:H7 strains also are negative on MUG tests (see above). Specific antisera are used to identify the O157:H7 strains. Assays for verotoxin are done in reference laboratories. Many cases of hemorrhagic colitis and its associated complications can be prevented by thoroughly cooking ground beef.

Enteroinvasive *E coli* (EIEC) produce a disease very similar to shigellosis. The disease occurs most commonly in children in developing countries and in travelers to these countries. Like *Shigella,* EIEC strains are nonlactose or late lactose fermenters and are nonmotile. EIEC produce disease by invading intestinal mucosal epithelial cells.

Enteroaggregative *E coli* (EAEC) cause acute and chronic diarrhea in persons in developing countries. They are characterized by their characteristic pattern of adherence to human cells. Very little is known about EAEC virulence factors and the epidemiology of the disease they cause.

3. Sepsis–When normal host defenses are inadequate, *E coli* may reach the bloodstream and cause sepsis. Newborns may be highly susceptible to *E coli* sepsis because they lack IgM antibodies. Sepsis may occur secondary to urinary tract infection.

4. Meningitis–*E coli* and group B streptococci are the leading causes of meningitis in infants. Approximately 75% of *E coli* from meningitis cases have the K1 antigen. This antigen cross-reacts with the group B capsular polysaccharide of *N meningitidis.* The mechanism of virulence associated with the K1 antigen is not understood.

B. *Klebsiella-Enterobacter-Serratia; Proteus-Morganella-Providencia;* and *Citrobacter:* The pathogenesis of disease caused by these groups of enteric gram-negative rods is similar to that of the nonspecific factors in disease caused by *E coli.*

1. *Klebsiella*–*K pneumoniae* is present in the respiratory tract and feces of about 5% of normal individuals. It causes a small proportion (about 3%) of bacterial pneumonias. *K pneumoniae* can produce extensive hemorrhagic necrotizing consolidation of the lung. It occasionally produces urinary tract infection and bacteremia with focal lesions in debilitated patients. Other enterics also may produce pneumonia. *K pneumoniae* and *Klebsiella oxytoca* cause hospital-acquired infections. Two other klebsiellae are associated with inflammatory conditions of the upper respiratory tract: *Klebsiella ozaenae* has been isolated from the nasal mucosa in ozena, a fetid, progressive atrophy of mucous membranes; and *Klebsiella rhinoscleromatis* from rhinoscleroma, a destructive granuloma of the nose and pharynx.

2. *Enterobacter aerogenes*–This organism has small capsules, may be found free-living as well as in the intestinal tract, and causes urinary tract infections and sepsis.

3. *Serratia*–*S marcescens* is a common opportunistic pathogen in hospitalized patients. *Serratia* (usually nonpigmented) causes pneumonia, bacteremia, and endocarditis—especially in narcotics addicts and hospitalized patients. *S marcescens* is often multiply resistant to aminoglycosides and penicillins; infections can be treated with third-generation cephalosporins.

4. *Proteus*–*Proteus* species produce infections in humans only when the bacteria leave the intestinal tract. They are found in urinary tract infections and produce bacteremia, pneumonia, and focal lesions in debilitated patients or those receiving intravenous infusions. *P mirabilis* causes urinary tract infections and occasionally other infections. *Proteus vulgaris* and *Morganella morganii* are important nosocomial pathogens.

Proteus species produce urease, resulting in rapid hydrolysis of urea with liberation of ammonia. Thus, in urinary tract infections with *Proteus,* the urine becomes alkaline, promoting stone formation and making acidification virtually impossible. The rapid motility of *Proteus* may contribute to its invasion of the urinary tract.

Motile strains of *Proteus* contain H antigen in addition to the somatic O antigen. Certain strains share specific polysaccharides with some rickettsiae and are agglutinated by sera from patients with rickettsial diseases (the now obsolete Weil-Felix test).

Strains of *Proteus* vary greatly in antibiotic sensitivity. *P mirabilis* is often inhibited by penicillins; the most active antibiotics for other members of the group are aminoglycosides and cephalosporins.

5. *Providencia*–*Providencia* species (*Providencia rettgeri, Providencia alcalifaciens,* and *Providencia stuartii*) are members of the normal intestinal flora.

All cause urinary tract infections and occasionally other infections and are often resistant to antimicrobial therapy.

6. *Citrobacter*–*Citrobacter* can cause urinary tract infections and sepsis.

Diagnostic Laboratory Tests

A. Specimens: Urine, blood, pus, spinal fluid, sputum, or other material, as indicated by the localization of the disease process.

B. Smears: The Enterobacteriaceae resemble each other morphologically. The presence of large capsules is suggestive of *Klebsiella.*

C. Culture: Specimens are plated on both blood agar and differential media. With differential media, rapid preliminary identification of gram-negative enteric bacteria is often possible (see Chapter 47).

Immunity

Specific antibodies develop in systemic infections, but it is uncertain whether significant immunity to the organisms follows. Antibodies against the core glycolipid of Enterobacteriaceae are associated with protection against the hemodynamic sequelae of bacteremia caused by gram-negative rods and also reduce the fever response and augment intravascular clearance of certain organisms.

Treatment

No single specific therapy is available. The sulfonamides, ampicillin, cephalosporins, chloramphenicol, tetracyclines, and aminoglycosides have marked antibacterial effects against the enterics, but variation in susceptibility is great, and laboratory tests for antibiotic susceptibility are essential. Multiple drug resistance is common and is under the control of transmissible plasmids.

Certain conditions predisposing to infection by these organisms require surgical correction, eg, relief of urinary tract obstruction, closure of a perforation in an abdominal organ, or resection of a bronchiectatic portion of lung.

Treatment of gram-negative bacteremia and impending septic shock requires rapid institution of antimicrobial therapy, restoration of fluid and electrolyte balance, and treatment of disseminated intravascular coagulation.

Various means have been proposed for the prevention of traveler's diarrhea, including daily ingestion of bismuth subsalicylate suspension (bismuth subsalicylate can inactivate *E coli* enterotoxin in vitro) and regular doses of tetracyclines or other antimicrobial drugs for limited periods. Because none of these methods are entirely successful or lacking in adverse effects, it is widely recommended that caution be observed in regard to food and drink in areas where environmental sanitation is poor and that early and brief treatment (eg, with ciprofloxacin or trimethoprim-sulfamethoxazole) be substituted for prophylaxis.

Epidemiology, Prevention, & Control

The enteric bacteria establish themselves in the normal intestinal tract within a few days after birth and from then on constitute a main portion of the normal aerobic (facultative anaerobic) microbial flora. *E coli* is the prototype. Enterics found in water or milk are accepted as proof of fecal contamination from sewage or other sources.

Control measures are not feasible as far as the normal endogenous flora is concerned. Enteropathogenic *E coli* serotypes should be controlled like salmonellae (see below). Some of the enterics constitute a major problem in hospital infection. It is particularly important to recognize that many enteric bacteria are "opportunists" which cause illness when they are introduced into debilitated patients. Within hospitals or other institutions, these bacteria commonly are transmitted by personnel, instruments, or parenteral medications. Their control depends on hand washing, rigorous asepsis, sterilization of equipment, disinfection, restraint in intravenous therapy, and strict precautions in keeping the urinary tract sterile (ie, closed drainage).

THE SHIGELLAE

The natural habitat of shigellae is limited to the intestinal tracts of humans and other primates, where they produce bacillary dysentery.

Morphology & Identification

A. Typical Organisms: Shigellae are slender gram-negative rods; coccobacillary forms occur in young cultures.

B. Culture: Shigellae are facultative anaerobes but grow best aerobically. Convex, circular, transparent colonies with intact edges reach a diameter of about 2 mm in 24 hours.

C. Growth Characteristics: All shigellae ferment glucose. With the exception of *Shigella sonnei,* they do not ferment lactose. The inability to ferment lactose distinguishes shigellae on differential media. Shigellae form acid from carbohydrates but rarely produce gas. They may also be divided into those that ferment mannitol and those that do not (Table 16–3).

Table 16–3. Pathogenic species of *Shigella.*

Present Designation	Group and Type	Mannitol	Ornithine Decarboxylase
S dysenteriae	A	−	−
S flexneri	B	+	−
S boydii	C	+	−
S sonnei	D	+	+

Antigenic Structure

Shigellae have a complex antigenic pattern. There is great overlapping in the serologic behavior of different species, and most of them share O antigens with other enteric bacilli.

The somatic O antigens of shigellae are lipopolysaccharides. Their serologic specificity depends on the polysaccharide. There are more than 40 serotypes. The classification of shigellae relies on biochemical and antigenic characteristics. The pathogenic species are shown in Table 16–3.

Pathogenesis & Pathology

Shigella infections are almost always limited to the gastrointestinal tract; bloodstream invasion is quite rare. Shigellae are highly communicable; the infective dose is on the order of 10^3 organisms (whereas it usually is 10^5–10^8 for salmonellae and vibrios). The essential pathologic process is invasion of the mucosal epithelial cells (eg, M cells) by induced phagocytosis, escape from the phagocytic vacuole, multiplication and spread within the epithelial cell cytoplasm, and passage to adjacent cells. Microabscesses in the wall of the large intestine and terminal ileum lead to necrosis of the mucous membrane, superficial ulceration, bleeding, and formation of a "pseudomembrane" on the ulcerated area. This consists of fibrin, leukocytes, cell debris, a necrotic mucous membrane, and bacteria. As the process subsides, granulation tissue fills the ulcers and scar tissue forms.

Toxins

A. Endotoxin: Upon autolysis, all shigellae release their toxic lipopolysaccharide. This endotoxin probably contributes to the irritation of the bowel wall.

B. *Shigella dysenteriae* Exotoxin: *S dysenteriae* type 1 (Shiga bacillus) produces a heat-labile exotoxin that affects both the gut and the central nervous system. The exotoxin is a protein that is antigenic (stimulating production of antitoxin) and lethal for experimental animals. Acting as an enterotoxin, it produces diarrhea as does the *E coli* verotoxin, perhaps by the same mechanism. In humans, the exotoxin also inhibits sugar and amino acid absorption in the small intestine. Acting as a "neurotoxin," this material may contribute to the extreme severity and fatal nature of *S dysenteriae* infections and to the central nervous system reactions observed in them (ie, meningismus, coma). Patients with *Shigella flexneri* or *Shigella sonnei* infections develop antitoxin that neutralizes *S dysenteriae* exotoxin in vitro. The toxic activity is distinct from the invasive property of shigellae in dysentery. The two may act in sequence, the toxin producing an early nonbloody, voluminous diarrhea and the invasion of the large intestine resulting in later dysentery with blood and pus in stools.

Clinical Findings

After a short incubation period (1–2 days), there is a sudden onset of abdominal pain, fever, and watery diarrhea. The diarrhea has been attributed to an exotoxin acting in the small intestine (see above). A day or so later, as the infection involves the ileum and colon, the number of stools increase; they are less liquid but often contain mucus and blood. Each bowel movement is accompanied by straining and tenesmus (rectal spasms), with resulting lower abdominal pain. In more than half of adult cases, fever and diarrhea subside spontaneously in 2–5 days. However, in children and the elderly, loss of water and electrolytes may lead to dehydration, acidosis, and even death. The illness due to *S dysenteriae* may be particularly severe.

On recovery, most persons shed dysentery bacilli for only a short period, but a few remain chronic intestinal carriers and may have recurrent bouts of the disease. Upon recovery from the infection, most persons develop circulating antibodies to shigellae, but these do not protect against reinfection.

Diagnostic Laboratory Tests

A. Specimens: Fresh stool, mucus flecks, and rectal swabs for culture. Large numbers of fecal leukocytes and some red blood cells often are seen microscopically. Serum specimens, if desired, must be taken 10 days apart to demonstrate a rise in titer of agglutinating antibodies.

B. Culture: The materials are streaked on differential media (eg, MacConkey's or EMB agar) and on selective media (Hektoen enteric agar or *Salmonella-Shigella* agar), which suppress other Enterobacteriaceae and gram-positive organisms. Colorless (lactose-negative) colonies are inoculated into triple sugar iron agar (see p 206). Organisms that fail to produce H_2S, that produce acid but not gas in the butt and an alkaline slant in triple sugar iron agar medium, and that are nonmotile should be subjected to slide agglutination by specific *Shigella* antisera.

C. Serology: Normal persons often have agglutinins against several *Shigella* species. However, serial determinations of antibody titers may show a rise in specific antibody. Serology is not used to diagnose *Shigella* infections.

Immunity

Infection is followed by a type-specific antibody response. Injection of killed shigellae stimulates production of antibodies in serum but fails to protect humans against infection. IgA antibodies in the gut may be important in limiting reinfection; these may be stimulated by live attenuated strains given orally as experimental vaccines. Serum antibodies to somatic *Shigella* antigens are IgM.

Treatxment

Ciprofloxacin, ampicillin, tetracycline, trimethoprim-sulfamethoxazole, and chloramphenicol are most commonly inhibitory for *Shigella* isolates and can suppress acute clinical attacks of dysentery and shorten the duration of symptoms. They may fail to eradicate the organisms from the intestinal tract. Multiple drug resistance can be transmitted by plasmids, and resistant infections are widespread. Many cases are self-limited. Opioids should be avoided in *Shigella* dysentery. A potent specific antitoxin against *S dysenteriae* exotoxin is available, but convincing proof of its clinical efficacy is lacking.

Epidemiology, Prevention, & Control

Shigellae are transmitted by "food, fingers, feces, and flies" from person to person. Most cases of *Shigella* infection occur in children under 10 years of age. *S dysenteriae* can spread widely. (In 1969 in Guatemala, there were 110,000 cases, with 8000 deaths.) Mass chemoprophylaxis for limited periods of time (eg, in military personnel) has been tried, but resistant strains of shigellae tend to emerge rapidly. Since humans are the main recognized host of pathogenic shigellae, control efforts must be directed at eliminating the organisms from this reservoir by (1) sanitary control of water, food, and milk; sewage disposal; and fly control; (2) isolation of patients and disinfection of excreta; and (3) detection of subclinical cases and carriers, particularly food handlers.

THE *SALMONELLA-ARIZONA* GROUP

Salmonellae are often pathogenic for humans or animals when acquired by the oral route. They are transmitted from animals and animal products to humans, where they cause enteritis, systemic infection, and enteric fever.

Morphology & Identification

Salmonellae vary in length. Most species except *Salmonella pullorum-gallinarum* are motile with peritrichous flagella. Salmonellae grow readily on simple media, but they almost never ferment lactose or sucrose. They form acid and sometimes gas from glucose and mannose. They usually produce H_2S. They survive freezing in water for long periods. Salmonellae are resistant to certain chemicals (eg, brilliant green, sodium tetrathionate, sodium deoxycholate) that inhibit other enteric bacteria; such compounds are therefore useful for inclusion in media to isolate salmonellae from feces.

Antigenic Structure

While salmonellae are initially detected by their biochemical characteristics, groups and species are identified by antigenic analysis. Like other Enterobacteriaceae, salmonellae possess several O antigens (from a total of more than 100) and different H antigens in one or both of two phases. Some salmonellae have capsular (K) antigens, referred to as Vi, which may interfere with agglutination by O antisera and are associated with invasiveness. Agglutination tests with absorbed antisera for different O and H antigens form the basis for serologic classification of the salmonellae.

Classification

The classification of the *Salmonella-Arizona* group is complex because the organisms are a continuum rather than defined species. One classification system had three primary species, *Salmonella typhi* (one serotype), *Salmonella choleraesuis* (one serotype), and *Salmonella enteritidis* (more than 1500 serotypes). Serotyping is based on the reactivity of the O antigens and the biphasic H antigens. On the basis of DNA hybridization studies, the formal taxonomic classification includes the genus *Salmonella* with subspecies and the genus *Arizona* with subspecies. Almost all the salmonellae that cause disease in humans and can be isolated from warm-blooded animals are in the *Salmonella choleraesuis* group; the others are predominantly isolated from cold-blooded animals and the environment. In practice, the formal species and subspecies names are not used. The simplified nomenclature considers the named serotypes as species. Laboratory reports typically list a specific serogroup, eg, *Salmonella* species serogroup C1; a serogroup may have many serotypes. Reports from reference laboratories that serotype isolates include the serotype name, eg, *Salmonella,* and the serotype, eg, *typhimurium,* which is shortened to *S typhimurium* (as if it were a genus-species designation).

Salmonellae that can and should be identified routinely because of their clinical significance include the following: *S typhi, S choleraesuis, S paratyphi* A, and *S paratyphi* B. These salmonellae can be identified by biochemical tests and serogrouping, with follow-up serotyping confirmation. Table 16–4 lists examples of a few named salmonellae and their antigenic formulas.

Variation

Organisms may lose H antigens and become nonmotile. Loss of O antigen is associated with a change from smooth to rough colony form. Vi antigen may be lost partially or completely. Antigens may be acquired (or lost) in the process of transduction.

Pathogenesis & Clinical Findings

S typhi, S choleraesuis, and perhaps *S paratyphi A* and *S paratyphi* B are primarily infective for humans,

Table 16–4. Representative antigenic formulas of salmonellae.

O Group	Serotype	Antigenic Formula[1]
D	*S typhi*	**9, 12** (Vi):d:—
A	*S paratyphi A*	**1, 2, 12**:a—
C_1	*S choleraesuis*	**6, 7**:c:1,5
B	*S typhimurium*	**1, 4, 5, 12**:i:1, 2
D	*S enteritidis*	**1, 9, 12**:g, m:—

[1]O antigens: boldface numerals.
(Vi): Vi antigen if present.
Phase 1 H antigen: lower-case letter.
Phase 2 H antigen: numeral.

and infection with these organisms implies acquisition from a human source. The vast majority of salmonellae, however, are chiefly pathogenic in animals that constitute the reservoir for human infection: poultry, pigs, rodents, cattle, pets (from turtles to parrots), and many others.

The organisms almost always enter via the oral route, usually with contaminated food or drink. The mean infective dose to produce clinical or subclinical infection in humans is 10^5–10^8 salmonellae (but perhaps as few as 10^3 *S typhi* organisms). Among the host factors that contribute to resistance to *Salmonella* infection are gastric acidity, normal intestinal microbial flora, and local intestinal immunity (see below).

Salmonellae produce three main types of disease in humans, but mixed forms are frequent (Table 16–5).

A. The "Enteric Fevers" (Typhoid Fever): This syndrome is produced by only a few of the salmonellae, of which *S typhi* (typhoid fever) is the most important. The ingested salmonellae reach the small intestine, from which they enter the lymphatics and then the bloodstream. They are carried by the blood to many organs, including the intestine. The organisms multiply in intestinal lymphoid tissue and are excreted in stools.

After an incubation period of 10–14 days, fever, malaise, headache, constipation, bradycardia, and myalgia occur. The fever rises to a high plateau, and the spleen and liver become enlarged. Rose spots, usually on the skin of the abdomen or chest, are seen briefly in rare cases. The white blood cell count is normal or low. In the preantibiotic era, the chief complications of enteric fever were intestinal hemorrhage and perforation, and the mortality rate was 10–15%. Treatment with antibiotics has reduced the mortality rate to less than 1%.

The principal lesions are hyperplasia and necrosis of lymphoid tissue (eg, Peyer's patches), hepatitis, focal necrosis of the liver, and inflammation of the gallbladder, periosteum, lungs, and other organs.

B. Bacteremia With Focal Lesions: This is associated commonly with *S choleraesuis* but may be caused by any *Salmonella* serotype. Following oral infection, there is early invasion of the bloodstream (with possible focal lesions in lungs, bones, meninges, etc), but intestinal manifestations are often absent. Blood cultures are positive.

C. Enterocolitis (Formerly "Gastroenteritis"): This is the most common manifestation of *Salmonella* infection. In the USA, *S typhimurium* is prominent, but enterocolitis can be caused by any of the 1500–2000 types of salmonellae. Eight to 48 hours after ingestion of salmonellae, there is nausea, headache, vomiting, and profuse diarrhea, with few leukocytes in the stools. Low-grade fever is common, but the episode usually resolves in 2–3 days.

Inflammatory lesions of the small and large intestine are present. Bacteremia is rare (2–4%) except in immunodeficient persons. Blood cultures are usually negative, but stool cultures are positive for salmonellae and may remain positive for several weeks after clinical recovery.

Diagnostic Laboratory Tests

A. Specimens: Blood for culture must be taken repeatedly. In enteric fevers and septicemias, blood cultures are often positive in the first week of the disease. Bone marrow cultures may be useful. Urine cultures may be positive after the second week.

Stool specimens also must be taken repeatedly. In enteric fevers, the stools yield positive results from the second or third week on; in enterocolitis, during the first week.

A positive culture of duodenal drainage establishes the presence of salmonellae in the biliary tract in carriers.

B. Bacteriologic Methods for Isolation of Salmonellae:

1. Differential medium cultures–EMB, MacConkey's, or deoxycholate medium permits rapid detection of lactose nonfermenters (not only salmonellae and shigellae but also *Proteus, Serratia, Pseudomonas,* etc). Gram-positive organisms are somewhat inhibited. Bismuth sulfite medium permits rapid detection of *S typhi,* which forms black colonies

Table 16–5. Clinical diseases induced by salmonellae.

	Enteric Fevers	Septicemias	Enterocolitis
Incubation period	7–20 days	Variable	8–48 hours
Onset	Insidious	Abrupt	Abrupt
Fever	Gradual, then high plateau, with "typhoidal" state	Rapid rise, then spiking "septic" temperature	Usually low
Duration of disease	Several weeks	Variable	2–5 days
Gastrointestinal symptoms	Often early constipation; later, bloody diarrhea	Often none	Nausea, vomiting, diarrhea at onset
Blood cultures	Positive in 1st–2nd weeks of disease	Positive during high fever	Negative
Stool cultures	Positive from 2nd week on; negative earlier in disease	Infrequently positive	Positive soon after onset

because of H_2S production. Many salmonellae produce H_2S.

2. Selective medium cultures–The specimen is plated on *Salmonella-Shigella* (SS) agar, Hektoen enteric agar, or deoxycholate-citrate agar, which favor growth of salmonellae and shigellae over other Enterobacteriaceae.

3. Enrichment cultures–The specimen (usually stool) also is put into selenite F or tetrathionate broth, both of which inhibit replication of normal intestinal bacteria and permit multiplication of salmonellae. After incubation for 1–2 days, this is plated on differential and selective media.

4. Final identification–Suspect colonies from solid media are identified by biochemical reaction patterns (Table 16–1) and slide agglutination tests with specific sera.

C. Serologic Methods: Serologic techniques are used to identify unknown cultures with known sera (see below) and may also be used to determine antibody titers in patients with unknown illness, although the latter is not very useful in diagnosis of *Salmonella* infections.

1. Rapid slide agglutination test–In this test, known sera and unknown culture are mixed on a slide. Clumping, when it occurs, can be observed within a few minutes. This test is particularly useful for rapid preliminary identification of cultures.

2. Tube dilution agglutination test (Widal test)–Serum agglutinins rise sharply during the second and third weeks of *Salmonella* infection. At least two serum specimens, obtained at intervals of 7–10 days, are needed to prove a rise in antibody titer. Serial (twofold) dilutions of unknown serum are tested against antigens from representative salmonellae. The results are interpreted as follows: (1) High or rising titer of O ($\geq$1:160) suggests that active infection is present. (2) High titer of H ($\geq$1:160) suggests past immunization or past infection. (3) High titer of antibody to the Vi antigen occurs in some carriers. Results of serologic tests for *Salmonella* infection must be interpreted cautiously. The possible presence of cross-reactive antibodies limits the use of serology in the diagnosis of *Salmonella* infections.

Immunity

Infections with *S typhi* or *S paratyphi* usually confer a certain degree of immunity. Reinfection may occur but is often milder than the first infection. Circulating antibodies to O and Vi are related to resistance to infection and disease. However, relapses may occur in 2–3 weeks after recovery in spite of antibodies. Secretory IgA antibodies may prevent attachment of salmonellae to intestinal epithelium.

Persons with S/S hemoglobin (sickle cell disease) are exceedingly susceptible to *Salmonella* infections, particularly osteomyelitis. Persons with A/S hemoglobin (sickle cell trait) may be more susceptible than normal individuals (those with A/A hemoglobin).

Treatment

While enteric fevers and bacteremias with focal lesions require antimicrobial treatment, the vast majority of cases of enterocolitis do not. Antimicrobial treatment of *Salmonella* enteritis in neonates is important. In enterocolitis, clinical symptoms and excretion of the salmonellae may be prolonged by antimicrobial therapy. In severe diarrhea, replacement of fluids and electrolytes is essential.

Antimicrobial therapy of invasive *Salmonella* infections is with ampicillin, trimethoprim-sulfamethoxazole, a third-generation cephalosporin, or chloramphenicol. Multiple drug resistance transmitted genetically by plasmids among enteric bacteria is a problem in *Salmonella* infections. Susceptibility testing is an important adjunct to selecting a proper antibiotic.

In most carriers, the organisms persist in the gallbladder (particularly if gallstones are present) and in the biliary tract. Some chronic carriers have been cured by ampicillin alone, but in most cases cholecystectomy must be combined with drug treatment.

Epidemiology

The feces of persons who have unsuspected subclinical disease or are carriers are a more important source of contamination than frank clinical cases that are promptly isolated, eg, when carriers working as food handlers are "shedding" organisms. Many animals, including cattle, rodents, and fowl, are naturally infected with a variety of salmonellae and have the bacteria in their tissues (meat), excreta, or eggs. The high incidence of salmonellae in commercially prepared chickens has been widely publicized. The incidence of typhoid fever has decreased, but the incidence of other *Salmonella* infections has increased markedly in the USA. The problem probably is aggravated by the widespread use of animal feeds containing antimicrobial drugs that favor the proliferation of drug-resistant salmonellae and their potential transmission to humans.

A. Carriers: After manifest or subclinical infection, some individuals continue to harbor salmonellae in their tissues for variable lengths of time (convalescent carriers or healthy permanent carriers). Three percent of survivors of typhoid become permanent carriers, harboring the organisms in the gallbladder, biliary tract, or, rarely, the intestine or urinary tract.

B. Sources of Infection: The sources of infection are food and drink that have been contaminated with salmonellae. The following sources are important:

1. Water–Contamination with feces often results in explosive epidemics.

2. Milk and other dairy products (ice cream, cheese, custard)–Contamination with feces and inadequate pasteurization or improper handling. Some outbreaks are traceable to the source of supply.

3. Shellfish–From contaminated water.

4. Dried or frozen eggs–From infected fowl or contaminated during processing.

5. Meats and meat products–From infected animals (poultry) or contamination with feces by rodents or humans.

6. "Recreational" drugs–Marihuana and other drugs.

7. Animal dyes–Dyes (eg, carmine) used in drugs, foods, and cosmetics.

8. Household pets–Turtles, dogs, cats, etc.

Prevention & Control

Sanitary measures must be taken to prevent contamination of food and water by rodents or other animals that excrete salmonellae. Infected poultry, meats, and eggs must be thoroughly cooked. Carriers must not be allowed to work as food handlers and should observe strict hygienic precautions.

Two injections of acetone-killed bacterial suspensions of *S typhi,* followed by a booster injection some months later, give partial resistance to small infectious inocula of typhoid bacilli but not to large ones. Oral administration of a live avirulent mutant strain of *S typhi* has given significant protection in areas of high endemicity. Vaccines against other salmonellae give less protection and are not recommended.

REFERENCES

Enterobacteriaceae

Ewing WH: *Edwards and Ewing's Identification of Enterobacteriaceae,* 4th ed. Elsevier, 1986.

Farmer JJ III et al: Biochemical identification of new species and biogroups of Enterobacteriaceae isolated from clinical specimens. J Clin Microbiol 1985;21:46.

Lipsky BA et al: *Citrobacter* infections in humans: Experience at the Seattle Veterans Administration Medical Center and a review of the literature. Rev Infect Dis 1980;2:746.

Meyer KS et al: Nosocomial outbreak of *Klebsiella* infection resistant to late-generation cephalosporins. Ann Intern Med 1993;119:353.

Saito H et al: *Serratia* bacteremia: Review of 118 cases. Rev Infect Dis 1989;11:912.

Yu VL: *Serratia marcescens:* Historical perspective and clinical review. N Engl J Med 1979;300:887.

Diarrheal Diseases

Banwell JG: Pathophysiology of diarrheal disorders. Rev Infect Dis 1990;12:S30.

Black RE: Epidemiology of traveler's diarrhea and relative importance of various pathogens. Rev Infect Dis 1990;12:S73.

Guerrant RL, Bobak DA: Bacterial and protozoal gastroenteritis. New Engl J Med 1991;325:327.

Guerrant RL et al: Diarrhea in developed and developing countries: Magnitude, special settings, and etiologies. Rev Infect Dis 1990;12:S41.

E coli

Donnenberg M, Kaper J: Minireview: Enteropathogenic *E coli.* Infect Immun 1992;60:3953.

Graham DY, Evans DG: Prevention of diarrhea caused by enterotoxigenic *Escherichia coli.* Rev Infect Dis 1990;12:S68.

Jann K, Jann B: The K antigens of *Escherichia coli.* Prog Allergy 1983;33:53.

Johnson JR: Virulence factors in *Escherichia coli* urinary tract infection. Clin Microbiol Rev 1991;4:80.

Karmali MA: Infection by verocytotoxin-producing *Escherichia coli.* Clin Microbiol Rev 1989;2:15.

Klemm P: Fimbrial adhesions of *Escherichia coli.* Rev Infect Dis 1985;7:321.

Levine MM: *Escherichia coli* that cause diarrhea: Enterotoxigenic, enteropathogenic, enteroinvasive, enterohemorrhagic, and enteroadherent. J Infect Dis 1987;155:377.

Nataro JP et al: Characterization of plasmids encoding the adherence factor of enteropathogenic *Escherichia coli.* Infect Immun 1987;55:2370.

Robins-Browne RM: Traditional enteropathogenic *Escherichia coli* of infantile diarrhea. Rev Infect Dis 1987;9:28.

Shigella

Bartlett AV III et al: Production of Shiga toxin and other cytotoxins by serogroups of *Shigella.* J Infect Dis 1986;154:996.

Blaser MJ, Pollard RA, Feldman RA: *Shigella* infections in the United States, 1974–1980. J Infect Dis 1983;147:771.

Goldberg MB, Sansonetti PJ: Minireview: *Shigella* subversion of the cellular cytoskeleton: A strategy for epithelial cell colonization. Infect Immun 1993;61:4941.

Lee LA et al: Hyperendemic shigellosis in the United States: A review of surveillance data for 1967–1988. J Infect Dis 1991;164:894.

O'Brien AD, Holmes RK: Shiga and Shiga-like toxins. Microbiol Rev 1987;51:206.

Salmonella

Blaser MJ, Newman LS: A review of human salmonellosis: 1. Infective dose. Rev Infect Dis 1982;4:1096.

Buchwald DS, Blaser MJ: A review of human salmonellosis: 2. Duration of excretion following infection with nontyphi *Salmonella.* Rev Infect Dis 1984;6:345.

Butler T et al: Patterns of morbidity and mortality in typhoid fever dependent on age and gender: Review of 552 hospitalized patients with diarrhea. Rev Infect Dis 1991;13:85.

Chalker RB, Blaser MJ: A review of human salmonellosis: 3. Magnitude of *Salmonella* infection in the United States. Rev Infect Dis 1988;10:111.

Edelman R, Levine MM: Summary of an international workshop on typhoid fever. Rev Infect Dis 1986;8:329.

Hornick RB et al: Typhoid fever: Pathogenesis and immunologic control. (Two parts.) N Engl J Med 1970;283:686, 739.

17 Pseudomonads, Acinetobacters, & Uncommon Gram-Negative Bacteria

The *Pseudomonas* and *Acinetobacter* species are widely distributed in soil and water. *Pseudomonas aeruginosa* sometimes colonizes humans and is the major human pathogen of the group. *P aeruginosa* is invasive and toxigenic, produces infections in patients with abnormal host defenses, and is an important nosocomial pathogen.

Gram-negative bacteria that rarely cause disease in humans are included in this chapter. Some of these bacteria (eg, chromobacteria and flavobacteria) are found in soil or water and are opportunistic pathogens for humans. Other gram-negative bacteria (eg, *Capnocytophaga, Eikenella corrodens, Kingella,* and *Moraxella*) are normal flora of humans and occur in a wide variety of infections; often they are unexpected causes of disease.

THE PSEUDOMONAS GROUP

The *Pseudomonas* group are gram-negative, motile, aerobic rods some of which produce water-soluble pigments. Pseudomonads occur widely in soil, water, plants, and animals. *P aeruginosa* is frequently present in small numbers in the normal intestinal flora and on the skin of humans and is the major pathogen of the group. Other *Pseudomonas* species infrequently cause disease. The classification of pseudomonads is based on rRNA/DNA homology and common culture characteristics. The medically important pseudomonads are listed in Table 17-1.

1. *PSEUDOMONAS AERUGINOSA*

P aeruginosa is widely distributed in nature and is commonly present in moist environments in hospitals. It can colonize normal humans, in whom it is a saprophyte. It causes disease in humans with abnormal host defenses.

Morphology & Identification

A. Typical Organisms: *P aeruginosa* is motile and rod-shaped, measuring about 0.6 × 2 μm. It is gram-negative and occurs as single bacteria, in pairs, and occasionally in short chains.

B. Culture: *P aeruginosa* is an obligate aerobe that grows readily on many types of culture media, sometimes producing a sweet or grape-like odor. Some strains hemolyze blood. *P aeruginosa* forms smooth round colonies with a fluorescent greenish color. It often produces the nonfluorescent bluish pigment **pyocyanin,** which diffuses into the agar. Other *Pseudomonas* species do not produce pyocyanin. Many strains of *P aeruginosa* also produce the fluorescent pigment **pyoverdin,** which gives a greenish color to the agar. Some strains produce the dark red pigment **pyorubin** or the black pigment **pyomelanin.**

P aeruginosa in a culture can produce multiple colony types, giving the impression of a culture of mixed species of bacteria. *P aeruginosa* from different colony types may also have different biochemical and enzymatic activities and different antimicrobial susceptibility patterns. Cultures from patients with cystic fibrosis often yield *P aeruginosa* organisms that form very mucoid colonies as a result of overproduction of alginate, an exopolysaccharide.

C. Growth Characteristics: *P aeruginosa* grows well at 37–42 °C; its growth at 42 °C helps differentiate it from other *Pseudomonas* species. It is **oxidase-positive.** It does not ferment carbohydrates, but many strains oxidize glucose. Identification is usually based on colonial morphology, oxidase positivity, the presence of characteristic pigments, and growth at 42 °C. Differentiation of *P aeruginosa* from other pseudomonads on the basis of biochemical activity requires testing with a large battery of substrates.

Antigenic Structure & Toxins

Pili (fimbriae) extend from the cell surface and promote attachment to host epithelial cells. Polysaccharide capsules are responsible for the mucoid colonies seen in cultures from patients with cystic fibrosis. The lipopolysaccharide, which exists in multiple immunotypes, is responsible for many of the endotoxic properties of the organism. *P aeruginosa* can be typed by lipopolysaccharide immunotype and by pyocin (bacteriocin) susceptibility. Most *P aeruginosa* isolates from clinical infections produce extracellular enzymes, including elastases, proteases, and two hemolysins: a heat-labile phospholipase C and a heat-stable glycolipid.

Table 17–1. Classification of pseudomonads that cause disease in humans.

rRNA Homology Group and Subgroup	Genus and Species
I. Fluorescent group	*Pseudomonas aeruginosa* *Pseudomonas fluorescens* *Pseudomonas putida*
Nonfluorescent group	*Pseudomonas stutzeri* *Pseudomonas mendocina* *Pseudomonas alcaligenes* *Pseudomonas pseudoalcaligenes*
II	*Pseudomonas pseudomallei* *Pseudomonas mallei* *Pseudomonas cepacia* *Pseudomonas picketti*
III and IV	Multiple species infrequently isolated from humans
V	*Xanthomonas maltophilia*

Many strains of *P aeruginosa* produce exotoxin A, which causes tissue necrosis and is lethal for animals when injected in purified form. The toxin blocks protein synthesis by a mechanism of action identical to that of diphtheria toxin, though the structures of the two toxins are not identical. Antitoxins to exotoxin A are found in some human sera, including those of patients who have recovered from serious *P aeruginosa* infections.

Pathogenesis

P aeruginosa is pathogenic only when introduced into areas devoid of normal defenses, eg, when mucous membranes and skin are disrupted by direct tissue damage; when intravenous or urinary catheters are used; or when neutropenia is present, as in cancer chemotherapy. The bacterium attaches to and colonizes the mucous membranes or skin, invades locally, and produces systemic disease. These processes are promoted by the pili, enzymes, and toxins described above. Lipopolysaccharide plays a direct role in causing fever, shock, oliguria, leukocytosis and leukopenia, disseminated intravascular coagulation, and adult respiratory distress syndrome.

P aeruginosa (and other species, eg, *Pseudomonas cepacia, Pseudomonas putida*) is resistant to many antimicrobial agents and therefore becomes dominant and important when more susceptible bacteria of the normal flora are suppressed.

Clinical Findings

P aeruginosa produces infection of wounds and burns, giving rise to blue-green pus; meningitis, when introduced by lumbar puncture; and urinary tract infection, when introduced by catheters and instruments or in irrigating solutions. Involvement of the respiratory tract, especially from contaminated respirators, results in necrotizing pneumonia. The bacterium is often found in mild otitis externa in swimmers. It may cause invasive (malignant) otitis externa in diabetic patients. Infection of the eye, which may lead to rapid destruction of the eye, occurs most commonly after injury or surgical procedures. In infants or debilitated persons, *P aeruginosa* may invade the bloodstream and result in fatal sepsis; this occurs commonly in patients with leukemia or lymphoma who have received antineoplastic drugs or radiation therapy and in patients with severe burns. In most *P aeruginosa* infections, the symptoms and signs are nonspecific and are related to the organ involved. Occasionally, verdoglobin (a breakdown product of hemoglobin) or fluorescent pigment can be detected in wounds, burns, or urine by ultraviolet fluorescence. Hemorrhagic necrosis of skin occurs often in sepsis due to *P aeruginosa;* the lesions, called **ecthyma gangrenosum,** are surrounded by erythema and often do not contain pus. *P aeruginosa* can be seen on Gram-stained specimens from ecthyma lesions, and cultures are positive. Ecthyma gangrenosum is uncommon in bacteremia due to organisms other than *P aeruginosa*.

Diagnostic Laboratory Tests

A. Specimens: Specimens from skin lesions, pus, urine, blood, spinal fluid, sputum, and other material should be obtained as indicated by the type of infection.

B. Smears: Gram-negative rods are often seen in smears. There are no specific morphologic characteristics that differentiate pseudomonads in specimens from enteric or other gram-negative rods.

C. Culture: Specimens are plated on blood agar and the differential media commonly used to grow the enteric gram-negative rods. Pseudomonads grow readily on most of these media, but they may grow more slowly than the enterics. *P aeruginosa* does not ferment lactose and is easily differentiated from the lactose-fermenting bacteria. Culture is the specific test for diagnosis of *P aeruginosa* infection.

Treatment

Clinically significant infections with *P aeruginosa* should not be treated with single-drug therapy, because the success rate is low with such therapy and because the bacteria can rapidly develop resistance when single drugs are employed. A penicillin active against *P aeruginosa*—ticarcillin, mezlocillin, and piperacillin—is used in combination with an aminoglycoside, usually gentamicin, tobramycin, or amikacin. Other drugs active against *P aeruginosa* include aztreonam, imipenem, and the newer quinolones, including ciprofloxacin. Of the newer cephalosporins, ceftazidime and cefoperazone are active against *P aeruginosa;* ceftazidime is used in primary therapy of *P aeruginosa* infections. The susceptibility patterns of *P aeruginosa* vary geographically, and susceptibility tests should be done as an adjunct to selection of antimicrobial therapy.

Epidemiology & Control

P aeruginosa is primarily a nosocomial pathogen, and the methods for control of infection are similar to those for other nosocomial pathogens. Since *Pseudomonas* thrives in moist environments, special attention should be paid to sinks, water baths, showers, hot tubs, and other wet areas. For epidemiologic purposes, strains can be typed by pyocins and by lipopolysaccharide immunotypes. Vaccine from appropriate types administered to high-risk patients provides some protection against *Pseudomonas* sepsis. Such treatment has been used experimentally in patients with leukemia, burns, cystic fibrosis, and immunosuppression.

2. *PSEUDOMONAS PSEUDOMALLEI*

P pseudomallei is a small, motile, aerobic, gram-negative bacillus. It grows well on standard bacteriologic media, forming colonies that vary from mucoid and smooth to rough and wrinkled (may take 72 hours) and in color from cream to orange. It grows at 42 °C and oxidizes glucose, lactose, and a variety of other carbohydrates. *P pseudomallei* causes **melioidosis,** an endemic glanders-like disease of animals and humans, primarily in Southeast Asia and Northern Australia. The organism is a natural saprophyte that has been cultured from soil, fresh water, rice paddies, and vegetable produce. Human infection probably originates from these sources by contamination of skin abrasions and possibly by ingestion or inhalation. Epizootic *P pseudomallei* infection occurs in sheep, goats, swine, horses, and other animals, though animals do not appear to be a primary reservoir for the organism.

Melioidosis may manifest itself as acute, subacute, or chronic infection. The incubation period can be as short as 2–3 days, but latent periods of months to years also occur. A localized suppurative infection can occur at the inoculation site where there is a break in the skin. This localized infection may lead to the acute septicemic form of infection with involvement of many organs. The signs and symptoms depend upon the major sites of involvement. The most common form of melioidosis is pulmonary infection, which may be a primary pneumonitis (*P pseudomallei* transmitted through the upper airway or nasopharynx) or subsequent to a localized suppurative infection and bacteremia. The patient may have fever and leukocytosis, with consolidation of the upper lobes. Subsequently, the patient may become afebrile, while upper lobe cavities develop, yielding an appearance similar to that of tuberculosis on chest x-ray films. Some patients develop chronic suppurative infection with abscesses in skin, brain, lung, myocardium, liver, bone, and other sites. Patients with chronic suppurative infections may be afebrile and have indolent disease. Latent infection is sometimes reactivated as a result of immunosuppression.

The diagnosis of melioidosis should be considered for a patient from an endemic area who has fulminant upper lobe pulmonary or unexplained systemic disease. A Gram stain of an appropriate specimen will show small gram-negative bacilli; bipolar staining (safety pin appearance) is seen with Wright's or methylene blue stains. A positive culture is diagnostic. A positive serologic test is diagnostically helpful and constitutes evidence of past infection.

Melioidosis has a high mortality rate if untreated. Surgical drainage of localized infection may be necessary. Antibiotic susceptibility testing is an important guide for treatment. *P pseudomallei* usually is susceptible to a variety of antibiotics, including tetracycline, sulfonamides, trimethoprim-sulfamethoxazole, chloramphenicol, amoxicillin or ticarcillin with clavulanic acid, piperacillin, imipenem, and third-generation cephalosporins. Patients with severe infections should be treated parenterally (eg, trimethoprim-sulfamethoxazole or a third-generation cephalosporin such as ceftazidime); combination therapy may be beneficial. Oral therapy for less severely ill patients can be with a tetracycline, trimethoprim-sulfamethoxazole, or chloramphenicol, often in combination. The duration of antimicrobial therapy should be at least 8 weeks; therapy for 6 months to 1 year should be considered for patients with extrapulmonary suppurative lesions. Relapses in melioidosis are common, and the optimal choice and duration of antibiotic therapy to prevent relapse have not been determined. There is no vaccine or specific preventive measures.

3. *PSEUDOMONAS MALLEI*

P mallei is a small, nonmotile, nonpigmented, aerobic, gram-negative rod that grows readily on most bacteriologic media. It causes **glanders,** a disease of horses, mules, and donkeys transmissible to humans. In horses, the disease has prominent pulmonary involvement, subcutaneous ulcerative lesions, and lymphatic thickening with nodules; systemic disease also occurs. Human infection, which can be fatal, usually begins as an ulcer of the skin or mucous membranes followed by lymphangitis and sepsis. Inhalation of the organisms may lead to primary pneumonia.

The diagnosis is based on rising agglutinin titers and culture of the organism from local lesions of humans or horses. Human cases can be treated effectively with a tetracycline plus an aminoglycoside.

The disease has been controlled by slaughter of infected horses and mules and at present is extremely rare. In some countries, laboratory infections are the only source of the disease.

4. OTHER PSEUDOMONADS

Some of the many *Pseudomonas* species are listed in Table 17–1; occasionally these pseudomonads are opportunistic pathogens. *Pseudomonas cepacia* is sometimes cultured from patients with cystic fibrosis. The diagnosis of infections caused by these pseudomonads is made by culturing the bacteria and identifying them by differential reactions on a complex set of biochemical substrates. Many of these pseudomonads have antimicrobial susceptibility patterns different from that of *P aeruginosa*.

5. *XANTHOMONAS MALTOPHILIA*

Xanthomonas maltophilia is the most widely accepted name for the organism previously called *Pseudomonas maltophilia. X maltophilia* is a free-living gram-negative rod that is widespread in the environment. On blood agar, colonies have a lavender-green or gray color. The organism is oxidase-negative and lysine decarboxylase-positive. *X maltophilia* generally does not produce the pigments and enzymes that are produced by *P aeruginosa* and which are associated with the virulence of *P aeruginosa.*

X maltophilia is an increasingly important cause of hospital-acquired infections in patients who are receiving antimicrobial therapy and in immunocompromised patients. It has been isolated from many anatomic sites including respiratory tract secretions, urine, skin wounds, and blood. The isolates are often part of mixed flora present in the specimens. When blood cultures are positive it is commonly in association with use of indwelling plastic intravenous catheters.

X maltophilia is usually susceptible to sulfamethoxazole-trimethoprim and resistant to other commonly used antimicrobials including cephalosporins, antipseudomonal penicillins, aminoglycosides, imipenem, and the quinolones. The widespread use of the drugs to which *X maltophilia* is resistant plays an important role in the increased frequency in which it causes disease.

ACINETOBACTER

Acinetobacter species are aerobic gram-negative bacteria that are widely distributed in soil and water and can occasionally be cultured from skin, mucous membranes, and secretions.

Acinetobacter baumannii was previously known as *Acinetobacter calcoaceticus* var *anitratus. Acinetobacter johnsonii* was previously known as *Acinitobacter calcoaceticus* var *lwoffii.* Other species include *Acinetobacter calcoaceticus, Acinetobacter haemolyticus, Acinetobacter junii,* and *Acinetobacter lwoffii.* Some isolates have not received species names. Acinetobacters were previously called by a number of different names, including *Mima polymorpha* and *Herellea vaginicola. A baumannii* is the most common species isolated.

Acinetobacters are usually coccobacillary or coccal in appearance; they resemble neisseriae on smears, because diplococcal forms predominate in body fluids and on solid media. Rod-shaped forms also occur, and occasionally the bacteria appear to be gram-positive. *Acinetobacter* grows well on most types of media used to culture specimens from patients. *Acinetobacter* recovered from meningitis and sepsis has been mistaken for *Neisseria meningitidis;* similarly, *Acinetobacter* recovered from the female genital tract has been mistaken for *Neisseria gonorrhoeae.* However, the neisseriae produce oxidase and *Acinetobacter* does not.

Acinetobacters often are commensals but occasionally cause nosocomial infection. *A baumannii* has been isolated from blood, sputum, skin, pleural fluid, and urine, usually in device-associated infections. *A johnsonii* is a nosocomial pathogen of low virulence and has been found in blood cultures of patients with plastic intravenous catheters. *Acinetobacter* encountered in nosocomial pneumonia often originates in the water of room humidifiers or vaporizers. In patients with *Acinetobacter* bacteremia, intravenous catheters are almost always the source of infection. In patients with burns or with immune deficiencies, *Acinetobacter* acts as an opportunistic pathogen and can produce sepsis. *Acinetobacter* strains are often resistant to antimicrobial agents, and therapy of infection can be difficult. Susceptibility testing should be done to help select the best antimicrobial drugs for therapy. *Acinetobacter* strains respond most commonly to gentamicin, amikacin, or tobramycin and to newer penicillins or cephalosporins.

UNCOMMON GRAM-NEGATIVE BACTERIA

Actinobacillus

Actinobacillus (Haemophilus) actinomycetemcomitans is a small, gram-negative, coccobacillary organism that grows slowly. As its name implies, it is often found in actinomycosis. It also causes severe periodontal disease in adolescents, endocarditis, abscesses, osteomyelitis, and other infections. It is treatable with tetracycline or chloramphenicol and sometimes with penicillin G, ampicillin, or erythromycin.

Alcaligenes

The *Alcaligenes* group includes four species of oxidase-positive gram-negative rods. They have peritrichous flagella and are motile, which differentiates them from the pseudomonads. They alkalinize citrate medium and oxidation-fermentation medium containing glucose and are urease-negative. They may be part of the normal human bacterial flora and have been isolated from respirators, nebulizers, and renal dialysis systems. They are occasionally isolated from urine, blood, spinal fluid, wounds, and abscesses. *Alcaligenes xylosoxidans* subsp *xylosoxidans* (*Achromobacter xylosoxidans*) has been isolated from many body sites but is very uncommon as a sole cause of infection.

Capnocytophaga

The *Capnocytophaga* species are slow-growing capnophilic, gram-negative, fusiform or filamentous bacilli. They are fermentative and facultative anaerobes that require CO_2 for aerobic growth. They may show **gliding motility,** which can be seen as outgrowths of colonies. They produce a substance that modifies polymorphonuclear cell chemotactic activity. *Capnocytophaga ochracea, Capnocytophaga sputigena,* and *Capnocytophaga gingivalis* are members of the normal oral flora of humans. They have been associated with severe periodontal disease in juveniles. They occasionally cause bacteremia and severe systemic disease in immunocompromised patients especially granulocytopenic patients with oral ulcerations. *Capnocytophaga canimorsis* (previously DF-2–dysgonic fermenter 2) are oral flora of dogs. When transmitted to humans, they occasionally cause fulminant infection in asplenic patients, alcoholics, and, rarely, healthy people. *Capnocytophaga cynodegmi* (DF-2-like) is associated with wound infections from dog or cat bites or scratches.

Cardiobacterium

Cardiobacterium hominis, another bacterium with a descriptive name, is a facultatively anaerobic, pleomorphic gram-negative rod that is part of the normal flora of the upper respiratory tract and bowel and occasionally causes endocarditis. Since it grows slowly in blood culture media, it may be necessary to observe the cultures for several weeks in order to diagnose infection.

Chromobacteria

Chromobacterium violaceum is a gram-negative bacillus resembling pseudomonads. The organism usually produces a violet pigment. It occurs in subtropical climates in soil and water and may infect animals and humans through breaks in the skin or via the gut. This may result in abscesses, diarrhea, and sepsis, with many deaths. Chromobacteria are often susceptible to chloramphenicol, tetracyclines, and aminoglycosides.

Eikenella corrodens

Eikenella corrodens is a small, fastidious, capnophilic gram-negative rod that is part of the gingival and bowel flora of 40–70% of humans. About 50% of isolates form pits in agar during the several days of incubation required for growth. *Eikenella* is oxidase-positive and does not ferment carbohydrates. It is found in mixed flora infections associated with contamination by oral mucosal or bowel flora; it is often present with streptococci. It occurs frequently in infections from human bites. *Eikenella* is uniformly resistant to clindamycin, which can be used to make a selective agar medium. *Eikenella* is susceptible to ampicillin and the newer penicillins and cephalosporins.

Flavobacterium

The *Flavobacterium* group includes at least five species. The organisms are long, thin, nonmotile gram-negative rods that are oxidase-positive, proteolytic, and weakly fermentative. They often form distinctive yellow colonies. Flavobacteria are commonly found in sink drains, faucets, and on medical equipment that has been exposed to contaminated water sources and not sterilized. Flavobacteria occasionally colonize the respiratory tract, and *Flavobacterium meningosepticum* rarely causes meningitis. They are often resistant to many antimicrobial drugs.

Kingella

The *Kingella* group includes three species, of which *Kingella kingae* is the most common. *K kingae,* previously known as a member of the genus *Moraxella,* is an oxidase-positive, nonmotile organism that is hemolytic when grown on blood agar. It is a gram-negative rod, but coccobacillary and diplococcal forms are common. It is part of the normal oral flora and occasionally causes infections of bone, joints, and tendons. The organism probably enters the circulation with minor oral trauma such as tooth brushing. It is susceptible to penicillin, ampicillin, erythromycin, and other antimicrobial drugs.

Moraxella

The *Moraxella* group includes six species. They are nonmotile, nonfermentative, and oxidase-positive. On staining, they appear as small gram-negative bacilli, coccobacilli, or cocci. They are members of the normal flora of the upper respiratory tract and occasionally cause bacteremia, endocarditis, conjunctivitis, meningitis, or other infections. Most of them are susceptible to penicillin and other antimicrobial drugs. *Moraxella catarrhalis* (previously *Branhamella catarrhalis*) often produces β-lactamase (Chapter 21).

REFERENCES

Pseudomonads

Anaissie E et al: *Pseudomonas putida:* Newly recognized pathogen in patients with cancer. Am J Med 1987;82:1191.

Barbaro DJ et al: *Pseudomonas testosteroni* infections: Eighteen recent cases and a review of the literature. Rev Infect Dis 1987;9:124.

Bodey GP et al: Infections caused by *Pseudomonas aeruginosa.* Rev Infect Dis 1983;5:279.

Chaowagul W et al: Relapse in melioidosis: Incidence and risk factors. J Infect Dis 1993;168:1181.

Kanaphun P et al: Serology and carriage of *Pseudomonas pseudomallei:* A prospective study in 1000 hospitalized patients in northeast Thailand. J Infect Dis 1993;167:230.

Khardori N et al: Nosocomial infections due to *Xanthomonas maltophilia* in patients with cancer. Rev Infect Dis 1990;12:997.

Marshall WF, et al: *Xanthomonas maltophilia:* An emerging nosocomial pathogen. Mayo Clin Proc 1989;64:1097.

McNeil MM et al: Nosocomial *Pseudomonas pickettii* colonization associated with a contaminated respiratory therapy solution in a special care nursery. J Clin Microbiol 1985;22:903.

Pier GB: Polysaccharide antigens of *Pseudomonas aeruginosa.* Rev Infect Dis 1988;10(Suppl 2):S337.

Pier GB: Pulmonary disease associated with *Pseudomonas aeruginosa* in cystic fibrosis: Current status of the host-bacterium interaction. J Infect Dis 1985;151:575.

Piggott JA, Hochholzer L: Human melioidosis: A histopathologic study of acute and chronic melioidosis. Arch Pathol 1970;90:101.

Pollack M: The role of exotoxin A in *Pseudomonas* disease and immunity. Rev Infect Dis 1983;5(Suppl 5):S979.

Taylor RF, Gaya H, Hodson ME: *Pseudomonas cepacia:* Pulmonary infection in patients with cystic fibrosis. Resp Med 1993;87:187.

Smith MA, Trowers NR, Klein RS: Cervical osteomyelitis caused by *Pseudomonas cepacia* in an intravenous-drug abuser. J Clin Microbiol 1985;21:445.

Woods DE, Iglewski BH: Toxins of *Pseudomonas aeruginosa:* New perspectives. Rev Infect Dis 1983;5(Suppl 4):S715.

Woods ML 2d: Neurological melioidosis: Seven cases from the Northern Territory of Australia. 1992;15:163.

Acinetobacter

Bouvet PJM, Grimont PAD. Taxonomy of the genus *Acinetobacter* with recognition of *Acinetobacter baumannii* sp. nov., *Acinetobacter haemolyticus* sp. nov., *Acinetobacter johnsonii* sp. nov., and *Acinetobacter junii* sp. nov. and emended descriptions of *Acinetobacter calcoaceticus* and *Acinetobacter lwoffii.* Int J Sys Bacteriol 1986;36:228.

Sherertz RJ, Sullivan ML: An outbreak of infections with *Acinetobacter calcoaceticus* in burn patients: Contamination of patients' mattresses. J Infect Dis 1985;151:252.

Seifert H, Baginski R: The clinical significance of *Acinetobacter baumanii* in blood cultures. Int J Med Microbiol 1992;277:210.

Seifert H et al: Vascular catheter-related bloodstream infection due to *Acinetobacter johnsonii* (formerly *Acinetobacter calcoaceticus* var. *lwoffii:* Report of 13 cases. Clin Infect Dis 1993;17:632.

Uncommon Gram-Negative Bacteria

Bilgrami S et al: *Capnocytophaga* bacteremia in a patient with Hodgkin's disease following bone marrow transplantation: Case report and review. Clin Infect Dis 1992;14:1045.

Goldstein EJ, Gombert ME, Agyare EO: Susceptibility of *Eikenella corrodens* to newer beta-lactam antibiotics. Antimicrob Agents Chemother 1980;18:832.

Goutzmanis JJ, Gonis G, Gilbert GL: *Kingella kingae* infection in children: Ten cases and a review of the literature. Ped Infect Dis J 1991;10:677.

Joshi N, O'Brien T, Applebaum PC: Pleuropulmonary infections caused by *Eikenella corrodens.* Rev Infect Dis 1991;13:1207.

Morrison VA, Wagner KF: Clinical manifestations of Kingella kingae infections: Case report and review. Rev Infect Dis 1989;11:776.

Parenti DM, Snydman DR: *Capnocytophagia* species: Infections in nonimmunocompromised and immunocompromised hosts. J Infect Dis 1985;151:140.

Ti TY et al: Nonfatal and fatal infections caused by *Chromobacterium violaceum.* Clin Infect Dis 1993;17:505.

Wormser GP, Bottone EJ: *Cardiobacterium hominis:* Review of microbiologic and clinical features. Rev Infect Dis 1983;5:680.

18 Vibrios, Campylobacters, *Helicobacter,* & Associated Bacteria

Vibrio, Aeromonas, Plesiomonas, Campylobacter, and *Helicobacter* species are gram-negative rods that are all widely distributed in nature. The vibrios are found in marine and surface waters. *Aeromonas* is found predominantly in fresh water and occasionally in cold-blooded animals. *Plesiomonas* exists in both cold- and warm-blooded animals. The campylobacters are found in many species of animals, including many domesticated animals. *Vibrio cholerae* produces an enterotoxin that causes cholera, a profuse watery diarrhea that can rapidly lead to dehydration and death. *Campylobacter jejuni* is a common cause of enteritis in humans. Less commonly, *Aeromonas*—and rarely, *Plesiomonas*—has been associated with diarrheal disease in humans. *Helicobacter pylori* has been associated with gastritis and duodenal ulcer disease.

THE VIBRIOS

Vibrios are among the most common bacteria in surface waters worldwide. They are curved aerobic rods and are motile, possessing a polar flagellum. They do not form spores. *V cholerae* serogroup O1 and related vibrios cause cholera in humans, while other vibrios may cause sepsis or enteritis. The medically important vibrios are listed in Table 18–1.

1. *VIBRIO CHOLERAE*

The epidemiology of cholera closely parallels the recognition of *V cholerae* transmission in water and the development of sanitary water systems.

Morphology & Identification

A. Typical Organisms: Upon first isolation, *V cholerae* is a comma-shaped, curved rod 2–4 μm long (Figure 18–1). It is actively motile by means of a polar flagellum. On prolonged cultivation, vibrios may become straight rods that resemble the gram-negative enteric bacteria.

B. Culture: *V cholerae* produces convex, smooth, round colonies that are opaque and granular in transmitted light. *V cholerae* and most other vibrios grow well at 37 °C on many kinds of media, including defined media containing mineral salts and asparagine as sources of carbon and nitrogen. *V cholerae* grows well on **thiosulfate-citrate-bile-sucrose (TCBS)** agar, on which it produces yellow colonies. Vibrios are oxidase-positive, which differentiates them from enteric gram-negative bacteria grown on blood agar. Characteristically, vibrios grow at a very high pH (8.5–9.5) and are rapidly killed by acid. Cultures containing fermentable carbohydrates therefore quickly become sterile.

In areas where cholera is endemic, direct cultures of stool on selective media such as TCBS, and enrichment cultures in alkaline peptone water are appropriate. However, routine stool cultures on special media such as TCBS generally are not necessary or cost-effective in areas where cholera is rare.

C. Growth Characteristics: *V cholerae* regularly ferments sucrose and mannose but not arabinose. A positive oxidase test is a key step in the preliminary identification of *V cholerae* and other vibrios. *Vibrio* species are susceptible to the compound O/129 (2,4-diamino-6,7-diisopropylpteridine phosphate), which differentiates them from *Aeromonas* species, which are resistant to O/129. Most *Vibrio* species are halotolerant, and NaCl often stimulates their growth. Some vibrios are halophilic, requiring the presence of NaCl to grow. Another difference between vibrios and *Aeromonas* is that vibrios grow on media containing 6% NaCl, whereas *Aeromonas* does not.

Antigenic Structure & Biologic Classification

Many vibrios share a single heat-labile flagellar H antigen. Antibodies to the H antigen are probably not involved in the protection of susceptible hosts.

V cholerae has O lipopolysaccharides that confer serologic specificity. There are more than 100 O antigen groups, depending upon the classification scheme. *V cholerae* strains of O group 1 cause classic cholera; occasionally non-O1 *V cholerae* cause cholera-like disease. Antibodies to the O antigens tend to protect laboratory animals against infections with *V cholerae.*

The *V cholerae* serogroup O1 antigen has determinants that make possible further typing; the main serotypes are Ogawa and Inaba. Two biotypes of epidemic *V cholerae* have been defined, classic and El

Table 18–1. The medically important vibrios.

	Human Disease
V cholerae serogroup O1 and O 139	Epidemic and pandemic cholera.
V cholerae serogroup non-O1	Choleralike diarrhea; mild diarrhea; rarely, extra-intestinal infection.
V parahaemolyticus	Gastroenteritis, possibly extra-intestinal infection.
Others (*V mimicus, V vulnificus, V hollisae, V fluvialis, V damsela, V alginolyticus, V metschnikovii*)	Ear, wound, soft tissue, and other extraintestinal infections, all uncommon.

Tor. The El Tor biotype produces a hemolysin, gives positive results on the Voges-Proskauer test, and is resistant to polymyxin B. Molecular techniques can also be used to type *V cholerae.* Typing is used for epidemiologic studies, and tests generally are done only in reference laboratories.

Vibrio cholerae Enterotoxin

V cholerae and related vibrios produce a heat-labile enterotoxin with a molecular weight of about 84,000, consisting of subunits A (MW 28,000) and B (see Chapter 10). Ganglioside G_{M1} serves as the mucosal receptor for subunit B, which promotes entry of subunit A into the cell. Activation of subunit A_1 yields increased levels of intracellular cAMP and results in prolonged hypersecretion of water and electrolytes. There is increased sodium-dependent chloride secretion, and absorption of sodium and chloride is inhibited. Diarrhea occurs—as much as 20–30 L/d—with resulting dehydration, shock, acidosis, and death. The genes for *V cholerae* enterotoxin are on the bacterial chromosome. Cholera enterotoxin is antigenically related to LT of *Escherichia coli* and can stimulate the production of neutralizing antibodies. However, the precise role of antitoxic and antibacterial antibodies in protection against cholera is not clear.

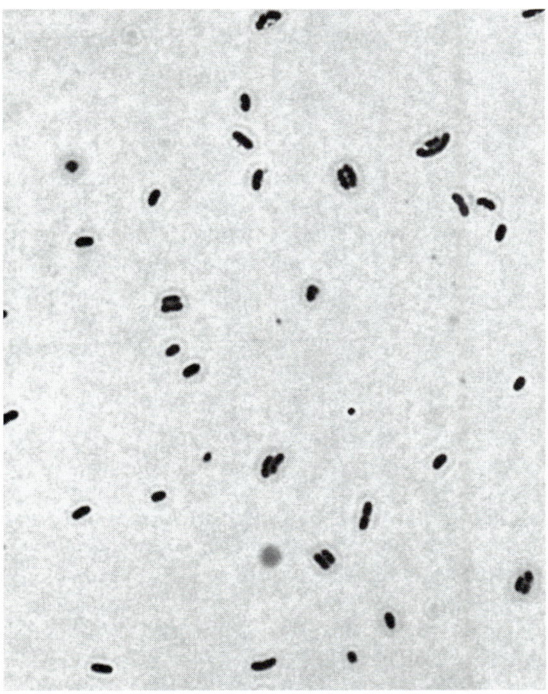

Figure 18–1. *Vibrio cholerae* grown in broth showing slightly curved gram-negative rods.

Pathogenesis & Pathology

Under natural conditions, *V cholerae* is pathogenic only for humans. A person may have to ingest 10^8–10^{10} organisms to become infected and develop disease—in contrast to salmonellosis or shigellosis, in which ingestion of 10^2–10^5 organisms can induce infection.

Cholera is not an invasive infection. The organisms do not reach the bloodstream but remain within the intestinal tract. Virulent *V cholerae* organisms attach to the microvilli of the brush border of epithelial cells. There they multiply and liberate cholera toxin and perhaps mucinases and endotoxin.

Clinical Findings

After an incubation period of 1–4 days, there is a sudden onset of nausea and vomiting and profuse diarrhea with abdominal cramps. Stools, which resemble "rice water," contain mucus, epithelial cells, and large numbers of vibrios. There is rapid loss of fluid and electrolytes, which leads to profound dehydration, circulatory collapse, and anuria. The mortality rate without treatment is between 25% and 50%. The diagnosis of a full-blown case of cholera presents no problem in the presence of an epidemic. However, sporadic or mild cases are not readily differentiated from other diarrheal diseases. The El Tor biotype tends to cause milder disease than the classic biotype.

Diagnostic Laboratory Tests

A. Specimens: Specimens for culture consist of mucus flecks from stools.

B. Smears: The microscopic appearance of smears made from stool samples is not distinctive. Dark-field or phase contrast microscopy may show the rapidly motile vibrios.

C. Culture: Growth is rapid in peptone agar, on blood agar with a pH near 9.0, or on TCBS agar, and typical colonies can be picked in 18 hours. For enrichment, a few drops of stool can be incubated for 6–8 hours in taurocholate-peptone broth (pH 8.0–9.0); organisms from this culture can be stained or subcultured.

D. Specific Tests: *V cholerae* organisms are further identified by slide agglutination tests using anti-O group 1 antiserum and by biochemical reaction patterns.

Immunity

Gastric acid provides some protection against cholera vibrios ingested in small numbers.

An attack of cholera is followed by immunity to reinfection, but the duration and degree of immunity are not known. In experimental animals, specific IgA antibodies occur in the lumen of the intestine. Similar antibodies in serum develop after infection but last only a few months. Vibriocidal antibodies in serum (titer $\geq$ 1:20) have been associated with protection against colonization and disease. The presence of antitoxin antibodies has not been associated with protection.

Treatment

The most important part of therapy consists of water and electrolyte replacement to correct the severe dehydration and salt depletion. Many antimicrobial agents are effective against *V cholerae*. Oral tetracycline tends to reduce stool output in cholera and shortens the period of excretion of vibrios. In some endemic areas, tetracycline resistance of *V cholerae* has emerged, carried by transmissible plasmids.

Epidemiology, Prevention, & Control

Worldwide epidemics of cholera occurred in the 1800s and early 1900s. The classic biotype was prevalent through the early 1960s; the El Tor biotype, discovered in 1905, became prevalent in the late 1960s and has caused the seventh pandemic of the disease in Asia, the Middle East, and Africa. Starting in 1991, the seventh pandemic spread to Peru and then to other countries of South America and Central America. Millions of people have had cholera in this pandemic. The disease has been rare in North America since the mid 1800s, but an endemic focus exists on the Gulf Coast of Louisiana and Texas.

Cholera is endemic in India and Southeast Asia. From these centers, it is carried along shipping lanes, trade routes, and pilgrim migration routes. The disease is spread by person-to-person contact involving individuals with mild or early illness and by water, food, and flies. In many instances, only 1–5% of exposed susceptible persons develop disease. The carrier state seldom exceeds 3–4 weeks, and true chronic carriers are rare. Vibrios survive in water for up to 3 weeks.

Control rests on education and on improvement of sanitation, particularly of food and water. Patients should be isolated, their excreta disinfected, and contacts followed up. Chemoprophylaxis with antimicrobial drugs may have a place. Repeated injection of a vaccine containing either lipopolysaccharides extracted from vibrios or dense *Vibrio* suspensions can confer limited protection to heavily exposed persons (eg, family contacts) but is not effective as an epidemic control measure. Very few countries require that travelers arriving from endemic areas have proof of immunization with these vaccines. The WHO vaccination certificate for cholera is only valid for 6 months.

2. *VIBRIO PARAHAEMOLYTICUS* & OTHER VIBRIOS

Vibrio parahaemolyticus is a halophilic bacterium that causes acute gastroenteritis following ingestion of contaminated seafood such as raw fish or shellfish. After an incubation period of 12–24 hours, nausea and vomiting, abdominal cramps, fever, and watery to bloody diarrhea occur. The mechanism of illness is not yet clear; fecal leukocytes are often observed. The enteritis tends to subside spontaneously in 1–4 days with no treatment other than restoration of water and electrolyte balance. No enterotoxin has yet been isolated from this organism. The disease occurs worldwide, with highest incidence in areas where people eat raw seafood. *V parahaemolyticus* does not grow well on some of the differential media used to grow salmonellae and shigellae, but it does grow well on blood agar. It also grows well on TCBS, where it yields green colonies. *V parahaemolyticus* is usually identified by its oxidase-positive growth on blood agar.

Vibrio vulnificus is also a halophilic vibrio from seawater. It can cause intense skin lesions in persons who have handled shellfish or other marine animals and can occasionally produce enteritis, bacteremia, and death in elderly or debilitated persons.

Several other vibrios also cause disease in humans: *Vibrio mimicus* causes diarrhea after ingestion of uncooked seafood, particularly raw oysters. *Vibrio hollisae* and *Vibrio fluvialis* also cause diarrhea. *Vibrio alginolyticus* causes eye, ear, or wound infection after exposure to seawater. *Vibrio damsela* also causes wound infections. Other vibrios are very uncommon causes of disease in humans.

AEROMONAS

Aeromonas species are free-living gram-negative rods found in fresh water and occasionally in reptiles, amphibians, or fish and in soil or food. Their primary importance in medical microbiology is in association with diarrhea. Occasionally they cause freshwater wound infections or infections in immunocompromised patients and, rarely, other nonintestinal infections.

The three most important species in humans are *Aeromonas hydrophila*, *Aeromonas sobria*, and *Aeromonas caviae*. Other species have been characterized, but there is a great deal of genetic complexity and biologic heterogeneity, so that there are different genospecies and phenospecies classifications. Aeromonads are 1–4 μm long and are motile. Their colony morphology is similar to that of enteric gram-negative rods (Chapter 16), and they produce large zones of hemolysis on blood agar. *Aeromonas* species cultured from stool specimens grow readily on the differential media used to culture enteric gram-negative rods and can easily be confused with enteric bacteria. *Aero-*

monas species are distinguished from the enteric gram-negative rods by finding a positive oxidase reaction in growth obtained from a blood agar plate. *Aeromonas* species are differentiated from vibrios by showing resistance to compound O/129 (see above) and lack of growth on media containing 6% NaCl.

Typically, aeromonads produce hemolysins. Some strains produce an enterotoxin. Cytotoxins and the ability to invade cells in tissue culture have been noted. However, none of these characteristics have been clearly shown to be associated with diarrheal disease in humans. Koch's postulates have not been satisfied, largely because there is no suitable animal model that reproduces human *Aeromonas*-associated diarrhea.

Aeromonas strains are susceptible to tetracyclines, aminoglycosides, and cephalosporins.

PLESIOMONAS

Plesiomonas shigelloides is a gram-negative rod with polar flagella. *Plesiomonas* is most common in tropical and subtropical areas. It has been isolated from freshwater fish and many animals. Most isolates from humans have been from stool cultures of patients with diarrhea. *Plesiomonas* grows on the differential media used to isolate *Salmonella* and *Shigella* from stool specimens (see Chapter 16). Some *Plesiomonas* strains share antigens with *Shigella sonnei,* and cross-reactions with *Shigella* antisera occur. *Plesiomonas* can be distinguished from shigellae in diarrheal stools by the oxidase test: *Plesiomonas* is oxidase-positive and shigellae are not. *Plesiomonas* is positive for DNase; this and other biochemical tests distinguish it from *Aeromonas.*

THE CAMPYLOBACTERS

Campylobacters were formerly grouped with vibrios and were known mainly as pathogens for various animals, in whom they caused sepsis, abortion, or enteritis. The widespread use of selective media greatly increased the recognition of *Campylobacter jejuni* as a common cause of diarrhea in humans. The medically important campylobacters are listed in Table 18–2.

Table 18–2. The medically important *Campylobacter* species.

Species	Reservoir	Primary Human Disease
Campylobacter jejuni	Birds and other animals	Diarrhea (common)
Campylobacter fetus subsp *fetus*	Cattle and sheep	Septicemia in debilitated and immunocompromised patients
Campylobacter coli	Pigs	Diarrhea
Campylobacter laridis	Birds and other animals	Diarrhea
Campylobacter (Helicobacter) cinaedi and *Campylobacter (Helicobacter) fennelliae;* others		Infections in homosexual men

1. CAMPYLOBACTER JEJUNI

Campylobacter jejuni has emerged as a common human pathogen, causing mainly enteritis and occasionally systemic invasion. The bacterium is at least as common as salmonellae and shigellae as a cause of diarrhea; an estimated 2 million cases occur in the USA each year.

Morphology & Identification

A. Typical Organisms: *C jejuni* and the other campylobacters are gram-negative rods with comma, S, or "gull-wing" shapes (Figure 18–2). They are motile, with a single polar flagellum, and do not form spores.

B. Culture: The culture characteristics are most important in the isolation and identification of *C jejuni* and the other campylobacters. Selective media are needed, and incubation must be in an atmosphere with reduced O_2 (5% O_2) with added CO_2 (10% CO_2). A relatively simple way to produce the incubation atmosphere is to place the plates in an anaerobe incubation jar without the catalyst and to produce the gas with a commercially available gas-generating pack or by gas exchange. Incubation of primary plates should be at 42–43 °C. Although *C jejuni* grows well at 36–37 °C, incubation at 42 °C prohibits growth of most of the other bacteria present in feces, thus simplifying the identification of *C jejuni.* Several selective media are in widespread use: Skirrow's medium incorporates vancomycin, polymyxin B, and trimethoprim; Campy BAP medium includes cephalothin as well. Both media (as well as other selective media) are suitable for isolation of *C jejuni* at 42 °C; when incubated at 36–37 °C, Skirrow's medium is helpful in isolating other campylobacters but Campy BAP medium is not, since many of the other campylobacters are susceptible to cephalothin. The colonies tend to be colorless or gray. They may be watery and spreading or round and convex, and both colony types may appear on one agar plate.

C. Growth Characteristics: Because of the selective media and incubation conditions for growth, an abbreviated set of tests is usually all that is necessary for identification. *C jejuni* and the other campylobacters pathogenic for humans are oxidase- and catalase-positive. Campylobacters do not oxidize or ferment

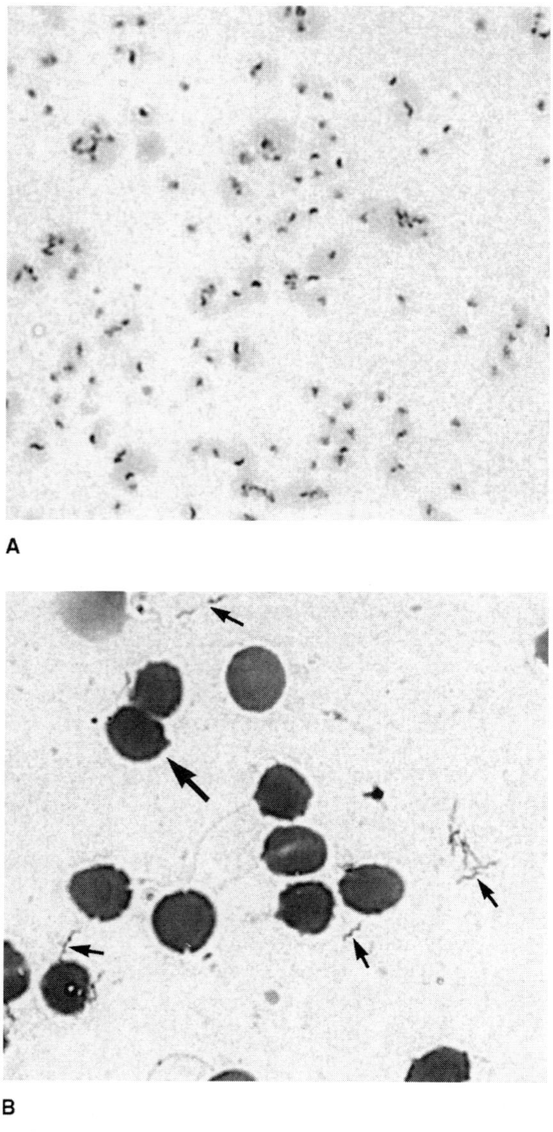

Figure 18–2. ***A: Campylobacter jejuni*** grown on solid medium showing "comma" or "gull wing"-shaped gram-negative bacilli. ***B:*** A *Campylobacter* species (small arrows) in a patient's blood culture; numerous red blood cells (large arrow) are also seen.

carbohydrates. Gram-stained smears show typical morphology. Nitrate reduction, hydrogen sulfide production, hippurate tests, and antimicrobial susceptibilities can be used for further identification of species.

Antigenic Structure & Toxins

The campylobacters have lipopolysaccharides with endotoxic activity. Cytopathic extracellular toxins and enterotoxins have been found, but the significance of the toxins in human disease is not well understood.

Pathogenesis & Pathology

The infection is acquired by the oral route from food, drink, contact with infected animals, or anal-genital-oral sexual activity. *C jejuni* is susceptible to gastric acid, and ingestion of about 10^4 organisms is usually necessary to produce infection. This inoculum is similar to that required for *Salmonella* and *Shigella* infection but less than that for *Vibrio* infection. The organisms multiply in the small intestine, invade the epithelium, and produce inflammation that results in the appearance of red and white blood cells in the stools. Occasionally, the bloodstream is invaded and a clinical picture of enteric fever develops. Localized tissue invasion coupled with the toxic activity appears to be responsible for the enteritis.

Clinical Findings

Clinical manifestations are acute onset of crampy abdominal pain, profuse diarrhea that may be grossly bloody, headache, malaise, and fever. Usually the illness is self-limited to a period of 5–8 days, but occasionally it continues longer. *C jejuni* isolates are usually susceptible to erythromycin, and therapy shortens the duration of fecal shedding of bacteria. Most cases resolve without antimicrobial therapy.

Diagnostic Laboratory Tests

A. Specimens: Diarrheal stool is the usual specimen. Campylobacters from other types of specimens are usually incidental findings or are found in the setting of known outbreaks of disease.

B. Smears: Gram-stained smears of stool may show the typical "gull wing"-shaped rods. Dark-field or phase contrast microscopy may show the typical darting motility of the organisms.

C. Culture: Culture on the selective media described above is the definitive test to diagnose *C jejuni* enteritis. If another species of *Campylobacter* is suspected, medium without cephalothin should be used and incubated at 36–37 °C.

Epidemiology & Control

Campylobacter enteritis resembles other acute bacterial diarrheas, particularly *Shigella* dysentery. The source of infection may be food (eg, milk), contact with infected animals or humans and their excreta, or oral-anal sexual contact. Outbreaks arising from a common source, eg, unpasteurized milk, may require public health control measures. Human carriers exist, but their role in transmission is unknown.

2. *CAMPYLOBACTER FETUS*

Campylobacter fetus subspecies *fetus* is an opportunistic pathogen that causes systemic infections in immunocompromised patients. It may occasionally cause diarrhea. The gastrointestinal tract may be the portal of entry when *C fetus* causes bacteremia and systemic infection. *C fetus* has several surface array proteins (S protein, MW 100,000–149,000) which form a capsule-like structure on the surface of the organism (as compared with the polysaccharide capsules of pathogens such as *Neisseria meningitidis* and *Streptococcus pneumoniae*). In a mouse model of *C fetus* infection, the presence of the S protein as a surface capsule correlated with the ability of the bacteria to cause bacteremia after oral challenge and cause death in a high percentage of the animals.

3. OTHER *CAMPYLOBACTER* SPECIES

Campylobacter species other than *C jejuni* are encountered infrequently. This is partially due to the standard methods used for isolation of campylobacters from stool specimens. *Campylobacter coli* occasionally causes diarrhea. *Campylobacter laridis* is often found in sea gulls and occasionally causes diarrhea in humans. A group of *Campylobacter*-like or *Helicobacter*-like organisms have been isolated from stool cultures from homosexual men and have been given species names.

HELICOBACTER PYLORI

Helicobacter pylori is a spiral-shaped gram-negative rod. *H pylori* is associated with antral gastritis, duodenal (peptic) ulcer disease, and possibly gastric ulcers and carcinoma.

Morphology & Identification

A. Typical Organisms: *H pylori* is a gram-negative spiral bacillus with many characteristics in common with *Campylobacter* species. *H pylori* have multiple flagella at one pole and are actively motile.

B. Culture: Culture sensitivity can be limited by prior therapy, contamination with other mucosal bacteria, and other factors. *H pylori* grows in 3–6 days when incubated at 37 °C in a microaerophilic environment, as for *C jejuni*. The media for primary isolation include Skirrow's medium with vancomycin, polymyxin B, and trimethoprim, chocolate medium, and other selective media with antibiotics (eg, vancomycin, nalidixic acid, amphotericin). The colonies are translucent and 1–2 mm in diameter.

C. Growth Characteristics: *H pylori* is oxidase-positive and catalase-positive, has a characteristic morphology, is motile, and is a strong producer of urease.

Pathogenesis & Pathology

H pylori grows optimally at a pH of 6.0–7.0 and would be killed or not grow at the pH within the gastric lumen. Gastric mucus is relatively impermeable to acid and has a strong buffering capacity. On the lumen side of the mucus, the pH is low—1.0–2.0—while on the epithelial side the pH is about 7.4. *H pylori* is found deep in the mucus layer near the epithelial surface where physiologic pH is present. *H pylori* also produces a protease that modifies the gastric mucus and further reduces the ability of acid to diffuse through the mucus. *H pylori* produces potent urease activity, which yields production of ammonia and further buffering of acid. *H pylori* is quite motile, even in mucus, and is able to find its way to the epithelial surface.

In human volunteers, ingestion of *H pylori* resulted in development of gastritis and hypochlorhydria. There is no direct evidence that *H pylori* causes duodenal ulcer disease, but there is a strong association between the presence of *H pylori* infection and duodenal ulceration. In therapeutic trials, antimicrobial therapy—compared with placebo—yielded clearing of *H pylori* and improvement of gastritis and duodenal ulcer disease.

The mechanisms by which *H pylori* causes mucosal inflammation and damage are not well defined. The bacteria invade the epithelial cell surface to a limited degree. Toxins and lipopolysaccharide may damage the mucosal cells, and the ammonia produced by the urease activity may directly damage the cells also.

Histologically, gastritis is characterized by chronic and active inflammation. Polymorphonuclear and mononuclear cell infiltrates are seen within the epithelium and lamina propria. Vacuoles within cells are often pronounced. Destruction of the epithelium is common, and glandular atrophy may occur.

Clinical Findings

The signs and symptoms are those of gastritis and duodenal ulcer disease. Many patients with *H pylori* infection are asymptomatic.

Diagnostic Laboratory Tests

A. Specimens: Gastric biopsy specimens can be used for histologic examination or minced in saline and used for culture. Blood is collected for determination of serum antibodies.

B. Smears: The diagnosis of gastritis and *H pylori* infection can be made histologically. A gastroscopy procedure with biopsy is required. Routine stains demonstrate gastritis, and Giemsa or special silver stains can show the curved or spiraled organisms.

C. Culture: As above.

D. Antibodies: Several assays have been developed to detect serum antibodies specific for *H pylori*. The serum antibodies persist even if the *H pylori* infection is eradicated, and the role of antibody tests in diagnosing active infection or following therapy is therefore limited.

E. Special Tests: Rapid tests to detect urease activity are widely used for presumptive identification of

H pylori in specimens. Gastric biopsy material can be placed onto a urea-containing medium with a color indicator. If *H pylori* is present, the urease rapidly splits the urea and the resulting shift in pH yields a color change in the medium. In vivo tests for urease activity can be done also. ^{13}C- or ^{14}C-labeled urea is ingested by the patient. If *H pylori* is present, the urease activity generates labeled CO_2 that can be detected in the patient's exhaled breath.

Immunity

Patients infected with *H pylori* develop an IgM antibody response to the infection. Subsequently, IgG and IgA are produced, and these persist, both systemically and at the mucosa, in high titer in chronically infected persons. Early antimicrobial treatment of *H pylori* infection blunts the antibody response; such patients are thought to be subject to repeat infection.

Treatment

Triple therapy with metronidazole and either bismuth subsalicylate or bismuth subcitrate plus either amoxicillin or tetracycline for 14 days eradicates *H pylori* infection in 70–95% of patients. Metronidazole is the essential feature of treatment.

Epidemiology & Control

H pylori is present on the gastric mucosa of less than 20% of persons under age 30 but increases in prevalence to 40–60% of persons age 60, including persons who are asymptomatic. In developing countries, the prevalence of infection may be 80% or higher in adults. Person-to-person transmission of *H pylori* is likely because intrafamilial clustering of infection occurs. Acute epidemics of gastritis suggest a common source for *H pylori*. The natural history of *H pylori* infection is not well defined, but it is likely that once acquired the infection persists for years or for life.

REFERENCES

Vibrio

Blake PA, Weaver RE, Hollis DG: Disease of humans (other than cholera) caused by vibrios. Annu Rev Microbiol 1980;34:341.

Centers for Disease Control and Prevention: Update: Cholera—Western Hemisphere, 1992. MMWR Morb Mortal Wkly Rep 199 1993;42:89.

Field M: Modes of action of enterotoxins from *Vibrio cholerae* and *Escherichia coli*. Rev Infect Dis 1979; 1:918.

Lowry PW et al: *Vibrio* gastroenteritis in Louisiana: A prospective study among attendees of a scientific congress in New Orleans. J Infect Dis 1989;160:978.

Morris JG Jr, Black RE: Cholera and other vibrioses in the United States. N Engl J Med 1985;312:343.

Tacket CO, Brenner F, Blake PA: Clinical features and an epidemiological study of *Vibrio vulnificus* infections. J Infect Dis 1984;149:558.

Wacksmuth IK et al: The molecular epidemiology of cholera in Latin America. J Infect Dis 1993;167: 621.

Wang F et al: The acidosis of cholera: Contributions of hyperproteinemia, lactic acidemia, and hyperphosphatemia to an increased serum anion gap. N Engl J Med 1986;315:1591.

Aeromonas & Plesiomonas

Holmberg SD et al: *Aeromonas* intestinal infections in the United States. Ann Intern Med 1986;105:683.

Holmberg SD et al: *Plesiomonas* enteric infections in the United States. Ann Intern Med 1986;105:690.

Janda JM: Recent advances in the study of the taxonomy, pathogenicity, and infectious syndromes associated with the genus *Aeromonas*. Clin Micrbiol Rev 1991; 4:397.

Campylobacter

Blaser MJ et al: *Campylobacter* enteritis in the United States: A multicenter study. Ann Intern Med 1983;98: 360.

Blaser MJ et al: Extraintestinal *Campylobacter jejuni* and *Campylobacter coli* infections: Host factors and strain characteristics. J Infect Dis 1986;153:552.

Korlath JA et al: A point-source outbreak of campylobacteriosis associated with consumption of raw milk. J Infect Dis 1985;152:592.

Taylor DE: Genetics of *Campylobacter* and *Helicobacter*. Ann Rev Microbiol 1992;46:35.

Wood RC et al: *Campylobacter* enteritis outbreaks associated with drinking raw milk during youth activities: A 10-year review of outbreaks in the United States. JAMA 1992;268:3228.

Helicobacter

Blaser MJ: *Helicobacter pylori* and the pathogenesis of gastroduodenal inflammation. J Infect Dis 1990;161: 626.

Blaser MJ: *Helicobacter pylori*: Its role in disease. Clin Infect Dis 1992;15:386.

Buck GE: *Campylobacter pylori* and gastroduodenal disease. Clin Microbiol Rev 1990;3:1.

Dooley CP et al: Prevalence of *Helicobacter pylori* infection and histologic gastritis in asymptomatic persons. New Engl J Med 1989;321:1562.

Drum B et al: Intrafamilial clustering of *Helicobacter pylori* infections. New Engl J Med 1990;322:359.

Haemophilus, Bordetella, & Brucella

19

THE *HAEMOPHILUS* SPECIES

This is a group of small, gram-negative, pleomorphic bacteria that require enriched media, usually containing blood or its derivatives, for isolation. *Haemophilus influenzae* type b is an important human pathogen; *Haemophilus ducreyi,* a sexually transmitted pathogen, causes chancroid; others are among the normal flora of mucous membranes.

1. *HAEMOPHILUS INFLUENZAE*

Haemophilus influenzae is found on the mucous membranes of the upper respiratory tract in humans. It is an important cause of meningitis in children and occasionally causes respiratory tract infections in children and adults.

Morphology & Identification

A. Typical Organisms: In specimens from acute infections, the organisms are short (1.5 μm) coccoid bacilli, sometimes occurring in pairs or short chains. In cultures, the morphology depends both on age and on the medium. At 6–8 hours in rich medium, coccobacillary forms predominate. Later there are longer rods, lysed bacteria, and very pleomorphic forms.

Organisms in young cultures (6–18 hours) on rich medium have a definite capsule. Capsule swelling tests are used for "typing" *H influenzae* (see below).

B. Culture: On brain-heart infusion agar with blood, small, round, convex colonies with a strong iridescence develop in 24 hours. The colonies on chocolate agar take 36–48 hours to develop diameters of 1 mm. IsoVitaleX in media enhances growth. There is no hemolysis. Around staphylococcal (or other) colonies, the colonies of *H influenzae* grow much larger ("satellite phenomenon").

C. Growth Characteristics: Identification of organisms of the *Haemophilus* group depends in part upon demonstrating the need for certain growth factors called X and V. Factor X acts physiologically as hemin; factor V can be replaced by nicotinamide adenine nucleotide (NAD) or other coenzymes. The requirements for X and V factors of various *Haemophilus* species are listed in Table 19–1. Carbohydrates are fermented poorly and irregularly.

D. Variation: In addition to morphologic variation, *H influenzae* has a marked tendency to lose its capsule and the associated type specificity. Nonencapsulated variant colonies lack iridescence.

E. Transformation: Under proper experimental circumstances, the DNA extracted from a given type of *H influenzae* is capable of transferring that type specificity to other cells (transformation). Resistance to ampicillin and chloramphenicol is controlled by genes on transmissible plasmids.

Antigenic Structure

Encapsulated *H influenzae* contains **capsular polysaccharides** (MW >150,000) of one of six types (a–f). The capsular antigen of type b is a polyribose-ribitol phosphate (PRP). Encapsulated *H influenzae* can be typed by a capsule swelling test with specific antiserum; this test is analogous to the quellung test for pneumococci. Comparable typing can be done by immunofluorescence as well. Most *H influenzae* organisms in the normal flora of the upper respiratory tract are not encapsulated.

The somatic antigens of *H influenzae* consist of outer membrane proteins. Lipooligosaccharides (endotoxins) share many structures with those of neisserriae.

Pathogenesis

H influenzae produces no exotoxin, and the role of its somatic antigen in natural disease is not clearly understood. The nonencapsulated organism is a regular member of the normal respiratory flora of humans. The capsule is antiphagocytic in the absence of specific anticapsular antibodies. The encapsulated forms of *H influenzae,* particularly type b, produce suppurative respiratory infections (sinusitis, laryngotracheitis, epiglottitis, otitis) and, in young children, meningitis. The blood of many persons over age 3–5 years is bactericidal for *H influenzae,* and clinical infections are less frequent in such individuals. However, bactericidal antibodies have been absent from 25% of adults in the USA, and clinical infections have occurred more often in adults. *H influenzae* that are untypable or not

Table 19–1. Characteristics and growth requirements of some *Haemophilus* species. (X = heme; V = nicotinamide-adenine dinucleotide.)

Species	Requires X	Requires V	Hemolysis
H influenzae (H aegyptius)	+	+	–
H parainfluenzae	–	+	–
H ducreyi	+	–	–
H haemolyticus	+	+	+
H parahaemolyticus	–	+	+
H aphrophilus	–	–	–

capsular type b commonly cause otitis media; the pathogenic mechanisms of these infections are not clear.

Clinical Findings

H influenzae type b enters by way of the respiratory tract. Other types rarely produce disease. There may be local extension with involvement of the sinuses or the middle ear. *H influenzae* type b and pneumococci are two of the most common etiologic agents of bacterial otitis media and acute sinusitis. The organisms may reach the bloodstream and be carried to the meninges or, less frequently, may establish themselves in the joints to produce septic arthritis. *H influenzae* has been the most common cause of bacterial meningitis in children age 5 months to 5 years in the USA. Clinically, it resembles other forms of childhood meningitis, and diagnosis rests on bacteriologic demonstration of the organism.

Occasionally, a fulminating obstructive laryngotracheitis with swollen, cherry-red epiglottis develops in infants and requires prompt tracheostomy or intubation as a lifesaving procedure. Pneumonitis and epiglottitis due to *H influenzae* may follow upper respiratory tract infections in small children and old or debilitated people. Adults may have bronchitis or pneumonia due to *H influenzae.*

Diagnostic Laboratory Tests

A. Specimens: Specimens consist of nasopharyngeal swabs, pus, blood, and spinal fluid for smears and cultures.

B. Direct Identification: When organisms are present in large numbers in specimens, they may be identified by immunofluorescence or mixed directly with specific rabbit antiserum (type b) for a capsule swelling test. Commercial kits are available for immunologic detection of *H influenzae* antigens in spinal fluid. A positive test indicates the fluid contains high concentrations of specific polysaccharide from *H influenzae* type b.

C. Culture: Specimens are grown on IsoVitaleX-enriched chocolate agar until typical colonies appear (24–48 hours). *H influenzae* is differentiated from related gram-negative bacilli by its requirements for X and V factors and by its lack of hemolysis on blood agar (Table 19–1).

Tests for X (heme) and V (nicotinamide-adenine dinucleotide) factor requirements can be done in several ways. The *Haemophilus* species that require V factor grow around paper strips or disks containing V factor placed on the surface of agar that has been autoclaved before the blood was added (V factor is heat-labile). Alternatively, a strip containing X factor can be placed in parallel with one containing V factor on agar deficient in these nutrients. Growth of *Haemophilus* in the area between the strips indicates requirement for both factors. A better test for X factor requirement is based on the inability of *H influenzae* (and a few other *Haemophilus* species) to synthesize heme from δ-aminolevulinic acid. The inoculum is incubated with the δ-aminolevulinic acid. *Haemophilus* organisms that do not require X factor synthesize porphobilinogen, porphyrins, protoporphyrin IX, and heme. The presence of red fluorescence under ultraviolet light (approximately 360 nm) indicates the presence of porphyrins and a positive test. *Haemophilus* species that synthesize porphyrins (and thus heme) are not *H influenzae.* (See Table 19–1.)

Immunity

Infants under age 3 months may have serum antibodies transmitted from the mother. During this time *H influenzae* infection is rare, but subsequently the antibodies are lost. Children often acquire *H influenzae* infections, which are usually asymptomatic but may be in the form of respiratory disease or meningitis. *H influenzae* has been the most common cause of bacterial meningitis in children from 5 months to 5 years of age. By age 3–5 years, many unimmunized children have naturally acquired anti-PRP antibodies that promote complement-dependent bactericidal killing and phagocytosis. Immunization of children with *H influenzae* type b conjugate vaccine induces the same antibodies.

There is a correlation between the presence of bactericidal antibodies and resistance to major *H influenzae* type b infections. However, it is not known whether these antibodies alone account for immunity. Pneumonia or arthritis due to *H influenzae* can develop in adults with such antibodies.

Treatment

The mortality rate of untreated *H influenzae* meningitis may be up to 90%. Many strains of *H influenzae* type b are susceptible to ampicillin, but up to 25% produce β-lactamase under control of a transmissible plasmid and are resistant. Most strains are susceptible to chloramphenicol, and essentially all strains are susceptible to the newer cephalosporins. Cefotaxime intravenously, may give excellent results. Prompt diagnosis and antimicrobial therapy are essential to minimize late neurologic and intellectual impairment. Prominent among late complications of influenzal meningitis is the development of a localized subdural accumulation of fluid that requires surgical drainage.

Epidemiology, Prevention, & Control

Encapsulated *H influenzae* type b is transmitted from person to person by the respiratory route. *H influenzae* type b disease can be prevented by administration of ***Haemophilus* b conjugate vaccine** to children. Children aged 2 months or older can be immunized with *H influenzae* type b vaccine conjugated with one of two carriers (HbOC with protein carrier CRM_{197} mutant *Corynebacterium diphtheriae* toxin protein; or *Neisseria meningitidis* outer membrane complex) with appropriate booster doses according to standard recommendations. Children aged 15 months or older can receive *H influenzae* type b vaccine conjugated with diphtheria toxoid (which is not immunogenic in younger children). The vaccine does not prevent the carrier state for *H influenzae*. Widespread use of *H influenzae* type b vaccine has greatly reduced the incidence of *H influenzae* type b meningitis in children.

Contact with patients suffering from *H influenzae* clinical infection poses little risk for adults but presents a definite risk for nonimmune siblings and other nonimmune children under age 4 years who are close contacts. Prophylaxis with rifampin is recommended for such children.

2. *HAEMOPHILUS AEGYPTIUS*

This organism was formerly called the Koch-Weeks bacillus; it is sometimes called *H influenzae* biotype III. It resembles *H influenzae* closely and has been associated with a highly communicable form of conjunctivitis. *H aegyptius* is the cause of Brazilian purpuric fever, a disease of children characterized by fever, purpura, shock, and death.

3. *HAEMOPHILUS APHROPHILUS*

This organism is sometimes encountered in infective endocarditis and pneumonia. It is present in the normal oral and respiratory tract flora. It is related to *Actinobacillus (Haemophilus) actinomycetemcomitans*.

4. *HAEMOPHILUS DUCREYI*

Haemophilus ducreyi causes chancroid (soft chancre), a sexually transmitted disease. Chancroid consists of a ragged ulcer on the genitalia, with marked swelling and tenderness. The regional lymph nodes are enlarged and painful. The disease must be differentiated from syphilis, herpes simplex infection, and lymphogranuloma venereum.

The small gram-negative rods occur in strands in the lesions, usually in association with other pyogenic microorganisms. *H ducreyi* requires X factor but not V factor. It is grown best from scrapings of the ulcer base on chocolate agar containing 1% IsoVitaleX and vancomycin, 3 µg/mL, and incubated in 10% CO_2 at 33 °C. There is no permanent immunity following chancroid infection. Treatment with intramuscular ceftriaxone, oral trimethoprim-sulfamethoxazole, or oral erythromycin often results in healing in 2 weeks.

5. OTHER *HAEMOPHILUS* SPECIES

Haemophilus haemoglobinophilus requires X factor but not V factor and has been found in dogs but not in human disease. *Haemophilus haemolyticus* is the most markedly hemolytic organism of the group in vitro; it occurs both in the normal nasopharynx and in association with rare upper respiratory tract infections of moderate severity in childhood. *Haemophilus parainfluenzae* resembles *H influenzae* and is a normal inhabitant of the human respiratory tract; it has been encountered occasionally in infective endocarditis and in urethritis. *H suis* resembles *H influenzae* bacteriologically and acts synergistically with swine influenza virus to produce the disease in hogs.

THE BORDETELLAE

There are three species of bordetellae. *Bordetella pertussis*, a highly communicable and important pathogen of humans, causes **whooping cough (pertussis).** *Bordetella parapertussis* and *Bordetella bronchiseptica* are much less common causes of disease.

1. *BORDETELLA PERTUSSIS*

Morphology & Identification

A. Typical Organisms: The organisms are short, gram-negative coccobacilli resembling *H influenzae*. With toluidine blue stain, bipolar metachromatic granules can be demonstrated. A capsule is present.

B. Culture: Primary isolation of *B pertussis* requires enriched media. Bordet-Gengou medium (potato-blood-glycerol agar) that contains penicillin G, 0.5 µg/mL, can be used; however, a charcoal-containing medium similar to that used for Legionella pneumophila is preferable. The plates are incubated at 35–37 °C for 3–7 days in a moist environment (eg, a sealed plastic bag). The small, faintly gram-negative rods are identified by immunofluorescence staining.

C. Growth Characteristics: The organism is a strict aerobe and forms acid but not gas from glucose and lactose. It does not require X and V factors on subculture. Hemolysis of blood-containing medium is associated with virulent *B pertussis*.

D. Variation: When isolated from patients and cultured on enriched media, *B pertussis* is in the hemolytic and pertussis toxin-producing virulent phase.

There are two mechanisms for *B pertussis* to shift to nonhemolytic, non-toxin-producing avirulent forms. Reversible phenotypic modulation occurs when *B pertussis* is grown under certain environmental conditions (eg, 28 °C versus 37 °C, the presence of $MgSO_4$, etc). Reversible phase variation follows a low-frequency mutation in the genetic locus that controls the expression of the virulence factors (see below). It is possible that these mechanisms play a role in the infectious process, but such a role has not been demonstrated clinically.

Antigenic Structure, Pathogenesis, & Pathology

B pertussis produces a number of factors that are involved in the pathogenesis of disease. Pili probably play a role in adherence of the bacteria to the ciliated epithelial cells of the upper respiratory tract. Five of the virulence factors are coordinately regulated by the *bvg* (*Bordetella* virulence gene) genetic locus (also called *vir*). The products of the A and C loci are similar to other prokaryotic regulatory proteins that respond to environmental stimuli. The **filamentous hemagglutinin** mediates adhesion to ciliated epithelial cells. **Pertussis toxin** promotes lymphocytosis, has a role in bacterial adhesion to ciliated epithelial cells, and has ADP ribosylating activity with a structure and mechanism of action similar to that of cholera toxin. The filamentous hemagglutinin and pertussis toxin are secreted proteins and are found outside of the *B pertussis* cells. **Adenylyl cyclase toxin, dermonecrotic toxin,** and **hemolysin** also are regulated by *bvg*. The **tracheal cytotoxin** inhibits DNA synthesis in ciliated cells and is not regulated by *bvg*. The lipopolysaccharide in the cell wall may also be important in causing damage to the epithelial cells of the upper respiratory tract.

B pertussis survives for only brief periods outside the human host. There are no vectors. Transmission is largely by the respiratory route from early cases and possibly via carriers. The organism adheres to and multiplies rapidly on the epithelial surface of the trachea and bronchi and interferes with ciliary action. The blood is not invaded. The bacteria liberate the toxins and substances that irritate surface cells, causing coughing and marked lymphocytosis. Later, there may be necrosis of parts of the epithelium and polymorphonuclear infiltration, with peribronchial inflammation and interstitial pneumonia. Secondary invaders like staphylococci or *H influenzae* may give rise to bacterial pneumonia. Obstruction of the smaller bronchioles by mucous plugs results in atelectasis and diminished oxygenation of the blood. This probably contributes to the frequency of convulsions in infants with whooping cough.

Clinical Findings

After an incubation period of about 2 weeks, the "catarrhal stage" develops, with mild coughing and sneezing. During this stage, large numbers of organisms are sprayed in droplets, and the patient is highly infectious but not very ill. During the "paroxysmal" stage, the cough develops its explosive character and the characteristic "whoop" upon inhalation. This leads to rapid exhaustion and may be associated with vomiting, cyanosis, and convulsions. The "whoop" and major complications occur predominantly in infants; paroxysmal coughing predominates in older children and adults. The white blood count is high (16,000–30,000/μL), with an absolute lymphocytosis. Convalescence is slow. Rarely, whooping cough is followed by the serious and potentially fatal complication of encephalitis. Several types of adenovirus and *Chlamydia pneumoniae* can produce a clinical picture resembling that caused by *B pertussis.*

Diagnostic Laboratory Tests

A. Specimens: A saline nasal wash is the preferred specimen. Nasopharyngeal swabs or cough droplets expelled onto a "cough plate" held in front of the patient's mouth during a paroxysm are used.

B. Direct Fluorescent Antibody (FA) Test: The FA reagent can be used to examine nasopharyngeal swab specimens. However, false-positive and false-negative results may occur; the sensitivity is about 50%. The FA test is most useful in identifying *B pertussis* after culture on solid media.

C. Culture: The saline nasal wash fluid is cultured on solid medium agar (see above). The antibiotics in the media tend to inhibit other respiratory flora but permit growth of *B pertussis*. Organisms are identified by immunofluorescence staining or by slide agglutination with specific antiserum.

D. Serology: Serologic tests on patients are of little diagnostic help, because a rise in agglutinating or precipitating antibodies does not occur until the third week of illness.

Immunity

Recovery from whooping cough or adequate vaccination is followed by immunity. Second infections may occur but are mild; reinfections occurring years later in adults may be severe. It is probable that the first defense against *B pertussis* infection is the antibody that prevents attachment of the bacteria to the cilia of the respiratory epithelium. Toxin-producing phase I cells are necessary to make pertussis vaccine.

Treatment

B pertussis is susceptible to several antimicrobial drugs in vitro. Administration of erythromycin during the catarrhal stage of disease promotes elimination of the organisms and may have prophylactic value. Treatment after onset of the paroxysmal phase rarely alters the clinical course. Oxygen inhalation and sedation may prevent anoxic damage to the brain.

Prevention

During the first year of life, every infant should receive three injections of pertussis vaccine. This crude suspension of bacteria, in proper concentration, is usually administered in combination with toxoids of diphtheria and tetanus (DTP). The *B pertussis* component is an effective immunogen but can lead to neurologic reactions similar to the encephalitis seen with pertussis. Should this happen, DTP should not be given again; instead, DT should be substituted. Vaccine quality and acceptance of the preparation are variable. When pertussis vaccination was discontinued in some areas, the number of clinical cases increased markedly. It is hoped that an acellular vaccine with purer antigen may be developed for universal use in the future.

Prophylactic administration of erythromycin for 5 days may also benefit unimmunized infants or heavily exposed adults.

Epidemiology & Control

Whooping cough is endemic in most densely populated areas worldwide and also occurs intermittently in epidemics. The source of infection is usually a patient in the early catarrhal stage of the disease. Communicability is high, ranging from 30 to 90%. Most cases occur in children under age 5 years; most deaths occur in the first year of life.

Control of whooping cough rests mainly on adequate active immunization of all infants.

2. *BORDETELLA BRONCHISEPTICA*

Bordetella bronchiseptica is a small gram-negative bacillus that inhabits the respiratory tracts of canines, in which it may cause "kennel cough" and pneumonitis. It grows on blood agar medium.

3. *BORDETELLA PARAPERTUSSIS*

This organism may produce a disease similar to whooping cough. The infection is often subclinical. *Bordetella parapertussis* grows more rapidly than typical *B pertussis* and produces larger colonies. It also grows on blood agar.

THE BRUCELLAE

The brucellae are obligate parasites of animals and humans and are characteristically located intracellularly. They are relatively inactive metabolically. *Brucella melitensis* typically infects goats; *Brucella suis*, swine; *Brucella abortus*, cattle; and *Brucella canis*, dogs. Other species are found only in animals. The disease in humans, brucellosis (undulant fever, Malta fever), is characterized by an acute bacteremic phase followed by a chronic stage that may extend over many years and may involve many tissues.

Morphology & Identification

A. Typical Organisms: The appearance in young cultures varies from cocci to rods 1.2 μm in length, with short coccobacillary forms predominating. They are gram-negative but often stain irregularly, and are aerobic, nonmotile, and non-spore-forming.

B. Culture: Small, convex, smooth colonies appear on enriched media in 2–5 days.

C. Growth Characteristics: Brucellae are adapted to an intracellular habitat, and their nutritional requirements are complex. Some strains have been cultivated on defined media containing amino acids, vitamins, salts, and glucose. Fresh specimens from animal or human sources are usually inoculated on trypticase-soy agar or blood culture media. *B abortus* requires 5–10% CO_2 for growth, whereas the other three species grow in air.

Brucellae utilize carbohydrates but produce neither acid nor gas in amounts sufficient for classification. Catalase and oxidase are produced by the four species that infect humans. Hydrogen sulfide is produced by many strains, and nitrates are reduced to nitrites.

Brucellae are moderately sensitive to heat and acidity. They are killed in milk by pasteurization.

D. Variation: Smooth, mucoid, and rough variants are recognized by colonial appearance and virulence. The typical virulent organism forms a smooth, transparent colony; upon culture, it tends to change to the rough form, which is avirulent.

The serum of susceptible animals contains a globulin and a lipoprotein that suppress growth of nonsmooth, avirulent types and favor the growth of virulent types. Resistant animal species lack these factors, so that rapid mutation to avirulence can occur. D-Alanine has a similar effect in vitro.

Antigenic Structure

Different species of brucellae cannot be differentiated by agglutination tests but can be distinguished by agglutinin absorption reactions. It is probable that two lipopolysaccharide antigens, A and M, are present in different proportions in the four species. In addition, a superficial L antigen has been demonstrated that resembles the Vi antigen of salmonellae.

Differentiation among the four *Brucella* species is made possible by their characteristic sensitivity to dyes and their production of H_2S (Table 19–2).

Pathogenesis & Pathology

Although each species of *Brucella* has a preferred host, all can infect a wide range of animals, including humans.

The common routes of infection in humans are the intestinal tract (ingestion of infected milk), mucous membranes (droplets), and skin (contact with infected tissues of animals). The organisms progress from the portal of entry, via lymphatic channels and regional lymph nodes, to the thoracic duct and the bloodstream, which distributes them to the parenchymatous organs.

Table 19–2. Characteristics of brucellae.

Organism	Preferred Host	CO_2 Requirement	H_2S Production	Growth in Presence of	
				Thionine (1:25,000)	Basic Fuchsin (1:50,000)
B abortus	Cattle	+	++	–	+
B melitensis	Goats, sheep	–	–	–	+
B suis	Swine	–	+	+	–
B canis	Dogs	–	–	+	–

Granulomatous nodules that may develop into abscesses form in lymphatic tissue, liver, spleen, bone marrow, and other parts of the reticuloendothelial system. In such lesions, the brucellae are principally intracellular. Osteomyelitis, meningitis, or cholecystitis also occasionally occurs. The main histologic reaction in brucellosis consists of proliferation of mononuclear cells, exudation of fibrin, coagulation necrosis, and fibrosis. The granulomas consist of epithelioid and giant cells, with central necrosis and peripheral fibrosis.

The four brucellae that infect humans have apparent differences in pathogenicity. *B abortus* usually causes mild disease without suppurative complications; noncaseating granulomas of the reticuloendothelial system are found. *B canis* also causes mild disease. *B suis* infection tends to be chronic with suppurative lesions; caseating granulomas may be present. *B melitensis* infection is more acute and severe.

Persons with active brucellosis react more markedly (fever, myalgia) than normal persons to injected *Brucella* endotoxin. Sensitivity to endotoxin thus may play a role in pathogenesis.

Placentas and fetal membranes of cattle, swine, sheep, and goats contain erythritol, a growth factor for brucellae. The proliferation of organisms in pregnant animals leads to placentitis and abortion in these species. There is no erythritol in human placentas, and abortion is not part of *Brucella* infection of humans.

Clinical Findings

The incubation period is 1–6 weeks. The onset is insidious, with malaise, fever, weakness, aches, and sweats. The fever usually rises in the afternoon; its fall during the night is accompanied by drenching sweat. There may be gastrointestinal and nervous symptoms. Lymph nodes enlarge, and the spleen becomes palpable. Hepatitis may be accompanied by jaundice. Deep pain and disturbances of motion, particularly in vertebral bodies, suggest osteomyelitis. These symptoms of generalized *Brucella* infection generally subside in weeks or months, although localized lesions and symptoms may continue.

Following the initial infection, a chronic stage may develop, characterized by weakness, aches and pains, low-grade fever, nervousness, and other nonspecific manifestations compatible with psychoneurotic symptoms. *Brucella*e cannot be isolated from the patient at this stage, but the agglutinin titer may be high. The diagnosis of "chronic brucellosis" is difficult to establish with certainty unless local lesions are present.

Diagnostic Laboratory Tests

A. Specimens: Blood should be taken for culture, biopsy material for culture (lymph nodes, bone, etc), and serum for serologic tests.

B. Culture: Blood or tissues are incubated in trypticase-soy broth and on thionine-tryptose agar. At intervals of several days, subcultures are made on solid media of similar composition. All cultures are incubated in 10% CO_2 and should be observed and subcultured for at least 3 weeks before being discarded as negative.

If organisms resembling brucellae are isolated, they are typed by H_2S production, dye inhibition, and agglutination by absorbed sera. As a rule, brucellae can be cultivated from patients only during the acute phase of the illness or during recurrence of activity.

C. Serology: IgM antibody levels rise during the first week of acute illness, peak at 3 months, and may persist during chronic disease. Even with appropriate antibiotic therapy, high IgM levels may persist for up to 2 years in a small percentage of patients. IgG antibody levels rise about 3 weeks after onset of acute disease, peak at 6–8 weeks, and remain high during chronic disease. IgA levels parallel the IgG levels. The usual serologic tests may fail to detect infection with *B canis*.

1. Agglutination test–To be reliable, agglutination tests must be performed with standardized heat-killed, phenolized, smooth *Brucella* antigens available from brucellosis centers and should be incubated at 37°C for 24 hours. IgG agglutinin titers above 1:80 indicate active infection. Individuals injected with cholera vaccine may develop agglutination titers to brucellae. If the serum agglutination test is negative in patients with strong clinical evidence of *Brucella* infection, tests must be made for the presence of "blocking" antibodies. These can be detected by adding antihuman globulin to the antigen-serum mixture. Brucellosis agglutinins are cross-reactive with tularemia agglutinins, and tests for both diseases should be done on positive sera; usually, the titer for one disease will be much higher than that for the other.

2. 2-Mercaptoethanol test–The addition of 2-mercaptoethanol destroys IgM and leaves IgG for agglutination reactions. The test is not as sensitive as the standard agglutination test, but the results correlate better with chronic active disease.

3. Blocking antibodies–These are IgA antibodies that interfere with agglutination by IgG and IgM and cause a serologic test to be negative in low serum dilutions (prozone) although positive in higher dilutions. These antibodies appear during the subacute stage of infection, tend to persist for many years independently of activity of infection, and are detected by the Coombs antiglobulin method.

D. Skin Test: When a protein *Brucella* extract is injected intradermally, erythema, edema, and induration develop within 24 hours in some infected individuals. The skin test is unreliable and is rarely used. Application of the skin test may stimulate the agglutinin titer.

Immunity

An antibody response occurs with infection, and it is probable that some resistance to subsequent attacks is produced. Immunogenic fractions from *Brucella* cell walls have a high phospholipid content, lysine predominates among eight amino acids, and there is no heptose (thus distinguishing the fractions from endotoxin).

Treatment

*Brucella*e may be susceptible to tetracyclines or ampicillin. Symptomatic relief may occur within a few days after treatment with these drugs is begun. However, because of their intracellular location, the organisms are not readily eradicated completely from the host. For best results, treatment must be prolonged. Combined treatment with streptomycin and a tetracycline may be considered.

Epidemiology, Prevention, & Control

Brucellae are animal pathogens transmitted to humans by accidental contact with infected animal feces, urine, milk, and tissues. The common sources of infection for humans are unpasteurized milk, milk products and cheese and occupational contact (eg, farmers, veterinarians, slaughterhouse workers) with infected animals. Occasionally the airborne route may be important. Because of occupational contact, *Brucella* infection is much more frequent in men. The majority of infections remain asymptomatic (latent).

Infection rates vary greatly with different animals and in different countries. In the USA, about 4% of cattle are infected, about 15% of cattle herds contain infected animals, and infection in hogs is common. In other countries, infection is much more prevalent. Eradication of brucellosis in cattle can be attempted by test and slaughter, active immunization of heifers with avirulent live strain 19, or combined testing, segregation, and immunization. Cattle are examined by means of agglutination tests.

Active immunization of humans against *Brucella* infection is experimental. Control rests on limitation of spread and possible eradication of animal infection, pasteurization of milk and milk products, and reduction of occupational hazards wherever possible.

REFERENCES

Haemophilus

Adams WG et al: Decline of childhood *Haemophilus influenzae* type b (Hib) disease in the Hib vaccine era. JAMA 1993;269:221.

Broome CV: Epidemiology of *Haemophilus influenzae* type b infections in the United States. Ped Infect Dis 1987;6:779.

Campos J et al: Genetic relatedness of antibiotic resistance determinants in multiply resistant *Hemophilus influenzae*. J Infect Dis 1989;160:810.

Morse SA: Chancroid and *Haemophilus ducreyi*. Clin Microbiol Rev 1989;2:137.

Musser JM et al: Global genetic structure and molecular epidemiology of encapsulated *Haemophilus influenzae*. Rev Infect Dis 1990;12:75.

Recommendations of the Advisory Committee on Immunization Practices (ACIP): Recommendations for use of *Haemophilus* b conjugate vaccines and a combined diphtheria, tetanus, pertussis, and *Haemophilus* b vaccine. MMWR Morb Mortal Wkly Rep 199 1993;42 (RR-13):1.

Bordetella

Arico B et al: Sequences required for expression of *Bordetella pertussis* virulence factors share homology with prokaryotic signal transduction proteins. Proc Natl Acad Sci USA 1989;86:6671.

Edwards KM: Acellular pertussis vaccines: A solution to the pertussis problem?. J Infect Dis 1993;168:15.

Koplan JP et al: Pertussis vaccine: An analysis of benefits, risks and costs. N Engl J Med 1979;301:906.

Long SS et al: Widespread silent transmission of pertussis in families: Antibody correlates of infection and symptomatology. J Infect Dis 1990;161:480.

Melton AR, Weiss AA: Environmental regulation of expression of virulence determinants in *Bordetella pertussis*. J Bacteriol 1989;171:6206.

Miller JF et al: Analysis of *Bordetella pertussis* virulence gene regulation by use of transcriptional fusions in *Escherichia coli*. J Bacteriol 1989;171:6345.

Mortimer EA Jr: Pertussis and its prevention: A family affair. J Infect Dis 1990;161:473.

Musser JM et al: Clonal diversity and host distribution in *Bordetella bronchiseptica*. J Bacteriol 1987;169: 2793.

Roy CR et al: The *bvg*A gene of *Bordetella pertussis* encodes a transcriptional activator required for coordinate regulation of several virulence genes. J Bacteriol 1989;171:6338.

Van Savage J et al: Natural history of pertussis antibody in the infant and effect on vaccine response. J Infect Dis 1990;161:487.

Brucella

Wise RI: Brucellosis in the United States: Past, present, and future. JAMA 1980;244:2318.

Young EJ: Human brucellosis. Rev Infect Dis 1983;5: 821.

Young EJ: Serologic diagnosis of human brucellosis: Analysis of 214 cases by aggglutinatioin tests and review of the literature. Rev Infect Dis 1991;13: 359.

Yersinia, Francisella, & Pasteurella 20

These organisms are short, pleomorphic, gram-negative rods that can exhibit bipolar staining. They do not form spores and are catalase-positive, oxidase-negative, and microaerophilic or facultatively anaerobic. Most have animals as their natural hosts, but they can produce serious disease in humans.

The genus *Yersinia* includes *Yersinia pestis,* the cause of plague; *Yersinia pseudotuberculosis* and *Yersinia enterocolitica,* important causes of human diarrheal diseases; and others. *Francisella tularensis* has vertebrate and invertebrate animal reservoirs and occasionally results in septic infections in humans. Several species of *Pasteurella* are primarily animal pathogens but can also produce human disease.

YERSINIA PESTIS & PLAGUE

Plague is an infection of wild rodents, transmitted from one rodent to another and occasionally from rodents to humans by the bites of fleas. Serious infection often results, which in previous centuries produced pandemics of "black death" with millions of fatalities.

Morphology & Identification

Y pestis is a plump gram-negative rod that exhibits striking bipolar staining with special stains (Figure 20–1). It is nonmotile. It grows as a facultative anaerobe on many bacteriologic media. Growth is more rapid in media containing blood or tissue fluids and fastest at 30 °C. In cultures on blood agar at 37 °C, colonies may be very small at 24 hours. A virulent inoculum, derived from infected tissue, produces gray and viscous colonies, but after passage in the laboratory the colonies become irregular and rough. The organism has little biochemical activity, and this is somewhat variable.

Antigenic Structure

All yersiniae possess lipopolysaccharides that have endotoxic activity when released. The organisms produce many antigens and toxins that act as virulence factors. The envelope contains a protein (fraction I) that is produced mainly at 37 °C, confers antiphagocytic properties, and activates complement. Virulent, wild-type *Y pestis* carries V-W antigens, which are encoded by genes on plasmids. A 72-kilobase plasmid is essential for virulence; avirulent strains lack this plasmid. Some stable, avirulent strains have served as live vaccines.

Y pestis produces a coagulase at 28 °C (the normal temperature of the flea) but not at 35 °C (transmission via fleas is low or absent in very hot weather).

Among several exotoxins produced, one is lethal for mice in amounts of 1 μg. This homogeneous protein (MW 74,000) produces beta-adrenergic blockade and is cardiotoxic in animals. Its role in human infection is unknown.

Y pestis also produces a bacteriocin (pesticin); the enzyme isocitrate lyase, which is said to be distinctive; and other products. Some antigens of *Y pestis* cross-react with other yersiniae; bacteriophages of *Y pestis* may lyse other yersiniae.

Pathogenesis & Pathology

When a flea feeds on a rodent infected with *Y pestis,* the ingested organisms multiply in the gut of the flea and, helped by the coagulase, block its proventriculus so that no food can pass through. Subsequently, the "blocked," hungry flea bites ferociously, and the aspirated blood, contaminated with *Y pestis* from the flea, is regurgitated into the bite wound. The inoculated organisms may be phagocytosed, but they can multiply intracellularly or extracellularly. They rapidly reach the lymphatics, and an intense hemorrhagic inflammation develops in the enlarged lymph nodes, which may undergo necrosis and become fluctuant. While the invasion may stop there, *Y pestis* often reach the bloodstream and become widely disseminated. Hemorrhagic and necrotic lesions may develop in all organs; meningitis, pneumonia, and serosanguineous pleuropericarditis are prominent.

Primary pneumonic plague results from inhalation of infective droplets (usually from a coughing patient), with hemorrhagic consolidation, sepsis, and death.

Clinical Findings

After an incubation period of 2–7 days, there is high fever and painful lymphadenopathy, commonly with greatly enlarged, tender nodes ("buboes") in the groin or axilla. Vomiting and diarrhea may develop with early sepsis. Later, disseminated intravascular coagu-

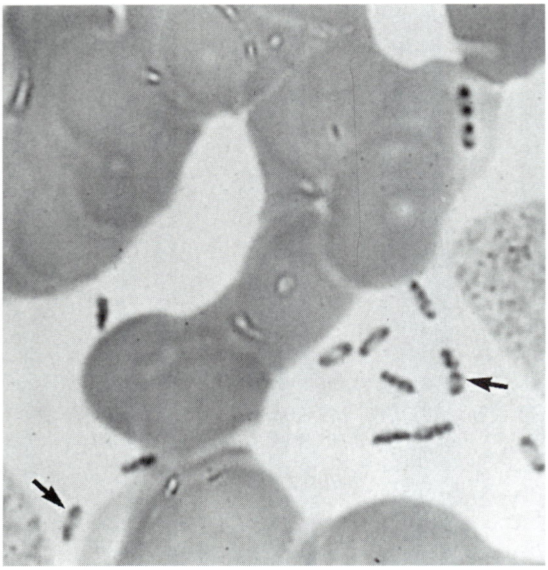

Figure 20–1. *Yersinia pestis* (arrows) in blood, Wright-Giemsa stain. Some of the *Y pestis* have bipolar staining, which gives them a hairpin-like appearance. (Courtesy of Dr Ken Gates, Plague Section, Centers for Disease Control and Prevention, Ft. Collins, Colorado.)

lation leads to hypotension, altered mental status, and renal and cardiac failure. Terminally, signs of pneumonia and meningitis can appear, and *Y pestis* multiplies intravascularly and can be seen in blood smears.

Diagnostic Laboratory Tests

Plague should be suspected in febrile patients who have been exposed to rodents in known endemic areas. Rapid recognition and laboratory confirmation of the disease are essential in order to institute lifesaving therapy.

A. Specimens: Blood is taken for culture and aspirates of enlarged lymph nodes for smear and culture. Acute and convalescent sera may be examined for antibody levels. In pneumonia, sputum is cultured; in possible meningitis, cerebrospinal fluid is taken for smear and culture.

B. Smears: Material from needle aspiration is examined after staining with Giemsa's stain and with specific immunofluorescent stains. With Wayson's stain, *Y pestis* may show a striking bipolar appearance. Spinal fluid and sputum smears should also be stained.

C. Culture: All materials are cultured on blood agar and MacConkey's agar plates and in infusion broth. Growth on solid media may be slow, but blood cultures are often positive in 24 hours. Cultures can be tentatively identified by biochemical reactions. Definite identification of cultures is best done by immunofluorescence (confirmation available through state health department laboratories and by consultation with the Centers for Disease Control and Prevention, Plague Branch, Fort Collins, CO 80522; telephone number: 303-221-6450).

All cultures are highly infectious and must be handled with extreme caution.

D. Serology: In patients who have not been previously vaccinated, a convalescent serum antibody titer of 1:16 or greater is presumptive evidence of *Y pestis* infection. A titer rise in two sequential specimens confirms the serologic diagnosis.

Treatment

Unless promptly treated, plague may have a mortality rate of nearly 50%; pneumonic plague, nearly 100%. The drug of choice is streptomycin. Tetracycline is an alternative drug and is sometimes given in combination with streptomycin. Drug resistance has not been noted in *Y pestis.*

Epidemiology & Control

Plague is an infection of wild rodents (field mice, gerbils, moles, skunks, and other animals) that occurs in many parts of the world. The chief enzootic areas are India, Southeast Asia (especially Vietnam), Africa, and North and South America. The western states of the USA and Mexico always contain reservoirs of infection. Epizootics with high mortality rates occur intermittently; at such times, the infection can spread to domestic rodents (eg, rats) and other animals (eg, cats), and humans can be infected by flea bites or by contact. The commonest vector of plague is the rat flea *(Xenopsylla cheopis),* but other fleas may also transmit the infection.

The control of plague requires surveys of infected animals, vectors, and human contacts. (In the USA this is done by county and state agencies with support from the Plague Branch of the Centers for Disease Control and Prevention) and by destruction of plague-infected animals. If a human case is diagnosed, health authorities must be notified promptly. All patients with suspected plague should be isolated, particularly if pulmonary involvement has not been ruled out. All specimens must be treated with extreme caution. Contacts of patients with suspected plague pneumonia should receive tetracycline, 0.5 g/d for 5 days, as chemoprophylaxis.

A formalin-killed vaccine is available for travelers to hyperendemic areas and for persons at special high risk.

YERSINIA ENTEROCOLITICA & *YERSINIA PSEUDOTUBERCULOSIS*

These are non-lactose-fermenting gram-negative rods that are urease-positive and oxidase-negative. They grow best at 25 °C and are motile at 25 °C but nonmotile at 37 °C. They are found in the intestinal tract of a variety of animals, in which they may cause disease, and are transmissible to humans, in whom they can produce a variety of clinical syndromes.

Y enterocolitica exists in more than 50 serotypes; most isolates from human disease belong to serotypes O3, O8, and O9. There are striking geographic differences in the distribution of *Y enterocolitica* serotypes. *Y pseudotuberculosis* exists in at least six serotypes, but serotype O1 accounts for most human infections. *Y enterocolitica* can produce a heat-stable enterotoxin, but the role of this toxin in diarrhea associated with infection is not well defined.

Y enterocolitica has been isolated from rodents and domestic animals (eg, sheep, cattle, swine, dogs, and cats) and waters contaminated by them. Transmission to humans probably occurs by contamination of food, drink, or fomites. *Y pseudotuberculosis* occurs in domestic and farm animals and birds, which excrete the organisms in feces. Human infection probably results from ingestion of materials contaminated with animal feces. Person-to-person transmission with either of these organisms is probably rare.

Pathogenesis & Clinical Findings

An inoculum of 10^8–10^9 yersiniae must enter the alimentary tract to produce infection. During the incubation period of 5–10 days, yersiniae multiply in the gut mucosa, particularly the ileum. This leads to inflammation and ulceration, and leukocytes appear in feces. The process may extend to mesenteric lymph nodes and, rarely, to bacteremia.

Early symptoms include fever, abdominal pain, and diarrhea. Diarrhea may be due to an enterotoxin or to the invasion of the mucosa, and it ranges from watery to bloody. At times, the abdominal pain is severe and located in the right lower quadrant, suggesting appendicitis. One to 2 weeks after onset some patients develop arthralgia, arthritis, and erythema nodosum, suggesting an immunologic reaction to the infection. Very rarely, *Yersinia* infection produces pneumonia, meningitis, or sepsis; in most cases, it is self-limited.

Diagnostic Laboratory Tests

A. Specimens: Specimens may be stool, blood, or material obtained at surgical exploration.

B. Smears: Stained smears are not contributory.

C. Culture: The number of yersiniae in stool may be small and can be increased by "cold enrichment": a small amount of feces or a rectal swab is placed in buffered saline, pH 7.6, and kept at 4 °C for 2–4 weeks; many fecal organisms do not survive, but *Y enterocolitica* will multiply. Subcultures made at intervals on MacConkey agar may yield yersiniae.

D. Serology: In paired serum specimens taken 2 or more weeks apart, a rise in agglutinating antibodies can be shown; however, cross reactions between yersiniae and other organisms (vibrios, salmonellae, brucellae) may confuse the results.

Treatment

Most *Yersinia* infections with diarrhea are self-limited, and the possible benefits of antimicrobial therapy are unknown. *Y enterocolitica* are generally susceptible to aminoglycosides, chloramphenicol, tetracycline, trimethoprim-sulfamethoxazole, piperacillin, third-generation cephalosporins, and fluoroquinolones; they typically are resistant to ampicillin, carbenicillin, and first-generation cephalosporins. Proved *Yersinia* sepsis or meningitis has a high mortality rate, but deaths occur mainly in immunocompromised patients. *Yersinia* sepsis can be successfully treated with third-generation cephalosporins (possibly in combination with an aminoglycoside) or a fluoroquinolone (possibly in combination with another antimicrobial). In cases where clinical manifestations strongly point to either appendicitis or mesenteric adenitis, surgical exploration has been the rule unless several simultaneous cases indicate that *Yersinia* infection is likely.

Prevention & Control

Contact with farm and domestic animals, their feces, or materials contaminated by them probably accounts for most human infections. Meat and dairy products have occasionally been indicated as sources of infection, and group outbreaks have been traced to contaminated food or drink. Conventional sanitary precautions are probably helpful. There are no specific preventive measures.

FRANCISELLA TULARENSIS & TULAREMIA

Francisella tularensis is widely found in animal reservoirs and is transmissible to humans by biting arthropods, direct contact with infected animal tissue, inhalation of aerosols, or ingestion of contaminated food or water. The resulting disease, tularemia, is rare in the USA, and its clinical presentation depends on the route of infection.

Morphology & Identification

A. Typical Organisms: *F tularensis* is a small, gram-negative, pleomorphic rod. It is rarely seen in smears of tissue.

B. Specimens: Blood is taken for serologic tests.

C. Culture: Growth does not occur in most ordinary bacteriologic media, but small colonies appear in 1–3 days on glucose cysteine blood agar or glucose blood agar incubated at 37 °C under aerobic conditions. The organism is usually identified by its growth requirements and immunofluorescence staining or agglutination by specific antisera. ***Caution:*** In order to avoid laboratory-acquired infection, *Francisella* should not be cultured in ordinary clinical laboratory facilities; this should be undertaken only with proper isolation facilities.

D. Serology: All isolates are serologically identical, possessing a polysaccharide antigen and one or more protein antigens that cross-react with brucellae.

However, there are two biologic categories of strains, called Jellison type A and type B. Type A occurs only in North America, is lethal for rabbits, produces severe illness in humans, ferments glycerol, and contains citrulline ureidase. Type B lacks these biochemical features, is not lethal for rabbits, produces milder disease in humans, and is isolated often from rodents or from water in Europe, Asia, and North America.

The usual antibody response consists of agglutinins developing 7–10 days after onset of illness.

Pathogenesis & Clinical Findings

F tularensis is highly infectious: penetration of the skin or mucous membranes or inhalation of 50 organisms can result in infection. Most commonly, organisms enter through skin abrasions. In 2–6 days, an inflammatory, ulcerating papule develops. Regional lymph nodes enlarge and may become necrotic, sometimes draining for weeks. Inhalation of an infective aerosol results in peribronchial inflammation and localized pneumonitis. Oculoglandular tularemia can develop when an infected finger or droplet touches the conjunctiva. Yellowish granulomatous lesions on the lids may be accompanied by preauricular adenopathy. In all cases, there is fever, malaise, headache, and pain in the involved region and regional lymph nodes.

Diagnostic Laboratory Tests

In general, smears and cultures are not contributory, and the diagnosis rests on serologic studies. Paired serum samples collected 2 weeks apart can show a rise in agglutination titer. A single serum titer of 1:160 is highly suggestive if the history and physical findings are compatible with the diagnosis. Because antibodies reactive in the agglutination test for tularemia also react in the test for brucellosis, both tests should be done for positive sera; the titer for the disease affecting the patient is usually fourfold greater than that for the other disease. A skin test (availability of the antigen is limited) may give a tuberculin-like response in the first week of illness, often before the agglutination titer rises.

Treatment

Streptomycin or gentamicin therapy for 10 days produces almost uniform rapid improvement. Tetracycline may be equally effective, but relapses occur more frequently. Ceftriaxone is not effective.

Prevention & Control

Humans acquire tularemia from handling infected rabbits or muskrats or from bites by an infected tick or deerfly. Less often, the source is contaminated water or food or contact with a dog or cat that has caught an infected wild animal. Avoidance is the key to prevention. The infection in wild animals cannot be controlled.

Persons at exceedingly high risk, particularly laboratory personnel, may be immunized by the administration of a live attenuated strain of *F tularensis*, available from the US Army Medical Research Institute of Infectious Diseases, Fort Detrick, Frederick, MD 21701. The vaccine is administered by multiple punctures through the skin. While not completely protective, it provides partial immunity. A similar live vaccine has been administered in Russia on a large scale.

THE PASTEURELLAE

Pasteurella species are primarily animal pathogens, but they can produce a range of human diseases. The generic term pasteurellae formerly included all yersiniae and *Francisella* as well as the pasteurellae discussed below.

Pasteurellae are nonmotile gram-negative coccobacilli with a bipolar appearance on stained smears. They are aerobes or facultative anaerobes that grow readily on ordinary bacteriologic media at 37 °C. They are all oxidase-positive and catalase-positive but diverge in other biochemical reactions.

Pasteurella multocida occurs worldwide in the respiratory and gastrointestinal tracts of many domestic and wild animals. It is perhaps the most common organism in human wounds inflicted by bites from cats and dogs. It is one of the common causes of hemorrhagic septicemia in a variety of animals, including rabbits, rats, horses, sheep, fowl, cats, and swine. It can also produce human infections in many systems and may at times be part of normal human flora.

Pasteurella hemolytica occurs in the upper respiratory tract of cattle, sheep, swine, horses, and fowl. It is a prominent cause of epizootic pneumonia in cattle and sheep and of fowl cholera in chickens and turkeys, causing major economic losses. Human infection appears to be rare.

Pasteurella pneumotropica is a normal inhabitant of the respiratory tract and gut of mice and rats and can cause pneumonia or sepsis when the host-parasite balance is disturbed. A few human infections have followed animal bites.

Pasteurella ureae has rarely been found in animals but occurs as part of a mixed flora in human chronic respiratory disease or other suppurative infections.

Clinical Findings

The most common presentation is an animal bite, with acute onset of redness, swelling, and pain within hours of the bite. Regional lymphadenopathy is variable, and fever is often low-grade. Sometimes *Pasteurella* infections present as bacteremia or chronic respiratory infection without an evident connection with animals.

REFERENCES

Yersinia pestis & Plague

Butler T et al: *Yersinia pestis* infection in VietNam. J Infect Dis 1976;133:493.

LD, Tempest B: Plague: A clinical review of 27 cases. Arch Int Med 1992;152:1253.

Straley SC: The low-Ca^{2+} response virulence regulon of human-pathogenic yersinae. Microb Pathogen 1991; 10:87.

von Reyn CF et al: Epidemiological and clinical features of an outbreak of bubonic plague in New Mexico. J Infect Dis 1977;136:489.

Williams JE, Cavanaugh DC: Measuring the efficacy of vaccination in affording protection against plague. Bull WHO 1979;57:309.

Yersinia enterocolitica & *Yersinia pseudotuberculosis*

Cover TL, Aber RC: *Yersinia enterocolitica.* N Engl J Med 1989;321:16.

Gayraud M et al: Antibiotic treatment of *Yersinia enterocolitica* septicemia: A retrospective review of 43 cases. Clin Infect Dis 1993;17:405.

Isberg RR, Falkow S: A single genetic locus encoded by *Yersinia pseudotuberculosis* permits invasion of cultured animal cells by *Escherichia coli* K12. Nature 1985;317:262.

Rabson AR et al: Generalized *Yersinia enterocolitica* infection. J Infect Dis 1975;131:447.

Franciscella tularensis & Tularemia

Cross JT, Jacobs RF: Tularemia: Treatment failures with outpatient use of ceftriaxone. Clin Infect Dis 1993;17: 976.

Evans ME et al: Tularemia: A 30-year experience with 88 cases. Medicine 1985;64:251.

Guerrant RL et al: Tickborne oculoglandular tularemia: Case report and review of seasonal and vectorial associations in 106 cases. Arch Intern Med 1976; 136:811.

Mason WL et al: Treatment of tularemia, including pulmonary tularemia, with gentamicin. Am Rev Respir Dis 1980;121:39.

Waag DM et al: Cell-mediated and humoral immune responses induced by scarification vaccination of human volunteers with a new lot of the live vaccine strain of *Franciscella tularensis.* J Clin Microbiol 1992;30:2256.

Pasteurella

Minton EJ: *Pasteurella pneumotropica:* meningitis following a dog bite. Postgrad Med J 1990;66:125.

Weber DJ et al: *Pasteurella multocida* infections: Report of 34 cases and review of the literature. Medicine 1984;63:133.

21 The Neisseriae

The family Neisseriaceae includes *Neisseria* species and *Moraxella (Branhamella) catarrhalis* as well as *Acinetobacter* and *Kingella* and other *Moraxella* species (see Chapter 17). The neisseriae are gram-negative cocci that usually occur in pairs. *Neisseria gonorrhoeae* (gonococci) and *Neisseria meningitidis* (meningococci) are pathogenic for humans and typically are found associated with or inside polymorphonuclear cells. Some neisseriae are normal inhabitants of the human respiratory tract, rarely if ever cause disease, and occur extracellularly. Members of the group are listed in Table 21–1.

Gonococci and meningococci are closely related, with 70% DNA homology, and are differentiated by a few laboratory tests and specific characteristics: meningococci have polysaccharide capsules, whereas gonococci do not, and meningococci rarely have plasmids whereas most gonococci do. Most importantly, the two species are differentiated by the usual clinical presentations of the diseases they cause: meningococci typically are found in the upper respiratory tract and cause meningitis, while gonococci cause genital infections. The clinical spectra of the diseases caused by gonococci and meningococci overlap, however. Study of the pathogenic neisseriae, especially the gonococci, has contributed greatly to our knowledge about the molecular basis of diseases caused by mucosal pathogens.

Morphology & Identification

A. Typical Organisms: The typical *Neisseria* is a gram-negative, nonmotile diplococcus, approximately 0.8 μm in diameter (Figures 21–1 and 21–2). Individual cocci are kidney-shaped; when the organisms occur in pairs, the flat or concave sides are adjacent.

B. Culture: In 48 hours on enriched media (eg, Mueller-Hinton, modified Thayer-Martin), gonococci and meningococci form convex, glistening, elevated, mucoid colonies 1–5 mm in diameter. Colonies are transparent or opaque, nonpigmented, and nonhemolytic. *Neisseria flavescens, Neisseria subflava,* and *Neisseria lactamica* have yellow pigmentation. *Neisseria sicca* produces opaque, brittle, wrinkled colonies. *M catarrhalis* produces nonpigmented or pinkish-gray opaque colonies.

C. Growth Characteristics: The neisseriae grow best under aerobic conditions, but some will grow in an anaerobic environment. They have complex growth requirements. Most neisseriae ferment carbohydrates, producing acid but not gas, and their carbohydrate fermentation patterns are a means of distinguishing them (Table 21–1). The neisseriae produce oxidase and give positive oxidase reactions; the oxidase test is a key test for identifying them. When bacteria are spotted on a filter paper soaked with tetramethylparaphenylenediamine hydrochloride (oxidase), the neisseriae rapidly turn dark purple.

Meningococci and gonococci grow best on media containing complex organic substances such as heated blood, hemin, and animal proteins and in an atmosphere containing 5% CO_2 (eg, candle jar). Growth is inhibited by some toxic constituents of the medium, eg, fatty acids or salts. The organisms are rapidly killed by drying, sunlight, moist heat, and many disinfectants. They produce autolytic enzymes that result in rapid swelling and lysis in vitro at 25 °C and at an alkaline pH.

NEISSERIA GONORRHOEAE (Gonococcus)

Gonococci ferment only glucose and differ antigenically from the other neisseriae. Gonococci usually produce smaller colonies than those of the other neisseriae. Gonococci that require arginine, hypoxanthine, and uracil (Arg^-, Hyx^-, Ura^- auxotype) tend to grow most slowly on primary culture. Gonococci isolated from clinical specimens or maintained by selective subculture have typical small colonies containing piliated bacteria. On nonselective subculture, larger colonies containing nonpiliated gonococci are also formed. Opaque and transparent variants of both the small and large colony types also occur; the opaque colonies are associated with the presence of a surface-exposed protein, Opa (protein II).

Antigenic Structure

N gonorrhoeae is antigenically heterogeneous and capable of changing its surface structures in vitro—and presumably in vivo—to avoid host defenses. Surface structures include the following:

Table 21–1. Biochemical reactions of the neisseriae.

	Growth on MTM, ML, or NYC Medium[1]	Acid Formed From				DNase
		Glucose	Maltose	Lactose	Sucrose or Fructose	
N gonorrhoeae	+	+	–	–	–	–
N meningitidis	+	+	+	–	–	–
N lactamica	+	+	+	+	–	–
N sicca	–	+	+	–	+	–
N subflava	–	+	+	–	±	–
N mucosa	–	+	+	–	+	–
N flavescens	–	–	–	–	–	–
N cinerea	±	–	–	–	–	–
M catarrhalis	–	–	–	–	–	+

[1]MTM = modified Thayer-Martin medium, ML = Martin-Lewis medium, NYC = New York City medium.

A. Pili: Pili are the hair-like appendages that extend up to several micrometers from the gonococcal surface. They enhance attachment to host cells and resistance to phagocytosis. They are made up of stacked pilin proteins (MW 17,000–21,000). The amino terminal of the pilin molecule, which contains a high percentage of hydrophobic amino acids, is conserved. The amino acid sequence near the mid portion of the molecule also is conserved; this portion of the molecule serves in attachment to host cells and is less prominent in the immune response. The amino acid sequence near the carboxyl terminal is highly variable; this portion of the molecule is most prominent in the immune response. The pilins of almost all strains of *N gonorrhoeae* are antigenically different, and a single strain can make many antigenically distinct forms of pilin.

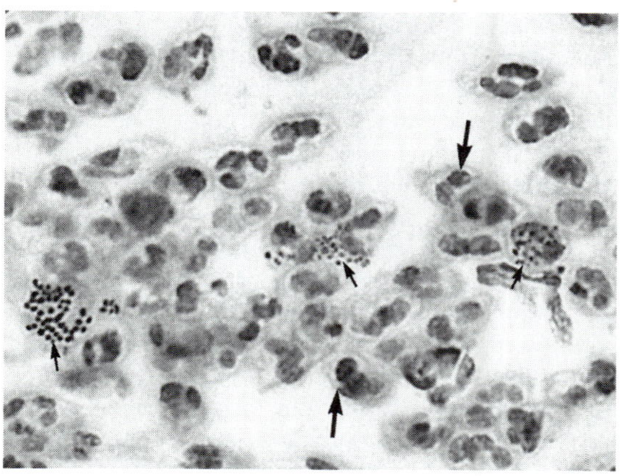

Figure 21–1. Gram stain of a urethral exudate of a patient with gonorrhea. Nuclei and cell membrane outlines of many polymorphonuclear cells are seen (two shown by large arrows). Intracellular gram-negative diplocccci *(Neisseria gonorrhoeae)* in clumps are marked by the small arrows.

B. Por (Protein I): Por extends through the gonococcal cell membrane. It occurs in trimers to form pores in the surface through which some nutrients enter the cell. The molecular weight of Por varies from 34,000 to 37,000. Each strain of gonococcus expresses only one type of Por, but the Por of different strains is antigenically different. Serologic typing of Por by agglutination reactions with monoclonal antibodies has distinguished 18 serovars of porA and 28 serovars of PorB. (Serotyping is done only in reference laboratories.)

C. Opa (Protein II): This protein functions in adhesion of gonococci within colonies and in attachment of gonococci to host cells. One portion of the Opa molecule is in the gonococcal outer membrane, and the rest is exposed on the surface. The molecular weight of Opa ranges from 24,000 to 32,000. A strain of gonococcus can express no, one, two, or occasionally three types of Opa, though each strain has ten or more genes for different Opas. Opa is present in gonococci from opaque colonies but may or may not be present in those from transparent colonies.

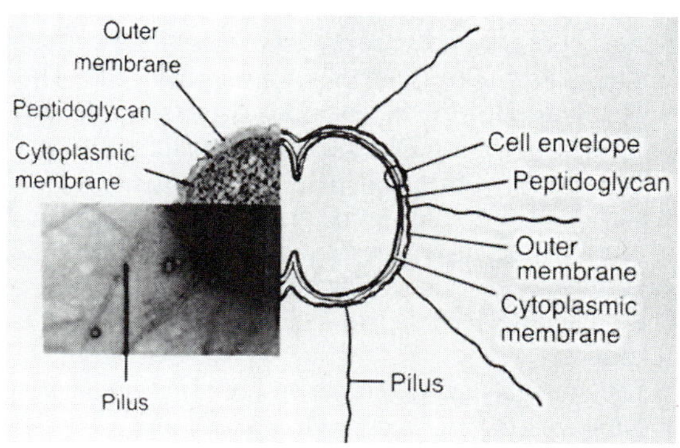

Figure 21–2. Collage and drawing of *N gonorrhoeae* showing pili and the three layers of the cell envelope.

D. Rmp (Protein III): This protein (MW about 33,000) is antigenically conserved in all gonococci. It is a reduction-modifiable protein (Rmp) and changes its apparent molecular weight when in a reduced state. It associates with Por in the formation of pores in the cell surface.

E. Lipooligosaccharide (LOS): In contrast to that of the enteric gram-negative rods (see Chapter 16), gonococcal LPS does not have long O-antigenic side chains and is sometimes called a lipooligosaccharide. Its molecular weight is 3000–7000. Gonococci can express more than one antigenically different LOS chain simultaneously. Toxicity in gonococcal infections is largely due to the endotoxic effects of LOS.

F. Other Proteins: Several antigenically constant proteins of gonococci have poorly defined roles in pathogenesis. **Lip (H8)** is a surface-exposed protein that is heat-modifiable like Opa. The **Fbp (iron-binding protein),** similar in molecular weight to Por, is expressed when the available iron supply is limited, eg, in human infection. Gonococci elaborate an **IgA1 protease** that splits and inactivates IgA1, a major mucosal immunoglobulin of humans. Meningococci, *Haemophilus influenzae,* and *Streptococcus pneumoniae* elaborate a similar IgA1 protease.

Table 21–2. Antigenic heterogeneity of *Neisseria gonorrhoeae.*

Antigen	Number of Types
Pilin	Hundreds
Por (protein I) (US system)	PorA with 18 subtypes PorB with 28 subtypes
Opa (protein II)	Many (perhaps hundreds)
Rmp (protein III)	One
Lipopolysaccharide	Six identified (probably more)
Fbp (iron-binding protein)	One
Lip (H8)	One
IgA1 protease	Two

Genetics & Antigenic Heterogeneity

Gonococci have evolved mechanisms for frequently switching from one antigenic form (pilin, Opa, or lipopolysaccharide) to another antigenic form of the same molecule. This switching takes place in one in every 10^3 gonococci, an extremely rapid rate of change for bacteria. Since pilin, Opa, and lipooligosaccharide are surface-exposed antigens on gonococci, they are important in the immune response to infection. The molecules' rapid switching from one antigenic form to another helps the gonococci elude the host immune system.

The switching mechanism for pilin, which has been the most thoroughly studied, is different from the mechanism for Opa.

Gonococci have multiple genes that code for pilin, but only one gene is inserted into the expression site. Gonococci can remove all or part of this pilin gene and replace it with all or part of another pilin gene. This mechanism allows gonococci to express many antigenically different pilin molecules over time.

The switching mechanism of Opa involves, at least in part, the addition or removal from the DNA of one or more of the pentameric coding repeats preceding the sequence that codes for the structural Opa gene. The switching mechanism of lipooligosaccharide is unknown.

The antigens and heterogeneity of types are shown in Table 21–2.

Gonococci contain several plasmids; 95% of strains have a small, "cryptic" plasmid (MW 2.4×10^6) of unknown function. Two other plasmids (MW 3.4×10^6 and 4.7×10^6) contain genes that code for β-lactamase production, which causes resistance to penicillin. These plasmids are transmissible by conjugation among gonococci; they are similar to a plasmid found in penicillinase-producing *Haemophilus* and may have been acquired from *Haemophilus* or other gram-negative organisms. Five to 20% of gonococci contain a plasmid (MW 24.5×10^6) with the genes that code for conjugation; the incidence is highest in geographic areas where penicillinase-producing gonococci are most common. High-level tetracycline resistance has developed in gonococci by the insertion of a streptococcal gene coding for tetracycline resistance into the conjugative plasmid.

Pathogenesis, Pathology, & Clinical Findings

Gonococci exhibit several morphologic types of colonies (see above), but only piliated bacteria from small colonies appear to be virulent. Gonococci that form opaque colonies and express Opa are isolated from men with symptomatic urethritis and from uterine cervical cultures at mid cycle. Gonococci that form transparent colonies are frequently isolated from men with asymptomatic urethral infection, from menstruating women, and from invasive forms of gonorrhea, including salpingitis and disseminated infection. In women, the colony type formed by a single strain of gonococcus changes during the menstrual cycle.

Gonococci attack mucous membranes of the genitourinary tract, eye, rectum, and throat, producing acute suppuration that may lead to tissue invasion; this is followed by chronic inflammation and fibrosis. In males, there is usually urethritis, with yellow, creamy pus and painful urination. The process may extend to the epididymis. As suppuration subsides in untreated infection, fibrosis occurs, sometimes leading to urethral strictures. Urethral infection in men can be asymptomatic. In females, the primary infection is in the endocervix and extends to the urethra and vagina, giving rise to mucopurulent discharge. It may then progress to the uterine tubes, causing salpingitis, fibrosis, and obliteration of the tubes. Infertility occurs in 20% of women with gonococcal salpingitis. Chronic gonococcal cervicitis or proctitis is often asymptomatic.

Gonococcal bacteremia leads to skin lesions (especially hemorrhagic papules and pustules) on the hands, forearms, feet, and legs and to tenosynovitis and suppurative arthritis, usually of the knees, ankles, and wrists. Gonococci can be cultured from blood or joint fluid of only 30% of patients with gonococcal arthritis. Gonococcal endocarditis is an uncommon but severe infection. Gonococci sometimes cause meningitis and eye infections in adults; these have manifestations similar to those due to meningococci.

Gonococcal ophthalmia neonatorum, an infection of the eye of the newborn, is acquired during passage through an infected birth canal. The initial conjunctivitis rapidly progresses and, if untreated, results in blindness. To prevent gonococcal ophthalmia neonatorum, instillation of tetracycline, erythromycin, or silver nitrate into the conjunctival sac of the newborn is compulsory in the USA.

Gonococci that produce localized infection are often serum-sensitive but relatively resistant to antimicrobial drugs. In contrast, gonococci that enter the bloodstream and produce disseminated infection are usually serum-resistant and may be quite susceptible to penicillin and other antimicrobial drugs.

Diagnostic Laboratory Tests

A. Specimens: Pus and secretions are taken from the urethra, cervix, rectum, conjunctiva, throat, or synovial fluid for culture and smear. Blood culture is necessary in systemic illness, but a special culture system is helpful, since gonococci (and meningococci) are susceptible to the polyanethol sulfonate present in standard blood culture media.

B. Smears: Gram-stained smears of urethral or endocervical exudate reveal many diplococci within pus cells. These give a presumptive diagnosis (Figure 21–1). Stained smears of the urethral exudate from men have a sensitivity of about 90% and a specificity of 99%. Stained smears of endocervical exudates have a sensitivity of about 50% and a specificity of about 95% when examined by an experienced microscopist. Cultures of urethral exudate from men are not necessary when the stain is positive, but cultures should be done for women. Stained smears of conjunctival exudates can also be diagnostic, but those of specimens from the throat or rectum are generally not helpful.

C. Culture: Immediately after collection, pus or mucus is streaked on enriched selective medium (eg, modified Thayer-Martin medium—Public Health Rep 1966;81:559) and incubated in an atmosphere containing 5% CO_2 (candle extinction jar) at 37 °C. To avoid overgrowth by contaminants, the culture medium should contain antimicrobial drugs (eg, vancomycin, 3 μg/mL; colistin, 7.5 μg/mL; amphotericin B, 1 μg/mL; and trimethoprim, 3 μg/mL). If immediate incubation is not possible, the specimen should be placed in a culture transport system. Forty-eight hours after culture, the organisms can be quickly identified by their appearance on a Gram-stained smear, by oxidase positivity, and by coagglutination, immunofluorescence staining, or other laboratory tests. The species of subcultured bacteria may be determined by fermentation reactions (Table 21–1). The neisserial isolates from anatomic sites other than the genital tract should be identified as to species.

D. Serology: Serum and genital fluid contain IgG and IgA antibodies against gonococcal pili, outer membrane proteins, and LOS. Some IgM of human sera is bactericidal for gonococci in vitro.

In infected individuals, antibodies to gonococcal pili and outer membrane proteins can be detected by immunoblotting, radioimmunoassay, and ELISA (enzyme-linked immunosorbent assay) tests. However, these tests are not useful as diagnostic aids for several reasons: gonococcal antigenic heterogeneity; the delay in development of antibodies in acute infection; and a high background level of antibodies in the sexually active population.

Immunity

Repeated gonococcal infections are common. Protective immunity to reinfection does not appear to develop as part of the disease process, because of the antigenic variety of gonococci. While antibodies can be demonstrated, including the IgA and IgG on mucosal surfaces, they either are highly strain-specific or have little protective ability.

Treatment

Since the development and widespread use of penicillin, gonococcal resistance to penicillin has gradually risen, owing to the selection of chromosomal mutants, so that many strains now require high concentrations of penicillin G for inhibition (MIC $\geq$ 1 μg/mL). Penicillinase-producing *N gonorrhoeae* (PPNG) also have increased in prevalence (see above). Chromosomally mediated resistance to tetracycline (MIC $\geq$ 1 μg/mL) is common, with 40% or more of gonococci resistant at this level. High-level resistance to tetracycline (MIC $\geq$ 32 μg/mL) also occurs. Spectinomycin resistance as well as resistance to other antimicrobials has been noted. Because of the problems with antimicrobial resistance in *N gonorrhoeae,* the United States Public Health Service recommends that uncomplicated genital or rectal infections be treated with ceftriaxone, intramuscularly as a single dose. Additional therapy with doxycycline is recommended for the possible concomitant chlamydial infection; erythromycin base is substituted for doxycycline in pregnant women. Modifications of these therapies are recommended for other types of *N gonorrhoeae* infection.

In urethritis in men, if clinical cure is apparent after treatment, it is not necessary to prove cure by culture.

In other forms of gonococcal infection, cure should be established by follow-up, including cultures from the involved sites. Since other sexually transmitted diseases may have been acquired at the same time, steps must also be taken to diagnose and treat these diseases (see discussions of chlamydiae, syphilis, etc).

Epidemiology, Prevention, & Control

Gonorrhea is worldwide in distribution, and its incidence has risen steadily since 1955. It is almost exclusively transmitted by sexual contact, often by women and men with asymptomatic infections. The infectivity of the organism is such that the chance of acquiring infection from a single exposure to an infected sexual partner is 20–30% for men and even greater for women. The infection rate can be reduced by avoiding multiple sexual partners, rapidly eradicating gonococci from infected individuals by means of early diagnosis and treatment, and finding cases and contacts through education and screening of populations at high risk. Mechanical prophylaxis (condoms) provides partial protection. Chemoprophylaxis is of limited value because of the rise in antibiotic resistance of the gonococcus.

PPNG first appeared in 1976. These totally penicillin-resistant gonococcal strains have appeared in many parts of the world, with the highest incidence in special populations, eg, 50% in some prostitute groups. Other areas with a high incidence of PPNG include areas in Asia, parts of sub-Saharan Africa, and some places in USA. Focal outbreaks of disease due to PPNG have occurred in many areas of the USA and elsewhere, and endemic foci are being established.

Gonococcal ophthalmia neonatorum is prevented by local application of 0.5% erythromycin ophthalmic ointment or 1% tetracycline ointment to the conjunctiva of newborns. Although instillation of silver nitrate solution is also effective and is the classic method for preventing ophthalmia neonatorum, silver nitrate is difficult to store and causes conjunctival irritation; its use has largely been replaced by use of erythromycin or tetracycline ointment.

NEISSERIA MENINGITIDIS (Meningococcus)

Antigenic Structure

At least 13 serogroups of meningococci have been identified by immunologic specificity of capsular polysaccharides. The most important serogroups associated with disease in humans are A, B, C, Y, and W-135. The group A polysaccharide is a polymer of N-acetylmannosamine phosphate, and that of group C is a polymer of N-acetyl-O-acetylneuraminic acid. Meningococcal antigens are found in blood and cerebrospinal fluid of patients with active disease. Outbreaks and sporadic cases in the Western Hemisphere in the last decade have been caused mainly by groups B, C, W-135, and Y; outbreaks in southern Finland and São Paulo, Brazil, were due to groups A and C; those in Africa were due mainly to group A. Group C and, especially, group A are associated with epidemic disease.

The outer membrane proteins of meningococci have been divided into classes on the basis of molecular weight. All strains have either class 1, class 2, or class 3 proteins; these are analogous to the Por proteins of gonococci and are responsible for the serotype specificity of meningococci. They help form pores in the meningococcal cell wall. As many as 20 serotypes have been defined; serotypes 2 and 15 have been associated with epidemic disease. The Opa (class 5) protein is comparable to Opa of the gonococci. Meningococci are piliated, but unlike gonococci, they do not form distinctive colony types indicating piliated bacteria. Meningococcal LOS is responsible for many of the toxic effects found in meningococcal disease.

Pathogenesis, Pathology, & Clinical Findings

Humans are the only natural hosts for whom meningococci are pathogenic. The nasopharynx is the portal of entry. There, the organisms attach to epithelial cells with the aid of pili; they may form part of the transient flora without producing symptoms. From the nasopharynx, organisms may reach the bloodstream, producing bacteremia; the symptoms may be like those of an upper respiratory tract infection. Fulminant meningococcemia is more severe, with high fever and hemorrhagic rash; there may be disseminated intravascular coagulation and circulatory collapse (Waterhouse-Friderichsen syndrome).

Meningitis is the most common complication of meningococcemia. It usually begins suddenly, with intense headache, vomiting, and stiff neck, and progresses to coma within a few hours.

During meningococcemia, there is thrombosis of many small blood vessels in many organs, with perivascular infiltration and petechial hemorrhages. There may be interstitial myocarditis, arthritis, and skin lesions. In meningitis, the meninges are acutely inflamed, with thrombosis of blood vessels and exudation of polymorphonuclear leukocytes, so that the surface of the brain is covered with a thick purulent exudate.

It is not known what transforms an asymptomatic infection of the nasopharynx into meningococcemia and meningitis, but this can be prevented by specific bactericidal serum antibodies against the infecting serotype. *Neisseria* bacteremia is favored by the absence of bactericidal antibody (IgM and IgG), inhibition of serum bactericidal action by a blocking IgA antibody, or a complement deficiency (C5, C6, C7, or C8). Meningococci are readily phagocytosed in the presence of a specific opsonin.

Diagnostic Laboratory Tests

A. Specimens: Specimens of blood are taken for culture, and specimens of spinal fluid are taken for smear, culture, and chemical determinations. Nasopharyngeal swab cultures are suitable for carrier surveys. Puncture material from petechiae may be taken for smear and culture.

B. Smears: Gram-stained smears of the sediment of centrifuged spinal fluid or of petechial aspirate often show typical neisseriae within polymorphonuclear leukocytes or extracellularly.

C. Culture: Culture media without sodium polyanethol sulfonate are helpful in culturing blood specimens. Cerebrospinal fluid specimens are plated on heated blood agar ("chocolate" agar) and incubated at 37 °C in an atmosphere of 5% CO_2 (candle jar). Freshly drawn spinal fluid can be directly incubated at 37 °C if agar culture media are not immediately available. A modified Thayer-Martin medium with antibiotics (vancomycin, colistin, amphotericin) favors the growth of neisseriae, inhibits many other bacteria, and is used for nasopharyngeal cultures. Presumptive colonies of neisseriae on solid media, particularly in mixed culture, can be identified by the oxidase test. Spinal fluid and blood generally yield pure cultures that can be further identified by carbohydrate fermentation reactions (Table 21–1) and agglutination with type-specific or polyvalent serum.

D. Serology: Antibodies to meningococcal polysaccharides can be measured by latex agglutination or hemagglutination tests or by their bactericidal activity. These tests are done only in reference laboratories.

Immunity

Immunity to meningococcal infection is associated with the presence of specific, complement-dependent, bactericidal antibodies in the serum. These antibodies develop after subclinical infections with different strains or injection of antigens and are group-specific, type-specific, or both. The immunizing antigens for groups A, C, Y, and W-135 are the capsular polysaccharides. For group B, an antigen suitable for use as a vaccine has not been defined. Infants may have passive immunity through IgG antibodies transferred from the mother. Children under the age of 2 years do not reliably produce antibodies when immunized with meningococcal or other bacterial polysaccharides.

Treatment

Penicillin G is the drug of choice for treating meningococcal disease. Either chloramphenicol or a third-generation cephalosporin such as cefotaxime or ceftriaxone is used in persons allergic to penicillins.

Epidemiology, Prevention, & Control

Meningococcal meningitis occurs in epidemic waves (eg, in military encampments; sub-Saharan Africa, Brazil, there were more than 15,000 cases in 1974) and a smaller number of sporadic interepidemic cases. Five to 30% of the normal population may harbor meningococci (often nontypable isolates) in the nasopharynx during interepidemic periods. During epidemics, the carrier rate goes up to 70–80%. A rise in the number of cases is preceded by an increased number of respiratory carriers. Treatment with oral penicillin does not eradicate the carrier state. Rifampin or minocycline, orally, can often eradicate the carrier state and serve as chemoprophylaxis for household and other close contacts. Since the appearance of many sulfonamide-resistant meningococci, chemoprophylaxis with sulfonamides is no longer reliable.

Clinical cases of meningitis present only a negligible source of infection, and isolation therefore has only limited usefulness. More important is the reduction of personal contacts in a population with a high carrier rate. This is accomplished by avoidance of crowding. Specific polysaccharides of groups A, C, Y, and W-135 can stimulate antibody response and protect susceptible persons against infection. Such vaccines are currently used in selected populations (eg, the military; civilian epidemics). Vaccines for group B are under clinical investigation.

OTHER NEISSERIAE

Neisseria lactamica very rarely causes disease but is important because it grows in the selective media (eg, modified Thayer-Martin medium) used for cultures of gonococci and meningococci from clinical specimens. *N lactamica* can be cultured from the nasopharynx of 3–40% of persons and most often is found in children. Unlike the other neisseriae, it ferments lactose.

Neisseria sicca, Neisseria subflava, Neisseria cinera, Neisseria mucosa, and *Neisseria flavescens* are also members of the normal flora of the respiratory tract, particularly the nasopharynx, and very rarely produce disease. *N cinera* sometimes resembles *N gonorrhoeae* because of its carbohydrate fermentation patterns.

Moraxella catarrhalis was previously named *Branhamella catarrhalis* and before that *Neisseria catarrhalis.* It is a member of the normal flora in 40–50% of normal school children. *M catarrhalis* causes bronchitis, pneumonia, sinusitis, otitis media, and conjunctivitis. It is also of concern as a cause of infection in immunocompromised patients. Most strains of *M catarrhalis* from clinically significant infections produce β-lactamase. *M catarrhalis* can be differentiated from the other neisseriae by its lack of carbohydrate fermentation and by its production of DNase. It produces butyrate esterase, which forms the basis for rapid fluorometric tests for identification.

REFERENCES

Britigan BE et al: Gonococcal infection: A model of molecular pathogenesis. N Engl J Med 1985;312:1683.

Catlin BW: *Branhamella catarrhalis*: An organism gaining respect as a pathogen. Clin Microbiol Rev 1990;3:293.

DeVoe IW: The meningococcus and mechanisms of pathogenicity. Microbiol Rev 1982;46:162.

Frasch CE et al: Serotype antigens of *Neisseria meningitidis* and a proposed scheme for designation of serotypes. Rev Infect Dis 1985;7:504.

Hook EW III, Holmes KK: Gonococcal infections. Ann Intern Med 1985;102:229.

Knapp JS et al: Characterization of *Neisseria cinerea,* a nonpathogenic species isolated on Martin-Lewis medium selective for pathogenic *Neisseria* spp. J Clin Microbiol 1984;19:63.

Mandrell RE, Apicella MA: Lipo-oligosaccharides (LOS) of mucosal pathogens: Molecular mimicry and host-modification of LOS. Immunobiology 1993;187:382.

Marchant CD: Spectrum of disease due to *Branhamella catarrhalis* in children with special reference to otitis media. Am J Med 1990;88 (Suppl 5A):15S.

Morse SA et al (editors): Perspectives on pathogenic neisseriae. Clin Microbiol Rev 1989;2(Suppl):S1.

1993 Sexually Transmitted Diseases Treatment Guidelines. MMWR Morb Mortal Wkly Rep 1993;48(RR-14):1.

Olyhoek T, Crowe BA, Achtman M: Clonal population structure of *Neisseria meningitidis* serogroup A isolated from epidemics and pandemics between 1915 and 1983. Rev Infect Dis 1987;9:665.

Powers D et al: Epidemic meningococcemia and purpura fulminans with induced protein C deficiency. Clin Infect Dis 1993;17:254.

Infections Caused by Anaerobic Bacteria

22

Medically important infections due to anaerobic bacteria are common. The infections are often polymicrobial—that is, the anaerobic bacteria are found in mixed infections with other anaerobes, facultative anaerobes, and aerobes (see the glossary of definitions). Anaerobic bacteria are found throughout the human body—on the skin, on mucosal surfaces, and in high concentrations in the mouth and gastrointestinal tract—as part of the normal flora (see Chapter 11). Infection results when anaerobes and other bacteria of the normal flora contaminate normally sterile body sites.

Several important diseases are caused by anaerobic *Clostridium* species from the environment or from normal flora: botulism, tetanus, gas gangrene, food poisoning, and pseudomembranous colitis. These diseases are discussed in Chapters 9 and 12 and briefly later in this chapter.

PHYSIOLOGY & GROWTH CONDITIONS FOR ANAEROBES

Anaerobic bacteria will not grow in the presence of oxygen and are killed by oxygen or toxic oxygen radicals (see below). pH and oxidation-reduction potential (E_h) are also important in establishing conditions that favor growth of anaerobes (Table 22–1). Anaerobes grow at a low or negative E_h.

Aerobes and facultative anaerobes often have the metabolic systems listed below, whereas anaerobic bacteria frequently do not.

(1) Cytochrome systems for the metabolism of O_2.

(2) Superoxide dismutase, which catalyzes the following reaction:

$$O_2^- + O_2^- + 2H^+ \rightarrow H_2O_2 + O_2$$

(3) Catalase, which catalyzes the following reaction:

$$2H_2O_2 \rightarrow 2H_2O + O_2 \text{ (gas bubbles)}$$

Anaerobic bacteria do not have cytochrome systems for oxygen metabolism. Less fastidious anaerobes may have low levels of superoxide dismutase (SOD) and may or may not have catalase. Most bacteria of the *Bacteroides fragilis* group—the most important anaerobic pathogens—have small amounts of both catalase and SOD. Relatively little is known about how anaerobic bacteria are killed or inhibited by oxygen. There appear to be multiple mechanisms for oxygen toxicity. Presumably, when anaerobes have SOD or catalase (or both), they are able to negate the toxic effect of oxygen radicals and hydrogen peroxide and thus tolerate oxygen. **Obligate anaerobes** usually lack superoxide dismutase and catalase and are susceptible to the lethal

GLOSSARY

Aerobic bacteria: Those that require oxygen as a terminal electron acceptor and will not grow under anaerobic conditions (ie, in the absence of O_2). Some *Micrococcus* species and *Nocardia asteroides* are obligate aerobes (ie, they must have oxygen to survive).

Anaerobic bacteria: Those that do not use oxygen for growth and metabolism but obtain their energy from fermentation reactions. A functional definition of anaerobes is that they require reduced oxygen tension for growth and fail to grow on the surface of solid medium in 10% CO_2 in ambient air. *Bacteroides* and *Clostridium* species are examples of anaerobes.

Capnophilic bacteria: Those that require carbon dioxide for growth.

Facultative anaerobes: Bacteria that can grow either oxidatively using oxygen as a terminal electron acceptor or anaerobically using fermentation reactions to obtain energy. Such bacteria are common pathogens. *Streptococcus* species and the Enterobacteriaceae (eg, *Escherichia coli*) are among the many facultative anaerobes that cause disease. Often, bacteria that are facultative anaerobes are called "aerobes."

Microaerophilic bacteria: Those that require oxygen as a terminal electron acceptor but fail to grow on the surface of solid medium in air and exhibit minimal (if any) growth under anaerobic conditions. Some streptococci are microaerophilic.

Table 22–1. Oxidation-reduction potential (E_h) related to anatomic location.

Millivolts	Location
+810	Oxygen electrode
+240	Human cell
+180	Venous blood
0	
−50	Periodontal pocket
−200	Dental plaque
−300	Colon
−420	Hydrogen electrode

effects of oxygen; such strict obligate anaerobes are infrequently isolated from human infections, and most anaerobic infections of humans are caused by **"moderately obligate anaerobes."**

The ability of anaerobes to tolerate oxygen or grow in its presence varies from species to species. Similarly, there is strain-to-strain variation within a given species (eg, one strain of *Prevotella melaninogenica* can grow at an O_2 concentration of 0.1% but not of 1%; another can grow at a concentration of 2% but not of 4%). Also, in the absence of oxygen some anaerobic bacteria will grow at a more positive E_h.

Facultative anaerobes grow as well or better under anaerobic conditions than they do under aerobic conditions. Bacteria that are facultative anaerobes are often termed "aerobes." When a facultative anaerobe such as *Escherichia coli* is present at the site of an infection (eg, abdominal abscess), it can rapidly consume all available oxygen and change to anaerobic metabolism, producing an anaerobic environment and low E_h and thus allow the anaerobic bacteria that are present to grow and produce disease.

ANAEROBIC BACTERIA FOUND IN HUMAN INFECTIONS

There are more than 30 genera and 200 species of anaerobes, and species names for many anaerobic bacteria have not yet been established. The classification and nomenclature of anaerobic bacteria change frequently; new publications may use different names for anaerobes than were used previously. (See Hofstad, 1990.) Because the classification of anaerobes is continually evolving, the nomenclature used in this chapter refers to genera of anaerobes frequently found in human infections and to certain species recognized as important pathogens of humans. Anaerobes commonly found in human infections are listed in Table 22–2.

Gram-Negative Anaerobes

A. Gram-Negative Bacilli:

1. *Bacteroides* species–The *Bacteroides* species are a very important anaerobes that cause human infection. They are a large group of non-spore-forming gram-enegative bacilli and may appear as slender rods or coccobacilli. Many species previously included in the genus *Bacteroides* have been reclassified into the genus *Prevotella* or the genus *Porphyromonas*.

Bacteroides species are normal inhabitants of the bowel an other sites. Normal stools contain 10^{11} *B fragilis* organisms per gram (compared to 10^8/g for facultative anaerobes). Most commonly isolated are members of the *B fragilis* group (*B fragilis, B ovatus, B distasonis, B vulgatus, B thetaiotaomicron,* and others), particularly from infections associated with contamination by the contents of the colon, where they may cause suppuration, eg, peritonitis after bowel injury. Classification is based on colonial and biochemical features and on characteristic short-chain fatty-acid patterns in gas chromatography.

In infections (eg, intra-abdominal abscess), *Bacteroides* species are often associated with other anaerobic organisms—particularly anaerobic cocci (*Peptostreptococcus*), anaerobic gram-positive rods (*Clostridium* and *Eubacterium* species)—as well as gram-positive and gram-negative facultative anaerobes that are part of the normal flora.

2. *Prevotella* species–The *Prevotella* species are non-spore-forming gram-negative bacilli and may appear as slender rods or coccobacilli. *Prevotella* includes newly named species and ones that were previously classified as *Bacteroides* species (eg, *Prevotella melaninogenica* was prevously named *Bacteroides melaninogenicus*). Most commonly isolated are *P melaninogenica, P bivia,* and *P disiens. P melaninogenica* and similar species are found in infections associated with the upper respiratory tract. *P bivia* and *P disiens* occur in the female genital tract. *Prevotella* species are found in brain and lung abscesses, in empyema, and in pelvic inflammatory disease and tubo-ovarian abscesses. In these infections the *Pre-*

Table 22–2. Anaerobic bacteria of clinical importance.

Genera	Anatomic Site
Bacilli (rods)	
Gram-negative	
Bacteroides fragilis group	Colon
Prevotella melaninogenica group	Mouth
Fusobacterium	Mouth, colon
Gram-positive	
Actinomyces	Mouth
Lactobacillus	Vagina
Propionibacterium	Skin
Eubacterium, Bifidobacterium, and *Arachnia*	Mouth, colon
Clostridium	Colon (also found in soil)
Cocci (spheres)	
Gram-positive	
Peptostreptococcus	Colon
Gram-negative	
Veillonella	Mouth, colon

votella are often associated with other anaerobic organisms that are part of the normal flora—particularly peptostreptococci, anaerobic gram-positive rods, and *Fusobacterium* species—as well as gram-positive and gram-negative facultative anaerobes that are part of the normal flora.

3. *Porphyromonas* species–The *Porphyromonas* species also are non-spore-forming gram-negative bacilli that are part of the normal oral flora and occur at other anatomic sites as well. The genus *Porphyromonas* includes newly named species and species that were previously included in the genus *Bacteroides*. *Porphyromonas* species can be cultured from gingival and periapical tooth infections and, more commonly, breast, axillary, perianal, and male genital infections.

4. Fusobacteria–The fusobacteria are pleomorphic gram-negative rods. Most species produce butyric acid and convert threonine to propionic acid. The *Fusobacterium* group includes several species frequently isolated from mixed bacterial infections caused by normal mucosal flora. Occasionally, a *Fusobacterium* species will be the only bacteria in an infection (eg, osteomyelitis).

B. Gram-Negative Cocci: *Veillonella* species are a group of small, anaerobic, gram-negative cocci that are part of the normal flora of the mouth, the nasopharynx, and probably the intestine. Previously known by various names, they are now collectively known as the veillonellae. Though occasionally isolated in polymicrobic anaerobic infections, they are rarely the sole cause of an infection.

Gram-Positive Anaerobes

A. Gram-Positive Bacilli:

1. *Actinomyces*–The *Actinomyces* group includes several species that cause actinomycosis, of which *Actinomyces israelii* is the most commonly encountered. On Gram stain, they vary considerably in length: they may be short and club-shaped or long, thin, beaded filaments. They may be branched or unbranched. Because they often grow slowly, prolonged incubation of the culture may be necessary before laboratory confirmation of the clinical diagnosis of actinomycosis can be made. Some strains produce colonies on agar that resemble molar teeth. Some *Actinomyces* species are oxygen-tolerant (aerotolerant) and grow in the presence of air; these strains may be confused with *Corynebacterium* species (diphtheroids; see Chapter 13). *Actinomyces* species are susceptible to penicillin G, erythromycin, and other antibiotics.

2. *Lactobacillus*–*Lactobacillus* species are major members of the normal flora of the vagina. The lactic acid product of their metabolism helps maintain the low pH of the normal adult female genital tract. They rarely cause disease.

3. *Propionibacterium*–*Propionibacterium* species are members of the normal flora of the skin and cause disease when they infect plastic shunts and appliances. Their metabolic products include propionic acid, from which the genus name derives. On Gram stain, they are highly pleomorphic, showing curved, clubbed, or pointed ends, long forms with beaded uneven staining, and occasionally coccoid or spherical forms. Propionibacteria participate in the genesis of acne. Because it is part of the normal skin flora, *Propionibacterium acnes* sometimes contaminates blood or cerebrospinal fluid cultures that are obtained by penetrating the skin. It is therefore important (but occasionally difficult) to differentiate a contaminated culture from one that is positive and indicates infection.

4. *Eubacterium, Bifidobacterium,* and *Arachnia*–These three genera of anaerobic, gram-positive rods are pleomorphic. There are several species. They are found in mixed infections associated with oropharyngeal or bowel flora.

5. *Clostridium*–Clostridia are gram-positive, spore-forming bacilli (see Chapter 12). There are more than 50 species. The major diseases associated with these bacteria are caused by exotoxins (see Chapter 9).

Spores of *Clostridium tetani*, which causes tetanus, are present throughout the environment. They germinate in devitalized tissue at an E_h of +10 mV (that of normal tissue is +120 mV). Once they are growing, the organisms elaborate the toxin tetanospasmin. Localized infection is often clinically insignificant. The toxin spreads along nerves to the central nervous system, where it binds to gangliosides, suppresses the release of inhibitory neurotransmitters, and causes muscle spasm. Death results from inability to breathe. Obviously, severe trauma may predispose to development of tetanus; however, more than 50% of tetanus cases follow minor injuries. Tetanus is totally preventable: active immunity is induced with tetanus toxoid (formalinized tetanus toxin). Tetanus toxoid is part of routine childhood DPT (diphtheria, tetanus, pertussis) immunizations; adults should be given boosters every 10 years.

Clostridium botulinum causes botulism (see Chapters 9 and 12). *C botulinum* is distributed throughout the environment. The spores find their way into preserved or canned foods with low oxygen levels, low E_h, and nutrients that support growth. The organisms germinate and elaborate the toxins as growth and lysis occur. Botulinus neurotoxins are the most potent toxins known but can be neutralized by specific antibodies. The toxins are heat-labile, so properly heated food does not transmit botulism. Preformed botulinus toxin is ingested and absorbed. The toxin acts on the peripheral nervous system by inhibiting the release of acetylcholine at cholinergic synapses, causing paralysis. Once the toxin is bound, the process is irreversible. The symptoms are associated with the anticholinergic action and include dysphagia, dry mouth, diplopia, and weakness or inability to breathe. Botulism should be treated with antitoxin. Infant botulism follows the ingestion of spores, germination of the spores, and toxin production; honey is a common vehicle for spread of the spores in infants.

Clostridium perfringens causes gas gangrene. There are at least 12 different soluble antigens, many of which are toxins. All types of *C perfringens* produce the alpha toxin, a necrotizing, hemolytic exotoxin that is a lecithinase. The other toxins have varying activities, including tissue necrosis and hemolysis. *C perfringens* is present throughout the environment. Gas gangrene occurs when a soft tissue wound is contaminated by *C perfringens,* as occurs in trauma, septic abortion, and war wounds. Bacteremia associated with *C perfringens* can be rapidly fatal. Milder forms of disease may also occur. Once infection is initiated, the organisms elaborate necrotizing toxins; CO_2, and H_2 accumulate in tissue and are clinically detectable as gas (eg, gas gangrene). Edema occurs and the circulation is impaired, promoting spread of the anaerobic infection. Therapy involves surgical removal of the infection and administration of penicillin G.

C perfringens is a common cause of food poisoning (but less so than *Staphylococcus aureus*). The disease is caused by an enterotoxin produced and released during sporulation. The incubation period for the abdominal pain, nausea, and acute diarrhea is 8–24 hours.

Clostridium difficile causes pseudomembranous colitis. *C difficile* is part of the normal gastrointestinal flora in 2–10% of humans. The organisms are relatively resistant to most commonly used antibiotics. Associated with or following antibiotic use, the normal gastrointestinal flora is suppressed and *C difficile* proliferates, producing cytopathic toxin and enterotoxins. Symptoms of the disease vary from diarrhea alone to marked diarrhea and necrosis of mucosa with accumulation of inflammatory cells and fibrin, which forms the pseudomembrane. The diagnosis is made by demonstrating neutralizable cytotoxin in the stool through its cytopathic effect in cell culture or by detecting enterotoxin by immunoassay.

Other *Clostridium* species are occasionally found in polymicrobial infections, particularly those associated with contamination of normal tissue by contents of the colon.

B. Gram-Positive Cocci: *Peptostreptococcus* species are gram-positive cocci of variable size and shape that are found on the skin and as part of the normal flora of mucous membranes. There are many species, including those previously called peptococci. They are frequently found in mixed infections due to normal flora. Occasionally, cultures from breast, brain, or pulmonary infections will be positive for only one species of these gram-positive cocci.

PATHOGENESIS OF ANAEROBIC INFECTIONS

Infections due to anaerobes commonly are due to combinations of bacteria that function in synergistic pathogenicity. Although studies of the pathogenesis of anaerobic infections have often focused on a single species, it is important to recognize that the anaerobic infections most often are due to several species of anaerobes acting together to cause infection.

B fragilis is the single most important pathogen among the anaerobes that are part of the normal flora. The pathogenesis of anaerobic infection has been most extensively studied with *B fragilis* using a rat model of intra-abdominal infection, which in many ways mimics human disease. A characteristic sequence occurs after colon contents (including *B fragilis* and a facultative anaerobe such as *E coli*) are placed via needle, gelatin capsule, or other means into the abdomen of rats. A high percentage of the study animals die of sepsis caused by the facultative anaerobe. However, if the animals are first treated with gentamicin, a drug effective against the facultative anaerobe but not *Bacteroides,* few of the animals die, and after a few days, the surviving animals develop intra-abdominal abscesses from the *Bacteroides* infection. Treatment of the animals with both gentamicin and clindamycin, a drug effective against *Bacteroides,* prevents both the initial sepsis and the later development of abdominal abscesses.

The capsular polysaccharides of *Bacteroides* are important virulence factors. When injected into the rat abdomen, purified capsular polysaccharides from *B fragilis* cause abscess formation, whereas those from other bacteria (eg, *Streptococcus pneumoniae* and *E coli*) do not. The mechanism by which the *B fragilis* capsule induces abscess formation is not well understood.

Bacteroides species have lipopolysaccharides (endotoxins; see Chapter 9) but lack the lipopolysaccharide structures with endotoxic activity (including β-hydroxymyristic acid). The lipopolysaccharides of *B fragilis* are much less toxic than those of other gram-negative bacteria. Thus, infection caused by *Bacteroides* does not directly produce the clinical signs of sepsis (eg, fever and shock) so important in infections due to other gram-negative bacteria. When these clinical signs appear in *Bacteroides* infection, they are a result of the inflammatory immune response to the infection.

B fragilis produces a superoxide dismutase and can survive in the presence of oxygen for days. When a facultative anaerobe such as *E coli* is present at the site of infection, it can consume all available oxygen and thereby produce an environment in which *Bacteroides* and other anaerobes can grow (see above).

Many anaerobic bacteria produce heparinase, collagenase, and other enzymes that damage or destroy tissue. It is likely that enzymes play a part in the pathogenesis of mixed anaerobic infections, although laboratory experiments have not been able to define specific roles.

IMMUNITY IN ANAEROBIC INFECTIONS

Relatively little is known about immunity in anaerobic infections. The most complete information has been obtained from studies of animal models of *B fragilis* infections.

Many anaerobes (including *Bacteroides, Propionibacterium,* and *Fusobacterium* species) produce serum-independent chemotactic factors that attract polymorphonuclear cells. The capsule of *B fragilis* is both antiphagocytic and inhibitory to complement-mediated bactericidal action. *Bacteroides* species are optimally phagocytosed by polymorphonuclear cells when the organisms are opsonized by both antibody and complement. Both animals and humans produce antibodies against *Bacteroides* antigens, including the capsular material. Passive transfer of antibodies from an immune animal to a nonimmune animal is protective against *Bacteroides* bacteremia but does not prevent abdominal abscess formation; in the rat model of infection, it is a T cell-dependent immune response that prevents abscess formation. Passive transfer of immune spleen cells or a low-molecular-weight cell-free factor prevents abdominal abscess formation in the rat model.

THE POLYMICROBIAL NATURE OF ANAEROBIC INFECTIONS

Most anaerobic infections are associated with contamination of tissue by normal flora of the mucosa of the mouth, pharynx, gastrointestinal tract, or genital tract. Typically, multiple species (5–6 species or more when standard culture conditions are used) are found, including both anaerobes and facultative anaerobes. Oropharyngeal, pleuropulmonary, abdominal, and female pelvic infections associated with contamination by normal mucosal flora have a relatively equal distribution of anaerobes and facultative anaerobes as causative agents: about 25% have anaerobes alone; about 25% have facultative anaerobes alone; and about 50% have both anaerobes and facultative anaerobes. Aerobic bacteria may also be present, but obligate aerobes are much less common than anaerobes and facultative anaerobes. Anaerobic bacteria and associated representative infections are listed in Table 22–3.

Table 22–3. Anaerobic bacteria and associated representative infections.

Brain abscesses: Peptostreptococci and others
Oropharyngeal infections: Oropharyngeal anaerobes; *Actinomyces, Prevotella melaninogenica, Fusobacterium* species
Pleuropulmonary infections: Peptostreptococci; *Fusobacterium* species: *P melaninogenica, B fragilis* in 20–25%; others
Intra-abdominal infections: Liver abscess: Mixed anaerobes in 40–90%; facultative organisms
Abdominal abscesses: *B fragilis;* other gastrointestinal flora
Female genital tract infections: Vulvar abscesses: Peptostreptococci and others
Tubo-ovarian and pelvic abscesses: *P bivia* and *P disiens*: peptostreptococci; others
Skin, soft tissue, and bone infections: Mixed anaerobic flora
Bacteremia: *B fragilis;* peptostreptococci; clostridia; propionibacteria; others
Endocarditis: *B fragilis*

DIAGNOSIS OF ANAEROBIC INFECTIONS

Clinical signs suggesting possible infection with anaerobes include the following:

(1) Foul-smelling discharge (due to short-chain fatty-acid products of anaerobic metabolism).

(2) Infection in proximity to a mucosal surface (anaerobes are part of the normal flora).

(3) Gas in tissues (production of CO_2 and H_2).

(4) Negative aerobic cultures.

Diagnosis of anaerobic infection is made by anaerobic culture of properly obtained and transported specimens (see Chapter 47). Anaerobes grow most readily on complex media such as trypticase soy agar base, Schaedler blood agar, *Brucella* agar, brain-heart infusion agar, and others—each highly supplemented (eg, with hemin, vitamin K_1, blood). A selective complex medium containing kanamycin is used in parallel. Kanamycin (like all aminoglycosides) does not inhibit the growth of obligate anaerobes; thus, it permits them to proliferate without being overshadowed by rapidly growing facultative anaerobes. Cultures are incubated at 35–37 °C in an anaerobic atmosphere containing CO_2.

Colony morphology, pigmentation, and fluorescence are helpful in identifying anaerobes. Biochemical activities and production of short-chain fatty acids as measured by gas-liquid chromatography are used for laboratory confirmation.

TREATMENT OF ANAEROBIC INFECTIONS

Treatment of mixed anaerobic infections is by surgical drainage (under most circumstances) plus antimicrobial therapy.

B fragilis group of organisms found in abdominal and other infections universally produce β-lactamase, as do many of the *P bivia* and *P disiens* strains found in upper genital tract infections in women. Therapy with antimicrobials (other than penicillin G) is necessary to treat infections with these organisms. About two-thirds of the *P melaninogenica* strains from pulmonary and oropharyngeal infections also produce β-lactamase; such infections have been successfully treated with penicillin G, but alternative antibiotic therapy is probably more efficacious.

The most active drugs for treatment of anaerobic infections are clindamycin and metronidazole. Clindamycin is preferred for infections above the diaphragm. Relatively few anaerobes are resistant to clindamycin and few, if any, are resistant to metronidazole. Alternative drugs include cefoxitin, cefotetan, some of the other newer cephalosporins, and mezlocillin and piperacillin, but these drugs are not as active as clindamycin and metronidazole. Penicillin G remains the drug of choice for treatment of anaerobic infections that do not involve β-lactamase-producing *Bacteroides* and *Prevotella* species.

REFERENCES

Baron EJ, Finegold SM: *Bailey and Scott's Diagnostic Microbiology,* 8th ed. Mosby, 1990.

Finegold SM, George WL (editors): *Anaerobic Infections in Humans.* Academic Press, 1989.

Finegold SM, Goldstein EJC: Proceedings of the first North American Congress on anaerobic bacteria and anaerobic infections. Clin Infect Dis 1993;16(Suppl 4):S159.

Hentges DJ: The anaerobic microflora of the human body. Clin Infect Dis 1993;16(Suppl 4):S175.

Hiller S, Moncla BJ: Anaerobic gram-positive nonsporeforming bacilli and cocci. In: *Manual of Clinical Microbiology,* 5th ed. Ballows A et al (editors). American Society for Microbiology, 1991.

Hofstad T: Current taxonomy of medically important nonsporing anaerobes. Rev Infect Dis 1990;12(Suppl 2):S122.

Johnson CC, Finegold SM: Uncommonly encountered, motile, anaerobic gram-negative bacilli associated with infection. Rev Infect Dis 1987;9:1150.

Jousimies-Somer HR, Finegold SM: Anaerobic gram-negative bacilli and cocci. In: *Manual of Clinical Microbiology,* 5th ed. Ballows A et al (editors). American Society for Microbiology, 1991.

Kasper DL, Onderdonk AB: International symposium on anaerobic bacteria and bacterial infections. Rev Infect Dis 1990;12(Suppl 2):S121.

Onderdonk AB et al: Use of a model of intraabdominal sepsis for studies of the pathogenicity of *Bacteroides fragilis.* Rev Infect Dis 1984;6(Suppl 1):S91.

Peraino VA, Cross SA, Goldstein EJ: Incidence and clinical significance of anaerobic bacteremia in a community hospital. Clin Infect Dis 1993;16(Suppl 4):S288.

Rotstein OD: Interactions between leukocytes and anaerobic bacteria in polymicrobial surgical infections. Clin Infect Dis 1993;16(Suppl 4):S190.

Shah HN, Gharbia SE: Ecophysiology and taxonomy of *Bacteroides* and related taxa. Clin Infect Dis 1993;16(Suppl 4):S160.

Shapiro ME et al: Cellular immunity to *Bacteroides fragilis* capsular polysaccharide. J Exp Med 1982;155:1188.

Styrt B, Gorbach SL: Recent developments in the understanding of the pathogenesis and treatment of anaerobic infections. (Two parts.) N Engl J Med 1989;321: 240, 298.

Summanen P: Recent taxonomic changes for anaerobic gram-positive and selected gram-negative organisms. Clin Infect Dis 1993;16(Suppl 4):S168.

Zaleznik DF et al: A soluble suppressor T cell factor protects against experimental intra-abdominal abscesses. J Clin Invest 1985;75:1023.

Legionellae & Unusual Bacterial Pathogens

23

LEGIONELLA PNEUMOPHILA & OTHER LEGIONELLAE

A widely publicized outbreak of pneumonia in persons attending an American Legion convention in Philadelphia in 1976 prompted investigations that defined *Legionella pneumophila* and the legionellae. Other outbreaks of respiratory illness caused by related organisms since 1947 have been diagnosed retrospectively. At least 22 species of *Legionella* exist, some with multiple serotypes. *L pneumophila* is the major cause of disease in humans; *Legionella micdadei* sometimes causes pneumonia. The other legionellae are rarely isolated from patients or have been isolated only from the environment.

Morphology & Identification

L pneumophila is the prototype bacterium of the group. Legionellae that cause disease in humans are listed in Table 23–1.

A. Typical Organisms: Legionellae are fastidious, aerobic gram-negative bacteria that are 0.5–1 μm wide and 2–50 μm long. They often stain poorly by Gram's method and are not seen in stains of clinical specimens. Gram-stained smears should be made for suspect *Legionella* growth on agar media. Basic fuchsin (0.1%) should be used as the counterstain, because safranin stains the bacteria very poorly.

B. Culture: Legionellae can be grown on complex media such as buffered charcoal-yeast extract agar (BCYE) with α-ketoglutarate, at pH 6.9, temperature 35 °C, and 90% humidity. Antibiotics can be added to make the medium selective for *Legionella.* A biphasic BCYE medium can be used for blood cultures.

Legionella grows slowly; visible colonies are usually present after 3 days of incubation. Colonies that appear after overnight incubation are not *Legionella.* Colonies are round or flat with entire edges. They vary in color from colorless to iridescent pink or blue and are translucent or speckled. Variation in colony morphology is common, and the colonies may rapidly lose their color and speckles. Many other genera of bacteria grow on BCYE medium and must be differentiated from *Legionella* by Gram-staining and other tests.

Legionella in blood cultures usually require 2 weeks or more to grow. Colonies can be seen on the agar surface of the biphasic medium.

C. Growth Characteristics: The legionellae are catalase-positive. *L pneumophila* is oxidase-positive; the other legionellae are variable in oxidase activity. *L pneumophila* hydrolyzes hippurate; the other legionellae do not. Most legionellae produce gelatinase and β-lactamase; *L micdadei* produces neither gelatinase nor β-lactamase.

Antigens & Cell Products

Antigenic specificity of *L pneumophila* is thought to be due to complex antigenic structures. There are more than ten serogroups of *L pneumophila*; serogroup 1 was the cause of the 1976 outbreak of Legionnaires' disease and remains the most common serogroup isolated from humans. *Legionella* species cannot be identified by serogrouping alone, because there is cross-reactive antigenicity among different *Legionella* species. Occasionally, *Bacteroides, Bordetella* and some *Pseudomonas* species also cross-react with *L pneumophila* antisera.

The legionellae produce distinctive 14- to 17-carbon branched-chain fatty acids. Gas-liquid chromatography can be used to help characterize and determine the species of legionellae.

The legionellae make proteases, phosphatase, lipase, DNase, and RNase. A hemolysin and cytotoxin have been described. The toxins and their mechanism of action are not well characterized.

Pathology & Pathogenesis

Legionellae are ubiquitous in warm moist environments. Infection of debilitated or immunocompromised humans commonly follows inhalation of the bacteria from aerosols generated from contaminated air-conditioning systems, shower heads, and similar sources. *L pneumophila* usually produces a lobar, segmental, or patchy pulmonary infiltration. Histologically, the appearance is similar to that produced by many other bacterial pathogens. Acute purulent pneumonia involving the alveoli is present with a dense intra-alveolar exudate of macrophages, polymorphonuclear leukocytes, red blood cells, and proteinaceous material. Most of the *Legionella* in the lesions are within phagocytic cells. There is little interstitial

Table 23–1. The *Legionella* species of primary medical importance.

Species	Pneumonia	Pontiac Fever
L pneumophila	+	Serogroups 1 and 6
L micdadei	+	
L gormanii	+	
L dumoffii	+	
L bozemanii	+	
L longbeachae	+	
L wadsworthii	+	
L jordanis	+	
L feeleii	+	+
L oakridgensis	+	

infiltration and little or no inflammation of the bronchioles and upper airways.

Knowledge of the pathogenesis of *L pneumophila* infection comes from study of isolated cells from humans and from study of susceptible animals such as guinea pigs.

L pneumophila readily enters and grows within human alveolar macrophages and monocytes and is not effectively killed by polymorphonuclear leukocytes. In vitro, when serum is present but there is no immune antibody, complement component C3 is deposited on the bacterial surface and the bacteria attach to complement receptors CR1 and CR3 on the phagocytic cell surface. Entry into the cell is by a phagocytic process involving coiling of a single pseudopod around the bacterium. When immune antibody is present, entry of the bacteria occurs by the more typical Fc-mediated phagocytosis. Once inside the cell, the individual bacteria are within phagosomal vacuoles, but the defense mechanisms of the macrophage cells stop at that point. Instead, the phagosomal vacuoles fail to fuse with lysosomal granules. The phagocyte oxidative metabolic burst is reduced. Phagosomes containing *L pneumophila* do not acidify as much as phagosomes containing other ingested particles. Ribosomes, mitochondria, and small vesicles accumulate around vacuoles containing the *L pneumophila.* The bacteria multiply within the vacuoles until they are numerous, the cells are destroyed, the bacteria are released, and infection of other macrophages then occurs. The presence of iron (transferrin-iron) is essential for the process of intracellular growth of the bacteria, but other factors important to the processes of growth, cell destruction, and tissue damage are not well understood.

Clinical Findings

Asymptomatic infection is common in all age groups, as shown by elevated titers of specific antibodies. The incidence of clinically significant disease is highest in men over age 55 years. Factors associated with high risk include smoking, chronic bronchitis and emphysema, steroid and other immunosuppressive treatment (as in renal transplantation), cancer chemotherapy, and diabetes mellitus. When pneumonia occurs in patients with these risk factors, *Legionella* should be investigated as the cause.

Infection may result in nondescript febrile illness of short duration or in a severe, rapidly progressive illness with high fever, chills, malaise, nonproductive cough, hypoxia, diarrhea, and delirium. Chest x-rays reveal patchy, often multilobar consolidation. There may be leukocytosis, hyponatremia, hematuria (and even renal failure), or abnormal liver function. During some outbreaks, the mortality rate has reached 10%. The diagnosis is based on the clinical picture and exclusion of other causes of pneumonia by laboratory tests. Demonstration of *Legionella* in clinical specimens can rapidly yield a specific diagnosis. The diagnosis can also be made by culture for *Legionella* or by serologic tests, but results of these tests are often delayed beyond the time when specific therapy must be started.

L pneumophila also produces a disease called "Pontiac fever," after the clinical syndrome that occurred in an outbreak in Pontiac, Michigan. The syndrome is characterized by fever and chills, myalgia, malaise, and headache that develop over 6–12 hours. Dizziness, photophobia, neck stiffness, and confusion also occur. Respiratory symptoms are much less prominent in Pontiac fever than in Legionnaires' disease and include mild cough and sore throat.

Diagnostic Laboratory Tests

A. Specimens: In human infections, the organisms can be recovered from bronchial washings, pleural fluid, lung biopsy specimens, or blood. Isolation of *Legionella* from sputum is more difficult because of the predominance of bacteria of the normal flora. *Legionella* is rarely recovered from other anatomic sites.

B. Smears: Legionellae are not demonstrable in Gram-stained smears of clinical specimens. Direct fluorescent antibody tests of specimens can be diagnostic, but the test has low sensitivity compared to culture. Silver stains are sometimes used on tissue specimens.

C. Culture: Specimens are cultured on BCYE agar (see above). Cultured organisms can be rapidly identified by immunofluorescence staining. BCYE agar containing antibiotics can be used to culture contaminated specimens.

D. Specific Tests: Sometimes *Legionella* antigens can be demonstrated in the patient's urine by immunologic methods.

E. Serologic Tests: Levels of antibodies to legionellae rise slowly during the illness. Serologic tests have a sensitivity of 60–80% and a specificity of 95–99%. Since fewer than 10% of all cases of pneumonia are due to *Legionella*, the predictive value of a positive serologic test in sporadic cases is low

(40–70%). Serologic tests are most useful in obtaining a retrospective diagnosis in outbreaks of *Legionella* infections.

Immunity

Infected patients make antibodies against *Legionella,* but the peak antibody response may not occur until 4–8 weeks after infection. The roles of antibodies and cell-mediated responses in protective immunity in humans have not been defined. Animals challenged with sublethal doses of virulent *L pneumophila,* avirulent *L pneumophila,* or a major secretory protein vaccine are immune to subsequent lethal doses of *L pneumophila.* Both humoral and cell-mediated immune responses occur. The cell-mediated response is important in protective immunity because of the intracellular infection and growth of *Legionella.*

Treatment

Legionellae are susceptible to erythromycin and some other drugs. The treatment of choice is erythromycin, which has been effective even in immunocompromised patients. Rifampin, 10–20 mg/kg/d, has been used in patients whose response to treatment was delayed. Assisted ventilation may be necessary, and management of shock is essential.

Epidemiology & Control

The legionellae are ubiquitous in the environment and worldwide in distribution. They commonly occur in soil and in freshwater lakes and streams and have been found in high numbers in air-conditioning systems and washing facilities, eg, shower stalls. The later sources have been responsible for outbreaks of human disease, especially in hospitals. Chlorination and heating of water and cleaning can help control the multiplication of *Legionella* in water and air-conditioning systems. Legionellae are not communicable from infected patients to others.

BACTERIA THAT CAUSE VAGINOSIS

Bacterial vaginosis is a common vaginal condition of women of reproductive age. It is associated with premature rupture of membranes and preterm labor and birth. Bacterial vaginosis has a complex microbiology; two organisms, *Gardnerella vaginalis* and *Mobiluncus* species, have been most specifically associated with the disease process.

Gardnerella vaginalis

Gardnerella vaginalis (formerly called *Corynebacterium vaginale* and *Haemophilus vaginalis*) is a serologically distinct organism isolated from the normal female genitourinary tract and also associated with vaginosis. In wet smears, this "nonspecific" vaginitis, or **bacterial vaginosis,** yields "clue cells," which are vaginal epithelial cells covered with many tiny rods, and there is an absence of other common causes of vaginitis such as *Trichomonas* or yeasts. Vaginal discharge often has a distinct "fishy" odor and contains many anaerobes in addition to *G vaginalis.* The pH of the vaginal secretions is over 4.5 (normal pH is < 4.5). The vaginitis attributed to this organism is suppressed by metronidazole, suggesting an association with anaerobes. Oral metronidazole is generally curative.

Mobiluncus

This genus comprises motile, curved, gram-negative, anaerobic rods isolated from **"bacterial vaginosis,"** which may be a clinical variant of "nonspecific vaginitis" associated with *G vaginalis.* It is possible that *Mobiluncus* may be part of the normal vaginal anaerobic flora in women, and it is likely that it is part of the anaerobic flora in bacterial vaginosis. The organisms are most commonly detected in Gram-stained smears of vaginal secretions, but they grow with difficulty in anaerobic cultures.

STREPTOBACILLUS MONILIFORMIS

Streptobacillus moniliformis is an aerobic, gram-negative, highly pleomorphic organism that forms irregular chains of bacilli interspersed with fusiform enlargements and large round bodies. It grows best at 37 °C in media containing serum protein, egg yolk, or starch but ceases to grow at 22 °C. L forms can easily be demonstrated in most cultures of the organism. Subculture of pure colonies of L forms in liquid media often yields the streptobacilli again. All strains of streptobacilli appear to be antigenically identical.

S moniliformis is a normal inhabitant of the throats of rats, and humans can be infected by rat bites. The human disease **(rat-bite fever)** is characterized by septic fever, blotchy and petechial rashes, and polyarthritis. Diagnosis rests on cultures of blood, joint fluid, or pus; on mouse inoculation; and on serum agglutination tests.

This organism can also produce infection after being ingested in milk—the disease is called Haverhill fever and has occurred in epidemics.

Penicillin and perhaps other antibiotics are therapeutically effective.

Rat-bite fever of somewhat different clinical appearance (sodoku) is caused by *Spirillum minor* (see Chapter 25).

BARTONELLA SPECIES

The three medically important species in the genus *Bartonella* are *Bartonella bacilliformis,* the cause of Oroya fever and verruga peruana; *Bartonella quintana,* the cause of trench fever of World War I and some cases of bacillary angiomatosis; and *Bartonella henselae,* which causes cat scratch disease and has also been associated with bacillary angiomatosis. These diseases have many common characteristics. *B quintana* and *B henselae* were previously named *Rochalimaea quintana* and *Rochalimaea henselae*.

The *Bartonella* species are gram-negative rods that are pleomorphic, slow growing, and difficult to isolate in the laboratory. They can be seen in infected tissues stained with the Warthin-Starry silver impregnation stain.

Bartonella bacilliformis

There are two stages of *Bartonella bacilliformis* infection: the initial stage is **Oroya fever,** a serious infectious anemia; and the eruptive stage, **verruga peruana,** which commonly begins 2–8 weeks later, though verrugae may also occr in the absence of Oroya fever.

Oroya fever is characterized by the rapid development of severe anemia due to red blood cell destruction, enlargement of the spleen and liver, and hemorrhage into the lymph nodes. Masses of bartonellae fill the cytoplasm of cells lining the blood vessels, and endothelial swelling may lead to vascular occlusion and thrombosis. The mortality rate of untreated Oroya fever is about 40%. The diagnosis is made by examining stained blood smears and blood cultures in semisolid medium.

Verruga peruana consists of vascular skin lesions that occur in successive crops; it lasts for about 1 year and produces little systemic reaction and no fatalities. Bartonellae can be seen in the granuloma; blood cultures are often positive, but there is no anemia.

B bacilliformis produces a protein that promotes deformity (indentation) of red blood cell membranes, and flagella provide the organisms with the mechanical force to invade red blood cells. *B bacilliformis* also invades endothelial cells and other types of human cells in vitro.

Bartonellosis is limited to the mountainous areas of the American Andes in tropical Peru, Colombia, and Ecuador and is transmitted by sandflies (*Phlebotomus* and *Lutzomyia*).

B bacilliformis grows in semisolid nutrient agar containing 10% rabbit serum and 0.5% hemoglobin. After 10 days or more of incubation at 28 °C, turbidity develops in the medium, and rod-shaped and granular organisms can be seen in Giemsa-stained smears.

Penicillin, streptomycin, and chloramphenicol are effective in Oroya fever and greatly reduce the mortality rate, particularly when blood transfusions are also given. Control of the disease depends upon elimination of the sandfly vectors: insecticides, insect repellents, and elimination of sandfly breeding areas are of value. Prevention with antibiotics may be useful.

Bartonella (Rochalimaea) henselae & Bartonella (Rochalimaea) quintana

A. Cat-Scratch Disease: Cat-scratch disease is usually a benign, self-limited illness manifested by fever and lymphadenopathy that develop about 2 weeks after contact with a cat (usually a scratch, lick, bite, or perhaps a flea bite). A primary skin lesion (papule or pustule) develops at the site 3–10 days after the contact. The patient usually appears well but may have low-grade fever and occasionally headache, sore throat, or conjunctivitis. The regional lymph nodes are markedly enlarged and sometimes tender, and they may not subside for several weeks or even months. They may suppurate and discharge pus. More than 20,000 cases a year are thought to occur in the United States.

The diagnosis of cat-scratch fever is based on (1) a suggestive history and physical findings; (2) aspiration of pus from lymph nodes that contain no bacteria culturable by routine methods; and (3) characteristic histopathologic findings with granulomatus lesions, which may include bacteria seen on silver-impregnated stains. A positive skin test has also been included as a criterion. A titer of 1:64 or greater in a single serum in the indirect fluorescent antibody test strongly supports the diagnosis, but development of a diagnostic titer may be delayed.

Cat scratch disease is caused by *B henselae,* a small, pleomorphic, gram-negative rod present mainly in the walls of capillaries near follicular hyperplasia or within microabscesses.* The organisms are seen best in tissue sections stained with Warthin-Starry silver impregnation stain; they may also be detected by immunofluorescent stains. Culture of *B henselae* is generally not recommended for this relatively benign disease.

The reservoir for *B henselae* is the domestic cat, and one-third of cats or more (and possibly their fleas) may be infected. Contact with infected cats through skin lesions is thought to communicate the infection.

Cat-scratch disease occurs commonly in immunocompetent people and is usually self-limited. Treatment is mainly supportive, with reassurance, hot moist soaks, and analgesics. Aspiration of pus or surgical removal of an excessively large lymph node may ameliorate symptoms. Tetracycline or erythromycin therapy may be helpful.

B. Bacillary Angiomatosis: Bacillary angiomatosis is a disease predominantly of immunosuppressed individuals, particularly AIDS patients. Rare cases occur in immunocompetent persons. Bacillary angiomatosis is characterized histopathologically as circumscribed lesions with lobular capillary proliferation and round, open vessels with cuboidal endothelial cells protruding into the vascular lumen. A prominent finding is epithelioid histiocytes surrounded by a loose fibromyxoid matrix. The pleomorphic bacilli can be seen in the subendothelial tissue when stained with the

*Early studies of the causes of cat-scratch disease incriminated the organism *Afipia felis,* but those initial observations have not been confirmed.

Warthin-Starry. The lesions may be infiltrated by polymorphonuclear leukocytes.

In its common form, bacillary angiomatosis presents as an enlarging red (cranberry-like) papule, often with surrounding scale and erythema. The lesions enlarge and may become several centimeters in diameter and ulcerate. There may be single or many lesions. The clinical appearance is often similar to that of Kaposi's sarcoma in AIDS patients, but the two diseases are different histologically. Bacillary angiomatosis occurs in virtually every organ. Involvement of the liver (and spleen) is characterized by a proliferation of cystic blood-filled spaces surrounded by a fibromyxoid matrix containing the bacteria; this form of the disease is called **peliosis hepatis** and is usually accompanied by fever, weight loss, and abdominal pain. A bacteremic form of infection with the nonspecific signs of malaise, fever, and weight loss also occurs.

The diagnosis is confirmed by the characteristic histopathologic findings and demonstration of the pleomorphic bacilli on silver-stained sections. *B henselae* and *B quintana* can be isolated by direct culture of biopsies of involved tissue carefully obtained so that no contaminating skin bacteria are present. The biopsy specimens are homogenized in supplemented tissue culture medium and inoculated onto fresh chocolate agar and heart infusion agar with 5% rabbit blood. Cultures of blood obtained by the lysis-centrifugation method can be inoculated onto the same media. The cultures should be incubated in 5% CO_2 at 36 °C for a minimum of 3 weeks. Specimens can also be cultured on eukaryotic tissue culture monolayers. Biochemically, *B henselae* and *B quintana* are relatively inert, including negative catalase and oxidase reactions and negative carbohydrate utilization tests. Enzyme activity can be seen with amino acid substrates by methods to test for preformed enzymes. Definitive identification is obtained by sequencing all or part of the 16S ribosomal RNA gene amplified by the polymerase chain reaction.

Bacillary angiomatosis is treated with oral erythromycin or doxycycline (plus gentamicin for very ill patients) for a minimum of 2 months. Relapses are common but can be treated by the same drugs used initially.

The reservoir for *B henselae* usually is the domestic cat, and patients with this organism as the etiology of bacillary angiomatosis often have contact with cats or histories of cat flea bites. The reservoir for *B quintana* is unknown.

CALYMMATOBACTERIUM (DONOVANIA) GRANULOMATIS

Calymmatobacterium granulomatis, related to the klebsiellae, causes **granuloma inguinale,** an uncommon sexually transmitted disease characterized by genital ulcers. The organism grows with difficulty on media containing egg yolk. Ampicillin or tetracycline is effective treatment.

WHIPPLE'S DISEASE

Whipple's disease is characterized by fever, abdominal pain, diarrhea, weight loss, and migratory polyarthralgia. The primary involvement is the small intestine and mesenteric lymph nodes, but any organ can be involved. Histologically, there is a prominent macrophage infiltration and fat deposition. There are characteristic vacuoles within the macrophage that stain with periodic acid-Schiff (PAS) stain, which is pathognomonic of the disease. The intracellular and extracellular PAS-positive material are bacilli, but cultures to isolate the organism have been unsuccessful. Polymerase chain reaction amplification of bacterial 16S ribosomal RNA allowed identification of a unique sequence from the bacteria in the lesions. Phylogenetic analysis has shown the organism is a gram-positive actinomycete not closely related to any known genus. The organism has tentatively been named *Tropheryma whippleii.*

REFERENCES

Legionella

Cianciotto N et al: Genetics and molecular pathogenesis of *Legionella pneumophila,* an intracellular parasite of macrophages. Mol Biol Med 1989;6:409.

Dowling JN et al: Virulence factors of the family Legionellaceae. Microbiol Rev 1992;56:32.

Kirby BD et al: Legionnaires' disease: Report of 65 nosocomially acquired cases and review of the literature. Medicine 1980;59:188.

Lowry PW, Tompkins LS: Nosocomial legionellosis: A review of pulmonary and extrapulmonary syndromes. Am J Infect Control 1993;21:21.

Thacker WL, Plikaytis BB, Wilkinson HW: Identification of 22 *Legionella* species and 33 serogroups with the slide agglutination test. J Clin Microbiol 1985;21:779.

Bacterial Vaginosis

Amsel R et al: Nonspecific vaginitis: Diagnostic criteria and microbial and epidemiologic association. Am J Med 1983;74:14.

Eschenbach DA: History and review of bacterial vaginosis. Am J Obstet Gyncol 1993;169(2 Part 2):441.

McGregor JA et al: Premature rupture of membranes and bacterial vaginosis. Am J Obstet Gyncol 1993;169(2 Part 2):463.

Roberts MC et al: Comparison of Gram stain, DNA probe, and culture for identification of species of *Mobiluncus* in female genital specimens. J Infect Dis 1985;152:74.

Spiegel CA et al: Anaerobic bacteria in nonspecific vaginitis. N Engl J Med 1980;303:601.

Streptobacillus Infections

Shanson DC et al: *Streptobacillus moniliformis* isolated from blood in four cases of Haverhill fever. Lancet 1983;2:92.

Bartonella (Rochalimaea) Infections

Cotell SL, Noskin GA: Bacillary angiomatosis: Clinical and histologic features, diagnosis, and treatment Arch Intern Med 1994;154:524.

Koehler JE, Tappero JW: Bacillary angiomatosis and bacillary peliosis in patients infected with human immunodeficiency virus. 1993;17:612.

Koehler JE et al: *Rochalimaea henselae* infection: A new zoonosis with the domestic cat as reservoir. JAMA 1994;271:531.

Scherer DC et al: Characterization of *Bartonella bacilliformis* flagella and effect of antiflagellin antibodies on invasion of human erythrocytes. Infect Immun 1993; 61:4962.

Schultz MG: A history of bartonellosis (Carrión's disease). Am J Trop Med Hyg 1968;17:503.

Schwartzman WA: Infections due to *Rochalimaea:* The expanding clinical spectrum. Clin Infect Dis 1992;15: 893.

Granuloma Inguinale

Kuberski T: Granuloma inguinale (donovanosis). Sex Transm Dis 1980;7:29.

Whipple's Disease

Relman DA et al: Identification of the uncultured bacillus of Whipple's disease. New Engl J Med 1992;327:293.

Relman DA: The identification of uncultured microbial pathogens. J Infect Dis 1993;168:1.

Mycobacteria

24

The mycobacteria are rod-shaped, aerobic bacteria that do not form spores. Although they do not stain readily, once stained they resist decolorization by acid or alcohol and are therefore called "acid-fast" bacilli. *Mycobacterium tuberculosis* causes tuberculosis and is a very important pathogen of humans. *Mycobacterium leprae* causes leprosy. *Mycobacterium avium-intracellulare* (*M avium* complex) and other **atypical mycobacteria** frequently infect patients with AIDS, are opportunistic pathogens in other immunocompromised persons, and occasionally cause disease in patients with normal immune systems. There are more than 50 *Mycobacterium* species, including many that are saprophytes. The mycobacteria that infect humans are listed in Table 24–1.

MYCOBACTERIUM TUBERCULOSIS

Morphology & Identification (Figure 24–1)

A. Typical Organisms: In tissue, tubercle bacilli are thin straight rods measuring about 0.4×3 μm. On artificial media, coccoid and filamentous forms are seen with variable morphology from one species to another. Mycobacteria cannot be classified as either gram-positive or gram-negative. Once stained by basic dyes they cannot be decolorized by alcohol, regardless of treatment with iodine. True tubercle bacilli are characterized by "acid-fastness"—ie, 95% ethyl alcohol containing 3% hydrochloric acid (acid-alcohol) quickly decolorizes all bacteria except the mycobacteria. Acid-fastness depends on the integrity of the waxy envelope. The **Ziehl-Neelsen technique** of staining is employed for identification of acid-fast bacteria. The method is detailed in Chapter 47. In smears of sputum or sections of tissue, mycobacteria can be demonstrated by yellow-orange fluorescence after staining with fluorochrome stains (eg, auramine, rhodamine).

B. Culture: The media for primary culture of mycobacteria should include a nonselective medium and a selective medium. Selective media contain antibiotics to prevent the overgrowth of contaminating bacteria and fungi. There are three general formulations that can be used for both the nonselective and selective media.

1. Semisynthetic agar media–These media (eg, Middlebrook 7H10 and 7H11) contain defined salts, vitamins, cofactors, oleic acid, albumin, catalase, glycerol, glucose, and malachite green; the 7H11 medium contains casein hydrolysate also. The albumin neutralizes the toxic and inhibitory effects of fatty acids in the specimen or medium. Large inocula yield growth on these media in several weeks. Because large inocula may be necessary these media may be less sensitive than other media for primary isolation of mycobacteria.

The semisynthetic agar media are used for observing colony morphology, for susceptibility testing, and, with added antibiotics, as selective media.

2. Inspissated egg media–These media (eg, Löwenstein-Jensen) contain defined salts, glycerol, and complex organic substances (eg, fresh eggs or egg yolks, potato flour, and other ingredients in various combinations). Malachite green is included to inhibit other bacteria. Small inocula in specimens from patients will grow on these media in 3–6 weeks.

These media with added antibiotics are used as selective media.

3. Broth media–Broth media (eg, Middlebrook 7H9 and 7H12) support the proliferation of small inocula. Ordinarily, mycobacteria grow in clumps or masses because of the hydrophobic character of the cell surface. If Tweens (water-soluble esters of fatty acids) are added, they wet the surface and thus permit dispersed growth in liquid media. Growth is often more rapid than on complex media.

The 7H12 medium with added antibiotics, supplements, and ^{14}C-palmitic acid is the basis for the BACTEC culture system for mycobacteria. During growth, the mycobacteria utilize the ^{14}C-palmitic acid, releasing $^{14}CO_2$, which is detected by the machine. Positive cultures can be detected with this system in an average of about 2 weeks.

C. Growth Characteristics: Mycobacteria are obligate aerobes and derive energy from the oxidation of many simple carbon compounds. Increased CO_2 tension enhances growth. Biochemical activities are not characteristic, and the growth rate is much slower than that of most bacteria. The doubling time of tubercle bacilli is about 18 hours. Saprophytic forms tend to grow more rapidly, to proliferate well at 22–33 °C, to

Table 24–1. Mycobacteria that infect humans.

	Species	Reservoir	Common Clinical Manifestations; Comment
Species always considered pathogens	*M tuberculosis*	Humans	Pulmonary and disseminated tuberculosis; millions of cases annually in the world
	M leprae	Humans	Leprosy
	M bovis	Humans, cattle	Tuberculosis-like disease; rare in North America; *M bovis* is closely related to *M tuberculosis*
Species potentially pathogenic in humans	**Moderately common causes of disease**		
	M avium-intracellulare complex	Soil, water, birds, fowl, swine, cattle, environment	Disseminated, pulmonary; very common in AIDS patients; occurs in other immunosuppressed patients; uncommon in patients with normal immune systems
	M kansasii	Water, cattle	Pulmonary, other sites
	Uncommon to very rare causes of disease		
	M africanum	Humans, monkeys	Pulmonary cultures; resembles *M tuberculosis;* rare
	M genavense	Humans?, pet birds?	Blood in AIDS patients; grows in liquid medium (BACTEC) and on solid medium supplemented with mycobactin j; grows in 2 to 8 weeks
	M haemophilum	Unknown	Subcutaneous nodules and ulcers primarily in AIDS patients; requires hemoglobin or hemin; grows at 28–32 °C; rare
	M malmoense	Unknown, environment`	Pulmonary, tuberculosis-like (adults), lymph nodes (children); most reported cases are from Sweden, but organism may be much more widespread; *M malmoense* is closely related to *M avium-intracellulare;* takes 8–12 weeks to grow
	M marinum	Fish, water	Subcutaneous nodules and abscesses, skin ulcers
	M scrofulaceum	Soil, water, moist foods	Cervical lymphadenitis; usually cured by incision, drainage, and removal of involved lymph nodes
	M simiae	Monkeys, water	Pulmonary, disseminated in AIDS patients; rare
	M szulgai	Unknown	Pulmonary, tuberculosis-like; rare
	M ulcerans	Humans, environment?	Subcutaneous nodules and ulcers; may be severe; *M ulcerans* is closely related to *M marinum;* takes 6 to 12 weeks to grow; optimal growth at 33 °C suggests environmental source; rare
	M xenopi	Water, birds	Pulmonary, tuberculosis-like with preexisting lung disease; rare
	Rapid growers		
	M fortuitum and *M chelonae*	Soil, water, animals, marine life	Cutaneous lesions most common, subcutaneous abscesses, disseminated infections; grow in ≤ 7 days; *M fortuitum* is more susceptible to antibiotics
Saprophytic species that very rarely cause disease in humans	*M gordonae* *M flavescens* *M fallax* *M gastri* *M smegmatis* *M terraetriviale*	Water Soil, water Soil, water Gastric washings Genital flora Soil, vegetables	These saprophytic *Mycobacterium* species are very uncommon causes of disease in humans. Positive cultures for these mycobacteria usually represent environmental contamination of specimens and not disease. Many of the saprophytic mycobacteria grow best at temperatures ≤ 33 °C. There are many other saprophytic *Mycobacterium* species not listed here that seldom if ever appear in cultures of patients' specimens.

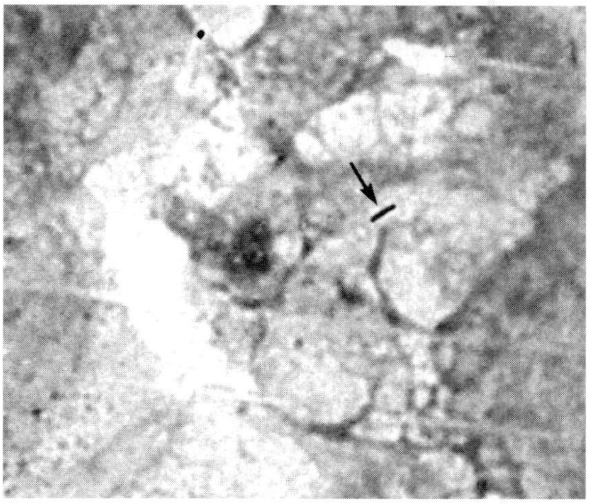

Figure 24–1. *Mycobacterium tuberculosis* (arrow) in a processed sputum specimen stained by Ziehl-Neelsen stain. The single *M tuberculosis* appeared red against a faint blue background.

produce more pigment, and to be less acid-fast than pathogenic forms.

D. Reaction to Physical and Chemical Agents: Mycobacteria tend to be more resistant to chemical agents than other bacteria because of the hydrophobic nature of the cell surface and their clumped growth. Dyes (eg, malachite green) or antibacterial agents (eg, penicillin) that are bacteriostatic to other bacteria can be incorporated into media without inhibiting the growth of tubercle bacilli. Acids and alkalies permit the survival of some exposed tubercle bacilli and are used to help eliminate contaminating organisms and for "concentration" of clinical specimens. Tubercle bacilli are resistant to drying and survive for long periods in dried sputum.

E. Variation: Variation can occur in colony appearance, pigmentation, virulence, optimal growth temperature, and many other cellular or growth characteristics.

F. Pathogenicity of Mycobacteria: There are marked differences in the ability of different mycobacteria to cause lesions in various host species. Humans and guinea pigs are highly susceptible to *M tuberculosis* infection, whereas fowl and cattle are resistant. *M tuberculosis* and *Mycobacterium bovis* are equally pathogenic for humans. The route of infection (respiratory versus intestinal) determines the pattern of lesions. In developed countries, *M bovis* has become very rare. Some "atypical" mycobacteria (eg, *Mycobacterium kansasii*) produce human disease indistinguishable from tuberculosis; others (eg, *Mycobacterium fortuitum*) cause only surface lesions or act as opportunists.

Constituents of Tubercle Bacilli

The constituents listed below are found mainly in cell walls. Mycobacterial cell walls can induce delayed hypersensitivity and some resistance to infection and can replace whole mycobacterial cells in Freund's adjuvant. Mycobacterial cell contents only elicit delayed hypersensitivity reactions in previously sensitized animals.

A. Lipids: Mycobacteria are rich in lipids. These include mycolic acids (long-chain fatty acids C78–C90), waxes, and phosphatides. In the cell, the lipids are largely bound to proteins and polysaccharides. Muramyl dipeptide (from peptidoglycan) complexed with mycolic acids can cause granuloma formation; phospholipids induce caseation necrosis. Lipids are to some extent responsible for acid-fastness. Their removal with hot acid destroys acid-fastness, which depends on both the integrity of the cell wall and the presence of certain lipids. Acid-fastness is also lost after sonication of mycobacterial cells. Analysis of lipids by gas chromatography reveals patterns that aid in classification of different species.

Virulent strains of tubercle bacilli form microscopic "serpentine cords" in which acid-fast bacilli are arranged in parallel chains. Cord formation is correlated with virulence. A "cord factor" (trehalose-6,6′-dimycolate) has been extracted from virulent bacilli with petroleum ether. It inhibits migration of leukocytes, causes chronic granulomas, and can serve as an immunologic "adjuvant."

B. Proteins: Each type of mycobacterium contains several proteins that elicit the tuberculin reaction. Proteins bound to a wax fraction can, upon injection, induce tuberculin sensitivity. They can also elicit the formation of a variety of antibodies.

C. Polysaccharides: Mycobacteria contain a variety of polysaccharides. Their role in the pathogenesis of disease is uncertain. They can induce the immediate type of hypersensitivity and can serve as antigens in reactions with sera of infected persons.

Pathogenesis

Mycobacteria in droplets 1–5 μm in diameter are inhaled and reach alveoli. The disease results from establishment and proliferation of virulent organisms and interactions with the host. Injected avirulent bacilli (eg, BCG) survive only for months or years in the normal host. Resistance and hypersensitivity of the host greatly influence the development of the disease.

Pathology

The production and development of lesions and their healing or progression are determined chiefly by (1) the number of mycobacteria in the inoculum and their subsequent multiplication, and (2) the resistance and hypersensitivity of the host.

A. Two Principal Lesions:

1. Exudative type–This consists of an acute inflammatory reaction, with edema fluid, polymorphonuclear leukocytes, and, later, monocytes around the tubercle bacilli. This type is seen particularly in lung tissue, where it resembles bacterial pneumonia. It may heal by resolution, so that the entire exudate becomes absorbed; it may lead to massive necrosis of tissue; or it may develop into the second (productive) type of lesion. During the exudative phase, the tuberculin test becomes positive.

2. Productive type–When fully developed, this lesion, a chronic granuloma, consists of three zones: (1) a central area of large, multinucleated giant cells containing tubercle bacilli; (2) a mid zone of pale epithelioid cells, often arranged radially; and (3) a peripheral zone of fibroblasts, lymphocytes, and monocytes. Later, peripheral fibrous tissue develops, and the central area undergoes caseation necrosis. Such a lesion is called a tubercle. A caseous tubercle may break into a bronchus, empty its contents there, and form a cavity. It may subsequently heal by fibrosis or calcification.

B. Spread of Organisms in the Host: Tubercle bacilli spread in the host by direct extension, through the lymphatic channels and bloodstream, and via the bronchi and gastrointestinal tract.

In the first infection, tubercle bacilli always spread from the initial site via the lymphatics to the regional lymph nodes. The bacilli may spread farther and reach the bloodstream, which in turn distributes bacilli to all organs (miliary distribution). The bloodstream can be invaded also by erosion of a vein by a caseating tubercle or lymph node. If a caseating lesion discharges its contents into a bronchus, they are aspirated and distributed to other parts of the lungs or are swallowed and passed into the stomach and intestines.

C. Intracellular Site of Growth: Once mycobacteria establish themselves in tissue, they reside principally intracellularly in monocytes, reticuloendothelial cells, and giant cells. The intracellular location is one of the features that makes chemotherapy difficult and favors microbial persistence. Within the cells of immune animals, multiplication of tubercle bacilli is greatly inhibited.

Primary Infection & Reaction Types of Tuberculosis

When a host has first contact with tubercle bacilli, the following features are usually observed: (1) An acute exudative lesion develops and rapidly spreads to the lymphatics and regional lymph nodes. The **"Ghon complex"** is the primary tissue lesion (usually in the lung) together with the involved lymph nodes. The exudative lesion in tissue often heals rapidly. (2) The lymph node undergoes massive caseation, which usually calcifies. (3) The tuberculin test becomes positive.

This primary infection type occurred in the past, usually in childhood but now frequently in adults who have remained free from infection and therefore tuberculin-negative in early life. In primary infections, the involvement may be in any part of the lung but is most often at the base.

The reactivation type is usually caused by tubercle bacilli that have survived in the primary lesion. Reactivation tuberculosis is characterized by chronic tissue lesions, the formation of tubercles, caseation, and fibrosis. Regional lymph nodes are only slightly involved, and they do not caseate. The reactivation type almost always begins at the apex of the lung, where the oxygen tension (Po_2) is highest.

The contrast between primary infection and reinfection is shown experimentally in **Koch's phenomenon.** When a guinea pig is injected subcutaneously with virulent tubercle bacilli, the puncture wound heals quickly, but a nodule forms at the site of injection in 2 weeks. This nodule ulcerates, and the ulcer does not heal. The regional lymph nodes develop tubercles and caseate massively. When the same animal is later injected with tubercle bacilli in another part of the body, the sequence of events is quite different: there is rapid necrosis of skin and tissue at the site of injection, but the ulcer heals rapidly. Regional lymph nodes either do not become infected at all or do so only after a delay.

These differences between primary infection and reinfection or reactivation are attributed to (1) resistance and (2) hypersensitivity induced by the first infection of the host with tubercle bacilli. It is not clear to what extent each of these components participates in the modified response in reactivation tuberculosis.

Immunity & Hypersensitivity

Unless a host dies during the first infection with tubercle bacilli, a certain resistance is acquired (see Koch's phenomenon, above), and there is an increased capacity to localize tubercle bacilli, retard their multiplication, limit their spread, and reduce lymphatic dissemination. This can be attributed to the development of cellular immunity during the initial infection, with evident ability of mononuclear phagocytes to limit the multiplication of ingested organisms and even to destroy them.

Antibodies form against a variety of the cellular constituents of the tubercle bacilli. The presence of antibodies can be determined by many different serologic tests. None of these serologic reactions bears any unequivocal relation to the immune state of the host, but high titers of IgG antibody to PPD, detectable by EIA test or precipitin reactions with polysaccharides, exist in many patients with active pulmonary tuberculosis.

In the course of primary infection, the host also acquires hypersensitivity to the tubercle bacilli. This is made evident by the development of a positive tuberculin reaction (see below). Tuberculin sensitivity can be induced by whole tubercle bacilli or by tuberculoprotein in combination with the chloroform-soluble wax D of the tubercle bacillus, but not by tuberculoprotein alone. Hypersensitivity and resistance appear to be distinct aspects of related cell-mediated reactions.

Tuberculin Test

A. Material: Old tuberculin is a concentrated filtrate of broth in which tubercle bacilli have grown for

6 weeks. In addition to the reactive tuberculoproteins, this material contains a variety of other constituents of tubercle bacilli and of growth medium. A purified protein derivative (PPD) is obtained by chemical fractionation of old tuberculin. PPD is standardized in terms of its biologic reactivity as "tuberculin units" (TU). By international agreement, the TU is defined as the activity contained in a specified weight of Seibert's PPD Lot No. 49608 in a specified buffer. This is PPD-S, the standard for tuberculin against which the potency of all products must be established by biologic assay—ie, by reaction size in humans. First-strength tuberculin has 1 TU; intermediate-strength has 5 TU; and second-strength has 250 TU. Bioequivalency of PPD products is not based on weight of the material but on comparative activity.

B. Dose of Tuberculin: A large amount of tuberculin injected into a hypersensitive host may give rise to severe local reactions and a flare-up of inflammation and necrosis at the main sites of infection (focal reactions). For this reason, tuberculin tests in surveys employ 5 TU; in persons suspected of extreme hypersensitivity, skin testing is begun with 1 TU. More concentrated material (250 TU) is administered only if the reaction to 5 TU is negative. The volume is usually 0.1 mL injected intracutaneously. The PPD preparation must be stabilized with polysorbate 80 to prevent adsorption to glass.

C. Reactions to Tuberculin: In an individual who has not had contact with mycobacteria, there is no reaction to PPD-S. An individual who has had a primary infection with tubercle bacilli develops induration, edema, erythema in 24–48 hours, and, with very intense reactions, even central necrosis. The skin test should be read in 48 or 72 hours. It is considered positive if the injection of 5 TU is followed by induration 10 mm or more in diameter. Positive tests tend to persist for several days. Weak reactions may disappear more rapidly.

The tuberculin test becomes positive within 4–6 weeks after infection (or injection of avirulent bacilli). It may be negative in the presence of tuberculous infection when "anergy" develops due to overwhelming tuberculosis, measles, Hodgkin's disease, sarcoidosis, or immunosuppression. A positive tuberculin test may occasionally revert to negative upon isoniazid treatment of a recent converter. After BCG vaccination, a positive test may last for only 3–7 years. Only the elimination of viable tubercle bacilli results in reversion of the tuberculin test to negative. However, persons who were PPD-positive years ago and are healthy may fail to give a positive skin test. When such persons are retested 2 weeks later, their PPD skin test—"boosted" by the recent antigen injection—will give a positive size of induration again. The reactivity to tuberculin can be transferred only by cells—not by serum—from a tuberculin-positive to a tuberculin-negative person.

D. Interpretation of Tuberculin Test: A positive tuberculin test indicates that an individual has been infected in the past and continues to carry viable mycobacteria in some tissue. It does not imply that active disease or immunity to disease is present. Tuberculin-positive persons are at risk of developing disease from reactivation of the primary infection, whereas tuberculin-negative persons who have never been infected are not subject to that risk, though they may become infected from an external source.

PPD preparations from other mycobacteria have been prepared. They exhibit some species specificity in low concentrations and marked cross-reaction in higher concentrations (see Other Mycobacteria, below).

Clinical Findings

Since the tubercle bacillus can involve every organ system, its clinical manifestations are protean. Fatigue, weakness, weight loss, and fever may be signs of tuberculous disease. Pulmonary involvement giving rise to chronic cough and spitting of blood usually is associated with far-advanced lesions. Meningitis or urinary tract involvement can occur in the absence of other signs of tuberculosis. Bloodstream dissemination leads to miliary tuberculosis with lesions in many organs and a high mortality rate.

Diagnostic Laboratory Tests

A positive tuberculin test does not prove the presence of active disease due to tubercle bacilli. Isolation of tubercle bacilli provides such proof.

A. Specimens: Specimens consist of fresh sputum, gastric washings, urine, pleural fluid, cerebrospinal fluid, joint fluid, biopsy material, blood, or other suspected material.

B. Decontamination and Concentration of Specimens: Specimens from sputum and other nonsterile sites should be liquefied with N-acetyl-L-cysteine, decontaminated with NaOH (kills many other bacteria and fungi), neutralized with buffer, and concentrated by centrifugation. Specimens processed in this way can be used for acid-fast stains and for culture. Specimens from sterile sites, such as cerebrospinal fluid, do not need the decontamination procedure but can be directly centrifuged, examined, and cultured.

C. Smears: Sputum, exudates, or other material is examined for acid-fast bacilli by Ziehl-Neelsen staining. Stains of gastric washings and urine generally are not recommended, because saprophytic mycobacteria may be present and yield a positive stain. Fluorescence microscopy with auramine-rhodamine stain is more sensitive than acid-fast stain; a confirmatory acid-fast stain is necessary if the fluorescent microscopy is positive. If acid-fast organisms are found in an appropriate specimen, this is presumptive evidence of mycobacterial infection.

D. Culture, Identification, and Susceptibility Testing: Processed specimens from nonsterile sites and centrifuged specimens from sterile sites can be cultured directly onto selective and nonselective media (see above). The selective broth culture often is the most sensitive method and provides results most rapidly. A selective agar media (eg, Löwenstein-Jensen or Middlebrook 7H10/7H11 biplate with antibiotics) should be inoculated in parallel with broth media cultures. Incubation is at 37 °C in 5–10% CO_2 for up to 8 weeks. If cultures are negative in the setting of a positive acid-fast stain or slowly growing atypical mycobacteria (see below) are suspected, then a set of inoculated media should be incubated at a lower temperature (eg, 24–33 °C) and both sets incubated for 12 weeks.

Blood for culture of mycobacteria (usually *M avium-intracellulare*) complex should be anticoagulated and processed by one of three methods: (1) commercially available lysis centrifugation system; (2) inoculation into commercially available broth media specifically designed for blood cultures; (3) centrifugation of the blood and inoculation of the white blood cell buffy coat layer, with or without deoxycholate lysis of the cells, into broth culture. Solid media can be used in parallel.

It is medically important to characterize and separate *M tuberculosis* from all the other species of mycobacteria. Isolated mycobacteria should be identified as to species. Conventional methods for identification of mycobacteria include observation of rate of growth, colony morphology, pigmentation, and biochemical profiles. The conventional methods often require 6–8 weeks for identification. Growth rate separates the rapid growers (growth in $\leq$ 7 days) from other mycobacteria (Table 24–1). **Photochromogens** produce pigment in light but not in darkness; **scotochromogens** develop pigment when growing in the dark; and **nonphotochromogens** develop various degrees of pigmentation unrelated to exposure to light (Runyon, Med Clin North Am 1959;43:273). Individual species or complexes are defined by additional biochemical characteristics (eg, positive niacin test as with *M tuberculosis*, reduction of nitrate, production of urease or catalase, arylsulfatase test, and many others). The conventional methods for classifying mycobacteria are rapidly becoming of historical interest because molecular probe methods are much faster and easier.

Molecular probes provide a rapid, sensitive, and specific method to identify mycobacteria. The probes can be used on mycobacterial growth from solid media or from broth cultures. DNA probes specific for rRNA sequences of the test organism are used in a hybridization procedure. There are approximately 10,000 copies of the rRNA per mycobacteria cell, providing a natural amplification system, enhancing detection. Double-stranded hybrids are separated from unhybridized single-stranded probes. The DNA probes are linked with chemicals that are activated in the hybrids and detected by chemiluminescence. Probes for the *M tuberculosis* complex (*M tuberculosis* and *M bovis*), *M avium-intracellulare* complex (*M avium, M intracellulare* and closely related mycobacteria), *M kansasii*, and *M gordonae* are in use and effectively identify most mycobacterial isolates in clinical laboratories. The use of these probes has shortened the time to identification of clinically important mycobacteria from several weeks to as little as 1 day.

High-performance liquid chromatography (HPLC) has been applied to speciation of many species of mycobacteria. The method is based on development of profiles of mycolic acids, which vary from one species to another. HPLC to speciate mycobacteria is available in reference laboratories.

Susceptibility testing of mycobacteria is an important adjunct in selecting drugs for effective therapy. A standardized radiometric broth culture technique can be used to test for susceptibility to first-line drugs. The complex and more arduous conventional agar-based technique usually is performed in reference laboratories; first- and second-line drugs can be tested by this method.

E. DNA Detection, Serology, and Antigen Detection: The polymerase chain reaction holds great promise for the rapid and direct detection of *M tuberculosis* in clinical specimens. The overall sensitivity is 80–85% with a specificity of about 99%. This method is under intense development for widespread application.

Enzyme immunoassays have been used to detect mycobacterial antigens, but the sensitivity and specificity are less than with other methods. Similar problems exist in application of EIA to detect antibodies to *M tuberculosis* antigens. Neither of these methods is adequate for routine diagnostic use.

Treatment

The primary treatment for mycobacterial infection is specific chemotherapy. The drugs for treatment of mycobacterial infection are discussed in Chapter 10. In the United States the most widely used antituberculosis drugs are isoniazid (INH), rifampin, ethambutol, and pyrazinamide. Second-line antituberculosis drugs include streptomycin, kanamycin, capreomycin, ethionamide, cycloserine, ofloxacin, and ciprofloxacin.

Between 1 in 10^6 and 1 in 10^8 tubercle bacilli are spontaneous mutants resistant to first-line antituberculosis drugs. When the drugs are used singly, the resistant tubercle bacilli emerge rapidly and multiply. Therefore, treatment regimens use drugs in combination to yield cure rates of > 95%. In the United States, initial therapy with three drugs is recommended for persons who have never been treated, do not reside in communities with a known high prevalence of drug-resistant tubercle bacilli, and who have no known risk factors for drug-resistant tuberculosis. A widely used regimen is isoniazid, rifampin, and pyrazinamide for 2 months until susceptibility test results are known, followed by isoniazid and rifampin for an additional 4 months. In AIDS patients, the isoniazid and rifampin are continued longer. Isoniazid and rifampin (without pyrazinamide) for 9 months also is effective. The sputum-positive patient becomes noninfective in 2–3 weeks after beginning effective chemotherapy.

A four-drug regimen of isoniazid, rifampin, pyrazinamide, and ethambutol is recommended for persons in the United States who have a slight to moderate risk for being infected with drug-resistant tubercle bacilli. The risk factors include recent emigration from Latin America or Asia; persons with HIV infections or who are at risk for HIV infection and live in an area with a low prevalence of multidrug-resistant tubercle bacilli; and persons who were previously treated with a regimen that did not include rifampin.

Multidrug-resistant *M tuberculosis* (resistant to both isoniazid and rifampin) is a major and increasing problem in tuberculosis treatment and control. Such strains are prevalent in certain geographic areas (eg, New York City) and certain populations (hospitals and prisons). There have been many outbreaks of tuberculosis with multidrug-resistant strains. They are particularly important in persons with HIV infections. Persons infected with multidrug-resistant organisms or who are at high risk for such infections, including exposure to another person with such an infection, should be treated according to susceptibility test results for the infecting strain. If susceptibility results are not available, the drugs should be selected according to the known pattern of susceptibility in the community and modified when the susceptibility test results are available. Therapy should include a minimum of three and preferably more than three drugs to which the organisms have demonstrated susceptibility.

Epidemiology

The most frequent source of infection is the human who excretes, particularly from the respiratory tract, large numbers of tubercle bacilli. Close contact (eg, in the family) and massive exposure (eg, in medical personnel) make transmission by droplet nuclei most likely.

Susceptibility to tuberculosis is a function of the risk of acquiring the infection and the risk of clinical disease after infection has occurred. For the tuberculin-negative person, the risk of acquiring tubercle bacilli depends on exposure to sources of infectious bacilli—principally sputum-positive patients. This risk is proportionate to the rate of active infection in the population, crowding, socioeconomic disadvantage, and inadequacy of medical care.

The development of clinical disease after infection may have a genetic component (proved in animals and suggested in humans by a higher incidence of disease in those with HLA-Bw15 histocompatibility antigen). It is influenced by age (high risk in infancy and in the elderly), by undernutrition, and by immunologic status, coexisting diseases (eg, silicosis, diabetes), and other individual host resistance factors.

Infection occurs at an earlier age in urban than in rural populations. Disease occurs only in a small proportion of infected individuals. In the USA at present, active disease has several epidemiologic patterns where individuals are at increased risk: minorities, predominantly African Americans and Hispanics; HIV-infected patients; homeless persons; and the very young and very old. The incidence of tuberculosis is especially high in minority persons with HIV infections. Primary infection can occur in any person exposed to an infectious source. Patients who have had tuberculosis can be infected exogenously a second time. Endogenous reactivation tuberculosis occurs most commonly among persons with AIDS and elderly malnourished or alcoholic destitute men.

Prevention & Control

(1) Prompt and effective treatment of patients with active tuberculosis and careful follow-up of their contacts with tuberculin tests, x-rays, and appropriate treatment are the mainstays of public health tuberculosis control. Resurgence of tuberculosis implies that these control measures have not been done adequately.

(2) Drug treatment of asymptomatic tuberculin-positive persons in the age groups most prone to develop complications (eg, children) and in tuberculin-positive persons who must receive immunosuppressive drugs greatly reduces reactivation of infection.

(3) Individual host resistance: Nonspecific factors may reduce host resistance, thus favoring the conversion of asymptomatic infection into disease. Such factors include starvation, gastrectomy, and suppression of cellular immunity by drugs (eg, corticosteroids) or infection. HIV infection is a major risk factor for tuberculosis.

(4) Immunization: Living avirulent tubercle bacilli, particularly BCG (bacillus Calmette-Guérin, an attenuated bovine organism), have been used to induce a certain amount of resistance in those heavily exposed to infection. Vaccination with these organisms is a substitute for primary infection with virulent tubercle bacilli without the danger inherent in the latter. The available vaccines are inadequate from many technical and biologic standpoints. Nevertheless, BCG is given to children in many countries. In the USA, the use of BCG is suggested only for tuberculin-negative persons who are heavily exposed (members of tuberculous families, medical personnel). Statistical evidence indicates that an increased resistance for a limited period follows BCG vaccination.

(5) The eradication of tuberculosis in cattle and the pasteurization of milk have greatly reduced *M bovis* infections.

OTHER MYCOBACTERIA

In addition to tubercle bacilli *(M tuberculosis, M bovis)*, other mycobacteria of varying degrees of pathogenicity have been grown from human sources in past decades. These "atypical" mycobacteria were initially grouped according to speed of growth at various temperatures and production of pigments (see above). Several are now identified using DNA probes. Most of them occur in the environment, are not readily transmitted from person to person, and are opportunistic pathogens (Table 24–1).

Species or complexes that are significant causes of disease are outlined below.

Mycobacterium avium-intracellulare Complex

The *M avium-intracellulare* complex are often called MAI or MAC (*Mycobacterium avium* complex). They grow optimally at 41 °C and produce smooth, soft, nonpigmented colonies. They are ubiquitous in the environment and have been cultured from water, soil, food, and animals, including birds.

MAI infrequently cause disease in immunocompetent humans. However, in the United States, disseminated MAI infection is the most common opportunistic infection of bacterial origin in AIDS patients. The risk of developing disseminated MAI infection in HIV-infected persons is greatly increased when the CD4-positive lymphocyte count declines to $< 100/\mu L$. Gender, race, ethnic group, and individual risk factors for HIV infection do not influence the development of disseminated MAI infection, but prior *Pneumocystis carinii* infection, severe anemia, and interruption of antiretroviral therapy may increase the risk.

At least 25% and perhaps as high as 50% of HIV-infected patients develop MAI bacteremia and disseminated infection during the course of AIDS. In the United States, laboratories often have many more cultures positive for MAI than for *M tuberculosis*.

Environmental exposure can led to MAI colonization of either the respiratory or gastrointestinal tract. Transient bacteremia occurs followed by invasion of tissues. Persistent bacteremia and extensive infiltration of tissues resulting in organ dysfunction result. Any organ can be involved. In the lung, nodules, diffuse infiltrates, cavities, and endobronchial lesions are common. Other manifestations include pericarditis, soft tissue abscesses, skin lesions, lymph node involvement, bone infection, and central nervous system lesions. The patients often present with nonspecific symptoms of fever, night sweats, abdominal pain, diarrhea, and weight loss.

The diagnosis is made by culturing MAI from blood or tissue. There is no standardized susceptibility test method and no good correlation of in vitro susceptibility test results with clinical outcome. Most information on drug therapy comes from clinical trials.

MAI routinely are resistant to first line antituberculosis drugs. Treatment with the new macrolides, either clarithromycin or azithromycin, plus ethambutol is a preferred initial therapy. Other drugs that may be useful are rifabutin (ansamycin), clofazimine, fluoroquinolones, and amikacin. Multiple drugs often are used in combination. Therapy should be continued for life. Therapy results in decreasing counts of MAI in blood and decrease or amelioration in clinical symptoms. Rifabutin prophylaxis decreases the incidence of bacteremia by about 50% and decreases the clinical symptoms when disseminated disease occurs.

Mycobacterium kansasii

M kansasii is a photochromogen that requires complex media for growth at 37 °C. It can produce pulmonary and systemic disease indistinguishable from tuberculosis, especially in patients with impaired immune responses. Sensitive to rifampin, it is often treated with the combination of rifampin, ethambutol, and isoniazid with good clinical response. The source of infection is uncertain, and communicability is low or absent.

Mycobacterium scrofulaceum

This is a scotochromogen occasionally found in water and as a saprophyte in adults with chronic lung disease. It causes chronic cervical lymphadenitis in children and, rarely, other granulomatous disease. Surgical excision of involved cervical lymph nodes may be curative, and resistance to antituberculosis drugs is common. (*Mycobacterium shulgai* and *Mycobacterium xenopi* are similar.)

Mycobacterium marinum & *Mycobacterium ulcerans*

These organisms occur in water, grow best at low temperature (31 °C), may infect fish, and can produce superficial skin lesions (ulcers, "swimming pool granulomas") in humans. Surgical excision, tetracyclines, rifampin, and ethambutol are sometimes effective.

Mycobacterium fortuitum-chelonae Complex

These are saprophytes found in soil and water that grow rapidly (3–6 days) in culture and form no pigment. They can produce superficial and systemic disease in humans on rare occasions. *Mycobacterium fortuitum* has contaminated porcine valves used as prostheses in human cardiac surgery. The organisms are often resistant to antimycobacterial drugs but may respond to amikacin, doxycycline, cefoxitin, erythromycin, or rifampin.

Other *Mycobacterium* Species

The high risk for mycobacterial infection in AIDS patients has resulted in increased awareness of mycobacterial infections in general. Species previously considered to be curiosities and extremely uncommon have been more widely recognized (Table 24–1). *Mycobacterium malmoense* has been reported mostly from Northern Europe. It causes a pulmonary tuberculosis-like disease in adults and lymphadenitis in children. *Mycobacterium haemophilum* and *Mycobacterium genavense* cause disease in AIDS patients.

The importance of these two species is not fully understood.

Saprophytic Mycobacteria Not Associated With Human Illness

Mycobacterium phlei is frequently found on plants, in soil, or in water. *Mycobacterium gordonae* is similar. *Mycobacterium smegmatis* occurs regularly in human sebaceous secretions and it might be confused with pathogenic acid-fast organisms. *Mycobacterium paratuberculosis* produces a chronic enteritis in cattle and may be associated with Crohn's disease (regional enteritis) in humans.

MYCOBACTERIUM LEPRAE

Although this organism was described by Hansen in 1873 (9 years before Koch's discovery of the tubercle bacillus), it has not been cultivated on nonliving bacteriologic media. It causes leprosy. There are more than 10 million cases of leprosy, mainly in Asia.

Typical acid-fast bacilli—singly, in parallel bundles, or in globular masses—are regularly found in scrapings from skin or mucous membranes (particularly the nasal septum) in lepromatous leprosy. The bacilli are often found within the endothelial cells of blood vessels or in mononuclear cells. The organisms have not been grown on artificial media. When bacilli from human leprosy (ground tissue nasal scrapings) are inoculated into footpads of mice, local granulomatous lesions develop with limited multiplication of bacilli. Inoculated armadillos develop extensive lepromatous leprosy, and armadillos naturally infected with leprosy have been found in Texas and Mexico. *M leprae* from armadillo or human tissue contains a unique *o*-diphenoloxidase, perhaps an enzyme characteristic of leprosy bacilli.

Clinical Findings

The onset of leprosy is insidious. The lesions involve the cooler tissue of the body: skin, superficial nerves, nose, pharynx, larynx, eyes, and testicles. The skin lesions may occur as pale, anesthetic macular lesions 1–10 cm in diameter; diffuse or discrete erythematous, infiltrated nodules 1–5 cm in diameter; or a diffuse skin infiltration. Neurologic disturbances are manifested by nerve infiltration and thickening, with resultant anesthesia, neuritis, paresthesia, trophic ulcers, and bone resorption and shortening of digits. The disfigurement due to the skin infiltration and nerve involvement in untreated cases may be extreme.

The disease is divided into two major types, lepromatous and tuberculoid, with several intermediate stages. In the lepromatous type, the course is progressive and malignant, with nodular skin lesions; slow symmetric nerve involvement; abundant acid-fast bacilli in the skin lesions; continuous bacteremia; and a negative lepromin (extract of lepromatous tissue) skin test. In lepromatous leprosy, cell-mediated immunity is markedly deficient and the skin is infiltrated with suppressor T cells. In the tuberculoid type, the course is benign and nonprogressive, with macular skin lesions, severe asymmetric nerve involvement of sudden onset with few bacilli present in the lesions, and a positive lepromin skin test. In tuberculoid leprosy, cell-mediated immunity is intact and the skin is infiltrated with helper T cells.

Systemic manifestations of anemia and lymphadenopathy may also occur. Eye involvement is common. Amyloidosis may develop.

Diagnosis

Scrapings with a scalpel from skin or nasal mucosa or from a biopsy of earlobe skin are smeared on a slide and stained by the Ziehl-Neelsen technique. Biopsy of skin or of a thickened nerve gives a typical histologic picture. No serologic tests are of value. Nontreponemal serologic tests for syphilis frequently yield false-positive results in leprosy.

Treatment

Several specialized sulfones (eg, dapsone, DDS; see Chapter 10) and rifampin suppress the growth of *M leprae* and the clinical manifestations of leprosy if given for many months. Sulfone resistance is beginning to emerge in leprosy. For this reason, initial treatment is with a combination of sulfone and rifampin. Clofazimine is an oral drug (100–300 mg/d) used in sulfone-resistant leprosy.

Epidemiology

Transmission of leprosy is most likely to occur when small children are exposed for prolonged periods to heavy shedders of bacilli. Nasal secretions are the most likely infectious material for family contacts. The incubation period is probably 2–10 years. Without prophylaxis, about 10% of exposed children may acquire the disease. Treatment tends to reduce and abolish the infectivity of patients. Naturally infected armadillos have been found in Texas and Mexico but probably play no role in transmission of leprosy to humans.

Prevention & Control

Identification and treatment of patients with leprosy is the key to control. Children of presumably contagious parents are given chemoprophylactic drugs until treatment of the parents has made them noninfectious. If any member of a domestic group has lepromatous leprosy, such prophylaxis is required for children in the group. Experimental BCG vaccination and an *M leprae* vaccine are also being explored for family contacts and possibly for community contacts in endemic areas.

REFERENCES

Alvarez S, McCabe WR: Extrapulmonary tuberculosis revisited. Medicine 1984;63:25.

Barnes PF, Barrows SA: Tuberculosis in the 1990s. Ann Intern Med 1993;119:400.

Carpenter JL et al: Disseminated disease due to *Mycobacterium chelonei* treated with amikacin and cefoxitin. Arch Intern Med 1984;144:2063.

Cohn DL et al: A 62 dose 6-month therapy for pulmonary and extrapulmonary tuberculosis. Ann Intern Med 1990; 112:407.

Combs DL et al: USPHS tuberculosis short-course chemotherapy trial 21. Ann Intern Med 1990;112:397.

Donta ST et al: Therapy of *Mycobacterium marinum* infections: Use of tetracyclines vs. rifampin. Arch Intern Med 1986;146:902.

Frieden TR et al: The emergence of drug-resistant tuberculosis in New York City. N Engl J Med 1993;328:521.

Goble M et al: Treatment of 171 patients with pulmonary tuberculosis resistant to isoniazid and rifampin. N Engl J Med 1993;328:527.

Iseman MD: Treatment of multidrug-resistant tuberculosis. N Engl J Med 1993;329:784.

Klein NC, Damsker B, Hirschman SZ: Mycobacterial meningitis: Retrospective analysis from 1970 to 1983. Am J Med 1985;79:29.

Lai KK et al: Mycobacterial cervical lymphadenopathy: Relation of etiologic agents to age. JAMA 1984;251:1286.

Lipsky BA et al: Factors affecting the clinical value of microscopy for acid-fast bacilli. Rev Infect Dis 1984;6:214.

Masur H (editor): Management of *Mycobacterium avium* complex in patients with HIV infection. Clin Infect Dis 1994;18(Suppl 5):S217.

Neill MA, Hightower AW, Broome CV: Leprosy in the United States 1971–1981. J Infect Dis 1985;152: 1064.

PHS Advisory Committee on Immunization Practices: BCG vaccines. MMWR Morb Mortal Wkly Rep 199 1979;28: 241.

Shepard CC: Leprosy today. N Engl J Med 1982;307:1640.

Snider DE: The tuberculin skin test. Am Rev Respir Dis 1982;125:108.

Stead WW et al: Tuberculosis as an endemic and nosocomial infection among the elderly in nursing homes. N Engl J Med 1985;312:1483.

Van Voorhis WC et al: The cutaneous infiltrates of leprosy: Cellular characteristics and the predominant T-cell phenotypes. N Engl J Med 1982;307:1593.

Wallace RJ et al: Spectrum of disease due to rapidly growing mycobacteria. Rev Infect Dis 1983;5:657.

Wallace RJ et al: Treatment of nonpulmonary infections due to *Mycobacterium fortuitum* and *M chelonei* on the basis of in vitro susceptibilities. J Infect Dis 1985;152: 500.

Yawalkar SJ et al: Once monthly rifampin plus daily dapsone in initial treatment of lepromatous leprosy. Lancet 1982; 1:1199.

Young LS: *Mycobacterium avium* complex infections. J Infect Dis 1988;157:863.

Spirochetes & Other Spiral Microorganisms

25

The spirochetes are a large, heterogeneous group of spiral, motile bacteria. One family (Spirochaetaceae) of the order Spirochaetales includes three genera of free-living, large spiral organisms. The other family (Treponemataceae) has genera whose members include human pathogens: (1) the *Treponema;* (2) the *Borrelia;* and, (3) the *Leptospira.*

The spirochetes have many structural characteristics in common, as typified by *Treponema pallidum* (Figure 25–1). They are long, slender, helically coiled, spiral or corkscrew-shaped, gram-negative bacilli. *T pallidum* has an **outer sheath** or glycosaminoglycan coating. Inside the sheath is the outer membrane which contains peptidoglycan and maintains the structural integrity of the organisms. **Endoflagella** (axial filaments) are the flagella-like organelles in the periplasmic space encased by the outer membrane. The endoflagella begin at each end of the organism and wind around it, extending to and overlapping at the midpoint. Inside the endoflagella is the inner membrane (cytoplasmic membrane) that provides osmotic stability and covers the protoplasmic cylinder. A series of cytoplasmic tubules (body fibrils) are inside the cell near the inner membrane. Treponemes reproduce by transverse fission.

TREPONEMA

The genus *Treponema* includes *Treponema pallidum* subsp *pallidum,* which causes syphilis; *Treponema pallidum* subsp *pertenue,* which causes yaws; *Treponema pallidum* subsp *endemicum,* which causes endemic syphilis (also called bejel); and *Treponema carateum,* which causes pinta.

TREPONEMA PALLIDUM & SYPHILIS

Morphology & Identification

A. Typical Organisms: Slender spirals measuring about 0.2 μm in width and 5–15 μm in length. The spiral coils are regularly spaced at a distance of 1 μm from one another. The organisms are actively motile, rotating steadily around their endoflagella even after attaching to cells by their tapered ends. The long axis of the spiral is ordinarily straight but may sometimes bend, so that the organism forms a complete circle for moments at a time, returning then to its normal straight position.

The spirals are so thin that they are not readily seen unless immunofluorescent stain or darkfield illumination is employed. They do not stain well with aniline dyes, but they can be seen in tissues when stained by a silver impregnation method.

B. Culture: Pathogenic *Treponema pallidum* has never been cultured continuously on artificial media, in fertile eggs, or in tissue culture. Nonpathogenic treponemes (eg, Reiter strain) can be cultured anaerobically in vitro. They are saprophytes antigenically related to *T pallidum.*

C. Growth Characteristics: *T pallidum* is a microaerophilic organism; it survives best in 1–4% oxygen. The saprophytic Reiter strain grows on a defined medium of 11 amino acids, vitamins, salts, minerals, and serum albumin.

In proper suspending fluids and in the presence of reducing substances, *T pallidum* may remain motile for 3–6 days at 25 °C. In whole blood or plasma stored at 4 °C, organisms remain viable for at least 24 hours, which is of potential importance in blood transfusions.

D. Reactions to Physical and Chemical Agents: Drying kills the spirochete rapidly, as does elevation of the temperature to 42 °C. Treponemes are rapidly immobilized and killed by trivalent arsenical, mercury, and bismuth (contained in drugs of historical interest in the treatment of syphilis. Penicillin is treponemicidal in minute concentrations, but the rate of killing is slow, presumably because of the metabolic inactivity and slow multiplication rate of *T pallidum* (estimated division time is 30 hours). Resistance to penicillin has not been demonstrated in syphilis.

Antigenic Structure

T pallidum cannot be cultured in vitro, which has markedly limited the characterization of its antigens. It is not clear if the glycosaminoglycan sheath is derived from host cells or made by the treponemes. The sheath

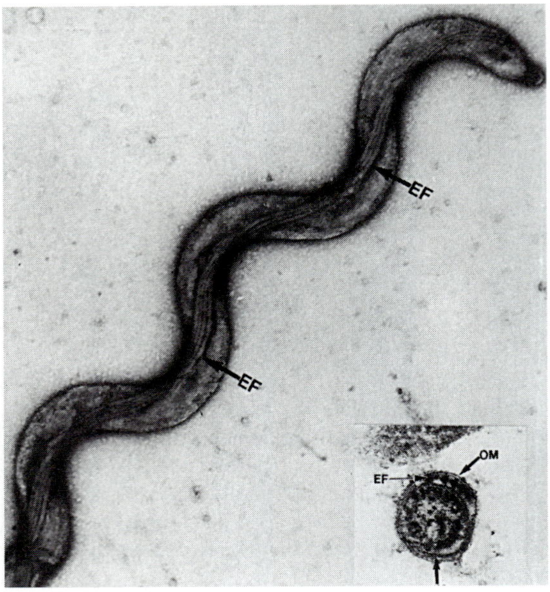

Figure 25–1. Electron micrograph of whole-mounted *Treponema pallidum* ssp *pallidum*. The endoflagella (EF) are clearly visible. Bar = 0.2 µm. ***Inset:*** Electron micrograph of thin-sectioned *Treponema pallidum*. Note the position of the endoflagella (EF) in the periplasmic space between the inner membrane (IM) and the outer membrane (OM). Bar = 50 nm. (Courtesy of Eldon M. Walker, University of Texas, Houston, Health Science Center.)

functions to inhibit the antibody- and complement-mediated killing of the organisms. There is sialic acid on the surface of the organism, which functions to inhibit activation of the alternative complement pathway. *T pallidum* subsp *pallidum* has hyaluronidase that breaks down the hyaluronic acid in the ground substance of tissue and presumably enhances the invasiveness of the organism. The protein profiles of *T pallidum* (all the subspecies) are indistinguishable; more than 100 protein antigens have been noted. The endoflagella are composed of three core proteins that are homologous to other bacterial flagellin proteins, plus an unrelated sheath protein. A group of lipoproteins are abundant and have unknown functions, though they appear to be important in the immune response. Cardiolipin is an important component of the treponemal antigens.

Humans with syphilis develop antibodies capable of staining *T pallidum* by indirect immunofluorescence, immobilizing and killing live motile *T pallidum* and fixing complement in the presence of a suspension of *T pallidum* or related spirochetes. The spirochetes also cause the development of a distinct antibody-like substance, reagin, which gives positive CF and flocculation tests with aqueous suspensions of cardiolipin extracted from normal mammalian tissues. Both reagin and antitreponemal antibody can be used for the serologic diagnosis of syphilis.

Pathogenesis, Pathology, & Clinical Findings

A. Acquired Syphilis: Natural infection with *T pallidum* is limited to the human host. Human infection is usually transmitted by sexual contact, and the infectious lesion is on the skin or mucous membranes of genitalia. In 10–20% of cases, however, the primary lesion is intrarectal, perianal, or oral. It may be anywhere on the body. *T pallidum* can probably penetrate intact mucous membranes, or it may enter through a break in the epidermis.

Spirochetes multiply locally at the site of entry, and some spread to nearby lymph nodes and then reach the bloodstream. In 2–10 weeks after infection, a papule develops at the site of infection and breaks down to form an ulcer with a clean, hard base ("hard chancre"). The inflammation is characterized by a predominance of lymphocytes and plasma cells. This "primary lesion" always heals spontaneously, but 2–10 weeks later the "secondary" lesions appear. These consist of a red maculopapular rash anywhere on the body, including the hands and feet, and moist, pale papules (condylomas) in the anogenital region, axillas, and mouth. There may also be syphilitic meningitis, chorioretinitis, hepatitis, nephritis (immune complex type), or periostitis. The secondary lesions also subside spontaneously. Both primary and secondary lesions are rich in spirochetes and highly infectious. Contagious lesions may recur within 3–5 years after infection, but thereafter the individual is not infectious. Syphilitic infection may remain subclinical, and the patient may pass through the primary or secondary stage (or both) without symptoms or signs yet develop tertiary lesions.

In about 30% of cases, early syphilitic infection progresses spontaneously to complete cure without treatment. In another 30%, the untreated infection remains latent (principally evident by positive serologic tests). In the remainder, the disease progresses to the "tertiary stage," characterized by the development of granulomatous lesions (gummas) in skin, bones, and liver; degenerative changes in the central nervous system (meningovascular syphilis, paresis, tabes); or cardiovascular lesions (aortitis, aortic aneurysm, aortic valve insufficiency). In all tertiary lesions, treponemes are very rare, and the exaggerated tissue response must be attributed to hypersensitivity to the organisms. However, treponemes can occasionally be found in the eye or central nervous system in late syphilis.

B. Congenital Syphilis: A pregnant syphilitic woman can transmit *T pallidum* to the fetus through the placenta beginning in the 10th to 15th weeks of gestation. Some of the infected fetuses die, and miscarriages result; others are stillborn at term. Others are born live but develop the signs of congenital syphilis in childhood: interstitial keratitis, Hutchinson's teeth, saddlenose, periostitis, and a variety of central nervous system anomalies. Adequate treatment of the mother during pregnancy prevents congenital syphilis. The reagin titer in the blood of the child rises with active infection but falls with time if antibody was passively transmitted from the mother. In congenital infection, the child makes IgM antitreponemal antibody.

C. Experimental Disease: Rabbits can be experimentally infected in the skin, testis, and eye with human *T pallidum.* The animal develops a chancre rich in spirochetes, and organisms persist in lymph nodes, spleen, and bone marrow for the entire life of the animal, although there is no progressive disease.

Diagnostic Laboratory Tests

A. Specimens: Tissue fluid expressed from early surface lesions for demonstration of spirochetes; blood serum for serologic tests.

B. Darkfield Examination: A drop of tissue fluid or exudate is placed on a slide and a coverslip pressed over it to make a thin layer. The preparation is then examined under oil immersion with darkfield illumination for typical motile spirochetes. (See Figure 2–1.)

Treponemes disappear from lesions within a few hours after the beginning of antibiotic treatment.

C. Immunofluorescence: Tissue fluid or exudate is spread on a glass slide, air dried, and sent to the laboratory. It is fixed, stained with a fluorescein-labeled antitreponeme serum, and examined by means of immunofluorescence microscopy for typical fluorescent spirochetes.

D. Serologic Tests for Syphilis (STS): These use either treponemal or nontreponemal antigens.

1. Nontreponemal antigen tests–The antigens employed are lipids extracted from normal mammalian tissue. The purified cardiolipin from beef heart is a diphosphatidylglycerol. It requires the addition of lecithin and cholesterol or other "sensitizers" to react with syphilitic "reagin." Reagin is a mixture of IgM and IgA antibodies directed against some antigens widely distributed in normal tissues. It is found in patients' serum after 2–3 weeks of untreated syphilitic infection and in spinal fluid after 4–8 weeks of infection. Two types of tests determine the presence of reagin.

a. Flocculation tests (VDRL Venereal Disease Research Laboratories; RPR rapid plasma reagin)–These tests are based on the fact that the particles of the lipid antigen (beef heart cardiolipin) remain dispersed with normal serum but form visible clumps when combining with reagin. Results develop within a few minutes, particularly if the suspension is agitated. The tests lend themselves to automation and to use for surveys because of their low cost. Positive VDRL or RPR tests revert to negative in 6–18 months after effective treatment of syphilis. VDRL and RPR tests can also be performed on spinal fluid. Antibodies do not reach the cerebrospinal fluid from the bloodstream but are probably formed in the central nervous system in response to syphilitic infection.

b. Complement fixation (CF) tests (Wassermann, Kolmer)–CF tests are based on the fact that reagin-containing sera fix complement in the presence of cardiolipin "antigen." It is necessary to ascertain that the serum is not "anticomplementary" (ie, that it does not destroy complement in the absence of antigen). This test is less widely used than the flocculation tests.

Both flocculation and CF tests can give quantitative results. An estimate of the amount of reagin present in serum can be made by performing the tests with twofold dilutions of serum and expressing the titer as the highest dilution that gives a positive result. Quantitative results are valuable in establishing a diagnosis, especially in neonates, and in evaluating the effect of treatment.

Nontreponemal tests are subject to false-positive results. Most commonly these are "biologic" false-positives attributable to the occurrence of "reagins" in a variety of human disorders. Prominent among the latter are other infections (malaria, leprosy, measles, infectious mononucleosis, etc), vaccinations, collagen-vascular diseases (systemic lupus erythematosus, polyarteritis nodosa, rheumatic disorders), and other conditions. Nontreponemal antibody tests may become negative spontaneously in progressive tertiary syphilis; thus, a negative VDRL does not rule out such disease activity.

2. Treponemal antibody tests–

a. Fluorescent treponemal antibody (FTA-ABS) test–A test employing indirect immunofluorescence (killed *T pallidum* + patient's serum + labeled antihuman gamma globulin) shows excellent specificity and sensitivity for syphilis antibodies if the patient's serum has been absorbed with sonicated Reiter spirochetes prior to the FTA test. The FTA-ABS test is the first to become positive in early syphilis, and it usually remains positive many years after effective treatment of early syphilis. The test cannot be used to judge the efficacy of treatment. The presence of IgM FTA in the blood of newborns is good evidence of in utero infection (congenital syphilis).

b. *Treponema pallidum* hemagglutination (TPHA) and microhemagglutination-*Treponema pallidum* tests–Red blood cells are treated to adsorb treponemes on their surface. When mixed with serum containing antitreponemal antibodies, the cells become clumped. This test is similar to the FTA-ABS test in specificity and sensitivity, but it becomes positive somewhat later in the course of infection.

c. TPI test–This test demonstrates *T pallidum* immobilization (TPI) by specific antibodies in the patient's serum after the second week of infection. Dilutions of serum are mixed with complement and with live, actively motile *T pallidum* extracted from the testicular chancre of a rabbit, and the mixture is observed microscopically. If specific antibodies are present, spirochetes are immobilized; in normal serum, active motion continues. The test requires live treponemes from infected animals and is difficult to perform, so it is now done rarely.

Immunity

A person with active or latent syphilis or yaws appears to be resistant to superinfection with *T pallidum.* However, if early syphilis or yaws is treated adequately and the infection is eradicated, the individual again becomes fully susceptible. The various immune responses usually fail to eradicate the infection or arrest its progression.

Treatment

Penicillin in concentrations of 0.003 unit/mL has definite treponemicidal activity, and penicillin is the treatment of choice. Syphilis of less than 1 year's duration is treated by a single injection of benzathine penicillin G intramuscularly. In older or latent syphilis, benzathine penicillin G intramuscularly is given three times at weekly intervals. In neurosyphilis, the same therapy is acceptable, but larger amounts of intravenous penicillin are sometimes recommended. Other antibiotics, eg, tetracyclines or erythromycin, can occasionally be substituted. Treatment of gonorrhea is thought to cure incubating syphilis. Prolonged follow-up is essential. In neurosyphilis, treponemes occasionally survive such treatment. Severe neurologic relapses of treated syphilis have occurred in patients with acquired immunodeficiency syndrome (AIDS) who are infected with both HIV and *T pallidum.* A typical Jarisch-Herxheimer reaction may occur within hours after treatment is begun. It is due to the release of toxic products from dying or killed spirochetes.

Epidemiology, Prevention, & Control

At present, the incidence of syphilis (and other sexually transmitted diseases) is rising in most parts of the world. With the exceptions of congenital syphilis and the rare occupational exposure of medical personnel, syphilis is acquired through sexual exposure. Reinfection in treated persons is common. An infected person may remain contagious for 3–5 years during "early" syphilis. "Late" syphilis, of more than 5 years' duration, is usually not contagious. Consequently, control measures depend on (1) prompt and adequate treatment of all discovered cases; (2) follow-up on sources of infection and contacts so they can be treated; (3) safe sex with condoms is highly recommended. Several sexually transmitted diseases can be transmitted simultaneously. Therefore, it is important to consider the possibility of syphilis when any one sexually transmitted disease has been found.

DISEASES RELATED TO SYPHILIS

These diseases are all caused by treponemes closely related to *T pallidum.* All give positive treponemal and nontreponemal serologic tests for syphilis, and some cross-immunity can be demonstrated in experimental animals and perhaps in humans. None are sexually transmitted diseases; all are commonly transmitted by direct contact. None of the causative organisms have been cultured on artificial media.

Bejel

Bejel (due to *T pallidum* subsp *endemicum*) occurs chiefly in Africa but also in the Middle East, in Southeast Asia, and elsewhere, particularly among children, and produces highly infectious skin lesions; late visceral complications are rare. Penicillin is the drug of choice.

Yaws

Yaws is endemic, particularly among children, in many humid, hot tropical countries. It is caused by *T pallidum* subsp *pertenue.* The primary lesion, an ulcerating papule, occurs usually on the arms or legs. Transmission is by person-to-person contact in children under age 15. Transplacental, congenital infection does not occur. Scar formation of skin lesions and bone destruction are common, but visceral or nervous system complications are very rare. It has been debated whether yaws represents a variant of syphilis adapted to transmission by nonsexual means in hot climates. There appears to be cross-immunity between yaws and syphilis. Diagnostic procedures and therapy are similar to those for syphilis. The response to penicillin treatment is dramatic.

Pinta

Pinta is caused by *Treponema carateum* and occurs endemically in all age groups in Mexico, Central and South America, the Philippines, and some areas of the Pacific. The disease appears to be restricted to dark-skinned races. The primary lesion, a nonulcerating papule, occurs on exposed areas. Some months later, flat, hyperpigmented lesions appear on the skin; depigmentation and hyperkeratosis take place years afterward. Late cardiovascular and nervous system involvement occurs very rarely. Pinta is transmitted by nonsexual means, either by direct contact or through the agency of flies or gnats. Diagnosis and treatment are the same as for syphilis.

Rabbit Syphilis

Rabbit syphilis (*Treponema cuniculi* infection) is a natural sexually transmitted infection of rabbits that produces minor lesions of the genitalia. The causative organism is morphologically indistinguishable from *T pallidum* and may lead to confusion in experimental work.

BORRELIA

BORRELIA RECURRENTIS

Morphology & Identification

A. Typical Organisms: *Borrelia recurrentis* is an irregular spiral 10–30 μm long and 0.3 μm wide. The distance between turns varies from 2 to 4 μm. The organisms are highly flexible and move both by rotation and by twisting. *B recurrentis* stains readily with bacteriologic dyes as well as with blood stains such as Giemsa's or Wright's stain.

B. Culture: The organism can be cultured in fluid media containing blood, serum, or tissue (Figure 25–2); but it rapidly loses its pathogenicity for animals when transferred repeatedly in vitro. Multiplication is rapid in chick embryos when blood from patients is inoculated onto the chorioallantoic membrane.

C. Growth Characteristics: Little is known of the metabolic requirements or activity of borreliae. At 4 °C, the organisms survive for several months in infected blood or in culture. In some ticks (but not in lice), spirochetes are passed from generation to generation.

D. Variation: The only significant variation of *Borrelia* is with respect to its antigenic structure.

Antigenic Structure

Isolates of *Borrelia* from different parts of the world, from different hosts, and from different vectors (ticks or lice) either have been given different species names or have been designated strains of *B recurrentis.* Biologic differences between these strains or species do not appear to be stable.

Agglutinins, CF antibodies, and lytic antibodies develop in high titer after infection with borreliae. Apparently the antigenic structure of the organisms changes in the course of a single infection. The antibodies produced initially may act as a selective factor that permits the survival only of antigenically distinct variants. The relapsing course of the disease appears to be due to the multiplication of such antigenic variants, against which the host must then develop new antibodies. Ultimate recovery (after three to ten relapses) is associated with the presence of antibodies against several antigenic variants.

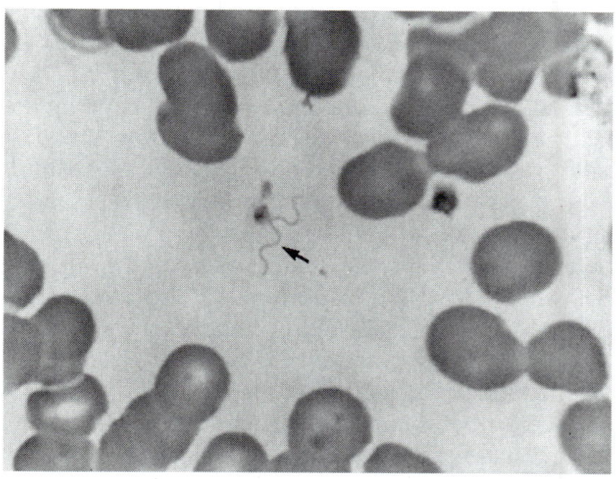

Figure 25–2. *Borrelia recurrentis* (arrow) in a peripheral blood smear of a patient with relapsing fever.

Pathology

Fatal cases show spirochetes in great numbers in the spleen and liver, necrotic foci in other parenchymatous organs, and hemorrhagic lesions in the kidneys and the gastrointestinal tract. Spirochetes have occasionally been demonstrated in the spinal fluid and brain of persons who have had meningitis. In experimental animals (guinea pigs, rats), the brain may serve as a reservoir of borreliae after they have disappeared from the blood.

Pathogenesis & Clinical Findings

The incubation period is 3–10 days. The onset is sudden, with chills and an abrupt rise of temperature. During this time, spirochetes abound in the blood. The fever persists for 3–5 days and then declines, leaving the patient weak but not ill. The afebrile period lasts 4–10 days and is followed by a second attack of chills, fever, intense headache, and malaise. There are from three to ten such recurrences, generally of diminishing severity. During the febrile stages (especially when the temperature is rising), organisms are present in the blood; during the afebrile periods, they are absent.

Antibodies against the spirochetes appear during the febrile stage, and the attack is probably terminated by their agglutinating and lytic effects. These antibodies may select out antigenically distinct variants that multiply and cause a relapse. Several distinct antigenic varieties of borreliae may be isolated from a single patient's sequential relapses, even following experimental inoculation with a single organism.

Diagnostic Laboratory Tests

A. Specimens: Blood obtained during the rise in fever, for smears and animal inoculation.

B. Smears: Thin or thick blood smears stained with Wright's or Giemsa's stain reveal large, loosely coiled spirochetes among the red cells.

C. Animal Inoculation: White mice or young rats are inoculated intraperitoneally with blood. Stained films of tail blood are examined for spirochetes 2–4 days later.

D. Serology: Spirochetes grown in culture can serve as antigens for CF tests, but the preparation of satisfactory antigens is difficult. Patients suffering from epidemic (louse-borne) relapsing fever may develop a positive VDRL.

Immunity

Immunity following infection is usually of short duration.

Treatment

The great variability of the spontaneous remissions of relapsing fever makes evaluation of chemotherapeutic effectiveness difficult. Tetracyclines, erythromycin, and penicillin are all believed to be effective. Treatment for a single day may be sufficient to terminate an individual attack.

Epidemiology, Prevention, & Control

Relapsing fever is endemic in many parts of the world. Its main reservoir is the rodent population, which serves as a source of infection for ticks of the genus *Ornithodorus.* The distribution of endemic foci and the seasonal incidence of the disease are largely determined by the ecology of the ticks in different areas. In the USA, infected ticks are found throughout the West, especially in mountainous areas, but clinical cases are rare. In the tick, *Borrelia* may be transmitted transovarially from generation to generation.

Spirochetes are present in all tissues of the tick and may be transmitted by the bite or by crushing the tick. The tick-borne disease is not epidemic. However, when an infected individual harbors lice, the lice become infected by sucking blood; 4–5 days later, they may serve as a source of infection for other individuals. The infection of the lice is not transmitted to the next generation, and the disease is the result of rubbing crushed lice into bite wounds. Severe epidemics may occur in louse-infected populations, and transmission is favored by crowding, malnutrition, and cold climate.

In endemic areas, human infection may occasionally result from contact with the blood and tissues of infected rodents. The mortality rate of the endemic disease is low, but in epidemics it may reach 30%.

Prevention is based on avoidance of exposure to ticks and lice and on delousing (cleanliness, insecticides). No vaccines are available.

BORRELIA BURGDORFERI & LYME DISEASE

Lyme disease is named after the town of Lyme, Connecticut, where clusters of cases were identified initially. It is caused by the spirochete *Borrelia burgdorferi* and is transmitted to humans by the bite of a small tick. The disease has early manifestations with a characteristic skin lesion along with flu-like symptoms, and late manifestations often with arthralgia and arthritis.

Morphology & Identification

A. Typical Organisms: *B burgdorferi* is a spiral organism 11–39 μm long and about 0.2 μm wide. The distance between turns varies from 2 μm to 4 μm. The organisms have variable numbers (7–11) of endoflagella and are highly motile. *B burgdorferi* stains readily with acid and aniline dyes and by silver impregnation techniques.

B. Culture and Growth Characteristics: *B burgdorferi* has been isolated from blood, cerebrospinal fluid, and skin lesions, but culture of the organism on solid or liquid media is a complex and specialized procedure with a low diagnostic yield. The organism is more readily cultured from ticks than from humans. On serial passage, the biologic properties of *B burgdorferi* change, and it becomes less virulent for animals.

Antigenic Structure & Variation

B burgdorferi has a structure similar to that of other spirochetes. It shows heterogeneity in morphology, proteins, plasmids, and DNA homology from one strain to another, but no accepted classification system for these characteristics has been developed.

Pathogenesis & Clinical Findings

The transmission of *B burgdorferi* to humans is by injection of the organism in tick saliva or by regurgitation of the ticks' midgut contents. Attachment of the tick for 24 hours or more is necessary before there is transmission of *B burgdorferi*. The organism adheres to proteoglycans on host cells, which is mediated by a borrelial glycosaminoglycan receptor. After injection by the tick, the organism migrates out from the site, producing the characteristic skin lesion. Dissemination occurs by lymphatics or blood to other skin and musculoskeletal sites and to many other organs.

Lyme disease, like other spirochetal diseases, occurs in stages with early and late manifestations. The initial stage is often marked by a unique skin lesion that begins 3 days to 4 weeks after a tick bite. The lesion, called **erythema chronicum migrans,** begins with a flat reddened area near the tick bite that slowly expands, with central clearing. With the skin lesion there is often a flu-like illness with fever, chills, myalgia, and headache. The second stage occurs weeks to months later and includes arthralgia and arthritis, neurologic manifestations, with meningitis, facial nerve palsy and painful radiculopathy, and cardiac disease, with conduction defects and myopericarditis. The third stage begins months to years later with chronic skin, nervous system, or joint involvement. Spirochetes have been isolated from all these sites, and it is likely that some of the late manifestations are caused by deposition of antigen-antibody complexes.

Diagnostic Laboratory Tests

In some symptomatic patients the diagnosis of early Lyme disease can be established clinically by observing the unique skin lesion erythema chronicum migrans. When this skin lesion is not present and at later stages of the disease, which must be differentiated from many other diseases, it is necessary to perform diagnostic laboratory tests. There is, however, no one test that is both sensitive and specific.

A. Specimens: Blood is obtained for serologic tests. Cerebrospinal fluid or joint fluid can be obtained, but culture usually is not recommended. These specimens and others can be used to detect *B burgdorferi* DNA by the polymerase chain reaction.

B. Smears: *B burgdorferi* has been found in sections of biopsy specimens, but examination of stained smears is an insensitive method to diagnose Lyme disease. *B burgdorferi* in tissue sections can sometimes be identified using antibodies and immunohistochemical methods.

C. Culture: *B burgdorferi* has been cultured from cerebrospinal fluid, joint fluid, and other specimens, but culture is generally not performed. Culture takes 6–8 weeks to complete, and the results lack sensitivity. An antigen capture assay can detect *B burgdorferi* antigens in urine or occasionally other body fluids.

D. Molecular Probes: The polymerase chain reaction assay has been applied to detection of *B burgdorferi* DNA in many body fluids. It is rapid (2 days), very sensitive, and specific, but it does not differentiate between DNA from live *B burgdorferi* in active disease and DNA from dead *B burgdorferi* in treated or inactive disease.

E. Serology: Serology has been the mainstay for the diagnosis of Lyme disease, but 3–5% of normal people and persons with other diseases (eg, rheumatoid arthritis, many infectious diseases) may be seropositive by some assays. Because the prevalence of Lyme disease is low, there is a much greater likelihood that a positive test is from a person who does not have Lyme disease than from a person who has the disease (a positive predictive value on the order of 1–2%). Thus, serology for Lyme disease should only be done when there are highly suggestive clinical findings, and a positive test in the absence of such clinical findings should not be used to diagnose Lyme disease. The most widely used tests are the indirect fluorescent antibody (IFA) and enzyme immunoassays (EIA or ELISA). Many variations of these assays using different antigen preparations, techniques, and end points have been marketed. The immunoblot (Western blot) assay is sometimes performed to confirm results obtained by other tests. *B burgdorferi* antigens are electrophoretically separated, transferred to a nitrocellulose membrane, and reacted with a patient's serum. The interpretation of the immunoblot is based on the number and molecular size of antibody reactions with the *B burgdorferi* proteins.

Immunity

Reactive IgM antibodies peak in titer 3–6 weeks after onset of illness. The IgM are directed primarily against a *B burgdorferi* flagellar protein. Reactive IgG titers rise slowly over months to years and appear to be directed sequentially against a series of *B burgdorferi* proteins. Early antimicrobial treatment decreases or aborts the antibody response, and such patients are susceptible to reinfection.

Treatment

Tetracycline or penicillin treatment relieves early symptoms and promotes resolution of skin lesions. Tetracyclines may be more effective than penicillins in preventing late manifestations. Established arthritis often responds to large doses of penicillin. In refractory cases, ceftriaxone has been effective. Nearly 50% of patients treated with a tetracycline or a penicillin early in the course of Lyme disease develop minor late complications (headache, joint pains, etc). Long-standing Lyme arthritis can be treated with doxycycline or amoxicillin plus probenecid for 30 days.

Epidemiology, Prevention, & Control

B burgdorferi is transmitted by a small tick of the genus *Ixodes*. The vector is *Ixodes dammini* in the Northeast and Midwest and *Ixodes pacificus* on the West Coast of the USA. In Europe, the vector is *Ixodes ricinus*, and other tick vectors appear to be important in other areas of the world. Mice and deer constitute the main animal reservoirs of *B burgdorferi* for ticks, but other rodents and birds may also be infected. In the eastern part of the USA, 10–50% of ticks are infected, while in the western states the infection rate in ticks is much lower, about 2%.

Most exposures are in May through July, when the nymphal stage of the ticks is most active; however, the larval stage (August and September) and adult stage (spring and fall) also feed on humans and can transmit *B burgdorferi*.

Prevention is based on avoidance of exposure to ticks. No vaccine is available.

LEPTOSPIRAE

LEPTOSPIROSIS

Morphology & Identification

A. Typical Organisms: Leptospirae are tightly coiled, thin, flexible spirochetes 5–15 μm long, with very fine spirals 0.1–0.2 μm wide. One end of the organism is often bent, forming a hook. There is active rotational motion, but no flagella have been discovered. Electron micrographs show a thin axial filament and a delicate membrane. The spirochete is so delicate that in the dark field it may appear only as a chain of minute cocci. It does not stain readily but can be impregnated with silver.

B. Culture: Leptospirae grow best under aerobic conditions at 28–30 °C in protein-rich semisolid media (Fletcher, others), where they produce round colonies 1–3 mm in diameter in 6–10 days. Leptospirae also grow on chorioallantoic membranes of embryonated eggs.

C. Growth Requirements: Leptospirae derive energy from oxidation of long-chain fatty acids and cannot use amino acids or carbohydrates as major energy sources. Ammonium salts are a main source of nitrogen. Leptospirae can survive for weeks in water, particularly at alkaline pH.

Antigenic Structure

The main strains ("serovars") of *Leptospira interrogans* isolated from humans or animals in different parts of the world (Table 25–1) are all serologically related and exhibit marked cross-reactivity in serologic tests. This indicates considerable overlapping in antigenic structure, and quantitative tests and antibody absorption studies are necessary for a specific serologic diagnosis. A serologically reactive lipopolysaccharide with group reactivity has been extracted from leptospirae.

Pathogenesis & Clinical Findings

Human infection results usually from ingestion of water or food contaminated with leptospirae. More rarely, the organisms may enter through mucous membranes or breaks in the skin. After an incubation period of 1–2 weeks, there is a variable febrile onset during which spirochetes are present in the bloodstream. They then establish themselves in the parenchymatous organs (particularly liver and kidneys), producing hemorrhage and necrosis of tissue and resulting in dysfunction of those organs (jaundice, hemorrhage, nitrogen retention). The illness is often biphasic. After an initial improvement, the second phase develops when the IgM antibody titer rises. It manifests itself often as "aseptic meningitis" with intense headache, stiff neck, and pleocytosis in the cerebrospinal fluid. Nephritis and hepatitis may also recur, and there may be skin, muscle, and eye lesions. During World War II, pretibial fever occurred at Fort Bragg, a US Army base, with patchy erythema on the lower legs or a generalized rash. The degree and distribution of organ involvement vary in the different diseases produced by different leptospirae in various parts of the world (Table 25–1). Many infections are mild or subclinical. Hepatitis is frequent in patients with leptospirosis. It is often associated with elevation of serum creatine phosphokinase, whereas that enzyme is present in normal concentrations in viral hepatitis.

Kidney involvement in many animal species is chronic and results in the shedding of large numbers of leptospirae in the urine; this is probably the main source of contamination and infection of humans. Human urine also may contain spirochetes in the second and third weeks of disease.

Agglutinating, CF, and lytic antibodies develop during the infection. Serum from convalescent patients protects experimental animals against an otherwise fatal infection. The immunity resulting from infection in humans and animals appears to be serovar-specific. Dogs have been artificially immunized with killed cultures of leptospirae.

Diagnostic Laboratory Tests

A. Specimens: Specimens consist of blood for microscopic examination, culture, and inoculation of young hamsters or guinea pigs; and serum for agglutination tests.

Table 25–1. Principal leptospiral diseases.

Leptospira interrogans Serovar[1]	Source of Infection	Disease in Humans	Clinical Findings	Distribution
autumnalis	?	Pretibial fever or Ft. Bragg fever	Fever, rash over tibia	USA, Japan
ballum	Mice	—	Fever, rash, jaundice	USA, Europe, Israel
bovis	Cattle, voles	—	Fever, prostration	USA, Israel, Australia
canicola	Dog urine	Infectious jaundice	Influenzalike illness, aseptic meningitis	Worldwide
grippotyphosa	Rodents, water	Marsh fever	Fever, prostration, aseptic meningitis	Europe, USA, Africa
hebdomadis	Rats, mice	Seven-day fever	Fever, jaundice	Japan, Europe
icterohaemorrhagiae	Rat urine, water	Weil's disease	Jaundice, hemorrhages, aseptic meningitis	Worldwide
mitis	Swine	Swineherd's disease	Aseptic meningitis	Australia
pomona	Swine, cattle	Swineherd's disease	Fever, prostration, aseptic meningitis	Europe, USA, Australia

[1]Formerly called species.

B. Microscopic Examination: Darkfield examination or thick smears stained by Giemsa's technique occasionally show leptospirae in fresh blood from early infections. Darkfield examination of centrifuged urine may also be positive.

C. Culture: Whole fresh blood or urine can be cultured in Fletcher's semisolid or Tween 80 albumin medium. Growth is slow, and cultures should be kept for several weeks.

D. Animal Inoculation: A sensitive technique for the isolation of leptospirae consists of the intraperitoneal inoculation of young hamsters or guinea pigs with fresh plasma or urine. Within a few days, spirochetes become demonstrable in the peritoneal cavity; on the death of the animal (8–14 days), hemorrhagic lesions with spirochetes are found in many organs.

E. Serology: Agglutinating antibodies attaining very high titers (1:10,000 or higher) develop slowly in leptospiral infection, reaching a peak 5–8 weeks after infection. Leptospiral antibody can be detected by macroscopic slide agglutination tests using killed leptospirae or by microscopic agglutination of live organisms. Cross-absorption of sera may permit identification of a serovar-specific antibody response. Agglutination of live suspensions is most specific for the serovar and may be followed by lysis. Passive hemagglutination of red blood cells with adsorbed leptospirae is sometimes used.

Immunity

A solid serovar-specific immunity follows infection, but reinfection with different serovars may occur.

Treatment

In very early infection, antibiotics (penicillin, tetracyclines) have some therapeutic effect but do not eradicate the infection. Doxycycline has marked prophylactic efficacy.

Epidemiology, Prevention, & Control

The leptospiroses are essentially animal infections; human infection is only accidental, following contact with water or other materials contaminated with the excreta of animal hosts. Rats, mice, wild rodents, dogs, swine, and cattle are the principal sources of human infection. They excrete leptospirae in urine and feces both during the active illness and during the asymptomatic carrier state. Leptospirae remain viable in stagnant water for several weeks; drinking, swimming, bathing, or food contamination may lead to human infection. Persons most likely to come in contact with water contaminated by rats (eg, miners, sewer workers, farmers, fishermen) run the greatest risk of infection. Children acquire the infection from dogs more frequently than do adults. Control consists of preventing exposure to potentially contaminated water and reducing contamination by rodent control. Doxycycline, 200 mg orally once weekly during heavy exposure, is effective prophylaxis. Dogs can receive distemper-hepatitis-leptospirosis vaccinations.

OTHER SPIROCHETAL DISEASES

SPIRILLUM MINOR (Spirillum morsus muris)

Spirillum minor causes one form of rat-bite fever (sodoku). This very small (3–5 μm) and rigid spiral organism is carried by rats all over the world. The organism is inoculated into humans through the bite of a rat and results in a local lesion, regional gland swelling, skin rashes, and fever of the relapsing type. The frequency of this illness depends upon the degree of contact between humans and rats. The *Spirillum* can be isolated by inoculation of guinea pigs or mice with material from enlarged lymph nodes or blood but has not been grown in bacteriologic media. In the USA and Europe, this disease has been recognized only infrequently. Several other motile gram-negative spiral aerobic organisms can produce spirillum fever.

SPIROCHETES OF THE NORMAL MOUTH & MUCOUS MEMBRANES

A number of spirochetes occur in every normal mouth. Some of them have been named (eg, *Borrelia buccalis*), but neither their morphology nor their physiologic activity permits definitive classification. On normal genitalia, a spirochete called *Borrelia refringens* is occasionally found that may be confused with *T pallidum*. These organisms are harmless saprophytes under ordinary conditions. Most of them are strict anaerobes that can be grown in petrolatum-sealed meat infusion broth tubes with tissue added.

FUSOSPIROCHETAL DISEASE

Under certain circumstances, particularly injury to mucous membranes, nutritional deficiency, or concomitant infection (eg, with herpes simplex virus) of the epithelium, the normal spirochetes of the mouth, together with anaerobic fusiform bacilli (fusobacteria), find suitable conditions for vast increase in numbers. This occurs in ulcerative gingivostomatitis (trench mouth), often called Vincent's stomatitis. When this type of process produces ulcerative tonsillitis and massive tissue involvement, it may be called Vincent's angina. It also occurs in lung abscesses where pyogenic microorganisms and *Bacteroides* species have broken down tissue; in bronchiectasis, where anatomic and physiologic disturbances interfere with normal drainage; in leg ("tropical") ulcers with mixed infection and venous stasis; and in bite wounds and similar situations.

In all of these instances, necrotic tissue provides the anaerobic environment required by the fusospirochetal flora. The anaerobic conditions in turn prevent rapid healing and may contribute to tissue breakdown. *Fusobacterium* species coexist with other anaerobes. The fusospirochetal flora is readily inhibited by antibiotics. Antibiotic therapy may thus control gingivostomatitis or angina. However, the fusospirochetal organisms are not primary pathogens. Effective treatment must direct itself against the initial cause of tissue breakdown.

Fusospirochetal disease is generally not transmissible through direct contact, since everyone carries the organisms in the mouth. However, outbreaks occur occasionally in children or young adults. This is attributed to the transmission of a viral agent (eg, herpes simplex virus) in a susceptible population group or to nutritional deficiency and poor oral hygiene ("trench mouth").

REFERENCES

Andriole VT (editor): Lyme disease and other spirochetal diseases. Rev Infect Dis 1989;(Suppl 6):S1433.

Barbour AG, Hayes SF: Biology of *Borrelia* species. Microbiol Rev 1986;50:381.

Burgdorfer W: Lyme borreliosis: Ten years after the discovery of the etiologic agent, *Borrelia burgdorferi*. Infection 1991;19:257.

Burke JP et al (editors): International symposium on yaws and other endemic treponematoses. Rev Infect Dis 1985; 7:S217.

Butler T et al: *Borrelia* recurrentis infection. J Infect Dis 1978;137:573.

Csonka G, Pace J: Endemic nonvenereal treponematosis (bejel) in Saudi Arabia. Rev Infect Dis 1985;7:S260.

Duffey PS, Salugsugan J: Serodiagnosis of Lyme disease. Clin Microbiol Rev 1993;15:81.

Feigin RD, Anderson DC: Human leptospirosis. CRC Crit Rev Clin Lab Sci 1974;5:413.

Fitzgerald TJ: Pathogenesis and immunology of *Treponema pallidum*. Annu Rev Microbiol 1981;35:29.

Hook WE III: Treatment of syphilis. Rev Infect Dis 1989; 11:S1511.

Malison MD: Relapsing fever. JAMA 1979;241:2819.

Rahn DW, Malawista SE: Lyme disease: Recommendations for diagnosis and treatment. Ann Intern Med 1991;114: 472.

Steere AC: Lyme disease. N Engl J Med 1989;321:586.

Watt G et al: Placebo-controlled trial of intravenous penicillin for severe and late leptospirosis. Lancet 1988;1: 433.

Mycoplasmas (Mollicutes) & Cell Wall–Defective Bacteria

26

MYCOPLASMAS (Mollicutes)

There are over 150 species in the class of cell wall-free bacteria known as Mollicutes. At least 15 of these species are thought to be of human origin, while others have been isolated from animals and plants. In humans, four species are of primary importance: *Mycoplasma pneumoniae* causes pneumonia and has been associated with joint and other infections. *Mycoplasma hominis* sometimes causes postpartum fever and has been found with other bacteria in uterine (fallopian) tube infections. *Ureaplasma urealyticum* is a cause of nongonococcal urethritis in men and is associated with lung disease in premature infants of low birth weight. *Mycoplasma genitalium* is closely related to *M pneumoniae* and has been associated with urethral and other infections. Other members of the genus *Mycoplasma* are pathogens of the respiratory and urogenital tracts and joints of animals.

The mollicutes evolved from gram-positive ancestors (certain clostridia) by reduction of genome size; the smallest genome of mycoplasmas is little more than twice the genome size of certain large viruses. Mycoplasmas are the smallest organisms that can be free-living in nature and self-replicating on laboratory media. They have the following characteristics: (1) The smallest mycoplasmas are 125–250 nm in size. (2) They are highly pleomorphic because they lack a rigid cell wall and instead are bounded by a triple-layered "unit membrane" that contains a sterol (mycoplasmas, but not all mollicutes, require sterols for growth). (3) They are completely resistant to penicillin because they lack the cell wall structures where penicillin acts, but they are inhibited by tetracycline or erythromycin. (4) They can reproduce in cell-free media; on agar, the center of the whole colony is characteristically embedded beneath the surface. (5) Growth is inhibited by specific antibody. (6) Mycoplasmas have an affinity for mammalian cell membranes.

Morphology & Identification

A. Typical Organisms: Mycoplasmas cannot be studied by the usual bacteriologic methods because of the small size of their colonies, the plasticity and delicacy of their individual cells (owing to the lack of a rigid cell wall), and their poor staining with aniline dyes. The morphology appears different according to the method of examination (eg, darkfield, immunofluorescence, Giemsa-stained films from solid or liquid media, agar fixation).

Growth in fluid media gives rise to many different forms, including rings, bacillary and spiral bodies, filaments, and granules. Growth on solid media consists principally of plastic protoplasmic masses of indefinite shape that are easily distorted. These structures vary greatly in size, ranging from 50 to 300 nm in diameter.

B. Culture: Many strains of mycoplasmas grow in heart infusion peptone broth with 2% agar (pH 7.8) to which about 30% human ascitic fluid or animal serum (horse, rabbit) has been added. Following incubation at 37 °C for 48–96 hours, there may be no turbidity; but Giemsa stains of the centrifuged sediment show the characteristic pleomorphic structures, and subculture on solid media yields minute colonies.

After 2–6 days on biphasic (broth over agar) and agar medium incubated in a Petri dish that has been sealed to prevent evaporation, isolated colonies measuring 20–500 μm can be detected with a hand lens. These colonies are round, with a granular surface and a dark center typically buried in the agar. They can be subcultured by cutting out a small square of agar containing one or more colonies and streaking this material on a fresh plate or dropping it into liquid medium. The organisms can be stained for microscopic study by placing a similar square on a slide and covering the colony with a cover-glass onto which an alcoholic solution of methylene blue and azure has been poured and then evaporated (agar fixation). Such slides can also be stained with specific fluorescent antibody.

C. Growth Characteristics: Mycoplasmas are unique in microbiology because of (1) their extremely small size and (2) their growth on complex but cell-free media.

Mycoplasmas pass through filters with 450-nm pore size and thus are comparable to chlamydiae or large viruses. However, parasitic mycoplasmas grow on cell-free media that contain lipoprotein and sterol. The sterol requirement for growth and membrane synthesis is unique. Mycoplasmas are resistant to thallium acetate in a concentration of 1:10,000, which can be used to inhibit bacteria.

Many mycoplasmas use glucose as a source of energy; ureaplasmas require urea.

Some human mycoplasmas produce peroxides and hemolyze red blood cells. In cell cultures and in vivo, mycoplasmas develop predominantly at cell surfaces. Many established animal and human cell culture lines carry mycoplasmas as contaminants.

D. Variation: The extreme pleomorphism of mycoplasmas is one of their principal characteristics.

Antigenic Structure

Many antigenically distinct species of mycoplasmas have been isolated from animals (eg, mice, chickens, turkeys). In humans, at least 15 species can be identified, including *M hominis, Mycoplasma salivarium, Mycoplasma orale, Mycoplasma fermentans, M pneumoniae, M genitalium, U urealyticum,* and others. The last two species are of pathogenic significance.

The species are classified by biochemical and serologic features. The CF antigens of mycoplasmas are glycolipids. Antigens for ELISA tests are proteins. Some species have more than one serotype.

Mycoplasma Infection

The mycoplasmas appear to be host-specific, being communicable and potentially pathogenic only within a single host species. In animals, mycoplasmas appear to be intracellular parasites with a predilection for mesothelial cells (pleura, peritoneum, synovia of joints). Several extracellular products can be elaborated (eg, hemolysins).

A. Infection of Humans: Mycoplasmas have been cultivated from human mucous membranes and tissues, particularly from the genital, urinary, and respiratory tracts. Mycoplasmas are part of the normal flora of the mouth and can be grown from normal saliva, oral mucous membranes, sputum, or tonsillar tissue. *M salivarium, Mycoplasma orale,* and other mycoplasmas can be recovered from the oral cavities of many healthy adults, but an association with clinical disease is uncertain. *M hominis* is found in the oropharynx of less than 5% of adults. *M pneumoniae* in the oropharynx is generally associated with disease (see below).

Some mycoplasmas are inhabitants of the genitourinary tract, particularly in females. In both men and women, genital carriage of mycoplasma is directly related to the number of lifetime sex partners. *M hominis* can be cultured from 1–5% of asymptomatic men and 30–70% of asymptomatic women; the rates increase to 20% and over 90% positive for men and women, respectively, in sexually transmitted disease clinics. *U urealyticum* is found in the genital tracts of 5–20% of sexually active men and 40–80% of sexually active women. Approximately 20% of women attending sexually transmitted disease clinics have *M genitalium* in their lower genital tracts. Other mycoplasmas also occur in the lower genital tract.

B. Infection of Animals: Bovine pleuropneumonia is a contagious, occasionally lethal disease of cattle associated with pneumonia and pleural effusion. The disease probably has an airborne spread. Mycoplasmas are found in inflammatory exudates.

Agalactia of sheep and goats in the Mediterranean area is a generalized infection with local lesions in the skin, eyes, joints, udder, and scrotum; it leads to atrophy of lactating glands in females. Mycoplasmas are present in blood early and in milk and exudates later.

In poultry, several economically important respiratory diseases are caused by mycoplasmas. The organisms can be transmitted from hen to egg to chick. Swine, dogs, rats, mice, and other species harbor mycoplasmas that can produce infection involving particularly the pleura, peritoneum, joints, respiratory tract, and eye. In mice, a *Mycoplasma* of spiral shape *(Spiroplasma)* can induce cataracts.

C. Infection of Plants: Aster yellows, corn stunt, and other plant diseases appear to be caused by mycoplasmas. They are transmitted by insects and can be suppressed by tetracyclines.

Diagnostic Laboratory Tests

A. Specimens: Specimens consist of throat swab, sputum, inflammatory exudates, and respiratory, urethral, or genital secretions.

B. Microscopic Examination: Direct examination of a specimen for mycoplasmas is useless. Cultures are examined as described above.

C. Cultures: The material is inoculated onto special solid media and incubated for 3–10 days at 37 °C with 5% CO_2 (under microaerophilic conditions), or into special broth and incubated aerobically. One or two transfers of media may be necessary before growth appears that is suitable for microscopic examination by staining or immunofluorescence. Colonies may have a "fried egg" appearance on agar.

D. Serology: Antibodies develop in humans infected with mycoplasmas and can be demonstrated by several methods. CF tests can be performed with glycolipid antigens extracted with chloroform-methanol from cultured mycoplasmas. HI tests can be applied to tanned red cells with adsorbed *Mycoplasma* antigens. Indirect immunofluorescence may be used. The test that measures growth inhibition by antibody is quite specific. When counterimmunoelectrophoresis is used, antigens and antibody migrate toward each other, and precipitin lines appear in 1 hour. With all these serologic techniques, there is adequate specificity for different human *Mycoplasma* species, but a rising antibody titer is required for diagnostic significance because of the high incidence of positive serologic tests in normal individuals. *M pneumoniae* and *M genitalium* are serologically cross-reactive.

Treatment

Many strains of mycoplasmas are inhibited by a variety of antimicrobial drugs, but most strains are resistant to penicillins, cephalosporins, and vancomycin. Tetracyclines and erythromycins are effective both in vitro and in vivo and are, at present, the drugs of choice in mycoplasmal pneumonia. Some ureaplasmas are resistant to tetracycline.

Epidemiology, Prevention, & Control

Isolation of infected livestock will control the highly contagious pleuropneumonia and agalactia in limited areas. No vaccines are available. Mycoplasmal pneumonia behaves like a communicable viral respiratory disease (see below).

Mycoplasma pneumoniae & Atypical Pneumonias

A. Causative Organisms: *M pneumoniae* is a prominent causative agent for pneumonia, especially in persons 5–20 years of age.

B. Pathogenesis: *M pneumoniae* is transmitted from person to person by means of infected respiratory secretions. Infection is initiated by attachment of the organism's tip to a receptor on the surface of respiratory epithelial cells (Figure 26–1). Attachment is mediated by a specific adhesin protein on the differentiated terminal structure of the organism. During infection, the organisms remain extracellular. The mechanism of cellular damage is unknown.

C. Clinical Findings: Mycoplasmal pneumonia is generally a mild disease. The clinical spectrum of *M pneumoniae* infection ranges from asymptomatic infection to serious pneumonitis, with occasional neurologic and hematologic (ie, hemolytic anemia) involvement and a variety of possible skin lesions. Bullous myringitis occurs in spontaneous cases and in experimentally inoculated volunteers.

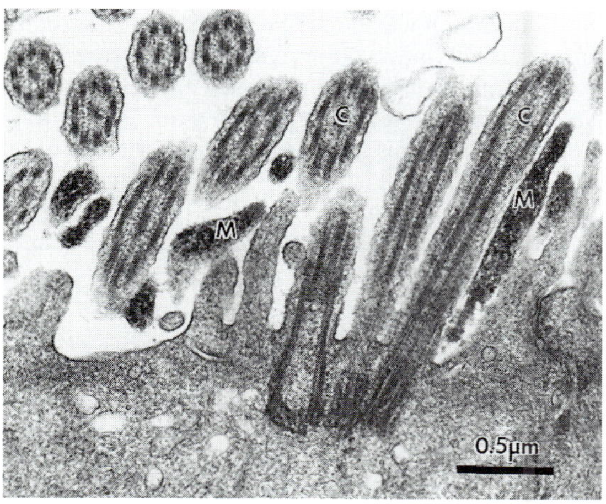

Figure 26–1. Electron micrograph of *Mycoplasma pneumoniae* attached to ciliated respiratory epithelial cells in a sputum sample from a patient with culture-proved *M pneumoniae* pneumonia. The *M pneumoniae* (M) are seen on the luminal border attached between cilia (C). (Courtesy of Albert M. Collier, Department of Pediatrics, University of North Carolina.)

The incubation period varies from 1 to 3 weeks. The onset is usually insidious, with lassitude, fever, headache, sore throat, and cough. Initially, the cough is nonproductive, but it is occasionally paroxysmal. Later there may be blood-streaked sputum and chest pain. Early in the course, the patient appears only moderately ill, and physical signs of pulmonary consolidation are often negligible compared to the striking consolidation seen on x-rays. Later, when the infiltration is at a peak, the illness may be severe. Resolution of pulmonary infiltration and clinical improvement occur slowly over 1–4 weeks. Although the course of the illness is exceedingly variable, death is very rare and is usually attributable to cardiac failure. Complications are uncommon, but hemolytic anemia may occur. The most common pathologic findings are interstitial and peribronchial pneumonitis and necrotizing bronchiolitis. Other diseases possibly related to *M pneumoniae* include erythema multiforme; central nervous system involvement, including meningitis, meningoencephalitis, and mono- and polyneuritis; myocarditis, pericarditis, arthritis, and pancreatitis.

D. Laboratory Findings: The following laboratory findings apply to *M pneumoniae* pneumonia: The white and differential counts are within normal limits. The causative *Mycoplasma* can be recovered by culture from the pharynx and from sputum. There is a rise in specific antibodies to *M pneumoniae* that is demonstrable by CF, immunofluorescence, passive hemagglutination, and growth inhibition tests.

A variety of nonspecific reactions can be observed. Cold hemagglutinins for group O human erythrocytes appear in about 50% of untreated patients, in rising titer, with the maximum reached in the third or fourth week after onset. A titer of 1:64 or more supports the diagnosis of *M pneumoniae* infection.

E. Treatment: Tetracyclines or erythromycins can produce clinical improvement but do not eradicate the mycoplasmas.

F. Epidemiology, Prevention, and Control: *M pneumoniae* infections are endemic all over the world. In populations of children and young adults, where close contact prevails, and in families, the infection rate may be high (50–90%), but the incidence of pneumonitis is variable (3–30%). For every case of frank pneumonitis, there exist several cases of milder respiratory illness. *M pneumoniae* is apparently transmitted mainly by direct contact involving respiratory secretions. Second attacks are infrequent. The presence of antibodies to *M pneumoniae* has been associated with resistance to infection but may not be responsible for it. Cell-mediated immune reactions occur. The pneumonic process may be attributed in part to an immunologic response rather than only to infection by mycoplasmas. Experimental vaccines have been prepared from agar-grown *M pneumoniae*. Several such killed vaccines have aggravated subsequent disease; a degree of protection has been claimed with the use of other vaccines, but none are available for clinical use.

Mycoplasma hominis

M hominis has been associated with a variety of diseases but is a demonstrated cause in only a few of them. The evidence for a causal relationship in disease is from culture and serologic studies. *M hominis* can be cultured from the upper urinary tract in about 10% of patients with pyelonephritis. *M hominis* is strongly associated with infection of the uterine tubes (salpingitis) and tubo-ovarian abscesses; the organism can be isolated from the uterine tubes of about 10% of patients with salpingitis but not from women with no signs of disease. Women with salpingitis more commonly have antibodies against *M hominis* than women with no disease. *M hominis* has been isolated from the blood of about 10% of women who have postabortal or postpartum fever and occasionally from joint fluid cultures of patients with arthritis.

Ureaplasma urealyticum

U urealyticum, like *M hominis*, has been associated with a variety of diseases but is a demonstrated cause in only a few of them. *U urealyticum*, which requires 10% urea for growth, probably causes nongonococcal urethritis in some men, but a majority of cases of nongonococcal urethritis are caused by *Chlamydia trachomatis* (Chapter 28). *U urealyticum* is common in the female genital tract, where the association with disease is weak. *U urealyticum* has been associated with lung disease in premature low-birth-weight infants who acquired the organism during birth. The evidence that *U urealyticum* is associated with involuntary infertility is at best marginal.

Mycoplasma genitalium

M genitalium was originally isolated from urethral cultures of two men with nongonococcal urethritis, but culture of *M genitalium* is difficult, and subsequent observations have been based on data obtained by using the polymerase chain reaction, molecular probes, and serologic tests. The data suggest that *M genitalium* is associated with some cases of acute as well as chronic nongonococcal urethritis.

CELL WALL–DEFECTIVE BACTERIA

L phase variants (L forms) are wall-defective microbial forms that can replicate serially as nonrigid cells and produce colonies on solid media. Some L phase variants are stable; others are unstable and revert to bacterial parental forms. Wall-defective forms are not genetically related to mycoplasmas. They can result from spontaneous mutation or from the effects of chemicals. Treatment of eubacteria with cell wall-inhibiting drugs or lysozyme can produce cell wall-defective microbial forms. **Protoplasts** are such forms usually derived from gram-positive organisms; they are osmotically fragile, with external surfaces free of cell wall constituents. **Spheroplasts** are cell wall-defective forms usually derived from gram-negative bacteria; they retain some outer membrane material.

There is no genetic relationship between mycoplasmas and cell wall-defective microbial forms or their parent bacteria. The characteristics of the cell wall-defective forms are similar to those of mycoplasmas, but by definition, mycoplasmas do not revert to parental bacterial forms or originate from them. Cell wall-defective forms continue to synthesize some antigens that are normally located in the cell wall of the parent bacteria (eg, streptococcal L forms produce M protein and capsular polysaccharide). Reversion of L forms to the parental bacterial form is enhanced by growth in the presence of 15–30% gelatin or 2.5% agar. Reversion is inhibited by inhibitors of protein synthesis.

It is uncertain whether cell wall-defective microbial forms cause tissue reactions resulting in disease. They may be important for the persistence of microorganisms in tissue and recurrence of infection after antimicrobial treatment, as in rare cases of endocarditis.

REFERENCES

Cassell GH, Cole BC: Mycoplasmas as agents of human disease. N Engl J Med 1981;304:80.

Cassell GH et al: Association of *Ureaplasma urealyticum* infection of the lower respiratory tract with chronic lung disease and death in very-low-birth-weight infants. Lancet 1988;1:240.

Cassell GH et al: Protein antigens of genital mycoplasmas. Rev Infect Dis 1988;10(Suppl 3):S391.

Cassell GH et al (editors): The changing role of mycoplasmas in respiratory disease and AIDS. Clin Infect Dis 1993;17(Suppl 1):S1.

Cimolai N et al: Immunological cross-reactivity of a *Mycoplasma pneumoniae* membrane-associated protein antigen with *Mycoplasma genitalium* and *Acholeplasma laidlawii*. J Clin Microbiol 1987;25:2136.

Collier AM: Attachment by mycoplasmas and its role in disease. Rev Infect Dis 1983;5(Suppl 4):S685.

Dallo SF et al: Identification of P1 gene domain containing epitope(s) mediating *Mycoplasma pneumoniae* cytadherence. J Exp Med 1988;167:718.

Kundsin RB et al: *Ureaplasma urealyticum* incriminated in perinatal morbidity and mortality. Science 1981;213:474.

Lin JS: Human mycoplasmal infections: Serologic observations. Rev Infect Dis 1985;7:216.

Lind K et al: Serological cross-reactions between *Myco-*

plasma genitalium and *Mycoplasma pneumoniae.* J Clin Microbiol 1984;20:1036.

McCormack WM et al: Vaginal colonization with *Mycoplasma hominis* and *Ureaplasma urealyticum.* Sex Transm Dis 1986;13:67.

Platt R et al: Infection with *Mycoplasma hominis* in postpartum fever. Lancet 1980;2:1217.

Romero R et al: Is genital colonization with *Mycoplasma hominis* or *Ureaplasma urealyticum* associated with prematurity/low birth weight? Obstet Gynecol 1989;73:532.

Sanchez PJ, Regan JA: *Ureaplasma urealyticum* colonization and chronic lung disease in low birth weight infants. Ped Infect Dis 1988;7:542.

Taylor-Robinson D, Furr PM, Hanna NF: Microbiological and serological study of nongonococcal urethritis with special reference to *Mycoplasma genitalium.* Genitourin Med 1985;61:319.

Taylor-Robinson D, McCormack WM: The genital mycoplasmas. (Two parts.) N Engl J Med 1980;302:1003, 1063.

Thompson SE III et al: The microbiology and therapy of acute pelvic inflammatory disease in hospitalized patients. Am J Obstet Gynecol 1980;136:179.

27 Rickettsial Diseases

Rickettsiae are small bacteria that are obligate intracellular parasites and—except for Q fever—are transmitted to humans by arthropods. At least four rickettsiae *(Rickettsia rickettsii, Rickettsia conorii, Rickettsia tsutsugamushi, Rickettsia akari)*—and perhaps others—are transmitted transovarially in the arthropod, which serves as both vector and reservoir. Rickettsial diseases (except Q fever and ehrlichiosis) typically exhibit fever, rashes, and vasculitis. They are grouped on the basis of clinical features, epidemiologic aspects, and immunologic characteristics (Table 27–1).

Properties of Rickettsiae

Rickettsiae are pleomorphic, appearing either as short rods, 600 × 300 nm in size, or as cocci, and they occur singly, in pairs, in short chains, or in filaments. When stained, they are readily visible under the light microscope. With Giemsa's stain, they appear blue; with Macchiavello's stain they appear red, in contrast with the blue-staining cytoplasm around them.

A wide range of animals are susceptible to infection with rickettsial organisms. Rickettsiae grow readily in the yolk sac of the embryonated egg (yolk sac suspensions contain up to 10^9 rickettsial particles per milliliter). Pure preparations of rickettsiae can be obtained by differential centrifugation of yolk sac suspensions. Many rickettsial strains also grow in cell culture. Isolation of rickettsiae should be done only in reference laboratories for reasons of biosafety.

Purified rickettsiae contain both RNA and DNA in a ratio similar to that in bacteria (3.5:1). Rickettsiae have cell walls that are made up of peptidoglycans containing muramic acid and diaminopimelic acid and thus resemble the cell walls of gram-negative bacteria. They divide like bacteria. In cell culture, the generation time is 8–10 hours at 34 °C.

Purified rickettsiae contain various enzymes concerned with metabolism. Thus they oxidize intermediate metabolites like pyruvic, succinic, and glutamic acids and can convert glutamic acid into aspartic acid. Rickettsiae lose their biologic activities when they are stored at 0 °C, or incubated for a few hours at 36 °C. This is due to the progressive loss of nicotinamide adenine dinucleotide (NAD). All of these properties can be restored by subsequent incubation with NAD.

Rickettsiae grow in different parts of the cell. Those of the typhus group are usually found in the cytoplasm; those of the spotted fever group, in the nucleus. Coxiellae grow only in cytoplasmic vacuoles. It has been suggested that rickettsiae grow best when the metabolism of the host cells is low. Thus, their growth is enhanced when the temperature of infected chick embryos is lowered to 32 °C. If the embryos are held at 40 °C, rickettsial multiplication is poor. Conditions that influence the metabolism of the host can alter its susceptibility to rickettsial infection.

Rickettsial growth is enhanced in the presence of sulfonamides, and rickettsial diseases are made more severe by these drugs. Tetracyclines or chloramphenicol inhibits the growth of rickettsiae and can be therapeutically effective.

In general, rickettsiae are quickly destroyed by heat, drying, and bactericidal chemicals. Although rickettsiae are usually killed by storage at room temperature, dried feces of infected lice may remain infective for months at room temperature.

The organism of Q fever is the rickettsial agent most resistant to drying. This organism may survive pasteurization at 60 °C for 30 minutes and can survive for months in dried feces or milk. This may be due to the formation of endospore-like structures by *Coxiella burnetii.*

Rickettsial Antigens & Antibodies

The direct immunofluorescent antibody test can be use to detect rickettsiae in ticks and sections of tissues. The test has been most useful to detect *R rickettsii* in skin biopsy specimens to aid in the early diagnosis of Rocky Mountain spotted fever; however, the test is performed in only a few reference laboratories.

Serologic evidence of rickettsial infection occurs no earlier than the second week of illness for any of the rickettsial diseases. Thus, serologic tests are useful only to confirm the diagnosis, which is based on clinical findings (eg, fever, headache, rash) and epidemiologic information (eg, tick bite). Therapy for potentially severe diseases, such as Rocky Mountain spotted fever and typhus, should be instituted before seroconversion occurs.

Traditionally, the **Weil-Felix reaction** was used to diagnose rickettsial diseases. Rickettsiae and *Proteus*

Table 27–1. Rickettsial and ehrlichial diseases.

Group	Organism	Disease	Geographic Distribution	Vector	Mammalian Reservoir	Clinical Features	Diagnostic Tests
Typhus group	*Rickettsia prowazekii*	Epidemic typhus (louseborne typhus), Brill-Zinsser disease	Worldwide: South America, Africa, Asia, ?North America	Louse	Humans	Fever, chills, myalgia, headache, rash (no eschar); severe illness if untreated	Serology
	Rickettsia typhi	Murine typhus, endemic typhus, flea-borne typhus	Worldwide (small foci)	Flea	Rodents	Fever, headache, myalgia, rash (no eschar); milder illness than epidemic typhus	Serology
	Rickettsia tsutsugamushi	Scrub typhus	Asia, South Pacific, Northern Australia	Mite	Rodents	Fever, headache, rash (50% have eschar), lymphadenopathy, atypical lymphocytes	Serology
Spotted fever group	Rickettsia rickettsii	Rocky Mountain spotted fever	Western Hemisphere (United States, South America)	Tick[1]	Rodents, dogs	Fever, headache, rash (no eschar); many systemic manifestations	Direct FA of rickettsiae in tissue; serology
	Rickettsia akari	Rickettsialpox	USA, Korea, Russia, South Africa	Mite[1]	Mice	Mild illness, fever, headache, vesicular rash (eschar)	Serology
	Rickettsia australis	Queensland tick typhus	Australia	Tick[1]	Rodents, marsupials	Fever, rash of trunk and limbs (eschar)	Serology
	Rickettsia canada	Canadian typhus	Northern USA, Canada	Tick[1]	Rodents	Fever, rash (eschar)	Serology
	Rickettsia conorii	Fièvre boutonneuse, Mediterranean spotted fever, Israeli spotted fever, South African tick fever, African (Kenya) tick typhus, Indian tick typhus	Mediterranean countries, Africa, Middle East, India	Tick[1]	Rodents, dogs	Fever, headache, rash, "tache noire" (eschar)	Direct FA of rickettsiae in tissue not sensitive; serology
	Rickettsia sibirica	Siberian tick typhus (North Asian tick typhus)	Siberia, Mongolia	Tick[1]	Rodents	Fever, rash (eschar)	Serology
Others	*Coxiella burnetii*	Q fever	Worldwide	None (transmission by airborne fomites)	Sheep, cattle, goats, others	Headache, fever, fatigue, pneumonia (no rash); can have major complications	Positive CF to phase I, II antigens
	Ehrlichia chaffeensis	Ehrlichiosis	Southeastern USA, ?other	Tick	?Humans	Fever, headache, atypical white blood cells	Inclusions in circulating white blood cells; indirect FA for antibodies

[1]Also serve as arthropod reservoir, by maintaining the rickettsiae through transovarian transmission.

organisms share certain antigens, and patients with rickettsial infections develop antibodies that variably agglutinate *Proteus vulgaris* strains OX19, OX2, and OXK. For example, strain OX19 is agglutinated strongly by sera from persons with epidemic or endemic typhus, weakly by sera from those with Rocky Mountain spotted fever, and not at all by those with Q fever. Convalescent sera from scrub typhus patients react most strongly with the strain OXK. However, the Weil-Felix reaction does not have good sensitivity and specificity and is primarily of historical interest.

A variety of other serologic tests have been used to diagnose rickettsial diseases. Most of these tests are performed only in reference laboratories because of the low incidence of rickettsial diseases. Antigens for the CF to diagnose Q fever are commercially available, but reagents for other tests are prepared only in public health or other reference laboratories. There is no single test that provides clear-cut advantages over others. The indirect fluorescent antibody technique may be the most widely used method, because of the availability of reagents and the ease with which it can be performed. The minimum titers that indicate a positive test differ for each of the tests and also from one laboratory to another.

A. Indirect Immunofluorescence Test With Rickettsial Antigens: The test is relatively sensitive, requires little antigen, and can be used to detect IgM and IgG. Rickettsiae partially purified from infected yolk sac material are tested with dilutions of a patient's serum. Reactive antibody is detected with a fluorescein-labeled antihuman globulin. The results indicate the presence of partly species-specific antibodies, but some cross-reactions are observed.

B. CF With Rickettsial Antigens: Detection of CF antibodies is commonly used to diagnose Q fever. Group-reactive soluble antigens can also be tested for the typhus group and the spotted fever group. These antigens originate in the cell wall. Some insoluble antigens may give species-specific reactions. A fourfold or greater antibody titer rise is usually required for the diagnosis of acute rickettsial infection. A minimal positive titer is 1:1 or 1:16, and convalescent titers often exceed 1:64.

C. Agglutination of Rickettsiae: Rickettsiae are agglutinated by specific antibodies. This reaction can be diagnostically useful when heavy rickettsial suspensions are available for microagglutination tests.

D. Indirect Hemagglutination and Latex Agglutination Tests: A substance obtained by alkali extraction of rickettsiae of the typhus or spotted fever groups is used to sensitize erythrocytes or latex particles, which can then be agglutinated by antibody.

E. EIA: Enzyme immunoassay (in the form of ELISA) tests are among the most sensitive tests to diagnose rickettsial diseases, particularly for detection of IgM early in the illness. The assays require large amounts of antigen and are most efficient when many specimens are tested simultaneously.

Pathology

Rickettsiae multiply in endothelial cells of small blood vessels and produce vasculitis. The cells become swollen and necrotic; there is thrombosis of the vessel, leading to rupture and necrosis. Vascular lesions are prominent in the skin, but vasculitis occurs in many organs and appears to be the basis of hemostatic disturbances. Disseminated intravascular coagulation and vascular occlusion may develop. In the brain, aggregations of lymphocytes, polymorphonuclear leukocytes, and macrophages are associated with the blood vessels of the gray matter; these are called typhus nodules. The heart shows similar lesions of the small blood vessels. Other organs may also be involved.

Immunity

In cell cultures of macrophages, rickettsiae are phagocytosed and replicate intracellularly even in the presence of antibody. The addition of lymphocytes from immune animals stops this multiplication in vitro. Infection in humans is followed by partial immunity to reinfection from external sources, but relapses occur (see Brill-Zinsser disease, below).

Clinical Findings

Except for Q fever, in which there is no skin lesion, rickettsial infections are characterized by fever, headache, malaise, prostration, skin rash, and enlargement of the spleen and liver.

A. Typhus Group:

1. Epidemic typhus–In epidemic typhus, systemic infection and prostration are severe, and fever lasts for about 2 weeks. The disease is more severe and is more often fatal in patients over 40 years of age. During epidemics, the case-fatality rate has been 6–30%.

2. Endemic typhus–The clinical picture of endemic typhus has many features in common with that of epidemic typhus, but the disease is milder and is rarely fatal except in elderly patients.

B. Spotted Fever Group: The spotted fever group resembles typhus clinically; however, unlike the rash in other rickettsial diseases, the rash of the spotted fever group usually appears first on the extremities, moves centripetally, and involves the palms and soles. Some, like Brazilian spotted fever, may produce severe infections; others, like Mediterranean fever, are mild. The case-fatality rate varies greatly. In untreated Rocky Mountain spotted fever, it is usually much greater in elderly persons (up to 50%) than in young adults or children.

Rickettsialpox is a mild disease with a rash resembling that of varicella. About a week before onset of fever, a firm red papule appears at the site of the mite bite and develops into a deep-seated vesicle that in turn forms a black eschar (see below).

C. Scrub Typhus: This disease resembles epidemic typhus clinically. One feature is the eschar, the punched-out ulcer covered with a blackened scab that indicates the location of the mite bite. Generalized lymphadenopathy and lymphocytosis are common. Cardiac and cerebral involvement may be severe.

D. Q Fever: This disease resembles influenza, nonbacterial pneumonia, hepatitis, or encephalopathy rather than typhus. There is a rise in the titer of specific antibodies (eg, microimmunofluorescence) to *Coxiella burnetii,* phase 2. Transmission results from inhalation of dust contaminated with rickettsiae from dried feces, urine, or milk or from aerosols in slaughterhouses.

Rarely, infective endocarditis develops in Q fever. Blood cultures for bacteria are negative, and there is a high titer of antibodies to *C burnetii,* phase 1. Virtually all patients have preexisting valve abnormalities. Continuous treatment with tetracycline for many months—occasionally with valve replacement—can provide prolonged survival.

Laboratory Findings

Isolation of rickettsiae is technically quite difficult and so is of only limited usefulness in diagnosis. Whole blood (or emulsified blood clot) is inoculated into guinea pigs, mice, or eggs. Rickettsiae are recovered most frequently from blood drawn soon after onset, but they have been found as late as the 12th day of the disease.

If the guinea pigs fail to show disease (fever, scrotal swellings, hemorrhagic necrosis, death), serum is collected for antibody tests to determine if the animal has had an inapparent infection.

Some rickettsiae can infect mice, and rickettsiae are seen in smears of peritoneal exudate. In Rocky Mountain spotted fever, skin biopsies taken from patients between the fourth and eighth days of illness may reveal rickettsiae by immunofluorescence stain.

The most widely used serologic tests are indirect immunofluorescence and CF (see above). An antibody rise should be demonstrated during the course of the illness.

Treatment

Tetracyclines and chloramphenicol are effective provided treatment is started early. Tetracycline or chloramphenicol, is given daily orally and continued for 3–4 days after defervescence. In severely ill patients, the initial doses can be given intravenously.

Sulfonamides enhance the disease and are contraindicated. Some fluoroquinolones (eg, ciprofloxacin) are effective in spotted fevers.

The antibiotics do not free the body of rickettsiae, but they do suppress their growth. Recovery depends in part upon the immune mechanisms of the patient.

Epidemiology

A variety of arthropods, especially ticks and mites, harbor *Rickettsia*-like organisms in the cells that line the alimentary tract. Many such organisms are not evidently pathogenic for humans.

The life cycles of different rickettsiae vary:

(1) *Rickettsia prowazekii* has a life cycle limited to humans and to the human louse (*Pediculus humanus corporis* and *Pediculus humanus capitis*). The louse obtains the organism by biting infected human beings and transmits the agent by fecal excretion on the surface of the skin of another person. Whenever a louse bites, it defecates at the same time. The scratching of the area of the bite allows the rickettsiae excreted in the feces to penetrate the skin. As a result of the infection the louse dies, but the organisms remain viable for some time in the dried feces of the louse. Rickettsiae are not transmitted from one generation of lice to another. Typhus epidemics have been controlled by delousing large proportions of the population with insecticides.

Brill-Zinsser disease is a recrudescence of an old typhus infection. The rickettsiae can persist for many years in the lymph nodes of an individual without any symptoms being manifest. The rickettsiae isolated from such cases behave like classic *R prowazekii;* this suggests that humans themselves are the reservoir of the rickettsiae of epidemic typhus. Epidemic typhus epidemics have been associated with war and the lowering of standards of personal hygiene, which in turn have increased the opportunities for human lice to flourish. If this occurs at the time of recrudescence of an old typhus infection, an epidemic may be set off. Brill-Zinsser disease occurs in local populations of typhus areas as well as in persons who migrate from such areas to places where the disease does not exist. Serologic characteristics readily distinguish Brill's disease from primary epidemic typhus. Antibodies arise earlier and are IgG rather than the IgM detected after primary infection. They reach a maximum by the tenth day of disease. The Weil-Felix reaction is usually negative. This early IgG antibody response and the mild course of the disease suggest that partial immunity is still present from the primary infection.

In the USA, *R prowazekii* has an extrahuman reservoir in the southern flying squirrel. In areas where southern flying squirrels are indigenous, human infections have occurred after bites by ectoparasites of this rodent.

(2) *Rickettsia typhi* has its reservoir in the rat, in which the infection is inapparent and long-lasting. Rat fleas carry the rickettsiae from rat to rat and sometimes from rat to humans, who develop endemic typhus. Cat fleas can serve as vectors. In endemic typhus, the flea cannot transmit the rickettsiae transovarially.

(3) *R tsutsugamushi* has its true reservoir in the mites that infest rodents. Rickettsiae can persist in rats for over a year after infection. Mites transmit the infection transovarially. Occasionally, infected mites or rat fleas bite humans, and scrub typhus results. The rickettsiae persist in the mite-rat-mite cycle in the scrub or secondary jungle vegetation that has replaced virgin jungle in areas of partial cultivation. Such areas may become infested with rats and trombiculid mites.

(4) *R rickettsii* may be found in healthy wood ticks *(Dermacentor andersoni)* and is passed transovarially. Vertebrates such as rodents, deer, and humans are occasionally bitten by infected ticks in the western USA. In order to be infectious, the tick carrying the rickettsiae must be engorged with blood, for this increases the number of rickettsiae in the tick. Thus, there is a delay of 45–90 minutes between the time of the attachment of the tick and its becoming infective. In the eastern USA, Rocky Mountain spotted fever is transmitted by the dog tick *Dermacentor variabilis.* Dogs are hosts to dog ticks and may serve as a reservoir for tick infection. Small rodents are another reservoir. Most cases of Rocky Mountain spotted fever in the USA now occur in the eastern and southeastern regions.

(5) *R akari* has its vector in bloodsucking mites of the species *Allodermanyssus sanguineus.* These mites may be found on the mice *(Mus musculus)* trapped in apartment houses in the USA where rickettsialpox has occurred. Transovarial transmission of the rickettsiae occurs in the mite. Thus the mite may act as a true reservoir as well as a vector. *R akari* has also been isolated in Korea.

(6) *C burnetii* is found in ticks, which transmit the agent to sheep, goats, and cattle. Workers in slaughterhouses and in plants that process wool and cattle hides have contracted the disease as a result of handling infected animal tissues. Occasionally, the source is a parturient cat. *C burnetii* is transmitted by the respiratory pathway rather than through the skin. There may be a chronic infection of the udder of the cow. In such cases the rickettsiae are excreted in the milk and rarely may be transmitted to humans by the ingestion of unpasteurized milk.

Infected sheep may excrete *C burnetii* in the feces and urine and heavily contaminate their skin and woolen coat. The placentas of infected cows, sheep, goats, and cats contain the rickettsiae, and parturition creates infectious aerosols. The soil may be heavily contaminated from one of the above sources, and the inhalation of infected dust leads to infection of humans and livestock. It has been proposed that endospores formed by *C burnetii* contribute to its persistence and dissemination. *Coxiella* infection is now widespread among sheep and cattle in the USA. *Coxiella* can cause endocarditis (with a rise in the titer of antibodies to *C burnetii,* phase 1) in addition to pneumonitis and hepatitis.

Geographic Occurrence

A. Epidemic Typhus: Potentially worldwide, it has disappeared from the USA, Britain, and Scandinavia. It is still present in the Balkans, Asia, Africa, Mexico, and the Andes. In view of its long duration in humans as a latent infection (Brill-Zinsser disease), it can flourish quickly under proper environmental conditions, as it did in Europe during World War II as a result of the deterioration of community hygiene.

B. Endemic, Murine Typhus: Worldwide, especially in areas of high rat infestation. It may exist in the same areas as—and may be confused with—epidemic typhus or scrub typhus.

C. Scrub Typhus: Far East, especially Burma, India, Ceylon, New Guinea, Japan, and Taiwan. The larval stage (chigger) of various trombiculid mites serves both as a reservoir, through transovarian transmission, and as a vector for infecting humans and rodents.

D. Spotted Fever Group: These infections occur around the globe, exhibiting as a rule some epidemiologic and immunologic differences in different areas. Transmission by a tick of the Ixodidae family is common to the group. The diseases that are grouped together include Rocky Mountain spotted fever and Colombian, Brazilian, and Mexican spotted fevers; Mediterranean (boutonneuse), South African tick, and Kenya fevers; North Queensland tick typhus; and North Asian tick-borne rickettsiosis.

E. Rickettsialpox: The human disease has been found among inhabitants of apartment houses in the northern USA. However, the infection also occurs in Russia, Africa, and Korea.

F. Q Fever: The disease is recognized around the world and occurs mainly in persons associated with goats, sheep, dairy cattle, or parturient cats. It has attracted attention because of outbreaks in veterinary and medical centers where large numbers of people were exposed to animals shedding *Coxiella.*

Seasonal Occurrence

Epidemic typhus is more common in cool climates, reaching its peak in winter and waning in the spring. This is probably a reflection of crowding, lack of fuel, and low standards of personal hygiene, which favor louse infestation.

Rickettsial infections that must be transmitted to the human host by vector reach their peak incidence at the time the vector is most prevalent—the summer and fall months.

Control

Control must rely on breaking the infection chain, treating patients with antibiotics, and immunizing when possible. Patients with rickettsial disease who are free from ectoparasites are not contagious and do not transmit the infection.

A. Prevention of Transmission by Breaking the Chain of Infection:

1. Epidemic typhus–Delousing with insecticide.

2. Murine typhus–Rat-proofing buildings and using rat poisons.

3. Scrub typhus–Clearing from campsites the secondary jungle vegetation in which rats and mites live.

4. Spotted fever–Similar measures for the spotted fevers may be used; clearing of infested land; personal prophylaxis in the form of protective clothing such as high boots, socks worn over trousers; tick repellents; and frequent removal of attached ticks.

5. Rickettsialpox–Elimination of rodents and their parasites from human domiciles.

B. Prevention of Transmission of Q Fever by Adequate Pasteurization of Milk: The presently recommended conditions of "high-temperature, short-time" pasteurization at 71.5 °C for 15 seconds are adequate to destroy viable *Coxiella.*

C. Prevention by Vaccination: Active immunization has been attempted with formalinized antigens prepared from the yolk sacs of infected chick embryos or from cell cultures. Such vaccines have been prepared for epidemic typhus *(R prowazekii),* Rocky Mountain spotted fever *(R rickettsii),* and Q fever *(C burnetii).* The *Coxiella* vaccine (formalinized phase 1) has benefited occupationally exposed abattoir workers in Australia. However, commercially produced vaccines are not available in the USA. Cell-culture-grown, inactivated suspensions of rickettsiae are under study as vaccines. A live vaccine (strain E) for epidemic typhus is effective and used experimentally but produces a self-limited disease.

D. Chemoprophylaxis: Chloramphenicol has been used as a chemoprophylactic agent against scrub typhus in endemic areas. Oral administration of 3-g doses at weekly intervals controls infection so that no disease occurs even though rickettsiae appear in the blood. The antibiotic must be continued for a month after the initiation of infection to keep the person well. Tetracyclines appear to be equally effective.

EHRLICHIOSIS

The ehrlichiae are obligate intracellular bacteria that are taxonomically grouped with the rickettsiae. *Ehrlichia chaffeensis* causes human ehrlichiosis, primarily in the southeastern United States; *Ehrlichia sennetsu* causes a similar disease in Japan and probably Malaysia. The clinical manifestations of ehrlichiosis in humans are nonspecific: fever, chills, headache, myalgia, nausea or vomiting, anorexia, and weight loss. The clinical manifestations are very similar to those of Rocky Mountain spotted fever without the rash. The ehrlichiae infect circulating leukocytes where they multiply within phagocytic vacuoles. The diagnosis is confirmed by observing typical inclusion bodies in the white blood cells and by finding a fourfold rise in antibody titer with an indirect fluorescent antibody test. The treatment is tetracycline. Most species of *Ehrlichia* are pathogens of animals. *Ehrlichia chaffeensis* is closely related to *Ehrlichia canis,* which causes pancytopenia and chronic disease in dogs. Other *Ehrlichia* species cause disease in large animals. The geographic distribution of human ehrlichial infection and those of animals is not well defined.

REFERENCES

Bretman LR et al: Rickettsialpox: Report of an outbreak and a contemporary review. Medicine 1981;60:363.

Clements ML et al: Reactogenicity, immunogenicity and efficacy of a chick embryo-cell derived vaccine for Rocky Mountain spotted fever. J Infect Dis 1983;148:922.

Dumler JS et al: Persistent infection with *Ehrlichia chaffeensis.* Clin Infect Dis 1993;17:903.

Hechemy KE: Laboratory diagnosis of Rocky Mountain spotted fever. N Engl J Med 1979;300:859.

Langley JM et al: Poker player's pneumonia: An urban outbreak of Q fever following exposure to a parturient cat. N Engl J Med 1988;319:354.

McDade JE: Ehrlichosis: A disease of animals and humans. J Infect Dis 1990;161:609.

McDonald JC, MacLean JD, Dade JE: Imported rickettsial diseases. Am J Med 1988;85:799.

Rauch AM et al: Sheep-associated outbreak of Q fever: Idaho. Arch Intern Med 1987;147:341.

Rikihisa Y: The tribe *Ehrlichieae* and ehrlichial diseases. Clin Microbiol Rev 1991;4:286.

Russo PK et al: Epidemic typhus *(R prowazekii)* in Massachusetts. N Engl J Med 1981;304:1166.

Salgo MP et al: A focus of Rocky Mountain spotted fever within New York City. N Engl J Med 1988; 318:1345.

Sawyer LA, Fishbein DB, McDade JE: Q fever: Current concepts. Rev Infect Dis 1987;9:935.

Sexton DJ et al: Spotted fever group rickettsial infections in Australia. Rev Infect Dis 1991;13:876.

Taylor JP, Betz TG, Rawlings JA: Epidemiology of murine typhus in Texas: 1980 through 1984. JAMA 1986;255: 2173.

28 Chlamydiae

Chlamydiae (Figure 28–1) are divided into three species, *Chlamydia trachomatis, Chlamydia pneumoniae,* and *Chlamydia psittaci,* on the basis of antigenic composition, intracellular inclusions, sulfonamide susceptibility, and disease production. All chlamydiae exhibit similar morphologic features, share a common group antigen, and multiply in the cytoplasm of their host cells by a distinctive developmental cycle. The Chlamydiae can be viewed as gram-negative bacteria that lack mechanisms for the production of metabolic energy and cannot synthesize ATP. This defect restricts them to an intracellular existence, where the host cell furnishes energy-rich intermediates. Thus, chlamydiae are **obligate intracellular parasites.**

Developmental Cycle

All chlamydiae have a common reproductive cycle. The environmentally stable infectious particle is a small cell **(elementary body)** about 0.3 µm in diameter with an electron-dense nucleoid. A heparin sulfate-like glycosaminoglycan on the surface of *C trachomatis* is required for attachment to host cells. Following attachment, the elementary body is taken by phagocytosis into the host cell in a vacuole derived from the host cell surface membranes. This elementary body is reorganized into a large one **(reticulate body),** measuring about 0.5–1 µm and devoid of an electron-dense nucleoid. Within the membrane-bound vacuole, the reticulate body grows in size and divides repeatedly by binary fission. Eventually, the entire vacuole becomes filled with elementary bodies derived by binary fission from reticulate bodies to form an **inclusion** in the host cell cytoplasm. The newly formed elementary bodies may be liberated from the host cell to infect new cells. The developmental cycle takes 24–48 hours.

Structure & Chemical Composition

Examination of highly purified suspensions of chlamydiae indicates the following: the outer **cell wall** resembles the cell wall of gram-negative bacteria. It has a relatively high lipid content. It is rigid but does not contain a typical bacterial peptidoglycan; perhaps it contains a tetrapeptide-linked matrix. Penicillin-binding proteins occur in chlamydiae, and chlamydial cell wall formation is inhibited by penicillins and other drugs that inhibit transpeptidation of bacterial peptidoglycan. Lysozyme has no effect on chlamydial cell walls. N-Acetylmuramic acid appears to be absent from chlamydial cell walls. Both DNA and RNA are present in elementary and reticulate bodies. The reticulate bodies contain about four times as much RNA as DNA, whereas the elementary bodies contain about equal amounts of RNA and DNA. In elementary bodies, most DNA is concentrated in the electron-dense central nucleoid. Most RNA exists in ribosomes. The circular genome of chlamydiae (MW 7×10^8) is similar to that of bacterial chromosomes.

A **toxic principle** is intimately associated with infectious chlamydiae. It kills mice after the intravenous administration of more than 10^8 particles. Toxicity is destroyed by heat but not by ultraviolet light.

Staining Properties

Chlamydiae have distinctive staining properties (similar to those of rickettsiae). Elementary bodies stain purple with Giemsa's stain—in contrast to the blue of host cell cytoplasm. The larger, noninfective reticulate bodies stain blue with Giemsa's stain. The Gram reaction of chlamydiae is negative or variable and is not useful in identification of the agents. Chlamydial particles and inclusions stain brightly by immunofluorescence, with group-specific, species-specific, or serovar-specific antibodies.

Fully formed, mature intracellular inclusions of *C trachomatis* are compact masses near the nucleus which are dark purple when stained with Giemsa's stain because of the densely packed mature particles. If stained with dilute Lugol's iodine solution, some of the inclusions of *C trachomatis* (but not *C pneumoniae* or *C psittaci*) appear brown because of the glycogen matrix that surrounds the particles. Inclusions of *C psittaci* are diffuse intracytoplasmic aggregates.

Antigens

Chlamydiae possess **shared group (genus)-specific antigens.** These are heat-stable lipopolysaccharides with 2-keto-3-deoxyoctonic acid as an immunodominant component. Antibody to these genus-specific antigens can be detected by CF and immunofluores-

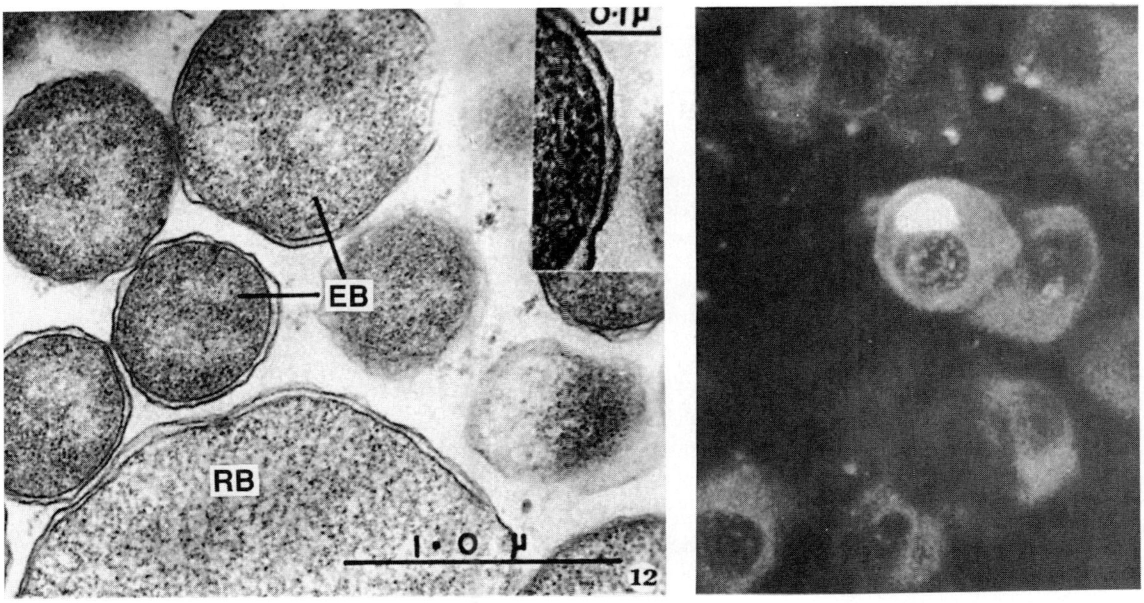

Figure 28–1. Chlamydiae. ***Left:*** Chlamydiae in various stages of intracellular development. (EB, elementary body particles with cell walls; RB, reticulate body.) ***Right:*** Fluorescent inclusion body of *C trachomatis* in epithelial cell (conjunctival scraping) stained with specific fluorescein-labeled antiserum.

cence. **Species-specific** or **serovar-specific** antigens are mainly outer membrane proteins. Specific antigens can best be detected by *immunofluorescence,* particularly using monoclonal antibodies. Specific antigens are shared by only a limited number of chlamydiae, but a given organism may contain several specific antigens. Fifteen **serovars** of *C trachomatis* have been identified (eg, A, B, Ba, C–K, L1–L3). Several serovars of *C psittaci* can be demonstrated by **complement fixation (CF)** and **microimmunofluorescence** tests. Only one serovar of *C pneumoniae* has been described.

Growth & Metabolism

Chlamydiae require an intracellular habitat, because they are unable to synthesize ATP and depend on the host cell for energy requirements. Chlamydiae grow in cultures of a variety of eukaryotic cells lines. Cells have attachment sites for chlamydiae. Removal of these sites prevents easy uptake of the organisms. McCoy cells treated with cycloheximide commonly are used to isolate chlamydiae. All types of chlamydiae proliferate in embryonated eggs, particularly in the yolk sac. Occasionally, mice are used to isolate chlamydiae.

Some chlamydiae have an endogenous metabolism like other bacteria. They can liberate CO_2 from glucose, pyruvate, and glutamate; they also contain dehydrogenases. Nevertheless, they require energy-rich intermediates from the host cell to carry out their biosynthetic activities.

Reactions to Physical & Chemical Agents

Chlamydiae are rapidly inactivated by heat. They lose infectivity completely after 10 minutes at 60 °C. They maintain infectivity for years at −70 °C to −50 °C. During the process of freeze-drying, much of the infectivity is lost. Some air-dried chlamydiae may remain infective for long periods. Chlamydiae are rapidly inactivated by ether (in 30 minutes) or by phenol (0.5% for 24 hours).

The replication of chlamydiae can be inhibited by many antibacterial drugs. Cell wall inhibitors such as penicillins and cephalosporins result in the production of morphologically defective forms but are not effective in clinical diseases. Inhibitors of protein synthesis (tetracyclines, erythromycins) are effective in most clinical infections. *C trachomatis* strains synthesize folates and are susceptible to inhibition by sulfonamides. Aminoglycosides are noninhibitory.

Characteristics of Host-Parasite Relationship

The outstanding biologic feature of infection by chlamydiae is the balance that is often reached between host and parasite, resulting in prolonged persistence of infection. Subclinical infection is the rule—and overt disease the exception—in the natural hosts of these agents. Spread from one species to another (eg, birds to humans, as in psittacosis) more frequently leads to disease. Antibodies to several antigens of chlamydiae are regularly produced by the infected host. These antibodies have little protective effect against reinfection. The infectious agent commonly persists in the presence of high antibody titers. Treatment with effective antimicrobial drugs (eg, tetracyclines) for prolonged periods may eliminate the chlamydiae from the infected host. Very early, intensive treatment may suppress antibody formation. Late treatment with antimicrobial drugs in moderate doses may suppress disease but permit persistence of the infecting agent in tissues.

The immunization of humans has been singularly unsuccessful in protecting against reinfection. Prior infection or immunization at most tends to result in milder disease upon reinfection, but at times the accompanying hypersensitization aggravates inflammation and scarring (eg, in trachoma).

Classification

Chlamydiae are arranged according to their pathogenic potential, host range, antigenic differences, and other methods. Three species have been characterized (see Table 28–1).

A. *C trachomatis*: This species produces compact intracytoplasmic inclusions that contain glycogen; it is usually inhibited by sulfonamides. It includes agents of human disorders such as trachoma, inclusion conjunctivitis, nongonococcal urethritis, salpingitis, cervicitis, pneumonitis of infants, and lymphogranuloma venereum and also mouse pneumonitis.

B. *C pneumoniae:* This species produces intracytoplasmic inclusions that lack glycogen; it is usually resistant to sulfonamides. It causes respiratory tract infections in humans.

C. *C psittaci:* This species produces diffuse intracytoplasmic inclusions that lack glycogen; it is usually resistant to sulfonamides. It includes agents of psittacosis in humans, ornithosis in birds, meningopneumonitis, feline pneumonitis, and other animal diseases.

CHLAMYDIA TRACHOMATIS: OCULAR, GENITAL, & RESPIRATORY INFECTIONS

Humans are the natural host for *C trachomatis.* Monkeys and chimpanzees can be infected in the eye and genital tract. All chlamydiae multiply in the yolk sacs of embryonated hens' eggs and cause death of the embryo when the number of particles becomes sufficiently high. *C trachomatis* also replicates in cells in tissue culture. *C trachomatis* of different serovars replicate differently. Isolates from trachoma do not grow as well as those from lymphogranuloma venereum or genital infections. Intracytoplasmic replication results in the formation of compact inclusions with a glycogen matrix in which elementary bodies are embedded.

A toxic factor is associated with *C trachomatis* provided the particles are viable. Neutralization of this toxic factor by immunotype-specific antisera permits typing of isolates that gives results analogous to those achieved by typing by microimmunofluorescence. The serovars specifically associated with endemic trachoma are A, B, Ba, and C; those associated with sexually transmitted disease are D–K; and those that cause lymphogranuloma venereum are L1, L2, and L3.

TRACHOMA

Trachoma is an ancient eye disease, well described in the Ebers Papyrus, which was written in Egypt 3800 years ago. It is a chronic keratoconjunctivitis that

Table 28–1. Characteristics of the chlamydiae.

	C trachomatis	*C pneumoniae*	*C psittaci*
Inclusion morphology	Round, vacuolar	Round, dense	Large, variable shape, dense
Glycogen in inclusions	Yes	No	No
Elementary body morphology	Round	Pear-shaped, round	Round
Susceptible to sulfonamides	Yes	No	No
DNA homology to *C pneumoniae*	< 10%	100%	< 10%
Plasmid	Yes	No	Yes
Serovars	15	1	≥ 4
Natural host	Humans	Humans	Birds
Mode of transmission	Person to person, mother to infant	Airborne person to person	Airborne bird excreta to humans
Major diseases	Trachoma, STDs, infant pneumonia, lymphogranuloma venereum	Pneumonia, bronchitis, pharyngitis, sinusitis	Psittacosis, pneumonia, fever of unexplained origin

begins with acute inflammatory changes in the conjunctiva and cornea and progresses to scarring and blindness.

Clinical Findings

In experimental human infections, the incubation period is 3–10 days. In endemic areas, initial infection occurs in early childhood, and the onset is insidious. Chlamydial infection is often mixed with bacterial conjunctivitis in endemic areas, and the two together produce the clinical picture. The earliest symptoms of trachoma are lacrimation, mucopurulent discharge, conjunctival hyperemia, and follicular hypertrophy. Microscopic examination of the cornea reveals epithelial keratitis, subepithelial infiltrates, and extension of limbal vessels into the cornea (pannus). As the pannus extends downward across the cornea, there is scarring of the conjunctiva, eyelid deformities (entropion, trichiasis), and added insult caused by eyelashes sweeping across the cornea. With secondary bacterial infection, loss of vision progresses over a period of years. There are, however, no systemic symptoms or signs of infection.

Laboratory Diagnosis

A. Culture: Typical cytoplasmic inclusions are found in epithelial cells of conjunctival scrapings stained with fluorescent antibody or by Giemsa's method. These occur most frequently in the early stages of the disease and on the upper tarsal conjunctiva.

Inoculation of conjunctival scrapings into cycloheximide-treated McCoy cell cultures permits growth of *C trachomatis* if the number of viable infectious particles is sufficiently large. Centrifugation of the inoculum into the cells increases the sensitivity of the method. The diagnosis can sometimes be made in the first passage after 2–3 days of incubation by looking for inclusions by immunofluorescence or staining with iodine or Giemsa's stain.

B. Serology: Infected individuals often develop both group antibodies and serovar-specific antibodies in serum and in eye secretions. Immunofluorescence is the most sensitive method for their detection. Neither ocular nor serum antibodies confer significant resistance to reinfection.

Treatment

In endemic areas, sulfonamides, erythromycins, and tetracyclines have been used to suppress chlamydiae and bacteria that cause eye infections. Periodic topical application of these drugs to the conjunctiva of all members of the community is sometimes supplemented with oral doses; the dosage and frequency of administration vary with the geographic area and the severity of endemic trachoma. Even a single monthly dose of 300 mg of doxycycline can result in significant clinical improvement, reducing the danger of blindness. Topical application of corticosteroids is not indicated and may reactivate latent trachoma. Chlamydiae can persist during and after drug treatment, and recurrence of activity is common.

Epidemiology & Control

It is believed that more than 400 million people throughout the world have trachoma and that 20 million are blinded by it. The disease is most prevalent in Africa, Asia, and the Mediterranean basin, where hygienic conditions are poor and water is scarce. In such hyperendemic areas, childhood infection may be universal, and severe, blinding disease (resulting from frequent bacterial superinfection) is common. In the USA, trachoma occurs sporadically in some areas, and endemic foci persist.

Control of trachoma depends mainly upon improvement of hygienic standards and drug treatment. When socioeconomic levels rise in an area, trachoma becomes milder and eventually may disappear. Experimental trachoma vaccines have not given encouraging results. Surgical correction of eyelid deformities may be necessary in advanced cases.

CHLAMYDIA TRACHOMATIS GENITAL INFECTIONS & INCLUSION CONJUNCTIVITIS

C trachomatis, serovars D–K, cause sexually transmitted diseases—especially in developed countries—and may also produce infection of the eye (inclusion conjunctivitis). In sexually active men, *C trachomatis* causes **nongonococcal urethritis** and, occasionally, **epididymitis.** In women, *C trachomatis* causes **urethritis, cervicitis,** and **pelvic inflammatory disease,** which can lead to **sterility** and predisposes to **ectopic pregnancy.** Any of these anatomic sites of infection may give rise to symptoms and signs, or the infection may remain asymptomatic but communicable to sex partners. Up to 50% of nongonococcal urethritis (men) or the urethral syndrome (women) is attributed to chlamydiae and produces dysuria, nonpurulent discharge, and frequency of urination. Genital secretions of infected adults can be self-inoculated into the conjunctiva, resulting in inclusion conjunctivitis, an ocular infection that closely resembles trachoma.

The newborn acquires the infection during passage through an infected birth canal. Probably 20–50% of infants of infected mothers acquire the infection, with 15–20% of infected infants manifesting eye symptoms and 10–20% manifesting respiratory tract involvement. **Inclusion conjunctivitis of the newborn** begins as a mucopurulent conjunctivitis 7–12 days after delivery. It tends to subside with erythromycin or tetracycline treatment, or spontaneously after weeks or months. Occasionally, inclusion conjunctivitis persists as a chronic chlamydial infection with a clinical picture indistinguishable from that of subacute or chronic childhood trachoma in nonendemic areas and usually not associated with bacterial conjunctivitis.

Laboratory Diagnosis

A. Culture: Scrapings of epithelial cells from the urethra, cervix, vagina, or conjunctiva and biopsy specimens from the salpinx or epididymis can be inoculated into cycloheximide-treated McCoy cell cultures for growth of *C trachomatis*. Isolates can be typed by immunofluorescence with specific sera. The same genital tract specimens can also be examined directly by immunofluorescence for chlamydial particles or by EIA for chlamydial antigens (Chapter 47). In neonatal—and sometimes adult—inclusion conjunctivitis, the cytoplasmic inclusions in epithelial cells are so dense that they are readily detected in conjunctival exudate and scrapings examined by immunofluorescence or Giemsa's stain.

B. Serology: Because of the relatively great antigenic mass of chlamydiae in genital tract infections, serum antibodies occur much more commonly than in trachoma and are of higher titer. A titer rise occurs during and after acute chlamydial infection. Because of the high prevalence of chlamydial genital tract infections in some societies, there is a high background of antichlamydial antibodies in the population; serologic tests to diagnose genital tract chlamydial infections generally are not useful.

In genital secretions (eg, cervical), antibody can be detected during active infection and is directed against the infecting immunotype (serovar).

Treatment

It is essential that chlamydial infections be treated simultaneously in both sex partners and in offspring to prevent reinfection. Tetracyclines (eg, doxycycline) are commonly used in nongonococcal urethritis and in nonpregnant infected females. Erythromycin is given to pregnant women. Topical tetracycline or erythromycin is used for inclusion conjunctivitis, sometimes in combination with a systemic drug.

Epidemiology & Control

Genital chlamydial infection and inclusion conjunctivitis are sexually transmitted diseases that are spread by contact with infected sex partners. Neonatal inclusion conjunctivitis originates in the mother's infected genital tract. Prevention of neonatal eye disease depends upon diagnosis and treatment of the pregnant woman and her sex partner. As in all sexually transmitted diseases, the presence of multiple etiologic agents (gonococci, treponemes, trichomonads, herpes, etc) must be considered. Instillation of erythromycin or tetracycline into the newborn's eyes does not prevent development of chlamydial conjunctivitis. The ultimate control of this—and all—sexually transmitted disease depends on safe sex practices and on early diagnosis and treatment of infected persons.

RESPIRATORY TRACT INVOLVEMENT WITH *CHLAMYDIA TRACHOMATIS*

Of newborns infected by the mother, 10–20% may develop respiratory tract involvement 2–12 weeks after birth, culminating in pneumonia. *C trachomatis* may be the most common cause of neonatal pneumonia. There is striking tachypnea, characteristic paroxysmal cough, absence of fever, and eosinophilia. Consolidation of lungs and hyperinflation can be seen by x-ray. The diagnosis should be suspected if pneumonitis develops in a newborn who has inclusion conjunctivitis and can be established by isolation of *C trachomatis* from respiratory secretions. In such neonatal pneumonia, an IgM antibody titer to *C trachomatis* of 1:32 or more is considered diagnostic. Systemic erythromycin is effective treatment in severe cases.

Adults with inclusion conjunctivitis often manifest upper respiratory tract symptoms (eg, otalgia, otitis, nasal obstruction, pharyngitis), presumably resulting from drainage of infectious chlamydiae through the nasolacrimal duct. Pneumonitis is infrequent in adults.

LYMPHOGRANULOMA VENEREUM

Lymphogranuloma venereum is a sexually transmitted disease caused by *C trachomatis* and characterized by suppurative inguinal adenitis; it is more common in tropical climates.

Properties of the Agent

The particles contain CF heat-stable chlamydial group antigens that are shared with all other chlamydiae. They also contain one of three serovar antigens (L1–L3), which can be defined by immunofluorescence. Infective particles contain a toxic principle.

Clinical Findings

Several days to several weeks after exposure, a small, evanescent papule or vesicle develops on any part of the external genitalia, anus, rectum, or elsewhere. The lesion may ulcerate, but usually it remains unnoticed and heals in a few days. Soon thereafter, the regional lymph nodes enlarge and tend to become matted and painful. In males, inguinal nodes are most commonly involved both above and below Poupart's ligament, and the overlying skin often turns purplish as the nodes suppurate and eventually discharge pus through multiple sinus tracts. In females and in homosexual males, the perirectal nodes are prominently involved, with proctitis and a bloody mucopurulent anal discharge. Lymphadenitis may be most marked in the cervical chains.

During the stage of active lymphadenitis, there are often marked systemic symptoms including fever, headaches, meningismus, conjunctivitis, skin rashes, nausea and vomiting, and arthralgias. Meningitis, arthritis, and pericarditis occur rarely. Unless effective antimicrobial drug treatment is given at that stage, the chronic inflammatory process progresses to fibrosis, lymphatic obstruction, and rectal strictures. The lymphatic obstruction may lead to elephantiasis of the penis, scrotum, or vulva. The chronic proctitis of women or homosexual males may lead to progressive rectal strictures, rectosigmoid obstruction, and fistula formation.

Laboratory Diagnosis

A. Smears: Pus, buboes, or biopsy material may be stained, but particles are rarely recognized.

B. Culture: Suspected material is inoculated into cell cultures; the organism also grows in the yolk sacs of embryonated eggs or the brains of mice. The inoculum can be treated with an aminoglycoside (but not with penicillin) to lessen bacterial contamination. The agent is identified by morphology and serologic tests.

C. Serology: Antibodies are commonly demonstrated by the CF reaction. The test becomes positive 2–4 weeks after onset of illness, at which time skin hypersensitivity can sometimes also be demonstrated. In a clinically compatible case, a rising antibody level or a single titer of more than 1:64 is good evidence of active infection. If treatment has eradicated the lymphogranuloma venereum infection, the CF titer falls. Serologic diagnosis of lymphogranuloma venereum can employ immunofluorescence, but the antibody is broadly reactive with many chlamydial antigens.

Immunity

Untreated infections tend to be chronic, with persistence of the agent for many years. Little is known about active immunity. The coexistence of latent infection, antibodies, and cell-mediated reactions is typical of many chlamydial infections.

Treatment

The sulfonamides and tetracyclines have been used with good results, especially in the early stages. In some drug-treated persons there is a marked decline in complement-fixing antibodies, which may indicate that the infective agent has been eliminated from the body. Late stages require surgery.

Epidemiology & Control

Although the highest incidence of lymphogranuloma venereum has been reported from subtropical and tropical areas, the infection occurs all over the world. The disease is most often spread by sexual contact, but not exclusively so. The portal of entry may sometimes be the eye (conjunctivitis with an oculoglandular syndrome). The genital tracts and rectums of chronically infected (but at times asymptomatic) persons serve as reservoirs of infection. Laboratory personnel exposed to aerosols of *C trachomatis* serovars L1–L3 can develop a chlamydial pneumonitis with mediastinal and hilar adenopathy. If the infection is recognized, treatment with tetracycline or erythromycin is effective.

The measures used for the control of other sexually transmitted diseases apply also to the control of lymphogranuloma venereum. Case-finding and early treatment and control of infected persons are essential.

CHLAMYDIA PNEUMONIAE & RESPIRATORY INFECTIONS

The first *C pneumoniae* (TWAR) strain was obtained in the 1960s in chick embryo yolk sac culture. Following the development of cell culture methods, this initial strain was thought to be a member of the species *C psittaci.* A second isolate was obtained in 1983. Subsequently, *C pneumoniae* has been firmly established as a new species that causes respiratory disease. Humans are the only known host.

Properties of the Agent

C pneumoniae produces round, dense, glycogen-negative inclusions that are sulfonamide-resistant, much like *C psittaci* (Table 28–1). The elementary bodies sometimes have a pear-shaped appearance. The genetic relatedness of *C pneumoniae* isolates is >95%. Only one serovar has been demonstrated.

Clinical Findings

Most infections with *C pneumoniae* are asymptomatic or associated with mild illness, but severe disease has been reported. There are no signs or symptoms that specifically differentiate *C pneumoniae* infections from those caused by many other agents. Both upper and lower airway disease occur. Pharyngitis is common. Sinusitis and otitis media may occur and be accompanied by lower airway disease. An atypical pneumonia similar to that caused by *Mycoplasma pneumoniae* is the primary recognized illness. Five to 20 percent of community-acquired pneumonia in young persons is thought to be caused by *C pneumoniae.*

Laboratory Diagnosis

A. Smears: Direct detection of elementary bodies in clinical specimens using fluorescent antibody techniques is relatively insensitive. Other stains do not effectively demonstrate the organism.

B. Culture: *C pneumoniae* grow in HeLa 229, HEp-2, and HL cells much better than in the McCoy cells used to isolate *C trachomatis;* they also grow in the yolk sacs of embryonated eggs. The sensitivity of cell culture is enhanced by pretreatment of the cells with diethylaminoethyl dextran. Growth is better at 35 °C than 37 °C. After 3 days' incubation, the cells are fixed and inclusions detected by fluorescent antibody staining with genus- or species-specific antibody. Giemsa staining is insensitive, and the glycogen-negative inclusions do not stain with iodine. It is moderately difficult to grow *C pneumoniae*—as evidenced by the number of isolates described compared with the incidence of infection.

C. Serology: Serology using the microimmunofluorescence test is the most sensitive method for diagnosis of *C pneumoniae* infection. The test is species-specific and can detect IgG or IgM antibodies by using the appropriate reagents. Primary infection yields IgM antibody after about 3 weeks followed by IgG antibody at 6–8 weeks. In reinfection, the IgM response may be absent or minimal and the IgG response occurs in 1–2 weeks. The following criteria have been suggested for the serologic diagnosis of *C pneumoniae* infection: a single IgM titer of >1:16; a single IgG titer of >1:512; and a fourfold rise in either the IgM or IgG titers.

The complement fixation test can be used, but it is group-reacting, does not differentiate *C pneumoniae* infection from psittacosis or lymphogranuloma venereum, and is less sensitive than the microimmunofluorescence test.

Immunity

Little is known about active or potentially protective immunity. Prolonged infections can occur with *C pneumoniae,* and asymptomatic carriage may be common.

Treatment

There is very limited information on the clinical efficacy of antimicrobial therapy for *C pneumoniae* infection. The organisms are susceptible to tetracyclines and erythromycins in vitro, and these drugs would presumably benefit patients. Optimal dosage and duration of treatment are undetermined; therapy for 3 weeks has been recommended.

Epidemiology

Infection with *C pneumoniae* is common. Worldwide, 30–50% of people have antibody to *C pneumoniae.* Few young children have antibody, but after the age of 6–8 years, the prevalence of antibody increases through young adulthood. Infection is both endemic and epidemic, with multiple outbreaks attributed to *C pneumoniae.* There is no known animal reservoir, and transmission is presumed to be from person to person, predominantly by the airborne route.

CHLAMYDIA PSITTACI & PSITTACOSIS (Ornithosis)

The term **"psittacosis"** is applied to the human *C psittaci* disease acquired from contact with birds and also the infection of psittacine birds (parrots, parakeets, cockatoos, etc). The term **"ornithosis"** is applied to infection with similar agents in all types of domestic birds (pigeons, chickens, ducks, geese, turkeys, etc) and free-living birds (gulls, egrets, petrels, etc). In humans, *C psittaci* produces a spectrum of clinical manifestations ranging from severe pneumonia and sepsis with a high mortality rate to a mild inapparent infection.

Properties of the Agent

C psittaci can be propagated in embryonated eggs, in mice and other animals, and in some cell cultures. In all these host systems, growth can be inhibited by tetracyclines. In animals and in humans, tetracyclines can suppress illness but may not be able to eliminate the infectious agent or end the carrier state. The heat-stable group-reactive CF antigen resists proteolytic enzymes and appears to be a lipopolysaccharide. Infected tissue contains a toxic principle, intimately associated with the agent, that rapidly kills mice upon intravenous or intraperitoneal infection. This toxic principle is active only in particles that are infective.

Treatment of *C psittaci* with deoxycholate and trypsin yields extracts that contain group-reactive CF antigens, whereas the cell walls retain the species-specific antigen. Antibodies to the species-specific antigen are able to neutralize toxicity and infectivity. Specific serovars characteristic for certain mammalian and avian species may be demonstrated by cross-neutralization tests of toxic effect. Neutralization of infectivity of the agent by specific antibody or cross-protection of immunized animals can also be used for serotyping, and the results parallel those of immunofluorescence typing.

Pathogenesis & Pathology

The agent enters through the respiratory tract, is found in the blood during the first 2 weeks of the disease, and may be found in the sputum at the time the lung is involved.

Psittacosis causes a patchy inflammation of the lungs in which consolidated areas are sharply demarcated. The exudate is predominantly mononuclear. Only minor changes occur in the large bronchioles and bronchi. The lesions are similar to those found in pneumonitis caused by some viruses and mycoplasmas. Liver, spleen, heart, and kidney are often enlarged and congested.

Clinical Findings

A sudden onset of illness taking the form of influenza or nonbacterial pneumonia in a person exposed to birds is suggestive of psittacosis. The incubation period averages 10 days. The onset is usually sudden, with malaise, fever, anorexia, sore throat, photophobia, and severe headache. The disease may progress no further, and the patient may improve in a few days. In severe cases, the signs and symptoms of bronchial pneumonia appear at the end of the first week of the disease. The clinical picture often resembles that of influenza, nonbacterial pneumonia, or typhoid fever. The mortality rate may be as high as 20% in untreated cases, especially in the elderly.

Laboratory Diagnosis

A. Culture: *C psittaci* can be isolated from blood or sputum of patients or from lung tissue in fatal cases. Specimens are inoculated into cell cultures, into the yolk sacs of embryonated eggs, and intra-abdominally into mice. Isolation is confirmed by the serial transmission of the infectious agent, its microscopic demonstration, and serologic identification of the recovered agent.

B. Serology: A variety of antibodies may develop in the course of infection. In humans, CF with group antigen is the most widely used diagnostic test. A single titer of 1:32 or higher in an illness compatible with this diagnosis is presumptive evidence of chlamydial pneumonia. For definitive diagnosis, acute and later phase sera should be run in the same test in order to establish an antibody rise. In birds, the indirect CF test may provide additional diagnostic information. Although antibodies usually develop within 10 days, the use of antibiotics may delay their development for 20–40 days or suppress it altogether.

Sera of patients with other chlamydial infections may fix complement in high titer with psittacosis antigen. In patients with psittacosis, the high titer persists for months or, in carriers, even for years. In live birds, infection is suggested by a positive CF test and an enlarged spleen or liver. This can be confirmed by demonstration of particles in smears or sections of organs and by passage of the agent in mice and eggs.

Immunity

Immunity in animals and humans is incomplete. A carrier state in humans can persist for 10 years after recovery. During this period, the agent may continue to be excreted in the sputum.

Live or inactivated vaccines induce only partial resistance in animals. They have not been used in humans.

Treatment

Tetracyclines are the drugs of choice and should be continued for 10 days after defervescence to prevent relapse. Psittacosis agents are not sensitive to aminoglycosides, and most strains are not susceptible to sulfonamides. Although antibiotic treatment may control the clinical evidence of disease, it may not free the patient from the agent, ie, the patient may become a carrier. Intensive antibiotic treatment may also delay the normal course of antibody development. Strains may become drug-resistant. With antibiotic therapy the mortality rate is 2% or less. Death occurs most frequently in patients over 40 years of age.

Epidemiology & Control

Outbreaks of human disease can occur whenever there is close and continued contact between humans and infected birds that excrete or shed large amounts of infectious agent. Birds often acquire infection as fledglings in the nest, may develop diarrheal illness or no illness, and often carry the infectious agent for their normal life span. When subjected to stress (eg, malnutrition, shipping), birds may become sick and die. The agent is present in tissues (eg, spleen) and is often excreted in feces by healthy birds. The inhalation of infected dried bird feces is a common method of human infection. Another source of infection is the handling of infected tissues (eg, in poultry rendering plants) and inhalation of an infected aerosol.

Birds kept as pets have been an important source of human infection. Foremost among these were the many imported psittacine birds. Latent infections often flared up in these birds during transport and crowding, and sick birds excreted exceedingly large quantities of infectious agent. Control of bird shipment, quarantine, testing of imported birds for psittacosis infection, and prophylactic tetracyclines in bird feed has helped to control this source. Pigeons kept for racing or as pets or raised for squab meat have been important sources of infection. Pigeons populating buildings and thoroughfares in many cities, if infected, shed relatively small quantities of agent.

Among the personnel of poultry farms involved in the dressing, packing, and shipping of ducks, geese, turkeys, and chickens, subclinical or clinical infection is relatively frequent. Outbreaks of disease among birds have at times resulted in heavy economic losses and have been followed by outbreaks in humans. Human-to-human transmission is rare.

Shipments of psittacine birds should be held in quarantine to ensure that there are no obviously sick birds in the lot. A proportion of each shipment should be tested for antibodies and examined for the agent. The incorporation of tetracyclines into bird feed has been used to reduce the number of carriers. The source of human infection should be traced, if possible, and infected birds should be killed.

REFERENCES

Bernstein DI et al: Mediastinal and supraclavicular lymphadenitis and pneumonitis due to *Chlamydia trachomatis,* serovars L_1 and L_2. N Engl J Med 1984;311:1543.

Brunham RC et al: Mucopurulent cervicitis: The counterpart in women of urethritis in men. N Engl J Med 1984;311:1.

Caldwell HD, Hitchcock PJ: Monoclonal antibody against a

genus-specific antigen of *Chlamydia:* Location of epitope on chlamydial lipopolysaccharide. Infect Immun 1984; 44:306.

Chernesky MA et al: Detection of *Chlamydia trachomatis* antigens by enzyme immunoassay and immunofluorescence in genital specimens from symptomatic and asymptomatic men and women. J Infect Dis 1986;154:141.

Fraiz J, Jones BR: Chlamydial infections. Annu Rev Med 1988;39:357.

Gnarpe J et al: Endemic prevalence of *Chlamydia pneumoniae* in subjectively healthy adults. Scand J Infect Dis 1991;23:387.

Grayston JT et al: A new respiratory tract pathogen: *Chlamydia pneumoniae* strain TWAR. J Infect Dis 1990;161: 618.

MacDonald AB: Antigens of *Chlamydia trachomatis.* Rev Infect Dis 1985;7:731.

McPhee SJ, Erb B, Harrington W: Psittacosis. West J Med 1987;146:91.

Schachter J: Chlamydiae.In: *Manual of Clinical Microbiology,* 5th ed. Balows A et al (editors). American Society for Microbiology, 1991.

Scieux C et al: Lymphogranuloma venereum: 27 cases in Paris. J Infect Dis 1989;160:662.

Stamm WE et al: Causes of the acute urethral syndrome in women. N Engl J Med 1980;303:409.

Wang SP et al: Immunotyping of *Chlamydia trachomatis* with monoclonal antibodies. J Infect Dis 1985;152:791.

Zhang JP, Stephens RS: Mechanism of *C trachomatis* attachment to host cells. Cell 1992;69:861.

General Properties of Viruses

29

INTRODUCTION TO VIRUSES

Viruses are the smallest infectious agents (20–300 nm in diameter), containing only one kind of nucleic acid (RNA or DNA) as their genome. The nucleic acid is encased in a protein shell, which may be surrounded by a lipid-containing membrane. The entire infectious unit is termed a virion. Viruses are inert in the extracellular environment. They replicate only in living cells, being parasites at the genetic level. The viral nucleic acid contains information necessary for programming the infected host cell to synthesize a number of virus-specific macromolecules required for the production of viral progeny. During the replicative cycle, numerous copies of viral nucleic acid and coat proteins are produced. The coat proteins assemble together to form the capsid, which encases and stabilizes the viral nucleic acid against the extracellular environment and facilitates the attachment and perhaps penetration by the virus upon contact with new susceptible cells.

The nucleic acid, once isolated from the virion, can be hydrolyzed by either ribo- or deoxyribonuclease, whereas the nucleic acid within the intact virus is not affected by such treatment. In contrast, viral antiserum will neutralize the virion because it reacts with the antigens of the protein coat. However, the same antiserum has no effect on the free infectious nucleic acid isolated from the virion.

The host range for a given virus may be broad or extremely limited. Viruses are known to infect unicellular organisms such as mycoplasmas, bacteria, and algae and all higher plants and animals. Details of the effects of viral infection on the host are considered in Chapter 30.

Much information on virus-host relationships has been obtained from studies on bacteriophages, the viruses that attack bacteria. This subject is discussed in Chapter 7. Properties of individual viruses are discussed in Chapters 31–44.

DEFINITIONS IN VIROLOGY (Figure 29–1)

Capsid: The protein shell, or coat, that encloses the nucleic acid genome. Empty capsids may be by-products of the replicative cycle of viruses with icosahedral symmetry.

Nucleocapsid: The capsid together with the enclosed nucleic acid.

Structural units: The basic protein building blocks of the coat. They are usually a collection of more than one nonidentical polypeptide.

Capsomers: Morphologic units seen in the electron microscope on the surface of icosahedral viral particles. Capsomers represent clusters of polypeptides, but the morphologic units do not necessarily correspond to the chemically defined structural units.

Envelope: A lipid-containing membrane that surrounds some viral particles. It is acquired during viral maturation by a budding process through a cellular membrane. Virus-encoded glycoproteins are exposed on the surface of the envelope.

Virion: The complete viral particle, which in some instances (adenoviruses, papovaviruses, picornaviruses) may be identical with the nucleocapsid. In more complex virions (herpesviruses, orthomyxoviruses), this includes the nucleocapsid plus a surrounding envelope. This structure, the virion, serves to transfer the viral nucleic acid from one cell to another.

Defective virus: A viral particle that is functionally deficient in some aspect of replication. Defective virus may interfere with the replication of normal virus.

EVOLUTIONARY ORIGIN OF VIRUSES

The origin of viruses is not known. Two likely hypotheses are as follows:

(1) Viruses may be derived from components of host cells that became autonomous. They resemble genes that have acquired the capacity to exist independent of the cell. Some viral sequences are related to portions of cellular genes encoding protein functional domains. The likelihood is great that most viruses evolved in this fashion.

(2) Viruses evolved from free-living cells. There is no evidence that viruses evolved from bacteria, al-

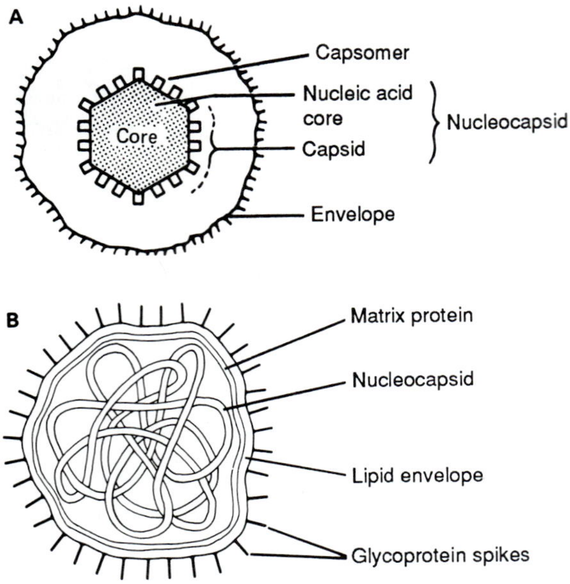

Figure 29–1. Schematic diagram illustrating the components of the complete viral particle (the virion). ***A:*** Enveloped virus with icosahedral symmetry. ***B:*** Virus with helical symmetry.

though the possibility exists that other obligatory intracellular organisms, eg, chlamydiae, did so. However, poxviruses are so large and complex that they might represent evolutionary products of some cellular ancestor.

CLASSIFICATION OF VIRUSES

Basis of Classification

The following properties, listed in order of importance, have been used as a basis for the classification of viruses. The amount of information available in each category is not uniform for all viruses. For some agents, knowledge is available for only a few of the properties listed.

(1) Nucleic acid type: RNA or DNA; single-stranded or double-stranded; strategy of replication.

(2) Size and morphology, including type of symmetry, number of capsomers, and presence or absence of membranes.

(3) Susceptibility to physical and chemical agents, especially ether.

(4) Presence of specific enzymes, particularly RNA and DNA polymerases concerned with genome replication, and neuraminidase necessary for release of certain viral particles (influenza) from the cells in which they were formed.

(5) Immunologic properties.

(6) Natural methods of transmission.

(7) Host, tissue, and cell tropisms.

(8) Pathology; inclusion body formation.

(9) Symptomatology.

Classification by Symptomatology

The oldest classification of viruses is based on the diseases they produce, and this system offers certain conveniences for the clinician. However, it is not satisfactory for the biologist because the same virus may appear in several groups if it causes more than one disease, depending upon the organ attacked.

A. Generalized Diseases: Diseases in which virus is spread throughout the body via the bloodstream and in which multiple organs are affected. Skin rashes may occur. These include vaccinia, measles, rubella, chickenpox, yellow fever, dengue, enteroviruses, and many others.

B. Diseases Primarily Affecting Specific Organs: The virus may reach the organ via the bloodstream, along peripheral nerves, or by other routes.

1. Diseases of the nervous system–Poliomyelitis, aseptic meningitis (polio-, coxsackie-, and echoviruses), rabies, arthropod-borne encephalitides, lymphocytic choriomeningitis, herpes simplex, meningoencephalitis of mumps, measles, vaccinia, and "slow" viral infections.

2. Diseases of the respiratory tract–Influenza, parainfluenza, respiratory syncytial viral pneumonia and bronchiolitis, adenovirus pharyngitis, and common cold (caused by many viruses).

3. Localized diseases of the skin or mucous membranes–Herpes simplex type 1 (usually oral) and type 2 (usually genital), molluscum contagiosum, warts, herpangina, herpes zoster, and others.

4. Diseases of the eye–Adenovirus conjunctivitis, herpes keratoconjunctivitis, and epidemic hemorrhagic conjunctivitis (enterovirus 70).

5. Diseases of the liver–Hepatitis type A (infectious hepatitis), type B (serum hepatitis), type C, and type E; yellow fever; and, in newborns, enteroviruses, herpesviruses, and rubella virus.

6. Diseases of the salivary glands–Mumps and cytomegalovirus.

7. Diseases of the gastrointestinal tract–Rotavirus, Norwalk virus, enteric adenoviruses.

8. Sexually transmitted diseases–Herpes simplex virus, hepatitis B virus, papillomaviruses, molluscum contagiosum virus, the retroviruses associated with acquired immunodeficiency syndrome (AIDS), and probably cytomegalovirus are all sexually transmitted pathogens.

Classification by Biologic, Chemical, & Physical Properties

Viruses can be clearly separated into major groupings, called families, on the basis of the type of nucleic acid genome and the size, shape, substructure, and mode of replication of the viral particle. Table 29–1 shows the standard scheme used for classifica-

Table 29–1. Classification of viruses into families based on chemical and physical properties.

Nucleic Acid Core	Capsid Symmetry	Virion: Enveloped or Naked	Ether Sensitivity	No. of Capsomers	Viral Particle Size (nm)[1]	Molecular Weight of Nucleic Acid in Virion ($\times 10^6$)	Physical Type of Nucleic Acid	No. of Genes (approx.)	Viral Family
DNA	Icosahedral	Naked	Resistant	32	18–26	1.5–2.2	ss	3–4	Parvoviridae
				72	45–55	3–5	ds circular	5–8	Papovaviridae
				252	70–90	20–30	ds	30	Adenoviridae
		Enveloped	Sensitive	162	100[2]	90–130	ds	160	Herpesviridae
	Complex	Complex coats	Resistant[3]		230 × 400	130–200	ds	300	Poxviridae
					42	1.6	ds circular[4]	4	Hepadnaviridae
RNA	Icosahedral	Naked	Resistant	32	20–30	2.3–2.8	ss	4–6	Picornaviridae
				32	35–39	2.6	ss	4–6	Caliciviridae
				[5]	60–80	12–15	ds segmented	10–12	Reoviridae
		Enveloped	Sensitive	32?	50–70	4	ss	10	Togaviridae
	Unknown or complex	Enveloped	Sensitive		45–50	4	ss	10	Flaviviridae
					50–300	3–5	ss segmented	10	Arenaviridae
					80–160	7	ss	30	Coronaviridae
					~100	7–10	ss diploid	4	Retroviridae
	Helical	Enveloped	Sensitive		90–100	6–15	ss segmented	>3	Bunyaviridae
					80–120	5	ss segmented	10	Orthomyxoviridae
					150–300	5–7	ss	>10	Paramyxoviridae
					75 × 180	4	ss	5	Rhabdoviridae

[1]Diameter, or diameter × length.

[2]The naked virus, ie, the nucleocapsid, is 100 nm in diameter; however, the enveloped virion varies up to 200 nm.

[3]The genus *Orthopoxvirus,* which includes the better studied poxviruses (eg, vaccinia, variola, cowpox, ectromelia, rabbitpox, monkeypox), is ether-resistant. Some of the poxviruses belonging to other genera are ether-sensitive.

[4]One strand has a constant length of 3182 bases, and the other varies between 1700 and 2800 bases.

[5]Reoviruses possess a double protein capsid shell in which the exact number and spatial arrangement of capsomers are difficult to determine.

ss = single-stranded

ds = double-stranded

tion. Diagrams of animal virus families are shown in Figure 29–4.

Within each family, subdivisions, called genera, are usually based on physicochemical or serologic differences. Properties of the major families of animal viruses are summarized in Table 29–1, are discussed briefly below, and are considered in greater detail in the chapters that follow.

Survey of DNA-Containing Viruses

A. Parvoviruses: Very small viruses with a particle size of about 20 nm. They contain single-stranded DNA and have cubic symmetry, with 32 capsomers. They have no envelope. Replication occurs only in actively dividing cells; capsid assembly takes place in the nucleus of the infected cell. Many parvoviruses replicate autonomously, but the adenoassociated satellite viruses are defective, ie, they require the presence of an adenovirus or herpesvirus as "helper." Some parvovirus infections occur in humans. (See Chapters 31 and 32.)

B. Papovaviruses: Small (45–55 nm), heat-stable, ether-resistant viruses containing double-stranded circular DNA and exhibiting cubic symmetry, with 72 capsomers. Known human papovaviruses are the papilloma (wart) viruses and agents isolated from brain tissue of patients with progressive multifocal leukoencephalopathy (JC virus) or from the urine of immunosuppressed renal transplant recipients (BK virus). In animals, there are papilloma, polyoma, and vacuolating viruses. These agents have a slow growth cycle, stimulate cell DNA synthesis, and replicate within the nucleus. Papovaviruses produce latent and chronic infections in their natural hosts, and all can induce tumors in some animal species. (See Chapters 42 and 43.)

C. Adenoviruses: Medium-sized (70–90 nm) viruses containing double-stranded DNA and exhibiting cubic symmetry, with 252 capsomers. They have no envelope. At least 41 types infect humans, especially in mucous membranes, and some types can persist in lymphoid tissue. Some adenoviruses cause acute respiratory diseases, pharyngitis, conjunctivitis, and gastroenteritis. Some human adenoviruses can induce tumors in newborn hamsters. There are many serotypes that infect animals. (See Chapters 32 and 43.)

D. Herpesviruses: Medium-sized viruses containing double-stranded DNA. The nucleocapsid is 100 nm in diameter, with cubic symmetry and 162 capsomers. It is surrounded by a lipid-containing envelope (150–200 nm in diameter). Latent infections may last for the life span of the host, usually in ganglial or lymphoblastoid cells. Human herpesviruses include herpes simplex types 1 and 2 (oral and genital lesions), varicella-zoster virus (shingles and chickenpox), cytomegalovirus, Epstein-Barr virus (infectious mononucleosis and association with human neoplasms), and human herpesviruses 6 and 7 (T lymphotropic). Other herpesviruses occur in many animals. (See Chapters 33 and 43.)

E. Poxviruses: Large brick-shaped or ovoid (230 × 400 nm) viruses containing double-stranded DNA, with a lipid-containing envelope. Poxviruses contain several enzymes within the virion, including a DNA-dependent RNA polymerase, and replicate entirely within the cell cytoplasm. All poxviruses tend to produce skin lesions. Some are pathogenic for humans (smallpox, vaccinia, molluscum contagiosum); others that are pathogenic for animals can infect humans, eg, cowpox, monkeypox. (See Chapter 34.)

F. Hepadnaviruses: Small (42 nm) viruses containing circular DNA molecules that are partially double-stranded. The virion carries a DNA polymerase able to make fully double-stranded molecules. The virus consists of a nucleocapsid core and a lipid-containing envelope. The surface protein is characteristically overproduced during replication of the virus, which takes place in the liver. Hepadnaviruses cause acute and chronic hepatitis; persistent infections are associated with a high risk of developing liver cancer. Three viral types that infect mammals (humans, woodchucks, and ground squirrels) and one type that infects ducks are known. (See Chapter 35.)

Survey of RNA-Containing Viruses

A. Picornaviruses: Small (20–30 nm), ether-resistant viruses containing single-stranded RNA and exhibiting cubic symmetry. The RNA genome is positive-sense, ie, it can serve as an mRNA. The groups infecting humans are rhinoviruses (more than 100 serotypes causing common colds) and enteroviruses (polio-, coxsackie-, and echoviruses). Rhinoviruses are acid-labile and have a high density; enteroviruses are acid-stable and have a lower density. Picornaviruses infecting animals include foot-and-mouth disease of cattle and encephalomyocarditis of rodents. (See Chapter 36.)

B. Caliciviruses: Similar to picornaviruses but slightly larger (35–39 nm). The genome is single-stranded, positive-sense RNA; the virion has no envelope. An important human pathogen is Norwalk virus, the cause of epidemic acute gastroenteritis; other agents infect cats, sea lions, and primates.

C. Reoviruses: Medium-sized (60–80 nm), ether-resistant viruses containing segmented double-stranded RNA and having cubic symmetry. Reoviruses of humans include rotaviruses, which have a distinctive wheel-shaped appearance and cause gastroenteritis. Antigenically similar reoviruses infect many animals. Orbiviruses constitute a distinct subgroup that includes arthropod-transmitted agents which infect insects and animals (such as bluetongue of cattle and sheep). The *Coltivirus* genus includes Colorado tick fever virus of humans. (See Chapter 37.)

D. Arboviruses: An ecologic grouping of viruses with diverse physical and chemical properties. All of these viruses (>350) have a complex cycle involving arthropods as vectors that transmit the viruses to vertebrate hosts by their bite. Viral replication does not seem to harm the infected arthropod. Arboviruses infect humans, mammals, birds, and snakes and use mosquitoes and ticks as vectors. Human pathogens include dengue, yellow fever, encephalitis viruses, and others. Arboviruses belong to several virus families, including toga-, flavi-, bunya-, rhabdo-, arena-, and reoviruses. (See Chapter 38.)

E. Togaviruses: Many arboviruses that are major human pathogens, as well as rubella virus, belong here. They have a lipid-containing envelope and are ether-sensitive, and their genome is single-stranded, positive-sense RNA. The enveloped virion measures 50–70 nm. The viral particles mature by budding from the host cell plasma membrane. (See Chapters 38 and 40.)

F. Flaviviruses: Enveloped viruses, 45–50 nm in diameter, containing single-stranded, positive-sense RNA. Mature virions accumulate within cisternae of the endoplasmic reticulum. This group of arboviruses includes yellow fever virus. Most members are transmitted by blood-sucking arthropods. Hepatitis C virus has no known vector.

G. Arenaviruses: RNA-containing, enveloped viruses ranging in size from 50 to 300 nm. The genome is single-stranded RNA that is negative-sense, ie, complementary to mRNA. The virions incorporate host cell ribosomes during maturation, which gives the particles a "sandy" appearance. Most members of this family are unique to tropical America (ie, the Tacaribe complex). All arenaviruses pathogenic for humans cause chronic infections in rodents. Lassa fever virus of Africa is one example. (See Chapter 38.)

H. Coronaviruses: Enveloped, 80- to 160-nm particles containing an unsegmented genome of single-stranded RNA; the nucleocapsid is probably helical, 11–13 nm in diameter. They resemble orthomyxoviruses, but coronaviruses have petal-shaped surface projections arranged in a fringe like a solar corona. Coronavirus nucleocapsids develop in the cytoplasm and mature by budding into cytoplasmic vesicles. Human coronaviruses have been isolated from acute upper respiratory tract illnesses—"colds." Toroviruses, which cause gastroenteritis, form a distinct genus in the coronavirus family. Coronaviruses of animals readily establish persistent infections and include avian infectious bronchitis virus. (See Chapter 41.)

I. Retroviruses: Enveloped viruses (90–120 nm in diameter) whose genome contains two copies of high-molecular-weight, single-stranded RNA of the same polarity as viral mRNA. The virion contains a reverse transcriptase (RNA → DNA). The virus is replicated from an integrated "provirus" DNA copy in infected cells. Hosts remain chronically infected. Leukemia and sarcoma viruses of animals and humans (see Chapter 43), foamy viruses of primates, and some "slow" viruses called lentiviruses (visna, maedi of sheep) (see Chapters 42 and 44) are included in this group. Retroviruses allowed the identification of cellular oncogenes (see Chapter 43). Retroviruses cause acquired immunodeficiency syndrome (AIDS) (see Chapter 44).

J. Bunyaviruses: Spherical, 90- to 100-nm particles that replicate in the cytoplasm and acquire an envelope by budding into the Golgi apparatus. The genome is made up of a triple-segmented, single-stranded, negative-sense RNA. The majority of these viruses are transmitted to vertebrates by arthropods (arboviruses). About 70 are antigenically related to Bunyamwera virus. Hantaviruses are transmitted not by arthropods but by rodents; they cause hemorrhagic fevers and nephropathy, as well as a severe pulmonary syndrome. (See Chapter 38.)

K. Orthomyxoviruses: Medium-sized, 80- to 120-nm enveloped viruses containing a segmented, single-stranded, negative-sense RNA genome and exhibiting helical symmetry. Particles are either round or filamentous. Orthomyxoviruses have surface projections that contain hemagglutinin or neuraminidase activity. The internal nucleoprotein helix measures 9–15 nm, and the RNA is made up of eight segments. During replication, the nucleocapsid is assembled in the nucleus, whereas the hemagglutinin and neuraminidase accumulate in the cytoplasm. The virus matures by budding at the cell membrane. All orthomyxoviruses are influenza viruses that infect humans or animals. The segmented nature of the viral genome permits ready genetic reassortment when two influenza viruses infect the same cell; this explains the high rate of natural variation among influenza viruses. (See Chapter 39.)

L. Paramyxoviruses: Similar to but larger (150–300 nm) than orthomyxoviruses. The internal nucleocapsid measures 18 nm, and the molecular weight of the single-stranded, nonsegmented, negative-sense RNA is greater than the sum of the RNA segments of the orthomyxoviruses. Both the nucleocapsid and the hemagglutinin are formed in the cytoplasm. Those infecting humans include mumps, measles, parainfluenza, and respiratory syncytial viruses. In contrast to influenza viruses, paramyxoviruses are genetically stable. (See Chapter 40.)

M. Rhabdoviruses: Enveloped virions resembling a bullet, flat at one end and round at the other, measuring about 75 × 180 nm. The envelope has 10-nm spikes. The genome is single-stranded, nonsegmented, negative-sense RNA. Particles are formed by budding from the cell membrane. Rabies virus is a member of this group. (See Chapter 42.)

N. Other Viruses: Insufficient information to permit classification. This applies to agents responsible for some immune complex diseases and for some "slow" or unconventional viral diseases, including degenerative neurologic disorders such as kuru or Creutzfeldt-Jakob disease, or scrapie of sheep (see Chapter 42), and to some viruses of gastroenteritis (see Chapter 37).

O. Viroids: Small infectious agents that cause diseases of plants. Viroids are agents that do not fit the definition of classic viruses. They are nucleic acid molecules (MW 70,000–120,000) without a protein coat. Plant viroids are single-stranded, covalently closed circular RNA molecules consisting of about 360 nucleotides and comprising a highly base-paired rod-like structure. Viroids replicate by an entirely novel mechanism. Viroid RNA does not encode any protein products; the devastating plant diseases induced by viroids occur by an unknown mechanism. To date, viroids have been detected only in plants; none have been demonstrated to exist in animals or humans.

PRINCIPLES OF VIRAL STRUCTURE

Knowledge of viral structure is necessary to understand the interaction of viral particles with cell surface receptors and neutralizing antibodies. It will be the basis for designing specific drugs capable of blocking viral attachment, uncoating, or both in susceptible cells.

Types of Symmetry of Viral Particles

Electron microscopy, cryoelectron microscopy, and x-ray diffraction techniques have made it possible to resolve fine differences in the basic morphology of viruses. The study of viral symmetry in the electron microscope requires the use of heavy metal stains (eg, potassium phosphotungstate) to emphasize surface structure. The heavy metal permeates the viral particle like a cloud and brings out the surface structure of viruses by virtue of "negative staining."

Viral architecture can be grouped into three types based on the arrangement of morphologic subunits: (1) those with cubic symmetry, eg, adenoviruses; (2) those with helical symmetry, eg, orthomyxoviruses; and (3) those with complex structures, eg, poxviruses. Genetic economy requires that a viral structure be made from many identical molecules of one or a few proteins.

A. Cubic Symmetry: All cubic symmetry observed with animal viruses to date is of the icosahedral pattern, the most efficient arrangement for subunits in a closed shell. Knowledge of rules guiding icosahedral symmetry makes it possible to determine the number of capsomers in a particle, an important characteristic in viral classification. The icosahedron has 20 faces (each an equilateral triangle), 12 vertices, and fivefold, threefold, and twofold axes of rotational symmetry. Capsomers can be arranged to comply with icosahedral symmetry in a limited number of ways, expressed by the formula $N = 10(n - 1)^2 + 2$, where N is the total number of capsomers and n the number of capsomers on one side of each equilateral triangle. Table 29–2 shows the number of capsomers in several viral groups, where n varies from 2 to 6.

Icosahedral structures can be built from one simple, asymmetric building unit, arranged as 12 pentamer (vertex) units and x number of hexamer units. The polypeptides that comprise the pentamers and hexamers of the capsid may be the same or different depending on the particular virus. The smallest and most basic capsid is that of the phage ϕX-174, which simply consists of 12 pentamer units.

Viruses exhibiting icosahedral symmetry can also be grouped according to their triangulation number, T, which is the number of small triangles formed on the single face of the icosahedron when all its adjacent morphologic subunits are connected by lines. The number of morphologic units (capsomers) is expressed by the formula $M = 10T + 2$. Table 29–2 shows the triangulation number for several viral groups. The total number of capsomers in a viral particle can be calculated if either the number of capsomers on one edge or the triangulation number of the particle can be determined from electron micrographs.

An example of icosahedral symmetry is seen in Figure 29–2. The adenovirus ($n = 6$) model illustrated shows the six capsomers along one edge (Figure 29–2[a]). Degradation of this virus with sodium lauryl sulfate releases the capsomers in groups of nine (Figure 29–2[b], [c]) and possibly groups of six. The groups of nine lie on the faces and include one capsomer from each of the three edges of the face, and the groups of six would be from the vertices. The groups of nine form the faces of the 20 triangular facets, which account for 180 subunits, and the groups of six that form the 12 vertices account for 72 capsomers; thus the total is 252 capsomers in the particle.

The viral nucleic acid is condensed within the isometric particles; virus-encoded "core" proteins or, in the case of papovaviruses, cellular histones are involved in condensation of the nucleic acid into a form suitable for packaging. The rules governing incorporation of nucleic acid into isometric particles are unknown; presumably a "packaging sequence" is involved in assembly, although in general, primary, secondary, and tertiary structures of the nucleic acid are not crucial. There are size constraints on the nucleic acid molecules that can be packaged into a given icosahedral capsid. Icosahedral capsids are formed in-

Table 29–2. Number of capsomers in several viral groups.

Viral Family	n	T	Capsomers
Phage (ϕX-174)	2	1	12
Picorna[1]	2	3	32
Papova[2]	3	7	72
Reo	4	9	92(?)
Herpes	5	16	162
Adeno	6	25	252

[1]Picornaviruses are a special case and, for $n = 2$, fit the formula $N = 30(n - 1)^2 + 2$.
[2]Capsomers in a skew arrangement.

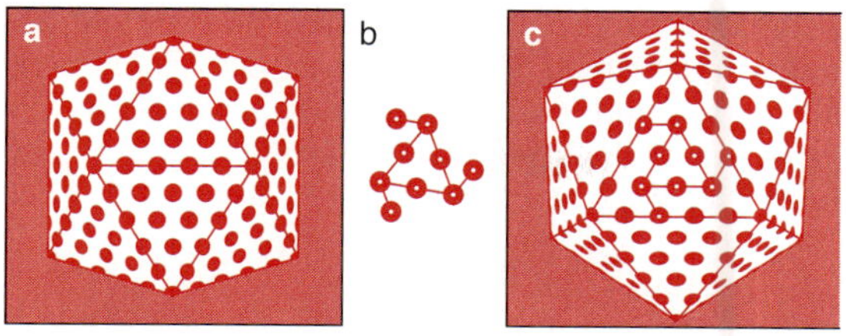

Figure 29–2. ***(a)*** Representation of the capsomer arrangement of an adenovirus particle, as viewed through the twofold axis of symmetry. ***(b)*** Arrangement of capsomer group of nine, obtained by treatment of an adenovirus with sodium lauryl sulfate. ***(c)*** Orientation of the capsomer group of nine on the adenovirus particle. If the model were marked to show the maximum number of small triangles formed on one face of the icosahedron by drawing a line between each adjacent morphologic subunit, it would yield the triangulation number of the adenovirus particle, which is 25.

dependent of nucleic acid. Most preparations of isometric viruses will contain some "empty" particles devoid of viral nucleic acid. Both DNA and RNA viral groups exhibit examples of cubic symmetry.

B. Helical Symmetry: In cases of helical symmetry, protein subunits are bound in a periodic way to the viral nucleic acid, winding it into a helix. The filamentous viral nucleic acid-protein complex (nucleocapsid) is then coiled inside a lipid-containing envelope. Thus, unlike the case with icosahedral structures, there is a regular, periodic interaction between capsid protein and nucleic acid in viruses with helical symmetry. It is not possible for "empty" helical particles to form.

An example of helical symmetry is shown in Figure 29–3. Tobacco mosaic virus, a plant virus, is most well-characterized with respect to the interaction between the viral RNA and capsid protein. However, it is a rigid rod. All known examples of animal viruses with helical symmetry contain RNA genomes and, with the exception of rhabdoviruses, have flexible nucleocapsids that are wound into a ball inside envelopes (Figures 29–1B and 29–4).

C. Complex Structures: Some viral particles do not exhibit simple cubic or helical symmetry but are more complicated in structure. For example, poxviruses are brick-shaped with ridges on the external surface and a core and lateral bodies inside (Figures 29–4 and 34–1).

Measuring the Sizes of Viruses

Small size and ability to pass through filters that hold back bacteria are classic attributes of viruses. However, because some bacteria may be smaller than the largest viruses, filterability is no longer regarded as a unique feature of viruses.

The following methods are used for determining the sizes of viruses and their components.

A. Direct Observation in the Electron Microscope: As compared with the light microscope, the electron microscope uses electrons rather than light waves and electromagnetic lenses rather than glass lenses. The electron beam obtained has a much shorter wavelength than that of light, so that objects much smaller than the wavelength of visible or ultraviolet light can be visualized. Viruses can be visualized in preparations from tissue extracts and in ultrathin sections of infected cells. Electron microscopy is the most widely used method for estimating particle size.

B. Filtration Through Membranes of Graded Porosity: Membranes are available with pores of different sizes. If the viral preparation is passed through a series of membranes of known pore size, the approximate size of any virus can be measured by determining which membranes allow the infective unit to pass and which hold it back. The size of the limiting APD (average pore diameter) multiplied by 0.64 yields the diameter of the viral particle. The passage of a virus through a filter will also depend on the physical structure of the virus; thus, only a very approximate estimate of size is obtained.

C. Sedimentation in the Ultracentrifuge: If particles are suspended in a liquid, they will settle to

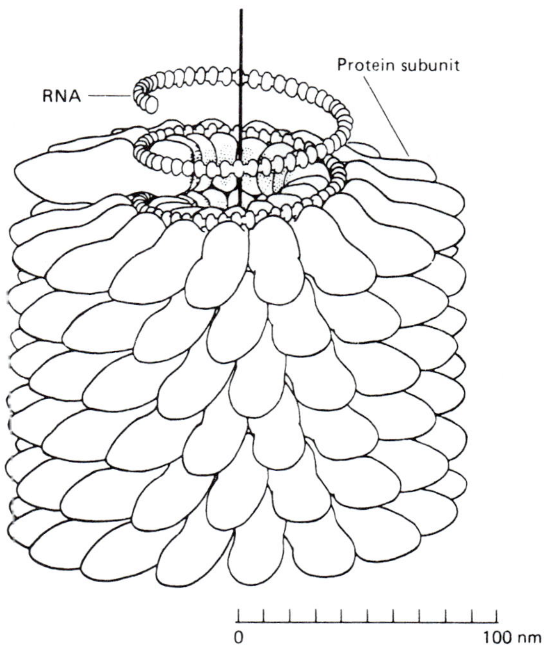

Figure 29–3. Schematic representation of tobacco mosaic virus. As can be seen in the cutaway section, the RNA helix is associated with protein molecules in the ratio of three nucleotides per protein molecule. (Reproduced, with permission, from Mattern CFT: Structure. Pages 707–715 in: *Medical Microbiology*. Baron S [editor]. Addison-Wesley, 1986. Modified from Caspar DLD: Adv Protein Chem 1963;18:37.)

the bottom at a rate that is proportionate to their size. In an ultracentrifuge, forces of more than 100,000 times gravity may be used to drive the particles to the bottom of the tube. The relationship between the size and shape of a particle and its rate of sedimentation permits determination of particle size. Once again, the physical structure of the virus will affect the size estimate obtained.

D. Comparative Measurements: (Table 29–1.) For purposes of reference, the following data should be recalled: (1) *Staphylococcus* has a diameter of about 1000 nm. (2) Bacterial viruses (bacteriophages) vary in size (10–100 nm). Some are spherical or hexagonal and have short or long tails. (3) Representative protein molecules range in diameter from serum albumin (5 nm) and globulin (7 nm) to certain hemocyanins (23 nm).

The relative sizes and morphology of various viral families are shown in Figure 29–4. Particles with a twofold difference in diameter have an eightfold difference in volume. Thus, the mass of a poxvirus is about 1000 times greater than that of the poliovirus particle, and the mass of a small bacterium is 50,000 times greater.

CHEMICAL COMPOSITION OF VIRUSES

Viral Protein

The structural proteins of viruses have several important functions. Their major purpose is to facilitate transfer of the viral nucleic acid from one host cell to another. They serve to protect the viral genome against inactivation by nucleases, participate in the attachment of the viral particle to a susceptible cell, and provide the structural symmetry of the viral particle.

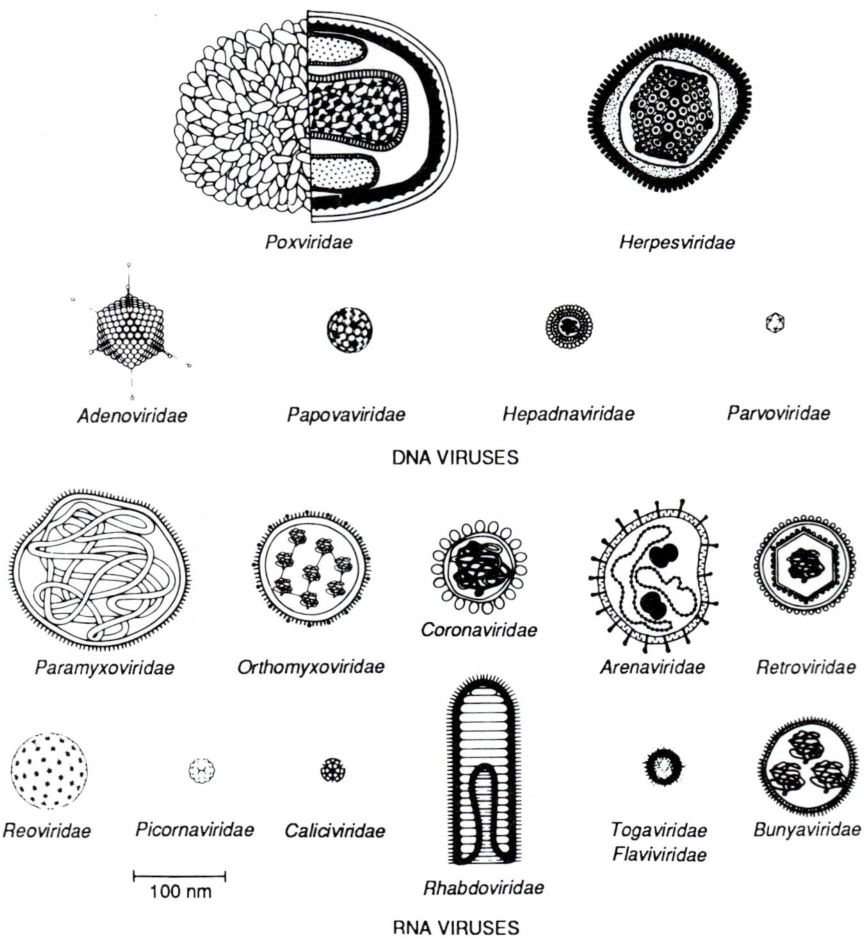

Figure 29–4. Shapes and relative sizes of animal viruses of families that include human pathogens. In some diagrams, certain internal structures of the particles are represented. (Reproduced, with permission, from White DO, Fenner FJ: *Medical Virology,* 3rd ed. Academic Press, 1986.)

The proteins determine the antigenic characteristics of the virus. The host's protective immune response is directed against antigenic determinants of proteins or glycoproteins exposed on the surface of the viral particle. Some surface proteins may also exhibit specific activities, eg, influenza virus hemagglutinin agglutinates red blood cells.

Some viruses carry enzymes (which are proteins) inside the virions. The enzymes are present in very small amounts and are probably not important in the structure of the viral particles; however, they are essential for the initiation of the viral replicative cycle when the virion enters a host cell. Examples include an RNA polymerase carried by viruses with negative-sense RNA genomes (eg, orthomyxoviruses, rhabdoviruses) that is needed to copy the first mRNAs, and reverse transcriptase, an enzyme in retroviruses that makes a DNA copy of the viral RNA, an essential step in replication and transformation. At the extreme in this respect are the poxviruses, the cores of which contain a transcriptional system; at least 15 different enzymes are packaged in poxvirus particles.

Viral Nucleic Acid

Viruses contain a single kind of nucleic acid, either DNA or RNA, that encodes the genetic information necessary for replication of the virus. The genome may be single-stranded or double-stranded, circular or linear, and segmented or nonsegmented. The type of nucleic acid, the strandedness, and the molecular weight are major characteristics used for classifying viruses into families (Table 29–1).

The molecular weight of the viral DNA genome ranges from 1.5×10^6 (parvoviruses) to 200×10^6 (poxviruses). The molecular weight of the viral RNA genome ranges from 2×10^6 (picornaviruses) to 15×10^6 (reoviruses).

Most viral genomes are quite fragile once they are removed from their protective protein capsid, but some nucleic acid molecules have been examined in the electron microscope without disruption, and their lengths have been measured. If linear densities of approximately 2×10^6 per µm for double-stranded nucleic acid and 1×10^6 per µm for single-stranded forms are used, molecular weights of viral genomes can be calculated from direct measurements (Table 29–1).

All major DNA viral groups in Table 29–1 have genomes that are single molecules of DNA and have a linear or circular configuration.

Viral RNAs exist in several forms. The RNA may be a single linear molecule (eg, picornaviruses). For other viruses (eg, orthomyxoviruses), the genome consists of several segments of RNA that may be loosely associated within the virion. The isolated RNA of picornaviruses and togaviruses, so-called positive-sense viruses, is infectious, and the entire molecule functions as an mRNA within the infected cell. The isolated RNA of the negative-sense RNA viruses, such as rhabdoviruses and orthomyxoviruses, is not infectious. For these viral families, the virions carry an RNA polymerase that in the cell transcribes the genome RNA molecules into several complementary RNA molecules, each of which may serve as an mRNA.

The sequence and composition of nucleotides of each viral nucleic acid are distinctive. One of the properties useful for characterizing a viral nucleic acid is its guanine-plus-cytosine content. DNA viral genomes can be analyzed and compared using restriction endonucleases, enzymes that cleave DNA at specific nucleotide sequences. Each genome will yield a characteristic pattern of DNA fragments after cleavage with a particular enzyme. Using molecularly cloned DNA copies of RNA, restriction maps also can be derived for RNA viral genomes. Molecular hybridization techniques (DNA to DNA, DNA to RNA, or RNA to RNA) permit the study of transcription of the viral genome within the infected cell as well as comparison of the relatedness of different viruses.

The number of genes in a virus can be approximated if one makes certain assumptions about (1) triplet code, (2) the molecular weight of the genome, and (3) the average size of a protein (Table 29–1). It must also be assumed in such calculations that there are no overlapping genes in the viral genome; this assumption has been proved incorrect for some viruses (papovaviruses, orthomyxoviruses). Many viral genomes have been sequenced. The number of proteins encoded by a virus can be estimated from the open reading frames deduced from the nucleic acid sequence. Although such estimates are not precise, the values serve to illustrate the varying complexities and relative coding capacities of different viral groups.

Viral Lipids

A number of different viruses contain lipid envelopes as part of their structure (eg, Sindbis virus; Figure 29–5). The lipid is acquired when the viral nucleocapsid buds through a cellular membrane in the course of maturation. Budding occurs only at sites where virus-specific proteins have been inserted into

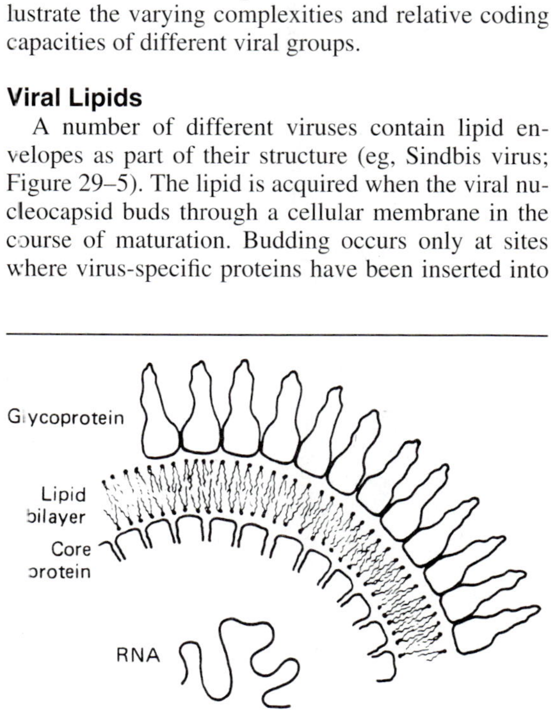

Figure 29–5. Proposed structure of Sindbis virus, an enveloped virus. (After B Harrison et al.)

the host cell membrane. The different ways in which various animal viruses acquire an envelope are suggested in Figure 29–6. The diagram serves to emphasize the diverse strategies that viruses have evolved in order to accomplish viral production by host cells.

The specific phospholipid composition of a virion envelope is determined by the specific type of cell membrane involved in the budding process. For example, herpesviruses bud through the nuclear membrane of the host cell, and the phospholipid composition of the purified virus reflects the lipids of the nuclear membrane. The acquisition of a lipid-containing membrane is an integral step in virion morphogenesis in some viral groups (see Replication of Viruses, below).

Lipid-containing viruses are sensitive to treatment with ether and other organic solvents (Table 29–1), indicating that disruption or loss of lipid results in loss of infectivity. Non-lipid-containing viruses are generally resistant to ether.

Viral Carbohydrates

Viral envelopes contain glycoproteins. In contrast to the lipids in viral membranes, which are derived from the host cell, the envelope glycoproteins are virus-encoded. However, the sugars added to viral glycoproteins often reflect the host cell in which the virus is grown.

It is the surface glycoproteins of an enveloped virus that attach the viral particle to a target cell by interacting with a cellular receptor. The glycoproteins are also important viral antigens. As a result of their position at the outer surface of the virion, they are frequently involved in the interaction of the viral particle with neutralizing antibody. The 3-dimensional structures of the externally exposed regions of both of the influenza virus membrane glycoproteins (hemagglutinin, neuraminidase) have been determined by x-ray crystallography (see Figure 39–2). Such studies are providing insights into the antigenic structure and functional activities of viral glycoproteins.

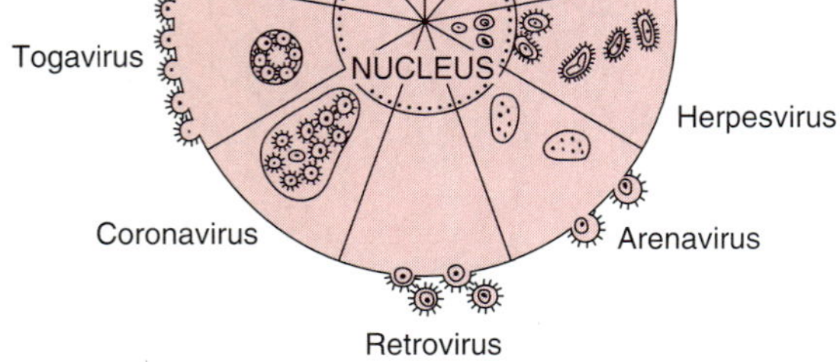

Figure 29–6. Diagram of relationships between several lipid-containing viruses and host cell membranes. (From Blough and Tiffany.)

CULTIVATION & ASSAY OF VIRUSES

Cultivation of Viruses

Many viruses can be grown in cell cultures or in fertile eggs under strictly controlled conditions. Growth of virus in animals is still used for the primary isolation of certain viruses and for studies of the pathogenesis of viral diseases and of viral oncogenesis. Diagnostic laboratories attempt to recover viruses from clinical samples to establish disease etiologies (see Chapter 47). Research laboratories cultivate viruses as the basis for detailed analyses of viral expression and replication.

The availability of cells grown in vitro has facilitated the identification and cultivation of newly isolated viruses and the characterization of previously known ones. There are three basic types of cell culture. Primary cultures are made by dispersing cells (usually with trypsin) from freshly removed host tissues. In general, they are unable to grow for more than a few passages in culture, as secondary cultures. Diploid cell lines are secondary cultures which have undergone a change that allows their limited culture (up to 50 passages) but which retain their normal chromosome pattern. Continuous cell lines are cultures capable of more prolonged, perhaps indefinite growth that have been derived from diploid cell lines or from malignant tissues. They invariably have altered and irregular numbers of chromosomes. The type of cell culture used for viral cultivation depends on the sensitivity of the cells to a particular virus.

A. Detection of Virus-Infected Cells: Multiplication of a virus can be monitored in a variety of ways:

1. Development of cytopathic effects, ie, morphologic changes in the cells. Types of virus-induced cytopathic effects include cell lysis or necrosis, inclusion formation, giant cell formation, and cytoplasmic vacuolization (Figure 29–7A, B, and C). Most viruses produce some obvious cytopathic effect in infected cells that is generally characteristic of the viral group.

2. Appearance of a virus-encoded protein, such as the hemagglutinin of influenza virus. Specific antisera can be used to detect the synthesis of viral proteins in infected cells.

3. Adsorption of erythrocytes to infected cells, called hemadsorption, due to the presence of virus-encoded hemagglutinin (parainfluenza, influenza) in cellular membranes. This reaction becomes positive before cytopathic changes are visible and in some cases occurs in the absence of cytopathic effects (Figure 29–7D).

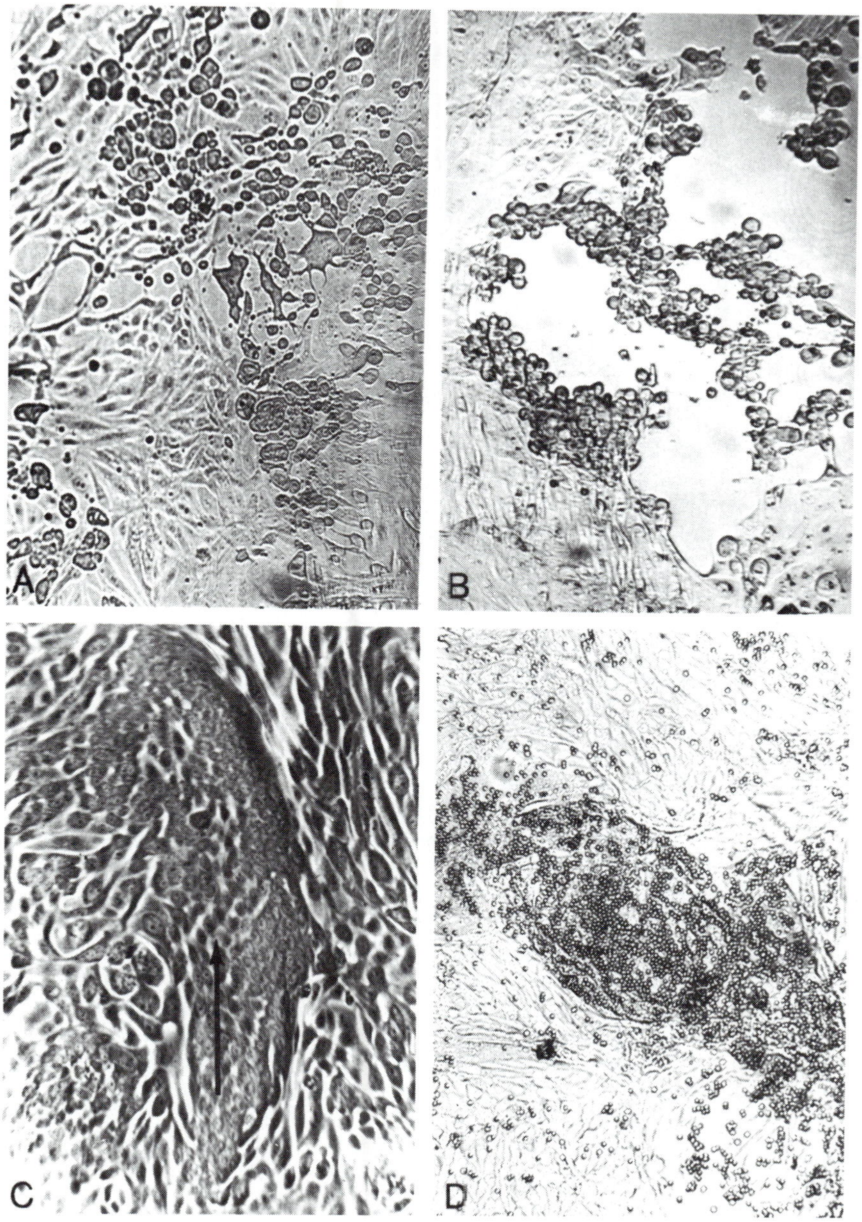

Figure 29–7. Cytopathic effects produced in monolayers of cultured cells by different viruses. The cultures are shown as they would normally be viewed in the laboratory, unfixed and unstained (60×). ***A:*** Enterovirus—rapid rounding of cells progressing to complete cell destruction. ***B:*** Herpesvirus—focal areas of swollen rounded cells. ***C:*** Paramyxovirus—focal areas of fused cells (syncytia). ***D:*** Hemadsorption. Erythrocytes adhere to those cells in the monolayer that are infected by a virus that causes a hemagglutinin to be incorporated into the plasma membrane. Many enveloped viruses that mature by budding from cytoplasmic membranes produce hemadsorption. (Courtesy I. Jack; reproduced from White DO, Fenner FJ: *Medical Virology,* 3rd ed. Academic Press, 1986.)

4. Interference by a noncytopathogenic virus (eg, rubella) with the replication and induction of cytopathic effects by a second, challenge virus (eg, echovirus) added as an indicator.

5. Morphologic transformation by an oncogenic virus (eg, Rous sarcoma virus), usually accompanied by the loss of contact inhibition and the piling up of cells into discrete foci (see Chapter 43).

Viral growth in an embryonated chick egg may result in death of the embryo (eg, encephalitis viruses), production of pocks or plaques on the chorioallantoic membrane (eg, herpes, smallpox, vaccinia), development of hemagglutinins in the embryonic fluids or tissues (eg, influenza), or development of infective virus (eg, poliovirus type 2).

B. Inclusion Body Formation: In the course of viral multiplication within cells, virus-specific structures called inclusion bodies may be produced. They become far larger than the individual viral particle and often have an affinity for acid dyes (eg, eosin). They may be situated in the nucleus (herpesvirus; see Figure 33–4), in the cytoplasm (poxvirus; see Figure 34–4), or in both (measles virus; see Figure 40–4). In many viral infections, the inclusion bodies are the site of development of the virions (the viral factories). In some infections (poxviruses, reoviruses), the inclusion body consists of masses of viral particles in the process of replication. In others (as in the intranuclear inclusion body of herpes), the virus multiplies earlier in the infection, and the inclusion body appears to be a remnant of viral multiplication. Variations in the appearance of inclusion material depend largely upon the tissue fixative used.

The presence of inclusion bodies may be of considerable diagnostic aid. The intracytoplasmic inclusion in nerve cells, the Negri body, is pathognomonic for rabies.

C. Chromosome Damage: One of the consequences of infection of cells by certain viruses is derangement of the karyotype. The changes observed are random. Breakage, fragmentation, rearrangement of the chromosomes, abnormal chromosomes, and changes in chromosome number may occur. To date, no pathognomonic chromosome alterations have been identified in virus-infected cells in humans.

Cells transformed by viruses also exhibit random chromosomal abnormalities. Particular chromosomal alterations, including translocations, inversions, and deletions, are frequently observed in human cancer cells, especially specific types of leukemia. More than 20 cellular oncogenes have been localized to specific human chromosomes; many are located at bands that are involved in translocations or deletions. The role of cellular oncogenes in human cancer is discussed in Chapter 43.

Quantitation of Viruses

A. Physical Methods: Viral particles can be counted directly in the electron microscope by comparison with a standard suspension of latex particles of similar small size. However, a relatively concentrated preparation of virus is necessary for this procedure, and infectious viral particles cannot be distinguished from noninfectious ones.

Certain viruses contain a protein (hemagglutinin) that has the ability to agglutinate red blood cells of humans or some animal. Hemagglutination assays are an easy and rapid method of quantitating these types of viruses (see Chapter 47). Both infective and noninfective particles give this reaction; thus, hemagglutination measures the total quantity of virus present.

A variety of serologic tests, such as radioimmunoassays (RIA) and enzyme-linked immunosorbent assays (ELISA; see Chapter 47), can be standardized to quantitate the amount of virus in a sample. Such tests do not distinguish infectious from noninfectious particles and sometimes detect viral proteins not assembled into particles.

B. Biologic Methods: End point biologic assays depend on the measurement of animal death, animal infection, or cytopathic effects in tissue culture at a series of dilutions of the virus being tested. The titer is expressed as the 50% infectious dose (ID_{50}), which is the reciprocal of the dilution of virus that produces the effect in 50% of the cells or animals inoculated. Precise assays require the use of a large number of test subjects.

The most widely used assay for infectious virus is the plaque assay. Monolayers of host cells are inoculated with suitable dilutions of virus and after adsorption are overlaid with medium containing agar or carboxymethylcellulose to prevent virus spreading throughout the culture. After several days, the cells initially infected have produced virus that spreads only to surrounding cells, producing a small area of infection, or plaque. Under controlled conditions, a single plaque can arise from a single infectious viral particle, termed a plaque-forming unit (PFU). The cytopathic effect of infected cells within the plaque can be distinguished from uninfected cells of the monolayer, with or without suitable staining, and plaques can usually be counted macroscopically (Figure 29–8). The ratio of the number of infectious particles to the total number of particles varies widely, from near unity to less than one per 1000.

Certain viruses, eg, herpes and vaccinia, form pocks when inoculated onto the chorioallantoic membrane of an embryonated egg. Such viruses can be quantitated by relating the number of pocks counted to the viral dilution inoculated.

PURIFICATION & IDENTIFICATION OF VIRUSES

Purification of Viral Particles

Pure virus must be available in order for meaningful studies on the properties and molecular biology of the agent to be carried out. For purification studies, the starting material is usually large volumes of tissue culture medium, body fluids, or infected cells. The first step frequently involves concentration of the viral particles by precipitation with ammonium sulfate, ethanol, or polyethylene glycol or by ultrafiltration. Hemagglutination and elution can be used to concentrate orthomyxoviruses (see Chapter 39). Once concentrated, virus can then be separated from host materials by differential centrifugation, density gradient centrifugation, column chromatography, and electrophoresis.

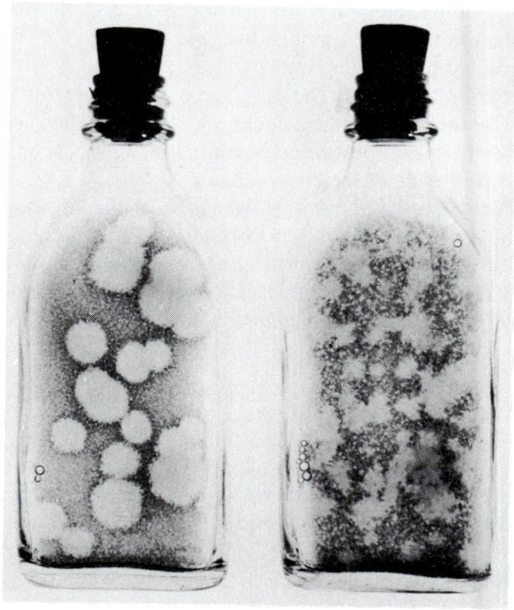

Figure 29–8. Plaques produced by poliovirus ***(left)*** and by an echovirus ***(right).*** Both viruses are cultivated in bottle cultures of monkey kidney cells. After the virus is inoculated, the cell sheet is covered with an agar overlay containing a vital dye (neutral red). As the cytopathic effect of the virus becomes manifest, the cells lose their vital stain and clear areas appear in the culture. The progeny of a single viral particle are located in each clear area. The plaque morphology of each of the viruses shown is sufficiently clear so that the two viral groups can readily be distinguished from each other by this method. (GD Hsiung and JL Melnick.)

More than one step is usually necessary to achieve adequate purification. A preliminary purification will remove most nonviral material. This first step may include centrifugation; the final purification step almost always involves density gradient centrifugation. In rate-zonal centrifugation, a sample of concentrated virus is layered onto a preformed linear density gradient of sucrose or glycerol, and during centrifugation, the virus sediments as a band at a rate determined primarily by the size and weight of the viral particle. Samples are collected by piercing a hole in the bottom of the centrifuge tube. The band of purified virus may be detected by optical methods, by following radioactivity if the virus is radiolabeled, or by assaying for infectivity.

Viruses can also be purified by high-speed centrifugation in density gradients of cesium chloride, potassium tartrate, potassium citrate, or sucrose. The gradient material of choice is the one that is least toxic to the virus. Viral particles migrate to an equilibrium position where the density of the solution is equal to their buoyant density and form a visible band. Viral bands are harvested by puncture through the bottom of the plastic centrifuge tube and are assayed for infectivity.

Additional methods for purification are based on the chemical properties of the viral surface. In column chromatography, virus is bound to a substance such as diethylaminoethyl or phosphocellulose and then eluted by changes in pH or salt concentration. Zone electrophoresis permits the separation of viral particles from contaminants on the basis of charge. Specific antisera also can be used to remove viral particles from host materials.

Icosahedral viruses are easier to purify than enveloped viruses. Because the latter usually contain variable amounts of envelope per particle, the viral population is heterogeneous in both size and density.

It is very difficult to achieve complete purity of viruses. Small amounts of cellular material tend to adsorb to particles and co-purify. The minimal criteria for purity are a homogeneous appearance in electron micrographs and the failure of additional purification procedures to remove "contaminants" without reducing infectivity.

Identification of a Particle as a Virus

When a characteristic physical particle has been obtained, it should fulfill the following criteria before it is identified as a viral particle:

(1) The particle can be obtained only from infected cells or tissues.

(2) Particles obtained from various sources are identical, regardless of the cellular species in which the virus is grown.

(3) The degree of infective activity of the preparation varies directly with the number of particles present.

(4) The degree of destruction of the physical particle by chemical or physical means is associated with a corresponding loss of viral activity.

(5) Certain properties of the particles and infectivity must be shown to be identical, such as their sedimentation behavior in the ultracentrifuge and their pH stability curves.

(6) The absorption spectrum of the purified physical particle in the ultraviolet range should coincide with the ultraviolet inactivation spectrum of the virus.

(7) Antisera prepared against the infective virus should react with the characteristic particle, and vice versa. Direct observation of an unknown virus can be accomplished by electron microscopic examination of aggregate formation in a mixture of antisera and crude viral suspension.

(8) The particles should be able to induce the characteristic disease in vivo (if such experiments are feasible).

(9) Passage of the particles in tissue culture should result in the production of progeny with biologic and serologic properties of the virus.

REACTION TO PHYSICAL & CHEMICAL AGENTS

Heat & Cold

There is great variability in the heat stability of different viruses. Icosahedral viruses tend to be stable, losing little infectivity after several hours at 37 °C. Enveloped viruses are much more heat-labile, rapidly dropping in titer at 37 °C. Viral infectivity is generally destroyed by heating at 50–60 °C for 30 minutes, although there are some notable exceptions (eg, hepatitis B virus, papovaviruses, scrapie agent).

Viruses can be preserved by storage at subfreezing temperatures, and some may withstand lyophilization and can thus be preserved in the dry state at 4 °C or even at room temperature. Viruses that withstand lyophilization are more heat-resistant when heated in the dry state. Enveloped viruses tend to lose infectivity after prolonged storage even at −90 °C and are particularly sensitive to repeated freezing and thawing.

Stabilization of Viruses by Salts

Many viruses can be stabilized by salts in concentrations of 1 mol/L, ie, the viruses are not inactivated even by heating at 50 °C for 1 hour. The mechanism by which the salts stabilize viral preparations is not known. Viruses are preferentially stabilized by certain salts. $MgCl_2$, 1 mol/L, stabilizes picorna- and reoviruses; $MgSO_4$, 1 mol/L, stabilizes orthomyxo- and paramyxoviruses; and Na_2SO_4, 1 mol/L, stabilizes herpesviruses.

The stability of viruses is important in the preparation of vaccines. The ordinary nonstabilized poliovaccine must be stored at freezing temperatures to preserve its potency. However, with the addition of salts for stabilization of the virus, potency can be maintained for weeks at ambient temperatures, even in the high temperatures of the tropics.

pH

Viruses are usually stable between pH values of 5.0 and 9.0. Some viruses (eg, enteroviruses) are resistant to acidic conditions. All viruses are destroyed by alkaline conditions. In hemagglutination reactions, variations of less than one pH unit may influence the result.

Radiation

Ultraviolet, x-ray, and high-energy particles inactivate viruses. The dose varies for different viruses. Infectivity is the most radiosensitive property, because replication requires expression of the entire genetic contents. Irradiated particles that are unable to replicate may still be able to express some specific functions in host cells.

Photodynamic Inactivation

Viruses are penetrable to a varying degree by vital dyes such as toluidine blue, neutral red, and proflavine. These dyes bind to the viral nucleic acid, and the virus then becomes susceptible to inactivation by visible light. Impenetrable viruses like poliovirus, when grown in the dark in the presence of vital dyes, incorporate the dye into their nucleic acid and are then susceptible to photodynamic inactivation. The coat antigen is unaffected by the process.

Neutral red is commonly used to stain plaque assays so that plaques are more readily seen. The assay plates must be protected from bright light once the neutral red has been added; otherwise, there is the risk that progeny virus will be inactivated and plaque development will cease.

Ether Susceptibility

Ether susceptibility can distinguish viruses that possess an envelope from those that do not. The following viruses are inactivated by ether: herpes-, orthomyxo-, paramyxo-, rhabdo-, corona-, retro-, arena-, toga-, flavi-, and bunyaviruses. The following viruses are resistant to ether: parvo-, papova-, adeno-, picorna-, and reoviruses. Poxviruses vary in sensitivity to ether.

Detergents

Nonionic detergents, eg, Nonidet P40 and Triton X-100, solubilize lipid constituents of viral membranes. The viral proteins in the envelope are released (undenatured). Anionic detergents, eg, sodium dodecyl sulfate, also solubilize viral envelopes; in addition, they disrupt capsids into separated polypeptides.

Formaldehyde

Formaldehyde destroys viral infectivity by reacting with nucleic acid. Viruses with single-stranded genomes are inactivated much more readily than those with double-stranded genomes. Formaldehyde has minimal adverse effects on the antigenicity of proteins and therefore has been used frequently in the production of inactivated viral vaccines.

Antibiotics & Other Antibacterial Agents

Antibacterial antibiotics and sulfonamides have no effect on viruses. Some antiviral drugs are available, however (see Chapter 30).

Quaternary ammonium compounds, in general, are not effective against viruses. Organic iodine compounds are also ineffective. Larger concentrations of chlorine are required to destroy viruses than to kill bacteria, especially in the presence of extraneous proteins. For example, the chlorine treatment of stools adequate to inactivate typhoid bacilli is inadequate to destroy poliomyelitis virus present in feces. Formalin destroys resistant poliomyelitis and coxsackieviruses. Alcohols, such as isopropanol and ethanol, are relatively ineffective against certain viruses, especially picornaviruses.

REPLICATION OF VIRUSES

Viruses multiply only in living cells. The host cell must provide the energy and synthetic machinery and the low-molecular-weight precursors for the synthesis of viral proteins and nucleic acids. The viral nucleic acid carries the genetic specificity to code for all the virus-specific macromolecules in a highly organized fashion.

The unique feature of viral multiplication is that, soon after interaction with a host cell, the infecting virion is disrupted and its measurable infectivity is lost. This phase of the growth cycle is called the **eclipse period**; its duration varies depending on both the particular virus and the host cell, and it ends with the formation of the first infectious progeny viral particles. The eclipse period is actually one of intense synthetic activity as the cell is redirected toward fulfilling the needs of the viral "pirate." In some cases, as soon as the viral nucleic acid enters the host cell, the cellular metabolism is redirected exclusively toward the synthesis of new viral particles. In other cases, the metabolic processes of the host cell are not altered significantly, although the cell synthesizes viral proteins and nucleic acids.

General Steps in Viral Replication Cycles

Viruses have evolved a variety of different strategies for accomplishing multiplication in parasitized host cells. Although the details vary from group to group, the general outline of the replication cycles is similar.

A. Attachment, Penetration, and Uncoating: The first step in viral infection is interaction of a virion with a specific receptor site on the surface of a cell. Receptor molecules differ for different viruses, being proteins in some cases (eg, picornaviruses) and oligosaccharides in others (eg, orthomyxoviruses and paramyxoviruses). The presence or absence of receptors plays an important determining role in cell tropism and viral pathogenesis; for example, poliovirus is able to attach only to cells in the central nervous system and intestinal tract of primates. Receptor binding is believed to reflect fortuitous configurational homologies between a virion surface structure and a cell surface component. For example, human immunodeficiency virus binds to the CD4 receptor on cells of the immune system, and it has been suggested that rabies virus interacts with acetylcholine receptors and that Epstein-Barr virus recognizes the receptor for the third component of complement on B cells. Each susceptible cell probably contains at least 100,000 receptor sites for a given virus.

After binding, the viral particle is taken up inside the cell. This step is referred to as penetration or engulfment. In some systems, this is accomplished by receptor-mediated endocytosis, with uptake of the ingested viral particles within endosomes. In other systems, the details of penetration are less clear. Uncoating occurs concomitant with or shortly after penetration. Uncoating is the physical separation of the viral nucleic acid (or, in some cases, internal nucleocapsids) from the outer structural components of the virion. The infectivity of the parental virus is lost at this point. Viruses are the only infectious agents for which dissolution of the infecting agent is an obligatory step in the replicative pathway.

B. Synthesis of Viral Components: The synthetic phase of the viral replicative cycle ensues after uncoating of the viral genome. The essential theme in viral replication is that specific mRNAs must be transcribed from the viral nucleic acid for successful expression and duplication of genetic information. Once this is accomplished, viruses use cell components to translate the mRNA. Various classes of viruses use different pathways to synthesize the mRNAs depending upon the structure of the viral nucleic acid. Some viruses (eg, rhabdo-, orthomyxo-, and paramyxoviruses) carry RNA polymerases to synthesize mRNAs. RNA viruses of this type are called negative-strand (negative-sense) viruses, since their single-strand RNA genome is complementary to mRNA, which is conventionally designated positive-strand (positive-sense). Table 29–3 summarizes the various pathways of transcription (but not necessarily those of replication) of the nucleic acids of different classes of viruses.

In the course of viral replication, all the virus-specified macromolecules are synthesized in a highly organized sequence. In some viral infections, notably those involving double-stranded, DNA-containing viruses, early viral proteins are synthesized soon after infection and late proteins are made only late in infection, after viral DNA synthesis. Early genes may or may not be shut off when late products are made. In contrast, most if not all of the genetic information of RNA-containing viruses is expressed at the same time. In addition to these temporal controls, quantitative controls also exist, since not all viral proteins are made in the same amounts. Virus-specific proteins may regulate the extent of transcription of the genome or the translation of viral mRNA.

Small animal viruses and bacteriophages are good models for studies of gene expression. Their small size has enabled the total nucleotide sequence of some viruses to be elucidated. This led to the discovery of overlapping genes in which some sequences in DNA are utilized in the synthesis of two different polypeptides, either by the use of two different reading frames or by two mRNA molecules using the same reading frame but different starting points. A viral system (adenovirus) first revealed the mRNA processing phenomenon called "splicing," whereby the mRNA sequences that code for a given protein are generated from separated sequences in the template, with noncoding intervening sequences spliced out of the transcript.

Table 29–3. Pathways of nucleic acid transcription for various viral classes.

Type of Viral Nucleic Acid	Intermediates	Type of mRNA	Example	Comments
± ds DNA	None	+ mRNA	Most DNA viruses (eg, herpesvirus, T4 bacteriophage)	
+ ss DNA	± ds DNA	+ mRNA	φX bacteriophage	See Chapter 7.
± ds RNA	None	+ mRNA	Reovirus	Virion contains RNA polymerase that transcribes each segment to mRNA.
+ ss RNA	± ds RNA	+ mRNA	Picornaviruses, togaviruses, flaviviruses	Viral nucleic acid is infectious and serves as mRNA. For togaviruses, smaller + mRNA is also formed for certain proteins.
− ss RNA	None	+ mRNA	Rhabdoviruses, paramyxoviruses, orthomyxoviruses	Viral nucleic acid is not infectious; virion contains RNA polymerase which forms + mRNAs smaller than the genome. For orthomyxoviruses, + mRNAs are transcribed from each segment.
+ ss RNA	− DNA, ± DNA	+ mRNA	Retroviruses	Virion contains reverse transcriptase; viral RNA is not infectious, but complementary DNA from transformed cell is.

ds = double-stranded
ss = single-stranded
− indicates negative strand
+ indicates positive strand
± indicates a helix containing a positive and a negative strand

The widest variation in strategies of gene expression is found among RNA-containing viruses (Table 29–4). Some virions carry polymerases (orthomyxoviruses, reoviruses); some systems utilize subgenomic messages, sometimes generated by splicing (orthomyxoviruses, retroviruses); and some viruses synthesize large polyprotein precursors that are processed and cleaved to generate the final gene products (picornaviruses, retroviruses).

The extent to which virus-specific enzymes are involved in these processes varies from group to group. The larger viruses (herpesviruses, poxviruses) are more independent of cellular functions than are the smaller viruses. This is one reason the larger viruses are more susceptible to antiviral chemotherapy (see Chapter 30), because more virus-specific processes are available as targets for drug action.

The intracellular sites where the different events in viral replication take place vary from group to group (Table 29–5). A few generalizations are possible. Viral protein is synthesized in the cytoplasm on polyribosomes composed of virus-specific mRNA and host cell

Table 29–4. Comparison of replication strategies of several important RNA viral families.

	Grouping Based on Genomic RNA[1]					
	Positive-Strand Viruses			Negative-Strand Viruses		Double-Stranded Viruses
Characteristic	Picornaviridae	Togaviridae	Retroviridae	Orthomyxoviridae	Paramyxo- and Rhabdoviridae	Reoviridae
Structure of genomic RNA	ss	ss	ss	ss	ss	ds
Sense of genomic RNA	Positive	Positive	Positive	Negative	Negative	
Segmented genome	0	0	0[2]	+	0	+
Genomic RNA infectious	+	+	0	0	0	0
Genomic RNA acts as messenger	+	+	+	0	0	0
Virion-associated polymerase	0	0	+[3]	+	+	+
Subgenomic messages	0	+	+	+	+	+
Polyprotein precursors	+	+	+	0	0	0

[1]Abbreviations used: ss = single-stranded, ds = double-stranded, positive = same sense as mRNA, negative = complementary to mRNA, + = indicated property applies to that viral family, 0 = indicated property does not apply to that viral family.
[2]Retroviruses contain a diploid genome (two copies of nonsegmented genomic RNA).
[3]Retroviruses contain a reverse transcriptase (RNA-dependent DNA polymerase).

Table 29–5. Summary of replication cycles of major viral families.

Viral Family	Type of Nucleic Acid Genome	Presence of Virion Envelope	Intracellular Location[1] Synthesis of Viral Proteins	Replication of Genome	Formation of Nucleocapsid	Virion Maturation	Duration of Multiplication Cycle (Hours)[2]
Papova	DNA	0	C	N	N	N	48
Adeno	DNA	0	C	N	N	N	25
Herpes	DNA	+	C	N	N	M	15–72
Pox	DNA	0	C	C	C	C	20
Picoma	RNA	0	C	C	C	C	6–8
Reo	RNA	0	C	C	C	C	15
Orthomyxo	RNA	+	C	N	N	M	15–30
Retro	RNA	+	C	N	C	M	
Toga	RNA	+	C	C	C	M	10–24
Paramyxo	RNA	+	C	C	C	M	10–48
Rhabdo	RNA	+	C	C	C	M	6–10
Bunya	RNA	+	C	C	C	M	24

[1]Abbreviations used: C = cytoplasm, N = nucleus, M = membranes.
[2]The values shown for duration of the multiplication cycle are approximate; ranges indicate that various members within a given family replicate with different kinetics. Different host cell types also influence the kinetics of viral replication.

ribosomes. Viral DNA is usually replicated in the nucleus. Viral genomic RNA is generally duplicated in the cell cytoplasm, although there are exceptions.

C. Morphogenesis and Release: Newly synthesized viral genomes and capsid polypeptides assemble together to form progeny viruses. Icosahedral capsids can condense in the absence of nucleic acid, whereas nucleocapsids of viruses with helical symmetry cannot form without viral RNA. There are no special mechanisms for the release of nonenveloped viruses; the infected cells eventually lyse and release the viral particles.

Enveloped viruses mature by a budding process. Virus-specific envelope glycoproteins are inserted into cellular membranes; viral nucleocapsids then bud through the membrane at these modified sites and, in so doing, acquire an envelope. Budding frequently occurs at the plasma membrane but may involve other membranes in the cell. Enveloped viruses are not infectious until they have acquired their envelopes. Therefore, infectious progeny virions typically do not accumulate within the infected cell.

Viral maturation is sometimes an inefficient process. Excess amounts of viral components may accumulate and be involved in the formation of inclusion bodies in the cell (see above). As a result of the profound deleterious effects of viral replication, cellular cytopathic effects eventually develop and the cell dies. However, there are instances in which the cell is not damaged by the virus and long-term, persistent infections evolve (see Chapter 30).

Examples of Viral Replication Cycles

The replicative cycle of a herpesvirus is summarized in Figure 29–9. Herpesviruses contain a DNA genome in an icosahedral capsid that obtains an envelope by budding through the nuclear membrane. The replication of picornaviruses is shown in Figure 29–10. Picornaviruses have an RNA genome in an icosahedral, nonenveloped capsid. The diagrams illustrate that steps in viral replication may involve different cellular compartments. Each virus effectively utilizes whichever cellular processes are necessary to achieve its multiplication and morphogenesis.

GENETICS OF ANIMAL VIRUSES

Genetic analysis is a powerful approach toward understanding the structure and function of the viral genome, its gene products, and their roles in infection and disease. Variation in viral properties is of great importance for human medicine. Viruses that have stable antigens on their surfaces (poliovirus, measles virus) can be controlled by vaccination. Other viruses that exist as many antigenic types (rhinoviruses) or change constantly (influenza virus A) are difficult to control by vaccination; viral genetics may help develop more effective vaccines. Some types of viral infections recur repetitively (parainfluenza viruses) or persist (retroviruses) in the presence of antibody and may be better controlled by antiviral drugs. Genetic analysis will help identify virus-specific processes that may be appropriate targets for the development of antiviral therapy.

The following terms are basic to a discussion of genetics: **Genotype** refers to the genetic constitution of an organism. **Phenotype** refers to the observable properties of an organism, which are produced by the genotype in cooperation with the environment. A **mutation** is a heritable change in the genotype. The **genome** is the sum of the genes of an organism.

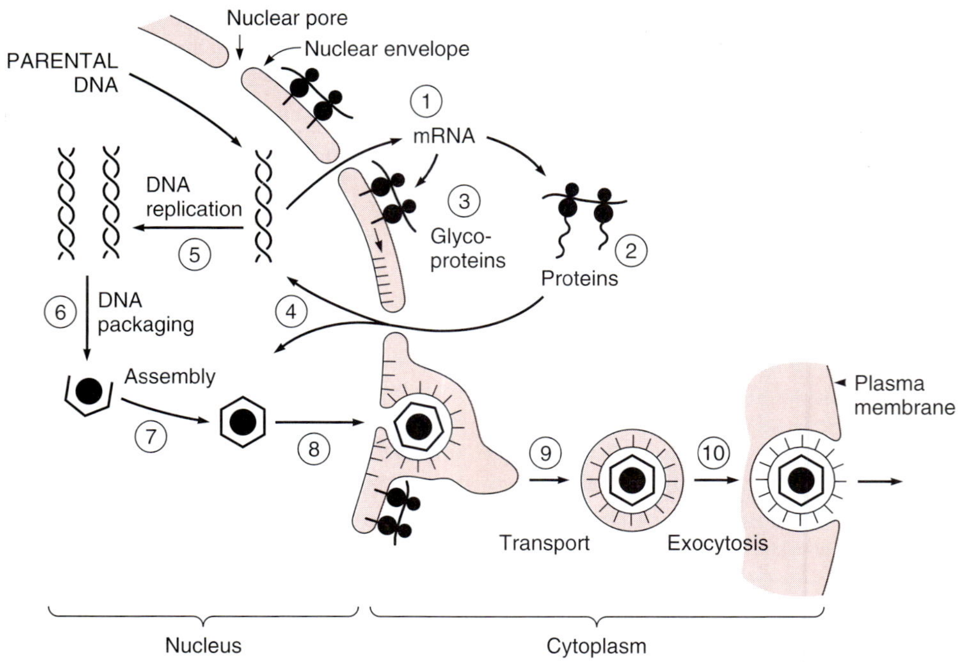

Figure 29–9. Herpesvirus replication and morphogenesis. Diagram begins with parental DNA (upper left) in nucleus of host cell. ***(1)*** Viral mRNAs are synthesized by host cell RNA polymerase on the viral DNA template. Messengers are exported from the nucleus and initiate the synthesis of viral proteins (free polyribosomes) ***(2)*** and glycoproteins (membrane-bound polyribosomes) ***(3).*** Viral proteins enter the nucleus ***(4),*** where they promote synthesis of additional classes of viral mRNAs. Viral DNA polymerase enters the nucleus and initiates viral DNA replication ***(5).*** DNA is cut into unit lengths, packaged into nucleoids ***(6),*** and encapsidated ***(7)*** within an icosahedral shell. The icosahedral shell buds through the nuclear membrane, acquiring a lipoprotein envelope containing viral glycoproteins ***(8).*** The mature virus is transported in vesicles to the plasma membrane ***(9).*** Fusion of the vesicle with the plasma membrane results in release of the virus into the extracellular space ***(10).*** (Reproduced, with permission, from Silverstein SC: Viral replication. Pages 94–100 in: *International Textbook of Medicine.* Vol 2: *Medical Microbiology and Infectious Diseases.* Braude AI [editor]. Saunders,

Mapping of Viral Genomes

Recent advances in animal viral genetics using restriction enzymes and other biochemical techniques have facilitated the identification of viral gene products and the mapping of these on the viral genome. Biochemical and physical mapping can usually be done much more rapidly than genetic mapping using classic genetic techniques.

The technique of reassortment mapping has been used with influenza A viruses, which have a genome of eight segments of RNA, each coding for one viral protein. Under suitable conditions, the RNA genome segments and the polypeptides of different influenza A viruses migrate at different rates in polyacrylamide gels, so that strains can be distinguished. By analyzing the recombinants (reassortants) formed between different influenza viruses, the RNA segment coding for each protein has been determined. Similar experiments with temperature-sensitive mutants have shown the biologic function of various polypeptides. Reassortants are being analyzed to determine which viral proteins are responsible for virulence in humans.

The use of restriction endonucleases for identification of specific strains or isolates of DNA viruses is illustrated in Figure 29–11. Viral DNA is isolated and incubated with a specific endonuclease until DNA sequences susceptible to the nuclease are cleaved. The fragments are then resolved on the basis of size by gel electrophoresis. The large fragments are most retarded by the sieving effect of the gel, so that an inverse relationship between size and migration is observed. The position of the DNA fragments can be determined by radioautography on x-ray film if the viral DNA is labeled. Such physical mapping techniques have been extremely useful in distinguishing viral types in systems in which the viruses cannot be cultured (eg, papillomaviruses).

Detailed physical maps can be prepared for DNA viruses by using a variety of restriction endonucleases. The position in the genome of given DNA sequences can be determined quite precisely.

Physical maps can be correlated with genetic maps if the latter are available. This allows viral gene products to be mapped to individual regions of the genome defined by the restriction enzyme fragments. Transcription of mRNAs throughout the replication cycle

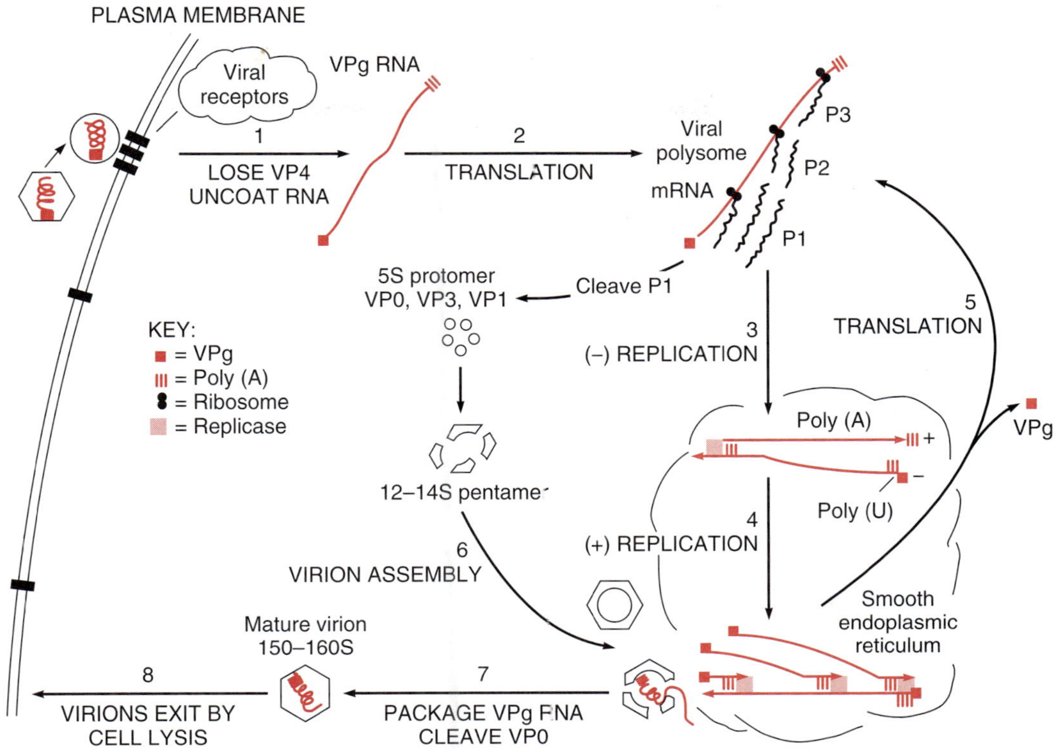

Figure 29–10. Overview of the picornavirus infection cycle. (Reproduced, with permission, from Rueckert RR: Picornaviridae and their replication. Pages 507–548 in: *Virology,* 2nd ed. Fields BN et al [editors]. Raven Press, 1990.)

can be assigned to specific DNA fragments. Using mutagens, it is also possible to alter isolated fragments of viral DNA in order to introduce mutations into defined regions of the genome. Viral genome fragments generated by polymerase chain reaction can be used in place of restriction enzyme fragments in mapping and mutagenesis studies.

Conditional-Lethal Mutants

Meaningful classic genetic studies with animal viruses depend on two factors. The first is a plaque assay for viral infectivity, a sensitive and accurate quantitative assay method. The second is stable genetic markers, which ideally should result from single mutations. "Stable markers" refers to the use of mutants of various viral genes that are recognizable by some change in an observable property of the parental virus. Some markers commonly used include plaque size, specific virus-induced antigens, drug resistance, host range, and inability to grow at high temperatures. Mutants with such markers are obtained either after spontaneous mutation or after treatment with a mutagen.

Conditional-lethal mutants are mutants that are lethal (in that no infectious virus is produced) under one set of conditions—termed nonpermissive conditions—but that yield normal infectious progeny under other conditions—termed permissive conditions. Conditional-lethal mutants include temperature-sensitive and host-range mutants. Temperature-sensitive mutants have been isolated from nearly all animal viruses; they grow at low (permissive) temperatures but not at high (nonpermissive) temperatures. Host-range mutants are able to grow and form plaques in one kind of cell (permissive cell), whereas abortive infection occurs in another type (nonpermissive cell). Host-range bacterial virus mutants may possess altered nucleic acid base sequences that are read as nonsense mutations by the nonpermissive host cell, resulting in polypeptide chain termination and consequently abortive infection. The permissive host cell, on the other hand, carries a transfer RNA that recognizes the altered sequence as a codon and inserts an amino acid, resulting in the formation of a functional polypeptide. It has not been established whether such a mechanism is also operative in host-range mutants of animal viruses. Following the induction and isolation of a set of conditional-lethal mutants, mixed infection studies with pairs of mutants under permissive and nonpermissive conditions can yield information concerning gene function, gene sequence (genetic mapping), and mechanisms of viral replication at the molecular level.

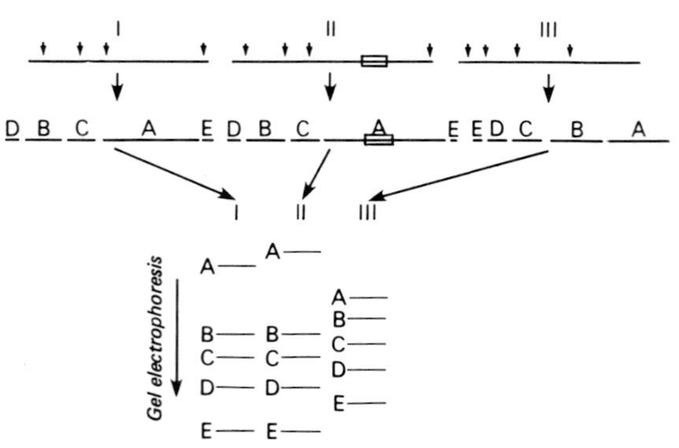

Figure 29–11. Illustration of principles of restriction endonuclease cleavage site analysis. The linear DNA (double-stranded) genomes of three hypothetical viruses to be compared are indicated as I, II, III. Suppose a specific nucleotide sequence, eg, GAATTC, the cleavage site for nuclease EcoRI, occurs at four sites in each genome as indicated by small arrows. Genomes I and II are identical except for a substantial DNA insertion mutation in genome II. Genome III has none of the sequences in question located in positions analogous to genomes I or II. Cleavage of these DNAs at the sites marked by arrows results in five fragments (A–E) in each case. If these DNA fragments are separated according to size in adjacent tracks in a gel electrophoresis experiment, the results will be as diagrammed: fragments B, C, D, and E of samples I and II will co-migrate and fragment A from each virus will differ. The fragments from genome III will co-migrate with none of those from genomes I and II. It should be noted that knowledge of the cleavage site maps at the top is not essential to be able to deduce the fact that genomes I and II are related to each other but not to genome III. (Reproduced, with permission, from Summers WC: Yale J Biol Med 1980;53:55.)

Defective Viruses

A defective virus is one that lacks one or more functional genes required for viral replication. Defective viruses require helper activity from another virus for some step in replication or maturation.

One type of defective virus lacks a portion of its genome (ie, deletion mutant). The extent of loss by deletion may vary from a short base sequence to a large amount of the genome. Deletion mutants may arise spontaneously or may be constructed in the laboratory using biochemical techniques.

Spontaneous deletion mutants frequently arise when viral stocks are passaged repeatedly at high multiplicity. Such defective viruses may interfere with the replication of homologous virus and are called defective interfering viral particles. Defective interfering particles have lost essential segments of genome but contain normal capsid proteins; they require infectious homologous virus as helper for replication, and they interfere with the multiplication of that homologous virus. This interference with standard helper virus probably results from successful competition by defective interfering particles for factors involved in genome replication. Defective particles do not accumulate if the parental virus is passaged at low multiplicity.

Defective interfering particles may be biologically important. It has been proposed that they may play a role in the establishment and maintenance of persistent infections.

Another category of defective virus requires an unrelated replication-competent virus as helper. Examples include the adenoassociated satellite viruses and hepatitis D virus (delta agent), which replicate only in the presence of co-infecting human adenovirus or hepatitis B virus, respectively. No nondefective isolates of this type of defective virus have been recovered. The essential helper function supplied by the helper virus varies, depending on the system.

Pseudovirions are a different type of defective particle. They contain only host cell DNA rather than the viral genome. During viral replication, the capsid sometimes encloses random pieces of host nucleic acid rather than viral nucleic acid. Such particles look like ordinary viral particles when observed by electron microscopy, but they do not replicate. Pseudovirions theoretically might be able to transduce cellular nucleic acid from one cell to another.

The transforming retroviruses are usually defective. A portion of the viral genome has been deleted and replaced with a piece of DNA of cellular origin that encodes a transforming protein. These viruses allowed the identification of cellular oncogenes (see Chapter 43). Another retrovirus is required as helper in order for the transforming virus to replicate.

Interactions Among Viruses

When two or more viral particles infect the same host cell, they may interact in a variety of ways. They must be sufficiently closely related, usually within the same viral family, for most types of interactions to occur. Genetic interaction results in some progeny that are heritably (genetically) different from either parent. Progeny produced as a consequence of nongenetic interaction are similar to the parental viruses. In genetic interactions the actual nucleic acid molecules interact, whereas the products of the genes are involved in nongenetic interactions.

A. Recombination: Recombination results in the production of progeny virus (recombinant) that carries traits not found together in either parent. The classic mechanism is that the nucleic acid strands break, and part of the genome of one parent is joined to part of the genome of the second parent. The recombinant virus is genetically stable, yielding progeny like itself upon replication. (See Chapter 39.) Viruses vary widely in the frequency with which they undergo recombination. Those with double-stranded DNA genomes recombine efficiently; most viruses with nonsegmented, single-stranded RNA genomes do not recombine. In the case of viruses with segmented genomes, eg, influenza virus, the formation of recombinants is due to reassortment of individual genome fragments rather than to an actual crossover event, and it occurs with ease.

B. Genetic Reactivation: This phenomenon represents a special case of recombination.

Marker rescue occurs between the genome of an active virion and the genome of a viral particle that has been inactivated in some way. A portion of the genome of the inactivated virus recombines with that of the active parent, so that certain markers of the inactivated parent are rescued and appear in the viable progeny. None of the progeny produced are identical to the inactivated parent. The progeny carrying the rescued markers of the inactivated parent are genetically stable.

Multiplicity reactivation occurs when many inactive viral particles interact in the same cell to generate a viable virus. This may occur when a heavily damaged viral preparation is used to infect cells at high multiplicity of infection. Recombination occurs between the damaged nucleic acids of the parents, producing a viable genome that can replicate. The greater the damage to the parental genomes, the larger the number of inactive particles required per cell to ensure the formation of a viable genome.

C. Complementation: This refers to the interaction of viral gene products in cells infected with two viruses, one or both of which may be defective. It results in the replication of one or both under conditions in which replication would not ordinarily occur. The basis for complementation is that one virus provides a gene product in which the second is defective, allowing the second virus to grow. The genotypes of the two viruses remain unchanged.

If both mutants are defective in the same gene product, they will not be able to complement each other's growth. Therefore, this test is routinely used to group conditional-lethal mutants of a virus as a prelude to detailed biochemical analyses of the gene functions represented by the mutants.

D. Phenotypic Mixing: A special case of complementation is phenotypic mixing, or the association of a genotype with a heterologous phenotype. This occurs when the genome of one virus becomes randomly incorporated within capsid proteins specified by a different virus or a capsid consisting of components of both viruses (Figure 29–12). If the genome is encased in a completely heterologous protein coat (third and fourth progeny from left), this extreme example of phenotypic mixing may be called "phenotypic masking" or "transcapsidation." Such mixing is not a stable genetic change because, upon replication, the phenotypically mixed parent will yield progeny encased in capsids homologous to the genotype.

Phenotypic mixing usually occurs between different members of the same viral family; the intermixed capsid proteins must be able to interact correctly to form a structurally intact capsid. However, phenotypic mixing also can occur between enveloped viruses, and in this case, the viruses do not have to be closely related. The nucleocapsid of one virus becomes encased within an envelope specified by another, a phenomenon designated "pseudotype formation." There are many examples of pseudotype formation among the RNA tumor viruses (see Chapter 43). The nucleocapsid of vesicular stomatitis virus, a rhabdovirus, has an unusual propensity for being involved in pseudotype formation with unrelated envelope material.

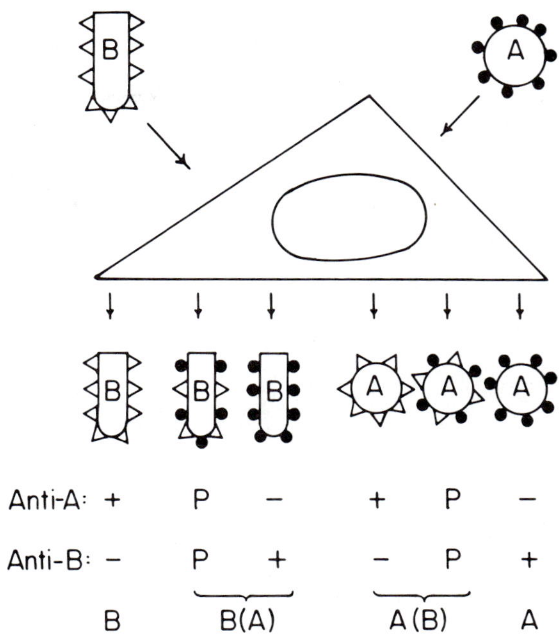

Figure 29–12. Schematic diagram of phenotypic mixing and neutralization of pseudotypes. (+, Viral lesions present: no neutralization. P, Partial neutralization: resistant fraction present or slower neutralization kinetics. −, No viral lesions: virus completely neutralized.) A and B are the pure viral types; A(B) is A genome with B envelope pseudotype; B(A) is B genome with A envelope pseudotype. (Reproduced, with permission, from Boettiger: Prog Med Virol 1979;25:37.)

E. Interference: Infection of either cell cultures or whole animals with two viruses often leads to an inhibition of multiplication of one of the viruses, an effect called interference. Interference in animals is distinct from specific immunity. Furthermore, interference does not occur with all viral combinations; two viruses may infect and multiply within the same cell as efficiently as in single infections.

Several mechanisms have been elucidated as causes of interference: (1) One virus may inhibit the ability of the second to adsorb to the cell, either by blocking its receptors (retroviruses, enteroviruses) or by destroying its receptors (orthomyxoviruses). (2) One virus may compete with the second for components of the replication apparatus (eg, polymerase, translation initiation factor). (3) The first virus may cause the infected cell to produce an inhibitor (interferon; see Chapter 30) that prevents replication of the second virus.

When this phenomenon occurs between unrelated viruses, it is called **heterologous** interference. When it occurs between related viruses, it is called **homologous** interference. Most viruses have the capability to interfere with their own replication (autointerference). In this case, defective interfering particles are produced at the expense of complete virus when high multiplicities of infection are used. Autointerference may have a role in the establishment of persistent viral infections.

Interference has been used as a basis for controlling outbreaks of infection with virulent strains of poliovirus by introducing into the population an attenuated poliovirus that interferes with the spread of the virulent virus. Interference between a preexisting viral infection and a superinfecting attenuated live-virus vaccine has sometimes been a problem in poliovirus vaccination programs.

Viral Genomes as Vectors

A. Recombinant DNA: The insertion of DNA fragments into plasmids of bacteria has given rise to a new technology that holds great promise for the production of biologic materials, hormones, vaccines, interferon, and other gene products. Viral genomes have been engineered to serve as replication and expression vectors for both viral and cellular genes. The SV40 system has been used most extensively, but papillomavirus, adenovirus, and retrovirus vectors are also useful. Correct transcriptional signals must be included in order for the cloned genes to be expressed. The principles of recombinant DNA technology are described and illustrated in Chapter 7. This approach offers the possibility of producing large amounts of a pure antigen for vaccine purposes.

B. Virus-Mediated Gene Transfer in Mammalian Cells: If external genetic information could be stably introduced into eukaryotic cells, this might permit repair of genetic defects. For instance, congenital galactosemia could be corrected by introducing the galactosidase gene into the patient's cells. There are encouraging results in some experimental systems, and studies aimed at repairing human genes are in pioneering stages.

Gene transfer in bacteria can be accomplished by transformation, phage transduction, and conjugation (see Chapter 7). In eukaryotic cells, gene transfer has been accomplished by transformation, microinjection, and transfection of DNA fragments or recombinant genomes. The most promising approach for gene therapy of human genetic defects is by the use of defective retrovirus vectors carrying cloned replacement genes. Retrovirus vectors will efficiently integrate a replacement gene into chromosomal DNA. Technical difficulties face the delivery of the vector to appropriate target cells. After that problem is surmounted, there will still exist the problems of possible immunologic incompatibility of new gene products, possible transfer of undesirable genes together with desired ones, deleterious side effects due to the site of integration of the vector, and altered regulation of gene expression that may turn out to be damaging.

NATURAL HISTORY (ECOLOGY) & MODES OF TRANSMISSION OF VIRUSES

Ecology is the study of interactions between living organisms and their environment. Different viruses have evolved ingenious and often complicated mechanisms for survival in nature and transmission from one host to the next. The mode of transmission utilized by a given virus depends on the nature of the interaction between the virus and the host.

Viruses may be transmitted in the following ways: (1) Direct transmission from person to person by contact. The major means of transmission may be by droplet or aerosol infection (eg, influenza, measles, smallpox); by the fecal-oral route (eg, enteroviruses, rotaviruses, infectious hepatitis A); by sexual contact (eg, hepatitis B, herpes simplex type 2, human immunodeficiency virus); by hand-mouth, hand-eye, or mouth-mouth contact (eg, herpes simplex, rhinovirus, Epstein-Barr virus); or by exchange of contaminated blood (eg, hepatitis B, human immunodeficiency virus). (2) Transmission from animal to animal, with humans an accidental host. Spread may be by bite (rabies) or by droplet or aerosol infection from rodent-contaminated quarters (eg, arenaviruses, hantaviruses). (3) Transmission by means of an arthropod vector (eg, arboviruses, now classified primarily as togaviruses, flaviviruses, and bunyaviruses).

At least three different transmission patterns have been recognized among the arthropod-borne viruses:

(1) Human-arthropod cycle: ***Examples:*** Urban yellow fever, dengue.

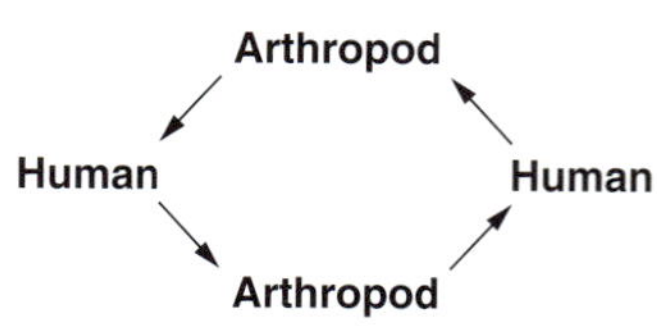

(2) Lower vertebrate-arthropod cycle with tangential infection of humans: ***Examples:*** Jungle yellow fever, St. Louis encephalitis. The infected human is a "dead-end" host. This is a more common transmission mechanism.

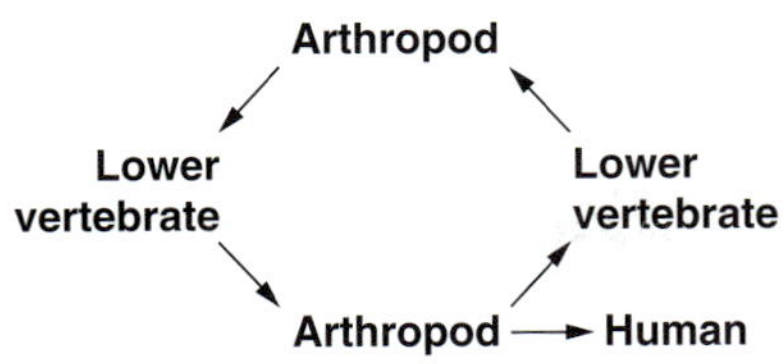

(3) Arthropod-arthropod cycle with occasional infection of humans and lower vertebrates: ***Examples:*** Colorado tick fever, LaCrosse encephalitis.

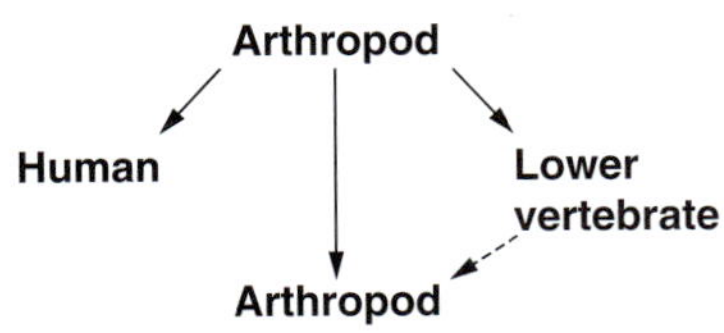

In this cycle, the virus may be transmitted from the adult arthropod to its offspring through the egg (transovarian passage); thus, the cycle may continue with or without intervention of a viremic vertebrate host.

In vertebrates, the invasion of most viruses evokes a violent reaction, usually of short duration. The result is decisive. Either the host succumbs or it lives through the production of antibodies that neutralize the virus. Regardless of the outcome, the sojourn of the active virus is usually short, although persistent or latent infections that last for months to years may occur (hepatitis B, herpes simplex, cytomegalovirus, retroviruses). In arthropod vectors of the virus, the relationship is usually quite different. The viruses produce little or no ill effect and remain active in the arthropod throughout the latter's natural life. Thus arthropods, in contrast to vertebrates, act as permanent hosts and reservoirs.

DIAGNOSIS OF VIRAL INFECTIONS

Information about approaches and methods used for diagnostic virology is included in Chapter 47 and in the chapters describing specific viral diseases (Chapters 31–44).

REFERENCES

Braciale TJ (guest editor): Viruses and the immune system. Semin Virol 1993;4:No. 2. [Entire issue.]

Cheville NF: *Cytopathology in Viral Diseases.* Vol 10 of: *Monographs in Virology.* Melnick JL (editor). Karger, 1975.

Ehrenfeld E (guest editor) Translational regulation. Semin Virol 1993;4:No. 4. [Entire issue.]

Fields BN et al (editors): *Virology,* 2nd ed. Raven Press, 1990.

Francki RIB et al (editors): Classification and nomenclature of viruses. Fifth report of the International Committee on Taxonomy of Viruses. Arch Virol 1991;(Suppl 2).

Hsiung GD et al: The use of electron microscopy for diagnosis of virus infections: An overview. Prog Med Virol 1979;25:133.

Koonin EV (guest editor): Evolution of viral genomes. Semin Virol 1992;3:No. 5. [Entire issue.]

Mims CA: Vertical transmission of viruses. Microbiol Rev 1981;45:267.

Nomoto A (guest editor): Cellular receptors for virus infection. Semin Virol 1992;3:No. 2. [Entire issue.]

Wilson TMA (guest editor): Early events in RNA virus infection. Semin Virol 1992;3:No. 6. [Entire issue.]

30 Pathogenesis & Control of Viral Diseases

PRINCIPLES OF VIRAL DISEASES

The fundamental process of viral infection is the expression of the viral replicative cycle (partial or complete) in a host cell. The cellular response to that infection may range from cytopathology with accompanying cell death to hyperplasia or cancer to no apparent effect.

Viral disease is some abnormality (structural or functional) that results from viral infection of the host organism. Viral infections that fail to produce any symptoms in the host are said to be inapparent (subclinical). Clinical disease in a host consists of overt signs and symptoms. A syndrome is a specific group of signs and symptoms.

More than 300 distinct viruses are known to infect humans and to cause as many as 50 different syndromes.

The following are important principles that pertain to viral disease: (1) Many viral infections are subclinical. (2) The same disease may be produced by a variety of viruses. (3) The same virus may produce a variety of diseases. (4) The disease produced bears no relationship to viral morphology. (5) The outcome in any particular case is determined by the genetic makeup of both the virus and the host.

Viral **pathogenesis** refers to the interaction of viral and host factors that leads to disease production. A virus is **pathogenic** for a particular host if it can infect and cause signs of disease in that host. A strain of a certain virus is more **virulent** than another strain if it commonly produces more severe disease in a host in which both strains are pathogenic. Viral virulence in intact animals should not be confused with cytopathogenicity for cultured cells; viruses highly cytocidal in vitro may be harmless in vivo, and, conversely, noncytocidal viruses may cause severe disease.

Important features of two general categories of acute viral diseases (local, systemic) are compared in Table 30–1.

PATHOGENESIS OF VIRAL DISEASES

To produce disease, viruses must enter a host, come in contact with susceptible cells, replicate, and produce cell injury. Much is still unknown about this process in many viral infections, but genetic and biochemical studies will eventually lead to an understanding of viral pathogenesis at the molecular level. Such understanding is necessary to design truly effective and specific antiviral strategies. Much of our knowledge of viral pathogenesis is based on animal models, because such systems can be more readily manipulated and studied.

Steps in Viral Pathogenesis

Specific steps involved in viral pathogenesis are the following: viral entry into the host, primary viral replication, viral spread, cellular injury, host immune response, viral clearance or establishment of persistent infection, and viral shedding.

A. Entry and Primary Replication: In order for host infection to occur, a virus must first attach to and enter cells of one of the body surfaces—skin, respiratory tract, gastrointestinal tract, urogenital tract, or conjunctiva (Figure 30–1). Most viruses enter their hosts through the mucosa of the respiratory or gastrointestinal tracts (Table 30–2). Major exceptions are those viruses that are introduced directly into the bloodstream by needles (hepatitis B, human immunodeficiency virus) or by insect vectors (arboviruses).

Viruses usually replicate at the primary site of entry. Some, such as influenza viruses (respiratory infections) and rotaviruses (gastrointestinal infections), produce disease at the portal of entry and have no necessity for further systemic spread. They spread locally over the epithelial surfaces, but there is no invasion of underlying tissues or spread to distant sites.

B. Viral Spread and Cell Tropism: Many viruses produce disease at sites distant from their point of entry (eg, enteroviruses, which enter through the gastrointestinal tract but produce central nervous system disease). After primary replication at the site of entry, these viruses then spread within the host (Figure 30–2). Mechanisms of viral spread vary, but the most common route is via the bloodstream or lymphatics. The presence of virus in the blood is called **viremia.** Virions may be free in the plasma (eg, enteroviruses, togaviruses) or associated with particular cell types (eg, measles virus). Some viruses even multiply within those cells. The viremic phase is short in many viral in-

Table 30–1. Important features of acute viral diseases.

	Local Infections	Systemic Infections
Specific disease example	Respiratory (rhinovirus)	Measles
Site of pathology	Portal of entry	Distant site
Incubation period	Relatively short	Relatively long
Viremia	Absent	Present
Duration of immunity	Variable—may be short	Usually lifelong
Role of secretory antibody (IgA) in resistance	Usually important	Usually not important

fections. In a few instances, neuronal spread is involved; this is apparently how rabies virus reaches the brain to cause disease and how herpes simplex virus moves to the ganglia to initiate latent infections.

Viruses tend to exhibit organ and cell specificities. Such tissue and cell tropism by a given virus usually reflects the presence of specific cell surface receptors for that virus. Receptors are components of the cell surface with which a region of the viral surface (capsid or envelope) can specifically interact and initiate infection. Receptors are cell constituents that function in normal cellular metabolism but also happen to have an affinity for a particular virus. The chemical nature of viral receptors is unknown in most cases.

A second mechanism dictating tissue tropism involves proteolytic enzymes. Certain paramyxoviruses are not infectious until an envelope glycoprotein undergoes proteolytic cleavage. Multiple rounds of viral replication will not occur in tissues that do not express the appropriate activating enzymes.

Viral spread may be determined in part by specific viral genes. Studies with reovirus have demonstrated that the extent of spread from the gastrointestinal tract is determined by one of the outer capsid proteins.

C. Cell Injury and Clinical Illness: Destruction of virus-infected cells in the target tissues and physiologic alterations produced in the host by the tissue injury are partly responsible for the development of disease. Some tissues, such as intestinal epithelium, can rapidly regenerate and withstand extensive damage better than others, such as the brain. Some physiologic effects may result from nonlethal impairment of specialized functions of cells, such as loss of hormone production. Clinical illness from viral infection is the result of a complex series of events, and many of the factors that determine degree of illness are unknown. An explanation for general symptoms associated with many viral infections, such as malaise and anorexia, is not available. Clinical illness is an insensitive indicator of viral infection; inapparent infections by viruses are very common.

D. Recovery From Infection: The host either succumbs or recovers from viral infection. Recovery mechanisms involve humoral and cell-mediated immunity, interferon and other lymphokines, and possibly other host defense factors. The relative importance of each component differs with the virus and the disease.

In acute infections, recovery is associated with viral clearance. However, there are times when the host remains persistently infected with the virus. Such long-term infections are described below.

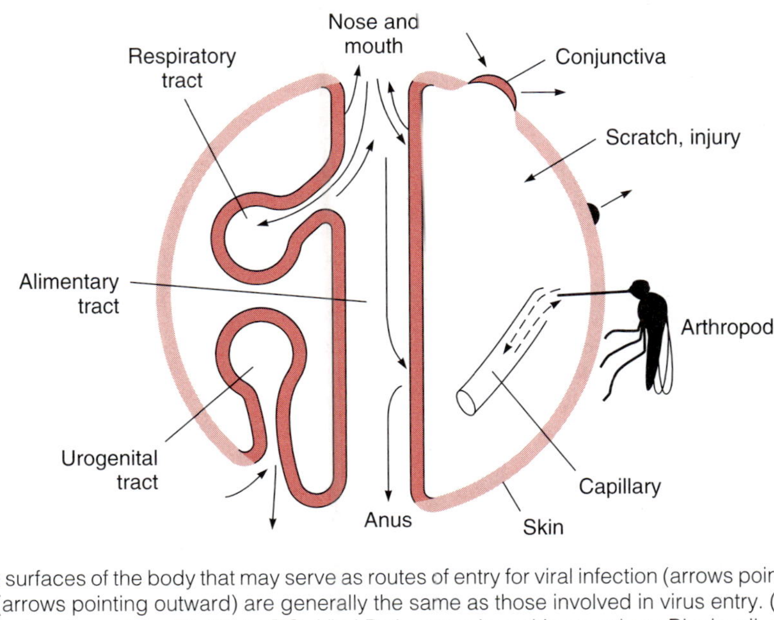

Figure 30–1. The surfaces of the body that may serve as routes of entry for viral infection (arrows pointing inward). Routes of viral shedding (arrows pointing outward) are generally the same as those involved in virus entry. (Modified and reproduced, with permission, from Mims CA, White DO: *Viral Pathogenesis and Immunology.* Blackwell, 1984.)

Table 30–2. Common routes of infection of humans by viruses.

Route of Entry	Virus Group	Produce Local Symptoms at Portal of Entry	Produce Generalized Infection Plus Specific Organ Disease
Respiratory tract	Adenovirus	Most species	—
	Herpesvirus	Epstein-Barr virus, herpes simplex	Varicella
	Poxvirus	—	Smallpox (extinct)
	Picornavirus	Rhinoviruses	Some enteroviruses
	Togavirus	—	Rubella
	Orthomyxovirus	Influenza	—
	Paramyxovirus	Parainfluenza viruses, respiratory syncytial virus	Mumps, measles
	Coronavirus	Most species	—
Mouth or intestinal tract	Adenovirus	Some species	—
	Herpesvirus	Epstein-Barr virus, herpes simplex	Cytomegalovirus
	Picornavirus	—	Some enteroviruses, including polio and hepatitis A
	Reovirus	Rotaviruses	—
Skin			
Mild trauma	Papovavirus	Papillomaviruses	—
	Herpesvirus	Herpes simplex	—
	Poxvirus	Molluscum contagiosum, orf	—
Injection	Herpesvirus	—	Epstein-Barr virus, cytomegalovirus
	Hepadnavirus	—	Hepatitis B
	Retrovirus	—	Human immunodeficiency virus
Bites	Rhabdovirus	—	Rabies
	Togavirus	—	Many species, eg, EEE[1]
	Flavivirus	—	Many species, eg, yellow fever

[1]EEE, eastern equine encephalitis.

E. Virus Shedding: The last stage in pathogenesis is the shedding of infectious virus into the environment. This is a necessary step to maintain a viral infection in populations of hosts. Shedding usually occurs from the body surfaces involved in viral entry (Figures 30–1 and 30–2). Shedding occurs at different stages of disease depending on the particular agent involved. It represents the time at which an infected individual is infectious to contacts. In some viral infections, such as rabies, humans represent dead-end infections, and shedding does not occur.

Host Immune Response

Both humoral and cellular components of the immune response are involved in control of viral infections. Viruses elicit a tissue response different from the response to pathogenic bacteria. Whereas polymorphonuclear leukocytes form the principal cellular response to the acute inflammation caused by pyogenic bacteria, infiltration with mononuclear cells and lymphocytes characterizes the inflammatory reaction of uncomplicated viral lesions.

Virus-encoded proteins, usually capsid proteins, serve as targets for the immune response. Virus-infected cells may be lysed by cytotoxic T lymphocytes as a result of recognition of viral polypeptides on the cell surface. Humoral immunity protects the host against reinfection by the same virus. This is the basis for viral vaccine programs. Neutralizing antibody blocks the initiation of viral infection, probably at the stage of attachment or uncoating. Secretory IgA antibody is important in protecting against infection by viruses through the respiratory or gastrointestinal tracts.

In addition to specific immunity, some nonspecific host defense mechanisms may be elicited by viral infection. The most prominent among the "nonimmune" responses is the induction of interferons (see below).

Special characteristics of certain viruses may have profound effects on the host's immune response. Some viruses infect and damage cells of the immune system. The most dramatic example is the human retrovirus associated with acquired immunodeficiency syndrome (AIDS) that infects T lymphocytes and destroys their ability to function (see Chapter 44).

Adverse effects of the immune response to viral infection are also known. Certain viruses do not invariably kill the cells they infect. The immunologic response of the host in such situations may be involved in the development of pathologic changes and clinical illness.

Another type of immunopathologic disorder was observed in humans immunized with vaccines containing killed measles or respiratory syncytial virus (no longer in use). A few persons developed unusual immune responses that gave rise to serious consequences when they later were exposed to the naturally occurring infective virus. Dengue hemorrhagic fever with shock syndrome, which develops in persons who

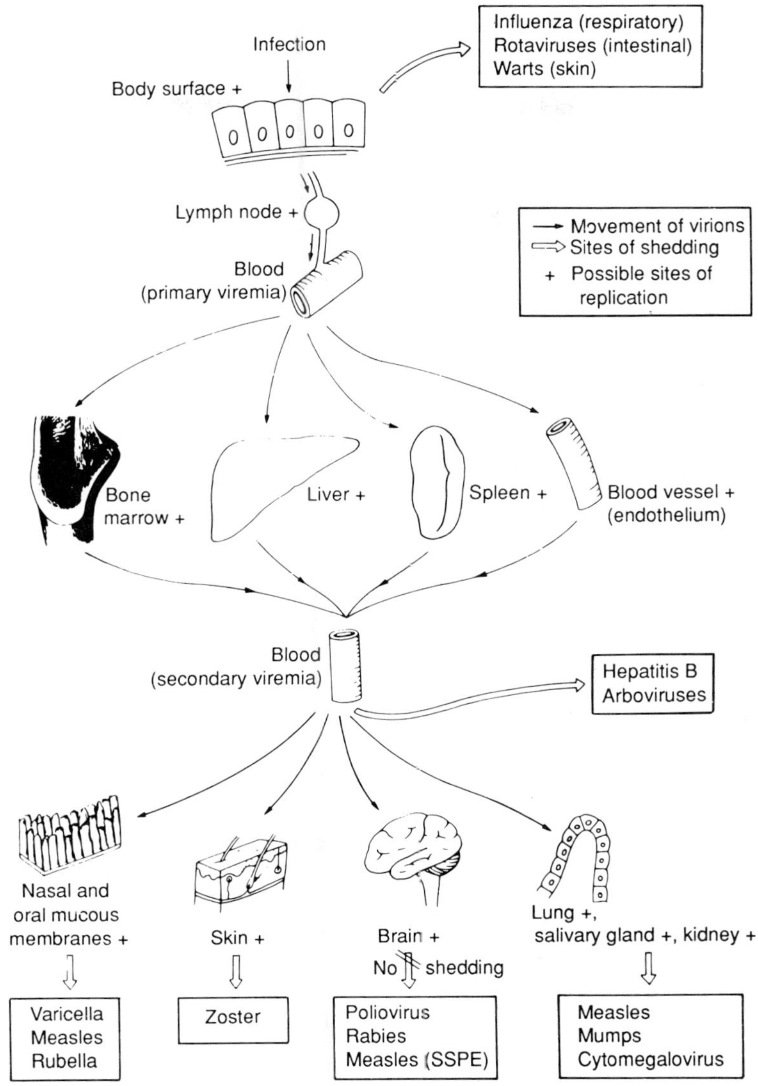

Figure 30–2. Mechanisms of spread of virus through the body in human viral infections. + indicates possible sites of viral replication; large arrows indicate sites of shedding of virus, with illustrative examples of diseases in which that route of excretion is important. Transfer from blood is by transfusion with hepatitis B and by mosquito bite in certain arboviral infections. (Modified and reproduced, with permission, from Mims CA, White DO: *Viral Pathogenesis and Immunology.* Blackwell, 1984.)

already have had at least one prior infection with another dengue serotype, may be a naturally occurring manifestation of the same type of immunopathology.

Another potential adverse effect of the immune response is the development of autoantibodies. If a viral antigen were to elicit antibodies that fortuitously recognized an antigenic determinant on a cellular protein in normal tissues, cellular injury or loss of function unrelated to viral infection might result. The magnitude of this potential problem in human disease is currently unknown.

Comparison of Pathogenesis of a Viral Disease of the Skin & of the Central Nervous System

The pathogenesis of mousepox, a disease of the skin, and of human poliomyelitis, a disease of the central nervous system, are outlined in Figure 30–3. Both viruses multiply at the primary site of entry prior to systemic spread to target organs.

In mousepox, the virus enters the body through minute abrasions of the skin and multiplies in the epidermal cells. At the same time, it is carried by the lym-

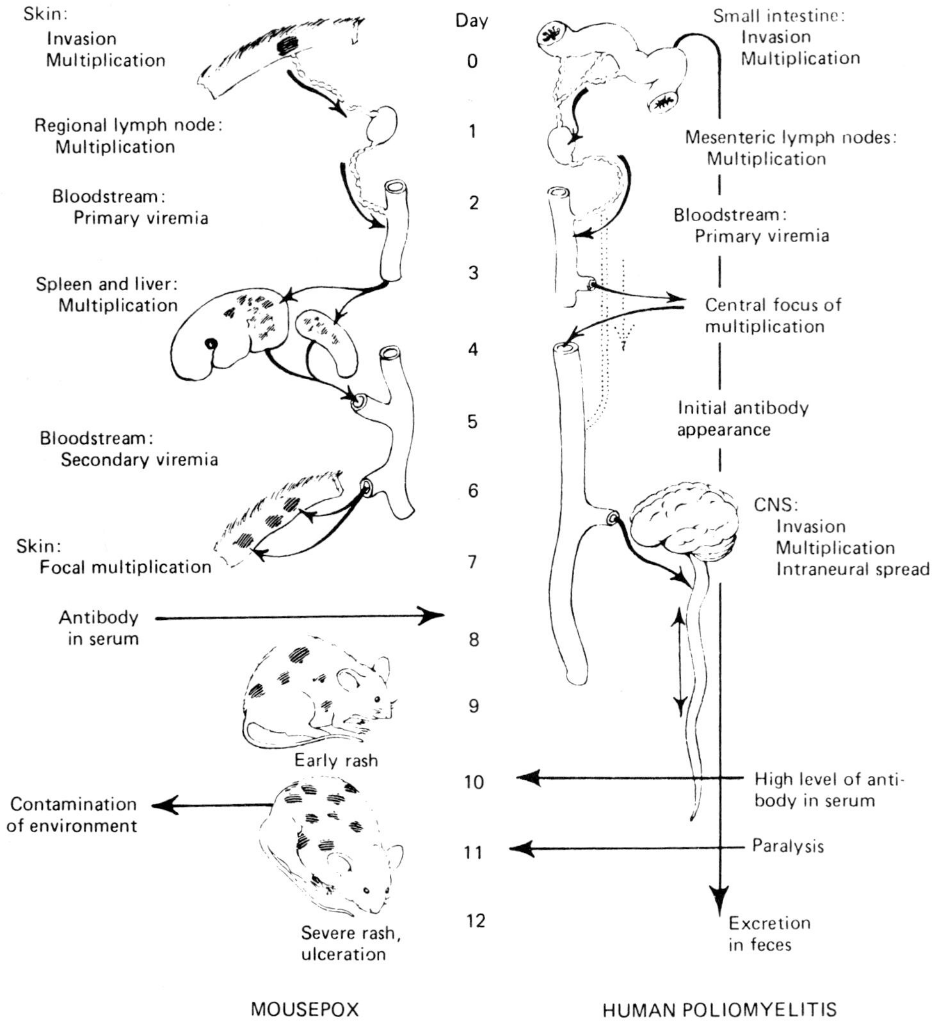

Figure 30–3. Schematic illustrations of the pathogenesis of mousepox and poliomyelitis. (Modified from F Fenner.)

phatics to the regional lymph nodes, where multiplication also occurs. The few viral particles entering the blood by way of the efferent lymphatics are taken up by the macrophages of the liver and spleen. The virus multiplies rapidly in both organs. Following release of virus from the liver and spleen, it moves by way of the bloodstream and localizes in the basal epidermal layers of the skin, in the conjunctival cells, and near the lymph follicles in the intestine. The virus may occasionally also localize in the epithelial cells of the kidney, lung, submaxillary gland, and pancreas. A primary lesion occurs at the site of entry of the virus. It appears as a localized swelling that rapidly increases in size, becomes edematous, ulcerates, and goes on to scar formation. A generalized rash follows that is responsible for the release of large quantities of virus into the environment.

In poliomyelitis, virus enters by way of the alimentary tract, multiplies locally at the initial sites of viral implantation (tonsils, Peyer's patches) or the lymph nodes that drain these tissues, and begins to appear in the throat and in the feces. Secondary viral spread occurs by way of the bloodstream to other susceptible tissues—specifically, other lymph nodes, brown fat, and the central nervous system. Within the central nervous system, the virus spreads along nerve fibers. If a high level of multiplication occurs as the virus spreads through the central nervous system, motor neurons are destroyed and paralysis occurs. The shedding of virus into the environment does not depend on secondary viral spread to the central nervous system. Spread to the central nervous system is readily interrupted by the presence of antibodies induced by prior infection or vaccination.

Viral Persistence: Chronic, Latent, & Slow Virus Infections

Viral infections are usually self-limiting. Sometimes, however, the virus persists for long periods of time in the host. Long-term virus-host interaction may take several forms. **Chronic infections** are those in which virus can be continuously detected; mild or no clinical symptoms may be evident. **Latent infections** are those in which the virus persists in an occult, or cryptic, form most of the time. There will be intermittent flare-ups of clinical disease; infectious virus can be recovered during flare-ups. **Slow virus infections** have a prolonged incubation period, lasting months or years, during which virus continues to multiply. Clinical symptoms are usually not evident during the long incubation period. **Inapparent or subclinical infection** refers to the many infections that give no overt sign of their presence at the host-parasite level.

Chronic infections occur with a number of animal viruses, and the persistence in certain instances depends upon the age of the host when infected. In humans, for example, rubella virus and cytomegalovirus infections acquired in utero characteristically result in viral persistence that is of limited duration, probably because of development of the immunologic capacity to react to the infection as the infant matures. Infants infected with hepatitis B virus frequently become persistently infected (chronic carriers); most carriers are asymptomatic (see Chapter 35). Animal studies have shown that in chronic infections the viral population often undergoes many genetic and antigenic changes.

Herpesviruses typically produce latent infections. Herpes simplex viruses enter the sensory ganglia and persist in a noninfectious state that is not understood at the molecular level (Figure 30–4). There may be periodic reactivations during which lesions containing infectious virus appear at peripheral sites (eg, fever blisters). Chickenpox virus (varicella-zoster) also becomes latent in sensory ganglia. Recurrences are rare and occur years later, usually following the distribution of a peripheral nerve (shingles). Other members of the herpesvirus family also establish latent infections, including cytomegalovirus and Epstein-Barr virus. All may be reactivated by immunosuppression. Consequently, reactivated herpesvirus infections may be a serious complication for persons receiving immunosuppressant therapy.

Persistent viral infections may play a far-reaching role in human disease. Persistent viral infections are associated with leukemias and sarcomas of chickens and mice (see Chapter 43) as well as with progressive degenerative diseases of the central nervous system of humans and animals (see Chapter 42).

Spongiform encephalopathies are a group of chronic, progressive, fatal infections of the central nervous system caused by unconventional, transmissible

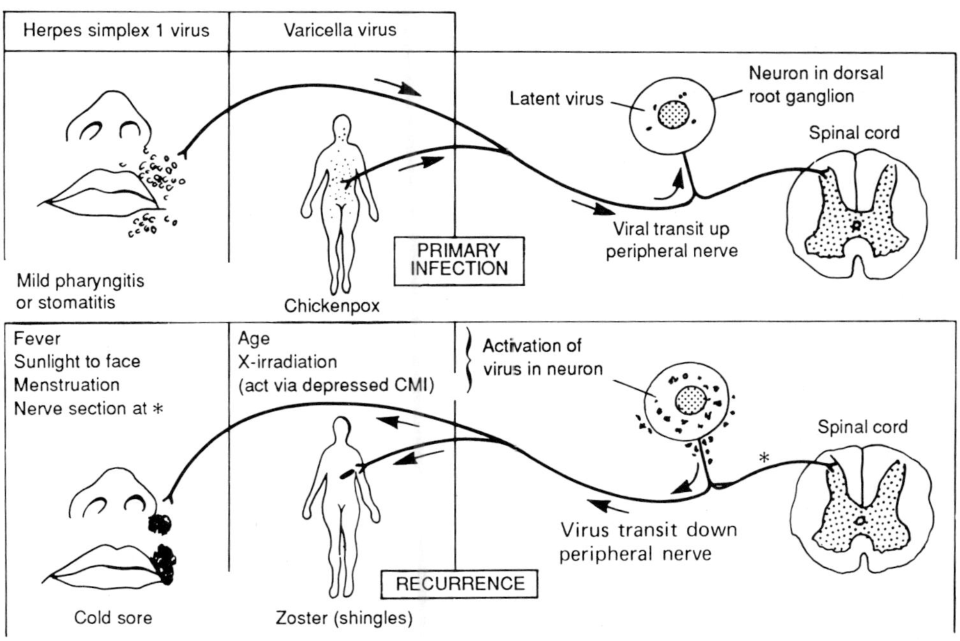

Figure 30–4. Latent infections by herpesviruses. Examples are shown for both herpes simplex and varicella-zoster viruses. Primary infections occur in childhood or adolescence, followed by establishment of latent virus in cerebral or spinal ganglia. Later activation causes recurrent herpes simplex or zoster. Recurrences are rare for zoster. (Reproduced, with permission, from Mims CA, White DO: *Viral Pathogenesis and Immunology.* Blackwell, 1984.)

agents (mentioned above). The best example of this type of "slow virus" infection is scrapie in sheep. Kuru and Creutzfeldt-Jakob disease occur in humans. The mechanism by which this baffling group of agents induce disease is unknown.

Examples of different types of persistent viral infections are presented in Figure 30–5.

Overview of Acute Viral Respiratory Infections

Many types of viruses gain access to the human body via the respiratory tract. This is the most frequent means of viral entry into the host. Successful infection occurs despite normal host protective mechanisms, including the mucus covering most surfaces, ciliary action, and alveolar macrophages. Many infections remain localized in the respiratory tract, although some viruses produce their disease symptoms following systemic spread (eg, chickenpox, measles, rubella; Table 30–2, Figure 30–2).

Disease symptoms exhibited by the host depend on whether the infection is concentrated in the upper or lower respiratory tract (Table 30–3). The most common viral cause of an acute respiratory infection will vary, depending on the particular case. Although definitive diagnosis requires isolation of the virus or demonstration of a rise in antibody titer, the specific viral disease can frequently be deduced by considering the major symptoms, the patient's age, the time of year, and any pattern of illness in the community.

The severity of respiratory infection can range from inapparent to overwhelming. The most severe illness is usually seen in infants infected with certain paramyxoviruses and in elderly or chronically ill adults infected with influenza virus.

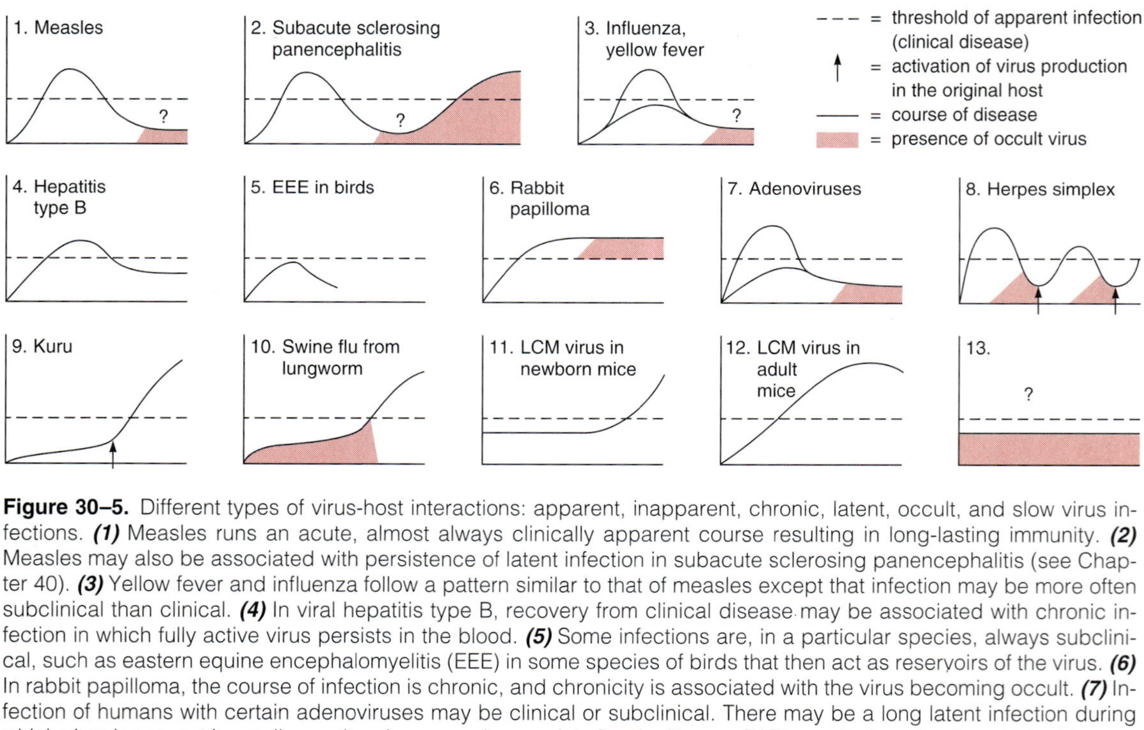

Figure 30–5. Different types of virus-host interactions: apparent, inapparent, chronic, latent, occult, and slow virus infections. ***(1)*** Measles runs an acute, almost always clinically apparent course resulting in long-lasting immunity. ***(2)*** Measles may also be associated with persistence of latent infection in subacute sclerosing panencephalitis (see Chapter 40). ***(3)*** Yellow fever and influenza follow a pattern similar to that of measles except that infection may be more often subclinical than clinical. ***(4)*** In viral hepatitis type B, recovery from clinical disease may be associated with chronic infection in which fully active virus persists in the blood. ***(5)*** Some infections are, in a particular species, always subclinical, such as eastern equine encephalomyelitis (EEE) in some species of birds that then act as reservoirs of the virus. ***(6)*** In rabbit papilloma, the course of infection is chronic, and chronicity is associated with the virus becoming occult. ***(7)*** Infection of humans with certain adenoviruses may be clinical or subclinical. There may be a long latent infection during which virus is present in small quantity; virus may also persist after the illness. ***(8)*** The periodic activation of latent herpes simplex virus, which may recur throughout life in humans, often follows an initial acute episode of stomatitis in childhood. ***(9)*** In many instances, infection is wholly latent for long periods of time before it is activated. Examples of such "slow" virus infections characterized by long incubation periods are scrapie in sheep and kuru in humans. ***(10)*** In pigs that have eaten virus-bearing lungworms, swine "flu" is occult until the appropriate stimulus induces viral production and, in turn, clinical disease. ***(11)*** Lymphocytic choriomeningitis (LCM) virus may be established in mice by in utero infection. A form of modified immunologic tolerance develops in which virus-specific T cells are not activated. Antibody is produced against viral proteins; this antibody and circulating lymphocytic choriomeningitis virus form antigen-antibody complexes that ultimately produce immune complex disease in the partially tolerant host. The presence of lymphocytic choriomeningitis virus in this chronic infection (circulating virus with little or no apparent disease) may be readily revealed by transmission to an indicator host, eg, adult mice from a virus-free stock. All adult mice develop classic acute symptoms of lymphocytic choriomeningitis and frequently die ***(12)***. ***(13)*** The possibility is shown of latent infection with an occult virus that is not readily activated. Proof of the presence of such a virus remains a difficult task which, however, is attracting the attention of cancer investigators (see Chapter 43).

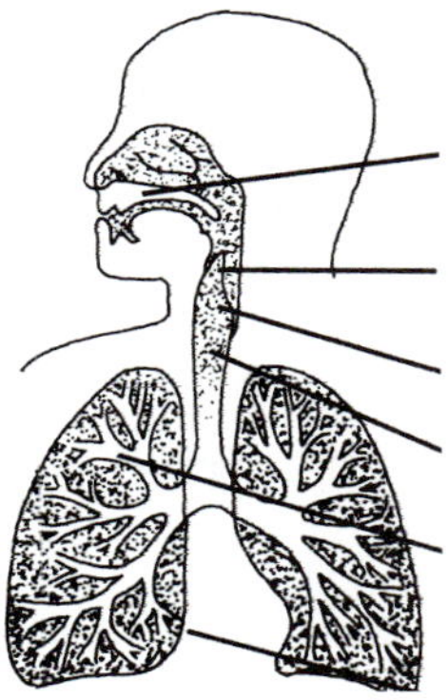

Table 30–3. Viral infections of the respiratory tract.

Syndromes	Main Symptoms	Most Common Viral Causes		
		Infants	**Children**	**Adults**
Common cold	Nasal obstruction, nasal discharge	Rhino Adeno	Rhino Adeno	Rhino Corona
Pharyngitis	Sore throat	Adeno Herpes simplex	Adeno Coxsackie	Adeno Coxsackie
Laryngitis/croup	Hoarseness, "barking" cough	Parainfluenza Influenza	Parainfluenza Influenza	Parainfluenza Influenza
Tracheobronchitis	Cough	Parainfluenza Influenza	Parainfluenza Influenza	Influenza Adeno
Bronchiolitis	Cough, dyspnea	Respiratory syncytial Parainfluenza	Rare	Rare
Pneumonia	Cough, chest pain	Respiratory syncytial Influenza	Influenza Parainfluenza	Influenza Adeno

Overview of Viral Infections of the Gastrointestinal Tract

Many viruses initiate infection via the alimentary tract. A few agents, such as herpes simplex virus and Epstein-Barr virus, probably infect cells in the mouth. Viruses are exposed in the intestinal tract to harsh elements involved in the digestion of food—acid, bile, and proteolytic enzymes. Consequently, viruses able to initiate infection by this route are all acid- and bile-resistant.

Acute gastroenteritis is the designation for short-term gastrointestinal disease with symptoms ranging from mild, watery diarrhea to severe febrile illness characterized by vomiting, diarrhea, and prostration. Rotaviruses, Norwalk viruses, and caliciviruses are major causes of gastroenteritis. Infants and children are affected most often.

Enteroviruses and adenoviruses also infect the gastrointestinal tract, but those infections are usually asymptomatic. Some enteroviruses, notably polioviruses and hepatitis A virus, are important causes of systemic disease but do not produce intestinal symptoms.

Overview of Viral Skin Infections

The skin is a tough and impermeable barrier to the entry of viruses. However, a few viruses are able to breach this barrier and initiate infection of the host (Table 30–2). Some obtain entry through small abrasions of the skin (poxviruses, papillomaviruses, herpes simplex viruses), others are introduced by the bite of arthropod vectors (arboviruses) or infected vertebrate hosts (rabies virus, herpes B virus), and still others are injected during blood transfusions or other manipulations involving contaminated needles (hepatitis B virus, human immunodeficiency virus, Ebola virus).

A few agents remain localized and produce lesions at the site of entry (papillomaviruses and molluscum contagiosum); most spread to other sites.

Many of the generalized skin rashes associated with viral infections develop because virus spreads to the skin via the bloodstream following replication at some other site. Such infections originate by another route (eg, measles virus infections occur via the respiratory tract), and the skin becomes infected from below.

Lesions in skin rashes are designated as macules, papules, vesicles, or pustules. Macules, which are caused by local dilation of dermal blood vessels, progress to papules if edema and cellular infiltration are present in the area. Vesicles occur if the epidermis is involved, and they become pustules if an inflammatory reaction delivers polymorphonuclear leukocytes to the lesion. Ulceration and scabbing follow. Hemorrhagic and petechial rashes occur when there is more severe involvement of the dermal vessels.

Skin lesions frequently play no role in viral transmission. Infectious virus is not shed from the maculopapular rash of measles or from rashes associated with arbovirus infections. In contrast, skin lesions are important in the spread of poxviruses and herpes simplex viruses. Infectious viral particles are present in high titers in the fluid of these vesiculopustular rashes, and they are able to initiate infection by direct contact with other hosts. However, even in these instances, it is believed that virions in oropharyngeal secretions may be more important to disease transmission than the skin lesions.

Overview of Viral Infections of the Central Nervous System

Invasion of the central nervous system by viruses is always a serious matter. Viruses can gain access to the brain by two routes: by the bloodstream (hematogenous spread) and by peripheral nerve fibers (neuronal spread). Access from the blood may occur by growth through the endothelium of small cerebral vessels, by passive transport across the vascular endothelium, or by passage through the choroid plexus to the cerebrospinal fluid. Once the blood-brain barrier is breached, more extensive spread throughout the brain and spinal cord is possible.

The other pathway to the central nervous system is via peripheral nerves. Virions can be taken up at sensory nerve or motor endings and be moved within axons, through endoneural spaces, or by Schwann cell infections. Herpesviruses travel in axons to be delivered to dorsal root ganglia neurons.

Many viruses, including herpes-, toga-, flavi-, entero-, rhabdo-, paramyxo-, and bunyaviruses, can infect the central nervous system and cause meningitis, encephalitis, or both. Encephalitis caused by herpes simplex virus is the most common cause of sporadic encephalitis in humans.

Pathologic reactions to cytocidal viral infections of the central nervous system include necrosis, inflammation, and phagocytosis by glial cells. The cause of symptoms in some other central nervous system infections, such as rabies, is unclear. The postinfectious encephalitis that occurs after measles infections (about one per 1000 cases) and more rarely after rubella infections is characterized by demyelination without neuronal degeneration and is probably an autoimmune disease.

There are several rare neurodegenerative disorders, called slow virus infections, that are uniformly fatal. Features of these infections include a long incubation period (months to years) followed by the onset of clinical illness and progressive deterioration, resulting in death in weeks to months; usually only the central nervous system is involved. Some slow virus infections, such as progressive multifocal leukoencephalopathy (human papovavirus) and subacute sclerosing panencephalitis (measles virus), are caused by typical viruses. In contrast, the subacute spongiform encephalopathies, typified by scrapie, are caused by unconventional agents. In those infections, characteristic neuropathologic changes occur, but no inflammatory or immune response is elicited.

Overview of Congenital Viral Infections

Few viruses produce disease in the human fetus. Most maternal viral infections do not result in viremia and fetal involvement. However, if the virus crosses the placenta and infection occurs in utero, serious damage may be done to the fetus.

Three principles involved in the production of congenital defects are (1) the ability of the virus to infect the pregnant woman and be transmitted to the fetus; (2) the stage of gestation at which infection occurs; and (3) the ability of the virus to cause damage to the fetus directly, by infection of the fetus, or indirectly, by infection of the mother resulting in an altered fetal environment (eg, fever). The sequence of events that may occur prior to and following viral invasion of the fetus is shown in Figure 30–6.

Rubella virus and cytomegalovirus are presently the primary agents responsible for congenital defects in humans (see Chapters 33 and 40). Congenital infections can also occur with herpes simplex, varicella-zoster, hepatitis B, measles, mumps, and some enteroviruses (Table 30–4).

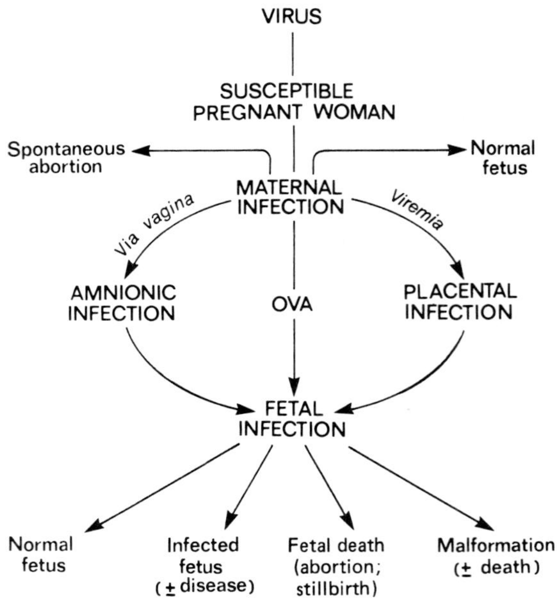

Figure 30–6. Viral infection of the fetus. (After Catalano and Sever.)

In utero infections may result in fetal death, premature birth, intrauterine growth retardation, or persistent postnatal infection. Developmental malformations, including congenital heart defects, cataracts, deafness, microcephaly, and limb hypoplasia, may result. Fetal tissue is rapidly proliferating. Viral infection and multiplication may destroy cells or alter cell function. Lytic viruses, such as herpes simplex, may result in fetal death. Less cytolytic viruses, such as rubella, may slow the rate of cell division. If this occurs during a critical phase in organ development, structural defects and congenital anomalies may result.

Many of the same viruses can produce serious disease in newborns (Table 30–4). Such infections may be contracted from the mother during delivery (natal) from contaminated genital secretions, stool, or blood. Less commonly, infections may be acquired during the first few weeks after birth (postnatal) from maternal sources, family members, hospital personnel, or blood transfusions.

Effect of Host Age

Host age is a factor in viral pathogenicity. More severe disease is often produced in newborn animals. In addition to maturation of the immune response with age, there seem to be age-related changes in the susceptibility of certain cell types to viral infection. Viral infections usually can occur in all age groups but may have their major impact at different times of life, from

Table 30–4. Acquisition of significant perinatal viral infections.

<table>
<tr><th rowspan="2">Virus</th><th colspan="3">Frequency of Time of Infection</th><th rowspan="2">Neonatal Incidence (per 1000 Live Births)</th></tr>
<tr><th>Prenatal (in Utero)</th><th>Natal (During Delivery)</th><th>Postnatal (After Delivery)</th></tr>
<tr><td>Rubella</td><td>+</td><td>–</td><td>Rare</td><td>0.1–0.7</td></tr>
<tr><td>Cytomegalo</td><td>+</td><td>++</td><td>+</td><td>5–25</td></tr>
<tr><td>Herpes simplex</td><td>+</td><td>++</td><td>+</td><td>0.03–0.5</td></tr>
<tr><td>Varicella-zoster</td><td>+</td><td>Rare</td><td>Rare</td><td>Rare</td></tr>
<tr><td>Hepatitis B</td><td>+</td><td>++</td><td>+</td><td>0–7</td></tr>
<tr><td>Entero</td><td>+</td><td>++</td><td>+</td><td>Uncommon</td></tr>
</table>

rubella, which is most serious during gestation, to St. Louis encephalitis, which is most serious in the elderly (Table 30–5).

PREVENTION & TREATMENT OF VIRAL INFECTIONS

Antiviral Chemotherapy

Unlike viruses, bacteria and protozoans do not rely on host cellular machinery for replication, so processes specific to these organisms provide ready targets for the development of antibacterial and antiprotozoal drugs. Because viruses are obligate intracellular parasites, antiviral agents must be capable of selectively inhibiting viral functions without damaging the host. Molecular virology studies have now succeeded in identifying virus-specific functions that can serve as realistic targets for inhibition. Theoretically, any stage in the viral replicative cycle (see Chapter 29) could be a target for antiviral therapy. The most amenable stages to target in viral infections include the stages of attachment of virus to host cells; of uncoating of the viral genome; of synthesis of virus-specific enzymes and coat proteins; of replication of viral nucleic acid; and of assembly and release of progeny viral particles. In reality, it has been very difficult to develop antivirals that can distinguish viral from host replicative processes. Compounds have been found that are of value in treatment of viral diseases (Figure 30–7 and Table 30–6). However, all are of use in only a limited number of situations and may be toxic to the host. Ideal antiviral agents remain to be developed.

A. Nucleoside Analogues: The majority of available antiviral agents are nucleoside analogues. Most are limited in inhibitory activity to use against herpesviruses or human immunodeficiency virus.

Analogues inhibit nucleic acid replication by inhibition of enzymes of the metabolic pathways for purines or pyrimidines or by inhibition of polymerases for nucleic acid replication. In addition, some analogues can be incorporated into the nucleic acid and block further synthesis or alter its function.

Table 30–5. Peak ages of incidence of serious viral diseases.[1]

<table>
<tr><th>Before Birth</th><th>At Birth</th><th>Infants</th><th>Children</th><th>Adolescents and Young Adults</th><th>Older Adults</th></tr>
<tr><td></td><td colspan="5">Herpes type 1</td></tr>
<tr><td></td><td>Herpes type 2</td><td>Respiratory syncytial disease</td><td>Rhinovirus colds</td><td>Herpes type 2</td><td></td></tr>
<tr><td colspan="2">Cytomegalovirus disease</td><td>Parainfluenza</td><td>Coronavirus disease</td><td>Hepatitis B</td><td></td></tr>
<tr><td>Rubella</td><td>Hepatitis B</td><td>Adenovirus disease</td><td colspan="2">Measles</td><td></td></tr>
<tr><td></td><td></td><td></td><td colspan="2">Rubella</td><td></td></tr>
<tr><td></td><td></td><td></td><td colspan="2">Mumps</td><td></td></tr>
<tr><td></td><td></td><td colspan="4">Influenza</td></tr>
<tr><td></td><td></td><td colspan="3">Polio and other enteroviral diseases</td><td></td></tr>
<tr><td></td><td></td><td>Rotavirus diarrhea</td><td>Hepatitis A</td><td>Infectious mononucleosis (Epstein-Barr virus)</td><td>St. Louis encephalitis</td></tr>
<tr><td></td><td></td><td></td><td colspan="3">Epidemic gastroenteritis (Norwalk virus)</td></tr>
<tr><td></td><td></td><td></td><td colspan="2">Varicella (chickenpox)</td><td>Herpes zoster (shingles)</td></tr>
</table>

[1]Adapted from Wilson EB: NIH Publication No. 80–433.

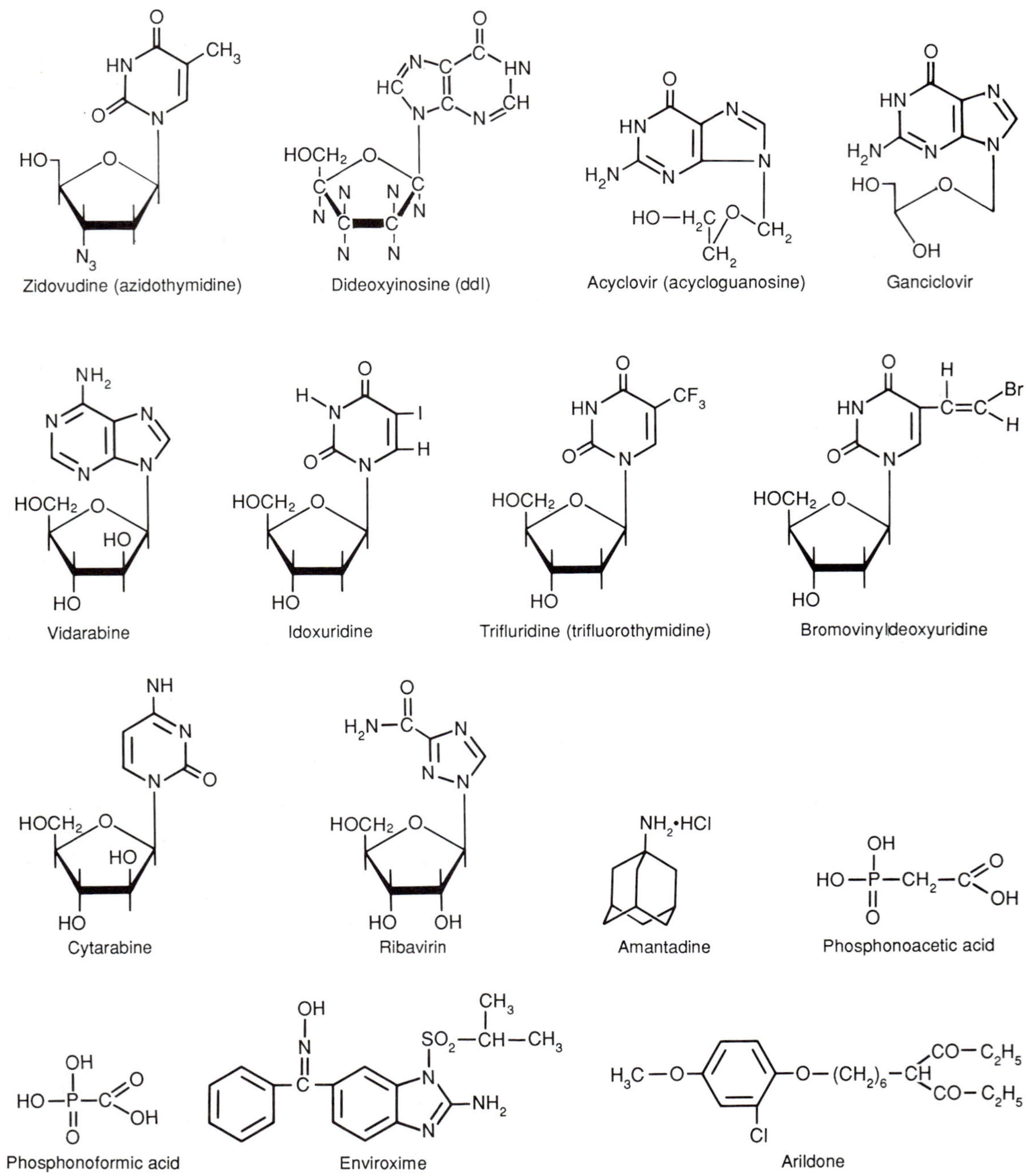

Figure 30–7. Structural formulas for antiviral compounds.

Analogues can inhibit cellular enzymes as well as virus-encoded enzymes. The clinical use of such compounds depends on a high therapeutic ratio, so that the benefit of viral inhibition outweighs the inherent toxicity. The new types of analogues are those able to specifically inhibit virus-encoded enzymes, with minimal inhibition of analogous host cell enzymes. Viral variants resistant to the drug usually arise over time.

Zidovudine (azidothymidine; 3-azido-3-deoxythymidine; AZT) is a synthetic thymidine analogue that inhibits the replication of human immunodeficiency virus by blocking the synthesis of proviral DNA. The reverse transcriptase of the virus is 100 times more sensitive than the cellular DNA polymerase to inhibition by AZT. AZT has been proved to reduce morbidity and mortality in patients with AIDS.

Table 30–6. Major antiviral compounds used for treatment of viral infections.

Drug	Nucleoside Analogue	Mechanism of Action	Viral Spectrum
Acyclovir	Yes	Viral polymerase inhibitor	Herpesviruses
Amantadine	No	Blocks viral uncoating	Influenza A
Didanosine (ddI)	Yes	Reverse transcriptase inhibitor	HIV-1, HIV-2[1]
Foscarnet	No	Viral polymerase inhibitor	Cytomegalovirus, herpes simplex, varicella-zoster, HIV-1
Ganciclovir	Yes	Viral polymerase inhibitor	Cytomegalovirus
Idoxuridine	Yes	Viral thymidine kinase inhibitor	Herpesvirus keratitis
Ribavirin	Yes	Perhaps blocks capping of viral mRNA	Respiratory syncytial virus, influenza A and B, Lassa fever
Trifluridine	Yes	—	Herpesvirus keratitis
Vidarabine	Yes	Viral polymerase inhibitor	Herpes simplex, varicella-zoster
Zalcitabine (ddC)	Yes	Reverse transcriptase inhibitor	HIV-1, HIV-2
Zidovudine (AZT)	Yes	Reverse transcriptase inhibitor	HIV-1, HIV-2

[1]HIV-1, HIV-2, human immunodeficiency virus types 1 and 2.

The drug causes a variety of toxic side effects, including bone marrow depression and neurotoxicity, and is quite expensive.

Didanosine (dideoxyinosine; 2′,3′-dideoxyinosine; ddI) is a dideoxynucleoside that inhibits the human immunodeficiency virus reverse transcriptase and blocks the synthesis of proviral DNA. Its immediate precursor, dideoxyadenosine (ddA), is readily deaminated to form ddI, and ddI can be metabolized to form ddA-5′ triphosphate, so the two drugs are almost identical. ddI causes relatively little bone marrow toxicity, but pancreatitis has been observed.

Zalcitabine (dideoxycytosine; ddC) is another nucleoside analogue that inhibits the reverse transcriptase of human immunodeficiency virus and blocks the synthesis of proviral DNA.

Acyclovir (9-[2-hydroxyethoxymethyl]guanine, acycloguanosine) is an analogue of guanosine or deoxyguanosine that strongly inhibits herpes simplex virus but has little effect on other DNA viruses or on host cells. The drug is phosphorylated by the virus-encoded thymidine kinase and causes a much greater inhibition of the virus-encoded DNA polymerase than of the corresponding host cell enzymes. Herpesviruses that encode for their own thymidine kinase (herpes simplex, varicella-zoster) are much more susceptible than those that do not (cytomegalovirus, Epstein-Barr virus). Mutants of herpesvirus that lack thymidine kinase fail to phosphorylate the drug and are resistant to it.

Acyclovir has activity in vivo in mice with herpes encephalitis and topically for treatment of herpetic lesions in the eyes of rabbits or skin lesions of guinea pigs. It has been effective topically in the control of herpetic eye lesions in humans and in the healing of primary but not recurrent herpetic skin lesions. Latent infections in the ganglia are not cured. Parenteral administration of acyclovir has prevented the reactivation of latent herpesvirus infections and has also been effective in the treatment of active herpetic lesions in patients undergoing immunosuppressive therapy.

Ganciclovir (9-[1,3-dihydroxy-2-propoxymethyl-guanine) is a methylguanine derivative related to acyclovir. It is more active in vitro against cytomegalovirus than is acyclovir, inhibiting viral DNA polymerase and blocking chain elongation. Significant clinical benefits have been achieved in transplant patients with severe cytomegalovirus infections. Patients with cytomegalovirus retinitis have responded well.

Vidarabine (9-β-D-arabinofuranosyladenine, ara-A, adenine arabinoside) is a purine analogue. Its precise mechanism of action is unclear, but it probably blocks viral DNA synthesis by inhibiting viral DNA polymerase. Vidarabine has been used topically to treat corneal lesions due to herpes simplex virus. The clinical effectiveness of parenteral vidarabine against herpes simplex and varicella-zoster infection in humans has been significant. Vidarabine has been replaced by acyclovir as the drug of choice in treating serious systemic infections with these viruses. It must be given early (before onset of coma) in herpesvirus encephalitis, making it essential that the early and reliable diagnosis of herpesvirus encephalitis be made. Vidarabine is relatively nontoxic but may cause nausea and phlebitis. It is not immunosuppressive.

Idoxuridine (5-iodo-2′-deoxyuridine), a halogenated pyrimidine, inhibits thymidine kinase and is incorporated into DNA. Drug-resistant mutants of viruses regularly emerge in the presence of idoxuridine. Topical administration of idoxuridine is used in humans in the treatment of corneal lesions due to herpes simplex virus. Because of its toxicity due to inhibition of cellular DNA synthesis and its lack of efficacy, it is not used in systemic herpes infections.

Idoxuridine was the first antiviral agent to be licensed for human use. It has been largely superseded by newer, less toxic analogues.

Trifluridine (trifluorothymidine, 5-trifluoromethyl-2′-deoxyuridine) has also been used successfully in the topical treatment of herpes keratitis. Trifluridine is effective against strains of herpesvirus that are resistant to idoxuridine.

Bromovinyldeoxyuridine ([E]-5-[2-bromovinyl]-2′-deoxyuridine) offers many advantages over idoxuridine. It is nontoxic, more active, and requires a virus-induced thymidine kinase for phosphorylation. It is even more active against varicella-zoster virus than against herpes simplex virus.

Cytarabine (1-β-D-arabinofuranosylcytosine monohydrochloride, ara-C, cytosine arabinoside), another pyrimidine analogue, inhibits cellular DNA synthesis and viral DNA synthesis about equally and, therefore, exhibits little viral specificity. Cytarabine is not effective as a systemic drug in viral infections and is immunosuppressive and cytotoxic.

Other halogenated pyrimidines, **5-fluoro-2′-deoxyuridine** and **5-bromo-2′-deoxyuridine,** inhibit viral DNA replication and have been useful for the study of viral replication but are not practical as chemotherapeutic agents.

Ribavirin (Virazole, 1-β-D-ribofuranosyl-1,2,4-triazole-3-carboxamide) is a synthetic nucleoside structurally related to guanosine that is effective to varying degrees against many DNA- and RNA-containing viruses in vitro. Its mechanism of action has not been defined, but it seems to interfere with an intracellular event, perhaps synthesis (capping) of viral mRNA. A small-particle aerosol delivery system has been devised to treat influenza and respiratory syncytial virus infections. The drug is approved for aerosol treatment of respiratory syncytial virus infections in infants. Intravenous ribavirin has also proved effective in the treatment of Lassa fever.

B. Other Types of Antiviral Agents: A number of other types of compounds have been shown to possess some antiviral activity under certain conditions.

Amantadine (Symmetrel, 1-aminoadamantane hydrochloride), a synthetic amine, specifically inhibits all influenza A viruses by blocking viral uncoating. When administered prophylactically, amantadine has a significant protective effect in experimental animals and humans against influenza A strains but not against influenza B or other viruses. **Rimantadine,** a derivative of amantadine, has the same spectrum of antiviral activity but is less toxic and has fewer side effects.

Phosphonoacetic acid and **phosphonoformic acid (trisodium phosphonoformate, foscarnet)** inhibit herpes simplex virus replication. They are potent inhibitors of herpes simplex virus-induced DNA polymerase and have little effect on known cellular DNA polymerases. Herpesvirus mutants resistant to the drugs arise easily. Phosphonoformic acid also inhibits to a lesser extent the polymerases of hepatitis B virus and retroviruses. Phosphonoacetic acid is very irritating when applied topically, whereas phosphonoformic acid is not. Both compounds accumulate in bone when given systemically.

Enviroxime (2-amino-1-[isopropylsulfonyl]-6-benzimidazole phenyl ketone oxime) inhibits rhinoviruses in cell culture. It markedly reduced common cold symptoms in treated volunteers. Another benzimidazole derivative, **2-(α-hydroxybenzyl)-benzimidazole,** inhibits the replication of many picornaviruses in vitro.

Methisazone (Marboran), or **N-methylisatin-β-thiosemicarbazone,** is of historical interest as an inhibitor of poxviruses. The drug is highly virus-specific and does not affect normal cell metabolism; it inhibits poxvirus replication if given soon after exposure. It blocks a late stage in viral replication, resulting in the formation of immature, noninfectious viral particles. Methisazone was the first antiviral agent to be described. However, since smallpox has been eradicated, the drug is not used.

Arildone (4-[6-(2-chloro-4-methoxy) phenoxyl]-hexyl-3,5-heptanedione), a phenoxyl diketone, is active in cultured cells against a number of DNA and RNA viruses. It appears to inhibit uncoating of viruses. Arildone is being tested for topical treatment of herpesvirus infections.

Interferons

Interferons are host-coded proteins that inhibit viral replication and are produced by intact animals or cultured cells in response to viral infection or other inducers. They are believed to be the body's first line of defense against viral infection. Interferons modulate humoral and cellular immunity and have broad cell-growth regulatory activities.

A. Properties of Interferons: There are multiple species of interferons that fall into three general groups, designated IFN-α, IFN-β, and IFN-γ (Table 30–7). The IFN-α family is large, being coded by at least 15 genes in the human genome plus several pseudogenes; the IFN-β and IFN-γ families are coded by one or a few genes each. Only the IFN-γ gene has been found to possess introns. The three multigene families have diverged so that the coding sequences now are not closely related.

The different interferons are similar in size, but the three classes are antigenically distinct. IFN-α and IFN-β are resistant to low pH. IFN-β and IFN-γ are glycosylated, but the sugars are not necessary for biologic activity, so cloned interferons produced in bacteria are biologically active.

B. Synthesis of Interferons: Interferons are produced by all vertebrate species. Normal cells do not generally synthesize interferon until they are induced to do so. Infection with viruses is a potent insult leading to induction; RNA viruses are stronger inducers of interferon than DNA viruses. Interferons also can be

Table 30–7. Properties of human interferons.

Property	Type		
	Alpha	Beta	Gamma
Current nomenclature	IFN-α	IFN-β	IFN-γ
Former designation	Leukocyte	Fibroblast	Immune
Number of genes that code for family	≥ 15	1	1
Principal cell source	Leukocytes	Fibroblasts	Lymphocytes
Inducing agent	Viruses; dsRNA	Viruses; dsRNA	Mitogens
Size of protein (MW)	17,000	17,000	17,000
Stability at pH 2.0	Stable	Stable	Labile
Glycosylated	No	Yes	Yes
Introns in genes	No	No	Yes
Homology with IFN-α	80–95%	30%	< 10%
Chromosomal location of genes	9	9	12
Size of secreted protein (number of amino acids)	143	145	146

induced by double-stranded RNA, bacterial endotoxin, and small molecules such as tilorone. IFN-γ is not produced in response to most viruses but is induced by mitogen stimulation.

The different classes of interferon are produced by different cell types. IFN-α is synthesized predominantly by leukocytes, IFN-β mainly by fibroblasts, and IFN-γ only by lymphocytes.

Because the amounts of interferon synthesized by induced cells are quite small, it was difficult to purify and characterize the proteins. With recombinant DNA techniques, cloned interferon genes are being expressed in large amounts in bacteria and in yeast, and the availability of genetically engineered interferons makes clinical studies feasible.

C. Antiviral Activity and Other Biologic Effects: Interferons were first recognized by their ability to interfere with viral infection in cultured cells. Interferons are produced soon (<48 hours) after viral infection in intact animals, and viral production then decreases (Figure 30–8). Antibody does not appear in the blood of the animal until several days after viral production has abated. This temporal relationship suggests that interferon plays a primary role in the defense of the host against viral infections. This conclusion is also supported by observations that agammaglobulinemic individuals usually recover from primary viral infections about as well as normal people.

The different types of interferon are roughly equivalent in antiviral activity. However, interferons also exhibit a wide variety of cell regulatory activities. They are actually cytokines involved in regulation of cell growth and differentiation. Observed anticellular activities of interferons include inhibition of cell growth, effects on differentiation, and modulation of the immune response (ie, increased expression of histocompatibility antigens, enhancement of natural killer cell activity). The cell regulatory activity of IFN-γ is much greater than that of IFN-α or IFN-β. Human IFN-β_2 is identical to B cell differentiation factor BSF-2 and to hybridoma growth factor and is no longer considered an interferon. IFN-γ and macrophage activating factor are identical. The multiplicity of effects of interferon upon host processes is summarized in Figure 30–9.

Interferons are almost always host species-specific in function. By contrast, interferon activity is not specific for a given virus; the replication of a wide variety of viruses can be inhibited. When interferon is added to cells prior to infection, there is marked inhibition of viral replication but nearly normal cell function. Interferons are extremely potent, so that very small amounts are required for function. It has been esti-

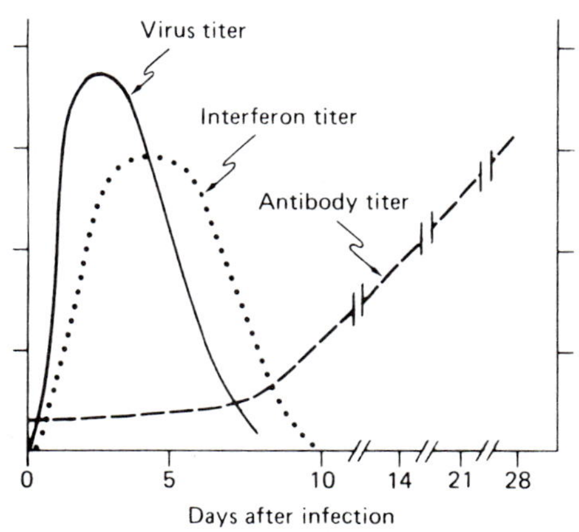

Figure 30–8. Illustration of kinetics of interferon and antibody synthesis after respiratory viral infection. The temporal relationships suggest that interferons are involved in the recovery process.

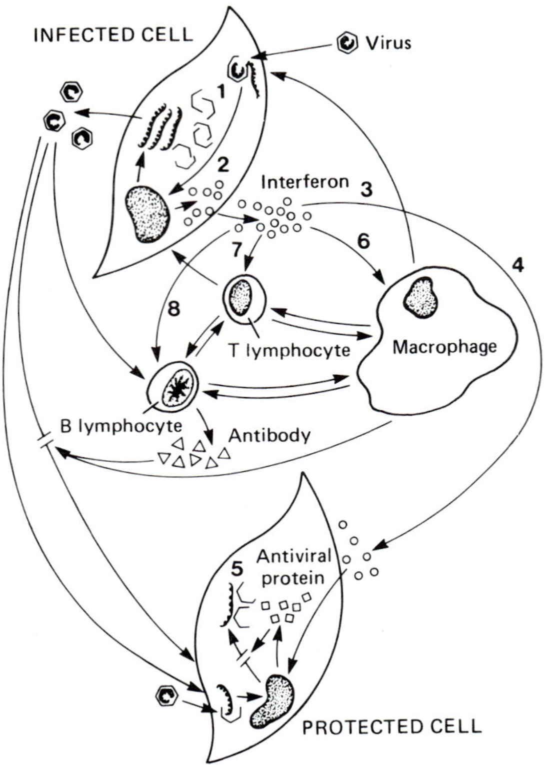

Figure 30–9. Overview of different sites of action of interferons. The original infected cell (1) produces interferon (2), which is released (3) and may interact with other cells (4), eliciting the synthesis of protective antiviral protein (5). The released interferon(s) (3) may also interact with components of the immune system (6, 7, 8) and modulate the immune response. Note that the original cell infected by virus produces interferon but is not protected by it. (Reprinted from Stringfellow DA [editor]: *Modern Pharmacology–Toxicology.* Vol 17: *Interferon and Interferon Inducers: Clinical Applications,* 1980. Courtesy of Marcel Dekker.)

mated that fewer than 50 molecules of interferon per cell are sufficient to induce the antiviral state.

The mechanism of interferon action is still poorly understood. However, it is clear that interferon is not the antiviral agent; rather, interferon induces an antiviral state by prompting the synthesis of other proteins that actually inhibit viral replication.

Interferon molecules bind to cell surface receptors, with IFN-α and IFN-β sharing a common receptor and IFN-γ recognizing a distinct receptor. This binding triggers tyrosine phosphorylation and activation of transcription factor subunits in the cytoplasm, which then translocate into the nucleus and mediate transcription. This results in the synthesis of several enzymes believed to be instrumental in the development of the antiviral state. These cellular enzymes subsequently block viral reproduction by inhibiting the translation of viral mRNA into viral protein. At least two enzymatic pathways appear to be involved: (1) a protein kinase phosphorylates and inactivates a cellular initiation factor and thus prevents formation of the initiation complex needed for viral protein synthesis, and (2) an oligonucleotide synthetase, 2-5A synthetase, which is needed for oligoadenylic acid, 2,5-oligoA, formation, activates a cellular endonuclease, RNase L, which, in turn, degrades mRNA. Interferons also may affect viral assembly, perhaps as a result of changes at the plasma membrane. These explanations, however, may not represent the key mechanisms of interferon action; they also fail to reveal why the antiviral state acts selectively against viral mRNAs and not cellular mRNAs.

D. Clinical Studies: It was originally hoped that interferons might be the answer to prevention of respiratory infections in which many different viruses may be involved. However, because high doses of interferons must be given frequently intranasally for several days prior to virus exposure to be effective, their use turns out to be impractical. Interferon treatment may be helpful in certain severe viral infections (rabies, hemorrhagic fever, herpes encephalitis) and in some persistent viral infections (hepatitis B, laryngeal papillomas, herpes zoster or varicella in lymphoma patients, cytomegalovirus in renal transplant recipients). Topical interferon in the eye may suppress herpetic keratitis and accelerate healing.

Large amounts of interferon are required for clinical trials, because million-unit injections are usually given daily. The availability of cloned interferon now permits large-scale testing of pure materials. Preliminary clinical trials testing interferons as anticancer agents (on the basis of their cell regulatory and immunomodulation properties) show limited but promising results. Surprisingly, IFN-α has displayed the most antitumor activity. IFN-γ would be expected to be most effective because of its higher anticellular activity in vitro, but it appears to be ineffective clinically.

Clinical studies using recombinant IFN-α showed that interferon therapy was effective in controlling hepatitis C viral infection of the liver (Chapter 35). Relapse after cessation of treatment was common.

Interferons exhibit toxic side effects, even when purified material is tested. Gastrointestinal and nervous system side effects proportionate to the dose given are common. Bone marrow suppression also may occur. Theoretically, interferon inducers could be administered therapeutically, but every inducer that has been carefully studied has also been found to be toxic.

Viral Vaccines

A. General Principles: Immunity to viral infection is based on the development of an immune response to specific antigens located on the surface of viral particles or virus-infected cells. For enveloped viruses, the important antigens are the surface glycoproteins. Although infected animals may develop antibodies against virion core proteins or nonstructural proteins involved in viral replication, that immune response is believed to play little or no role in the development of resistance to infection.

Vaccines are available for the prevention of several significant human diseases. Currently available vaccines, described in detail in the chapters dealing with specific virus families and diseases, are summarized in Table 30–8. Certain general principles apply to most viral vaccines for use in the prevention of human disease.

The pathogenesis of a particular viral infection influences the objectives of immunoprophylaxis. Mucosal immunity (local IgA) is important in resistance to infection by viruses that replicate exclusively in mucosal membranes (rhinoviruses, influenza viruses, rotaviruses). Viruses that have a viremic mode of spread (polio, hepatitis, measles) are controlled by serum antibodies. Cell-mediated immunity also is involved in protection against systemic infections (measles, herpes).

Neither vaccination nor recovery from natural infection always results in total protection against a later

Table 30–8. Principal vaccines used in prevention of viral diseases of humans.

Disease	Source of Vaccine	Condition of Virus	Route of Administration
Immunization Recommended for General Public			
Poliomyelitis	Tissue culture (human diploid cell line, monkey kidney)	Live attenuated	Oral
		Killed	Subcutaneous
Measles[1]	Tissue culture (chick embryo)	Live attenuated[2]	Subcutaneous[3]
Mumps[1]	Tissue culture (chick embryo)	Live attenuated	Subcutaneous
Rubella[1,4]	Tissue culture (duck embryo, rabbit, or human diploid)	Live attenuated	Subcutaneous
Immunization Recommended Only Under Certain Conditions (Epidemics, Exposure, Travel, Military)			
Smallpox[5]	Lymph from calf or sheep (glycerolated, lyophilized) Chorioallantois, tissue cultures (lyophilized)	Live vaccinia	Intradermal: multiple pressure, multiple puncture
Yellow fever	Tissue cultures and eggs (17D strain)	Live attenuated	Subcutaneous or intradermal
Hepatitis type B	Purified HBsAg from "healthy" carriers; HBsAg from recombinant DNA in yeast	Subunit	Intramuscular
Influenza	Highly purified or subunit forms of chick embryo allantoic fluid (formalinized or UV-irradiated)	Killed	Intramuscular
Rabies	Duck embryo or human diploid cells	Killed	Intramuscular
Adenovirus[6]	Human diploid cell cultures	Live attenuated	Oral, by enteric-coated capsule
Japanese B encephalitis[7]	Mouse brain (formalinized), tissue culture	Killed	Subcutaneous
Venezuelan equine encephalomyelitis[8]	Guinea pig heart cell culture	Live attenuated	Subcutaneous
Eastern equine encephalomyelitis[7]	Chick embryo cell culture	Killed	Subcutaneous
Western equine encephalomyelitis[7]	Chick embryo cell culture	Killed	Subcutaneous
Russian spring-summer encephalitis[7]	Mouse brain (formalinized)	Killed	Subcutaneous

[1]Available also as combined vaccines.

[2]Killed measles vaccine was available for a short period. However, a serious delayed hypersensitivity reaction sometimes occurred when children who had received primary immunization with killed measles vaccine were later exposed to live measles virus. Because of this complication, killed measles vaccine is no longer used.

[3]With less attenuated strains, immune globulin USP is given in another limb at the time of vaccination.

[4]Neither monovalent rubella vaccine nor combination vaccines incorporating rubella should be administered to a postpubertal susceptible woman unless she is not pregnant and understands that it is imperative not to become pregnant for at least 3 months after vaccination. (The time immediately postpartum has been suggested as a safe period for vaccination.)

[5]Since smallpox virus has been totally eradicated from the world, vaccination is no longer recommended. However, stocks of vaccine are held in depots if cases should reappear.

[6]Licensed but recommended only for military populations in which epidemic respiratory disease caused by adenovirus is a frequent occurrence. Types 4 and 7 are available as vaccines.

[7]Not available in the USA except for the armed forces or for investigative purposes.

[8]Available for use in domestic animals (from the US Department of Agriculture) and for investigative purposes.

infection with the same virus. This situation holds true for diseases for which successful control measures are available, including polio, smallpox, influenza, rubella, measles, mumps, and adenovirus infections. Control can be achieved by limiting the multiplication of virulent virus upon subsequent exposure and preventing its spread to target organs where the pathologic damage is done (eg, polio and measles viruses must be kept from the brain and spinal cord; rubella virus must be kept from the embryo). Recently, Marek's disease, a widespread lymphoproliferative tumor caused by a herpesvirus of domestic chickens, has been brought under control by an attenuated live-virus vaccine. The vaccine results in a lifelong active infection of the chicken. It does not prevent superinfection of the vaccinated animal with the virulent virus, but it does prevent the appearance of the tumor. This is the first practical cancer vaccine that has been developed. A second cancer vaccine—hepatitis B vaccine to prevent primary hepatocellular carcinoma in areas with high chronic carrier rates—is now in use.

Certain characteristics of a virus or of a viral disease may complicate the generation of an effective vaccine. The existence of many serotypes, as with rhinoviruses, and of large animal reservoirs, as with influenza virus, makes vaccine production difficult. Other hurdles include the integration of viral DNA into host chromosomal DNA (retroviruses), transmission of infection by cells that may not express viral antigen (human immunodeficiency virus), and infection of cells of the host's immune system (human immunodeficiency virus).

B. Killed-Virus Vaccines: Killed-virus vaccines are made by purifying viral preparations to a certain extent and then inactivating viral infectivity in a way that does minimal damage to the viral structural proteins; mild formalin treatment is frequently used.

Killed-virus vaccines prepared from whole virions generally stimulate the development of circulating antibody against the coat proteins of the virus, conferring some degree of resistance. For some diseases, killed-virus vaccines are currently the only ones available.

The following disadvantages apply to killed-virus vaccines:

(1) Extreme care is required in their manufacture to make certain that no residual live virulent virus is present in the vaccine.

(2) The immunity conferred is often brief and must be boosted, which not only involves the logistic problem of repeatedly reaching the persons in need of immunization but also has caused concern about the possible effects (hypersensitivity reactions) of repeated administration of foreign proteins.

(3) Parenteral administration of killed-virus vaccine, even when it stimulates circulating antibody (IgM, IgG) to satisfactory levels, has sometimes given limited protection because local resistance (IgA) is not induced adequately at the natural portal of entry or primary site of multiplication of the wild virus infection—eg, nasopharynx for respiratory viruses, alimentary tract for poliovirus (see Figure 30–10 and Chapters 36 and 39).

(4) The cell-mediated response to inactivated vaccines is generally poor.

(5) Some killed-virus vaccines have induced hypersensitivity to subsequent infection, perhaps owing to an unbalanced immune response to viral surface antigens that fails to mimic infection with natural virus.

C. Attenuated Live-Virus Vaccines: Live-virus vaccines utilize viral mutants that antigenically overlap with wild-type virus but are restricted in some step in the pathogenesis of disease.

The development of viral strains suitable for live-virus vaccines previously was done chiefly by selecting naturally attenuated strains or by cultivating the virus serially in various hosts and cultures in the hope of deriving an attenuated strain fortuitously. The search for such strains is now being approached by laboratory manipulations aimed at specific, planned, genetic alterations in the virus (eg, rabies, influenza, respiratory syncytial viruses).

Attenuated live-virus vaccines have the advantage of acting like the natural infection with regard to their effect on immunity. They multiply in the host and tend to stimulate longer-lasting antibody production, to induce a good cell-mediated response, and to induce antibody production and resistance at the portal of entry (Figure 30–10).

The disadvantages of attenuated live-virus vaccines include the following:

(1) The risk of reversion to greater virulence during multiplication within the vaccinee. Although reversion

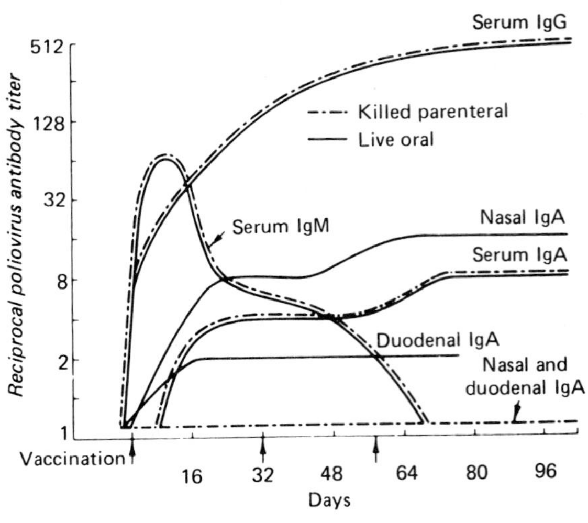

Figure 30–10. Serum and secretory antibody response to orally administered, live attenuated poliovaccine and to intramuscular inoculation of killed poliovaccine. (Reproduced, with permission, from Ogra et al: Rev Infect Dis 1980;2:352.)

has not proved to be a problem in practice, its potential exists.

(2) Unrecognized adventitious agents latently infecting the culture substrate (eggs, primary cell cultures) may enter the vaccine stocks. Viruses found in vaccines have included avian leukosis virus, simian papovavirus SV40, and simian cytomegalovirus. The problem of adventitious contaminants may be circumvented through the use of normal cells serially propagated in culture (eg, human diploid cell lines) as substrates for cultivation of vaccine viruses. Vaccines prepared in such cultures have been in use for years.

(3) There is the potential problem that the live vaccine virus may produce persistent infections in the vaccinee. The actual risk of this is unknown, but it appears to be very low.

(4) The storage and limited shelf life of attenuated vaccines present problems, but this can be overcome in some cases by the use of viral stabilizers (eg, $MgCl_2$ for poliovaccine).

(5) Interference by coinfection with a naturally occurring, wild-type virus may inhibit replication of the vaccine virus and decrease its effectiveness. This has been noted with the vaccine strains of poliovirus, which can be inhibited by concurrent infections by various enteroviruses.

D. Proper Use of Present Vaccines: One fact cannot be overemphasized: An effective vaccine does not protect against disease until it is administered in the proper dosage to susceptible individuals. Failure to reach all sectors of the population with complete courses of immunization is reflected in the continued occurrence of paralytic poliomyelitis and measles in unvaccinated persons. Preschool children in poverty areas are the least adequately vaccinated group in the USA.

There was a theoretical possibility that antibody response might be diminished or that interference might occur if two or more live-virus vaccines were given at the same time. In practice, however, simultaneous administration of live-virus vaccines can be safe and effective. Trivalent live oral poliovaccine (when given in three doses) or a combined live measles, mumps, and rubella vaccine, given by injection, is effective. Antibody response to each component of these combination vaccines is comparable with antibody response to the individual vaccines given separately.

As indicated in Table 30–8, certain viral vaccines are recommended for use by the general public. Other vaccines are recommended only for use by persons at special risk due to occupation, travel, or life-style.

E. Future Prospects: Molecular biology and modern technologies are combining to make possible novel approaches to vaccine development. The ultimate success of these new approaches remains to be determined.

1. Attenuation of viruses by genetic manipulation–This is being utilized to produce recombinants or mutants that can serve as live-virus vaccines.

The introduction of deletion mutations that damage the virus but do not completely inactivate it should yield a vaccine candidate unlikely to revert to virulence.

2. Use of avirulent viral vectors–The concept is to use recombinant DNA techniques to insert the gene coding for the protein of interest into the genome of an avirulent virus that can be administered as the vaccine. The prototype vector under study is vaccinia virus. Other viral vectors possessing large genomes (eg, herpesvirus) are also under study.

3. Purified proteins produced using cloned genes–Viral genes can now be easily cloned into plasmids. This cloned DNA can then be expressed in prokaryotic or eukaryotic cells if appropriately engineered constructions are used. The immunizing antigens of hepatitis B virus, rabies virus, herpes simplex virus, foot-and-mouth disease virus, and influenza virus have been successfully synthesized in bacteria or yeast cells. If the bacteria can be made to produce the antigen in sufficient quantity and immunogenicity, the production of a purified vaccine containing only the immunizing antigen will be facilitated. Interestingly, it is apparent that the glycosylation of viral surface glycoproteins is not always essential for antigenicity. Unglycosylated herpesvirus proteins synthesized in bacteria have been able to induce neutralizing antibodies in test animals.

4. Synthetic peptides–Viral nucleic acids can be readily sequenced and the amino acid sequence of the gene products predicted. It is now technically possible to synthesize short peptides that correspond to antigenic determinants on a viral protein.

Antigenically active polypeptides synthesized for hepatitis B, influenza, and polioviruses have produced neutralizing antibodies in animals. The possibility of producing synthetic immunizing antigens for human vaccination is now being explored. Chemical synthesis would preclude exposure of vaccinees to viral nucleic acid, thereby avoiding any possibility of reversion to virulence. The problem of contaminating cellular proteins also would be avoided.

Although this approach holds promise, there are several obstacles to be overcome. The immune response induced by synthetic peptides is considerably weaker than that induced by intact protein or inactivated virus. It is not easy to identify peptide sequences able to induce a protective immune response. A single peptide representing a single epitope may not be able to induce resistance against a viral protein containing multiple antigenic determinants. Finally, not all antigenic determinants are sequential; it may be very difficult to simulate conformational determinants (ie, those determined by the tertiary configuration of the protein, which juxtaposes amino acids that may be widely separated in the primary sequence).

5. Subunit vaccines–Subviral components are being obtained by breaking apart the virion to include in the vaccine only those viral components needed to stimulate protective antibody. This approach, coupled with better purification procedures, can eliminate nonviral proteins and reduce the possibility of adverse reactions to the vaccine. Purified material can be administered in more concentrated form, containing greatly increased amounts of the specifically desired antigen.

6. Naked DNA vaccines–An unexpectedly effective approach involves the use of gene vaccines, or antigen-encoding DNAs. Cells take up the DNA and produce the immunizing protein. Efficient immunization has been achieved in animals using a "gene gun" to deliver DNA-coated gold beads to the epidermis. Many questions remain to be answered about this novel approach to vaccine production, but naked DNA holds the promise of being a simple, cheap, and safe vaccine.

7. Local administration of vaccine–Intranasally administered aerosol vaccines are being developed, particularly for respiratory disease viruses and also for measles virus. It is hoped that they will stimulate local antibody at the portal of entry.

8. Conventional vaccines–While these new approaches are being pursued, efforts also continue to develop more conventional vaccines in certain systems.

Considerable success has been claimed for a varicella-zoster vaccine developed in Japan and currently undergoing testing in the USA. There is some concern about the possibility of vaccinated subjects contracting zoster in later life. Vaccines are also under development for cytomegalovirus and Epstein-Barr virus. A vaccine is also being tested for respiratory syncytial virus.

REFERENCES

Advisory Committee on Immunization Practices: General recommendations on immunization. Morb Mortal Wkly Rep 1994;43(Suppl RR-1).

Arnon R (editor): *Synthetic Vaccines.* CRC Press, 1987.

Davis GL et al: Treatment of chronic hepatitis C with recombinant interferon alfa: A multicenter, randomized, controlled trial. N Engl J Med 1989;321:1501.

Fields BN et al (editors): *Virology,* 2nd ed. Raven Press, 1990.

Fynan EF et al: DNA vaccines: Protective immunizations by parenteral, mucosal, and gene-gun inoculations. Proc Natl Acad Sci USA 1993;90:11478.

Hermans PE, Cockerill FR III: Antiviral agents. Mayo Clin Proc 1987;62:1108.

Marsden HS (guest editor): Antiviral therapies. Semin Virol 1992;3:No. 1. [Entire issue.]

Smith GL, Mackett M, Moss B: Infectious vaccinia virus recombinants that express hepatitis B virus surface antigen. Nature 1983;302:490.

Taylor JL, Grossberg SE: Recent progress in interferon research: Molecular mechanisms of regulation, action, and virus circumvention. Virus Res 1990;15:1.

White DO: *Antiviral Chemotherapy, Interferons and Vaccines.* Vol 16 of: *Monographs in Virology.* Melnick JL (editor). Karger, 1984.

Yarchoan R et al: Clinical pharmacology of 3′-azido-2′,3′-dideoxythymidine (zidovudine) and related dideoxynucleosides. N Engl J Med 1989;321:726.

Parvoviruses 31

Parvoviruses are the simplest DNA animal viruses. Because of the small coding capacity of their genome, viral replication is dependent on functions supplied by replicating host cells or by coinfecting helper viruses. One human parvovirus is the cause of aplastic crisis; of erythema infectiosum ("fifth disease"), a common childhood exanthem; of a polyarthralgia syndrome in normal adults; and of fetal death.

PROPERTIES OF PARVOVIRUSES

Important properties of parvoviruses are listed in Table 31–1.

Structure & Composition

The icosahedral, nonenveloped particles are 18–26 nm in diameter (Figure 31–1). Virions contain two coat proteins which are encoded by a common DNA sequence. The minor VP1 protein (83 kDa) is identical in sequence to the major VP2 protein (58 kDa) except that VP1 contains an additional 227 residues. The genome is a 5.6 kb, linear, single-stranded DNA. An autonomous virus, H1, contains 5176 bases, whereas a defective parvovirus, AAV-2, contains 4675 bases. Autonomous parvoviruses usually encapsidate only DNA strands complementary to viral mRNA; defective viruses tend to encapsidate DNA strands of both polarities with equal frequency into separate virions.

Classification

The genus *Parvovirus* is able to replicate autonomously in rapidly dividing cells. Human parvovirus B19 belongs to this genus, as do feline panleukopenia virus and canine parvovirus, both serious pathogens of veterinary diseases. The genus *Dependovirus* contains members that are defective and depend on a helper virus (usually an adenovirus) for replication. Human "adenoassociated viruses" have not been linked with any disease.

PARVOVIRUS INFECTIONS IN HUMANS

Pathogenesis & Pathology

Human parvovirus B19 has been implicated as the causative agent of several diseases. Nondefective parvoviruses require dividing host cells in order to replicate, and known parvovirus diseases reflect that target specificity. Immature cells in the erythroid lineage are targets for human B19 parvovirus. Viral replication causes cell death, interrupting red cell production. In immunocompromised patients, persistent B19 infections occur, resulting in chronic anemia. In cases of fetal death, chronic infections may have caused severe anemia in the fetus. Several pathogenic parvoviruses of animals replicate in intestinal mucosal cells and cause enteritis.

B19 can be found in blood and respiratory secretions of infected patients. Transmission is presumably by the respiratory route. The virus can be transmitted parenterally by blood transfusions or by infected blood products and vertically from mother to fetus. The rash associated with erythema infectiosum may be immune complex-mediated.

In cell cultures, defective parvoviruses of humans (adenoassociated viruses) establish latent infections in which adenoassociated virus DNA is integrated into the cellular genome. When the cell is superinfected with a helper virus, the adenoassociated virus genome is readily rescued. Integration of parvovirus DNA has no observable effect on the phenotype of the cell, but it allows the biologic survival of the defective viral genome until an appropriate helper virus becomes available for replication. Adenoassociated viruses are not known to cause disease.

Clinical Findings

A. Erythema Infectiosum (Fifth Disease): The most common manifestation of human parvovirus B19

Table 31–1. Important properties of parvoviruses.

Virion: Icosahedral, 18–26 nm in diameter, 32 capsomers.
Composition: DNA (20%), protein (80%).
Genome: Single-stranded DNA, linear, 5.6 kb, MW 1.5–2.2 million.
Proteins: Two coat proteins.
Envelope: None.
Replication: Nucleus, dependent on functions of dividing host cells.
Outstanding characteristics: Very simple viruses; one genus is replication-defective and requires a helper virus.

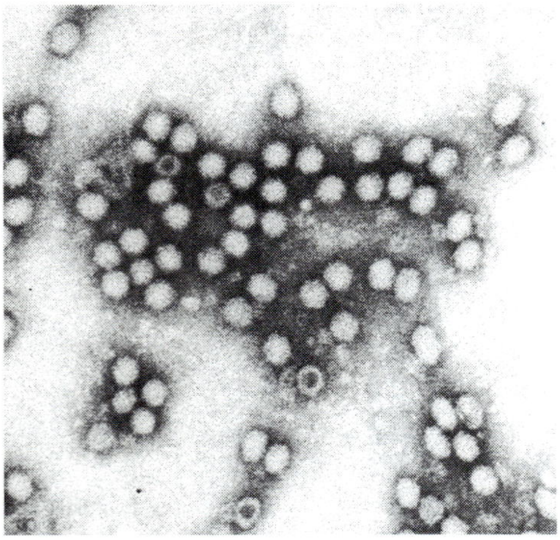

Figure 31–1. Electron micrograph of parvovirus particles. (Courtesy of FA Murphy and EL Palmer.)

infection is erythema infectiosum, or fifth disease. This erythematous illness is most common in children of early school age and occasionally affects adults. Mild constitutional symptoms may accompany the rash, which has a typical "slapped-cheek" appearance. Joint involvement is a prominent feature in adult cases; joints in the hands and the knees are most frequently affected. Both sporadic cases and epidemics have been described.

The incubation period is usually 4–14 days but may extend to 20 days. Viremia occurs 1 week after infection and persists for about 5 days. During the period of viremia, virus is present in nasal washes and gargle specimens, identifying the upper respiratory tract—most probably the pharynx—as the site of viral shedding. The first phase of illness occurs at the end of the first week; symptoms include fever, malaise, myalgia, chills, and itching. The first episode of illness coincides in time with viremia and, more particularly, with detection of circulating IgM-parvovirus immune complexes. After an incubation period of about 17 days, a second phase of illness begins. The appearance of an erythematous facial rash and a lace-like rash on the limbs or trunk may be accompanied by joint symptoms, especially in adults. The illness is short-lived, with the rash fading after 2 or 3 days, although the joint symptoms may persist longer.

B. Transient Aplastic Crisis: Parvovirus B19 is the cause of transient aplastic crisis that may complicate chronic hemolytic anemia, eg, in patients with sickle cell disease. The infection lowers production of erythrocytes, causing a reduction in the hemoglobin level of peripheral blood. The temporary arrest of production of red blood cells becomes apparent only in patients with chronic hemolytic anemia because of the short life span of their erythrocytes; a 7-day interruption in erythropoiesis would not be expected to cause detectable anemia in a normal person. Few anemia patients have a rash.

C. Infection in Immunodeficient Patients: B19 may cause chronic suppression of bone marrow and chronic anemia in immunocompromised patients.

D. Infection During Pregnancy: Maternal infection with B19 virus may pose a serious risk to the fetus, resulting in hydrops fetalis and fetal death. The overall risk of human parvovirus infection during pregnancy is low; fetal loss occurs in less than 10% of primary maternal infections. Fetal death occurs most commonly before the 20th week of pregnancy. There is no evidence that B19 infection causes congenital anomalies.

Laboratory Diagnosis

The most sensitive test for viral detection is nucleic acid hybridization. B19 DNA has been detected in serum, white blood cells, tissue samples, and respiratory secretions.

Detection of B19 IgM antibody is indicative of recent infection. B19 IgG antibody persists for years, though antibody may not be found in immunodeficient patients with chronic B19 infections.

The virus is difficult to grow. Diagnostic tests are currently available only in a few laboratories.

Epidemiology

The B19 virus is widespread. Infections can occur throughout the year, in all age groups, and as outbreaks or as sporadic cases. Infections are most commonly seen as outbreaks in schools. Parvovirus infection is common in childhood; antibody most often develops between the ages of 5 and 19 years; up to 60% of adults are seropositive.

Infection seems to be transmitted via the respiratory tract. Many infections are subclinical. Estimates of attack rates in susceptible contacts range from 20% to 40%.

Transmission of B19 from patients with aplastic crisis to members of the hospital staff has been documented. Patients with aplastic crisis are likely to be infectious during the course of their illness, whereas patients with fifth disease are probably no longer infectious by the time of onset of rash.

Prevention & Control

There is no vaccine against human parvovirus.

Infection control practices should be followed to prevent transmission of B19 to health care workers from patients with aplastic crisis and from immunodeficient patients with chronic B19 infection.

ANIMAL MODEL OF IMMUNE COMPLEX DISEASE

Aleutian Disease of Mink

In a number of the human progressive degenerative disorders of suspected viral cause, the immunologic response of the host to the virus may be responsible for the pathologic changes and for the clinical illness. Aleutian disease of mink is a model for this type of pathogenesis. Aleutian disease of mink is a chronic immune complex disease initiated by a parvovirus. Virus circulates from the acute stage of infection onward and can be found in many organs and in serum and urine. Antibody is produced in large quantity, so there is IgG hyperglobulinemia. The virus complexes with the antibody without being neutralized. Virus-antibody complexes circulate and then deposit in glomeruli, leading to renal failure and death. The failure of viral neutralization and elimination by the excess antibody is not entirely understood.

REFERENCES

Anand A et al: Human parvovirus infection in pregnancy and hydrops fetalis. N Engl J Med 1987;316:183.

Anderson MJ et al: Experimental parvoviral infection in humans. J Infect Dis 1985;152:257.

Bansal GP et al: Candidate recombinant vaccine for human B19 parvovirus. J Infect Dis 1993;167:1034.

Centers for Disease Control: Risks associated with human parvovirus B19 infection. Morb Mortal Wkly Rep 1989; 38:81.

Frickhofen N, Young NS: Persistent parvovirus B19 infections in humans. Microbial Pathogen 1989;7:319.

Umene K, Nunoue T: Partial nucleotide sequencing and characterization of human parvovirus B19 genome DNAs from damaged human fetuses and from patients with leukemia. J Med Virol 1993;39:333.

32 Adenoviruses

Adenoviruses can replicate and produce disease in the eye and in the respiratory, gastrointestinal, and urinary tracts. Many adenovirus infections are subclinical, and virus may persist in the host for months. About one-third of the 41 known human serotypes are responsible for most cases of human adenovirus disease. A few types serve as models for cancer induction in animals. Adenoviruses are especially valuable systems for molecular and biochemical studies of eukaryotic cell processes.

PROPERTIES OF ADENOVIRUSES

Important properties of adenoviruses are listed in Table 32–1.

Structure & Composition

Adenoviruses are 70–90 nm in diameter and display icosahedral symmetry, with capsids composed of 252 capsomers. There is no envelope. Adenoviruses contain 13% DNA and 87% protein. The particle has an estimated molecular weight of 175×10^6. Adenoviruses are unique among icosahedral viruses in that they have a structure called a "fiber" projecting from each of the 12 vertices, or penton bases (Figure 32–1 and Table 32–2). The rest of the capsid is composed of 240 hexon capsomers. The hexons, pentons, and fibers constitute the major adenovirus antigens important in viral classification and disease diagnosis.

The DNA (MW $20–30 \times 10^6$) is linear and double-stranded. The guanine-plus-cytosine content of the DNA is lowest (48–49%) in group A (types 12, 18, and 31) adenoviruses, the most strongly oncogenic types, and ranges as high as 61% in other types. This is one criterion used in grouping human isolates. Viral DNA contains a virus-encoded protein that is covalently linked to each 5′ end of the linear genome. The DNA can be isolated in an infectious form, and the relative infectivity of that DNA is reduced at least 100-fold if the terminal protein is removed by proteolysis. The entire DNA sequence of the genome of adenovirus type 2 (≈35,000 base-pairs) is known.

Molecular characterization of viral DNA from 41 human adenovirus serotypes shows that they can be divided into six groups on the basis of genome homology. The DNA is condensed in the core of the virion in an arrangement resembling 12 large spheres packed tightly together. A virus-encoded protein, polypeptide VII (Table 32–2), is important in forming the core structure.

The major adenovirus antigens, their sizes, and their structural positions in the virion are shown in Table 32–2. Three structural proteins, produced in large excess, constitute "soluble antigens" designated "alpha," "beta," and "gamma." The hexons that form a majority of capsomers possess a group-reactive antigen (alpha). All human adenoviruses display this common hexon antigenicity. Pentons occur at the 12 vertices of the capsid and have fibers protruding from them. The penton base carries a toxin-like activity that causes rapid appearance of cytopathic effects and detachment of cells from the surface on which they are growing. Another group-reactive antigen (beta) is exhibited by the penton base. The fibers contain the type-specific antigens (gamma) that are important in serotyping. Fibers are associated with hemagglutinating activity. Because the hemagglutinin is type-specific, HI tests are commonly used for typing isolates.

Classification

Adenoviruses have been recovered from a wide variety of species and grouped into two genera: one that infects birds (aviadenoviruses) and another that infects mammals (mastadenoviruses). All mammalian adenoviruses share a common antigen detectable by complement fixation. At least 41 distinct antigenic types have been isolated from humans and many other types from various animals.

Human adenoviruses are divided into six groups (A–F) on the basis of their physical, chemical, and biologic properties (Table 32–3). Adenoviruses of a given group have fibers of a characteristic length, display considerable DNA homology (>90%, as compared to <20% with members of other groups), and exhibit similar capacities to agglutinate erythrocytes from either monkeys or rats. Members of a given adenovirus group resemble one another in the guanine-plus-cytosine content of their DNA and in their potential to produce tumors in newborn rodents. Importantly, viruses within a group tend to behave similarly with respect to epidemiologic spread and disease association.

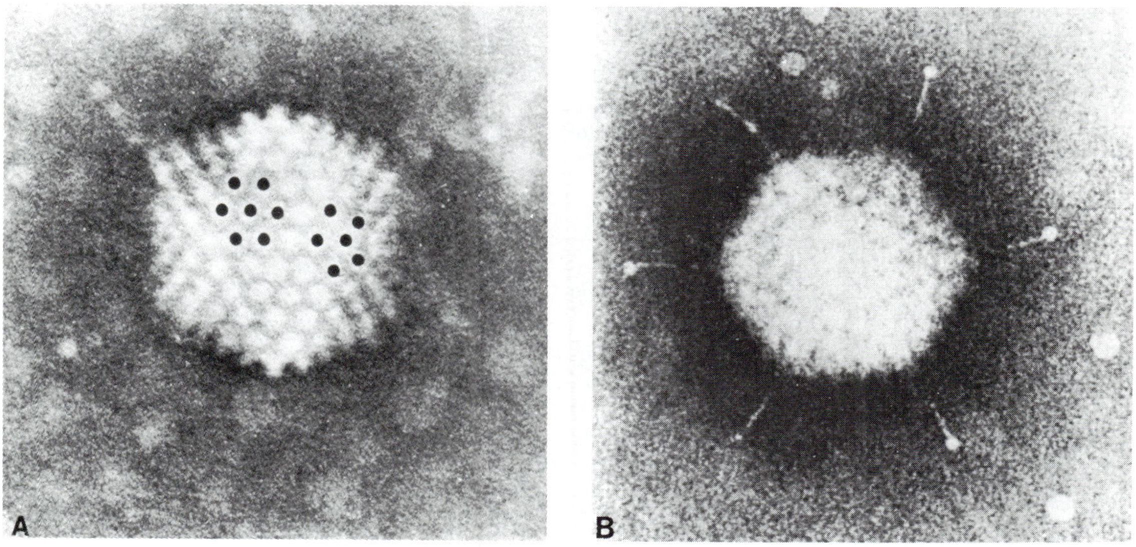

Figure 32–1. Electron micrographs of adenovirus. ***A:*** The viral particle displays cubic symmetry and is nonenveloped. A hexon capsomer (surrounded by six identical hexons) and a penton capsomer (surrounded by five hexons) are marked with dots. ***B:*** Note the fiber structures projecting from the vertex penton capsomers (285,000×). (Reproduced, with permission, from Valentine RC, Pereira HG: Antigens and structure of the adenovirus. J Mol Biol 1965;13:13.)

Adenovirus Replication

Adenoviruses replicate well only in cells of epithelial origin. The replicative cycle is sharply divided into early and late events. The carefully regulated expression of sequential events in the adenovirus cycle is summarized in Figure 32–2.

A. Virus Attachment, Penetration, and Uncoating: The virus attaches to cells via the fiber structures. There are about 100,000 fiber receptors per cell. The viral particle is internalized; the interaction of the penton base with cellular integrins following attachment promotes the internalization step. Uncoating commences in the cytoplasm and is completed in the nucleus. Uncoating is an organized, sequential process that systematically breaks down the stabilizing interactions that were established during maturation of the viral particle. Both proteolytic degradation and selective dissociation are involved in the disassembly process.

Table 32–1. Important properties of adenoviruses.

Virion: Icosahedral, 70–90 nm in diameter, 252 capsomers; fiber projects from each vertex.
Composition: DNA (13%), protein (87%).
Genome: Double-stranded DNA, linear, MW 20–30 million, protein-bound to termini, infectious.
Proteins: Important antigens (hexon, penton base, fiber) are associated with the major outer capsid proteins.
Envelope: None.
Replication: Nucleus.
Outstanding characteristic: Excellent models for molecular studies of eukaryotic cell processes.

B. Early Events: The steps that occur before the onset of viral DNA synthesis are defined as early events. Soon after infection, host macromolecular synthesis is inhibited by an unknown mechanism involving early gene products of the virus. The cessation of host protein synthesis is particularly rapid and is undoubtedly part of the reason infected cells are killed. The E1B region encodes proteins that block cell death (apoptosis) that occurs due to E1A functions; this is necessary to prevent premature cell death that would adversely affect virus yields.

The early ("E") transcripts come from seven widely separated regions of the viral genome and from both viral DNA strands (Figure 32–3). The E1A gene is especially important; it must be expressed in order for the other early regions to be transcribed. The E1A/E1B regions contain the only adenovirus genes involved in cell transformation. More than 20 early proteins, many of which are nonstructural and are involved in viral DNA replication, are synthesized in adenovirus-infected cells. The early proteins are represented by the 75K DNA-binding protein shown in Figure 32–2. The E3 region is nonessential for viral growth in tissue culture but presumably performs some necessary function during viral infection of human hosts.

C. Replication of Viral DNA and Late Events: Viral DNA replication takes place in the nucleus. The virus-encoded, covalently linked terminal protein functions as a primer for initiation of viral DNA synthesis.

Late events begin concomitantly with the onset of viral DNA synthesis. Late ("L") genes coding for viral structural proteins (Figure 32–3) are transcribed, processed, and transported to the cytoplasm, where the viral proteins are synthesized. Although host genes

Table 32–2. Comparative data on adenovirus type 2 morphological and antigenic subunits and protein components.

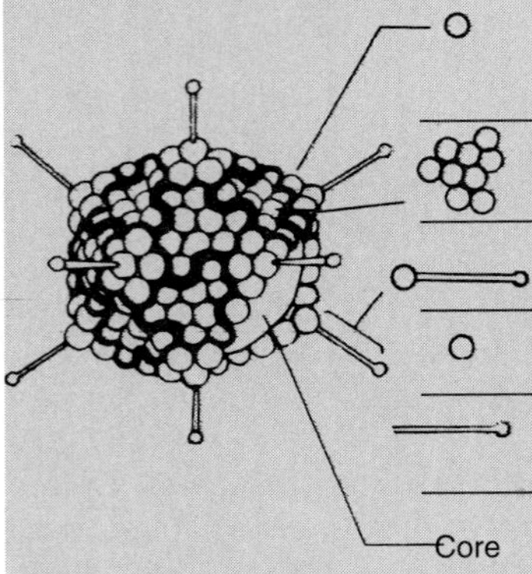

	Morphologic Subunits			Antigenic Subunits		
Appearance	**Name**	**Number Per Virion**	**Molecular Weight**	**Antigen**	**Specificity**	**Protein Components**
Virion	DNA		23,000,000			
	Protein		150,000,000			
	Hexon	240	210,000 400,000 320,000 360,000	Alpha Epsilon	Group Type	II
	Hexons	20	3,600,000			II, VIII, IX
	Penton	12	280,000 1,100,000			III, IV
	Penton base	12	210,000	Beta	Group	III
	Fiber	12	70,000	Gamma Delta	Type Intragroup	IV
Core	DNA	1	23,000,000			
	Protein		29,000,000			V, VI, VII
	Protein		13,000			VII, IX
	Protein		7,500			X

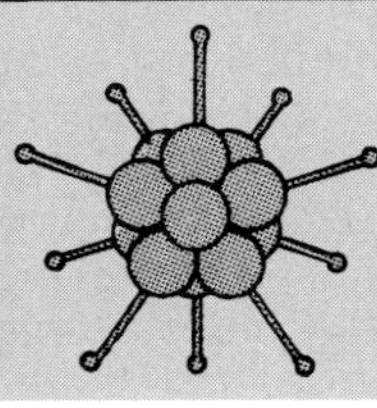

Dodecon: Hemagglutinin made up of 12 pentons with their fibers.

continue to be transcribed in the nucleus late in the course of infection, few host genetic sequences are transported to the cytoplasm. Studies with adenovirus hexon mRNA led to the profound discovery that eukaryotic mRNAs are usually not colinear with their genes but are spliced products of separated coding regions in the genomic DNA. Very large amounts of viral structural proteins are made.

Table 32–3. Classification schemes for human adenoviruses.

		Hemagglutination			Oncogenic Potential	
Group	**Serotypes**	**Group**	**Result**	**Percentage G + C[1] in DNA**	**Tumorigenicity in Vivo[2]**	**Transformation of Cells**
A	12, 18, 31	IV	None	47–49	High	+
B	3, 7, 11, 14, 16, 21, 34, 35	I	Monkey (complete)	50–52	Weak	+
C	1, 2, 5, 6	III	Rat (partial)	57–59	None	+
D	8–10, 13, 15, 17, 19, 20, 22–30, 32, 33, 36–39	II	Rat (complete)	57–60	None	+
E	4	III	Rat (partial)	57	None	+
F	40, 41	III	Rat (partial)			+

[1]G + C, guanine-plus-cytosine.
[2]Tumor induction in newborn hamsters.

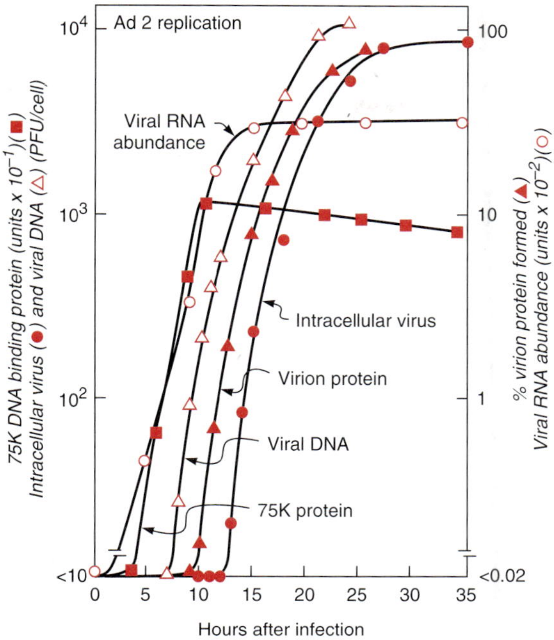

Figure 32–2. Time course of adenovirus replication cycle. The time between infection and the first appearance of progeny virus is the eclipse period. Note the sequential regulation of specific events in the virus replication cycle. "PFU" means "plaque-forming unit," a measure of infectious virus. (From M Green.)

D. Viral Maturation: Virion morphogenesis occurs in the nucleus, but the initial step in the assembly process begins in the cytoplasm. Newly synthesized polypeptides assemble into capsomers in the cytoplasm. Each hexon capsomer is a trimer of identical polypeptides. The penton is composed of five penton base polypeptides and three fiber polypeptides. A virus-encoded "scaffold protein" assists in the aggregation of hexon polypeptides but is not part of the final structure.

Capsomers self-assemble into empty-shell capsids in the nucleus. Naked DNA then enters the preformed capsid by an unknown mechanism, followed by precursor core proteins. Finally, precursor core proteins are cleaved, which allows the particle to tighten its configuration, and several or all of the pentons are added. The mature particle is then stable, infectious, and resistant to nucleases. The assembly process is inefficient, producing some empty particles devoid of DNA and leaving many structural proteins unused in the cell. Structural proteins associated with mature viral particles are catalogued in Table 32–2.

E. Virus Effects on Cells: Adenoviruses are cytopathic for human cell cultures, particularly primary kidney and continuous epithelial cells. Growth of virus in tissue culture is associated with a stimulation of acid production (increased glycolysis) in the early stages of infection. The cytopathic effect usually consists of marked rounding, enlargement, and aggregation of affected cells into grape-like clusters. The infected cells do not lyse even though they round up and leave the glass surface on which they have been grown.

In cells infected with some adenovirus types, rounded intranuclear inclusions containing DNA are seen (Figure 32–4). Such nuclear inclusions may be mistaken for those of cytomegalovirus, but adenovirus infections do not induce syncytia or multinucleated giant cells. Although the cytologic changes are not pathognomonic for adenoviruses, they are helpful for diagnostic purposes in tissue culture and biopsy specimens.

Viral particles in the nucleus frequently exhibit crystalline arrangements (Figure 32–5). Cells infected with group B viruses also contain crystals composed of protein without nucleic acid. About 7000 viral particles are produced per infected cell, and most of them remain within the cell after the cycle is complete and the cell is dead. Crude infected cell lysates show huge quantities of capsomers, sometimes partially assembled into viral components.

Human adenoviruses exhibit a narrow host range. When cells derived from species other than humans are infected, the human adenoviruses usually undergo an abortive replication cycle. Adenovirus early antigens, mRNA, and DNA are all synthesized, but not all capsid proteins and no infectious progeny are produced.

Gene Therapy

There is growing interest in the potential use of adenoviruses as gene-delivery vehicles for gene therapy. Adenoviruses are attractive because replication-defective virus is able to lyse the endosome after internalization and release DNA into the cytoplasm. Efficient delivery of foreign DNA has been achieved by chemically coupling the DNA of interest with adenovirus particles.

Adenovirus Interactions With Other Viruses

A. Defective Parvoviruses: In some adenovirus preparations, small 20-nm particles have been found (Figure 32–6). These have proved to be parvoviruses that cannot replicate unless adenovirus (or sometimes herpesvirus) is present as a helper (see Chapter 31). Adenoassociated viruses contain single-stranded DNA (MW 1.6×10^6) and are serologically unrelated to adenovirus. Although adenoassociated virus can infect cells in the absence of an adenovirus helper and induce a latent infection, it is not involved in the production of any known adenovirus-induced human disease.

B. Adenovirus-SV40 "Hybrids": Human adenovirus replication in monkey kidney cells can be achieved by coinfection with SV40. In the 1960s, certain adenovirus vaccine strains grown in monkey kidney cell cultures inadvertently became "contaminated" with SV40. Some SV40 sequences became covalently linked to the adenovirus DNA, so that sta-

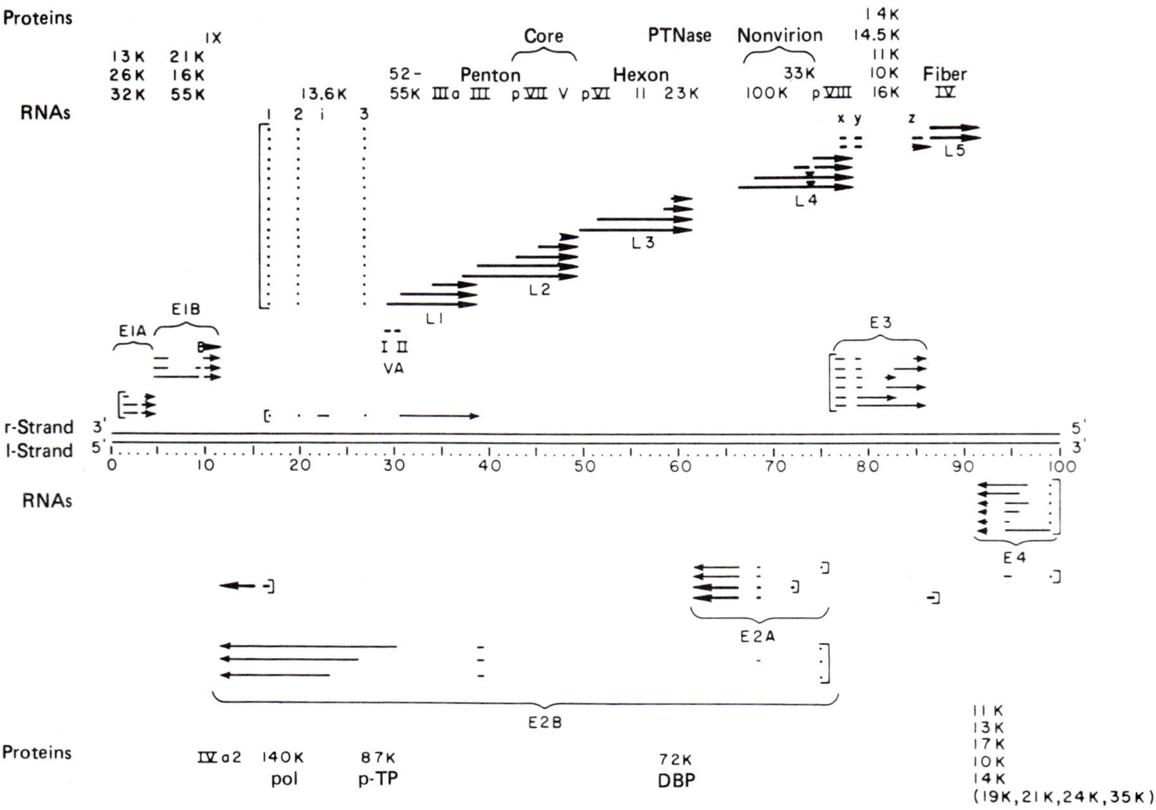

Figure 32–3. Transcription and translation map of adenovirus type 2. The early mRNAs are designated E, and the late mRNAs are labeled L. All late transcripts contain the tripartite leader, denoted 1, 2, and 3. Polypeptides designated by roman numerals are part of the virion; proteins identified in kilodaltons (K) are nonstructural translation products. (Reproduced, with permission, from Broker TR: Animal virus RNA processing. In: *Processing of RNA*. Apirion D [editor]. CRC Press, 1984.)

ble "hybrids" were formed. These hybrids have been very useful in genetic analyses but have no manifest medical relevance.

Animal Susceptibility & Transformation of Cells

Most laboratory animals are not readily infected with human adenoviruses, though newborn hamsters sustain a fatal infection with type 5. Several serotypes, especially types 12, 18, and 31, are able to induce tumors when inoculated into newborn hamsters (Table 32–3). All adenoviruses can morphologically transform cells in culture, regardless of their oncogenic potential in vivo (see Chapter 43). Only a small part (<20%) of the adenovirus genome is present in most transformed cells.

The transforming genes of human adenoviruses are located in the early region (E1A/E1B) at the left-hand end of the viral genome (Figure 32–3). Studies of adenovirus transforming genes have revealed cellular growth control mechanisms that are altered in many types of cancer cells.

The highly oncogenic nature of adenovirus type 12 may be related to the observation that one effect of its early region is to turn off the synthesis of class I major histocompatibility antigens (H2 or HLA) in infected and transformed cells.

Adenovirus DNA or mRNA has never been found in human tumors.

ADENOVIRUS INFECTIONS IN HUMANS

Pathogenesis

Adenoviruses infect epithelial cells of the pharynx, conjunctiva, small intestine, and occasionally other organ systems. They usually do not spread beyond the regional lymph nodes. Group C viruses persist as latent infections for years in adenoids and tonsils and are shed in the feces for many months after the initial infection. Long-term culture of the cells in vitro permits the viruses to grow, but they cannot be isolated directly from suspensions of such tissues. In fact, the

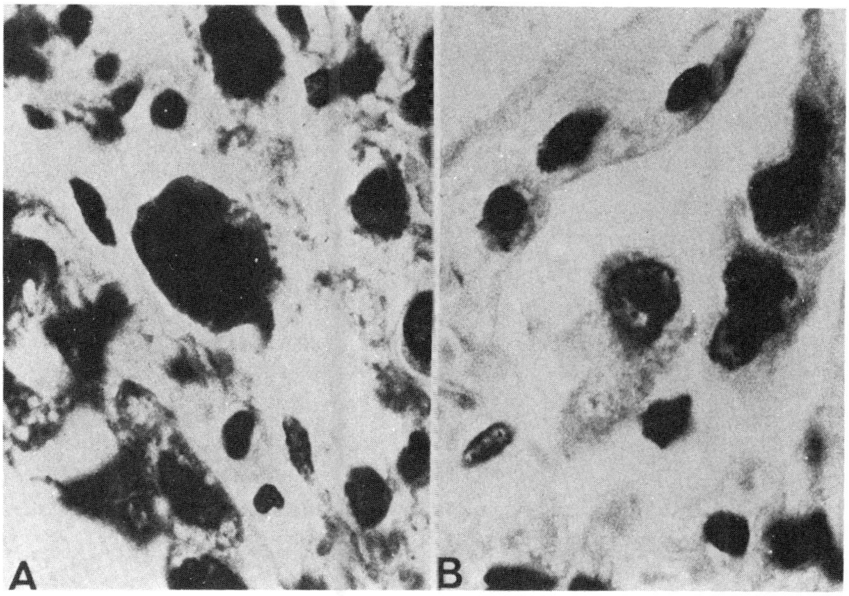

Figure 32–4. Adenovirus cytopathology in human tissue. ***A:*** Lung tissue from a fatal case of adenovirus pneumonia. In the center of the field is a desquamated alveolar lining cell with a basophilic inclusion body filling the entire nucleus and obliterating the nuclear membrane ("smudge cell"). ***B:*** A desquamated cell with less advanced adenovirus cytopathology; there is a smaller nuclear inclusion body, highlighted by a clear halo that is contained within the nuclear membrane (800×). (Reproduced, with permission, from Myerowitz RL et al: Fatal disseminated adenovirus infection in a renal transplant recipient. Am J Med 1975;59:591.)

name "adenovirus" reflects the recovery of the initial isolate from explants of human adenoids.

Most human adenoviruses grow in intestinal epithelium after ingestion but usually produce subclinical infections rather than symptoms or lesions.

Clinical Findings

The association of human adenoviruses with clinical diseases is listed in Table 32–4. About one-third of the known human serotypes are commonly associated with human illness. It should be noted that a single serotype may cause different clinical diseases and, conversely, that more than one type may cause the same clinical illness. Adenoviruses 1–7 are the most common types worldwide and account for most instances of adenovirus-associated illness.

Adenoviruses are responsible for about 5% of acute respiratory disease in young children, but they account for much less in adults. The viruses occasionally cause disease in other organs, particularly the eye and the gastrointestinal tract.

A. Respiratory Diseases: Typical symptoms include cough, nasal congestion, headache, and coryza, but these may be accompanied by systemic symptoms of fever, chills, malaise, and myalgia. Four different syndromes of respiratory infection have been linked to adenoviruses.

1. Acute febrile pharyngitis–Most commonly manifested in infants and children, this syndrome usually involves group C viruses. Symptoms include cough, stuffy nose, fever, and sore throat. Some of these cases are difficult to distinguish from other mild viral respiratory infections that may exhibit similar symptoms.

2. Pharyngoconjunctival fever–The symptoms are similar to those of acute febrile pharyngitis, but conjunctivitis is also present. Pharyngoconjunctival fever tends to occur in outbreaks, such as at children's summer camps ("swimming pool conjunctivitis"). Group B viruses, principally types 3, 7, and 14, are most often implicated.

3. Acute respiratory disease–This syndrome is characterized by pharyngitis, fever, cough, and malaise. It occurs in epidemic form among young military recruits under conditions of fatigue and crowding soon after induction. This disease is caused by types 4 and 7 and occasionally by type 3.

4. Pneumonia–Adenoviral pneumonia is a complication of acute respiratory disease in military recruits. Children may also develop severe and sometimes fatal pneumonia following infection with common types, particularly types 3 and 7. Adenoviral pneumonia has been reported to have an 8–10% mortality rate in the very young.

B. Eye Infections: Mild ocular involvement may be part of the respiratory-pharyngeal syndromes caused by adenoviruses. Complete recovery with no lasting sequelae is the common outcome. Swimming

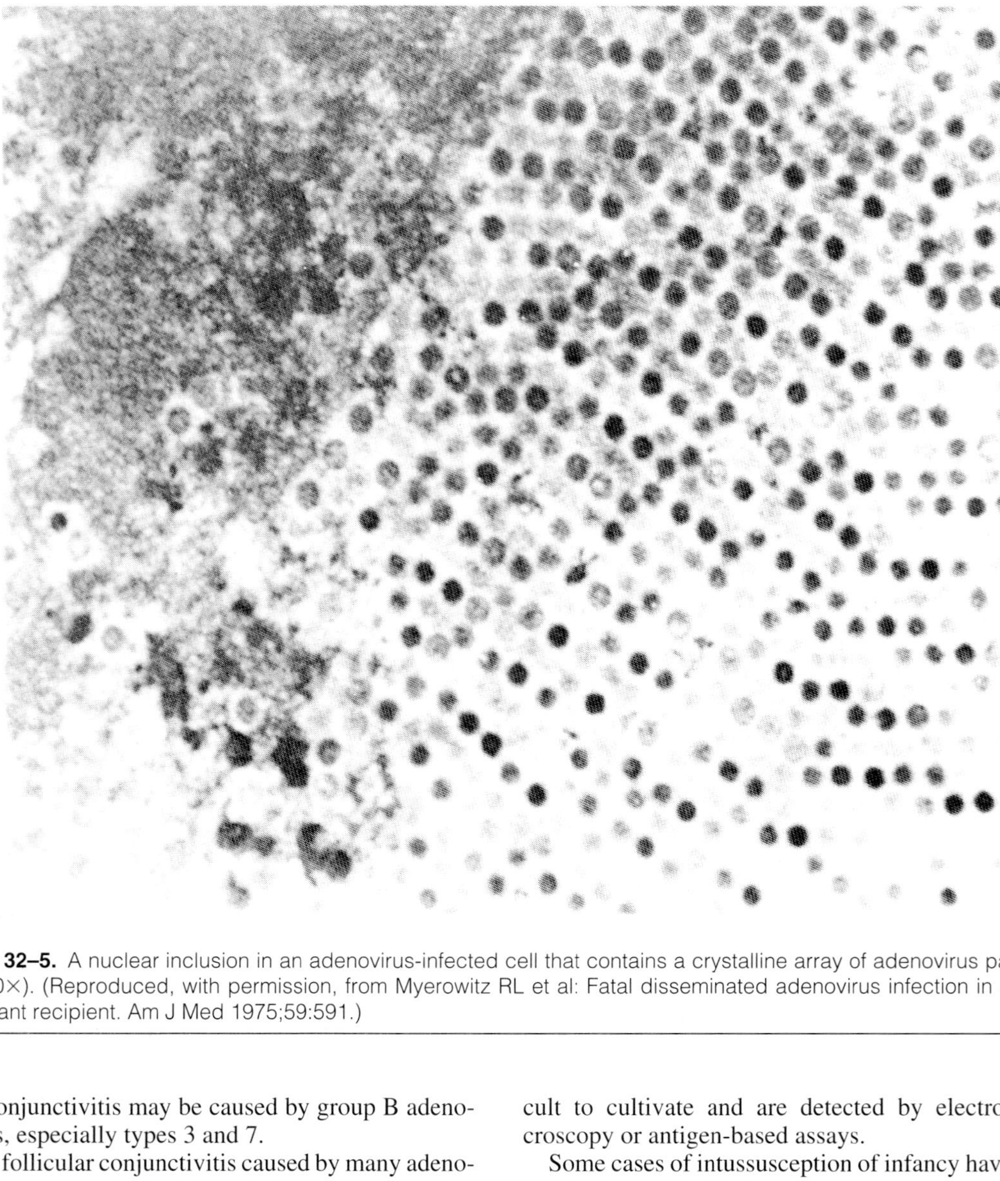

Figure 32–5. A nuclear inclusion in an adenovirus-infected cell that contains a crystalline array of adenovirus particles (59,500×). (Reproduced, with permission, from Myerowitz RL et al: Fatal disseminated adenovirus infection in a renal transplant recipient. Am J Med 1975;59:591.)

pool conjunctivitis may be caused by group B adenoviruses, especially types 3 and 7.

The follicular conjunctivitis caused by many adenovirus types resembles chlamydial conjunctivitis (see Chapter 28) and is self-limited.

A more serious disease is epidemic keratoconjunctivitis. This disease is highly contagious and characterized by acute conjunctivitis, with enlarged, tender preauricular nodes, followed by keratitis that leaves round subepithelial opacities in the cornea for up to 2 years. It is caused by types 8, 19, and 37.

C. Gastrointestinal Disease: Many adenoviruses replicate in intestinal cells and are present in stools, but the presence of the common types is not associated with gastrointestinal disease. However, two serotypes (types 40 and 41) have been etiologically associated with infantile gastroenteritis and may account for 5–15% of cases of viral gastroenteritis in young children. These viruses are abundantly present in diarrheic stools. The enteric adenoviruses are very difficult to cultivate and are detected by electron microscopy or antigen-based assays.

Some cases of intussusception of infancy have been ascribed to group C adenoviruses.

D. Other Diseases: Types 11 and 21 may cause acute hemorrhagic cystitis in children, especially boys. Virus commonly occurs in the urine of such patients. Type 37 occurs in cervical lesions and in male urethritis and may be sexually transmitted.

Immunocompromised patients may suffer from adenovirus infections, though not as often as from herpesvirus infections. The most common problem caused by adenovirus infection in transplant patients is severe pneumonia, which may be fatal (usually types 1–7). Children receiving liver transplants may develop adenovirus hepatitis in the allograft. In one study involving 262 pediatric transplant recipients, 22 patients developed adenovirus infections and 5 of those included adenovirus hepatitis (caused by type 5). Two died of liver failure. Patients with acquired immuno-

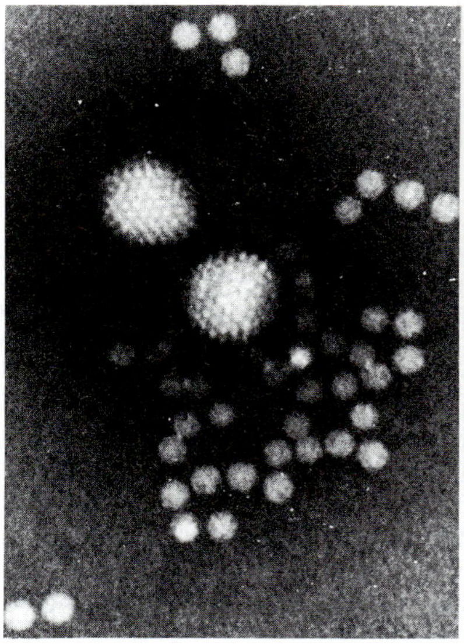

Figure 32–6. A group of adenoassociated satellite viruses surrounding two adenovirions that function as helpers for the defective parvoviruses (250,000×). (HD Mayor, L Jordan, and JL Melnick.)

deficiency syndrome (AIDS) may suffer adenovirus infections, often with type 35.

Immunity

In contrast to most respiratory agents, the adenoviruses induce effective and long-lasting immunity against reinfection. This may reflect the fact that adenoviruses also infect the regional lymph nodes and lymphoid cells in the gastrointestinal tract. Resistance to clinical disease appears to be directly related to the presence of circulating neutralizing antibodies. Although type-specific neutralizing antibodies may protect against disease symptoms, they may not always prevent reinfection. (Infections with adenoviruses are frequently induced without the production of overt illness.)

Maternal antibodies usually protect infants against severe adenovirus respiratory infections. Neutralizing antibodies against one or more types have been detected in over 50% of infants 6–11 months old. Normal, healthy adults generally have antibodies to several types. Neutralizing antibodies to types 1, 2, and 5 occur in 40–60% of individuals aged 6–15 years, but antibodies to types 3 and 4 are less prevalent. Neutralizing antibodies probably persist for life.

The CF test measures a group-reactive antibody response, different from the type-specific neutralizing antibody. Complement-fixing antibodies are not protective and decline with time. Such antibodies do not reveal the serotypes of previous viral infections. Young children sometimes do not develop complement-fixing antibodies during adenovirus infections. Older individuals with neutralizing antibodies to four or more strains frequently give completely negative complement-fixing reactions. The incidence of infection in military recruits (especially due to types 3 and 4) is not influenced by the presence of group complement-fixing antibodies.

Table 32–4. Illnesses associated with human adenoviruses.

Group	Principal Types	Disease
B	3, 7, 14 7, 14, 21 3, 7 11, 21 34, 35	Pharyngoconjunctival fever. Acute respiratory disease. Pneumonia. Hemorrhagic cystitis. Pneumonia with dissemination; persistence in urinary tract.
C	1, 2, 5, 6	Acute febrile pharyngitis in small children, latent infection in lymphatic tissue.
D	8, 19, 37	Epidemic keratoconjunctivitis, cervicitis, urethritis.
E	4	Acute respiratory disease with fever, pneumonia.
F	40, 41	Gastroenteritis.

Laboratory Diagnosis

A. Isolation and Identification of Virus: Depending on the clinical disease, virus may be recovered from stool or urine or from a throat, conjunctival, or rectal swab. Viral isolation in a cell culture requires human cells. Primary human embryonic kidney cells are most susceptible but usually unavailable. Established human epithelial cell lines, such as HeLa and KB, are sensitive but are difficult to maintain without degeneration for the length of time (28 days) required to detect some slow-growing natural isolates. The development of characteristic cytopathic effects—rounding and clustering of swollen cells—indicates the presence of adenovirus in inoculated cultures. Adenoviruses cause increased glycolysis in cells, so the growth medium tends to become highly acidic on infected cultures.

Isolates can be identified as adenoviruses by using fluorescent antibody or CF tests to detect group-specific antigens. This is done using an antihexon antibody and culture fluid from infected cells. HI and Nt tests measure type-specific antigens and can be used to identify specific serotypes.

Characterization of viral DNA by hybridization or by restriction endonuclease digestion patterns can identify an isolate as an adenovirus and group it. These approaches are especially useful for types that are difficult to cultivate.

The fastidious enteric adenoviruses can be detected by direct examination of fecal extracts by electron microscopy or by ELISA. With difficulty, they can be isolated in a line of human embryonic kidney cells transformed with a fragment of adenovirus 5 DNA (293 cells).

Since adenoviruses can persist in the gut and in lymphoid tissue for long periods and since recrudescent viral shedding can be precipitated by other infections, the significance of a viral isolation must be interpreted with caution. Viral recovery from the eye, lung, or genital tract is diagnostic of current infection. Isolation of virus from throat secretions of a patient with respiratory illness can be considered relevant to the clinical disease. Viral isolation from fecal specimens is inconclusive unless one of the fastidious types is recovered from a patient with gastroenteritis.

B. Serology: Infection of humans with any adenovirus type stimulates a rise in complement-fixing antibodies to adenovirus group antigens shared by all types. The CF test is an easily applied method for detecting infection by any member of the adenovirus group. A fourfold or greater rise in complement-fixing antibody titer between acute-phase and convalescent-phase sera indicates current infection with an adenovirus, though it gives no clue about the specific type involved.

If specific identification of a patient's serologic response is required, Nt or HI tests can be used. In most cases, the neutralizing antibody titer of infected persons shows a fourfold or greater rise against the adenovirus type recovered from the patient.

Epidemiology

Adenoviruses exist in all parts of the world. They are present year-round and do not cause community outbreaks of disease. Adenoviruses are spread predominantly by the fecal-oral route but may also be transmitted by respiratory droplets or by contaminated fomites.

Infections with types 1, 2, 5, and 6 occur chiefly during the first years of life and are associated with fever and pharyngitis or asymptomatic infection. These are the types most frequently obtained from the adenoids and tonsils.

In prospective surveillance studies of family groups, adenovirus infections have been found to be predominantly enteric. They may be abortive or invasive and followed by persistent intermittent excretion of virus for months to years after initial infection. Such excretion is most characteristic of types 1, 2, 3, and 5, which are usually endemic. Infection rates are highest among infants, but siblings who introduce the infection into a household are more effective in spreading the disease than are infants. Adenoviruses contributed 3–5% of all infectious illness in the children studied, based on virus-positive infections only. These family studies document that many adenovirus infections are completely asymptomatic.

While adenoviruses cause only 2–5% of all respiratory illness in the general population, respiratory disease due to types 3, 4, 7, 14, and 21 is common among military recruits. Adenovirus disease causes great morbidity when large numbers of persons are being inducted into the armed forces; consequently, its greatest impact is during periods of mobilization. During a 1-year study, 10% of recruits in basic training were hospitalized for respiratory illness caused by an adenovirus. During the winter, adenovirus accounted for 72% of all respiratory illnesses. However, adenovirus disease is not a problem in seasoned troops. The exceptional susceptibility of new recruits to these viruses remains unexplained.

Eye infections can be transmitted in several ways, but hand-to-eye transfer is particularly important. Outbreaks of swimming pool conjunctivitis are presumably waterborne, usually occur in the summer, and are commonly caused by types 3 and 7. Epidemic keratoconjunctivitis is a highly contagious and serious disease. Caused by type 8, the disease spread in 1941 from Australia via the Hawaiian Islands to the Pacific Coast. It spread rapidly through the shipyards (hence the name "shipyard eye") and across the USA. In the USA, the incidence of neutralizing antibody to type 8 in the general population is very low (about 1%), whereas in Japan it is more than 30%. More recently, adenovirus types 19 and 37 have caused epidemics of typical epidemic keratoconjunctivitis. Outbreaks of conjunctivitis traced to ophthalmologists' offices were presumably caused by contaminated ophthalmic solutions or diagnostic equipment.

The observed incidence of adenovirus infection in patients undergoing marrow transplantation is about 5%, an underestimate of the true incidence of infection because of the lack of serologic studies and sensitive methods for routine viral isolation. The distribution of serotypes found in transplant patients resembles that found in community surveys, but the illness may be more serious. Types 34 and 35 are found most often in renal transplant recipients and in the urine of patients with AIDS. The most likely source of infection in transplant patients is endogenous viral reactivation.

Prevention & Control

Attempts to control adenovirus infections in the military have focused on vaccines. Live attenuated virus, grown in human diploid cells, is encased in gelatin-coated capsules and given orally. In this way it bypasses the respiratory tract, where it could cause disease, and is released in the intestine, where it produces a subclinical infection that confers a high degree of immunity against wild strains. It does not spread from a vaccinated person to contacts. Such live-virus vaccines against types 4 and 7 are licensed but are recommended only for immunization of military populations. When both virus types are administered simultaneously, vaccinees respond with neutralizing antibodies against both.

Human cells have replaced monkey cells in the preparation of these vaccines. A trivalent vaccine was prepared by growing type 3, 4, and 7 viruses in monkey kidney cultures and then inactivating the viruses with formalin. However, it was found that the vaccine strains were contaminated genetically with SV40 DNA sequences, and the vaccine was subsequently withdrawn from use. It was later found that most adenovirus strains do not replicate in monkey cells unless SV40 is present as a helper virus.

In addition to vaccination, other methods of prevention and control are available. The risk of waterborne outbreaks of conjunctivitis can be minimized by chlorination of swimming pools and wastewater. Rigid asepsis during eye examinations, coupled with adequate sterilization of equipment, is essential for the control of epidemic keratoconjunctivitis.

REFERENCES

Adrian T et al: Genome type analysis of adenovirus 37 isolates. J Med Virol 1988;25:77.

Cristiano RJ et al: Hepatic gene therapy: Efficient gene delivery and expression in primary hepatocytes utilizing a conjugated adenovirus–DNA complex. Proc Natl Acad Sci USA 1993;90:11548.

D'Angelo LJ et al: Epidemic keratoconjunctivitis caused by adenovirus type 8: Epidemiologic and laboratory aspects of a large outbreak. Am J Epidemiol 1981;113: 44.

Flomenberg PR et al: Molecular epidemiology of adenovirus type 35 infections in immunocompromised hosts. J Infect Dis 1987;155:1127.

Fox JP, Hall CE, Cooney MK: The Seattle Virus Watch. 7. Observations of adenovirus infections. Am J Epidemiol 1977;105:362.

Greber UF et al: Stepwise dismantling of adenovirus 2 during entry into cells. Cell 1993;75:477.

Hierholzer JC, Wigand R, de Jong JC: Evaluation of human adenoviruses 38, 39, 40, and 41 as new serotypes. Intervirology 1988;29:1.

Kemp MC et al: The changing etiology of epidemic keratoconjunctivitis: Antigenic and restriction enzyme analyses of adenovirus types 19 and 37 isolated over a 10-year period. J Infect Dis 1983;148:24.

Koneru B et al: Adenoviral infections in pediatric liver transplant recipients. JAMA 1987;258:489.

McPherson RA, Ginsberg HS, Rose JA: Adeno-associated virus helper activity of adenovirus DNA binding protein. J Virol 1982;44:666.

Shields AF et al: Adenovirus infections in patients undergoing bone-marrow transplantation. N Engl J Med 1985; 312:529.

Takafuji ET et al: Simultaneous administration of live, enteric-coated adenovirus types 4, 7, and 21 vaccines: Safety and immunogenicity. J Infect Dis 1979;140:48.

Wadell G: Molecular epidemiology of human adenoviruses. Curr Top Microbiol Immunol 1984;110:191.

Wadell G et al: Molecular epidemiology of adenoviruses: Global distribution of adenovirus 7 genome types. J Clin Microbiol 1985;21:403.

Wold WSM, Gooding LR: Region E3 of adenovirus: A cassette of genes involved in host immunosurveillance and virus-cell interactions. Virology 1991;184:1.

33 Herpesviruses

The herpesvirus family contains several of the most important human pathogens. Clinically, the herpesviruses exhibit a spectrum of diseases. Some have a wide host-cell range, whereas others have a narrow host-cell range. The outstanding property of herpesviruses is their ability to establish lifelong persistent infections in their hosts and to undergo periodic reactivation. Their frequent reactivation in immunosuppressed patients causes serious health complications. Curiously, the reactivated infection may be clinically quite different from the disease caused by the primary infection. Herpesviruses possess a large number of genes, some of which have proved to be susceptible to antiviral chemotherapy.

There are seven herpesviruses that commonly infect humans: herpes simplex virus types 1 and 2, varicella-zoster virus, cytomegalovirus, Epstein-Barr virus, and human herpesviruses 6 and 7. There are nearly 100 viruses of the herpes group that infect many different animal species.

PROPERTIES OF HERPESVIRUSES

Important properties of herpesviruses are summarized in Table 33-1.

Structure & Composition

Herpesviruses are large viruses. Different members of the group share architectural details and are indistinguishable by electron microscopy (Figure 33–1). All herpesviruses have a core of double-stranded DNA, in the form of a toroid, surrounded by a protein coat that exhibits icosahedral symmetry and has 162 capsomers. The nucleocapsid is surrounded by an envelope that is derived from the nuclear membrane of the infected cell and contains viral glycoprotein spikes about 8-nm long. An amorphous, sometimes asymmetrical structure between the capsid and envelope is designated the tegument. The enveloped form measures 120–200 nm; the "naked" virion, 100 nm.

The double-stranded DNA genome (MW 95–150 $\times$ 10^6; 120–230 kbp) is linear. A striking feature of herpesvirus DNAs is their sequence arrangement (Figure 33–2). Herpesvirus genomes possess terminal and internal repeated sequences. Some members, such as the herpes simplex viruses, undergo genome rearrangements, giving rise to different genome "isomers." The biologic significance of these novel arrangements is unknown. Spontaneous deletions occur, and defective viral particles are common among herpesviruses. The base composition of herpesvirus DNAs varies from 31% to 75% (guanine-plus-cytosine). There is little DNA homology among different herpesviruses except for herpes simplex types 1 and 2, which show 50% sequence homology, and human herpesviruses 6 and 7, which display limited (30–50%) sequence homology. Treatment with restriction endonucleases yields characteristically different cleavage patterns for herpesviruses and even for different strains of each type. This "fingerprinting" of strains allows epidemiologic tracing of a given strain, whereas in the past the ubiquitousness of herpes simplex virus made such investigations impossible.

The herpesvirus genome is large enough to code for at least 100 different proteins. Of these, more than 35 polypeptides are involved in the structure of the viral particle; some are part of the viral envelope (Figure 33–3). Several virus-specific enzymes (DNA polymerase, thymidine kinase) are synthesized in infected cells, but no enzymes appear to be incorporated into viral particles.

Classification

Classification of the numerous members of the herpesvirus family is complicated. A useful division into subfamilies is based on biologic properties of the agents (Table 33–2). Alphaherpesviruses are fast-growing, cytolytic viruses that tend to establish latent infections in neurons; herpes simplex virus and varicella-zoster virus are members. Betaherpesviruses are slow-growing and cytomegalic (massive enlargements of infected cells) and become latent in secretory glands and kidneys; cytomegalovirus is classified here. Gammaherpesviruses, exemplified by Epstein-Barr virus, infect and become latent in lymphoid cells. The

Table 33–1. Important properties of herpesviruses.

Virion: Spherical, 120–200 nm in diameter (icosahedral capsid, 100 nm).
Genome: Double-stranded DNA, linear, MW 95–150 million, 120–240 kbp, reiterated sequences.
Proteins: More than 35 proteins in virion.
Envelope: Contains viral glycoproteins, Fc receptors.
Replication: Nucleus, bud from nuclear membrane.
Outstanding characteristics: Establish latent infections; persist indefinitely in infected hosts; are frequently reactivated in immunosuppressed hosts.

newest human herpesviruses, designated human herpesvirus 6 and 7, are difficult to classify. By biologic criteria, they should be classified as gammaherpesviruses, because they infect lymphocytes (T lymphotropic). However, molecular analyses of their genomes suggest that they are more closely related to the betaherpesviruses.

Many herpesviruses infect animals, the most notable being B virus and herpesviruses saimiri, aotus, and ateles of monkeys; marmoset herpesvirus; pseudorabies virus of pigs; and infectious bovine rhinotracheitis virus of cattle.

There is little antigenic relatedness among members of the herpesvirus group. Only herpes simplex viruses type 1 and type 2 share a significant number of common antigens. This is not surprising, since there is approximately 50% homology between those two viral genomes. Human herpesviruses 6 and 7 exhibit a few cross-reacting epitopes.

Herpesvirus Replication

The virus enters the cell by fusion with the cell membrane after binding to specific cellular receptors via an envelope glycoprotein. Several herpesviruses bind to cell surface glycosaminoglycans, principally heparan sulfate. The capsid is transported through the cytoplasm to a nuclear pore; uncoating occurs; and the DNA becomes associated with the nucleus. The viral DNA forms a circle immediately upon release from the capsid. Expression of the viral genome is tightly regulated and sequentially ordered in a cascade fashion. Immediate-early genes are expressed, yielding "alpha" proteins. These proteins permit expression of the early set of genes, which are translated into "beta" proteins. Viral DNA replication begins, and late transcripts are produced that give rise to "gamma" proteins. More than 50 different proteins are synthesized in herpesvirus-infected cells. Many alpha and beta proteins are enzymes or DNA-binding proteins; most of the gamma proteins are structural components.

Viral DNA is transcribed throughout the replicative cycle by cellular RNA polymerase II but with the participation of viral factors. Viral DNA is synthesized by

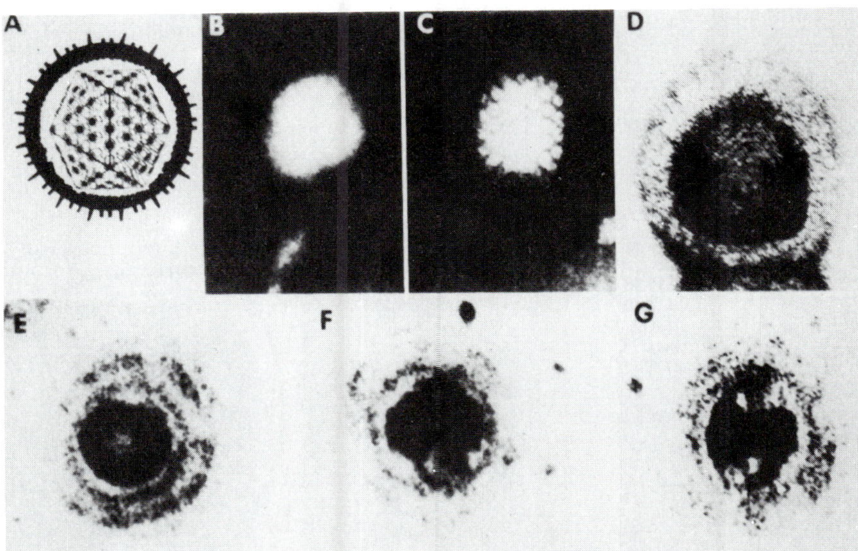

Figure 33–1. Morphology of herpesviruses. ***A:*** Schematic diagram of a herpesvirion seen through a cross section of the envelope with spikes projecting from its surface. An irregular tegument lies between the icosahedral capsid and the envelope. ***B:*** An intact, negatively stained HSV-1 virion. The intact envelope is not permeable to negative stain. ***C:*** HSV-1 capsid exposed to negative stain. Structural details are now visible. ***D:*** HSV-1 capsid containing DNA permeated with uranyl acetate stain. The electron micrograph shows thread-like structures on the surface of the core. ***E, F, G:*** Electron micrographs of thin sections of HSV-1 virions showing the core cut at different angles. The DNA core appears as a toroid with an outer diameter of 70 nm and an inner diameter of 18 nm. The toroid is seen looking down the hole ***(E),*** in cross section ***(F),*** and from the side ***(G).*** (Reproduced, with permission, from Roizman B: Herpesviridae: A brief introduction. Pages 1787–1793 in: *Virology,* 2nd ed. Fields BN et al [editors]. Raven Press, 1990.)

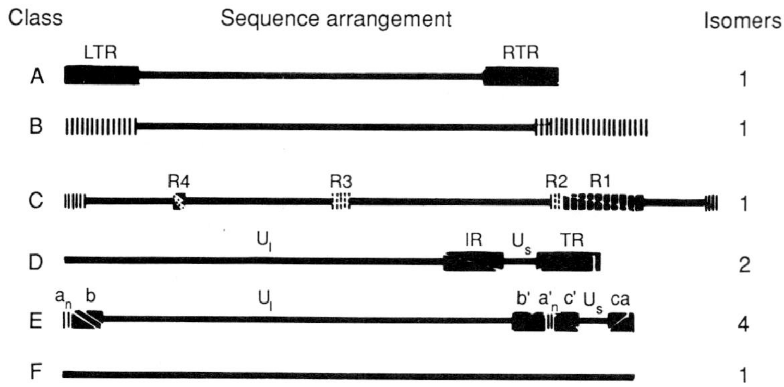

Figure 33–2. Schematic diagram of sequence arrangements of herpesvirus DNAs. Genome classes A, B, C, D, E, and F are exemplified by channel catfish virus, herpesvirus saimiri, Epstein-Barr virus, varicella-zoster virus, herpes simplex viruses, and tupaia herpesvirus, respectively. Horizontal lines represent unique regions. Reiterated domains are shown as rectangles: left and right terminal repeats (LTR and RTR) for class A; repeats R1 to R4 for internal repeats of class C; and internal and terminal repeats (IR and TR) of class D. In class B, terminal sequences are reiterated numerous times at both termini. The termini of class E consist of two elements. The terminal sequences (ab and ca) are inserted in an inverted orientation separating the unique sequences into long (U_l) and short (U_s) domains. Genomes of class F have no terminal reiterations. The components of the genomes in classes D and E invert. In class D (varicella-zoster virus), the short component inverts relative to the long, and the DNA forms two populations (isomers) differing in the orientation of the short component. In class E (herpes simplex virus), both the short and long components can invert, and viral DNA consists of four isomers. (Reproduced, with permission, from Roizman B: Herpesviridae: A brief introduction. Pages 1787–1793 in: *Virology,* 2nd ed. Fields BN et al [editors]. Raven Press, 1990.)

a rolling-circle mechanism. Herpesviruses differ from other nuclear DNA viruses in that they encode a large number of enzymes involved in DNA synthesis. (These enzymes are good targets for antiviral drugs.) Newly synthesized viral DNA is packaged into preformed empty nucleocapsids in the cell nucleus.

Maturation occurs by budding of nucleocapsids through the altered inner nuclear membrane. En-

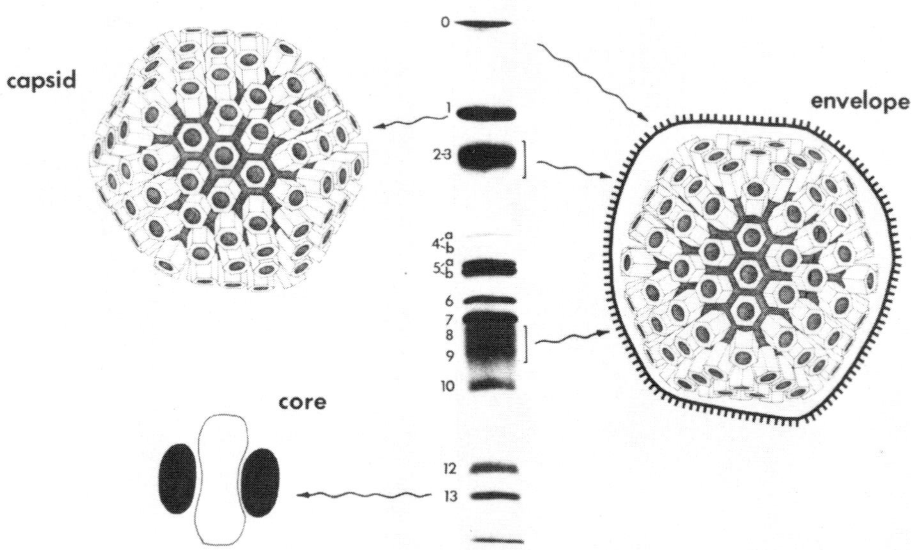

Figure 33–3. Herpesvirus. Several of the many proteins in the virion have been identified. The protein in band 1 by gel electrophoresis is associated with the viral capsid; the glycoproteins present in bands 0, 2–3, 8, and 9 are associated with the envelope; and a DNA-binding protein (band 13) is associated with the internal core. (KL Powell and DJM Purifoy.)

Table 33–2. Classification of human herpesviruses.

Subfamily	Biologic Properties			Examples	
	Growth Cycle	Cyto-pathology	Latent Infections	Official Name	Common Name
Alphaherpesvirinae	Short	Cytolytic	Neurons	Human herpesvirus 1 Human herpesvirus 2 Human herpesvirus 3	Herpes simplex virus type 1 Herpes simplex virus type 2 Varicella-zoster virus
Betaherpesvirinae	Long	Cytomegalic	Glands, kidneys	Human herpesvirus 5	Cytomegalovirus
Gammaherpesvirinae	Variable	Lympho-proliferative	Lymphoid tissue	Human herpesvirus 4 Human herpesvirus 6[1] Human herpesvirus 7[1]	Epstein-Barr virus Human herpesvirus 6 Human herpesvirus 7

[1]Human herpesviruses 6 and 7 are difficult to classify. They infect lymphocytes (predominantly T cells), but their genomes resemble that of cytomegalovirus (betaherpesvirus).

veloped viral particles are then released from the cell through tubular structures that are continuous with the outside of the cell or from vacuoles that release their contents at the surface of the cell (see Figure 29–9).

The length of the replication cycle varies from about 18 hours for herpes simplex virus to over 70 hours for cytomegalovirus. Cells productively infected with herpesviruses are invariably killed. Host macromolecular synthesis is shut off early in infection; normal cellular DNA and protein synthesis virtually stop as viral replication begins. Cytopathic effects induced by human herpesviruses are quite distinct (Figure 33–4).

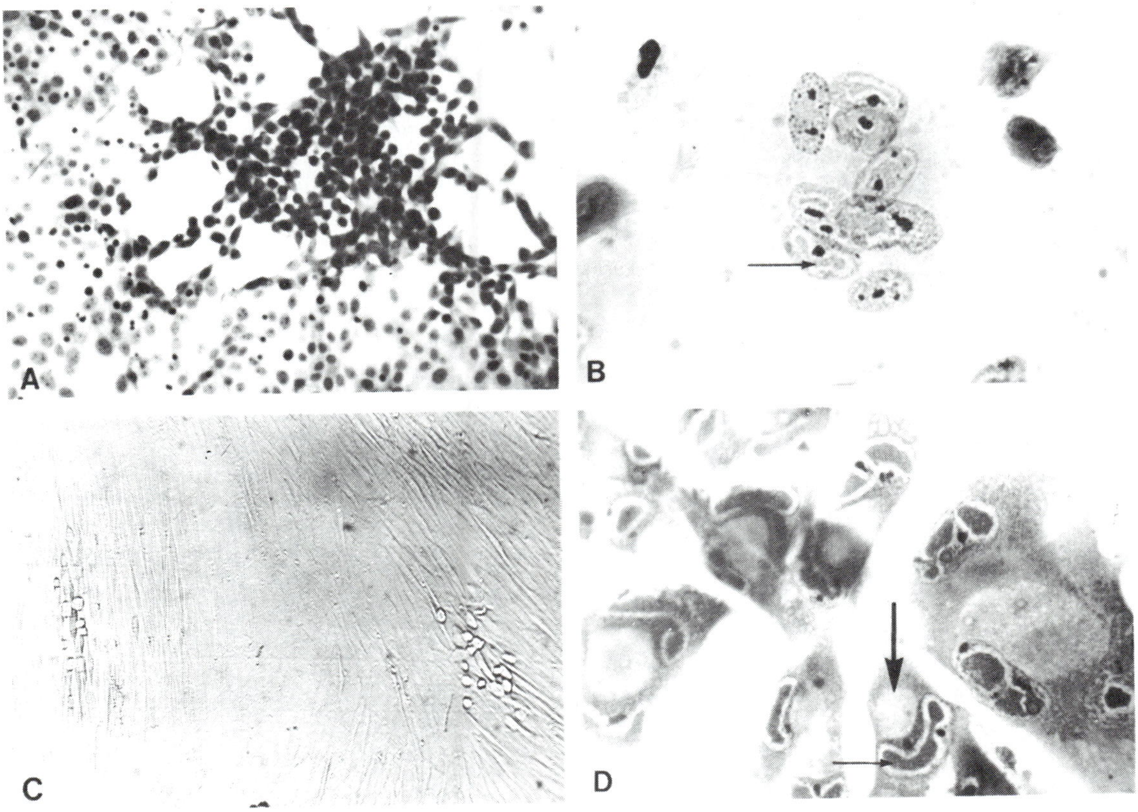

Figure 33–4. Cytopathic effects induced by herpesviruses. ***A:*** Herpes simplex virus in HEp-2 cells (H&E stain, 57 ×), with early focus of swollen, rounded cells. ***B:*** Varicella-zoster virus in human kidney cells (H&E stain, 228 ×), with multinucleated giant cell containing acidophilic intranuclear inclusions (arrow). ***C:*** Cytomegalovirus in human fibroblasts (unstained, 35 ×) with two foci of slowly developing cytopathic effect. ***D:*** Cytomegalovirus in human fibroblasts (H&E stain, 228 ×), showing giant cells with acidophilic inclusions in the nuclei (small arrow) and cytoplasm (large arrow), the latter being characteristically large and round. (Courtesy of I Jack; reproduced, with permission, from White DO, Fenner FJ: *Medical Virology*, 3rd ed. Academic Press, 1986.)

Overview of Herpesvirus Diseases

A wide variety of diseases are associated with infection by herpesviruses. Primary infection and reactivated disease by a given virus may involve different cell types and present different clinical pictures.

Herpes simplex virus types 1 and 2 infect epithelial cells and establish latent infections in neurons. Type 1 is classically associated with oropharyngeal lesions and causes recurrent attacks of "fever blisters." Type 2 primarily infects the genital mucosa and is mainly responsible for genital herpes. Both viruses also cause neurologic disease. Herpes simplex virus type 1 is the leading cause of sporadic encephalitis in the USA. Both type 1 and type 2 can cause neonatal infections which are often severe.

Varicella-zoster virus causes chickenpox (varicella) on primary infection and establishes latent infection in neurons. Upon reactivation, the virus causes zoster (shingles). Adults who are infected for the first time with varicella-zoster virus are apt to develop serious viral pneumonia.

Cytomegalovirus replicates in epithelial cells of the respiratory tract, salivary glands, and kidneys and persists in lymphocytes. It causes an infectious mononucleosis (heterophil-negative). In newborns, cytomegalic inclusion disease may occur. Cytomegalovirus is an important cause of congenital defects and mental retardation.

Epstein-Barr virus replicates in epithelial cells of the oropharynx and parotid gland and establishes latent infections in lymphocytes. It causes infectious mononucleosis (heterophil test-positive) and appears to be the cause of two human cancers, one a lymphoma and the other a carcinoma.

Human herpesvirus 6 infects T lymphocytes. It is typically acquired in early infancy and causes exanthem subitum (roseola infantum). Target cells for latent infections and the consequences of reactivations are not known. Human herpesvirus 7, also a T-lymphotropic virus, has not yet been linked to any specific disease.

Herpes B virus of macaque monkeys can infect humans. Such infections are rare, but those that occur usually result in severe neurologic disease and are frequently fatal.

Human herpesviruses are frequently reactivated in immunosuppressed patients (eg, transplant recipients, cancer patients) and may cause severe disease, such as pneumonia or lymphomas.

Herpesviruses have been linked with malignant diseases in humans and lower animals: Epstein-Barr virus with Burkitt's lymphoma of African children and with nasopharyngeal carcinoma; herpes simplex virus type 2 with cervical and vulvar carcinoma; Lucké virus with renal adenocarcinomas of the frog; Marek's disease virus with a lymphoma of chickens; and a number of primate herpesviruses with reticulum cell sarcomas and lymphomas in monkeys.

HERPESVIRUS INFECTIONS IN HUMANS

HERPES SIMPLEX VIRUSES

Herpes simplex viruses are extremely widespread in the human population. They exhibit a broad host range, being able to replicate in many types of cells and to infect many different animals. They grow rapidly and are highly cytolytic. The herpes simplex viruses are responsible for a spectrum of diseases, ranging from gingivostomatitis to keratoconjunctivitis, encephalitis, genital disease, and infections of newborns. The herpes simplex viruses establish latent infections in nerve cells; recurrences are common.

Properties of the Viruses

There are two distinct herpes simplex viruses: type 1 and type 2 (HSV-1, HSV-2) (Table 33–3). Their genomes are similar in organization and exhibit substantial sequence homology. However, they can be distinguished by restriction enzyme analysis of viral DNA. The two viruses cross-react serologically, but some unique proteins exist for each type. They differ in their mode of transmission; HSV-1 is spread by contact, usually involving infected saliva, whereas HSV-2 is transmitted sexually or from a maternal genital infection to a newborn. This results in different clinical features of human infections.

The HSV growth cycle proceeds rapidly, requiring 8–16 hours for completion. The alpha (immediate-early) genes are expressed soon after infection. Those genes are transcribed in the absence of viral protein synthesis and are responsible for the initiation of replication. The beta (early) genes are then expressed; they require functional alpha gene products for expression. They are mostly enzymes and replication proteins. Beta gene expression coincides with a decrease in transcription of alpha genes and an irreversible shutoff of host cell protein synthesis, foretelling the ultimate death of the cell. Gamma (late) gene products are then produced and include most of the structural proteins of the virus.

At least eight viral glycoproteins are made. One (gD) is the most potent inducer of neutralizing antibodies. Glycoprotein C is a complement (C3b)-binding protein, and gE is an Fc receptor, binding to the Fc portion of IgG. Glycoprotein G is type-specific and allows for antigenic discrimination between HSV-1 (gG-1) and HSV-2 (gG-2).

The HSV genome is large (MW≈100 million) and can encode at least 70 polypeptides; the functions of most of those proteins in replication or latency are not known.

Table 33–3. Comparison of herpes simplex virus type 1 and type 2.[1]

Characteristics	HSV-1	HSV-2
Biochemical		
Viral DNA base composition (guanine-plus-cytosine)	67%	69%
Buoyant density of DNA (g/cm^3)	1.726	1.728
Buoyant density of virions (g/cm^3)	1.271	1.267
Homology between viral DNAs	~50%	~50%
Biologic		
Animal vectors or reservoirs	None	None
Site of latency	Trigeminal ganglia	Sacral ganglia
Epidemiologic		
Age of primary infection	Young children	Young adults
Transmission	Contact (often saliva)	Sexual
Clinical		
Primary infection:		
Gingivostomatitis	+	−
Pharyngotonsillitis	+	−
Keratoconjunctivitis	+	−
Neonatal infections	±	+
Recurrent infection:		
Cold sores, fever blisters	+	−
Keratitis	+	−
Primary or recurrent infection:		
Cutaneous herpes		
Skin above the waist	+	−
Skin below the waist	−	+
Hands or arms	+	+
Herpetic whitlow	+	+
Eczema herpeticum	+	−
Genital herpes	±	+
Herpes encephalitis	+	−
Herpes meningitis	±	+

[1]Modified from Oxman MN: Herpes stomatitis. Pages 752–772 in: *Infectious Diseases and Medical Microbiology,* 2nd ed. Braude AI, Davis CE, Fierer J (editors). Saunders, 1986.

Pathogenesis & Pathology

A. Pathology: Because HSV causes cytolytic infections, pathologic changes are due to necrosis of infected cells together with the inflammatory response. Lesions induced in the skin and mucous membranes by HSV-1 and HSV-2 are the same and resemble those of varicella-zoster virus. Changes induced by HSV are similar for primary and recurrent infections but vary in degree, reflecting the extent of viral cytopathology.

Characteristic histopathologic changes include ballooning of infected cells, production of Cowdry type A intranuclear inclusion bodies, margination of chromatin, and formation of multinucleated giant cells. The early inclusions virtually fill the nucleus but later condense and are separated by a halo from the chromatin at the nuclear margin. Cell fusion provides an efficient method for cell-to-cell spread of HSV, even in the presence of neutralizing antibody.

Edema fluid accumulates between the epidermis and dermal layer. This vesicular fluid contains large amounts of cell-free virus, cell debris, and inflammatory cells. In the skin the fluid is absorbed, scabs form, and lesions heal without scarring. In mucous membrane sites, the vesicles rupture rapidly and shallow ulcers form.

In other organs, such as in cases of disseminated neonatal herpes, perivascular cuffing and areas of hemorrhagic necrosis may be prominent. Mononuclear cell infiltrates can be detected in infected tissues.

B. Primary Infection: HSV is transmitted by contact of a susceptible person with an individual excreting virus. The virus must encounter mucosal surfaces or broken skin in order for an infection to be initiated (unbroken skin is resistant). HSV-1 infections are usually limited to the oropharynx, and virus is spread by respiratory droplets or by direct contact with infected saliva. HSV-2 is usually transmitted by genital routes. Viral replication occurs first at the site of infection. Virus then invades local nerve endings and is transported by retrograde axonal flow to dorsal root ganglia, where, after further replication, latency is established. Oropharyngeal HSV-1 infections result in latent infections in the trigeminal ganglia, whereas genital HSV-2 infections lead to latently infected sacral ganglia.

Primary HSV infections are usually mild; in fact, most are asymptomatic. Only rarely does systemic disease develop. Widespread organ involvement can result when an immunocompromised host is not able to limit viral replication and viremia ensues.

C. Latent Infection: Virus resides in latently infected ganglia in a nonreplicating state; only a very few viral genes are expressed. Viral persistence in latently infected ganglia lasts for the lifetime of the host. No virus can be recovered between recurrences at or near the usual site of recurrent lesions. Proper provocative stimuli can reactivate virus from the latent state; the virus follows axons back to the peripheral site; and replication proceeds at the skin or mucous membranes. Spontaneous reactivations occur in spite of HSV-specific humoral and cellular immunity in the host. However, this immunity limits local viral replication, so that recurrent infections are less extensive and less severe. Many recurrences are asymptomatic, reflected only by viral shedding in secretions. When symptomatic, episodes of recurrent HSV-1 infection are usually manifested as cold sores (fever blisters) near the lip. The molecular basis of reactivation is not known; effective inducing stimuli include axonal injury, fever, physical or emotional stress, and exposure to ultraviolet light. More than 80% of the human population harbors HSV-1 in a latent form, but only a small portion experience recurrences. It is not known why some individuals suffer reactivations and others do not.

Clinical Findings

Herpes simplex virus types 1 and 2 may cause many clinical entities, and the infections may be primary or recurrent (Table 33–3). Primary infections occur in persons without antibodies and in most individuals are clinically inapparent but result in antibody production and establishment of latent infections in sensory ganglia. Recurrent lesions are common.

A. Oropharyngeal Disease: Primary HSV-1 infections are usually asymptomatic. Symptomatic disease occurs most frequently in small children (1–5 years of age) and involves the buccal and gingival mucosa of the mouth. The incubation period is short (about 3–5 days, with a range of 2–12 days), and clinical illness lasts 2–3 weeks. Symptoms include fever, sore throat, vesicular and ulcerative lesions, edema, gingivostomatitis, submandibular lymphadenopathy, anorexia, and malaise. Gingivitis (swollen, tender gums) is the most striking and common lesion. Primary infections in adults commonly cause pharyngitis and tonsillitis. Localized lymphadenopathy may occur.

Recurrent disease is characterized by a cluster of vesicles most commonly localized at the border of the lip. Intense pain occurs at the outset but fades over 4–5 days. Lesions progress through the pustular and crusting stages, and healing without scarring is usually complete in 8–10 days. The lesions may recur, repeatedly and at various intervals, in the same location. The frequency of recurrences varies widely among individuals.

B. Keratoconjunctivitis: The initial infection with HSV-1 may be in the eye, producing severe keratoconjunctivitis. Recurrent lesions of the eye are common and appear as dendritic keratitis or corneal ulcers or as vesicles on the eyelids. With recurrent keratitis, there may be progressive involvement of the corneal stroma, with permanent opacification and blindness. HSV-1 infections are second only to trauma as a cause of corneal blindness in the USA.

C. Genital Herpes: Genital disease is usually caused by HSV-2, although HSV-1 can also cause clinical episodes of genital herpes. Primary genital herpes infections can be severe, with illness lasting about 3 weeks. Genital herpes is characterized by vesiculoulcerative lesions of the penis of the male or of the cervix, vulva, vagina, and perineum of the female. The lesions are very painful and may be associated with fever, malaise, dysuria, and inguinal lymphadenopathy. Systemic complaints are common in both sexes. Complications include extragenital lesions (≈20% of cases) and aseptic meningitis (≈10% of cases). Viral excretion persists for about 3 weeks.

An initial HSV-2 infection in a person already immune to HSV-1 tends to be less severe symptomatically. Healing occurs more rapidly, and less virus is shed. Because of the antigenic cross-reactivity between HSV-1 and HSV-2, preexisting immunity provides some protection against heterotypic infection.

Recurrences of genital herpetic infections are common and tend to be mild. A limited number of vesicles appear and heal in about 10 days. Virus is shed for only a few days. Some recurrences are asymptomatic. Whether a recurrence is symptomatic or asymptomatic, a person shedding virus can transmit the infection to sexual partners. It has been shown that susceptible females are at high risk for contracting HSV infection from infected males. Whereas most episodes of recurrent disease are due to reactivation of virus latent in sacral ganglia, a recurrence may occasionally represent a sexually acquired infection with a new HSV-2 strain.

D. Skin Infections: Intact skin is resistant to HSV, so cutaneous HSV infections are uncommon in healthy persons. Localized lesions caused by HSV-1 or HSV-2 may occur in abrasions that become contaminated with the virus (traumatic herpes). These lesions are seen on the fingers of dentists and hospital personnel (herpetic whitlow) and on the bodies of wrestlers (herpes gladiatorum).

Cutaneous infections are often severe and life-threatening when they occur in individuals with disorders of the skin, such as eczema or burns, that permit extensive local viral replication and spread. Eczema herpeticum is a primary infection, usually with HSV-1, in a person with chronic eczema. There may be extensive vesiculation of the skin over much of the body and high fever. In rare instances, the illness may be fatal.

E. Encephalitis: A severe form of encephalitis may be produced by herpesvirus. HSV-1 infections are considered the most common cause of sporadic, fatal encephalitis in the USA. In older children and in adults, the neurologic manifestations suggest a lesion in the temporal lobe. Pleocytosis (chiefly of lymphocytes) is present in the cerebrospinal fluid; however, definitive diagnosis during the illness can usually be made only by isolation of the virus from brain tissue obtained by biopsy or at postmortem examination. The disease carries a high mortality rate, and those who survive often have residual neurologic defects. The source of virus for brain infections is not clear. About half of patients with HSV encephalitis appear to have primary infections, and the rest appear to have recurrent infection.

F. Neonatal Herpes: HSV infection of the newborn may be acquired in utero, during birth, or after birth. Neonatal herpes is estimated to occur in about one in 5000 deliveries per year. The newborn infant seems to be unable to limit the replication and spread of HSV and has a propensity to develop severe disease.

The most common route of infection ($\approx$75% of cases) is for HSV to be transmitted to the newborn during birth by contact with herpetic lesions in the birth canal. To avoid infection, delivery by cesarean section has been used in pregnant women with genital herpes lesions. To be effective, cesarean section must be performed before rupture of the membranes. However, many fewer cases of neonatal HSV infection occur than cases of recurrent genital herpes, even when virus is present at term.

Neonatal herpes can be acquired postnatally by exposure to either HSV-1 or HSV-2. Sources of infection include family members and hospital personnel who are shedding virus.

About 75% of neonatal herpes infections are caused by HSV-2. There do not appear to be any differences between the nature and severity of neonatal herpes in premature or full-term infants, in infections caused by HSV-1 or HSV-2, or in disease when virus is acquired during delivery or postpartum.

Neonatal herpes infections are almost always symptomatic. The overall mortality rate of untreated disease is 50%. Babies with neonatal herpes exhibit three categories of disease: (1) lesions localized to the skin, eye, and mouth; (2) encephalitis with or without localized skin involvement; and (3) disseminated disease involving multiple organs, including the central nervous system. The worst prognosis (mortality rate about 80%) applies to infants with disseminated infection, many of whom develop encephalitis. The cause of death of babies with disseminated disease is usually viral pneumonitis or intravascular coagulopathy. Many survivors of severe infections are left with permanent neurologic impairment.

Transplacental infection of the fetus with HSV may cause congenital malformations, but this phenomenon is very rare. On occasions, the fetus may be spontaneously aborted.

G. Infections in Immunocompromised Hosts: Immunocompromised patients are at increased risk of developing severe HSV infections. These include patients immunosuppressed by disease or therapy (especially those with deficient cellular immunity) and individuals with malnutrition. Renal, cardiac, and bone marrow transplant recipients are at particular risk for severe herpes infections. Patients with hematologic malignancies and patients with AIDS suffer more frequent and more severe HSV infections. Herpes lesions may spread and involve the respiratory tract, esophagus, and intestinal mucosa. Malnourished children are prone to fatal disseminated HSV infections. In most cases, the disease reflects reactivation of latent HSV infection.

Immunity

Many newborns acquire passively transferred maternal antibodies. These antibodies are lost during the first 6 months of life, and the period of greatest susceptibility to primary herpes infection occurs between ages 6 months and 2 years. Transplacentally acquired antibodies from the mother are not totally protective against infection of newborns, but they seem to ameliorate infection if not prevent it. HSV-1 antibodies begin to appear in the population in early childhood; by adolescence, they are present in most persons. Antibodies to HSV-2 rise during the age of adolescence and sexual activity.

During primary infections, IgM antibodies appear transiently and are followed by IgG and IgA antibodies that persist for long periods. The more severe the primary infection or the more frequent the recurrences, the greater the level of antibody response. However, the pattern of antibody response has not correlated with the frequency of disease recurrence. Cell-mediated immunity and nonspecific host factors (natural killer cells, interferon) are important in controlling both primary and recurrent HSV infections.

After recovery from a primary infection (inapparent, mild, or severe), the virus is carried in a latent state in the presence of antibodies. These antibodies do not prevent reinfection or reactivation of latent virus but may modify subsequent disease.

Laboratory Diagnosis

A. Isolation and Identification of Virus: Virus isolation remains the definitive diagnostic approach. Virus may be isolated from herpetic lesions (skin, cornea, or brain). It may also be found in throat washings, cerebrospinal fluid, and stool, both during primary infection and during asymptomatic periods. Therefore, the isolation of HSV is not in itself sufficient evidence to indicate that the virus is the causative agent of a disease under investigation.

Inoculation of tissue cultures is used for viral isolation. Because HSV has a wide host range, many cell culture systems are susceptible. The appearance of typical cytopathic effects in cell culture in 2–3 days suggests the presence of HSV. The agent is then identified by Nt test or immunofluorescence staining with specific antiserum. Typing of HSV isolates may be done using specific antisera or by restriction endonuclease analysis of viral DNA, but such tests are not widely available.

Scrapings or swabs from the base of herpetic lesions contain multinucleated giant cells. These are indicative but not diagnostic of HSV infection.

Since the only hope for treatment of HSV encephalitis lies in early diagnosis, a rapid means of diagnosis is needed. The fluorescent antibody test using brain biopsy material is currently the method of choice. Hybridization using labeled DNA probes or DNA amplification assays will one day provide routine, rapid tests.

B. Serology: Antibodies appear in 4–7 days after infection; they can be measured by Nt, CF, ELISA, radioimmunoassay, or immunofluorescence and reach a peak in 2–4 weeks. They persist with minor fluctuations for the life of the host.

The diagnostic value of serologic assays is limited by the multiple antigens shared by HSV-1 and HSV-2. There may also be some heterotypic anamnestic responses to varicella-zoster virus in persons infected with HSV, and vice versa. The use of HSV type-specific antibodies, available in some laboratories, allows more meaningful serologic tests.

Epidemiology

Herpes simplex viruses are worldwide in distribution. No animal reservoirs or vectors are involved with the human viruses. Transmission is by contact with infected secretions. The epidemiology of type 1 and type 2 herpes simplex virus differs.

HSV-1 is probably more constantly present in humans than any other virus. Primary infection occurs early in life and is usually asymptomatic; occasionally, it produces oropharyngeal disease (gingivostomatitis in young children, pharyngitis in young adults). Antibodies develop, but the virus is not eliminated from the body; a carrier state is established that lasts throughout life and is punctuated by transient recurrent attacks of herpes.

The highest incidence of HSV-1 infection occurs among children 6 months to 3 years of age. By adulthood, 70–90% of persons have type 1 antibodies. Middle-class individuals in developed countries acquire antibodies later in life than those in lower socioeconomic populations. Presumably this reflects more crowded living conditions and poorer hygiene among the latter.

The virus is spread by direct contact with infected saliva or through utensils contaminated with the saliva of a virus shedder. The source of infection for children is usually an adult with a symptomatic herpetic lesion or with asymptomatic viral shedding in saliva.

The frequency of recurrent HSV-1 infections varies widely among individuals. At any given time, 1–5% of normal adults will be excreting virus, often in the absence of clinical symptoms.

HSV-2 is usually acquired as a sexually transmitted disease, so antibodies to this virus are seldom found before puberty. It is estimated that approximately 500,000 new cases of genital herpes occur each year and that there are about 60 million infected individuals in the USA. Antibody prevalence studies have been complicated by the cross-reactivity between HSV types 1 and 2. Surveys using type-specific glycoprotein antigens recently determined that 20% of white adults and 65% of black adults in the USA possess HSV-2 antibodies.

Recurrent genital infections may be symptomatic or asymptomatic. Either situation provides a reservoir of virus for transmission to susceptible persons. HSV-2 tends to recur more often than HSV-1, irrespective of the site of infection. The molecular basis of this phenomenon is unknown.

Maternal genital HSV infections pose risks to both mother and fetus. Rarely, pregnant women may develop disseminated disease after primary infection, with a high mortality rate. Primary infection before 20 weeks of gestation has been associated with spontaneous abortion. The fetus may acquire infection as a result of viral shedding from recurrent lesions in the mother's birth canal at the time of delivery. Estimates of the frequency of cervical shedding of virus among pregnant women vary widely. However, the majority of infants (≈70%) who develop neonatal disease are born to women who do not have a history of genital herpes and are asymptomatic at the time of delivery.

Treatment

Several antiviral drugs have proved effective against HSV infections. All are inhibitors of viral DNA synthesis. The drugs inhibit herpesvirus replication and may suppress clinical manifestations. However, HSV remains latent in sensory ganglia, and the rate of relapse is similar in drug-treated and untreated individuals. Drug-resistant virus strains may emerge.

Acyclovir (acycloguanosine) must be activated by an initial phosphorylation event by virus-encoded thymidine kinase, conferring high selectivity on the drug for infected cells. It appears to be remarkably nontoxic in patients. Intravenous acyclovir is the drug of choice for treating herpes encephalitis diagnosed by biopsy. Best results are obtained if treatment is begun early in the disease, before coma sets in. Acyclovir also reduces the mortality rate in neonatal herpes. Acyclovir administered systemically will suppress the activation of latent herpes infections in immunosuppressed patients. As therapy for reactivated infections in immunocompromised persons, acyclovir has shortened durations of viral shedding, of lesion pain, and of time to healing.

Acyclovir is effective treatment for genital herpes infections. Topical, intravenous, and oral formulations are all useful against primary infections. The severity and duration of clinical symptoms are reduced. However, acyclovir does not prevent establishment of latency. The drug is also effective in reducing recurrent outbreaks of genital herpes and appears to be safe for long-term administration.

Vidarabine (adenine arabinoside, ara-A) is also effective against neonatal herpes and HSV encephalitis. However, it is more toxic and difficult to administer than acyclovir. It may be of use in treatment of infections caused by acyclovir-resistant isolates of HSV.

Topically applied idoxuridine (5-iodo-2′-deoxyuridine), trifluridine (trifluorothymidine), vidarabine, and acyclovir have been used for treatment of herpetic keratitis.

Prevention & Control

Newborns and persons with eczema should be protected from exposure to persons with active herpetic lesions.

Experimental vaccines of various types are being developed. One approach is to use purified glycoprotein antigens found in the viral envelope, expressed in some recombinant system, or synthetic peptides to these glycoproteins. Another approach has been through the development of modified vaccinia virus into which a herpesvirus gene coding for an immunizing glycoprotein is inserted. Infection by the modified vaccinia virus allows the herpesvirus DNA to be expressed. A genetically engineered HSV deletion mutant is also being evaluated as a candidate vaccine. Such vaccines should be helpful for the prevention of primary infections. However, as herpes recurs in the presence of circulating antibody, a vaccine would seem to be of little use in a person who already had recovered from a primary infection.

VARICELLA-ZOSTER VIRUS

Varicella (chickenpox) is a mild, highly contagious disease, chiefly of children, characterized clinically by a generalized vesicular eruption of the skin and mucous membranes. The disease may be severe in adults and in immunocompromised children.

Zoster (shingles) is a sporadic, incapacitating disease of adults or immunocompromised individuals that is characterized by a rash limited in distribution to the skin innervated by a single sensory ganglion. The lesions are similar to those of varicella.

Both diseases are caused by the same virus. Varicella is the acute disease that follows primary contact with the virus, whereas zoster is the response of the partially immune host to reactivation of varicella virus present in latent form in sensory ganglia.

Properties of the Virus

Varicella-zoster virus is morphologically identical to herpes simplex virus. The virus propagates in cultures of human embryonic tissue and produces typical intranuclear inclusion bodies (Figure 33–4). Cytopathic changes are more focal and spread much more slowly than those induced by HSV. Infectious virus remains strongly cell-associated, and serial propagation is more easily accomplished by passage of infected cells than of tissue culture fluids. Varicella-zoster virus has not been propagated in laboratory animals.

The same virus causes chickenpox and zoster. Viral isolates from the vesicles of chickenpox or zoster patients exhibit no significant differences at the DNA level. Inoculation of zoster vesicle fluid into children produces chickenpox. Contacts of such children often develop typical varicella. Children who have recovered from zoster virus-induced infection are resistant to varicella.

Pathogenesis & Pathology

A. Varicella: The route of infection is the mucosa of the upper respiratory tract or the conjunctiva. The virus circulates in the blood, undergoes multiple cycles of replication, and eventually localizes in the skin. Focal cutaneous and mucosal lesions are initiated by viral infection of capillary endothelial cells. Swelling of epithelial cells, ballooning degeneration, and the accumulation of tissue fluids result in vesicle formation (Figure 33–5). Eosinophilic inclusion bodies are found in the nuclei of infected cells.

Varicella lesions that may develop in other organs in neonatal disease or in complicated varicella-zoster virus infection of adults are similar. The lung is usually the most severely involved; multinuclear giant cells are common.

Varicella-zoster virus replication and spread is limited by host humoral and cellular immune responses. Interferon may also be involved.

B. Zoster: The skin lesions of zoster are histopathologically identical to those of varicella. There is also an acute inflammation of the sensory nerves and ganglia. Often only a single ganglion may be involved. As a rule, the distribution of lesions in the skin corresponds closely to the areas of innervation from an individual dorsal root ganglion. Lesions of disseminated zoster are identical to those seen in fatal varicella.

It is not clear what triggers reactivation of latent varicella-zoster virus infections in ganglia. It is believed that waning immunity allows viral replication to occur in a ganglion, causing intense inflammation and pain. Virus travels down the nerve to the skin and induces vesicle formation. Cell-mediated immunity is probably the most important host defense in containment of varicella-zoster virus. Reactivations are sporadic and recur infrequently.

Clinical Findings

A. Varicella: Subclinical varicella is unusual. The incubation period of typical disease is 14–21 days. Malaise and fever are the earliest symptoms, soon followed by the rash, first on the trunk and then on the face, the limbs, and the buccal and pharyngeal mucosa in the mouth. Successive fresh vesicles appear in crops during the next 2–4 days, so that all stages of macules, papules, vesicles, and crusts may be seen at one time.

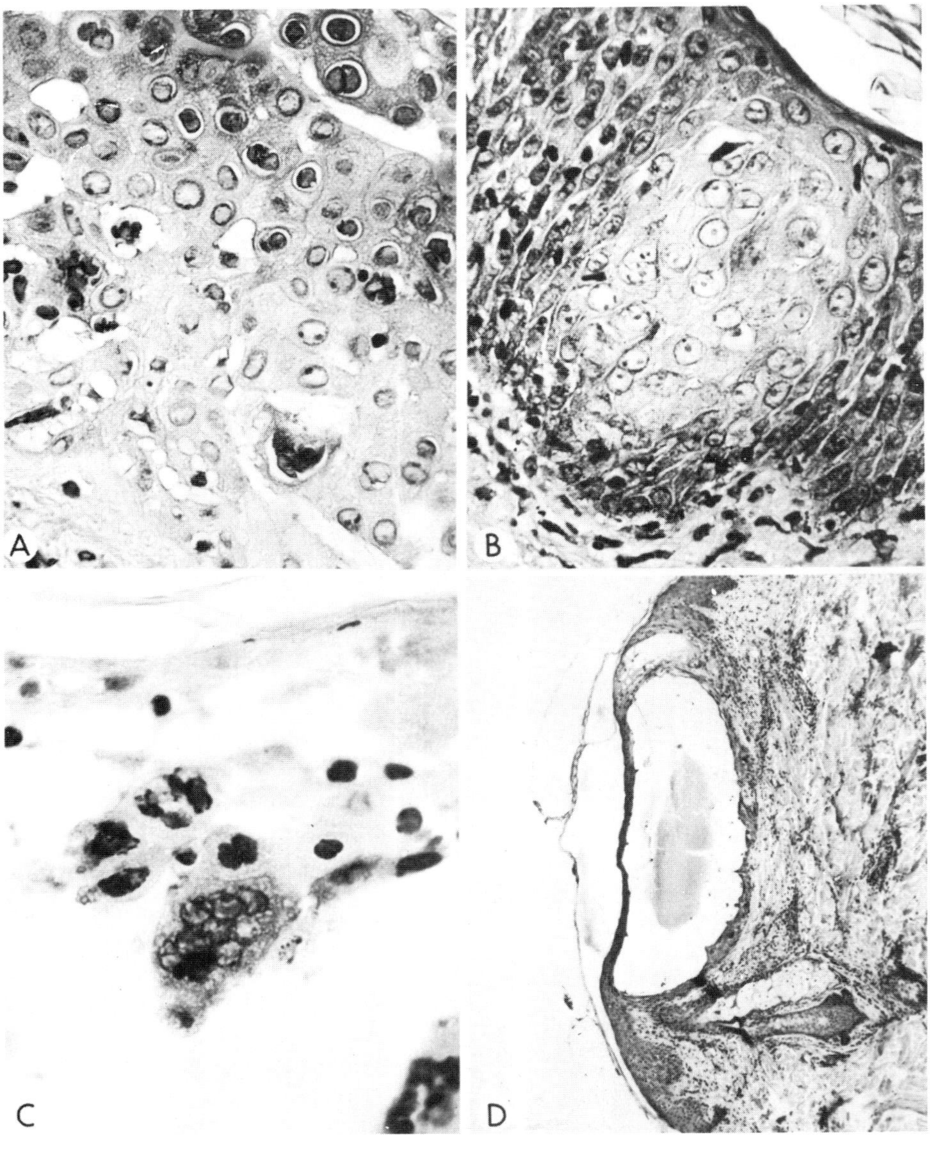

Figure 33–5. Characteristic histologic changes of varicella-zoster virus infection. Punch biopsies of varicella-zoster virus vesicles were fixed and stained with hematoxylin-eosin. ***A:*** Early infection showing "balloon degeneration" of cells with basophilic nuclei and marginated chromatin (reduced from 480×). ***B:*** Later infection showing eosinophilic intranuclear inclusions surrounded by wide clear zones (reduced from 480×). ***C:*** Multinucleated giant cell in the roof of a varicella vesicle (reduced from 480×). ***D:*** Low-power view of an early vesicle showing separation of the epidermis (acantholysis), dermal edema, and mononuclear cell infiltration (reduced from 40×). (Reproduced, with permission, from Gelb LD: Varicella-zoster virus. Pages 2011–2054 in: *Virology,* 2nd ed. Fields BN et al [editors]. Raven Press, 1990.)

The fever persists as long as new lesions appear and is proportionate to the severity of the rash.

Complications are rare in normal children, and the mortality rate is very low. Encephalitis does occur in about one case per thousand. In neonatal varicella, the infection is contracted from the mother just before or just after birth but without sufficient maternal antibody to modify the disease. Virus is often widely disseminated, and the infant fatality rate can exceed 30%. Survivors of varicella encephalitis may be left with permanent sequelae.

Varicella pneumonia is rare in children but is the most common complication in adults with primary varicella-zoster virus infections. The mortality rate ranges from 10% to 40%.

Immunocompromised patients are at increased risk of various complications of varicella. Children with leukemia are especially prone to develop severe, disseminated varicella-zoster virus disease. Progressive varicella in immunocompromised children has a mortality rate of about 20%.

B. Zoster: The disease usually starts with severe pain in the area of skin or mucosa supplied by one or more groups of sensory nerves and ganglia. Within a few days after onset, a crop of vesicles appears over the skin supplied by the affected nerves. The eruption is usually unilateral; the trunk, head, and neck are most commonly involved. The duration and severity of cutaneous eruption are generally proportionate to the age of the patient. Zoster involves the ophthalmic division of the trigeminal nerve fairly commonly (10–15% of cases). Lymphocytic pleocytosis in the cerebrospinal fluid may be present.

In patients with localized zoster and no underlying disease, vesicle interferon levels peak early during infection (by the sixth day). Peak interferon levels are followed by clinical improvement within 48 hours. Vesicles pustulate and crust, and dissemination is halted.

The most common complication of zoster in the elderly is postherpetic neuralgia. The pain may continue for weeks to months. It is especially common after ophthalmic zoster.

Zoster tends to disseminate and be more severe when there is underlying disease, especially in patients with cancer, those with immune defects, and those receiving immunosuppressive therapy. Many patients with Hodgkin's disease eventually develop zoster. Visceral disease, especially pneumonia, is responsible for a significant number of deaths in immunosuppressed patients with zoster.

Immunity

Varicella and zoster viruses are identical, the two diseases being the result of differing host responses. Previous infection with varicella is believed to confer lifelong immunity to varicella. However, zoster can occur in the presence of relatively high levels of neutralizing antibody to varicella.

The development of varicella-zoster virus-specific cell-mediated immunity seems important in recovery from both varicella and zoster. Appearance of local interferon may also contribute to recovery.

Laboratory Diagnosis

In stained smears of scrapings or swabs of the base of vesicles, multinucleated giant cells are seen (Figure 33–5). These are absent in nonherpetic vesicles. Intracellular viral antigens can be demonstrated by immunofluorescence staining of similar smears.

Virus can be isolated from vesicle fluid using cultures of human cells in 3–7 days, although cytopathic effects sometimes develop more slowly. Varicella-zoster virus in vesicle fluid is very labile, and cell cultures should be inoculated promptly. It does not infect laboratory animals or eggs. Isolates are identified by immunofluorescence or other immunologic tests with specific antisera.

Rapid diagnostic procedures are clinically useful for varicella-zoster virus. Herpesviruses can be differentiated from poxviruses by the morphologic appearance of particles in vesicular fluids examined by electron microscopy (Figure 33–6). Varicella-zoster virus-specific antigens or viral DNA can be detected in vesicle fluid, in extracts of crusts, or in biopsy material.

A rise in specific antibody titer can be detected in the patient's serum by various tests, including CF, Nt (in cell culture), indirect immunofluorescence, and enzyme immunoassay. The choice of assay to use depends on the purpose of the test and the laboratory facilities available. Cell-mediated immunity is important, but difficult to demonstrate.

Epidemiology

Varicella and zoster occur worldwide. Varicella (chickenpox) is a common epidemic disease of childhood (peak incidence in children age 2–6 years). Adult cases do occur. It is much more common in winter and spring than in summer in temperate climates. Almost 200,000 cases are reported annually in the USA, but that is probably an underestimate. Zoster occurs sporadically, chiefly in adults and without seasonal prevalence. Ten to 20 percent of adults will experience at least one zoster attack during their lifetime.

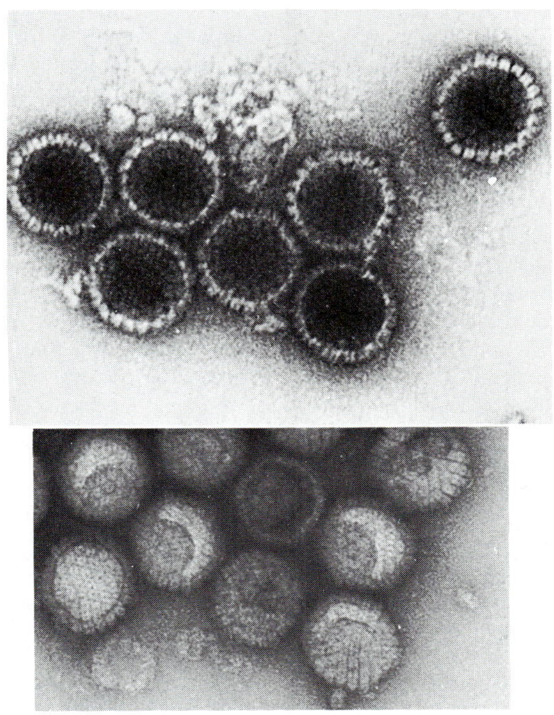

Figure 33–6. ***Top:*** Herpesvirus particles from human vesicle fluid, stained with uranyl acetate to show DNA core (140,000×). ***Bottom:*** Virions stained to show protein capsomers of the virus coat (140,000×). (KO Smith and JL Melnick.)

Varicella spreads readily, presumably by airborne droplets and, less importantly, by contact with skin eruptions. A varicella patient is probably infectious (capable of transmitting the disease) from shortly before the appearance of vesicles to about 5 days later. Contact infection is less common in zoster, perhaps because the virus is absent from the upper respiratory tract in typical cases. Zoster patients can be the source of varicella in susceptible children and can initiate large outbreaks. Varicella-zoster virus DNA has been detected, using a polymerase chain reaction amplification method, in air samples from hospital rooms of patients with active varicella (82%) and zoster (70%) infections.

Uncomplicated varicella is a mild disease. Very few patients require hospitalization; less than 1% of those die, usually from central nervous system or lung complications. The mortality rate may approach 30% in leukemic children infected with varicella in the absence of treatment.

Treatment

Varicella in normal children is a mild disease and requires no treatment. In contrast, varicella in neonates, immunocompromised patients, and some adults is potentially fatal, and treatment attempts are warranted.

Gamma globulin of high varicella-zoster virus antibody titer (varicella-zoster immune globulin) can be used to prevent the development of the illness in immunocompromised patients exposed to varicella. It has no therapeutic value once varicella has started. Standard immune globulin USP is without value because of the low titer of varicella antibodies.

Three antiviral compounds have been shown in carefully controlled studies to be effective against varicella: acyclovir, vidarabine, and leukocyte interferon. Acyclovir can prevent the development of systemic disease in varicella-infected immunosuppressed children and can halt the progression of zoster in adults. Acyclovir does not appear to prevent postherpetic neuralgia. Vidarabine is beneficial in adults with severe varicella pneumonia, immunocompromised children with varicella, and adults with disseminated zoster. Leukocyte interferon treatment has been beneficial against varicella in children with cancer, but its use is associated with fever and other side effects. Acyclovir is currently the treatment of choice.

Idoxuridine and cytarabine inhibit replication of varicella-zoster virus in vitro but are too toxic for systemic treatment of patients.

Prevention & Control

No measures are available for prevention or control of varicella and zoster in the general population.

Varicella may spread rapidly among patients. As varicella in immunosuppressed children poses the serious threat of pneumonia, encephalitis, or death, efforts should be made to prevent their exposure to varicella. Varicella-zoster immune globulin may be used to modify the disease in such children who have been exposed to varicella; it must be given before disease develops. Treatment with antiviral drugs such as acyclovir may also help control varicella in immunodeficient children.

A live attenuated varicella vaccine has been developed and tested successfully in hospitalized immunosuppressed children who were exposed to varicella. The vaccine is particularly useful in preventing the spread of varicella in children at high risk. A similar vaccine has been used successfully in Japan for about 20 years. The vaccine may soon be available for general use in the USA.

CYTOMEGALOVIRUS

Cytomegaloviruses are ubiquitous herpesviruses that are common causes of human disease. The name for the classic cytomegalic inclusion disease derives from the propensity for massive enlargement of cytomegalovirus-infected cells.

Cytomegalic inclusion disease is a generalized infection of infants caused by intrauterine or early postnatal infection with the cytomegaloviruses. The disease causes severe congenital anomalies in about 3000–6000 infants in the USA per year. Cytomegalovirus poses an important public health problem because of its high frequency of congenital infections. Inapparent infection is common during childhood and adolescence. Severe cytomegalovirus infections are frequently found in adults who are immunosuppressed.

Properties of the Virus

Cytomegalovirus has the largest genetic content of the human herpesviruses. Its DNA genome (MW 150 $\times 10^6$, 240 kbp) is significantly larger than that of HSV. Only a few of the many proteins encoded by the virus have been characterized. One, a cell surface glycoprotein, acts as an Fc receptor that can nonspecifically bind the Fc portion of immunoglobulins. This may help infected cells evade immune elimination by providing a protective coating of irrelevant host immunoglobulins.

Many genetically different strains of cytomegalovirus are circulating in the human population. The strains are sufficiently related antigenically, however, so that strain differences are probably not important determinants in human disease.

Cytomegaloviruses are very species-specific and cell type-specific. All attempts to infect animals with human cytomegalovirus have failed. A number of animal cytomegaloviruses exist, all of them species-specific.

Human cytomegalovirus replicates in vitro only in human fibroblasts, although the virus is often isolated from epithelial cells of the host. The virus can transform human and hamster cells in culture, but whether it is oncogenic in vivo is unknown.

Cytomegalovirus produces a characteristic cytopathic effect (Figure 33–4). Perinuclear cytoplasmic inclusions form in addition to the intranuclear inclusions typical of herpesviruses. Multinucleated cells are seen. Many affected cells become greatly enlarged. Inclusion-bearing cytomegalic cells can be found in samples from infected individuals (Figure 33–7).

Cytomegalovirus replicates very slowly in cultured cells, with growth proceeding more slowly than that of HSV or varicella-zoster virus. Very little virus becomes cell-free; infection is spread primarily cell-to-cell. It may take several weeks for an entire monolayer to become involved. Many defective viral particles appear to be produced.

Pathogenesis & Pathology

A. Normal Hosts: Cytomegalovirus may be transmitted person-to-person in several different ways, all requiring close contact with virus-bearing material. There is a 4- to 8-week incubation period in normal older children and adults after viral exposure. The disease is an infectious mononucleosis-like syndrome. Most cytomegalovirus infections are subclinical. Like all herpesviruses, cytomegalovirus establishes lifelong latent infections. Virus can be shed intermittently from the pharynx and in the urine for months to years after primary infection (Figure 33–8). Prolonged cytomegalovirus infection of the kidney does not seem to be deleterious in normal persons but is suspected of contributing to renal dysfunction in kidney transplant patients. Salivary gland involvement is common and is probably chronic.

Cell-mediated immunity is depressed with primary cytomegalovirus infections (Figure 33–8). It may take several months for cellular responses to recover. This may contribute to the persistence of viral infection.

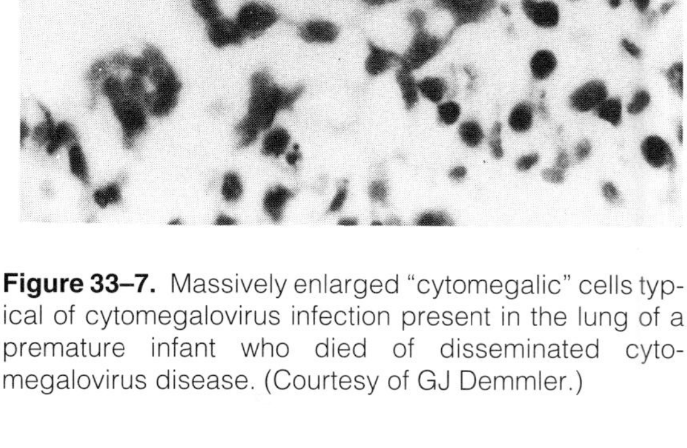

Figure 33–7. Massively enlarged "cytomegalic" cells typical of cytomegalovirus infection present in the lung of a premature infant who died of disseminated cytomegalovirus disease. (Courtesy of GJ Demmler.)

B. Immunosuppressed Hosts: Primary cytomegalovirus infections in immunosuppressed hosts are much more severe than in normal hosts. The individuals at greatest risk for cytomegalovirus disease are those receiving organ transplants, those with malignant tumors who are receiving chemotherapy, and especially those with AIDS. Viral excretion is increased and prolonged, and the infection is more apt to become disseminated. Pneumonia is the most common complication.

The host immune response presumably maintains cytomegalovirus in a latent state in seropositive individuals. Reactivated infections are associated with disease much more often in immunocompromised patients than in normal hosts. Although usually less severe, reactivated infections may be as virulent as primary infections, depending on the circumstances of immunosuppression.

Cytomegalovirus involvement can be detected in many organ systems in severe disseminated disease, based on the distribution of typical cytomegalic inclusion cells. However, the number of cytomegalic cells does not reflect the extent of functional disturbance in diseased organs. Ductal epithelial cells are usually infected rather than fibroblasts—this despite the fact that growth of cytomegalovirus in vitro is restricted to fibroblasts.

C. Congenital and Perinatal Infections: Fetal and newborn infections with cytomegalovirus may be severe. About 1% of live births annually in the USA have congenital cytomegalovirus infections (30,000–35,000 infants). About 10% of those will suffer cytomegalic inclusion disease. A high percentage of babies with this disease will exhibit developmental defects and mental retardation.

The virus can be transmitted in utero with both primary and reactivated maternal infections. Generalized cytomegalic inclusion disease results most often from primary maternal infections. In contrast to the situation with rubella, there is no evidence that gestational age at the time of maternal infection affects expression of disease in the fetus. Fetal damage seldom results from reactivated maternal infections; the infection of the infant remains subclinical though chronic (Figure 33–8).

The most common cause of congenital infection is believed to be transmission of reactivated virus in utero. Intrauterine transmission occurs in no more than 50% of cases. Cytomegalovirus can also be acquired by the infant from exposure to virus in the mother's genital tract during delivery and from maternal breast milk. In these cases, the infants usually have received some maternal antibody, and the perinatally acquired cytomegalovirus infections tend to be subclinical. Transfusion-acquired cytomegalovirus infections in newborns will vary, depending on the amount of virus received and the serologic status of the blood donor.

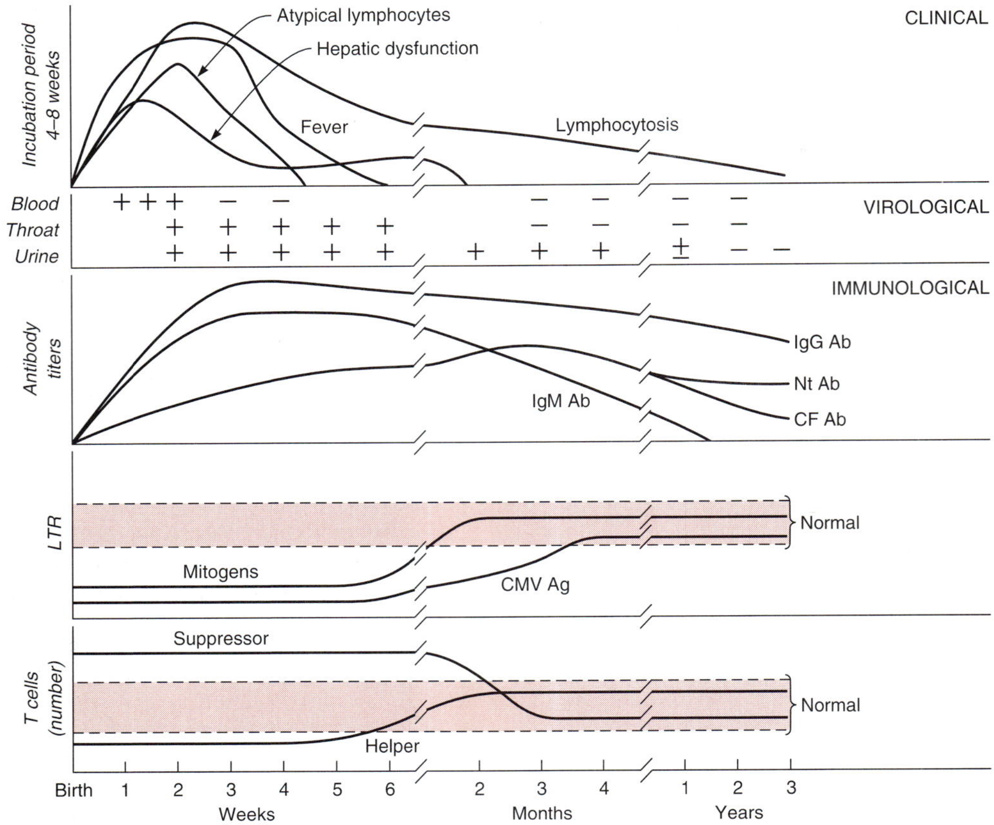

A

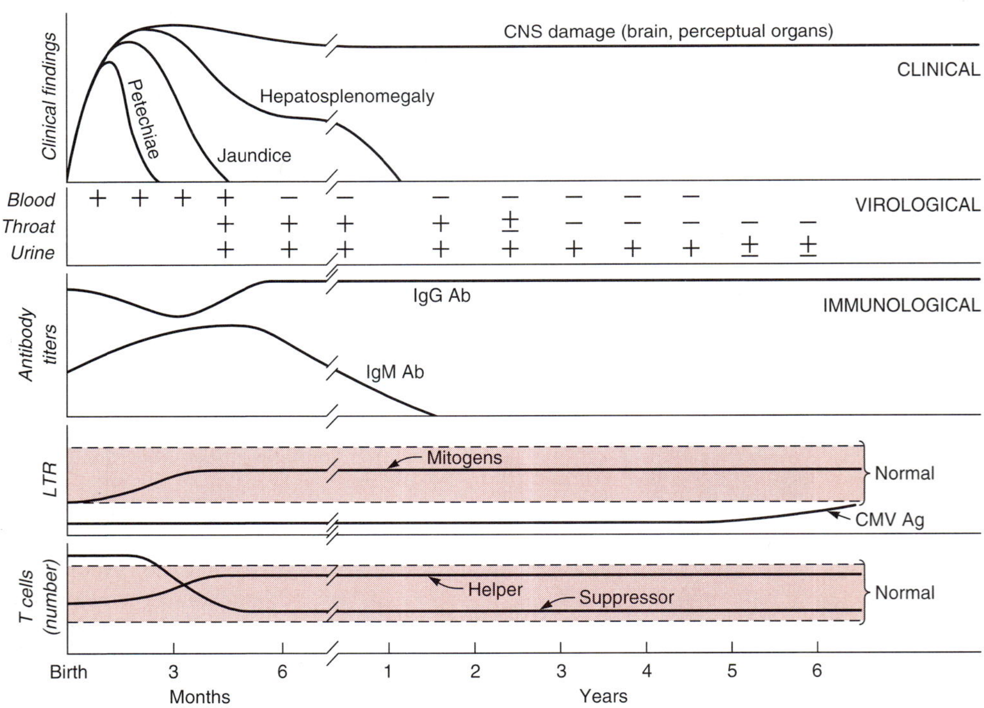

B

Figure 33–8. Clinical, virologic, and immunologic features of cytomegalovirus (CMV) infection in normal individuals ***(A)*** and in congenitally infected infants ***(B).*** LTR, lymphocyte transformation response. (Reproduced, with permission, from Alford CA, Britt WJ: Cytomegalovirus. Pages 1981–2010 in: *Virology,* 2nd ed. Fields BN et al [editors]. Raven Press, 1990.)

Whether cytomegalovirus is acquired in utero or perinatally, a more chronic infection results—with respect to viral excretion—than when the virus is acquired later in life (Figure 33–8).

Clinical Findings

A. Normal Hosts: Primary cytomegalovirus infection of older children and adults causes a spontaneous infectious mononucleosis syndrome. The disease is characterized by malaise, myalgia, protracted fever, liver function abnormalities, and lymphocytosis with an excess of atypical lymphocytes in the absence of a reactive heterophile test. Cytomegalovirus is estimated to cause 20–50% of heterophil-negative (non-Epstein-Barr virus) mononucleosis cases.

Cytomegalovirus mononucleosis is a mild disease, and complications are rare. Subclinical hepatitis is common. In younger children (<7 years old), hepatosplenomegaly is frequently observed.

B. Immunocompromised Hosts: Both morbidity and mortality rates are increased with primary and recurrent cytomegalovirus infections in immunocompromised individuals. Pneumonia is a frequent complication. Interstitial pneumonia caused by cytomegalovirus is the leading cause of death in bone marrow transplant recipients. Cytomegalovirus often causes disseminated disease in AIDS patients; gastroenteritis and chorioretinitis are common problems, the latter often leading to progressive blindness. The colon is most often the site of gastrointestinal tract involvement.

C. Congenital and Perinatal Infections: Congenital infection may result in death of the fetus in utero. Cytomegalic inclusion disease of newborns is characterized by involvement of the central nervous system and the reticuloendothelial system. Mortality rates can approach 30%. About 90% of infants with cytomegalic inclusion disease will develop significant central nervous system defects within 2 years; severe hearing loss, ocular abnormalities, and mental retardation are common. About 10% of infants with subclinical congenital cytomegalovirus infection will develop deafness. It has been estimated that one in every 1000 infants born in the USA is seriously retarded as a result of congenital cytomegalovirus infection.

Many women infected previously with cytomegalovirus show reactivation and begin to excrete the virus from the cervix during pregnancy. At the time of delivery through the infected birth canal, infants may become infected, though they possess high titers of maternal antibody acquired transplacentally. These infants begin to shed virus at about 8–12 weeks of age. They continue to excrete the virus for several years but remain healthy.

Acquired infection with cytomegalovirus is common and usually inapparent. The virus is shed in the saliva and urine of infected individuals for weeks or months.

Cytomegalovirus may be a cause of isolated pneumonia in infants less than 6 months of age.

Immunity

Antibodies to cytomegalovirus occur in most human sera. Cytomegalovirus-specific antibodies of the IgM, IgA, and IgG classes have all been detected. Reactivation of latent infection occurs in the presence of humoral immunity. The presence of antibody in breast milk does not prevent transmission of infection to breast-feeding infants. Maternal antibody protects more against development of serious disease in the infant than viral transmission. Seroconversion using appropriate tests distinguishes primary from recurrent cytomegalovirus infections in immunosuppressed persons.

Laboratory Diagnosis

A. Isolation of Virus: The best means of diagnosing cytomegalovirus infection is viral isolation. The virus can be recovered most readily from throat washings and urine. Other body fluids, as well as biopsy materials, sometimes yield cytomegalovirus. In cultures, 1–2 weeks are usually needed for the appearance of cytologic changes, consisting of small foci of swollen, translucent cells with large intranuclear inclusions. Cell degeneration progresses slowly, and the virus stays cell-associated.

Cell culture methods of viral isolation are too slow to be useful in guiding therapy, particularly in immunosuppressed patients. Rapid diagnostic methods that have been developed include observation of inclusion bodies in tissue or in desquamated cells found in urine, direct detection of viral antigen, visualization of virus by electron microscopy, and DNA hybridization.

Viral isolation, coupled with seroconversion, is the best indication of primary cytomegalovirus infection in normal hosts.

B. Serology: Antibodies may be detected by Nt, CF, radioimmunoassay, or immunofluorescence tests. Such tests may be useful in detecting congenitally infected infants with no clinical manifestations of disease. Serologic techniques cannot distinguish strain differences among clinical isolates. Restriction enzyme analysis of cytomegalovirus DNAs may prove more useful.

Epidemiology

Cytomegalovirus is endemic in all parts of the world; epidemics are unknown. It is present throughout the year, with no seasonal variation seen in infection rates.

The prevalence of infection varies with socioeconomic status, living conditions, and hygienic practices. Antibody prevalence may be moderate (40–80%) in adults in high socioeconomic groups in developed countries—in contrast to a prevalence of 90–100% in children and adults in developing nations and in low socioeconomic groups in developed countries.

Humans are the only known host for cytomegalovirus. Transmission requires close person-to-person contact. Virus may be shed in urine, saliva, semen, breast milk, and cervical secretions and is carried in circulating white blood cells. Oral and respiratory spread are probably the dominant routes of cytomegalovirus transmission. It can also be spread transplacentally, by blood transfusion, by organ transplantation, and by sexual contact.

New infections are almost always asymptomatic. After infection, virus is shed from multiple sites. Viral shedding may continue for years, often intermittently, as latent virus becomes reactivated. Thus, exposures to cytomegalovirus are widespread and common.

Intrauterine infection may produce serious disease in the newborn. About 1% of infants born in the USA are infected with cytomegalovirus. The majority have subclinical but chronic infections; 10% have cytomegalic inclusion disease with attendant developmental defects. Mortality rates are high (up to 30%) among those with cytomegalic inclusion disease. Congenital infections, whether subclinical or clinically apparent, result in chronic infections, with viral shedding detectable for years. Some infections are acquired during birth by exposure to virus in the mother's genital tract. Many more infants (8–60%) become infected with cytomegalovirus in the first months of life, often from infected breast milk or by nursery spread. Most of these infections are subclinical but are usually chronic, with viral shedding persisting for years.

Primary maternal infections during pregnancy are responsible for most cases of cytomegalic inclusion disease. Infants and children with subclinical cytomegalovirus infections are the major source of exposure. Other congenital infections are due to reactivations of latent maternal infections. Genital shedding of cytomegalovirus increases during pregnancy, reaching about 13% in women near term.

Cytomegalovirus can be transmitted by blood transfusion. Estimated risk varies widely but is probably about 3% per unit of whole blood.

Cytomegalovirus infections are markedly increased in immunosuppressed populations. More than 90% of bone marrow or kidney transplant recipients develop infections, most of which are due to reactivations of their own latent virus. Close to 100% of AIDS patients are seropositive for cytomegalovirus and are at high risk for cytomegalovirus-induced disease.

Treatment & Control

Ganciclovir, a nucleoside structurally related to acyclovir, has been used successfully to treat life-threatening cytomegalovirus infections in immunosuppressed patients. Viral replication often recurs when therapy is discontinued. The severity of cytomegalovirus retinitis, esophagitis, and colitis is reduced by ganciclovir. In addition, early treatment with ganciclovir reduces the incidence of cytomegalovirus pneumonia in bone marrow allograft recipients. Acyclovir, vidarabine, and interferon have also been tested as treatments for cytomegalic diseases. Acyclovir has shown some benefits.

Specific control measures are not available to prevent cytomegalovirus spread. Isolation of newborns with generalized cytomegalic inclusion disease from other newborns is advisable.

Screening of transplant donors and recipients for cytomegalovirus antibody may prevent some transmissions of primary cytomegalovirus. The cytomegalovirus-seronegative transplant recipient population represents a high-risk group for cytomegalovirus infections. Administration of human IgG prepared from plasma pools obtained from healthy persons with high titers of cytomegalovirus antibodies (cytomegalovirus immune globulin) effectively decreases the incidence of viral infections in transplant recipients. Cytomegalovirus immune globulin is in limited supply.

The use of blood from seronegative donors has been recommended when infants will require multiple transfusions. This approach would eliminate transfusion-acquired cytomegalovirus infections, but it is difficult to implement.

A live cytomegalovirus "vaccine" has been developed by extended passage in human cells and has had some preliminary clinical trials. In contrast to natural infections, neither viral shedding nor reactivation of latent infections has been detected with the vaccine virus. However, the use of live cytomegalovirus vaccines remains controversial because of safety concerns. Another approach to immunization (that avoids the use of live virus) involves purified cytomegalovirus polypeptides able to induce neutralizing antibodies.

EPSTEIN-BARR VIRUS

Epstein-Barr virus (EB virus) is a ubiquitous herpesvirus that is the causative agent of acute infectious mononucleosis and a factor in the development of nasopharyngeal carcinoma, Burkitt's lymphoma, and other lymphoproliferative disorders in immunodeficient individuals.

Properties of the Virus

EB virus is distinct from all other human herpesviruses. Its DNA genome contains about 172 kbp and has a guanine-plus-cytosine content of 59%.

No classification system exists for EB virus isolates. However, many different viral strains have been detected, based on variation in genome structure, antigen expression, and biologic properties. Most isolates are "transforming," but some are unable to immortalize lymphocytes.

A. Biology of EB Virus: One target cell for EB virus is the B lymphocyte. When human B lymphocytes are infected with EB virus, continuous cell lines can be established, indicating that cells have been immortalized by the virus. Very few of the immortalized cells produce infectious virus. Laboratory studies of EB virus are hampered by the lack of a fully permissive cell system able to propagate the virus.

EB virus initiates infection of B cells by binding to the viral receptor, which is also the receptor for the C3d component of complement (CR2 or CD21). EB virus directly enters a latent state in the lymphocyte without undergoing a period of complete viral replication.

The efficiency of B cell immortalization by EB virus is quite high. When virus binds to the cell surface, cells are activated to enter the cell cycle. Subsequently, some EB virus genes are expressed, and the cells are able to proliferate indefinitely. The linear EB virus genome forms a circle and is amplified; the majority of viral DNA in the immortalized cells exists as circular episomes, though some EB virus DNA has been detected integrated into the cellular genome.

EB virus-immortalized B lymphocytes express differentiated functions, such as secretion of immunoglobulin. B cell activation products (eg, CD23) are also expressed. At least ten viral gene products are expressed in immortalized cells, including six different EB virus nuclear antigens (EBNA1–6) and two latent membrane proteins (LMP1, LMP2).

At any given time, very few cells (<10%) in an immortalized population release viral particles. Latency can be disrupted and the EB virus genome activated to replicate in a cell by a variety of stimuli, including in vitro cultivation of cells and chemical inducing agents. Host-determined differences that are not understood also influence the frequency of transition from latency to viral synthesis.

EB virus replicates in vivo in epithelial cells of the oropharynx, parotid gland, and uterine cervix; it is found in epithelial cells of some nasopharyngeal carcinomas. Although epithelial cells in vivo do contain an EB virus receptor, the receptor is lost from cultured cells.

B. Viral Antigen Systems: EB virus antigens are divided into three classes, based on the phase of the viral life cycle in which they are expressed: (1) Latent phase antigens are synthesized by latently infected cells. These include the EBNAs and the LMPs. Their expression reveals that an EB virus genome is present. Only EBNA1, needed to maintain the viral DNA episomes, is invariably expressed; expression of the other latent phase antigens may be regulated in different cells. LMP2 expression appears to block reactivation from latency. The latent phase antigens represent the membrane target for cytotoxic T cells. (2) Early antigens are nonstructural proteins whose synthesis is not dependent on viral DNA replication. The expression of early antigens indicates the onset of productive viral replication. (3) Late antigens are the structural components of the viral capsid (viral capsid antigen) and viral envelope (membrane antigen). They are produced abundantly in cells undergoing productive viral infection.

C. Experimental Animal Infections: EB virus is quite species-specific. However, several types of New World primates have been infected. Cotton-top marmosets inoculated with EB virus frequently develop fatal malignant lymphomas. Cultured lymphoblastoid cells from such monkeys contain higher levels of viral capsid antigen and release more extracellular virus than do human cells.

Pathogenesis & Pathology

A. Infectious Mononucleosis: EB virus is commonly transmitted by infected saliva and initiates infection in the oropharynx. Viral replication occurs in epithelial cells of the pharynx and salivary glands. Many people shed low levels of virus for weeks to months after infection. Following replication in epithelial cells, the virus infects B lymphoid cells, where it persists in a latent state. In normal individuals, most virus-infected cells are eliminated, but small numbers of infected lymphocytes persist for the lifetime of the host.

EB virus-infected B cells synthesize immunoglobulin; IgA and IgG are commonly found, whereas IgM synthesis is rare. Mononucleosis is a polyclonal transformation of B cells. Autoantibodies are typical of the disease. Heterophile antibody that reacts with antigens on sheep erythrocytes is the classic autoantibody. In addition, many autoantibodies react with cytoskeletal components. EB virus infection causes activation of many B cells that are not infected, and these may be the source of autoantibodies.

Reactivations of EB virus latent infections can occur (evidenced by increased levels of virus in saliva) but are usually clinically silent. Treatment with immunosuppressive drugs is known to reactivate infection, sometimes with serious consequences.

B. Burkitt's Lymphoma: EB virus is associated with the development of Burkitt's lymphoma (a tumor of the jaw in African children and young adults). (See Chapter 43.) Most African tumors (>90%) contain EB virus DNA and EBNA antigen. In other parts of the world, only about 20% of Burkitt's lymphomas contain EB virus DNA. It is speculated that EB virus may be involved at an early stage in Burkitt's lymphoma by immortalizing B cells. Malaria, suspected of being a cofactor, may foster enlargement of the pool of EB virus-transformed cells. Finally, there are characteristic chromosome translocations that involve immunoglobulin genes and result in deregulation of expression of the c-*myc* proto-oncogene. It is unknown how Burkitt's lymphoma cells escape immune elimination by the host.

C. Nasopharyngeal Carcinoma: This cancer of epithelial cells is common in males of Chinese origin. EB virus DNA is regularly found in nasopharyngeal carcinoma cells, and patients have high levels of antibody to EB virus. There are no consistent chromosomal changes in nasopharyngeal carcinoma (as seen in Burkitt's lymphoma). The tumors are poorly differentiated, aggressive, and infiltrated with lymphocytes. Genetic and environmental factors are believed to be important also in the development of nasopharyngeal carcinoma.

D. Lymphoproliferative Diseases in Immunodeficient Hosts: Immunodeficient patients are susceptible to EB virus-induced lymphoproliferative diseases that may be fatal. Lymphomas are often multiclonal and do not show the Burkitt's lymphoma-like chromosome abnormalities. Pathologically, the tumors are different from Burkitt's lymphoma. Lymphoproliferative disease is apt to develop following primary infection of individuals suffering from either congenital or drug-induced immunodeficiency. AIDS patients are susceptible to several EB virus-associated lesions—diffuse polyclonal lymphomas, lymphocytic interstitial pneumonitis, and hairy oral leukoplakia of the tongue. Not all Burkitt's lymphomas occurring in AIDS patients are associated with EB virus.

Clinical Findings

Most primary infections in children are asymptomatic. In adolescents and young adults, the classic syndrome associated with primary infection is infectious mononucleosis (35–75% of infections).

A. Infectious Mononucleosis: After an incubation period of 30–50 days, symptoms of headache, malaise, fatigue, and sore throat occur. Fever lasts about 10 days. Enlarged lymph nodes and spleen are characteristic. Some patients develop signs of hepatitis. A rash occurs in a small percentage of cases.

The typical illness is self-limited and lasts 2–4 weeks. During the disease, there is an increase in the number of circulating white blood cells, with a predominance of lymphocytes. Many of these are large, atypical T lymphocytes. Antigen-reactive T cells develop that can lyse EB virus genome-positive target cells. Part of the infectious mononucleosis syndrome may reflect a rejection reaction against virally converted lymphocytes.

Low-grade fever and malaise may persist for weeks to months after acute illness in some individuals. Complications are rare in normal hosts but include splenic rupture and a number of hematologic syndromes, such as thrombocytopenia and hemolytic anemia. Neurologic manifestations include encephalitis and aseptic meningitis. Fatalities associated with infectious mononucleosis are rare but may occur in patients with underlying immune defects.

B. Chronic EB Virus Infections: A few patients may develop a severe syndrome following EB virus infection that includes pneumonitis, hepatitis, and hematologic abnormalities. There is a prolonged, relapsing course, sometimes ending in death.

EB virus has been proposed to be linked with a confusing syndrome called "chronic fatigue syndrome." Symptoms include extreme fatigue not cured by rest, low-grade fever, sore throat, painful lymph nodes, muscle weakness, and decreased memory. The syndrome can last for months. There is no credible evidence that chronic fatigue syndrome is caused by chronic EB virus infection.

C. Tumors: EB virus appears to be etiologically important in Burkitt's lymphoma and nasopharyngeal carcinoma, a malignancy of epithelial cells. Sera from such patients contain elevated levels of antibody to virus-specific antigens, and the tumor tissues contain EB virus DNA and express viral antigens. EB virus-associated B cell lymphomas may develop in immunodeficient patients.

EB virus DNA has been detected in Reed-Sternberg cells in biopsies from some patients with Hodgkin's disease and in nasal T cell lymphomas in patients with lethal midline granuloma. EB virus-positive T lymphocytes have also been detected in a case of Kawasaki disease (thought to be an immunologically mediated vasculitis). The significance of EB virus in these latter diseases is unknown.

Immunity

EB virus infections elicit an intense immune response consisting of antibodies against many virus-specific proteins, a number of cell-mediated responses, and secretion of lymphokines. Cytotoxic cells that are induced include T cells that react with the EB virus lymphocyte-detected membrane antigen in a histocompatibility (HLA)-restricted fashion, as well as natural killer cells. Both alpha and gamma interferons seem to be involved in control of EB virus infection. The exact role played by antibodies in the process is not known, but the combination of humoral and cell-mediated immune responses appears to suppress B cell proliferation and depress (but not eliminate) oropharyngeal replication of the virus.

Serologic testing to determine the pattern of specific antibodies to different classes of EB virus antigens is the usual means of ascertaining a patient's status with regard to EB virus infection.

Laboratory Diagnosis

A. Isolation and Identification of Virus: EB virus can be isolated from saliva, peripheral blood, or lymphoid tissue by immortalization of normal human lymphocytes, usually obtained from umbilical cord blood. This assay is laborious and time-consuming (6–8 weeks), requires specialized facilities, and is seldom performed. It is also possible to culture "spontaneously transformed" B lymphocytes from EB virus-infected patients. Any recovered immortalizing agent is confirmed as EB virus by detection of EB virus-specific antigens in the immortalized lymphocytes.

EB virus is present in the saliva of many immunosuppressed patients. Up to 20% of healthy adults will also yield virus-positive throat washings.

Nucleic acid hybridization is the most sensitive means of detecting EB virus in patient materials. Viral antigens can be demonstrated directly in lymphoid tissues, in nasopharyngeal carcinomas, and sometimes in peripheral blood cells. During the acute phase of infection, about 1% of circulating lymphocytes will contain EB virus markers; after recovery from infection, about one in 1 million B lymphocytes will carry the virus.

B. Serology: The most common serologic procedure for detection of EB virus antibodies is the indirect immunofluorescence test using smears of EB virus-positive lymphoid cells. ELISA tests are also used.

The typical pattern of antibody responses to EB virus-specific antigens after a primary infection is shown in Figure 33–9. Early in acute disease, a transient rise in IgM antibodies to viral capsid antigen occurs, replaced within weeks by IgG antibodies to this antigen, which persist for life. Slightly later, antibodies to the early antigen develop that persist for several months. Several weeks after acute infection, antibodies to EBNA and the membrane antigen arise and persist throughout life.

The less specific heterophile agglutination test is often used to diagnose EB virus infections. In the course of infectious mononucleosis, most patients develop transient heterophile antibodies that agglutinate sheep cells. There is a comparable horse erythrocyte agglutination test. Commercially available spot tests are convenient. The accidental antigenic relationships that provide for the specificity of this heterophile reaction are not well understood.

C. Interpretation of Results: Serologic tests for EB virus antibodies require some interpretation. Current infection is usually detected by a rise in antibody titer to one of the EB virus antigen systems. The presence of antibody of the IgM type to the viral capsid antigen is also suggestive of current infection. Antibody of the IgG type to the viral capsid antigen is a marker of past infection and indicates immunity to mononucleosis. Early antigen antibodies are generally evidence of current viral infection, though such antibodies are often found in patients with Burkitt's lymphoma or nasopharyngeal carcinoma. Antibodies to the EBNA antigens reveal past infection with EB virus, though detection of a rise in anti-EBNA antibody would suggest a primary infection. Not all persons develop antibody to EBNA. Detection of serum IgA antibodies to EB virus capsid antigen appears to be a useful screening test for early detection of nasopharyngeal carcinoma.

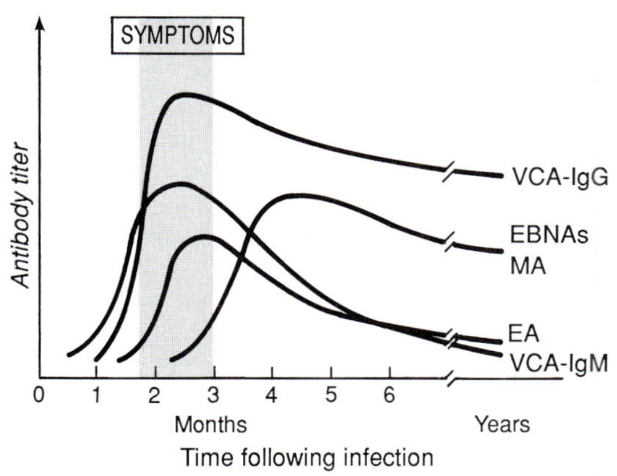

Figure 33–9. Typical pattern of antibody formation to EB virus-specific antigens after a primary infection. Individuals with recent infection have IgM and IgG antibodies to the viral capsid antigen (VCA-IgM, VCA-IgG); only the IgG antibodies persist for years. Antibodies to early antigens (EA) develop in many patients and persist for several months. Several weeks after acute infection, antibodies to EB virus nuclear-associated antigens (EBNAs) and membrane antigen (MA) appear and persist for life. (Modified by permission of the publisher from Straus SE, Smith HA: Cytomegalovirus, varicella-zoster virus, and Epstein-Barr virus. Pages 401–416 in: *Clinical Virology Manual.* Specter S, Lancz GJ [editors]. Copyright 1986 by Elsevier Science Publishing Co.)

Epidemiology

A. Primary Infections: EB virus is common in all parts of the world. In developing areas, infections occur early in life; more than 90% of children are infected by age 6. These infections in early childhood usually occur without any recognizable disease. The inapparent infections result in permanent immunity to infectious mononucleosis. In industrialized nations, more than 50% of EB virus infections are delayed until late adolescence and young adulthood. Again, many of these adult infections are asymptomatic, but in almost half of cases the infection is manifested by heterophil-positive infectious mononucleosis.

B. Burkitt's Lymphoma: Burkitt's lymphoma occurs throughout the world, but sections of equatorial Africa are high-incidence areas. In these endemic regions, which are coincident geographically with universal malaria infections, Burkitt's lymphoma is the most common childhood cancer. The median age of patients with Burkitt's lymphoma is similar worldwide (7.7–10.5 years).

The association of EB virus with African Burkitt's lymphoma is based on two findings: EB virus genomes are present in more than 90% of Burkitt's lymphoma biopsies, and patients with Burkitt's lymphoma have markedly higher titers to EB virus capsid antigen and early antigen than do children without the tumor. In other parts of the world, EB virus is present in about 20% of cases of Burkitt's lymphoma.

C. Nasopharyngeal Carcinoma: This is a rare tumor of adults aged 20–50 years except in the southern provinces of China, where the annual incidence may reach 10 per 100,000. Male cases outnumber female cases 2:1. Both genetic susceptibility and environmental factors are believed to be involved in development of nasopharyngeal carcinoma. EB virus DNA is found in the epithelial cells in nasopharyngeal carcinoma specimens from different parts of the world. Patients with nasopharyngeal carcinoma have elevated levels of IgG antibodies to EB virus capsid antigen and early antigen. In addition, these patients have serum IgA antibodies against both antigens, perhaps reflecting local immune response in the nasopharynx.

Prevention, Treatment, & Control

There is no EB virus vaccine available for use, though candidate vaccines are under study.

Acyclovir reduces EB virus shedding from the oropharynx during the period of drug administration, but it does not affect the number of EB virus-immortalized B cells. Acyclovir has no effect on the symptoms of mononucleosis and is of no proved benefit in the treatment of EB virus-associated lymphomas in immunocompromised patients.

Malaria eradication has been associated with decreased incidence of Burkitt's lymphoma in endemic areas in Africa.

Mass screening programs in China for serum IgA antibody against EB virus antigen appear useful in early diagnosis of nasopharyngeal carcinoma. About 20% of those with elevated IgA to viral capsid antigen who were biopsied were found to have nasopharyngeal carcinoma.

HUMAN HERPESVIRUS 6

The T-lymphotropic human herpesvirus 6 was first recognized in 1986. Initial isolations were made from cultures of peripheral blood mononuclear cells from patients with lymphoproliferative disorders.

Properties of the Virus

The viral DNA is about 160–170 kbp in size and has a mean composition of 43–44% (guanine-plus-cytosine). The genetic arrangement of the human herpesvirus 6 genome resembles that of human cytomegalovirus more closely than it does the lymphotropic gammaherpesviruses.

Very little is known about human herpesvirus 6-specific proteins. However, human herpesvirus 6 appears to be unrelated antigenically to the other known human herpesviruses, except for some limited cross-reactivity with human herpesvirus 7. Isolates of human herpesvirus 6 seem to segregate into two closely related but distinct antigenic groups.

The virus grows well in peripheral blood mononuclear cells, apparently in immature T cells. Other cell types also support viral replication, including B cells and cells of glial, fibroblastoid, and megakaryocyte origin. It is not known which cells in the body become latently infected.

Epidemiology & Clinical Findings

Seroepidemiologic studies using immunofluorescence tests have shown that human herpesvirus 6 is widespread in the population. It is estimated that 60–80% of children and adults in the USA, Japan, and England are seropositive.

Infections with human herpesvirus 6 typically occur in early infancy. This primary infection causes exanthem subitum (roseola infantum, or "sixth disease"), the mild common childhood disease characterized by high fever and skin rash. Viral isolations and seroconversion correlate with this disease in affected infants.

The consequences of primary infections in adulthood or of persistent or reactivated infections remain to be determined. There is evidence it may be involved in idiopathic pneumonitis in immunocompromised individuals. Also, there are suggestions that human herpesvirus 6 may be associated with persistent lymphadenopathy and, perhaps, with occasional cases of hepatitis. Although proteins encoded by human herpesvirus 6 can transactivate the expression of human immunodeficiency virus, there is no evidence to support a role for human herpesvirus 6 in activation of human immunodeficiency virus or progression of human immunodeficiency virus-positive patients to AIDS.

The mode of transmission of human herpesvirus 6 is not known. The fact that it is a ubiquitous agent suggests that it must be shed into the environment from an infected carrier. The virus has been isolated from saliva of normal adults and from a kidney biopsy, so the possibility of salivary transmission and urinary shedding should be considered.

HUMAN HERPESVIRUS 7

The newest T-lymphotropic human herpesvirus, designated human herpesvirus 7, was first isolated in 1990 from activated T cells from peripheral blood lymphocytes of a healthy individual.

Human herpesvirus 7 is immunologically distinct from human herpesvirus 6, though they share limited homology at the DNA level. There are also some genetic similarities with cytomegalovirus.

Human herpesvirus 7 appears to be a ubiquitous agent, with most infections occurring in childhood but later than the very early age of infection noted with human herpesvirus 6. Any association of human herpesvirus 7 with disease remains to be established.

B VIRUS

Herpes B virus of Old World monkeys is highly pathogenic for humans. Transmissibility of virus to humans is limited, but those infections that do occur are associated with a high mortality rate. B virus disease of humans is an acute, usually fatal ascending myelitis and encephalomyelitis.

Properties of the Virus

B virus is a typical herpesvirus that is indigenous to Old World monkeys. B virus is enzootic in rhesus, cynomolgus, and other macaque monkeys (genus *Macaca*). It is currently designated cercopithecine herpesvirus 1, replacing the older name of *Herpes simiae*. As with all herpesviruses, B virus establishes latent infections in infected hosts.

Viral DNA is about 162 kbp in size (MW 107 × 10^6), with a high guanine-plus-cytosine content (75%). B virus shares some antigenic determinants with herpes simplex viruses. It is relatively stable upon storage at 4 °C or frozen (−70 °C).

The virus grows well in cultures of monkey kidney, rabbit kidney, and human cells as well as in chick embryos. The growth cycle is short; both extracellular and intracellular virus levels are maximal within about 24 hours. Cytopathic effects induced by B virus are similar to those of herpes simplex virus. Cells fuse into multinucleated giant cells, and intranuclear inclusions form.

Pathogenesis & Pathology

A. Animal Infections: B virus infections seldom cause disease in rhesus monkeys. Vesicular lesions of the oropharynx may occur and resemble those induced in humans by herpes simplex virus. Many rhesus monkeys carry latent B virus infections that may be reactivated by conditions of stress. The virus has been recovered from monkey saliva, brain, and spinal cord and from preparations of monkey kidney cells.

The virus is transmissible to other monkeys, rabbits, guinea pigs, rats, and mice. The rabbit model is preferred for isolation and characterization of virus. Rabbits routinely develop fatal infections after B virus inoculation by any route.

B. Human Infections: B virus infections in humans usually result from a monkey bite, though infection by the respiratory route is possible. The striking feature of B virus infections in humans is the very strong propensity to cause neurologic disease.

The virus enters through the skin and localizes at the site of the monkey bite, producing vesicles and then necrosis of the area. From the site of the skin lesion, the virus enters the central nervous system by way of the peripheral nerves. Several days after exposure, the patient develops vesicular lesions at the site; regional lymphangitis and lymphadenitis follow. About 7 days later, motor and sensory abnormalities occur; this is followed by acute ascending paralysis, involvement of the respiratory center, and death. Virus can be recovered from the brain and spinal cord of fatal cases. Other tissues and organs can be involved also, depending on the route of inoculation.

Epidemiology & Clinical Findings

B virus is transmitted by direct contact with virus or virus-containing material. Transmission occurs among *Macaca* monkeys and between monkeys and humans. Virus may be present in saliva, conjunctival and vesicular fluids, and, perhaps, feces of monkeys. Respiratory transmission can occur.

Infection in the natural host is rarely associated with obvious disease. Serologic surveys are the basis of knowledge about B virus epidemiology. Infections with B virus are very common in colonies of rhesus monkeys. Seroprevalence is directly correlated with animal age and extent of crowding. More than 70% of adult animals have antibodies against B virus. As latent infections may be reactivated, seropositive animals are reservoirs for transmission of B virus infections. The frequency of excretion of B virus by monkeys is probably no more than 3%.

Transmission to humans is rare, even by monkey bites. Other sources of infection include direct contact with infected materials and animal cages and with infected monkey cell cultures. Direct person-to-person transmission of B virus has been proved.

Only 22 cases of B virus infection in humans have been documented. Of these, 20 individuals developed encephalitis, and 75% died. Most survivors are left with severe neurologic impairment.

Subclinical or mild infections of humans have not been well documented. Serologic studies to detect human B virus infections are difficult because of the extensive cross-reactivity between B virus and herpes simplex virus antigens (and most adults possess herpes simplex virus antibodies). If asymptomatic human infections are more common than suspected, the potential for B virus disease induced by reactivation of latent infection would exist.

Animal workers and persons handling macaque monkeys are at risk of acquiring B virus infection. Individuals having intimate contact with animal workers exposed to the monkeys are also at some risk.

Treatment & Control

There is no specific treatment once the clinical disease is manifest. However, treatment with acyclovir is recommended immediately after exposure. Gamma globulin has not proved to be effective treatment for human B virus infections.

An experimental inactivated B virus vaccine has been tested in monkeys, but it is not available for use in humans.

The risk of B virus infections can be reduced by proper procedures in the laboratory and in the handling and management of macaque monkeys. Guidelines were formulated by the Centers for Disease Control in 1987 for preventing infection by B virus.

REFERENCES

Adler SP: Cytomegalovirus and child day care. Evidence for an increased infection rate among day-care workers. N Engl J Med 1989;321:1290.

Asano Y et al: Viremia and neutralizing antibody response in infants with exanthem subitum. J Pediatrics 1989; 114:535.

Berneman ZN et al: Human herpesvirus 7 is a T-lymphotropic virus and is related to, but significantly different from, human herpesvirus 6 and human cytomegalovirus. Proc Natl Acad Sci USA 1992;89:10552.

Cone RW et al: Human herpesvirus 6 in lung tissue from patients with pneumonitis after bone marrow transplantation. N Engl J Med 1993;329:156.

Fields BN et al (editors): Herpesviridae. Chapters 64–73 in: *Virology,* 2nd ed. Raven Press, 1990.

Gershon AA et al: Live attenuated varicella vaccine. Efficacy for children with leukemia in remission. JAMA 1984; 252:355.

Handsfield HH et al: Cytomegalovirus infection in sex partners: Evidence for sexual transmission. J Infect Dis 1985; 151:344.

Kaplan JE: Herpesvirus simiae (B virus) infection in monkey handlers. J Infect Dis 1988;157:1090.

Masucci MG, Ernberg I: Epstein-Barr virus: Adaptation to a life within the immune system. Trends Microbiol 1994; 2:125.

Onorato IM et al: Epidemiology of cytomegaloviral infections: Recommendations for prevention and control. Rev Infect Dis 1985;7:479.

Rowley AH et al: Rapid detection of herpes-simplex-virus DNA in cerebrospinal fluid of patients with herpes simplex encephalitis. Lancet 1990;335:440.

Sawyer MH et al: Detection of varicella-zoster virus DNA in air samples from hospital rooms. J Infect Dis 1994; 169:91.

Spector SA et al: Detection of human cytomegalovirus in clinical specimens by DNA-DNA hybridization. J Infect Dis 1984;150:121.

Stanberry LR: Genital and neonatal herpes simplex virus infections: Epidemiology, pathogenesis and prospects for control. Rev Med Virol 1993;3:37.

Straus SE: Clinical and biological differences between recurrent herpes simplex virus and varicella-zoster virus infections. JAMA 1989;262:3455.

Whitley RJ: Herpes simplex virus infections of women and their offspring: Implications for a developed society. Proc Natl Acad Sci USA 1994;91:2441.

Whitley RJ, Gnann JW Jr: Acyclovir: A decade later. N Engl J Med 1992;327:782.

World Health Organization: Prevention and control of herpesvirus diseases. (Two parts.) Bull WHO 1985;63:185, 427.

Poxviruses

34

Poxviruses are the largest and most complex of viruses. The family encompasses a large group of agents that are morphologically similar and share a common nucleoprotein antigen. Infections with most poxviruses are characterized by a rash, although lesions induced by some members of the family are markedly proliferative. The group includes variola virus, the etiologic agent of smallpox, the viral disease that has most affected humans throughout recorded history until its elimination in 1977.

Even though smallpox has been declared eradicated from the world after an intensive campaign coordinated by the World Health Organization, there is a continuing need to be familiar with vaccinia virus (used for smallpox vaccinations) and its possible complications in humans. It is also necessary to be aware of other poxvirus diseases that may resemble smallpox and must be differentiated from it by laboratory means. Lastly, vaccinia virus is under intensive study as a vector for introducing active immunizing genes as live-virus vaccines for a variety of viral diseases of humans and domestic animals.

PROPERTIES OF POXVIRUSES

Important properties of the poxviruses are listed in Table 34–1.

Structure & Composition

Poxviruses are large enough to be seen as featureless particles by light microscopy. By electron microscopy, they appear to be brick-shaped or ellipsoid particles measuring about 400 × 230 nm. Their structure is complex and conforms to neither icosahedral nor helical symmetry displayed by other viruses. The external surface of particles contains ridges. There is an outer lipoprotein membrane, or envelope, that encloses a core and two structures of unknown function called lateral bodies (Figure 34–1). The core contains the large viral genome of linear double-stranded DNA (MW 85–150 × 10^6). The DNA contains inverted terminal repeats of variable length, and the strands are connected at the ends by terminal hairpin loops. The DNA is rich in adenine and thymine bases.

The chemical composition of a poxvirus resembles that of a bacterium. Vaccinia virus is composed predominantly of protein (90%), lipid (5%), and DNA (3%). More than 100 structural polypeptides have been detected. A number of the proteins are glycosylated or phosphorylated. The lipids are cholesterol and phospholipids.

The virion contains a multiplicity of enzymes, including a transcriptional system that can synthesize, polyadenylate, cap, and methylate viral mRNA.

Classification

Poxviruses are divided into two subfamilies, based on vertebrate or insect host range. The vertebrate poxviruses fall into six genera, with the members of a given genus displaying similar morphology and host range, as well as some antigenic relatedness.

Most of the poxviruses that can cause disease in humans are contained in the *Orthopoxvirus* and *Parapoxvirus* genera; there are also several that are currently unclassified (Table 34–2).

The orthopoxviruses have a broad host range, affecting several vertebrates. They include ectromelia (mousepox), rabbitpox, cowpox, monkeypox, vaccinia, and variola (smallpox) viruses. The last four are infectious for humans. Vaccinia virus differs in only minor morphologic respects from variola and cowpox viruses. It is the prototype of poxviruses in terms of structure and replication. Monkeypox can infect both monkeys and humans and may resemble smallpox clinically.

Some poxviruses have a restricted host range and infect only rodents (fibroma and myxoma) or only birds. Others infect mainly sheep and goats (sheeppox, goatpox) or cattle (eg, milker's node).

Parapoxviruses are morphologically distinctive. Compared to the orthopoxviruses, parapoxviruses are somewhat smaller particles (260 × 160 nm), and their surfaces exhibit a crisscross pattern (Figure 34–2). Their genomes are smaller (MW 85 × 10^6) and have a higher guanine-plus-cytosine content (63%) than those of the orthopoxviruses (MW 110–140 × 10^6; guanine-plus-cytosine, 30–40%).

All vertebrate poxviruses share a common nucleoprotein antigen in the inner core. There is serologic cross-reactivity among viruses within a given genus but very limited reactivity across genera. Conse-

Table 34–1. Important properties of poxviruses.

Virion: Complex structure, oval or brick-shaped, 400 nm in length × 230 nm in diameter; external surface shows ridges; contains core and lateral bodies.
Composition: DNA (3%), protein (90%), lipid (5%).
Genome: Double-stranded DNA, linear, MW 85–150 million; has terminal loops; has low guanine-plus-cytosine content (30–40%) except for *Parapoxvirus* (63%).
Proteins: Virions contain more than 100 polypeptides; many enzymes are present in core, including transcriptional system.
Envelope: Outer membrane of virion is synthesized by virus; some particles acquire an additional envelope from the cell (not required for infectivity).
Replication: Cytoplasmic factories.
Outstanding characteristics: Largest and most complex viruses; very resistant to inactivation. Smallpox was the first viral disease eradicated from the world.

quently, immunization with vaccinia virus affords no protection against disease induced by parapoxviruses or the unclassified poxviruses.

Poxvirus Replication

The replication cycle of vaccinia virus is summarized in Figure 34–3. Poxviruses are unique among DNA viruses in that the entire multiplication cycle takes place in the cytoplasm of infected cells. They are further distinguished from all other animal viruses by the fact that the uncoating step requires a newly synthesized, virus-encoded protein.

A. Viral Attachment, Penetration, and Uncoating: Viral particles establish contact with the cell surface and are then engulfed in phagocytic vacuoles of the cell. First-stage uncoating takes place by means of hydrolytic enzymes in the vacuole. This releases the viral core into the cytoplasm. Among the several enzymes inside the poxvirus particle, there is a viral RNA polymerase that transcribes about half the viral genome into early mRNA. These mRNAs are transcribed within the viral core and are then released into the cytoplasm. Because the necessary enzymes are contained within the viral core, early transcription is not affected by inhibitors of protein synthesis. The "uncoating" protein that acts on the cores is among the more than 50 polypeptides made early after infection. The second-stage uncoating step liberates viral DNA from the cores; it requires both RNA and protein synthesis. The synthesis of host cell macromolecules is inhibited at this stage.

Poxviruses inactivated by heat can be reactivated either by viable poxviruses or by poxviruses inactivated by nitrogen mustards (which inactivate the DNA). This process is called **nongenetic reactivation** and is due to the action of the uncoating protein. Heat-inactivated virus alone cannot cause second-stage uncoating because of the heat lability of the RNA polymerase. Any vertebrate poxvirus can reactivate any other vertebrate poxvirus.

B. Replication of Viral DNA and Synthesis of Viral Proteins: Among the early proteins made after vaccinia virus infection are enzymes involved in DNA replication, including a DNA polymerase and thymidine kinase. Viral DNA replication starts soon after the release of viral DNA in the second stage of uncoating. It occurs from 2 to 6 hours after infection in discrete

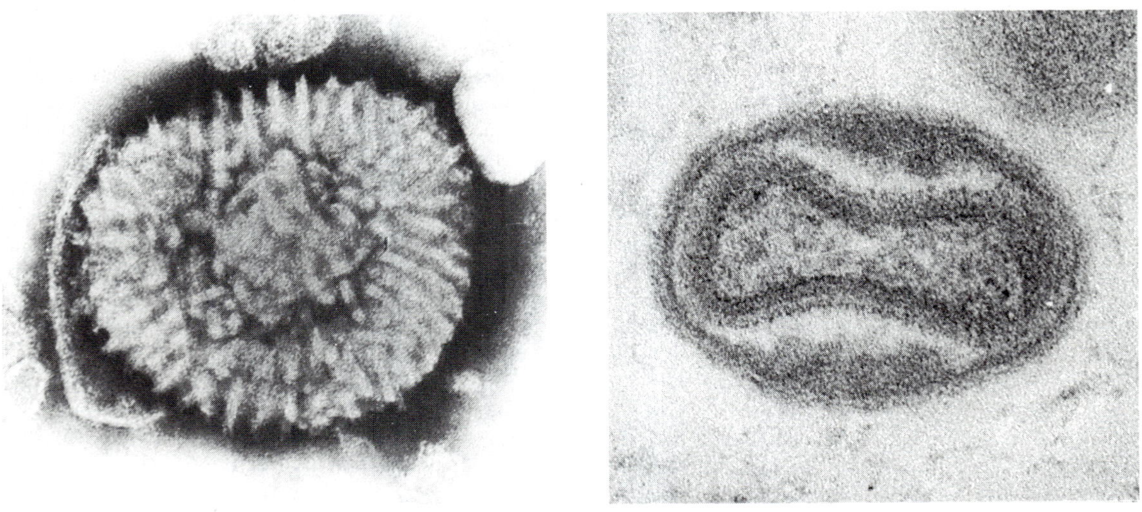

A. B.

Figure 34–1. Electron micrographs of vaccinia *(Orthopoxvirus)* virions. ***A:*** Negatively stained particle showing ridges or tubular elements covering the surface (228,000×). (Reproduced, with permission, from Dales S: J Cell Biol 1963;18:51.) ***B:*** Thin section of vaccinia virion showing a central biconcave core, two lateral bodies, and an outer membrane (220,000×). (Reproduced, with permission, from Pogo BGT, Dales S: Proc Natl Acad Sci USA 1969;63:820.)

Table 34–2. Poxviruses causing disease in humans.

Genus	Virus	Primary Host	Disease
Orthopoxvirus	Variola	Humans	Smallpox (now extinct).
	Vaccinia	Humans	Used for smallpox vaccination.
	Monkeypox	Monkeys	Human infections rare, generalized disease.
	Cowpox	Cows	Human infections rare, localized ulcerating lesion.
Parapoxvirus	Orf	Sheep	Human infections rare, localized lesion.
	Milker's node	Cows	
Unclassified	Molluscum contagiosum	Humans	Many benign skin nodules.
	Tanapox	Monkeys	Human infections rare, localized lesion.
	Yabapox	Monkeys	Human infections very rare and accidental, localized skin tumors.

areas of the cytoplasm, which appear as "factories" or inclusion bodies (Figure 34–4) in electron micrographs. Inclusion bodies can form anywhere in the cytoplasm. The number observed per cell is proportionate to the multiplicity of infection, suggesting that each infectious particle can induce a "factory."

The pattern of viral gene expression changes markedly with the onset of replication of viral DNA. The synthesis of many of the early proteins is inhibited. Late viral mRNA is translated into large amounts of structural proteins and small amounts of other viral proteins and enzymes. DNA replication then ceases.

C. Maturation: The assembly of the viral particle from the manufactured components is a complex process. Poxviruses are unique in that de novo formation of viral membranes occurs (Figure 34–5). Mature virions appear in electron micrographs as a DNA-containing core encased in double membranes, surrounded by protein, and all enclosed within two outer membranes. Some of the particles are released from the cell by budding and gain a cell-related envelope. This second envelope is not required for infectivity. However, the majority of poxvirus particles remain within the host cell. About 10,000 viral particles are produced per cell.

Two antiviral drugs affect the morphogenesis of poxvirus particles. Rifampin can block the formation and assembly of the vaccinia virus envelope. Methisazone interferes with the formation of late proteins and assembly of the particle. (See Chapter 30.)

D. Virus-Encoded Growth Factor: A 140-residue polypeptide encoded by one of the early genes of vaccinia virus is closely related to epidermal growth factor and to transforming growth factor-alpha. The vaccinia growth factor can enhance epithelial wound healing in vivo. Production of growth factors similar to epidermal growth factor by virus-infected cells could account for the proliferative diseases associated with members of the poxvirus family such as Shope fibroma, Yaba tumor, and molluscum contagiosum viruses. Another viral gene product is a secretory polypeptide related to complement control proteins (which can function to block complement-mediated induction of the inflammatory response).

POXVIRUS INFECTIONS IN HUMANS: VACCINIA & VARIOLA

Control & Eradication of Smallpox

Control of smallpox by deliberate infection with mild forms of the disease was practiced for centuries.

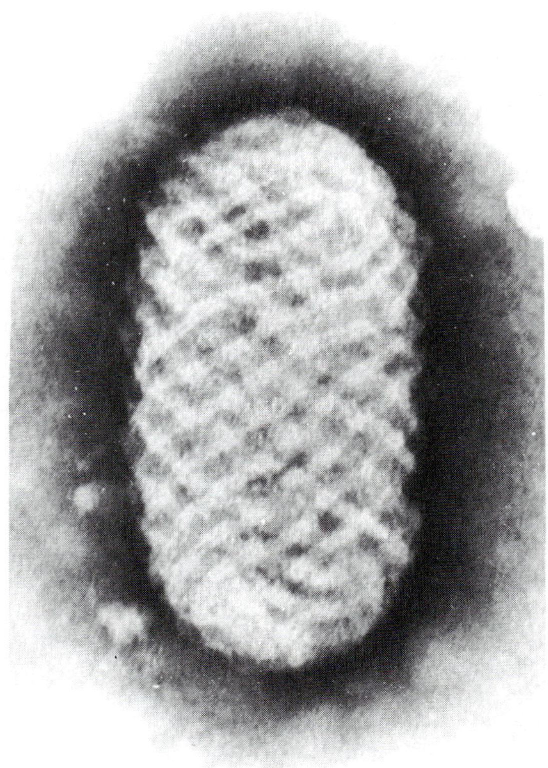

Figure 34–2. Electron micrograph of orf virus *(Parapoxvirus)*. Note distinctive crisscross pattern of surface of virion (200,000×). (Courtesy of FA Murphy and EL Palmer.)

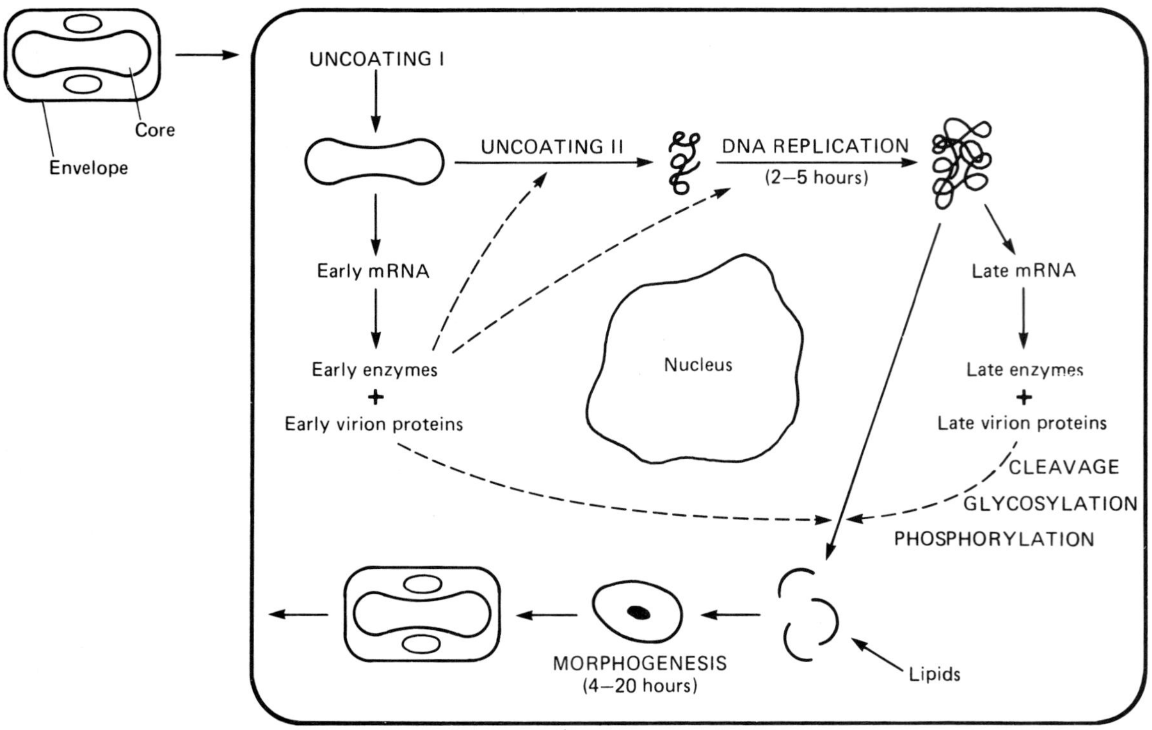

Figure 34–3. Outline of replication cycle of vaccinia virus. (Reproduced, with permission, from Moss B: Replication of poxviruses. Pages 685–703 in: *Virology*. Fields BN et al [editors]. Raven Press, 1985.)

This process, called variolation, was dangerous but decreased the disastrous effects of major epidemics, reducing the case-fatality rate from 25% to 1%. Jenner introduced vaccination with live vaccinia virus in 1798.

In 1967, the World Health Organization introduced a worldwide campaign to eradicate smallpox. Epidemiologic features of the disease (described below) made it feasible to attempt total eradication. At that time, there were 33 countries with endemic smallpox and 10–15 million cases per year. The last Asiatic case occurred in Bangladesh in 1975, and the last natural victim was diagnosed in Somalia in 1977. Smallpox was officially declared eliminated in 1980. There were three main reasons for this outstanding success: The vaccine was easily prepared, stable, and safe; it could be given simply by personnel in the field; and mass vaccination of the world population was not necessary. Cases of smallpox were traced, and contacts of the patient and those in the immediate area were vaccinated.

Even though there has been no evidence of smallpox transmission anywhere in the world, the World Health Organization coordinated the investigation of 173 possible cases of smallpox between 1979 and 1984. All were diseases other than smallpox, most commonly chickenpox or other illnesses that produce a rash. Even so, a suspected case of smallpox becomes a public health emergency and must be promptly investigated by means of clinical evaluation, collection of laboratory specimens, and preliminary laboratory diagnosis.

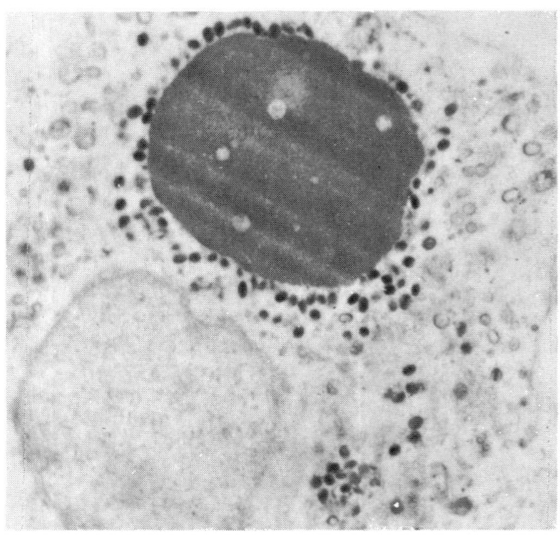

Figure 34–4. Mousepox virus within the infected cell (7400×). Nucleus at lower left; above it can be seen a dark cytoplasmic inclusion body surrounded by viral particles. A group of viral particles in the process of development is located to the right of the nucleus. (WH Gaylord and JL Melnick.)

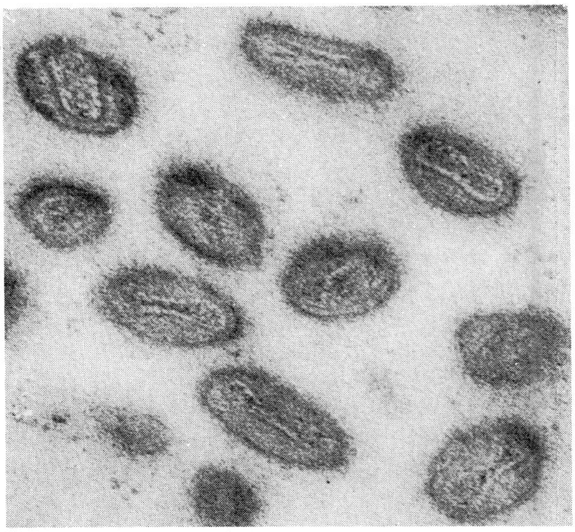

Figure 34–5. Ultrathin section of vaccinia virus particles within the cytoplasm of an infected cell (74,000×). The internal structure of the mature virus is evident. (C Morgan, HM Rose, and DH Moore.)

The presence of stocks of virulent smallpox virus in laboratories is of concern because of the danger of laboratory infection and subsequent spread into the community. Variola virus stocks have been destroyed in all laboratories except two World Health Organization collaborating centers (one in Atlanta and one in Moscow) that pursue diagnostic and research work on variola-related poxviruses. There is debate as to whether these remaining stocks should be destroyed. There is still no understanding of what made variola so virulent.

Comparison of Vaccinia & Variola Viruses

Vaccinia virus, the agent used for smallpox vaccination, is a distinct species of *Orthopoxvirus.* Restriction endonuclease maps of the genome of vaccinia virus are distinctly different from those of cowpox virus, which was believed to be its ancestor. Vaccinia virus may be the product of genetic recombination, a new species derived from cowpox virus or variola virus by serial passage, or the descendant of a now extinct viral genus.

Variola has a narrow host range (only humans and monkeys), whereas vaccinia has a broad host range that includes rabbits and mice. Both vaccinia and variola viruses grow on the chorioallantoic membrane of the 10- to 12-day-old chick embryo, but the latter produces much smaller pocks. Both grow in several types of chick and primate cell lines.

The nucleotide sequences of variola (186 kb) and vaccinia (192 kb) are similar, with the most divergence in terminal regions of the genomes. Of 187 putative proteins, 150 were markedly similar in sequence between the two viruses; the remaining 37 diverged or were variola-specific and may represent potential virulence determinants. The sequences do not reveal variola virus origins or explain its strict human host range or its particular virulence.

Pathogenesis & Pathology of Smallpox

Although smallpox has been eradicated, the pathogenesis of the disease (described here in the past tense) is instructive for other poxvirus infections. The pathogenesis of mousepox is illustrated in Figure 30–3.

The portal of entry of variola virus was the mucous membranes of the upper respiratory tract. After viral entry, the following are believed to have taken place: (1) primary multiplication in the lymphoid tissue draining the site of entry; (2) transient viremia and infection of reticuloendothelial cells throughout the body; (3) a secondary phase of multiplication in those cells, leading to (4) a secondary, more intense viremia; and (5) the clinical disease.

In the preeruptive phase, the disease was barely infective. By the sixth to ninth days, lesions in the mouth tended to ulcerate and discharge virus. Thus, early in the disease, infectious virus originated in lesions in the mouth and upper respiratory tract. Later, pustules broke down and discharged virus into the environment of the smallpox patient.

The skin lesion followed the localization of virus in the epidermis from the bloodstream. The virus could be isolated from the blood in the first few days of the disease. Clinical improvement followed the development of the skin eruption, perhaps owing to the appearance of antibodies. Pustulation of the skin lesions sometimes gave rise to a secondary fever; this may have been due to absorption of the products of cell necrosis rather than to secondary bacterial infection.

Skin pustules could become contaminated, usually with staphylococci, sometimes leading to bacteremia and sepsis.

Histopathologic examination of the skin showed proliferation of the prickle-cell layer. Those proliferated cells contained many cytoplasmic inclusions. There was infiltration with mononuclear cells, particularly around the vessels in the corium. Epithelial cells of the malpighian layer became swollen through distention of cytoplasm and underwent "ballooning degeneration." The vacuoles in the cytoplasm enlarged. The cell membrane broke down and coalesced with neighboring, similarly affected cells, resulting in the formation of vesicles. The vesicles enlarged and then became filled with white cells and tissue debris. All the layers of the skin were involved, and there was actual necrosis of the corium. Thus, scarring occurred after variola infection. Similar histopathology is seen with vaccinia.

Vaccinia virus ordinarily causes localized pustular lesions at the site of inoculation.

Clinical Findings

The incubation period of variola (smallpox) was about 12 days. The onset was usually sudden. One to 5 days of fever and malaise preceded the appearance of the exanthems, which were papular for 1–4 days, vesicular for 1–4 days, and pustular for 2–6 days, forming crusts that fell off 2–4 weeks after the first sign of the lesion and leaving pink scars that faded slowly. In each affected area, the lesions were generally found in the same stage of development (in contrast to chickenpox). Body temperature fell within 24 hours after the rash appeared.

Rash distribution was characteristic. Lesions were most abundant on the face and less so on the trunk. The nature and extent of the rash were functions of the severity of the disease. In severe cases, the rash was hemorrhagic. The case-fatality rate varied from 5 to 40%. In mild variola, called variola minor, or in vaccinated persons, the mortality rate was under 1%.

Variola minor gave rise to a mild disease in contacts, whereas modified variola major in immunized persons often caused severe smallpox in contacts. Vaccinated contacts could develop a febrile illness without rash that progressed no further. A "Smallpox Recognition Card" prepared by the World Health Organization shows the typical rash (Figure 34–6).

Immunity

An attack of smallpox gave complete protection against reinfection. Vaccination with vaccinia induced immunity against variola virus for at least 5 years and sometimes longer. Neonates of vaccinated, immune mothers receive maternal antibody transplacentally, which persists for several months. After that time, artificial immunity can be produced by vaccination (see below). Immunity is demonstrable 8–9 days following vaccination, reaches its maximum within 2–3 weeks, and is maintained at an appreciable level for a few years.

All viruses within the *Orthopoxvirus* genus are so closely related antigenically that they cannot be easily differentiated serologically. Infection with one induces an immune response that reacts with all other members of the group.

In addition to structural antigens, poxviruses produce soluble antigens and hemagglutinins. The structural antigens are the viral nucleoproteins and virion surface tubule proteins. The soluble antigens are re-

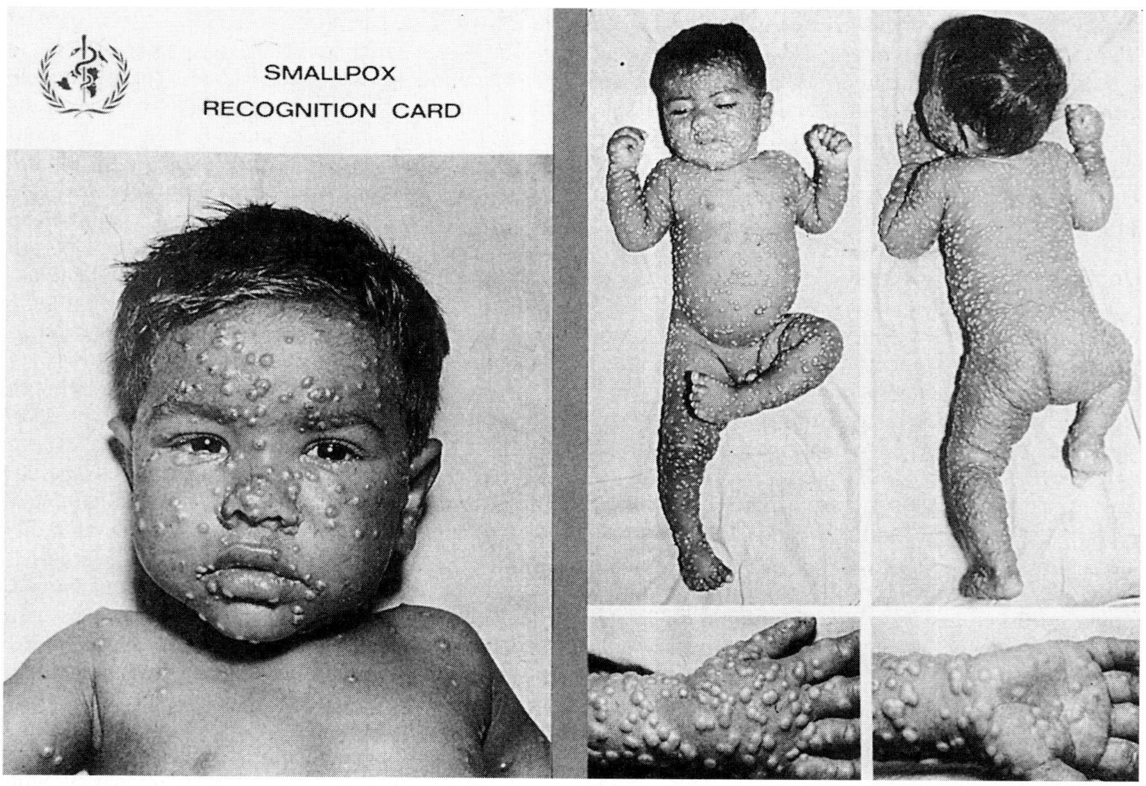

Figure 34–6. Smallpox rash. A "Smallpox Recognition Card" from the World Health Organization illustrates the distribution and nature of the typical rash of smallpox in an unvaccinated child. (Courtesy of Frank Fenner and the World Health Organization.)

leased from infected cells during the infection. The hemagglutinin of vaccinia or variola virus is not an integral part of the virion. It is a lipoprotein complex associated with a small subviral particle.

Antibodies alone are not sufficient for recovery from primary poxvirus infection. In the human host, neutralizing antibodies develop within a few days after onset of smallpox but do not prevent progression of lesions, and patients may die in the pustular stage with high antibody levels. Cell-mediated immunity is probably more important than circulating antibody. Patients with hypogammaglobulinemia generally react normally to vaccination and develop immunity despite the apparent absence of antibody. Immunity is accompanied by delayed cutaneous hypersensitivity to vaccinia. Patients who have defects in both cellular immune response and antibody response develop a progressive, usually fatal disease upon vaccination.

Production of interferon (see Chapter 30) is another possible immune mechanism. Irradiated animals without detectable antibody or delayed hypersensitivity recovered from vaccinia infection as rapidly as untreated control animals.

Laboratory Diagnosis

Several tests are available to confirm the diagnosis of smallpox. Now that the disease is presumably eradicated, it is important to diagnose any cases that resemble smallpox. The tests depend upon direct microscopic examination of material from skin lesions, recovery of virus from the patient, identification of viral antigen from the lesion, and least importantly, demonstration of antibody in the blood.

A. Isolation and Identification of Virus: Skin lesions are the specimen of choice for viral isolation. Poxviruses are stable and will remain viable in specimens for weeks, even without refrigeration.

Direct examination of clinical material in the electron microscope is used for rapid identification of viral particles (in about 1 hour) and can readily differentiate a poxvirus infection from chickenpox (the latter is caused by a herpesvirus). Orthopoxviruses cannot be distinguished from one another by electron microscopy, because they are similar in size and morphology. However, they can be easily differentiated from tanapoxvirus and parapoxviruses.

Viral isolation is carried out by inoculation of vesicular fluid onto the chorioallantoic membrane of chick embryos. This is the most reliable laboratory test. It is the easiest way of distinguishing cases of smallpox from generalized vaccinia, for the lesions produced by these viruses on the membrane differ markedly. In 2–3 days, vaccinia pocks are large with necrotic centers whereas variola pocks are much smaller. Cowpox and monkeypox produce distinctive hemorrhagic lesions. The parapoxviruses, molluscum contagiosum virus, and tanapoxvirus do not grow on the membrane.

Cell cultures can also be used for viral isolation. Human and nonhuman primate cells are most susceptible. The orthopoxviruses grow well in cultured cells; parapoxviruses and tanapoxvirus grow less well, and molluscum contagiosum virus has not yet been grown in cell culture.

Viral antigen can be detected by agar gel precipitation in material collected from skin lesions. The test identifies orthopoxviruses as a group. It is a good substitute if electron microscopy is not available. Stained smears of lesion material were used in the past to look for poxvirus inclusion bodies, but electron microscopy has made this method obsolete.

B. Serology: Viral isolation is necessary for quick and accurate identification of poxvirus infections. However, antibody assays can be used to confirm a diagnosis. Antibodies appear after the first week of infection that can be detected by HI, Nt, ELISA, RIA, or immunofluorescence tests. None of these tests will distinguish among the orthopoxviruses.

Differential Diagnosis

Smallpox may be confused with varicella, pustular acne, meningococcemia, blood dyscrasias, drug rashes, and other illnesses associated with a skin eruption, but none of these illnesses yields materials that give positive laboratory tests for poxviruses.

The use of restriction enzyme cleavage of viral DNA and the analysis of polypeptides in poxvirus-infected cells can demonstrate distinct characteristics for variola, vaccinia, monkeypox, and cowpox. This is important because smallpox-like illnesses must be identified to ascertain that variola has indeed been eradicated.

Treatment

Vaccinia immune globulin is prepared from blood provided by revaccinated military personnel. Indications for use of vaccinia immune globulin are accidental inoculation of vaccine in the eye or eczema vaccinatum.

Methisazone (Marboran) is the only chemotherapeutic agent of any value against poxviruses. It is effective as prophylaxis but is not useful in treatment of established disease (see Chapter 30). It may be beneficial in severe cases of eczema vaccinatum that do not quickly respond to vaccinia immune globulin. Rifampin inhibits the replication of vaccinia virus in cell culture, but it was not effective against smallpox in field trials.

Epidemiology

Transmission of smallpox could usually be traced to contact between cases. Smallpox was highly contagious. The virus was stable in the extracellular environment but was most commonly transmitted by respiratory spread. The dried virus in crusts from skin lesions could survive on clothes or other materials and result in infections.

Patients could be infectious during the incubation period. Virus was isolated from throat swabs obtained from family contacts of patients with smallpox. Respiratory droplets were infectious earlier than skin lesions.

The following epidemiologic features made smallpox amenable to total eradication: There was no known nonhuman reservoir. There was one stable serotype. There was an effective vaccine. Subclinical infectious cases did not occur. Chronic, asymptomatic carriage of the virus did not occur. Since virus in the environment of the patient derived from lesions in the mouth and throat (and later in the skin), patients with infection sufficiently severe to transmit the disease were likely to be so ill that they quickly reached the attention of medical authorities. The close contact requisite for effective spread of the disease generally made for ready identification of a patient's contacts so that specific control measures could be instituted to interrupt the cycle of transmission.

The World Health Organization was successful in eradicating smallpox by using a surveillance-containment program. The source of each outbreak was determined, and all susceptible contacts were identified and vaccinated.

Vaccination With Vaccinia

Vaccinia virus for vaccination is prepared from vesicular lesions ("lymph") produced in the skin of calves or sheep, or it can be grown in chick embryos. The final product contains 40% glycerol to stabilize the virus and 0.4% phenol to destroy bacteria. World Health Organization standards require that smallpox vaccines have a potency of no fewer than 10^8 pock-forming units per milliliter.

Calf-lymph vaccine is kept frozen until issued to physicians. It can then be stored for some weeks in a refrigerator without significant loss of potency, but when removed to room temperature it must be used promptly. Deterioration of vaccine is a problem in tropical countries. There, a stable lyophilized vaccine prepared from infected chorioallantoic membranes of embryonated eggs ("avianized vaccine") has been used.

The success of smallpox eradication has meant that routine vaccination is no longer recommended. The following summary of vaccination is given because vaccinia virus continues to be administered to millions of persons in military and other populations, and complications from such use continue to occur. In addition, vaccinia virus is under consideration as a vector for introducing foreign genes for immunization purposes.

A. Time of Vaccination: Complications of vaccination (see below) occur most commonly under the age of 1 year. Therefore, vaccinating between 1 and 2 years of age is preferable to vaccinating in the first year of life. Infants suffering from skin diseases or those with siblings who have skin diseases should not be vaccinated because the vaccinia virus may localize in the lesions of the vaccinated child or of the contact (eczema vaccinatum). Revaccination has been done at 3-year intervals.

B. Technique: The methods used are multiple pressure, multiple puncture, or jet injection. In all techniques, inoculation should be intradermal, never subcutaneous.

C. Reactions and Interpretations:

1. Primary take–In the fully susceptible person, a papule surrounded by hyperemia appears on the third or fourth day. The papule increases in size until vesiculation appears (on the fifth or sixth day). The vesicle reaches its maximum size by the ninth day and then becomes pustular, usually with some tenderness of the axillary nodes. Desiccation follows and is complete in about 2 weeks, leaving a depressed pink scar that ultimately turns white. The reading of the result is usually done on the seventh day. If this reaction is not observed, vaccination should be repeated.

2. Revaccination–A successful revaccination shows in 6–8 days a vesicular or pustular lesion or an area of palpable induration surrounding a central lesion, which may be a scab or an ulcer. Only this reaction indicates with certainty that viral multiplication has taken place. **Equivocal reactions** may represent immunity but may also represent merely allergic reactions to a vaccine that has become inactivated. When an equivocal reaction occurs, the revaccination should be repeated using a new lot of vaccine known to give "takes" in other persons.

D. Complications of Vaccination: Smallpox vaccination is associated with a definite measurable risk. In the USA, the risk of death from all complications was 1 per million for primary vaccinees and 0.1 per million for revaccinees. For children under 1 year of age, the risk of death was 5 per million primary vaccinations. Among primary vaccinees, the combined incidence of postvaccinal encephalitis and vaccinia necrosum was 3.8 per million in persons of all ages. In revaccinees, these two complications occurred at a rate of 0.7 per million.

Even though routine smallpox vaccination of children in the USA was stopped in 1971, more than four million doses of smallpox vaccine were administered in 1978. Severe complications of vaccination occurred in conjunction with immunodeficiency, immunosuppression, hematologic or other malignancies, and pregnancy.

1. Generalized vaccinia–This is manifested by the occurrence of crops of vaccinial lesions over the surface of the body. Following vaccination, children suffering from eczema may develop vaccinial lesions on the eczematous areas (eczema vaccinatum). Children with a current or prior history of eczema should not be vaccinated, since the mortality rate in untreated generalized vaccinia is 30–40%. Neither should children who have siblings with eczema be vaccinated, because of the danger of transmitting the virus and producing generalized vaccinia in the siblings. Generalized vaccinia can occur in the absence of eczema, but this is rare. The use of vaccinia immune globulin has reduced the mortality rate of eczema vaccinatum from 40% to 7%.

2. Postvaccinal encephalitis–The mortality rate of this serious complication may be as high as 40%. The incidence in the USA was about 3 per million among primary vaccinees of all ages. The onset is sudden and occurs about 12 days after vaccination. There is a pleocytosis of the cerebrospinal fluid. Focal lesions are widely distributed throughout the gray and white matter of the brain and cord. Perivascular infiltrations of mononuclear cells and areas of demyelination are the chief histologic lesions.

The cause is not clear. Several possibilities exist: (1) Vaccinia virus may invade the central nervous system. (2) Vaccination may activate a latent virus of the nervous system. (3) The reaction may be due to an antigen-antibody reaction that is allergic in character. Similar demyelinating disease has been reported after infection with variola, measles, and varicella and after vaccination against rabies.

3. Vaccinia necrosum or progressive vaccinia–This results from inability to make antibody or to develop cellular resistance and may be fatal. Treatment with vaccinia immune globulin or methisazone may be of value.

4. Fetal vaccinia–Very rarely, a woman vaccinated late in pregnancy has transmitted vaccinia virus to the fetus and stillbirth has resulted. Therefore, vaccination should be avoided in pregnancy.

MONKEYPOX INFECTIONS

Monkeypox virus is a species of *Orthopoxvirus*. The disease was first recognized in captive monkeys in 1958. Human infections with this virus were discovered in the early 1970s in west and central Africa after the eradication of smallpox from the region.

The disease is a rare zoonosis that has been detected only in remote villages in tropical rain forests, particularly in Zaire. It is probably acquired by direct contact with wild animals killed for food and skins. The primary reservoir host is not known but may be a rodent.

The clinical features of human monkeypox have been established, based on an examination of 282 infected patients in Zaire from 1980 to 1985. Patients were of all ages, but the majority (90%) were less than 15 years old. Clinical symptoms were similar to ordinary and modified forms of smallpox. "Cropping" of the rash occurred in some patients, posing a diagnostic problem with chickenpox. Pronounced lymphadenopathy occurred in most patients, a feature not seen with smallpox or chickenpox.

Complications were common and often serious. These were generally pulmonary distress and secondary bacterial infections. In unvaccinated patients, the fatality rate was about 11%. Vaccination with vaccinia either protects against monkeypox or lessens the severity of disease.

Human monkeypox infection is not easily transmitted from person to person. It is estimated that only about 15% of susceptible family contacts acquire monkeypox from patients.

Human monkeypox infections are rare, but they are probably the most important orthopoxvirus infections now occurring in humans.

COWPOX INFECTIONS

Cowpox virus is another species of *Orthopoxvirus*. This disease of cattle is milder than the pox diseases of other animals, the lesions being confined to the teats and udders. Infection of humans occurs by direct contact during milking, and the lesion in milkers is usually confined to the hands. The disease is more severe in unvaccinated persons than in those vaccinated with vaccinia virus. The local lesion is associated with fever and lymphadenitis.

Cowpox virus is similar to vaccinia virus immunologically and in host range. It is also closely related immunologically to variola virus. Jenner observed that those who have had cowpox are immune to smallpox. Cowpox virus can be distinguished from vaccinia virus by the deep red hemorrhagic lesions that cowpox virus produces on the chorioallantoic membrane of the chick embryo.

The natural reservoir of cowpox seems to be a rodent, and both cattle and humans are only accidental hosts. Domestic cats also are susceptible to cowpox virus. More than 50 cases in felines have been reported from the United Kingdom, but transmission from cats to humans is believed to be uncommon. Cowpox is no longer enzootic in cattle, although bovine and associated human cases occasionally occur. Feline cowpox is sporadic, and transmission is probably from a small wild rodent. Human cases (with hemorrhagic skin lesions, fever, and general malaise) may occur without any known animal contact and may not be diagnosed.

ORF VIRUS INFECTIONS

The virus of orf is a species of *Parapoxvirus*. It causes a disease in sheep and goats that is prevalent worldwide. The disease is also called contagious pustular dermatitis or sore mouth.

Orf is transmitted to humans by direct contact with an infected animal. It is an occupational disease of sheep handlers. Infection of humans occurs usually as a single lesion on a finger, hand, or forearm but may appear on the face or neck. The infection is seldom generalized. Healing takes several weeks.

MOLLUSCUM CONTAGIOSUM

Molluscum contagiosum is a benign epidermal tumor that occurs only in humans. The causative agent is an unclassified member of the poxvirus group.

The virus has not been transmitted to animals and has not been grown in tissue culture. It has been studied in the human lesion by electron microscopy. The purified virus is oval or brick-shaped and measures 230 × 330 nm; it resembles vaccinia. Antibodies to the virus do not cross-react with any other poxviruses.

The lesions of this disease are small, pink, wart-like tumors on the face, arms, back, and buttocks. They are rarely found on the palms, soles, or mucous membranes. The disease occurs throughout the world, in both sporadic and epidemic forms, and is more frequent in children than in adults. It is spread by direct and indirect contact (eg, by barbers, common use of towels, swimming pools).

The incidence of molluscum contagiosum as a sexually transmitted disease in young adults is increasing. It is seen also in some patients with AIDS. Although the typical lesion is an umbilicated papule, lesions in moist genital areas may become inflamed or ulcerated and may be confused with those produced by herpes simplex virus (HSV). Specimens from such lesions are often submitted to viral diagnostic laboratories for isolation of HSV (see below).

The incubation period may extend for up to 6 months. Lesions may itch, leading to autoinoculation. The lesions may persist for up to 2 years but will eventually regress spontaneously. The virus is a poor immunogen; about one-third of patients never produce antibodies against the virus. Second attacks are common.

Although molluscum contagiosum virus has not been serially propagated in cell culture, it can infect human and primate cells and undergo an abortive infection. Uncoating occurs to produce cores, followed by a transient characteristic cytopathic effect. The cellular changes can be mistaken for those produced by HSV; thus, isolates from specimens suspected to contain HSV should be specifically identified by immunologic methods. In a 1985 study of 137 specimens cultured for HSV with the use of human fibroblast cells, 49 contained HSV; six others produced cytopathic effects but were negative for HSV antigens. Electron microscopy confirmed the presence of molluscum contagiosum virus in those HSV-negative, cytopathic-effect-positive samples.

The diagnosis of molluscum contagiosum can usually be made clinically. However, a semi-solid caseous material can be expressed from the lesions and used for laboratory diagnosis. Electron microscopy will detect poxvirus particles.

TANAPOX & YABA MONKEY TUMOR POXVIRUS INFECTIONS

Tanapox is a fairly common skin infection in parts of Africa, mainly in Kenya and Zaire. It is thought to be spread from infected animals to humans by contaminated arthropods. Its natural host is probably monkeys.

Tanapox and Yaba monkey tumor viruses are serologically related to each other but are distinct from all other poxviruses. They are morphologically similar to orthopoxviruses. The viruses grow only in cultures of monkey and human cells, with cytopathic effects. They do not grow on the chorioallantoic membrane of embryonated eggs.

Tanapox begins with a febrile period of 3–4 days and can include severe headache and prostration. There are usually only one or two skin lesions; pustulation never occurs. Healing may take 4–7 weeks.

Yaba monkey tumor poxvirus causes benign histiocytomas 5–20 days after subcutaneous or intramuscular administration to monkeys. The tumors regress after about 5 weeks. Intravenous administration of the virus causes the appearance of multiple histiocytomas in the lungs, heart, and skeletal muscles. True neoplastic changes do not occur. The virus is easily isolated from tumor tissue, and characteristic inclusions are found in the tumor cells. Monkeys of various species and humans are susceptible to the cellular proliferative effects of the virus, but other laboratory animals are insusceptible. Although animal handlers have become infected, Yaba virus infections of humans have not been observed naturally in Africa.

REFERENCES

Baxby D: Identification and interrelationships of the variola/vaccinia subgroup of poxviruses. Prog Med Virol 1975;19:215.

Breman JG, Arita I: The confirmation and maintenance of smallpox eradication. N Engl J Med 1980;303:1263.

Brown JP et al: Vaccinia virus encodes a polypeptide homologous to epidermal growth factor and transforming growth factor. Nature 1985;313:491.

Committee on Orthopoxvirus Infections: Smallpox: Posteradication vigilance continues. WHO Chron 1982; 36:87.

Dennis J, Oshiro LS, Bunter JW: Molluscum contagiosum, another sexually transmitted disease: Its impact on the clinical virology laboratory. (Letter.) J Infect Dis 1985; 151:376.

Fenner F: Portraits of viruses: The poxviruses. Intervirology 1979;11:137.

Ježek Z et al: Human monkeypox: Clinical features of 282 patients. J Infect Dis 1987;156:293.

Johnson GP, Goebel SJ, Paoletti E: An update on the vaccinia virus genome. Virology 1993;196:381.

Massung RF et al: Potential virulence determinants in terminal regions of variola smallpox virus genome. Nature 1993;366:748.

Moss B: Vaccinia virus: A tool for research and vaccine development. Science 1991;252:1662.

Hepatitis Viruses

35

Viral hepatitis is a systemic disease primarily involving the liver. Most cases of acute viral hepatitis in children and adults are caused by one of the following agents: hepatitis A virus (HAV), the etiologic agent of viral hepatitis type A (infectious hepatitis or short incubation hepatitis); hepatitis B virus (HBV), which is associated with viral hepatitis B (serum hepatitis or long incubation hepatitis); hepatitis C virus (HCV); or hepatitis E virus (HEV), the agent of enterically transmitted hepatitis. Other viruses are associated with hepatitis that cannot be ascribed to HAV, HBV, or HCV, and the associated disease is designated non-A, non-B (NANB) hepatitis. Additional well-characterized viruses that can cause sporadic hepatitis, such as yellow fever virus, cytomegalovirus, Epstein-Barr virus, herpes simplex virus, rubella virus, and the enteroviruses, are discussed in other chapters. Hepatitis viruses produce acute inflammation of the liver, resulting in a clinical illness characterized by fever, gastrointestinal symptoms such as nausea and vomiting, and jaundice. Regardless of the virus type, identical histopathologic lesions are observed in the liver during acute disease.

PROPERTIES OF HEPATITIS VIRUSES

The characteristics of the five known hepatitis viruses are shown in Table 35–1. Nomenclature of the hepatitis viruses, antigens, and antibodies is presented in Table 35–2.

Hepatitis Type A

HAV is a distinct member of the picornavirus family (see Chapter 36). HAV is a 27- to 32-nm spherical particle with cubic symmetry, containing a linear single-stranded RNA genome with a size of 7.8 kb. Although it was first provisionally classified as enterovirus 72, the nucleotide and amino acid sequences of HAV are sufficiently distinct to assign it to a new picornavirus genus, *Heparnavirus.* Only one serotype is known. There is no antigenic cross-reactivity with HBV or with the other hepatitis viruses. Important properties of the picornavirus family are listed in Table 36–1.

HAV is stable to treatment with ether, acid, and heat (60 °C for 1 hour), and its infectivity can be preserved for at least 1 month after being dried and stored at 25 °C and 42% relative humidity or for years at −20 °C. The virus is destroyed by autoclaving (121 °C for 20 minutes), by boiling in water for 5 minutes, by dry heat (180 °C for 1 hour), by ultraviolet irradiation (1 minute at 1.1 watts), by treatment with formalin (1:4000 for 3 days at 37 °C), or by treatment with chlorine (10–15 ppm for 30 minutes). The relative resistance of HAV to disinfection procedures emphasizes the need for extra precautions in dealing with hepatitis patients and their products.

HAV initially was identified in stool and liver preparations by employing immune electron microscopy as the detection system (Figure 35–1). The addition of specific hepatitis A antisera from convalescent patients to fecal specimens obtained from patients early in the incubation period of their illness prior to the onset of jaundice permitted concentration and visibility of viral particles by the formation of antigen-antibody aggregates. More sensitive serologic assays, such as the microtiter solid-phase immunoradiometric assay and immune adherence, have made it possible to detect HAV in stools, liver homogenates, and bile and to measure specific antibody in serum.

Chimpanzees and two South American monkeys, the white-moustached *(Saguinus mystax)* and rufiventer marmosets, are susceptible to HAV and have provided laboratories with a source of virus for experimentation and for preparation of diagnostic reagents. HAV from marmoset-adapted material and from extracts of patients' feces has been cultivated serially in primary explant cultures of adult *Saguinus labiatus* marmoset livers and in cell cultures of primate origin. A noncytopathic infection occurs, which is identified by immunofluorescence and by radioimmunoassay.

Hepatitis Type B

HBV, the cause of serum hepatitis, is classified as a hepadnavirus (Table 35–3). HBV establishes chronic infections, especially in those infected as infants; it is a major factor in the eventual development of liver disease and hepatocellular carcinoma in those individuals.

Table 35–1. Characteristics of hepatitis viruses.

Virus	Hepatitis A	Hepatitis B	Hepatitis C	Hepatitis D	Hepatitis E
Family	Picornaviridae	Hepadnaviridae	Flaviviridae	Unclassified	Caliciviridae
Genus	*Heparnavirus*	*Orthohepadnavirus*	*Hep-c-virus*	*Deltavirus*	*Hepevirus*
Virion	27 nm, icosahedral	42 nm, spherical	30–60 nm, spherical	35 nm, spherical	27–34 nm, icosahedral
Envelope	No	Yes (HBsAg)	Yes	Yes (HBsAg)	No
Genome	ssRNA	dsDNA	ssRNA	ssRNA	ssRNA
Genome size	7.8 kb	3.2 kb	9.4 kb	1.7 kb	7.5 kb
Stability	Heat- and acid-stable	Acid-sensitive	Ether-sensitive	Acid-sensitive	Heat-stable
Transmission	Fecal-oral	Parenteral	Parenteral	Parenteral	Fecal-oral
Prevalence	High	High	Moderate	Low, regional	Regional
Fulminant disease	Rare	Rare	Rare	Frequent	In pregnancy
Chronic disease	Never	Often	Often	Often	Never
Oncogenic	No	Yes	Yes	?	No

A. Structure and Composition: Electron microscopy of HBsAg-reactive serum reveals three morphologic forms (Figures 35–2 and 35–3). The most numerous are spherical particles measuring 22 nm in diameter (Figure 35–4). These small particles are made up exclusively of HBsAg—as are tubular or filamentous forms, which have the same diameter but may be over 200 nm long—and result from overproduction of HBsAg. Larger, 42-nm spherical virions (originally referred to as Dane particles) are less frequently observed (Figure 35–2). The outer surface, or envelope, contains HBsAg and surrounds a 27-nm inner nucleocapsid core that contains HBcAg (Figure 35–5). The variable length of a single-stranded region of the circular DNA genome results in genetically heterogeneous particles with a wide range of buoyant densities.

The viral genome (Figure 35–6) consists of partially double-stranded circular DNA with a molecular weight of approximately 2×10^6, 3200 bp in length. Different HBV isolates share 90–98% nucleotide sequence homology. The full-length DNA minus strand is complementary to all HBV mRNAs; the positive strand is variable and between 50 and 80% of unit length.

There are four open reading frames that encode seven polypeptides. These include structural proteins of the virion surface and core, a small transcriptional transactivator (X), and a large polymerase (P) protein that includes DNA polymerase, reverse transcriptase, and RNase H activities. The S gene has three in-frame initiation codons and encodes the major HBsAg, as well as polypeptides containing in addition pre-S2 or pre-S1 and pre-S2 sequences. The C gene has two in-frame initiation codons and encodes HBcAg plus the HBe protein, which is processed to produce soluble HBeAg.

The stability of HBsAg does not always coincide with that of the infectious agent. However, both are stable at −20 °C for over 20 years and stable to repeated freezing and thawing. The virus also is stable at 37 °C for 60 minutes and remains viable after being dried and stored at 25 °C for at least 1 week. HBV (but not HBsAg) is sensitive to higher temperatures (100 °C for 1 minute) or to longer incubation periods (60 °C for 10 hours) depending on the amount of virus present in the sample. HBsAg is stable at pH 2.4 for up to 6 hours, but HBV infectivity is lost. Sodium hypochlorite, 0.5% (eg, 1:10 chlorine bleach), destroys antigenicity within 3 minutes at low protein concentrations, but undiluted serum specimens require higher concentrations (5%). HBsAg is not destroyed by ultraviolet irradiation of plasma or other blood products, and viral infectivity may also resist such treatment. HBV is unevenly distributed during Cohn ethanol fractionation of plasma. Most of the virus is retained in fraction I (fibrinogen, factor VIII) or III (prothrombin complex), whereas HBsAg is relegated to fractions II (gamma globulin) and IV (plasma protein).

B. Replication of Hepatitis B Virus: The infectious virion attaches to cells and becomes uncoated (Figure 35–7). In the nucleus, the partially double-stranded viral genome is converted to covalently closed circular double-stranded DNA (cccDNA). The cccDNA serves as template for all viral transcripts, including a 3.5-kb pregenome RNA. The pregenome RNA becomes encapsidated with newly synthesized HBcAg. Within the cores, the viral polymerase synthesizes by reverse transcription a negative strand DNA copy. The polymerase starts to synthesize the positive DNA strand, but the process is not completed. Cores may bud from the cell, acquiring HBsAg-containing envelopes. Alternatively, cores may be reimported into the nucleus and initiate another round of replication in the same cell.

Table 35–2. Nomenclature and definitions of hepatitis viruses, antigens, and antibodies.

Disease	Component of System	Definition
Hepatitis A	HAV	Hepatitis A virus. Etiologic agent of infectious hepatitis. A picornavirus, originally classified as enterovirus 72, now considered to be prototype of a new genus, *Heparnavirus.*
	Anti-HAV	Antibody to HAV. Detectable at onset of symptoms; lifetime persistence.
	IgM anti-HAV	IgM class antibody to HAV. Indicates recent infection with hepatitis A; positive up to 4–6 months after infection.
Hepatitis B	HBV	Hepatitis B virus. Etiologic agent of serum hepatitis (long-incubation hepatitis). A hepadnavirus.
	HBsAg	Hepatitis B surface antigen. Surface antigen(s) of HBV detectable in large quantity in serum; several subtypes identified.
	HBeAg	Hepatitis B e antigen. Soluble antigen; associated with HBV replication, with high titers of HBV in serum, and with infectivity of serum.
	HBcAg	Hepatitis B core antigen. No test available for routine use.
	Anti-HBs	Antibody to HBsAg. Indicates past infection with and immunity to HBV, presence of passive antibody from HBIG, or immune response from HBV vaccine.
	Anti-HBe	Antibody to HBeAg. Presence in serum of HBsAg carrier suggests lower titer of HBV.
	Anti-HBc	Antibody to HBcAg. Indicates infection with HBV at some undefined time in the past.
	IgM anti-HBc	IgM class antibody to HBcAg. Indicates recent infection with HBV; positive for 4–6 months after infection.
Hepatitis C	HCV	Hepatitis C virus, a common etiologic agent of posttransfusion hepatitis. A flavivirus; previously classified among the non-A, non-B hepatitis agents.
	Anti-HCV	Antibody to HCV.
Hepatitis D	HDV	Hepatitis D virus. Etiologic agent of delta hepatitis; causes infection only in presence of HBV.
	HDAg	Delta antigen (delta-Ag). Detectable in early acute HDV infection.
	Anti-HDV	Antibody to delta-Ag (anti-delta). Indicates past or present infection with HDV.
Hepatitis E	HEV	Hepatitis E virus. Enterically transmitted hepatitis virus, previously classified with the non-A, non-B hepatitis agents. Causes large epidemics in Asia and North Africa; fecal-oral or waterborne transmission.
Non-A, non-B hepatitis	NANB	Non-A, non-B hepatitis virus. Diagnosis by exclusion. At least two viruses in group. Epidemiology parallels that of hepatitis B.
Immune globulins	IG	Immune globulin USP (previously called ISG, immune serum globulin, or gamma globulin). Contains antibodies to HAV, low titers of antibodies to HBV.
	HBIG	Hepatitis B immune globulin. Contains high titers of antibodies to HBV.

Hepatitis Type C

Clinical and epidemiologic studies and cross-challenge experiments in chimpanzees had suggested that there were three NANB hepatitis agents which, based on serologic tests, were not related to HAV or HBV. One of these agents has been identified as hepatitis C virus (HCV). HCV proved to be a positive-stranded RNA virus, now classified as a flavivirus. The genome is 9.4 kb in size and is thought to encode a core protein and two envelope glycoproteins (Figure 35–8). The expression of cDNA clones of HCV in yeast led to the development of serologic tests for antibodies to HCV. At least 50% of patients previously diagnosed as having posttransfusion NANB hepatitis have tested positive for anti-HCV. The addition of anti-HCV testing to the screening of blood donors should significantly reduce the risk of transfusion-associated hepatitis. The test can be carried out by ELISA or radioimmunoassay.

About half of HCV patients develop chronic hepatitis, and it appears that many of these cases continue into cirrhosis. In some countries, as in Japan, HCV infection often leads to hepatocellular carcinoma. About 25,000 individuals die annually of chronic liver disease and cirrhosis in the USA; HCV appears to be a major contributor to this burden.

Tests are under development to detect HCV in liver and plasma. The tests depend on finding HCV RNA by a cDNA-based polymerase chain reaction. HCV RNA has been detected in some patients and in experimentally infected chimpanzees at a time when they were negative for anti-HCV, presumably early in the infection.

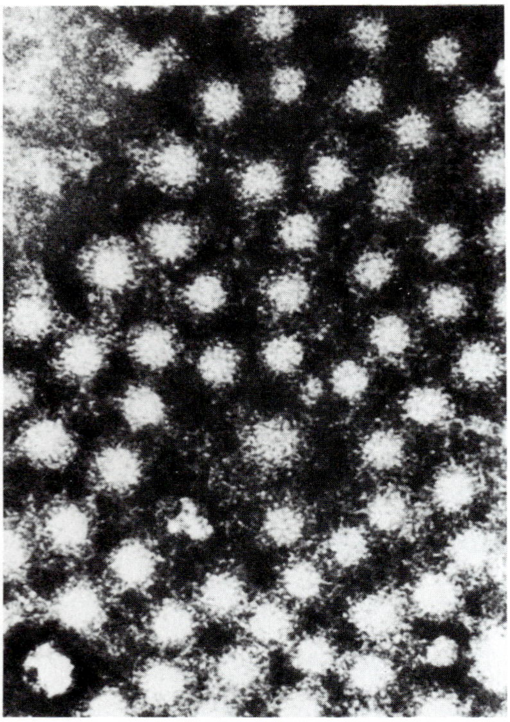

Figure 35–1. Electron micrograph of 27-nm hepatitis A virus aggregated with antibody (222,000×). Note the presence of an antibody "halo" around each particle. (DW Bradley, CL Hornbeck, and JE Maynard.)

Hepatitis Type D (Delta Hepatitis)

An antigen-antibody system termed the delta antigen (delta-Ag) and antibody (anti-delta) is detected in some HBV infections. The antigen is found within certain HBsAg particles. In blood, HDV (delta agent) contains delta-Ag (HDAg) surrounded by an HBsAg envelope. It has a particle size of 35–37 nm and a buoyant density of 1.24–1.25 g/mL. The genome of HDV consists of RNA, 1.7 kb in size. No homology exists with the HBV genome. HDAg is coded for by HDV RNA and is distinct from the antigenic determinants of HBV. HDV is a defective virus that acquires an HBsAg coat for transmission.

HDAg has been subjected to chemical and enzymatic treatment. No loss of activity occurred following treatment with ethylenediaminetetraacetic acid, detergents, ether, nucleases, glycosidases, or acid; but partial or complete loss of activity was detected after treatment with alkali, thiocyanate, guanidine hydrochloride, trichloracetic acid, and proteolytic enzymes.

Table 35–3. Important properties of hepadnaviruses.[1]

Virion: About 42 nm in diameter overall (nucleocapsids, 18 nm).
Genome: One molecule of double-stranded DNA, circular, MW about 2.3×10^6; contains 3200 nucleotides. In virion, negative DNA strand is full length and positive DNA strand is partially complete. The gap must be completed at beginning of replication cycle.
Proteins: Two major polypeptides (one glycosylated) are present in HBsAg; one polypeptide is present in HBcAg.
Envelope: Contains HBsAg and lipid.
Replication: By means of an intermediate RNA copy of the DNA genome (HBcAg in nucleus; HBsAg in cytoplasm). Both mature virus and 22-nm spherical particles consist of HBsAg secreted from the cell surface.
Outstanding characteristics: Family is made up of many types that infect humans and lower animals (eg, woodchucks, squirrels, ducks); cause acute and chronic hepatitis, often progressing to permanent carrier states and hepatocellular carcinoma.

[1]For HAV, see properties of picornaviruses (Table 36–1). For HCV, see description of flaviviruses (Table 38–1).

Hepatitis Type E

Another virus originally classified as a NANB agent has been identified as hepatitis E virus (HEV). It is different from the other hepatitis viruses in that it is transmitted enterically and occurs in epidemic form in developing countries, where water supplies are sometimes fecally contaminated. It was first documented in samples collected during the New Delhi, India, outbreak of 1955, when 29,000 cases of icteric hepatitis occurred after sewage contamination of the city's drinking water supply. Pregnant women may have a high (20%) mortality rate. Outbreaks involving thousands of persons have occurred in Soviet and Southeast Asia, in Africa, and in the Americas.

Hepatitis E has been transmitted to nonhuman primates by a virus obtained from human stools, and the agent can be recovered from the infected animals. The available data support a viral diameter of 32–34 nm with biophysical properties of a calicivirus. The viral genome has been cloned and is a positive-sense, single-strand RNA 7.5 kb in size.

HEPATITIS VIRUS INFECTIONS IN HUMANS

Pathology

Microscopically, there is spotty parenchymal cell degeneration, with necrosis of hepatocytes, a diffuse lobular inflammatory reaction, and disruption of liver cell cords. These parenchymal changes are accompanied by reticuloendothelial (Kupffer) cell hyperplasia, periportal infiltration by mononuclear cells, and cell degeneration. Localized areas of necrosis with ballooning or acidophilic bodies are frequently observed. Later in the course of the disease, there is an accumulation of macrophages containing lipofuscin near degenerating hepatocytes. Disruption of bile canaliculi or blockage of biliary excretion may occur following liver cell enlargement or necrosis. Preservation of the reticulum framework allows hepatocyte regeneration so that the highly ordered architecture of the liver lob-

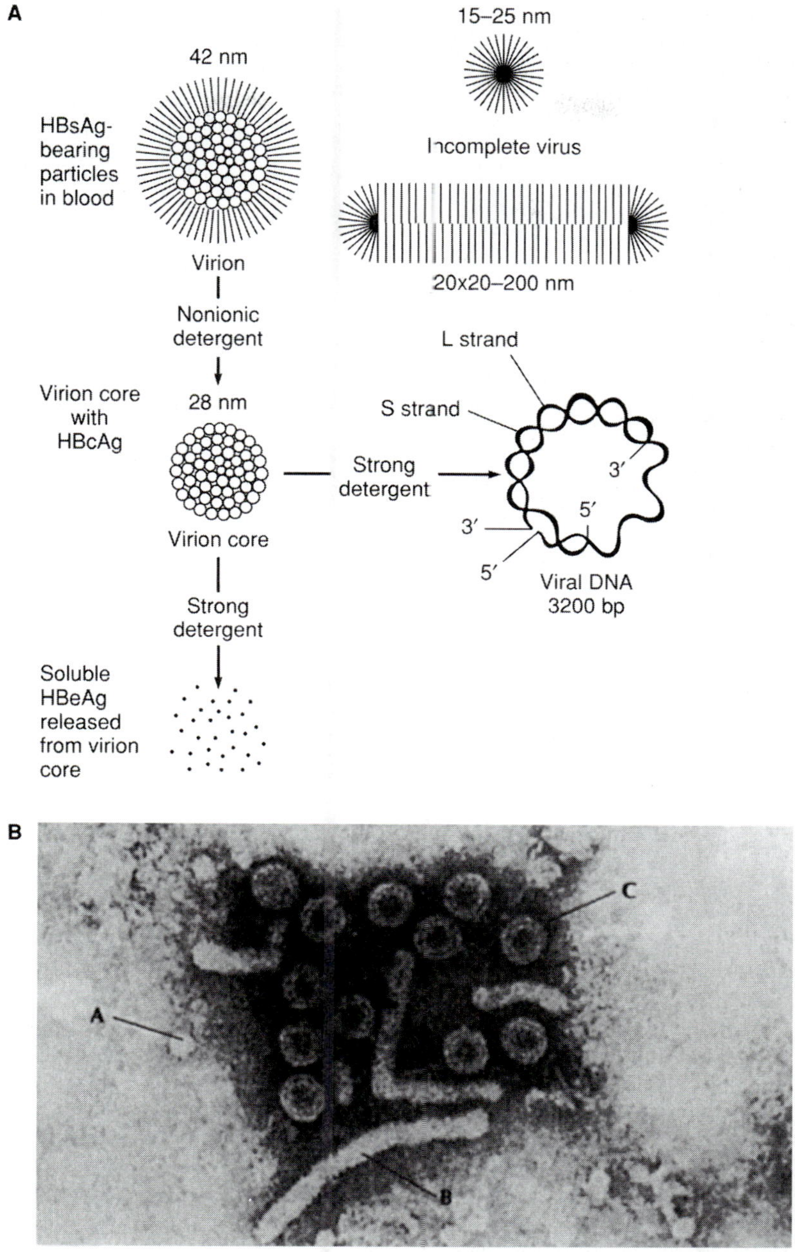

Figure 35–2. Hepatitis B viral and subviral forms. ***A:*** Schematic representation of three HBsAg-containing forms that can be identified in serum from HBV carriers. The 42-nm spherical Dane particle can be disrupted by nonionic detergents to release the 28-nm core that contains the partially double-stranded viral DNA genome. A soluble antigen, termed HBeAg, may be released from core particles by treatment with strong detergent. ***B:*** Electron micrograph showing three distinct HBsAg-bearing forms: 20-nm pleomorphic spherical particles (A), filamentous forms (B), and 42-nm spherical Dane particles, the infectious form of HBV (C). (Reprinted by permission of Wiley-Liss, a Division of John Wiley and Sons, Inc., from Robinson WS, Klote L, Aoki N: Hepadnaviruses in cirrhotic liver and hepatocellular carcinoma. J Med Virol 1990;31:18.)

ule can be ultimately regained. The damaged hepatic tissue is usually restored in 8–12 weeks.

In 5–15% of patients, the initial lesion consists of confluent (bridging) hepatic necrosis with impaired regeneration, resulting in collapsed stroma. The occurrence of this lesion in patients over age 40 years frequently presages a precarious clinical course leading to fibrosis, cirrhosis, and death.

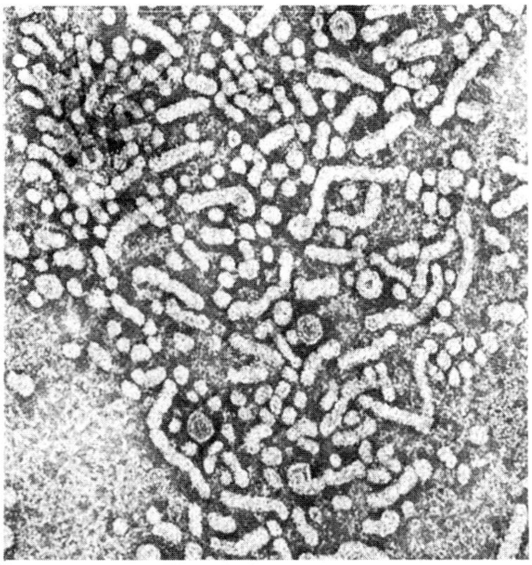

Figure 35–3. Unfractionated HBsAg-positive human plasma. Filaments, 22-nm spherical particles, and a few 42-nm virions are shown (77,000×).

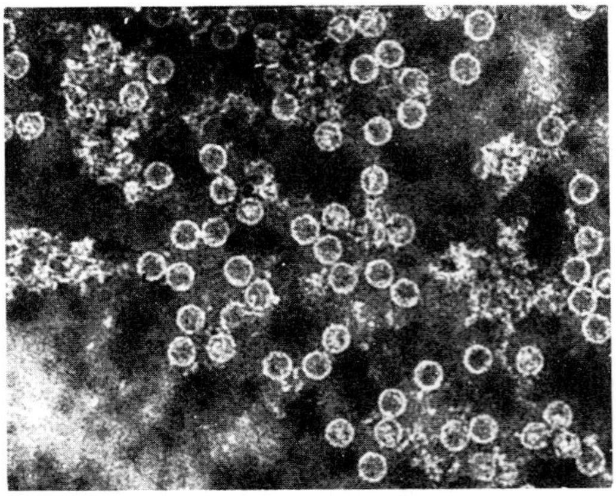

Figure 35–5. HBcAg purified from infected liver nuclei (122,400×). The diameter of the core particles is 27 nm. (HA Fields, GR Dreesman, and G Cabral.)

Chronic carriers of HBsAg may or may not have demonstrable evidence of liver disease. Persistent (unresolved) viral hepatitis, a mild benign disease that may follow acute hepatitis B in 8–10% of adult patients, is characterized by sporadically abnormal transaminase values and hepatomegaly. Histologically, the lobular architecture is preserved, with portal inflammation, swollen and pale hepatocytes (cobblestone arrangement), and slight to absent fibrosis. This lesion is frequently observed in asymptomatic carriers, usually does not progress toward cirrhosis, and has a favorable prognosis.

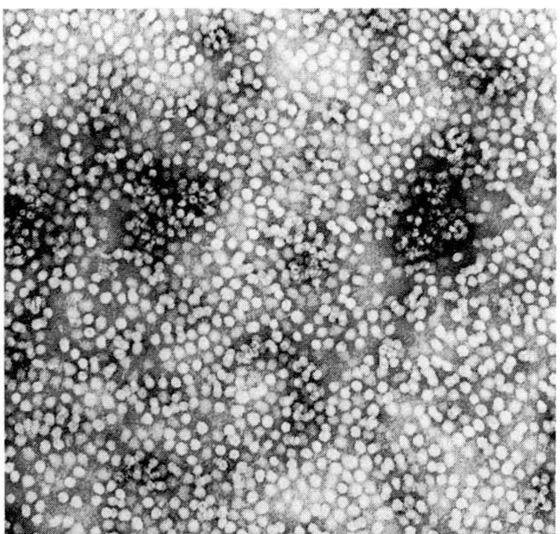

Figure 35–4. Purified hepatitis B surface antigen (HBsAg) (55,000×). (RM McCombs and JP Brunschwig.)

Chronic active (aggressive) hepatitis features a spectrum of histologic changes from inflammation and necrosis to collapse of the normal reticulum framework with bridging between the portal triads or terminal hepatic veins. HBsAg is observed in 10–50% of these patients. The prognosis is guarded, with progression to macronodular cirrhosis frequently occurring.

Occasionally during acute viral hepatitis, more extensive damage may occur that prevents orderly liver cell regeneration. Such fulminant or massive hepatocellular necrosis is seen in 1–2% of jaundiced patients with hepatitis B but is less common in hepatitis A.

In hepatitis B patients, electron microscopic studies have revealed in liver cell nuclei 27-nm particles that are morphologically similar to the inner core of the virus. Correspondingly, immunofluorescence studies indicate that during HBV infection HBcAg is found primarily in the nucleus, whereas HBsAg is localized in the cytoplasm. HBsAg and HBcAg are rarely found in the same cell, and there appears to be an inverse relationship between the severity of the lesion and the abundance of HBsAg. Hepatocytes with a ground-glass appearance are laden with cytoplasmic HBsAg and are often found in biopsy specimens from patients with persistent viral hepatitis. Nuclear HBcAg predominates in patients whose immune systems are compromised.

HBV DNA sequences have been detected in bone marrow cells and in peripheral blood lymphocytes of patients who may or may not be positive for HBs antigenemia. Patients with acquired immunodeficiency syndrome (AIDS) may have HBV DNA sequences in bone marrow, semen, and lymph nodes as well as in mononuclear blood cells, even in the absence of serologic markers of HBV. Thus, HBV may play a role as one of many cofactors in the pathogenesis of AIDS, as well as its direct role in hepatitis and primary hepato-

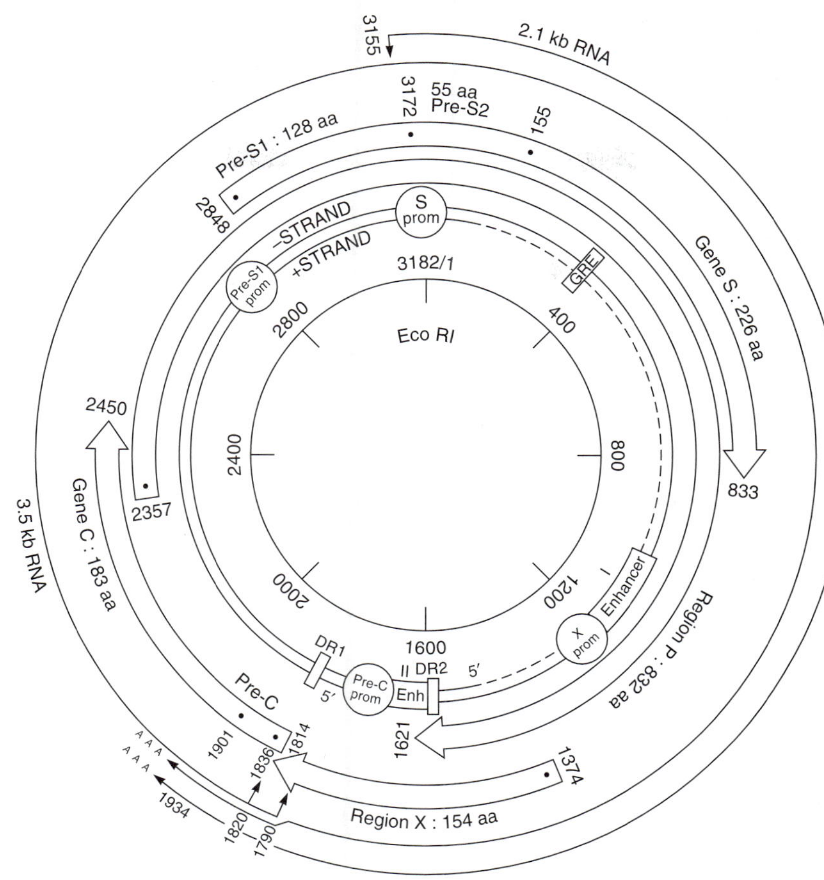

Figure 35–6. Genetic organization of the HBV genome. Four open reading frames encoding seven peptides are indicated by large arrows. Regulatory sequences (promoters [prom], enhancers [Enh], and glucocorticoid responsive element [GRE]) are marked. Only the two major transcripts (core/pre-genome and S mRNAs) are represented. DR1 and DR2 are two directly repeated sequences of 11 bp at the 5′ extremities of the minus- and plus-strand DNA. (Reproduced, with permission, from Buendia MA: Hepatitis B viruses and hepatocellular carcinoma. Adv Cancer Res 1992;59:167. Academic Press, Inc., 1992.)

cellular carcinoma. HCV also plays a role in hepatocellular carcinoma in some areas (Asia).

Clinical Findings (Table 35–4)

In individual cases, it is not possible to make a reliable clinical distinction among cases caused by the hepatitis viruses. Other viral diseases that may present as hepatitis are infectious mononucleosis, yellow fever, cytomegalovirus infection, herpes simplex, rubella, and some enterovirus infections. Hepatitis may occasionally occur as a complication of leptospirosis, syphilis, tuberculosis, toxoplasmosis, and amebiasis, all of which are susceptible to specific drug therapy. Noninfectious causes include biliary obstruction, primary biliary cirrhosis, Wilson's disease, drug toxicity, and drug hypersensitivity reactions.

In viral hepatitis, onset of jaundice is often preceded by gastrointestinal symptoms such as nausea, vomiting, severe anorexia, and fever that may mimic influenza. Jaundice may appear within a few days of the prodromal period, but anicteric hepatitis is more common.

Extrahepatic manifestations of viral hepatitis (primarily type B) include (1) a transient serum sickness-like prodrome consisting of urticaria, rash, and nonmigratory polyarthralgia or arthritis occurring 1–6 weeks prior to the onset of hepatitis in 15–20% of patients; (2) polyarteritis nodosa; and (3) glomerulonephritis. Circulating immune complexes have been suggested as the cause of these syndromes. Mixed cryoglobulinemia is a syndrome characterized by purpura, arthralgia, and weakness, often with renal involvement. Vasculitis and immune complex deposition are common. In most cases, the cryoprecipitates contain either HBsAg or anti-HBs.

Complete recovery occurs in most hepatitis A cases and in more than 85% of type B hepatitis cases. Hepatitis A is more severe in adults than in children, in

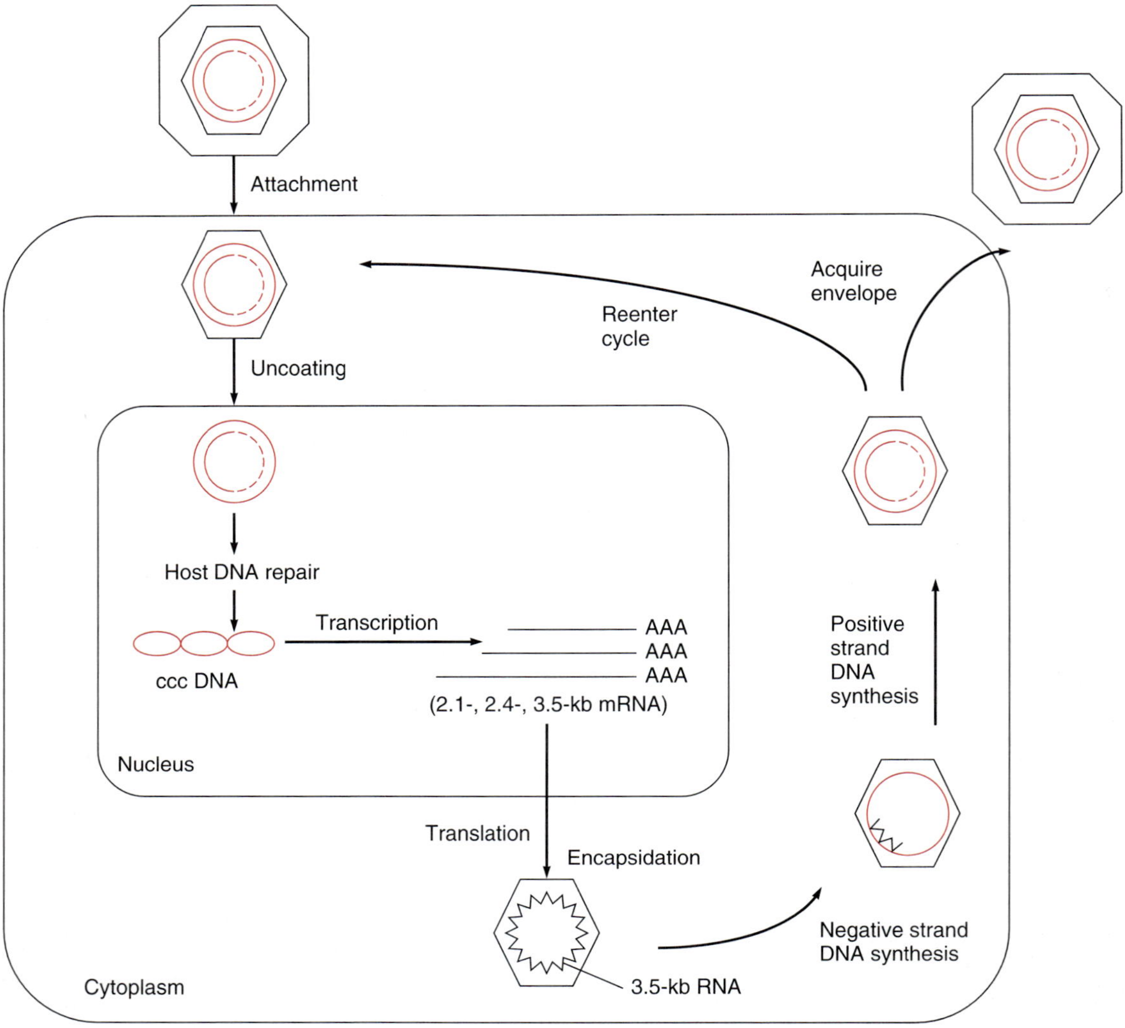

Figure 35–7. HBV replication cycle. HBV attachment to a receptor on the surface of hepatocytes occurs via a portion of the pre-S region of HBsAg. After uncoating of the virus, unidentified cellular enzymes convert the partially double-stranded DNA to ccc DNA that can be detected in the nucleus. The ccc DNA serves as the template for the production of HBV mRNAs and the 3.5-kb RNA pregenome. The pregenome is encapsidated by a packaging signal located near the 5′ end of the RNA into newly synthesized core particles, where it serves as template for the HBV reverse transcriptase encoded within the polymerase gene. An RNase H activity of the polymerase removes the RNA template as the negative-strand DNA is being synthesized. Positive-strand DNA synthesis does not proceed to completion within the core, resulting in replicative intermediates consisting of full-length minus-strand DNA plus variable length (20–80%) positive-strand DNA. Core particles containing these DNA replicative intermediates can either bud from the cell (acquiring HBsAg in the process) or reenter the intracellular infection cycle. (Courtesy of BL Slagle.)

whom it often goes unnoticed. Approximately 3% of patients with acute icteric type B hepatitis ultimately develop chronic active hepatitis. Case-fatality rates appear to vary with age and may reflect underlying conditions rather than any increased virulence of the specific causative agent. For the epidemiologic years 1973–1974, the case-fatality rate for hepatitis B among persons age 29 years or younger was 0.5–0.6%; for the age group 30 years and older, it was 2%. The rates are highest for transfusion-associated cases (2.7%). Fulminant hepatitis is lethal in 60–90% of cases and is highly correlated with age. In most patients who survive, complete restoration of the hepatic parenchyma and normal liver function is the rule. Patients who develop confluent (bridging) hepatic necrosis (submassive hepatic necrosis) also have a poor prognosis, and 15–30% of those who survive develop chronic active hepatitis.

The potential courses of acute viral hepatitis have been discussed in the section on pathology. Uncom-

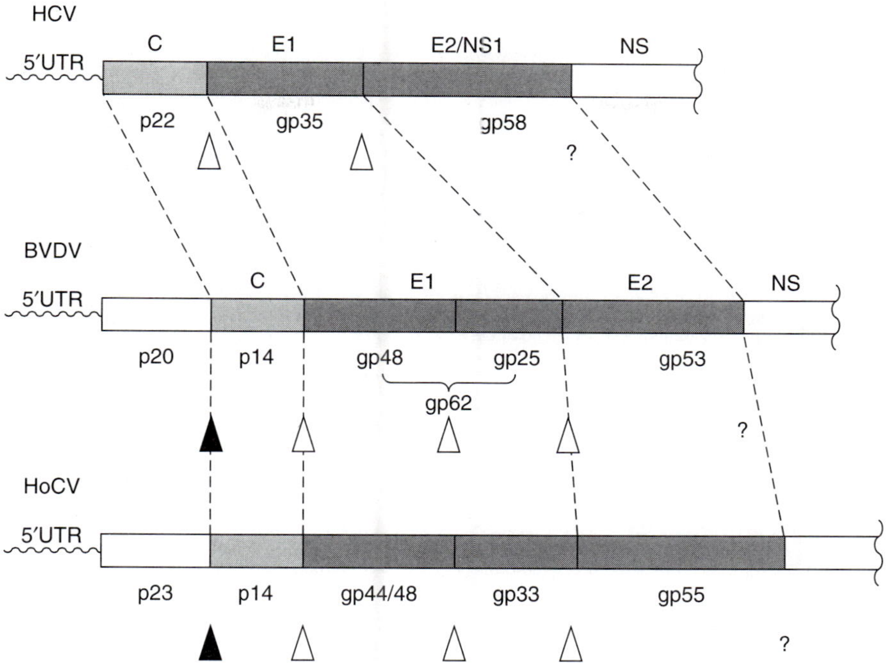

Figure 35–8. Coding regions of viral structural proteins of HCV and the pestiviruses bovine viral diarrhea virus (BVDV) and hog cholera virus (HoCV). Open boxes, nonstructural proteins; dotted boxes, core proteins; shaded boxes, envelope proteins. Open triangles, cleavage sites for cellular signalase; filled triangles, cleavage sites for viral protease. (Reproduced, with permission, from Miyamura T, Matsuura Y: Structural proteins of hepatitis C virus. Trends Microbiol 1993;1:229. Elsevier Science Publishers, 1993.)

plicated viral hepatitis rarely continues for more than 10 weeks without improvement. Relapses occur in 5–20% of cases and are manifested by abnormalities in liver function with or without the recurrence of clinical symptoms. A posthepatitis syndrome may occur, especially in postmenopausal women. It is characterized by repeated episodes of anorexia, irritability, lethargy, weakness, headaches, and right upper quadrant pain. This syndrome is due to interference with normal estrogen metabolism in the liver and can be successfully treated with estrogens and progesterone in women.

Hepatitis C is usually clinically mild, with only minimal to moderate elevation of liver enzymes. Hospitalization is unusual, and jaundice occurs in less than 25% of patients. Despite the mild nature of the disease, 30–50% of cases progress to chronic liver disease. Most patients are asymptomatic, but histologic evaluation often reveals evidence of chronic active hepatitis, especially in those whose disease is acquired following transfusion.

Laboratory Features

Attempts to isolate HBV in a cell or organ culture system have generally not been successful. However, successful transmission of HBV to chimpanzees has been achieved. The infection results in serologic, biochemical, and histologic evidence of type B hepatitis. Immunofluorescence and electron microscopy reveal HBsAg in the cytoplasm and virus-like particles with HBcAg in the nuclei of hepatocytes. Serial passage has been successful. No evidence for hepatitis B transmission from chimpanzees to humans has been reported.

Liver biopsy permits a tissue diagnosis of hepatitis. Tests for abnormal liver function, such as serum alanine aminotransferase (ALT; formerly SGPT) and bilirubin, supplement the clinical, pathologic, and epidemiologic findings. Transaminase values in acute hepatitis range between 500 and 2000 units and are almost never below 100 units. ALT values are usually higher than serum aspartate transaminase (AST; formerly SGOT) values. A sharp rise in ALT with a short duration (3–19 days) is more indicative of viral hepatitis A, whereas a gradual rise with prolongation (35–200 days) appears to characterize viral hepatitis B and C infections.

Leukopenia is typical in the preicteric phase and may be followed by a relative lymphocytosis. Large atypical lymphocytes such as are found in infectious mononucleosis may occasionally be seen but do not exceed 10% of the total lymphocyte population.

Further evidence of liver dysfunction and host response is reflected in decreased serum albumin and increased serum globulin levels. Elevation of gamma

Table 35–4. Epidemiologic and clinical features of viral hepatitis types A, B, and C.

	Viral Hepatitis Type A	Viral Hepatitis Type B	Viral Hepatitis Type C
Incubation period	15–45 days (avg, 25–30).	50–180 days (avg, 60–90).	40–120 days.
Principal age distribution	Children,[1] young adults.	15–29 years.[2]	Adults.[2]
Seasonal incidence	Throughout the year but tends to peak in autumn.	Throughout the year.	Throughout the year.
Route of infection	Predominantly fecal-oral.	Predominantly parenteral.	Predominantly parenteral.
Occurrence of virus			
Blood	2 weeks before to ≤ 1 week after jaundice.	Months to years.	Months to years.
Stool	2 weeks before to 2 weeks after jaundice.	Absent.	Probably absent.
Urine	Rare.	Absent.	Probably absent.
Saliva, semen	Rare (saliva).	Frequently present.	Unknown.
Clinical and laboratory features			
Onset	Abrupt.	Insidious.	Insidious.
Fever > 38 °C (100.4 °F)	Common.	Less common.	Less common.
Duration of aminotransferase elevation	1–3 weeks.	1–6+ months.	1–6+ months.
Immunoglobulins (IgM levels)	Elevated.	Normal to slightly elevated.	Normal to slightly elevated.
Complications	Uncommon, no chronicity.	Chronicity in 5–10%.	Chronicity in 30–50%.
Mortality rate (icteric cases)	< 0.5%.	< 1–2%.	0.5–1%.
HBsAg	Absent.	Present.	Absent.
Immunity			
Homologous	Yes.	Yes.	?
Heterologous	No.	No.	No.
Duration	Probably lifetime.	Probably lifetime.	?
Gamma globulin (immune globulin USP) prophylaxis	Regularly prevents jaundice.	Prevents jaundice only if gamma globulin is of sufficient potency against HBV.	?

[1]Nonicteric hepatitis A is common in children.
[2]Among the 15–29 year age group, hepatitis B and C are often associated with drug abuse or promiscuous sexual behavior. Patients with transfusion-associated HBV or HCV are generally over age 29.

globulin and serum transaminase is frequently used to gauge chronicity and activity of liver disease. In many patients with hepatitis A, an abnormally high level of IgM is found that appears 3–4 days after the ALT begins to rise. Hepatitis B patients have normal to slightly elevated IgM levels.

The clinical, virologic, and serologic events following exposure to HAV are shown in Figure 35–9. Viral particles have been detected by immune electron microscopy in fecal extracts of hepatitis A patients (Figure 35–1). Virus appears early in the disease and disappears within 3 weeks following the onset of jaundice.

By means of radioimmunoassay, the HAV antigen has been detected in the liver, stool, bile, and blood of naturally infected humans and experimentally infected chimpanzees and marmosets. Detection of HAV in the blood of infected chimpanzees and humans supports previous epidemiologic evidence of viremia during the acute stage of the disease. Peak titers of HAV are detected in the stool about 1–2 weeks prior to the first detectable liver enzyme abnormalities.

Anti-HAV appears in the IgM fraction during the acute phase, peaking about 3 weeks after elevation of liver enzymes. During convalescence, anti-HAV is in the IgG fraction, where it persists for decades. Thus, detection of IgM-specific anti-HAV in the blood of an acutely infected patient confirms the diagnosis of hepatitis A. The methods of choice for measuring HAV antibodies are radioimmunoassay, ELISA, and immune adherence hemagglutination.

The most sensitive and specific methods for detecting HBsAg or anti-HBs are radioimmunoassay and ELISA. These assays and the red cell agglutination technique, which employs anti-HBs-coated cells in a microtiter system, have replaced counterelectrophoresis as the methods of choice for detecting HBsAg.

The particles containing HBsAg are antigenically complex. Each contains a group-specific antigen, *a,* in addition to two pairs of mutually exclusive subdeter-

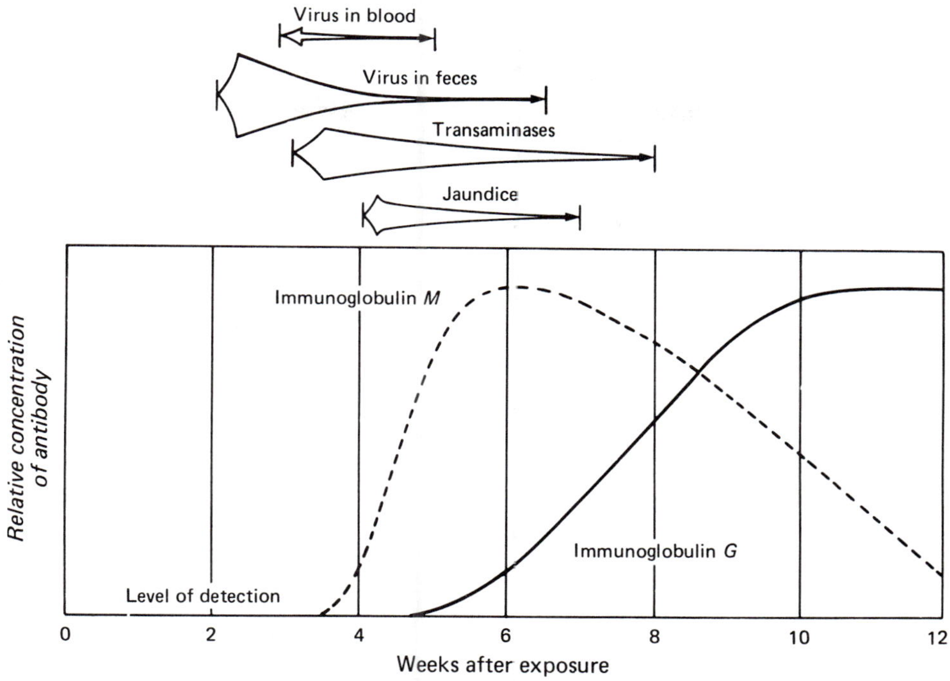

Figure 35–9. Immunologic and biologic events associated with viral hepatitis type A. (From Hollinger FB, Dienstag JL: *Manual of Clinical Microbiology,* 4th ed. American Society for Microbiology, 1985.)

minants, *d/y* and *w/r*. Thus, four phenotypes of HBsAg have been observed: *adw, ayw, adr,* and *ayr.* In the USA, *adw* is the predominant subtype, although *ayw* is also commonly seen, especially among parenteral drug abusers. These virus-specific markers are useful in epidemiologic investigations, since secondary cases have the same subtype as the index case. These antigenic determinants are the phenotypic expression of HBV genotypes and are not determined by host factors.

Clinical and serologic events following exposure to HBV are depicted in Figure 35–10 and Table 35–5. DNA polymerase activity, which is representative of the viremic stage of hepatitis B, occurs early in the incubation period, shortly after the first appearance of HBsAg. The latter is usually detectable 2–6 weeks in advance of clinical and biochemical evidence of hepatitis and persists throughout the clinical course of the disease but typically disappears by the sixth month after exposure. A diagnosis of chronic hepatitis is entertained in those patients in whom HBsAg persists for more than 6 months. In patients destined to become carriers the initial illness may be mild or inapparent, manifested only by an elevated transaminase level.

Anti-HBc is frequently detected at the onset of clinical illness approximately 2–4 weeks after HBsAg reactivity appears. Because this antibody is directed against the internal core component of HBV, its appearance in the serum is indicative of viral replication. In the typical case of acute type B hepatitis, high titers of IgM-specific anti-HBc are detected. In contrast, low titers of IgM anti-HBc are found in the sera of most chronic HBsAg carriers. Antibody to HBsAg is first detected at a variable period after the disappearance of HBsAg. It is present in low concentrations usually detectable only by the most sensitive methods.

The anti-HBc test is of limited clinical value when the HBsAg test is positive. However, in perhaps 5% of the acute cases of hepatitis B, and more frequently during early convalescence, HBsAg may be undetectable in the serum. Examination of these sera for high titers of IgM-specific anti-HBc may help establish the correct diagnosis. In the absence of anti-HBc and HBsAg, active hepatitis B can be excluded. In contrast, the presence of anti-HBc alone is presumptive evidence for an active HBV infection. However, this relationship is not infallible, and some patients who have recovered from hepatitis B with the development of anti-HBs and anti-HBc eventually lose one or the other antibody.

Another antigen-antibody system of importance involves HBeAg and its antibody. If the specimen contains HBsAg, certain situations may warrant further testing of the serum for HBeAg or anti-HBe. These include assessing the risk of transmission of HBV following exposure to contaminated blood and advising health care professionals who are chronically infected. Specimens positive for HBeAg (or positive for HBsAg at a dilution of 1:10,000) are considered to be very infectious, ie, they contain high concentrations of HBV.

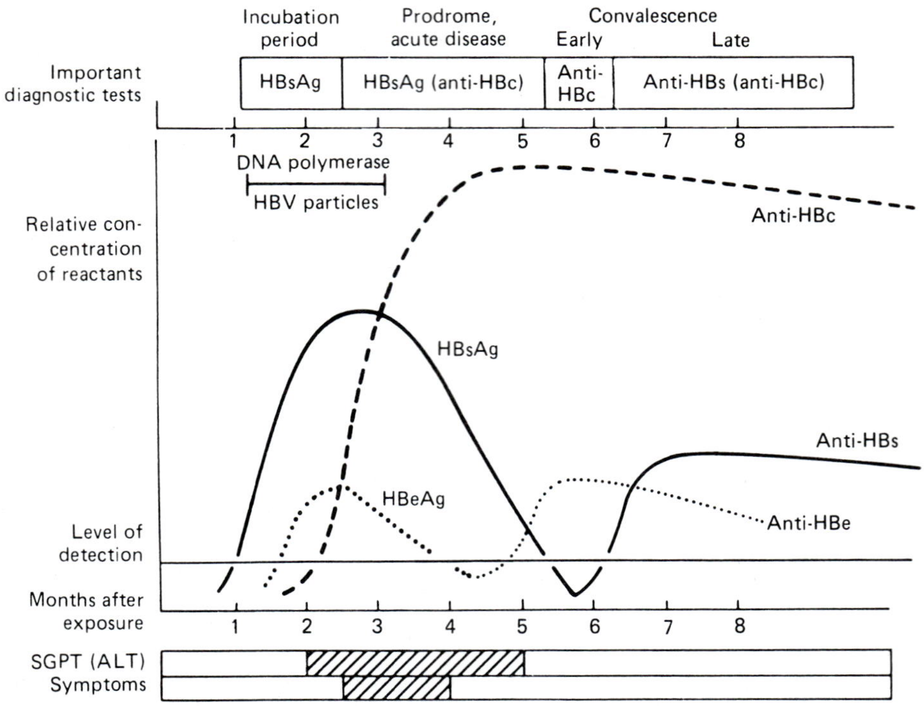

Figure 35–10. Clinical and serologic events occurring in a patient with hepatitis B. The common diagnostic tests and their interpretation are presented in Table 35–5. (From Hollinger FB, Dienstag JL: *Manual of Clinical Microbiology,* 4th ed. American Society for Microbiology, 1985.)

Infectivity is reduced but probably not eliminated in specimens containing anti-HBe (or low titers of HBsAg).

Interpretation of Serologic Tests in the Diagnosis of Acute Viral Hepatitis

The availability of a test for IgM-specific anti-HBc has greatly increased the accuracy of diagnostic tests for acute viral hepatitis. This test, which is specific for recent HBV infection, may be combined with previously available tests for HBsAg and IgM-specific anti-HAV (specific for acute hepatitis A) to identify the cause of an episode of acute hepatitis. A test for anti-HDV detects HDV coinfection with HBV or superinfection of an HBV carrier.

Table 35–6 summarizes the interpretation of the four basic diagnostic tests that are necessary for cases of viral hepatitis. The cause of disease is usually a single virus: hepatitis A (IgM anti-HAV positive); hepatitis B (total anti-HBc positive); or hepatitis C (anti-HCV positive). However, combinations of acute

Table 35–5. Common serologic tests for HBV and their interpretation.

Positive Tests	Interpretation
HBsAg (surface antigen)	Active hepatitis B infection, either acute or chronic.
Anti-HBs (in absence of HBsAg)	Protection against reinfection (immunity). Remains for years.
Anti-HBc (in absence of anti-HBs)	Active HBV infection cannot be excluded. A recent HBV infection can be confirmed by examining the sample for high titers of IgM anti-HBc.
HBeAg[1]	Active hepatitis infection, acute or chronic. Found in presence of HBsAg. Indicates specimens that exhibit potential for enhanced infectivity.
Anti-HBe	When present in HBsAg carrier, blood is potentially less infectious.

[1]Other HBV serologic markers that may be present at the same time include HBV (Dane particles), observable by electron microscopy. Core antigen and viral DNA polymerase can be measured by disrupting HBV.

Table 35–6. Interpretation of current serodiagnostic test results for acute symptomatic hepatitis.

	Tests					Most Likely Clinical Diagnosis
	HBsAg	Total Anti-HBc	Anti-HCV	IgM Anti-HAV	Anti-HDV[1]	
Single virus	–	–	–	+		Hepatitis A
	+	+	–	–	–	Acute hepatitis B[2]
	–	–	+	–		Hepatitis C
Combined viruses	+	+	–	+		Hepatitis A and B[2]
	+	+	–	–	+	Hepatitis B and D coinfection[3]
	–	+	–	–	+	
	+	–	+	–	–	Hepatitis B and C coinfection[2]

[1]Testing should only be done when serologic evidence of HBV infection exists.
[2]To distinguish acute from chronic HBV, obtain IgM anti-HBc.
[3]Consider coinfection if IgM anti-HBc is positive. A superinfection presumably exists if IgM anti-HBc is negative.

infection with these viruses may be inferred from certain test results, and superinfection of HBV carriers with HAV, HCV, or HDV may be inferred from others. In persons with proved acute or chronic HBV infection, testing for anti-HDV may show that HDV is a contributing factor.

Virus-Host Immune Reactions

Currently there is evidence for at least five hepatitis viruses—types A, B, C, D, and E. A single infection with any is believed to confer homologous but not heterologous protection against reinfection. Infection with HBV of a specific subtype, eg, HBsAg/*adw*, appears to confer immunity to other HBsAg subtypes, probably because of their common group *a* specificity.

Most cases of hepatitis type A presumably occur without jaundice during childhood, and by late adulthood there is a widespread resistance to reinfection. However, serologic studies in the USA indicate that the incidence of infection among certain populations may be declining as a result of improvements in sanitation commensurate with a rise in the standard of living. It has been estimated that as many as 60–90% of young middle- to upper-income adults in the USA may be susceptible to type A hepatitis. Younger people who live in poorer circumstances or crowded institutions (eg, military forces) are at increased risk.

The immunopathogenetic mechanisms that result in viral persistence and hepatocellular injury in type B hepatitis remain to be elucidated. Since the virus is not believed to be cytopathic, it is postulated that hepatocellular injury during acute disease represents T cell lysis of HBV-infected hepatocytes, whereas piecemeal necrosis may be a reflection of an autoimmune response to native liver membrane antigens induced by the virus. It is not known which of the various HBV-specified antigens are being recognized by the immunocompetent T cells. The degree of cell-mediated immunologic activity attained and the effects of immunoregulatory lipoprotein molecules generated by the infection may be responsible for continuation of the disease and for focal distribution of the hepatic necrosis. The role of antibody-dependent, complement-mediated cytolysis; defective suppressor cell function; and humoral immune mechanisms in the pathogenesis of this disease are also unclear at present.

Various host responses, immunologic and genetic, have been proposed to account for the frequency of HBsAg persistence, which has been observed to be higher in infants and children than in adults. About 95% of newborns infected at birth become chronic carriers of virus, often for life (Table 35–7). This risk decreases steadily with time, so that the risk of infected adults becoming carriers decreases to 10%. Hepato-

Table 35–7. Transmission of hepatitis B virus and spectrum of outcomes to infection.

Transmission[1]	Vertical (Asia)	Contact (Africa)	Parenteral, Sexual
Age at infection	Newborns, infants	Young children	Teenagers, adults
Recovery from acute infection	5%	20%	90–95%
Progression to chronic infection	95%	80%	5–10%
Chronic carriers[2] (% of total population)	10–20%	10–20%	0.5%

[1]Vertical and contact-associated transmission occurs in endemic countries; parenteral and sexual transmission are main modes in nonendemic countries.
[2]At high risk of developing hepatocellular carcinoma.

cellular carcinoma is most likely to occur in adults who experienced HBV infection at a very early age and became carriers. Therefore, for vaccination to be maximally effective against the carrier state, cirrhosis, and hepatoma, it must be carried out during the first week of life. (See Prevention by Vaccination, below.)

Also at high risk of infection are patients in certain disease states, eg, Down's syndrome, leukemia (acute and chronic lymphocytic), leprosy, thalassemia, and chronic renal insufficiency. In comparison with other mentally retarded patients, patients with Down's syndrome are particularly prone to persistent antigenemia. This does not imply that patients with Down's syndrome have an increased susceptibility to HBV. On the contrary, among equally exposed patients who are residents within the same institution, the total serologic evidence of HBV infection is similar except that the antigen carrier rate is low and the antibody prevalence rate is high in patients who do not have Down's syndrome. An immunologic difference in the host response to the infectious virus is apparently responsible for this serologic dichotomy.

Persistent antigenemia and mild or subclinical infections are more frequently observed in individuals who have been infected with low doses of virus. Correspondingly, an inverse relationship between virus dose and time of appearance of HBsAg or an abnormal ALT value has been reported—ie, the incubation period becomes longer as the dose of virus diminishes.

The frequency of the chronic HBsAg carrier state following acute type B hepatitis is about 10%. More than half these patients continue to exhibit biochemical and histologic evidence of chronic liver disease, ie, chronic persistent or chronic active hepatitis.

Treatment

Treatment of patients with hepatitis is directed at allowing hepatocellular damage to resolve and repair itself under optimal conditions. In previously healthy young military recruits, ad libitum ward privileges or strenuous exercise did not appear to alter the acute course of viral hepatitis.

Interferon-α has a role in the treatment of viral hepatitis, particularly in patients with chronic hepatitis C. Recombinant interferon-α produced a prompt decrease in levels of serum aminotransferase to normal values in about half the patients. Not all who responded clinically and biochemically had histologic improvement, and many relapsed after cessation of treatment. Although interferon-α and interferon-β have been successful in reducing the level of HBV markers, the response has been temporary in most instances, with resumption of viral replication after discontinuance of the drug. Corticosteroids and acyclovir have proved ineffective in treatment of viral hepatitis.

Epidemiology

The incidence of reported hepatitis in the USA had varied from 26 to 33 cases per 100,000 population, with about 70% categorized as hepatitis A, until 1983, when cases of hepatitis B exceeded those of hepatitis A. In 1985, of 60,000 reported hepatitis cases, 39% were hepatitis A, 45% hepatitis B, 7% NANB, and 9% unspecified hepatitis. The actual incidence is undoubtedly much higher, because many persons contract so mild a form of hepatitis that they do not seek treatment, and physicians report only 10–20% of the cases they see. To permit more accurate hepatitis surveillance and to identify epidemiologic trends, all acute cases and confirmed carriers of type B hepatitis should be reported promptly to the local or state health department as required by law. The incidence of hepatitis A and B is highest in persons in the 20- to 29-year-old age group. Since the identification of hepatitis C in 1989, the epidemiology of the disease is undergoing elucidation.

As shown in Table 35–4, there are marked differences in the epidemiologic features of hepatitis A, B, and C infections.

A. Viral Hepatitis Type A (Short Incubation Hepatitis): Outbreaks of type A hepatitis are common in families and institutions, summer camps, and especially among troops. The most likely mode of transmission under these conditions is by the fecal-oral route through close personal contact. Intestinal carriers probably do not exist. The clinical disease is most often manifest in children and young adults, with the highest rates in those between 15 and 30 years of age. The ratio of anicteric to icteric cases in adults is about 1:3; in children, it may be as high as 12:1.

Sudden, explosive epidemics of type A hepatitis usually result from fecal contamination of a single source (eg, drinking water, food, or milk). The consumption of raw oysters or improperly steamed clams obtained from water polluted with sewage has also resulted in several outbreaks of hepatitis.

Other identified sources of potential infection are nonhuman primates. There have been more than 35 outbreaks in which primates, usually chimpanzees, have infected humans in close personal contact with them. These animals probably acquire the infection after arrival and transmit the virus to their caretakers. A persistent carrier state is unlikely, since the number of new cases diminishes with residence.

HAV is seldom transmitted by the use of contaminated needles and syringes or through the administration of blood. Hemodialysis plays no role in the spread of hepatitis A infections to either patients or staff. The prevalence of anti-HAV is identical in persons with prior histories of multiple blood transfusions or accidental inoculations with blood-contaminated instruments and in those from the same socioeconomic background without such exposures. About 30–60% of adults in the USA possess antibodies, with a higher prevalence in those from lower socioeconomic groups.

B. Viral Hepatitis Type B (Long Incubation Hepatitis): HBV is worldwide in distribution. Transmission modes and response to infection vary, depending on the age at time of infection (Table 35–7). Most individuals infected as infants develop chronic infections. As adults they are subject to liver disease and are at high risk of developing hepatocellular carcinoma. There are more than 250 million carriers, of whom about 1 million live in the USA; 25% of carriers develop chronic active hepatitis. Each year in the USA, about 4000 persons die of HBV-associated cirrhosis and 800 die of HBV-related primary hepatocellular carcinoma. Worldwide, one million deaths a year are attributed to HBV-related liver disease and hepatocellular carcinoma.

There is no seasonal trend and no high predilection for any age group, although there are definite high-risk groups such as parenteral drug abusers, institutionalized persons, health care personnel, individuals who have recently received blood transfusions, hemodialysis patients and staff, highly promiscuous persons, and newborn infants born to mothers with hepatitis B. The incidence of hepatitis B among recipients of blood transfusions is about 1%. Since mandatory screening of blood donors for HBsAg was instituted and commercial donors are being replaced with all-volunteer donor sources, the number of icteric cases of transfusion-associated hepatitis has been substantially reduced. At present, hepatitis C accounts for the majority of transfusion-associated hepatitis cases in the USA.

Cases of hepatitis B appear sporadically and are often associated with the parenteral inoculation of infective human blood (or its products), usually obtained from an apparently healthy carrier. Thousands of cases have occurred following parenteral administration of human serum, plasma, whole blood or blood products, or vaccines that contained human serum. Many persons have been infected by improperly sterilized syringes, needles, or scalpels or even by tattooing or ear piercing. The estimated ratio of anicteric to icteric infections is reported to be as high as 4:1.

Other modes of transmission of hepatitis B exist. Volunteers who ingested infectious plasma developed infection. HBsAg can be detected in saliva, nasopharyngeal washings, semen, menstrual fluid, and vaginal secretions as well as in blood. Transmission from carriers to close contacts by the oral route or by sexual or other intimate exposure occurs. There is particularly strong evidence of transmission from persons with subclinical cases and carriers of HBsAg to homosexual and heterosexual long-term partners, although the precise mechanism of transmission is not clear. Transmission by the fecal-oral route has not been documented.

Health care personnel (surgeons, pathologists, and other physicians, dentists, nurses, laboratory technicians, and blood bank personnel) have a higher incidence of hepatitis and prevalence of detectable HBsAg or anti-HBs than those who have no occupational exposure to patients or blood products. The risk that these apparently healthy HBsAg carriers (especially medical and dental surgeons) represent to the patients under their care remains to be determined but is probably small.

Hepatitis B infections are common among patients and staff of hemodialysis units. Family contacts are also at increased risk. As many as 50% of the renal dialysis patients who contract hepatitis B may become chronic carriers of HBsAg compared with 2% of the staff group, emphasizing differences in the host immune response.

The incubation period of hepatitis B is 50–180 days, with a mean between 60 and 90 days. It appears to vary with the dose of HBV administered and the route of administration, being prolonged in patients who receive a low dose of virus or who are infected by a nonpercutaneous route.

Immune (gamma) globulin and albumin are blood products that appear free from the risk of hepatitis B. Their method of preparation includes cold ethanol fractionation. In addition, albumin is heated to 60 °C for 10 hours.

C. Viral Hepatitis Type C: In the 1980s, NANB hepatitis accounted for 6% of all reported cases of hepatitis in the USA but for 90% of the cases of transfusion-associated hepatitis, now known to be caused by HCV. In addition, up to 25% of sporadic hepatitis cases may be caused by HCV. The incubation period ranges from 5 to 10 weeks, though both shorter (2 weeks) and longer (4 months) intervals have been observed. Serologic markers for active HAV, HBV, or other viral agents occasionally associated with hepatitis are absent, but anti-HCV can be detected. Studies in the past identified other risk factors associated with this disease. The most meaningful predictor of disease in a blood donor was a high alanine aminotransferase (ALT [SGPT]) value. Transfusion of a donor unit with an elevated ALT level of ≥ 45 IU/L significantly increases the recipient's risk of contracting type C hepatitis.

HCV is probably transmitted in somewhat the same way as HBV. It has been shown that HCV can be vertically transmitted from mother to infant. The risk of transmission seems to be related to the level of HCV in the mother.

D. Hepatitis D (Delta Agent): HDV is found throughout the world, but its highest prevalence has been reported in Italy, the Middle East, Africa, and South America. Persons who have received multiple transfusions, intravenous drug abusers, and their close contacts are at high risk. The primary routes of transmission are believed to be similar to those of HBV. Infection is dependent on HBV replication with synthesis of HBsAg. HBV provides an HBsAg envelope for HDV. Once infection is established, HDV interferes with the expression of HBV gene products and reduces the concentration of hepatitis B markers associated with infectivity. The incubation period varies from 2 to 12 weeks, being shorter in HBV carriers who are superinfected with the agent than in susceptible persons who are simultaneously infected with both HBV and

HDV. Infection with HDV can be diagnosed by identifying an IgM anti-HDV response during the acute or chronic stage of the disease. Persons who have recovered from delta infection are immune to rechallenge with that agent or with HBV.

Two epidemiologic patterns of delta infection have been identified. In Mediterranean countries (northern Africa, southern Europe, and the Middle East), delta infection is endemic among persons with hepatitis B, and most infections are thought to be transmitted by intimate contact. In nonendemic areas, such as the USA and northern Europe, delta infection is confined to persons exposed frequently to blood and blood products, primarily drug addicts and hemophiliacs. Whether in endemic or nonendemic countries, the only persons with any appreciable risk of transfusion-associated delta hepatitis are those who receive pooled blood derivatives obtained from thousands of donors. This group includes persons with inherited or acquired coagulation problems who are receiving commercial clotting factor concentrates. The same demographic factors that increase the likelihood of hepatitis B and C in commercial blood donors also contribute to their enhanced risk of exposure to HDV.

Delta hepatitis was not found in Swedish drug addicts before 1973. In the ensuing decade, its incidence in that population increased to about 75% of all addicts who were hepatitis B carriers; the disease involved their intimate contacts as well. Delta hepatitis also may occur in explosive outbreaks and affect entire localized pockets of hepatitis B carriers. Outbreaks of severe, often fulminant and chronic delta hepatitis have occurred for decades in isolated populations in the Orinoco and Amazon basins of South America and have been given such exotic names as "Labrea fever" and "hepatitis of the Sierra Nevada de Santa Marta." Severe outbreaks of delta hepatitis are not confined to isolated, remote regions of developing countries. In the USA, HDV has been found to participate in 20–30% of cases of chronic hepatitis B, acute exacerbations of chronic hepatitis B, and fulminant hepatitis B; and 3–12% of blood donors with serum HBsAg have antibodies to HDV. Delta hepatitis is not a new disease, because globulin lots prepared from plasma collected in the USA 40 years ago contain antibodies to HDV.

Prevention by Vaccination

A vaccine for hepatitis B has been available since 1982. Vaccine can be prepared by purifying HBsAg associated with the 22-nm particles from healthy HBsAg-positive carriers and treating the particles with virus-inactivating agents (formalin, urea, heat). Protection is conferred by antibody to the *a* antigen, an antigen common to all subtypes. Preparations containing intact 22-nm particles have been highly effective in reducing HBV infection in hemodialysis patients and staff, among homosexuals, and in newborns born to HBV-infected mothers. Other sources of immunogen have been developed: (1) HBsAg produced by a recombinant DNA in yeast cells or in continuous mammalian cell lines into which a plasmid containing the gene for HBsAg has been incorporated; (2) polypeptides derived from the 22-nm particles; and (3) a recombinant of live vaccinia virus and the HBsAg gene. All of these new sources have been used successfully in immunizing chimpanzees, and new vaccines now compete with the plasma-derived vaccine.

A product made from yeast is the second-generation vaccine. The HBsAg is expressed in yeast as particles 15–30 nm in diameter, with the morphologic characteristics of free surface antigen in plasma. In contrast to HBsAg from human plasma, the polypeptide antigen produced by recombinant yeast is not glycosylated. The vaccine formulated using this purified material has proved to be immunogenic for animals and for humans, with a potency similar to that of vaccine made from plasma-derived antigen. In addition, chimpanzees immunized with this yeast recombinant hepatitis B vaccine (HBsAg, subtype *adw*) were protected when challenged with virus of subtype *adr* or *ayw*, whereas nonimmunized animals were infected when challenged with live virus.

Sources of large amounts of HAV have become available, and inactivated virus vaccines are now licensed in Europe and expected to be licensed soon in the USA. Until all susceptible at-risk groups are immunized, prevention and control of hepatitis must be directed toward interrupting the chain of transmission and using passive immunization.

Control Measures

A. Viral Hepatitis Type A: The appearance of hepatitis in camps or institutions is often an indication of poor sanitation and poor personal hygiene. Control measures are directed toward the prevention of fecal contamination of food, water, or other sources by the individual. Reasonable hygiene—such as hand washing after bowel movements or before meals, the use of disposable plates and eating utensils, and the use of 0.5% sodium hypochlorite (eg, 1:10 dilution of chlorine bleach) as a disinfectant—is essential in preventing the spread of HAV during the acute phase of the illness. Extraordinarily conservative measures, such as the use of gowns, masks, and gloves, are usually unnecessary unless there is exposure to feces or fecally contaminated items. Infectivity studies indicate that the risk of transmitting hepatitis A is greatest from 2 weeks before to 1 week after onset of jaundice. Transmission by the aerosol route appears relatively unimportant.

Immune (gamma) globulin (IG) is prepared from large pools of normal adult plasma and confers passive protection in about 90% of those exposed when given within 1–2 weeks after exposure to hepatitis A. Its prophylactic value decreases with time, and its administration more than 4 weeks after exposure or after onset of clinical symptoms is probably not indicated.

In the doses generally prescribed, IG does not prevent infection but rather makes the infection mild or subclinical and permits active immunity to develop. For ordinary exposure, the dose is 0.02 mL/kg given once intramuscularly during the incubation period. HAV vaccine produces a more enduring immunity and should replace the use of IG.

B. Viral Hepatitis Type B: Persons who have had hepatitis probably should not be used as blood donors. Even persons without a history of hepatitis and with normal liver function tests may be carriers of the virus. In addition, HBV or HBcAg carriers may develop acute hepatitis A and the underlying condition may go unrecognized. Sensitive methods for detecting HBsAg in blood donors are now being employed by all blood banks to avoid administering HBsAg-positive blood. Nevertheless, cases of posttransfusion hepatitis B continue to occur, although at a reduced frequency. Since the incidence of posttransfusion hepatitis (both B and C) is higher among recipients of commercial (paid donor) blood or blood from first-time donors, the establishment of an all-volunteer population who donate periodically is an important measure for eliminating transfusion-associated hepatitis. However, registries of minimal-risk donors who are known to be in good health should also provide satisfactory sources of blood, even if such persons are paid.

Proper donor selection and the development of a central registry for identification of carriers can lower the incidence of transfusion-associated hepatitis. In addition, blood or its products should be used only when necessary, since the risk of hepatitis appears to increase with the number of units administered. HBV may be transmitted to personnel in blood transfusion laboratories, but there is no evidence for transmission of infection from members of the staff to blood or blood products.

Patients with acute type B hepatitis generally need not be isolated so long as blood and instrument precautions are stringently observed, both in the general patient care areas and in the laboratories. Staff members should always follow universal precautions when in contact with blood or blood-contaminated objects. Because spouses and intimate contacts of persons with acute type B hepatitis are at risk of acquiring clinical type B hepatitis, they need to be warned about practices that might increase the risk of infection or transmission.

There is no justification for removing HBsAg-positive carriers from patient contact in the absence of evidence of disease transmission. The use of gloves should reduce the potential for HBV transmission. There is no evidence that asymptomatic HBsAg-positive food handlers pose a health risk to the general public.

The resistance of HBV to physical and chemical agents makes it difficult to treat human blood and its products to render them safe for human inoculation. Autoclaving and the use of ethylene oxide gas are both acceptable methods for disinfecting metal objects, instruments, or heat-sensitive equipment. Another useful germicide is 2% activated glutaraldehyde.

Since as little as 0.0001 mL of plasma can transmit the disease, a single carrier of hepatitis B virus might "infect" a large batch of pooled plasma. It has been recommended, therefore, that pooled plasma not be used. If pools must be used, they should be made from blood from no more than five donors and each unit tested for HBsAg by one of the more sensitive methods (eg, radioimmunoassay) prior to pooling. Pooled plasma should be used only in cases of emergency because of the possibility of transmitting hepatitis B to a patient who is already ill.

Studies on passive immunization using specific hepatitis B immune globulin (HBIG) have been encouraging. Studies that have compared placebo with IG containing anti-HBs have indicated a protective effect if the latter is given soon after exposure. However, the concentration of antibody required for protection has not been adequately ascertained. The incubation period of hepatitis B was prolonged significantly in volunteers receiving a high-titer IG preparation. Administration of specific HBIG (or conventional IG with titers of anti-HBs $>$ 1:256) to spouses of patients with acute type B hepatitis has been shown to be effective in preventing not only symptomatic type B hepatitis but the infection itself. However, passive-active immunity appeared to occur more frequently in susceptible individuals receiving conventional IG.

Prevention of transfusion-associated hepatitis by the administration of standard IG has not been consistently demonstrated in carefully conducted trials. Therefore, although HBIG has been officially released for clinical use in exposure to small amounts of HBV, such as might occur with an accidental prick with a contaminated needle or direct mucous membrane contact arising from a splash or pipetting accident, its routine administration to recipients of blood transfusions is not recommended.

Women who are HBV carriers or who acquire type B hepatitis while pregnant can transmit the disease to their infants. The risk of transmission is increased during the third trimester and the postpartum period. Infants who become HBsAg-positive generally do so within 1–2 months, but testing should continue at monthly intervals for at least 6 months. Most develop persistent antigenemia, especially if the mother is also HBeAg-positive. The effectiveness of hepatitis vaccine and HBIG in preventing hepatitis B in infants born to these HBV-positive mothers has been substantiated in several studies. If vaccine is not available at the time of birth, it should be given within the next 7 days. Optimally, a second dose of vaccine should be given at 1 month and a third dose at 6 months of age. Infants are given 0.5 mL of HBIG plus 10 μg of vaccine concurrently but at a different site within a few hours of birth. Reduction in the cost of vaccine to about $1 per dose for public health programs has made vaccination of newborns feasible in areas of high endemicity. The high cost of HBIG precludes its use in most countries.

Table 35–8. Hepatitis B virus postexposure recommendations.[1]

Exposure	HBIG		Vaccine	
	Dose	**Recommended Timing**	**Dose**	**Recommended Timing**
Perinatal	0.5 mL IM	Within 12 hours of birth.	0.5 mL (10 μg) IM	Within 12 hours of birth;[2] repeat at 1 and 6 months.
Sexual	0.06 mL/kg IM	Single dose within 14 days of last sexual contact.	[3]	—

[1]Based on recommendations of the Immunization Practices Advisory Committee. MMWR (February) 1990;39 (No. RR-2):1.
[2]The first dose can be given at the same time as the HBIG dose but at a different site.
[3]Vaccine is recommended for homosexual men and for regular sexual contacts of HBV carriers and is optional in initial treatment of heterosexual contacts of persons with acute HBV.

Preexposure prophylaxis with a commercially available hepatitis B vaccine currently is recommended by the World Health Organization, the Centers for Disease Control, and the Advisory Committee on Immunization Practices for all susceptible, at-risk groups. The human-plasma-derived vaccine (Heptavax-B) has been administered in many countries, with extensive follow-up of vaccinees. The product has been shown to be safe, immunogenic, and effective in preventing hepatitis B.

The plasma-derived hepatitis B vaccine became available in the USA in mid 1982, but by mid 1987 most of those vaccinated (85%) were health care workers. As might have been expected, there was no decrease in incidence of acute hepatitis B. About 30,000 cases were reported in 1985, with the estimated number of cases at 300,000. Apparently the high-risk groups—with the exception of health care workers—were not taking the vaccine.

Chimpanzee studies have shown that pre-S2 and pre-S1 specific antibodies can protect against HBV infections. It is believed that antibody responses against the pre-S sequences may make a vaccine more efficacious. It is possible that these sequences may be included in future vaccines.

In the USA, perinatal transmission of HBV is uncommon. When it does occur, there follows the same highly associated morbidity and mortality, including chronic hepatitis, cirrhosis, and liver cancer, that occur in other parts of the world. Routine screening of pregnant women for HBsAg and anti-HBc should be conducted even in the USA, and infants born at risk should be immunized, beginning in the perinatal period, with either the plasma-derived or recombinant vaccine. A new program of hepatitis B control has been recommended for many countries, including the USA, in which HB vaccine will be administered to all children as part of their regular immunization schedule.

HBV vaccination in hemodialysis patients has not always been successful. Seroconversion rates vary with the intensity of their cell-mediated immune response as determined by the skin reaction to dinitrochlorobenzene. Patients with a strong skin reaction react as well as healthy persons to the vaccine, but those with a weak skin reaction need higher doses of vaccine.

Guidelines for postexposure prophylaxis have been established by the Center for Infectious Diseases, Centers for Disease Control (Tables 35–8 and 35–9). Per-

Table 35–9. Recommendations for hepatitis B prophylaxis following percutaneous exposure.[1]

Source	Exposed Person	
	Unvaccinated	**Vaccinated**
HBsAg-positive	1. HBIG once immediately.[2] 2. Initiate HB vaccine[3] series.	1. Test exposed person for anti-HBs. 2. If inadequate antibody,[4] HBIG once immediately plus HB vaccine booster dose.
Known source High-risk HBsAg-positive	1. Initiate HB vaccine series. 2. Test source for HBsAg. If positive, HBIG once.	1. Test source for HBsAg only if exposed person is vaccine nonresponder; if source is HBsAg-positive, give HBIG once immediately plus HB vaccine booster dose.
Low-risk HBsAg-positive	Initiate HB vaccine series.	Nothing required.
Unknown source	Initiate HB vaccine series.	Nothing required.

[1]Based on recommendations of the Immunization Practices Advisory Committee. MMWR (February) 1990;39 (No. RR-2):1.
[2]HBIG dose 0.06 mL/kg IM.
[3]HB vaccine dose 20 μg IM for adults; 10 μg IM for infants or children under 10 years of age. First dose within 1 week; second and third doses, 1 and 6 months later.
[4]Fewer than 10 sample ratio units by radioimmunoassay, negative by enzyme immunoassay.

sons exposed to HBV percutaneously or by contamination of the mucosal surfaces should immediately receive both HBIG and HBsAg vaccine administered simultaneously at different sites to provide immediate protection with passively acquired antibody followed by active immunity generated by the vaccine. IG or HBsAg vaccine is of no demonstrable benefit in the treatment of HBsAg carriers.

Delta hepatitis can be prevented by vaccinating HBV-susceptible persons with hepatitis B vaccine. However, vaccination does not protect hepatitis B carriers from superinfection by HDV.

REFERENCES

Blumberg BS: Australia antigen and the biology of hepatitis B. Science 1977;197:17.

Bradley DW (guest editor): Human hepatitis viruses. Semin Virol 1993;4:No. 5. [Entire issue.]

Buendia MA: Hepatitis B viruses and hepatocellular carcinoma. Adv Cancer Res 1992;59:167.

Choo QL et al: Isolation of a cDNA clone derived from a blood-borne non-A, non-B viral hepatitis genome. Science 1989;244:359.

Davis GL et al: Treatment of chronic hepatitis C with recombinant interferon alfa: A multicenter randomized, controlled trial. N Engl J Med 1989;321:1501.

Hadler SC et al: Long-term immunogenicity and efficacy of hepatitis B vaccine in homosexual men. N Engl J Med 1986;315:209.

Hollinger FB: Hepatitis B virus. In: *Virology,* 2nd ed. Fields BN et al (editors). Raven Press, 1990.

Hollinger FB: Non-A, non-B hepatitis viruses. In: *Virology,* 2nd ed. Fields BN et al (editors). Raven Press, 1990.

Hollinger FB, Ticehurst J: Hepatitis A virus. In: *Virology,* 2nd ed. Fields BN et al (editors). Raven Press, 1990.

Krugman S, Giles JP: Viral hepatitis, type B (MS-2 strain): Further observations on natural history and prevention. N Engl J Med 1973;288:755.

Kurosaki M et al: Rapid sequence variation of the hypervariable region of hepatitis C virus during the course of chronic infection. Hepatology 1993;18:1293.

Lettau LA et al: Outbreak of severe hepatitis due to delta and hepatitis B viruses in parenteral drug abusers and their contacts. N Engl J Med 1987;317:1256.

Melnick JL: Hepatocellular carcinoma caused by hepatitis B virus. In: *Viral Infections of Humans: Epidemiology and Control,* 3rd ed. Evans AS (editor). Plenum Press, 1989.

Miyamura T et al: Detection of antibody against antigen expressed by molecularly cloned hepatitis C virus cDNA: Application to diagnosis and blood screening for post-transfusion hepatitis. Proc Natl Acad Sci USA 1990; 87:983.

Nassal M, Schaller H: Hepatitis B virus replication. Trends Microbiol 1993;1:221.

Ohto H et al: Transmission of hepatitis C virus from mothers to infants. N Engl J Med 1994;330:744.

Purcell RH, Gerin JL: Hepatitis delta virus. In: *Virology,* 2nd ed. Fields BN et al (editors). Raven Press, 1990.

Zuckerman AJ (editor): *Viral Hepatitis and Liver Disease.* Alan R. Liss, 1988.

36 Picornaviruses (Enterovirus & Rhinovirus Groups)

Picornaviruses represent a very large virus family with respect to the number of members but one of the smallest in terms of virion size. They include two major groups: **enteroviruses** and **rhinoviruses.**

Many picornaviruses cause diseases in humans ranging from severe paralysis to aseptic meningitis, pleurodynia, myocarditis, vesicular and exanthematous skin lesions, mucocutaneous lesions, respiratory and intestinal illnesses, undifferentiated febrile illness, and conjunctivitis. However, subclinical infection is far more common than clinically manifest disease. Different viruses may produce the same syndrome; conversely, the same picornavirus may cause more than a single syndrome. Furthermore, some clinical symptoms produced by enteroviruses cannot be distinguished from those caused by some nonenteroviruses. Hence, laboratory tests are required to establish etiology.

PROPERTIES OF PICORNAVIRUSES

Important properties of picornaviruses are shown in Table 36–1.

Structure & Composition

The virion of enteroviruses and rhinoviruses consists of a capsid shell of 60 subunits, each of four proteins (VP1–VP4) arranged with icosahedral symmetry around a genome made up of a single strand of positive-sense RNA (Figure 36–1).

By means of x-ray diffraction studies, the molecular structures of poliovirus and rhinovirus have been determined. The three largest viral proteins, VP1–VP3, have a very similar core structure, in which the peptide backbone of the protein loops back on itself to form a barrel of eight strands held together by hydrogen bonds (the beta barrel). The amino acid chain between the beta barrel and the N and C terminal portions of the protein contains a series of loops. These loops include the main antigenic sites that are found on the surface of the virion and are involved in the neutralization of viral infection.

There is a prominent cleft or canyon around each pentameric vertex on the surface of the viral particle. The receptor binding site used to attach the virion to a host cell is thought to be located near the floor of the canyon. This location would protect the crucial cell attachment site from structural variation influenced by antibody selection in hosts, as the canyon is too narrow to permit deep penetration of antibody molecules (Figure 36–1).

Enteroviruses are stable at acid pH (3.0–5.0) for 1–3 hours, whereas rhinoviruses are acid-labile. Enteroviruses and some rhinoviruses are stabilized by magnesium chloride against thermal inactivation. Enteroviruses and rhinoviruses differ in buoyant density. Enteroviruses have a buoyant density in cesium chloride of about 1.34 g/mL; human rhinoviruses, about 1.4 g/mL.

Classification

Enteroviruses of human origin include the following: (1) polioviruses, types 1–3; (2) coxsackieviruses of group A, types 1–24 (there is no type 23); (3) coxsackieviruses of group B, types 1–6; (4) echoviruses, types 1–34 (no types 10 or 28); and (5) enteroviruses, types 68–71 (Table 36–2). Since 1969, new enterovirus types have been assigned enterovirus type numbers rather than being subclassified as coxsackieviruses or echoviruses. The vernacular names of the previously identified enteroviruses have been retained. Hepatitis A virus was originally classified as enterovirus type 72 but is now assigned to a new genus. Enteroviruses also exist in many animals, including cattle, pigs, and mice.

Human rhinoviruses include more than 100 antigenic types. Rhinoviruses of other host species include those of horses and cattle.

Other picornaviruses are foot-and-mouth disease virus of cattle *(Aphthovirus)* and encephalomyocarditis virus of rodents *(Cardiovirus)*.

Enteroviruses are transient inhabitants of the human alimentary tract and may be isolated from the throat or lower intestine. Rhinoviruses, on the other hand, are isolated chiefly from the nose and throat. Among the enteroviruses that are cytopathogenic (polioviruses, echoviruses, and some coxsackieviruses), growth can be readily obtained at 36–37 °C in primary cultures of human and monkey kidney cells and certain cell lines (such as HeLa); in contrast, most rhinovirus strains can be recovered only in cells of human origin

Table 36–1. Important properties of picornaviruses.

Virion: Icosahedral, about 27 nm in diameter; contains 60 subunits.
Composition: RNA (30%), protein (70%).
Genome: Single-stranded RNA, linear, positive-sense, MW 2.5 million, infectious.
Proteins: Four major polypeptides cleaved from a large precursor polyprotein. Surface proteins VP1 and VP3 are major antibody-binding sites. Internal protein VP4 is associated with viral RNA.
Envelope: None.
Replication: Cytoplasm.
Outstanding characteristics: Family is made up of many enterovirus and rhinovirus types that infect humans and lower animals; cause various illnesses ranging from poliomyelitis to aseptic meningitis to the common cold.

(embryonic human kidney or lung, human diploid cell strains) at 33 °C.

The host range of picornaviruses varies greatly from one type to the next and even among strains of the same type. They may readily be induced, by laboratory manipulation, to yield variants that have host ranges and tissue tropisms different from those of certain wild strains; this has led to the development of attenuated poliovirus strains now used as vaccines.

ENTEROVIRUS GROUP

POLIOMYELITIS

Poliomyelitis is an acute infectious disease that in its serious form affects the central nervous system. The destruction of motor neurons in the spinal cord results in flaccid paralysis. However, most poliovirus infections are subclinical.

Properties of the Virus

A. General Properties: Poliovirus particles are typical enteroviruses (see above). They are inactivated when heated at 55 °C for 30 minutes, but Mg^{2+}, 1 mol/L, prevents this inactivation. Milk or ice cream is also protective, but proper pasteurization inactivates the virus. While purified poliovirus is inactivated by a chlorine concentration of 0.1 ppm, much higher concentrations of chlorine are required to disinfect sewage containing virus in fecal suspensions and in the presence of other organic matter. In contrast to arboviruses, which may be prevalent at the same time of year, polioviruses are not affected by ether or sodium deoxycholate.

B. Animal Susceptibility and Growth of Virus: Polioviruses have a very restricted host range. Most strains will infect monkeys when inoculated directly into the brain or spinal cord. Chimpanzees and cynomolgus monkeys can also be infected by the oral route; in chimpanzees, the infection thus produced is usually asymptomatic. The animals become intestinal carriers of the virus; they also develop a viremia that is quenched by the appearance of antibodies in the circulating blood. Unusual strains have been transmitted to mice or chick embryos.

Most strains can be grown in primary or continuous cell line cultures derived from a variety of human tissues or from monkey kidney, testis, or muscle, but not in cells of lower animals.

Poliovirus requires a primate-specific membrane receptor for infection, and the absence of this receptor on the surface of nonprimate cells makes them virus-resistant. This restriction can be overcome by introducing poliovirus into resistant cells by means of synthetic lipid vesicles called liposomes. More recently, introduction of the functioning receptor gene has been achieved, and this maneuver also converts resistant cells to susceptible cells. Once inside the cell, poliovirus replicates normally. Transgenic mice harboring the primate receptor gene have been developed; they are susceptible to human polioviruses.

C. Viral Replication: After attaching to viral receptors (which seem to be controlled in humans by genes on chromosome 19), poliovirus undergoes replication as diagrammed in Figure 29–10. Poliovirus RNA serves both as its own messenger RNA and as the source of the genetic information.

D. Antigenic Properties: There are three antigenic types. Complement-fixing antigens for each type may be prepared from tissue culture or infected central nervous system specimens. Inactivation of the virus by formalin, heat, or ultraviolet light liberates a soluble complement-fixing antigen. This antigen is cross-reactive and fixes complement with heterotypic poliomyelitis antibodies. A type-specific precipitin reaction occurs when concentrated virus is used with immune animal or convalescent human sera. Two type-specific antigens are contained in poliovirus preparations and can be detected by ELISA and CF tests. They are the D and C antigens. The D form can be converted to the C form by heating. The D form represents full particles containing RNA; the C form, empty particles. C antigens of different viral types are cross-reactive, but D antigens are not.

Pathogenesis & Pathology

The mouth is the portal of entry of the virus, and primary multiplication takes place in the oropharynx or intestine. The virus is regularly present in the throat and in the stools before the onset of illness. One week after onset there is little virus in the throat, but virus continues to be excreted in the stools for several weeks, even though high antibody levels are present in the blood.

The virus may be found in the blood of patients with abortive and nonparalytic poliomyelitis and in orally

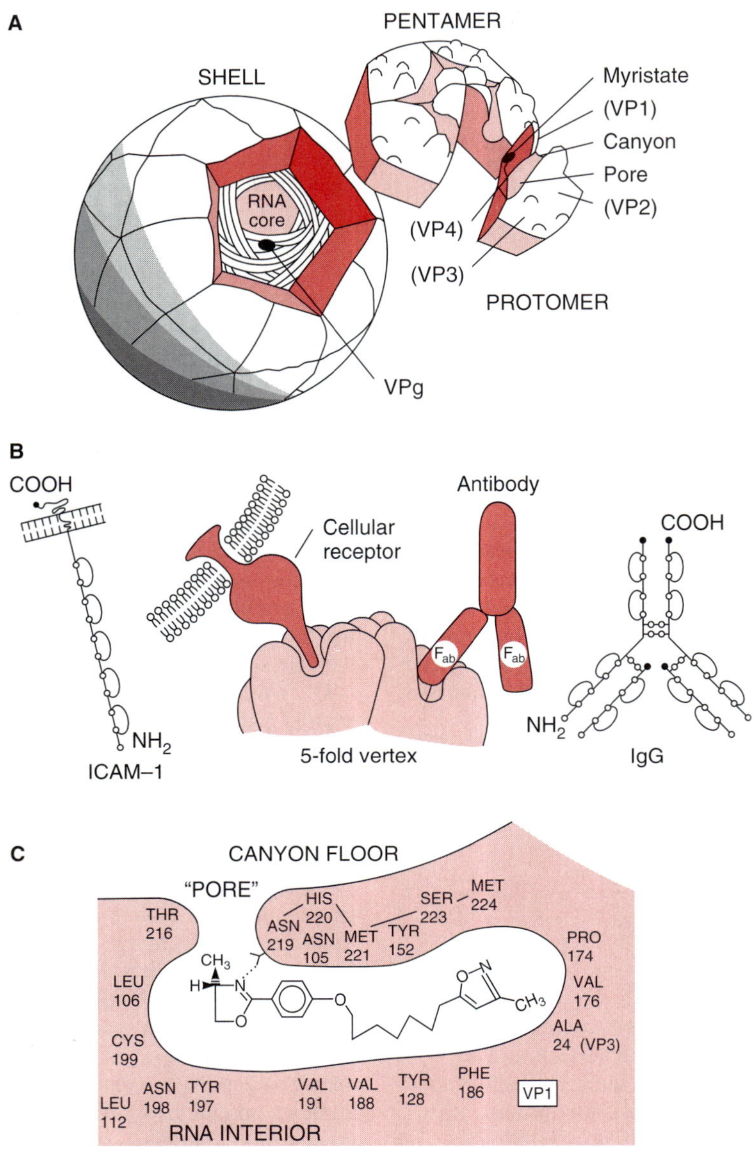

Figure 36–1. Structure of a typical picornavirus. ***A:*** Exploded diagram showing internal location of the RNA genome surrounded by capsid composed of pentamers of proteins VP1, VP2, VP3, and VP4. Note the "canyon" depression surrounding the vertex of the pentamer. ***B:*** Binding of cellular receptor to the floor of the canyon. The major rhinovirus receptor (ICAM-1 molecule) has a diameter roughly half that of an IgG antibody molecule. ***C:*** Location of a drug binding site in VP1 of a rhinovirus. The antiviral drug shown, WIN 52084, prevents viral attachment by deforming part of the canyon floor. (Reproduced, with permission, from Rueckert RR: Picornaviridae and their replication. In: *Virology,* 2nd ed. Fields BN et al [editors]. Raven Press, 1990.)

infected monkeys and chimpanzees in the preparalytic phase of the disease. Antibodies to the virus appear early in the disease, usually before paralysis occurs.

Viremia is also associated with immunization with type 2 oral vaccine. Free virus is usually present in the blood between days 2 and 5 after vaccination, and virus is bound to antibody for an additional few days. Bound virus is detected by acid treatment, which inactivates the antibody and liberates active virus.

These findings have led to the view that the virus first multiplies in the tonsils, the lymph nodes of the neck, Peyer's patches, and the small intestine. The central nervous system may then be invaded by way of the circulating blood. In monkeys infected by the oral

Table 36–2. Characteristics of human picornaviruses.

Property	Enteroviruses					Rhinoviruses
		Coxsackie				
	Polio	A	B	Echo	Entero[1]	
Serotypes	1–3	1–24	1–6	1–34	68–71	> 100
Acid pH	Stable	Stable	Stable	Stable	Stable	Labile
Density (g/mL)	1.34	1.34	1.34	1.34	1.34	1.4
Optimal temperature for growth	37 °C	37 °C	37 °C	37 °C	37 °C	33 °C
Common sites of isolation from humans						
Nose	0	0	0	0	0	+
Throat	+	+	+	+	+	+
Lower intestine	+	+	+	+	+	0
Infect newborn mice[2]	0	+	+	0		0

[1]Since 1969, new enteroviruses have been assigned a number rather than being subclassified as coxsackieviruses or echoviruses.
[2]Some variability exists in this property.

route, small amounts of antibody prevent the paralytic disease, whereas large amounts are necessary to prevent passage of the virus along nerve fibers. In humans also, antibody in the form of pooled human gamma globulin (immune globulin USP) may prevent paralysis if given before exposure to the virus.

Poliovirus can spread along axons of peripheral nerves to the central nervous system, where it continues to progress along the fibers of the lower motor neurons to increasingly involve the spinal cord or the brain. Operations on the oropharynx and tonsillectomy enhance the likelihood of central nervous system involvement during prevalence of polioviruses in the community. This may be attributable to the access of cut nerve fibers to virus in the pharynx or to the removal of immunologically active lymphoid tissue.

Poliovirus invades certain types of nerve cells, and in the process of its intracellular multiplication it may damage or completely destroy these cells. The anterior horn cells of the spinal cord are most prominently involved, but in severe cases the intermediate gray ganglia and even the posterior horn and dorsal root ganglia are often involved. In the brain, the reticular formation, vestibular nuclei, and deep cerebellar nuclei are most often affected. The cortex is virtually spared, with the exception of the motor cortex along the precentral gyrus.

Poliovirus does not multiply in muscle in vivo. The changes that occur in peripheral nerves and voluntary muscles are secondary to the destruction of nerve cells. Changes occur rapidly in nerve cells, from mild chromatolysis to neuronophagia and complete destruction. Some cells that lose their function may recover completely. Inflammation occurs secondary to the attack on the nerve cells; the focal and perivascular infiltrations are chiefly lymphocytes, with some polymorphonuclear cells, and microglia.

In addition to pathologic changes in the nervous system, there may be myocarditis, lymphatic hyperplasia, ulceration of Peyer's patches, prominence of follicles, and enlargement of lymph nodes.

Clinical Findings

When an individual susceptible to infection is exposed to the virus, one of the following responses may occur: (1) inapparent infection without symptoms, (2) mild illness, (3) aseptic meningitis, (4) paralytic poliomyelitis. As the disease progresses, one response may merge with a more severe form, often resulting in a biphasic course: a minor illness, followed first by a few days free of symptoms and then by the major, severe illness. Only about 1% of infections are recognized clinically.

The incubation period is usually 7–14 days, but it may range from 3 to 35 days.

A. Abortive Poliomyelitis: This is the most common form of the disease. The patient has only the minor illness, characterized by fever, malaise, drowsiness, headache, nausea, vomiting, constipation, and sore throat in various combinations. The patient recovers in a few days. The diagnosis of abortive poliomyelitis can be made only when the virus is isolated or antibody development is measured.

B. Nonparalytic Poliomyelitis (Aseptic Meningitis): In addition to the above symptoms and signs, the patient with the nonparalytic form has stiffness and pain in the back and neck. The disease lasts 2–10 days, and recovery is rapid and complete. In a small percentage of cases, the disease advances to paralysis. Poliovirus is only one of many viruses that produce aseptic meningitis.

C. Paralytic Poliomyelitis: The major illness usually follows the minor illness described above, but it may occur without the antecedent first phase. The predominating complaint is flaccid paralysis resulting from lower motor neuron damage. However, incoordination secondary to brain stem invasion and painful spasms of nonparalyzed muscles may also occur. The amount of damage varies greatly. Muscle involvement is usually maximal within a few days after the paralytic phase begins. Maximal recovery usually occurs within 6 months, with residual paralysis lasting much longer.

D. Progressive Postpoliomyelitis Muscle Atrophy: A recrudescence of paralysis and muscle wasting has been repeatedly observed in individuals decades after their experience with paralytic poliomyelitis. This phenomenon had been first observed a century ago, but only in recent years have there been sequential studies to follow the progression of neurologic deficit. Many of the recently reported cases have been in the USA, where in 1993 there were approximately 300,000 persons with a history of poliomyelitis. Although progressive postpoliomyelitis muscle atrophy is rare, it is a specific syndrome. It does not appear to be a consequence of persistent infection but rather a result of physiologic and aging changes in paralytic patients already burdened by loss of neuromuscular functions.

Laboratory Diagnosis

A. Cerebrospinal Fluid: The cerebrospinal fluid contains an increased number of leukocytes—usually 10–200/μL, seldom more than 500/μL. In the early stage of the disease, the ratio of polymorphonuclear cells to lymphocytes is high, but within a few days the ratio is reversed. The total cell count slowly subsides to normal levels. The protein content of the cerebrospinal fluid is elevated (average, about 40–50 mg/dL), but high levels may occur and persist for weeks. The glucose content is normal.

B. Recovery of Virus: Cultures of human or monkey cells may be used. The virus may be recovered from throat swabs taken soon after onset of illness and from rectal swabs or feces collected for longer periods. The virus has been found in about 80% of patients during the first 2 weeks of illness but in only 25% during the third 2-week period. No permanent carriers are known. Poliovirus is uncommonly recovered from the cerebrospinal fluid, unlike some coxsackieviruses and echoviruses.

In fatal cases, the virus should be sought in the cervical and lumbar enlargements of the spinal cord, in the medulla, and in the colon contents. Histologic examination of the spinal cord and parts of the brain should be performed. If paralysis has lasted 4–5 days, it is difficult to recover the virus from the cord.

Specimens should be kept frozen during transit to the laboratory. After treatment with antibiotics, cell cultures are inoculated, incubated, and observed. Cytopathogenic effects appear in 3–6 days. An isolated virus is identified and typed by neutralization with specific antiserum.

C. Serology: Paired serum specimens are required to show a rise in antibody titer.

During poliomyelitis infection, complement-fixing C antibodies form before D antibodies (see Antigenic Properties, above). The level of C antibodies declines first. Early acute stage sera thus contain C antibodies only; 1–2 weeks later, both antibodies are present; in late convalescent sera, only D antibodies are present. Only first infection with poliovirus produces strictly type-specific complement-fixing responses. Subsequent infections with heterotypic polioviruses recall or induce antibodies, mostly against the heat-stable group antigen shared by all three types of poliovirus.

Neutralizing antibodies appear early and are usually already detectable at the time of hospitalization. If the first specimen is taken sufficiently early, a rise in titer can be demonstrated during the course of the disease.

Immunity

Immunity is permanent to the type causing the infection. There may be a low degree of heterotypic resistance induced by infection, especially between type 1 and type 2 polioviruses.

Passive immunity is transferred from mother to offspring. The maternal antibodies gradually disappear during the first 6 months of life. Passively administered antibody lasts only 3–5 weeks.

Virus-neutralizing antibody forms soon after exposure to the virus, often before the onset of illness, and apparently persists for life. Its formation early in the disease implies that viral multiplication occurs in the body before the invasion of the nervous system. As the virus in the brain and spinal cord is not influenced by high titers of antibodies in the blood (which are found in the preparalytic stage of the disease), immunization is of value only if it precedes the onset of symptoms referable to the nervous system.

The VP1 surface protein of poliovirus contains several virus-neutralizing epitopes, each of which may contain fewer than ten amino acids. Each epitope is capable of inducing virus-neutralizing antibodies.

Treatment

Treatment involves reduction of pain and muscle spasm and maintenance of respiration and hydration. When the fever subsides, early mobilization and active exercise are begun. There is no role for antiserum.

Epidemiology

Poliomyelitis occurs worldwide—year-round in the tropics and during summer and fall in the temperate zones. Winter outbreaks are rare.

The disease occurs in all age groups, but children are usually more susceptible than adults because of the acquired immunity of the adult population. In isolated populations (Arctic Eskimos), poliomyelitis attacks all ages equally. In developing areas, where conditions favor the wide dissemination of virus, poliomyelitis continues to be a disease of infancy. In developed countries, before the onset of vaccination, the age distribution shifted so that most patients were over age 5 and 25% were over age 15 years. With rising levels of hygiene and sanitation, a similar trend has been noted in developing countries.

The case-fatality rate is variable. It is highest in the oldest patients and may reach 5–10%.

Humans are the only known reservoir of infection. Under conditions of poor hygiene and sanitation in warm areas, where almost all children become immune early in life, polioviruses maintain themselves by continuously infecting a small part of the population. In temperate zones with high levels of hygiene, epidemics have been followed by periods of little spread of virus, until sufficient numbers of susceptible children have grown up to provide a pool for transmission in the area. Warm weather favors the spread of virus by increasing human contacts, the susceptibility of the host, or the dissemination of virus by extrahuman sources. Virus can be recovered from the pharynx and intestine of patients and healthy carriers. The prevalence of infection is highest among household contacts. When the first case is recognized in a family, all susceptibles in the family are already infected, the result of rapid dissemination of virus.

During periods of wide prevalence of poliovirus in an area, flies become contaminated and may distribute virus to food. The role of flies in disease transmission is unsettled. Virus is present in sewage during such periods and can serve as a source of contamination of flies or water used for drinking, bathing, or irrigation.

In temperate climates, infection with enteroviruses, including polio, occurs mainly during the summer. There is a direct correlation between poor hygiene, sanitation, and crowding and the acquisition of infection and antibodies at an early age.

Prevention & Control

Both live-virus and killed-virus vaccines are available. Formalinized vaccine (Salk) is prepared from virus grown in monkey kidney cultures. At least four inoculations over a period of 1–2 years have been recommended in the primary series. Periodic booster immunizations have been necessary to maintain immunity. Killed-virus vaccine induces humoral antibodies, but, upon exposure, virus is still able to multiply in the gut.

Oral vaccines contain live attenuated virus grown in primary monkey or human diploid cell cultures. The vaccine can be stabilized by magnesium chloride, 1 mol/L, so that it can be kept without losing potency for a year at 4 °C and for weeks at moderate room temperature (about 25 °C). Nonstabilized vaccine must be kept frozen until used.

The live poliovaccine multiplies, infects, and thus immunizes. In the process, infectious progeny of the vaccine virus are disseminated in the community. Although the viruses, particularly types 2 and 3, mutate in the course of their multiplication in vaccinated children, only extremely rare cases of paralytic poliomyelitis have occurred in recipients of oral poliovaccine or their close contacts. Repeat vaccinations are important to establish permanent immunity. The vaccine produces not only IgM and IgG antibodies in the blood but also secretory IgA antibodies in the intestine, which then becomes resistant to reinfection (see Figure 30–10).

A potential limiting factor for oral vaccine is interference. If the alimentary tract of a child is infected with another enterovirus at the time the vaccine is given, the establishment of polio infection and immunity may be blocked. This may be an important problem in areas (particularly in tropical regions) where enterovirus infections are common.

Trivalent oral poliovaccine is generally used in the USA. The American Academy of Pediatrics recommends that primary immunization of infants begin at 2 months of age simultaneously with the first diphtheria-tetanus-pertussis inoculation. The second and third doses should be given at 2-month intervals thereafter, and a fourth dose at 1½ years of age. The multiple doses are recommended to maximize immunity for all three serotypes. A trivalent vaccine booster is recommended for all children entering elementary school. No further boosters are presently recommended.

Adults residing in the continental USA have only a small risk of exposure. However, adults who are at increased risk because of contact with a patient or who are anticipating travel to an endemic or epidemic area should be immunized. Pregnancy is neither an indication for nor a contraindication to required immunization.

Before the beginning of vaccination campaigns in the USA, there were about 21,000 cases of paralytic poliomyelitis per year. In 1977, only 18 such cases occurred. Twelve cases of type 1 poliomyelitis occurred in the USA in 1979—all among unvaccinated religious groups. The disease failed to spread to surrounding vaccinated communities. No wild virus has been isolated in the USA since 1979, and the disease has almost vanished in all industrialized countries. There have been no cases caused by a wild poliovirus in the entire Western Hemisphere since 1989. However, there is a continuing need for adequate vaccination programs in all population groups in order to limit the spread of wild viruses. This is particularly important when wild viruses are introduced from some developing countries, where thousands of cases continue to occur.

Both killed-virus and live-virus vaccines induce antibodies and protect the central nervous system from subsequent invasion by wild virus. Low levels of antibody resulting from killed-virus vaccine have little effect on intestinal carriage of virus. The gut develops a far greater degree of resistance after administration of live-virus vaccine, which seems to be dependent on the extent of initial vaccine virus multiplication in the alimentary tract rather than on serum antibody level.

Live-virus vaccine should not be administered to immunodeficient or immunosuppressed individuals. Only killed-virus (Salk) vaccine is to be used.

On very rare occasions, a live-virus vaccine strain can induce neurologic or paralytic disease in persons who are not evidently immunodeficient. Such cases are carefully studied by public health agencies, and it is estimated that there has been no more than one vaccine-associated case for every million persons vaccinated.

In the 1980s, great strides were made in understanding the molecular biology of poliovirus, particularly through knowledge of its complete genome sequence and the detailed structure of the virion. Studies with synthetic peptides that contain neutralizing epitope residues revealed that they are weak immunogens. Consequently, when a nonliving antigen is required, killed-virus poliovaccine is used. (It has given excellent results in the field when administered in sufficient numbers of injections.)

The application of recombinant DNA technology may permit the development of a live poliovirus that cannot mutate to increased neurovirulence. A key technologic advance was the construction of infectious cDNA clones that made possible the manipulation of nucleotide sequences in order to generate poliovirus mutants with specific and desirable alterations in the genome. Recombinant viruses have been constructed from parental viruses belonging to different poliovirus serotypes and between virulent and attenuated strains of the same serotype. Sequences in the viral genome that are responsible for an attenuated phenotype have been identified.

The type 1 vaccine virus, which is extremely stable genetically, has been used as a vector for type 2 and type 3 nucleotide sequences encoding immunogenic regions of their VP1 proteins. The new "chimeric" strains have the desired biologic characteristics of type 1 but the immunogenic properties of type 2 or type 3, respectively. A poliovirus chimera has been constructed that carries a short nucleotide sequence of type 3 inserted into the type 1 genome. The chimeric virus expressed a fusion protein containing eight amino acids of type 3 VP1 and induced antibodies to both type 1 and type 3 viruses.

These advances may lead to a more genetically stable type 3 vaccine. However, it will be difficult to field-test such a new vaccine candidate, as it will be necessary to prove that the new vaccine produces fewer than one vaccine-associated case per million susceptible recipients.

Immune globulin USP (gamma globulin), 0.3 mL/kg, can provide protection for a few weeks against the paralytic disease but does not prevent subclinical infection. Gamma globulin is effective only if given shortly before infection; it is of no value after clinical symptoms develop.

The prevention of poliomyelitis depends on vaccination. Quarantine of patients or intimate contacts is ineffective in controlling the spread of the disease. This is understandable in view of the large number of inapparent infections that occur.

During epidemic periods (defined now as two or more local cases caused by the same type in any 4-week period), children with fever should be placed at bed rest. Undue exercise or fatigue, elective nose and throat operations, and dental extractions should be avoided. Food and human excrement should be protected from flies. Oral poliovaccine should be administered to susceptible persons in the population.

Patients with poliomyelitis can be admitted to general hospitals provided appropriate isolation precautions are employed. All pharyngeal and bowel discharges are considered infectious and should be disposed of quickly and safely.

COXSACKIEVIRUSES

Coxsackieviruses, a large subgroup of the enteroviruses, are divided into two groups, A and B, having different pathogenic potentials for mice. They produce a variety of illnesses in humans. Herpangina, hand-foot-and-mouth disease, and acute hemorrhagic conjunctivitis are caused by certain coxsackievirus group A serotypes; pleurodynia (devil's grip), myocarditis, pericarditis, and meningoencephalitis are caused by some group B coxsackieviruses. In addition to these, a number of group A and B serotypes can give rise to aseptic meningitis, respiratory and undifferentiated febrile illnesses, hepatitis, and paralysis. Generally, paralysis produced by nonpolio enteroviruses is incomplete and reversible. Coxsackie B viruses are the most commonly identified causative agents of viral heart disease in humans (Table 36–3). The coxsackieviruses tend to be more pathogenic than the echoviruses.

Properties of the Virus

A. General Properties: Coxsackieviruses are typical enteroviruses (see above).

B. Animal Susceptibility and Growth of Virus: Coxsackieviruses are highly infective for newborn mice. Certain strains (B1–6, A7, 9, 16, and 24) also grow in monkey kidney cell culture. Some group A strains grow in human amnion and human embryonic lung fibroblast cells. Chimpanzees and cynomolgus monkeys can be infected subclinically; virus appears in the blood and throat for short periods and is excreted in the feces for 2–5 weeks. Type A14 produces poliomyelitis-like lesions in adult mice and in monkeys, but in suckling mice this type produces only myositis. Type A7 strains produce paralysis and severe central nervous system lesions in monkeys.

Group A viruses produce widespread myositis in the skeletal muscles of newborn mice, resulting in flaccid paralysis without other observable lesions. Group B viruses may produce focal myositis, encephalitis, and, most typically, necrotizing steatitis involving mainly fetal fat lobules. The genetic makeup of inbred strains of mice determines their susceptibility to coxsackie B viruses. Some B strains also produce pancreatitis, myocarditis, endocarditis, and hepatitis in both suckling and adult mice. Normal adult mice tolerate

Table 36–3. Human enteroviruses and commonly associated clinical syndromes.

		Coxsackievirus			
Syndrome	Poliovirus Types 1–3	Group A Types 1–24	Group B Types 1–6	Echovirus Types 1–34	Enterovirus Types 68–71
Neurologic					
Aseptic meningitis	1–3	Many	1–6	Many	71
Paralysis	1–3	4, 7, 9	2–5	2, 4, 6, 9, 11, 30	70, 71
Encephalitis		2, 5–7, 9	1–5	2, 6, 9, 17, 19	71
Skin and mucosa					
Herpangina		2–6, 8, 10			
Hand-foot-and-mouth disease		5, 9, 10, 16			71
Exanthems		Many	1, 3, 5	2, 4, 6, 9, 11, 16, 18	
Cardiac and muscular					
Pleurodynia		9	1–5	1, 6, 9	
Myocarditis		4, 16	1–5	1, 6, 9, 19	
Ocular					
Acute hemorrhagic conjunctivitis		24			70
Respiratory					
Colds		21, 24	1, 3, 4, 5	4, 9, 11, 20, 25	
Pneumonia			4, 5		68
Gastrointestinal					
Diarrhea		18, 20–22, 24		18, 20	
Hepatitis		4, 9	5	4, 9	
Other					
Undifferentiated febrile illness	1–3		1–6		
Generalized disease of infants			1–5	3, 6, 9, 11, 17, 19	
Diabetes			4		

infections with group B coxsackieviruses. However, severely malnourished or immunodeficient mice have greatly enhanced susceptibility to overt disease.

C. Antigenic Properties: At least 29 different immunologic types of coxsackieviruses are now recognized; 23 are listed as group A and six as group B types.

Pathogenesis & Pathology

Virus has been recovered from the blood in the early stages of natural infection in humans and of experimental infection in chimpanzees. Virus is also found in the throat for a few days early in the infection and in the stools for up to 5–6 weeks. Virus distribution is similar to that of the other enteroviruses.

Group B coxsackieviruses may cause acute fatal encephalomyocarditis in infants. This appears to be a generalized systemic disease with viral replication and lesions in the central nervous system, heart muscle, and other organs.

Clinical Findings

The incubation period of coxsackievirus infection ranges from 2 to 9 days. The clinical manifestations of infection with various coxsackieviruses are diverse and may present as distinct disease entities (Table 36–3). The examples shown are not all-inclusive; different serotypes may be associated with a particular outbreak.

A. Neurologic: Aseptic meningitis is caused by all types of group B coxsackieviruses and by many group A coxsackieviruses, most commonly A7 and A9. Fever, malaise, headache, nausea, and abdominal pain are common early symptoms. Signs of meningeal irritation, stiff neck or back, and vomiting may appear 1–2 days later. The disease sometimes progresses to mild muscle weakness suggestive of paralytic poliomyelitis. Patients almost always recover completely from nonpoliovirus paresis. Early in aseptic meningitis, the cerebrospinal fluid shows pleocytosis (up to 500 cells/μL) with up to 50% polymorphonuclear neutrophils.

B. Skin and Mucosa: Herpangina is a severe febrile pharyngitis. It is caused by certain group A viruses (2–6, 8, 10). It has nothing to do with herpesviruses, despite the name. There is an abrupt onset of fever and sore throat. The pharynx is usually hyperemic, and characteristic discrete vesicles occur on the posterior half of the palate, pharynx, tonsils, or tongue. The illness is self-limited and most frequent in small children.

Hand-foot-and-mouth disease is characterized by oral and pharyngeal ulcerations and a vesicular rash of the palms and soles that may spread to the arms and legs. Vesicles heal without crusting, which clinically differentiates them from the vesicles of herpes- and poxviruses. This disease has been associated particularly with coxsackievirus A16, but A5, A9, and A10 have also been implicated. Virus may be recovered not only from the stool and pharyngeal secretions but also from vesicular fluid. It is not to be confused with foot-

and-mouth disease of cattle, caused by an unrelated picornavirus that does not infect humans.

C. Cardiac and Muscular Disease: Pleurodynia (also known as epidemic myalgia or Bornholm disease) is caused by group B viruses. Fever and stabbing chest pain are usually abrupt in onset but are sometimes preceded by malaise, headache, and anorexia. The chest pain may be located on either side or substernally, is intensified by movement, and may last from 2 days to 2 weeks. Abdominal pain occurs in approximately half of cases, and in children this may be the chief complaint. The illness is self-limited and recovery is complete, though relapses are common.

Myocarditis is a serious disease. It is an acute inflammation of the heart or its covering membranes (pericarditis). Coxsackievirus B infections are a cause of primary myocardial disease in adults as well as children. About 5% of all symptomatic coxsackievirus infections induce heart disease. The virus may affect the endocardium, pericardium, myocardium, or all three. Infections may be fatal in neonates or may cause permanent heart damage at any age. Acute myocardiopathies have been shown to be caused by coxsackieviruses A4, A16, B1–5, and several echovirus types.

In experimental animals, the severity of acute viral myocardiopathy is greatly increased by vigorous exercise, hydrocortisone, alcohol consumption, pregnancy, and undernutrition and is greater in males than in females. In human illnesses, these factors may similarly increase the severity of the disease.

D. Ocular: Acute hemorrhagic conjunctivitis was recognized as a new disease in 1969. It is usually caused by enterovirus 70 (see below) but may also be caused by a variant of the prototypic coxsackievirus A24.

E. Respiratory Infections: A number of the enteroviruses have been associated with **common colds;** among these are coxsackieviruses A21, A24, B1, and B3–5.

F. Gastrointestinal: Although the gastrointestinal tract is the primary site of replication for the enteroviruses, they do not cause marked disease there. Certain group A coxsackieviruses have been associated with **diarrhea** in children, but causality is unproved.

G. Other: Undifferentiated febrile illnesses are acute bouts of short duration that occur during the summer or fall and are without distinctive features. Group B coxsackieviruses are often isolated from these patients.

Generalized disease of infants is an extremely serious disease in which the infant is overwhelmed by simultaneous viral infections of multiple organs, including heart, liver, and brain. The clinical course may be rapidly fatal, or the patient may recover completely. The disease is caused by group B coxsackieviruses. In severe cases, myocarditis or pericarditis can occur within the first 8 days of life; it may be preceded by a brief episode of diarrhea and anorexia. The disease may sometimes be acquired transplacentally.

Serologic studies suggest an association of type 1 **diabetes** with past infection by coxsackievirus B4. Finally, the agent of **swine vesicular disease** is an enterovirus antigenically related to coxsackievirus B5. The swine virus can also infect humans.

Laboratory Diagnosis

A. Recovery of Virus: The virus is isolated readily from throat washings during the first few days of illness and from stools during the first few weeks. In coxsackievirus A21 infections, the largest amount of virus is found in nasal secretions. In cases of aseptic meningitis, strains have been recovered from the cerebrospinal fluid as well as from the alimentary tract. In hemorrhagic conjunctivitis cases, A24 virus is isolated from conjunctival swabs, throat swabs, and feces.

Specimens are inoculated into tissue cultures and also into suckling mice. In tissue culture, a cytopathic effect appears within 5–14 days. In suckling mice, signs of illness appear usually within 3–8 days with group A strains and 5–14 days with group B strains. The virus is identified by the pathologic lesions it produces and by immunologic means.

B. Serology: Neutralizing antibodies, which are detected as shown in Figure 36–2, appear early during the course of infection. Neutralizing antibodies tend to be specific for the infecting virus and persist for years. Complement-fixing antibodies exhibit cross-reactions and disappear in 6 months. Serologic tests are difficult to evaluate (because of the multiplicity of types) unless the antigen used in the test has been isolated from a specific patient or during an epidemic outbreak.

Serum antibodies can also be detected and titrated by the immunofluorescence technique, using infected cell cultures on coverslips as antigens. These can be preserved frozen for years.

Immunity

In humans, neutralizing and complement-fixing antibodies are transferred passively from mother to fetus. Adults have antibodies against more types of coxsackieviruses than do children, which indicates that multiple experience with these viruses is common and increases with age.

Epidemiology

Viruses of the coxsackie group have been encountered around the globe. Isolations have been made mainly from human feces, pharyngeal swabbings, sewage, and flies. Antibodies to various coxsackieviruses are found in serum collected from persons all over the world and in pooled gamma globulin.

Coxsackieviruses are recovered much more frequently in summer and early fall. Also, children develop neutralizing and complement-fixing antibodies in summer, indicating infection by coxsackieviruses during this period. Such children have much higher incidence rates for acute, febrile minor illnesses during

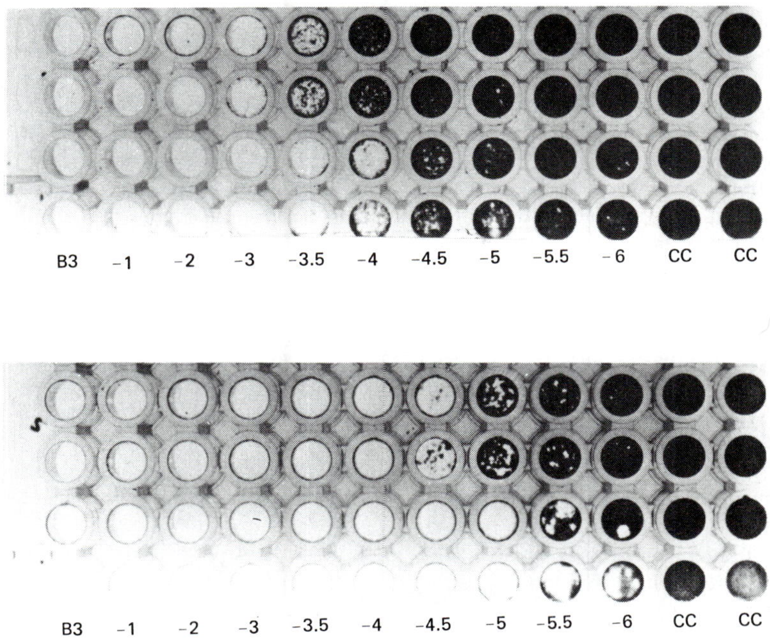

Figure 36–2. Titration of coxsackievirus B3 in the presence of antibody and control medium. From left to right, as the viral dilution increases, complete cytopathic effect, incomplete cytopathic effect, and then individual plaques are seen. The last two rows on the right side are cell controls (CC). B3 line shows 0.5 $\log_{10}$ dilutions of virus. ***Top:*** Assayed 48 hours postinfection. **Bottom:** Assayed 72 hours postinfection; further progression of cytopathic effect is evident. (From Randhawa AS et al: J Clin Microbiol 1977;5:535.)

the summer than children who fail to develop coxsackievirus antibodies.

Familial exposure is important in the acquisition of infections with coxsackieviruses. Once the virus is introduced into a household, all susceptible persons usually become infected, although all do not develop clinically apparent disease.

In herpangina, only about 30% of infected persons within households develop faucial lesions. Others may present a mild febrile illness without throat lesions. Virus has been found in 85% of patients with herpangina, in 65% of their neighbors, in 40% of family contacts, and in 4% of all persons in the community.

The coxsackieviruses share many properties with the echo- and polioviruses. Because of their epidemiologic similarities, various enteroviruses may occur together in nature, even in the same human host or the same specimens of sewage or flies.

ECHOVIRUSES

Echoviruses (*e*nteric *c*ytopathogenic *h*uman *o*rphan viruses) are grouped together because they infect the human enteric tract and because they can be recovered from humans only by inoculation of certain tissue cultures. More than 30 serotypes are known, but not all cause human illness. Aseptic meningitis, febrile illnesses with or without rash, common colds, and acute hemorrhagic conjunctivitis are among the diseases caused by echoviruses.

Properties of the Virus

A. General Properties: Echoviruses are typical enteroviruses (see above).

B. Growth of Virus: Monkey kidney cell culture is the method of choice for the isolation of these agents. Some also multiply in human amnion cells and cell lines such as HeLa.

Initially, echoviruses were distinguished from coxsackieviruses by their failure to produce pathologic changes in newborn mice, but echovirus 9 can produce paralysis in newborn mice. Conversely, strains of some coxsackievirus types (especially A9) lack mouse pathogenicity and thus resemble echoviruses. This variability in biologic properties is the chief reason why new enteroviruses are no longer being subclassified as echoviruses or coxsackieviruses.

C. Antigenic Properties: More than 30 different antigenic types have been identified. The different types may be separated on the basis of cross-Nt or cross-CF tests. Variants exist that do not behave exactly like the prototypes. After human infections, neutralizing antibodies persist longer than complement-fixing antibodies.

D. Animal Susceptibility: To be included in the echovirus group, prototype strains must not produce disease in suckling mice, rabbits, or monkeys. In the chimpanzee, no apparent illness is produced, but infection can be demonstrated by the presence and persistence of virus in the throat and in the feces and by the type-specific antibody responses.

Pathogenesis & Pathology

The pathogenesis of the alimentary infection is similar to that of the other enteroviruses. Virus may be recovered from the throat and stools; in certain types associated with aseptic meningitis, the virus has been recovered from the cerebrospinal fluid.

Clinical Findings

To establish etiologic association of echovirus with disease, the following criteria are used: (1) There is a much higher rate of recovery of virus from patients with the disease than from healthy individuals of the same age and socioeconomic level living in the same area at the same time. (2) Antibodies against the virus develop during the course of the disease. If the clinical syndrome can be caused by other known agents, then virologic or serologic evidence must be negative for concurrent infection with such agents. (3) The virus is isolated from body fluids or tissues manifesting lesions, eg, from the cerebrospinal fluid in cases of aseptic meningitis.

Many echoviruses have been associated with aseptic meningitis. Rashes are common in types 4, 9, 16 ("Boston exanthem disease"), and 18. Rashes are commonest in young children. Occasionally, there is conjunctivitis, muscle weakness, and spasm (types 6, 9, and others). Infantile diarrhea may be associated with some types (eg, 18, 20). Echovirus type 28 isolated from upper respiratory illness causes "colds" in volunteers and has been reclassified as rhinovirus type 1. For many echoviruses (and some coxsackieviruses), no disease entities have been defined.

With the virtual elimination of poliomyelitis in developed countries, the central nervous system syndromes associated with echoviruses and coxsackieviruses have assumed greater prominence. The latter in children under age 1 year may lead to neurologic sequelae and mental impairment. This does not appear to happen in older children.

Laboratory Diagnosis

It is impossible in an individual case to diagnose an echovirus infection on clinical grounds. However, in the following epidemic situations, echoviruses must be considered: (1) summer outbreaks of aseptic meningitis; (2) summer epidemics, especially in young children, of a febrile illness with rash; and (3) outbreaks of diarrheal disease in young infants from whom no pathogenic enterobacteria can be recovered.

The diagnosis is dependent upon laboratory tests. The procedure of choice is isolation of virus from throat swabs, stools, rectal swabs, and, in aseptic meningitis, cerebrospinal fluid. Certain echoviruses agglutinate human group O erythrocytes. Serologic tests are impractical—because of the many different viral types—except when a virus has been isolated from a patient or during an outbreak of typical clinical illness. Neutralizing and hemagglutination-inhibiting antibodies are type-specific and may persist for years. Complement-fixing antibodies give many heterotypic responses.

If an agent is isolated in tissue culture, it is tested against different pools of antisera against enteroviruses. Determination of the type of virus present depends upon neutralization by a single serum. Infection with two or more enteroviruses may occur simultaneously.

Epidemiology

The epidemiology of echoviruses is similar to that of other enteroviruses. They occur in all parts of the globe. Unlike the enterobacteria, which are constantly present in the intestinal tract, the enteroviruses produce only transitory infections. They are more apt to be found in the young than in the old. In the temperate zone, infections occur chiefly in summer and autumn and are about five times more prevalent in children of lower-income families than in those living in more favorable circumstances.

Studies of families into which enteroviruses were introduced demonstrate the ease with which these agents spread and the high frequency of infection in persons who had formed no antibodies from earlier exposures. This is true for all enteroviruses.

Wide dissemination is the rule. In a period when 149 inhabitants of a city of 740,000 were hospitalized with echo 9 disease, approximately 6% of the population, or 45,000 persons, had a compatible illness.

Control

Avoidance of contact with patients exhibiting acute febrile illness, especially those with a rash, is advisable for very young children. Members of institutional staffs responsible for caring for infants should be tested to determine whether they are carriers of enteroviruses. This is particularly important during outbreaks of diarrheal disease among infants.

OTHER ENTEROVIRUS TYPES

Four enteroviruses (types 68–71) grow in monkey kidney cultures, and three of them cause human disease.

Enterovirus 68 has been isolated from the respiratory tracts of children with bronchiolitis or pneumonia.

Enterovirus 70 is the chief cause of acute hemorrhagic conjunctivitis. It was isolated from the conjunctiva of patients with this striking eye disease, which occurred in pandemic form in 1969–1971 in Africa and Southeast Asia. It was not diagnosed in the USA until its importation into Florida in 1981. Acute hemorrhagic conjunctivitis has a sudden onset of subconjunctival hemorrhage ranging from small petechiae to large blotches covering the bulbar conjunctiva. There may also be epithelial keratitis and occasionally lumbar radiculomyelopathy. The disease is most common in adults, with an incubation period of 1 day and a duration of 8–10 days. Complete recovery is the rule. The virus is highly communicable and spreads rapidly under crowded or unhygienic conditions. There is no effective treatment.

Enterovirus 71 has been isolated from patients with meningitis, encephalitis, and paralysis resembling poliomyelitis. It continues to be one of the main causes of central nervous system disease, sometimes fatal, around the world. In some areas, particularly in Japan and Sweden, the virus has caused outbreaks of hand-foot-and-mouth disease.

RHINOVIRUS GROUP

Rhinoviruses are the common cold viruses. They are usually isolated from the nose and throat but very rarely from feces. These viruses, as well as coronaviruses and some reoviruses, adenoviruses, enteroviruses, parainfluenza viruses, and influenza viruses, cause upper respiratory tract infections, including the common cold.

Properties of the Virus

A. General Properties: Rhinoviruses are picornaviruses similar to enteroviruses but differ from them in having a buoyant density in cesium chloride of 1.40 g/mL and in being acid-labile.

B. Animal Susceptibility and Growth of Virus: These viruses are infectious only for humans and chimpanzees. They have been grown in cultures of human embryonic lung fibroblasts (WI-38) and in organ cultures of ferret and human tracheal epithelium. They are grown best at 33 °C, which is similar to the temperature of the nasopharynx in humans.

C. Antigenic Properties: More than 100 serotypes are known. Some cross-react (eg, types 9 and 32).

Pathogenesis & Pathology

The virus enters via the upper respiratory tract. High titers of virus in nasal secretions—which can be found as early as 2–4 days after exposure—are associated with maximal illness. Thereafter, viral titers fall, although illness persists.

Histopathologic changes are limited to the submucosa and surface epithelium. These include engorgement of blood vessels, edema, mild cellular infiltration, and desquamation of surface epithelium, which is complete by the third day. Nasal secretion increases in quantity and in protein concentration.

Experiments under controlled conditions have shown that chilling, including the wearing of wet clothes, does not produce a cold or increase susceptibility to the virus. Chilliness is an early symptom of the common cold.

Clinical Findings

The incubation period is brief, from 2 to 4 days, and the acute illness usually lasts for 7 days although a nonproductive cough may persist for 2–3 weeks. The average adult has 1–2 attacks each year. Usual symptoms in adults include irritation in the upper respiratory tract, nasal discharge, headache, mild cough, malaise, and a chilly sensation. There is little or no fever. The nasal and nasopharyngeal mucosa become red and swollen, and the sense of smell becomes less keen. Mild hoarseness may be present. Prominent cervical adenopathy does not occur. Secondary bacterial infection may produce acute otitis media, sinusitis, bronchitis, or pneumonitis, especially in children. Type-specific antibodies appear or rise with each infection.

Immunity

Natural immunity may exist but may be brief. Only 30–50% of volunteers can be infected with infectious material; yet the "resistant" volunteers may catch colds of the same serotype at other times. It has also been observed that older adults experience fewer colds than young adults and children. One 3-year study of acute respiratory tract illness in college and medical students showed that the same serotype was never isolated from separate illnesses in any student who had two or more illnesses.

Work with human volunteers has shown that resistance to the common cold is independent of measurable serum antibody but perhaps is related to specific antibody in the nasal secretions. These secretory antibodies are primarily 11S IgA immunoglobulins, produced locally in the mucosa and not a transudate from the serum. These 11S IgA antibodies do not persist as long as those in serum, and this could explain the paradox of reinfection in a person with adequate serum antibodies.

Volunteers infected with one rhinovirus serotype resist challenge with both homologous and heterologous virus for 2–16 weeks after the initial infection. Resistance to homologous challenge is complete during this period, whereas resistance to heterologous challenge is incomplete. This nonspecific resistance may be a factor in the control of naturally occurring colds.

Epidemiology

The disease occurs throughout the world. In the temperate zones, the attack rates are highest in early fall and winter, declining in the late spring. Members of isolated communities form highly susceptible groups.

The virus is believed to be transmitted through close contact, by large droplets. The fingers of a person with a cold are usually contaminated because of frequent contact with the virus-shedding nose. Transmission to susceptible persons then occurs by hand to hand or hand to object (eg, doorknob) to hand contamination. Self-inoculation after hand contamination may be a more important mode of spread than that by airborne particles.

Colds in children spread more easily to others than do colds in adults. Adults in households with a child in school have twice as many colds as adults in households without schoolchildren.

In a single community, many rhinovirus serotypes cause outbreaks of disease in a single season, and different serotypes predominate during different respiratory disease seasons.

Treatment & Control

No specific treatment is available. The development of a potent rhinovirus vaccine is unlikely because of the difficulty in growing rhinoviruses to high titer in culture, the fleeting immunity, and the many serotypes causing colds. In addition, many rhinovirus serotypes are present during single respiratory disease outbreaks and may recur only rarely in the same area. Injection of purified vaccines has shown that the high levels of serum antibody are frequently not associated with similar elevation of local secretory antibody, which may be the most significant factor in disease prevention.

A 7-day course of intranasal interferon-α has been shown to be effective in preventing the spread of rhinoviruses from an index case within families. In field studies, the use of virucidal paper tissues (containing 3.5 mg of citric acid, 1.7 mg of malic acid, and 0.7 mg of sodium lauryl sulfate per square inch) markedly reduced hand contamination by rhinoviruses during nose blowing and also lessened the infectiousness of the virus shedder.

X-ray diffraction studies have given the search for antiviral drugs for rhinoviruses a new impetus. Drugs are being designed that prevent the uncoating of viral RNA by inserting themselves into the hydrophobic interim of the VP1 beta barrel and covering the entrance to the ion channel on the floor of the viral "canyon" (Figure 36–1). Another approach to the control of rhinoviruses is to block the cellular receptor sites by using monoclonal antibodies or other agents.

FOOT-AND-MOUTH DISEASE (Aphthovirus of Cattle)

This highly infectious disease of cattle, sheep, pigs, and goats is rare in the USA but endemic in Mexico and Canada. It may be transmitted to humans by contact or ingestion. In humans, the disease is characterized by fever, salivation, and vesiculation of the mucous membranes of the oropharynx and of the skin of the palms, soles, fingers, and toes.

The disease in animals is highly contagious in the early stages of infection when viremia is present and when vesicles in the mouth and on the feet rupture and liberate large amounts of virus. Excreted material remains infectious for long periods. The mortality rate in animals is usually low but may reach 70%. Infected animals become poor producers of milk and meat. Many cattle serve as foci of infection for up to 8 months.

The virus is a typical picornavirus, measuring 24 nm in diameter, and is acid-labile, with a buoyant density in cesium chloride of 1.43 g/mL. There are at least seven types with more than 50 subtypes.

Immunity after infection is adequate but of short duration.

A variety of animals are susceptible to infection. The typical disease can be reproduced by inoculating the virus into the pads of the foot. The reaction in infant mice inoculated with the virus of foot-and-mouth disease is similar to their reaction to inoculation with coxsackieviruses: paralysis results as a consequence of myositis. The virus grows readily in tissue culture of cattle tongue or hamster BHK-21 cells. Formalin-treated vaccines have been prepared from virus grown in such tissue cultures. However, such vaccines do not produce a long-lasting immunity, and frequent booster inoculations are necessary. New vaccines are being developed by two techniques: recombinant DNA in bacteria *(Escherichia coli),* and synthetic peptides representing immunogenic epitopes.

The methods of control of the disease are dictated by its high degree of contagiousness and the resistance of the virus to inactivation. Should a focus of infection occur in the USA, all exposed animals are slaughtered and their carcasses destroyed. Strict quarantine is established, and the area is not presumed to be safe until susceptible animals fail to develop symptoms within 30 days. Another method is to quarantine the herd and vaccinate all unaffected animals. Other countries have successfully employed systematic vaccination schedules. Some nations (eg, the USA and Australia) forbid the importation of potentially infective materials such as fresh meat, and the disease has been eliminated in these areas. Even so, migrating birds may play a role in carrying the virus from one country to another, as from France and Holland to England.

REFERENCES

Banatvala JE: Insulin-dependent (juvenile-onset, type 1) diabetes mellitus: Coxsackie B viruses revisited. Prog Med Virol 1987;34:33.

Evans AS: Criteria for control of infectious diseases with poliomyelitis as an example. Prog Med Virol 1984;29:141.

Furione M et al: Polioviruses with natural recombinant genomes isolated from vaccine-associated paralytic poliomyelitis. Virology 1993;196:199.

Hogle JM, Chow M, Filman DJ: Three-dimensional structure of poliovirus at 2.9 Å resolution. Science 1985;229:1358.

Kandolf R et al: Molecular pathogenesis of enterovirus-induced myocarditis: Virus persistence and chronic inflammation. Intervirology 1993;35:140.

McBean AM, Modlin JF: Rationale for the sequential use of inactivated poliovirus vaccine and live attenuated poliovirus vaccine for routine poliomyelitis immunization in the United States. Ped Infect Dis J 1987;6:881.

Melnick JL, Horaud F (guest): Homage to Albert B. Sabin. Biologicals 1993;21:No. 4. [Entire issue.]

Melnick JL: Enteroviruses: Polioviruses, coxsackieviruses, echoviruses, and newer enteroviruses. In: *Virology,* 2nd ed. Fields BN et al (editors). Raven Press, 1990.

Melnick JL, Wenner HA, Phillips CA: Enteroviruses. In: *Diagnostic Procedures for Viral, Rickettsial, and Chlamydial Infections,* 5th ed. Lennette EH, Schmidt NJ (editors). American Public Health Association, 1979.

Minor PD: The molecular biology of poliovaccines. J Gen Virol 1992;73:3065.

Racaniello VR: Poliovirus neurovirulence. Adv Virus Res 1988;34:217.

Sabin AB: Oral poliovirus vaccine: History of its development and use and current challenge to eliminate poliomyelitis from the world. J Infect Dis 1985;151:420.

Smith TJ et al: The site of attachment in human rhinovirus 14 for antiviral agents that inhibit uncoating. Science 1986; 233:1286.

Yin-Murphy M: Acute hemorrhagic conjunctivitis. Prog Med Virol 1984;29:23.

37 Reoviruses & Rotaviruses

Reoviruses are medium-sized viruses with a double-stranded, segmented RNA genome. The family includes human rotaviruses, the most important cause of infantile gastroenteritis around the world (Figure 37–1). Acute gastroenteritis is a very common disease with significant public health impact. In developing countries it is estimated to cause as many as 3.5 million deaths of preschool children annually. In the USA, acute gastroenteritis is second only to acute respiratory infections as a cause of disease in families.

In addition to rotaviruses, some unclassified viral agents are associated with gastroenteritis. These are considered briefly at the end of this chapter.

Of the other major groups in this family, reoviruses are not known to be an important cause of any disease, and orbiviruses are of more significance to veterinary disease than to human illness. Humans are an accidental host for Colorado tick fever virus, classified as a *Coltivirus.*

PROPERTIES OF REOVIRUSES

Important properties of reoviruses are summarized in Table 37–1.

Structure & Composition

The virions measure 60–80 nm in diameter and possess two concentric capsid shells, each of which is icosahedral. There is no envelope. Single-shelled viral particles that lack the outer capsid exhibit rough outer edges and are 50–60 nm in diameter. The inner core of the particles is 33–40 nm in diameter (Figure 37–2). The inner capsids of all genera display sharply defined subunits; the outer capsids of rotaviruses and orbiviruses lack visible subunit structures. The double-shelled particle is the infectious form of the virus.

The genome consists of double-stranded RNA in 10–12 discrete segments (total MW 12–15 $\times$ 10^6), depending on the genus. The virion core contains several enzymes needed for transcription and capping of viral RNAs.

Reoviruses are unusually stable to heat, to range of pH, and to lipid solvents, but they are inactivated by 70% ethanol. Limited treatment with proteolytic enzymes increases infectivity.

Classification

The family **Reoviridae** is divided into eight genera. Four of the genera are able to infect humans and animals: *Orthoreovirus, Rotavirus, Coltivirus,* and *Orbivirus.* Four other genera infect only plants and insects.

There are at least two major subgroups and six serotypes of human rotaviruses. Only three different serotypes of reovirus are recognized. There are about 100 different orbivirus serotypes. There are two known serotypes for coltiviruses.

Rotaviruses contain 11 genome segments of double-stranded RNA, whereas orthoreoviruses and orbiviruses each possess ten segments and coltiviruses have 12 segments.

Reovirus Replication

Viral particles attach to specific receptors on the cell surface. The cell attachment protein for reoviruses is the viral hemagglutinin (σ1 protein), a minor component of the outer capsid. The receptor-binding protein for rotaviruses remains to be determined.

After attachment and penetration, uncoating of viral particles occurs in lysosomes in the cell cytoplasm. Only the outer shell of the virus is removed, and a core-associated RNA transcriptase is activated. This transcriptase transcribes mRNA molecules from the minus strand of each genome double-stranded RNA segment contained in the intact core. The functional mRNA molecules correspond in size to the genome segments. Reovirus cores contain all enzymes necessary for transcribing, capping, and extruding the mRNAs from the core, leaving the double-stranded RNA genome segments inside.

Once extruded from the core, the mRNAs are translated into primary gene products. Some of the full-length transcripts are encapsidated to form immature viral particles. A viral replicase is responsible for synthesizing negative-sense strands to form the double-stranded genome segments. Apparently, this replication to form progeny double-stranded RNA occurs in partially completed core structures. The mechanisms that ensure assembly of the correct complement of genome segments into a developing viral core are unknown. Viral polypeptides probably self-assemble to form the inner and outer capsid shells.

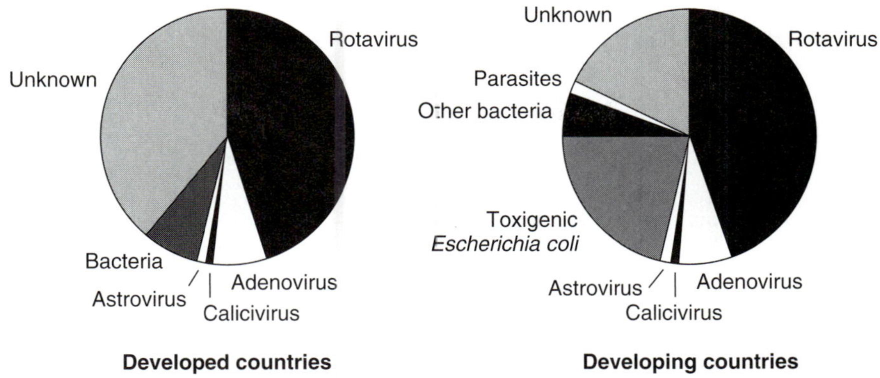

Figure 37–1. An estimate of the role of etiologic agents in severe diarrheal illnesses requiring hospitalization of infants and young children in developed countries (left) and in developing countries (right). (Reproduced, with permission, from Kapikian AZ: Viral gastroenteritis. JAMA 1993;269:627.)

Reoviruses produce inclusion bodies in the cytoplasm in which viral particles are found. These viral factories are closely associated with tubular structures (microtubules and intermediate filaments). Rotavirus morphogenesis involves budding of single-shelled particles into the rough endoplasmic reticulum. The "pseudoenvelopes" so acquired are then removed and the outer capsids are added (Figure 37–3). This unusual pathway is utilized because the major outer capsid protein is glycosylated.

Cell lysis results in release of progeny virions.

ROTAVIRUSES

Rotaviruses are a major cause of diarrheal illness in human infants and young animals, including calves and piglets. Infections in adult humans and animals are also common. Among rotaviruses are the agents of human infantile diarrhea, Nebraska calf diarrhea, epizootic diarrhea of infant mice, and SA11 virus of monkeys.

Rotaviruses are closely related to reoviruses in terms of morphology and strategy of replication.

Table 37–1. Important properties of reoviruses.

Virion: Icosahedral, 60–80 nm in diameter, double capsid shell.
Composition: RNA (15%), protein (85%).
Genome: Double-stranded RNA, linear, segmented (10–12 segments), total MW 12–15 million.
Proteins: Nine structural proteins; core contains several enzymes.
Envelope: None. (Transient pseudoenvelope is present during rotavirus particle morphogenesis.)
Replication: Cytoplasm; virions not completely uncoated.
Outstanding characteristics: Genetic reassortment occurs readily. Rotaviruses are the major cause of infantile diarrhea; reoviruses are good models for molecular studies of viral pathogenesis.

Classification & Antigenic Properties

Rotaviruses possess common antigens located on the inner capsid. These can be detected by immunofluorescence, CF, and ELISA. Two major antigenic subgroups of rotaviruses have been identified. Type-specific antigens are located on the outer capsid; VP7 is the predominant antigen for neutralizing activity. These type-specific antigens differentiate among rota-

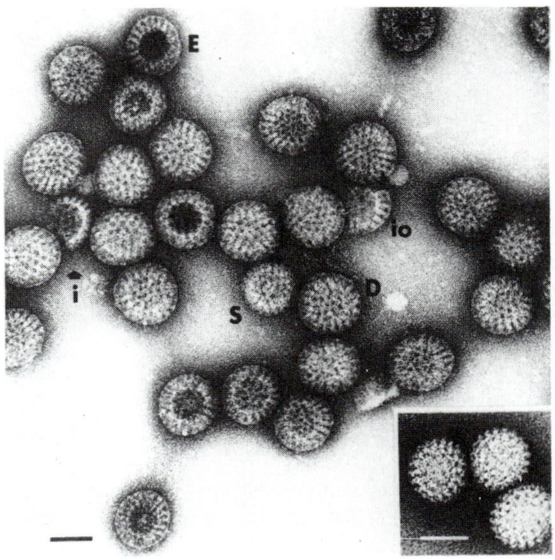

Figure 37–2. Electron micrograph of a negatively stained preparation of human rotavirus. (D, double-shelled particles; S, single-shelled particles; E, empty capsids; i, fragment of inner shell; io, fragments of a combination of inner and outer shell.) **Inset:** single-shelled particles obtained by treatment of the viral preparation with sodium dodecyl sulfate, 100 µg/mL, immediately prior to processing for electron microscopy. Bars, 50 nm. (J Esparza and F Gil.)

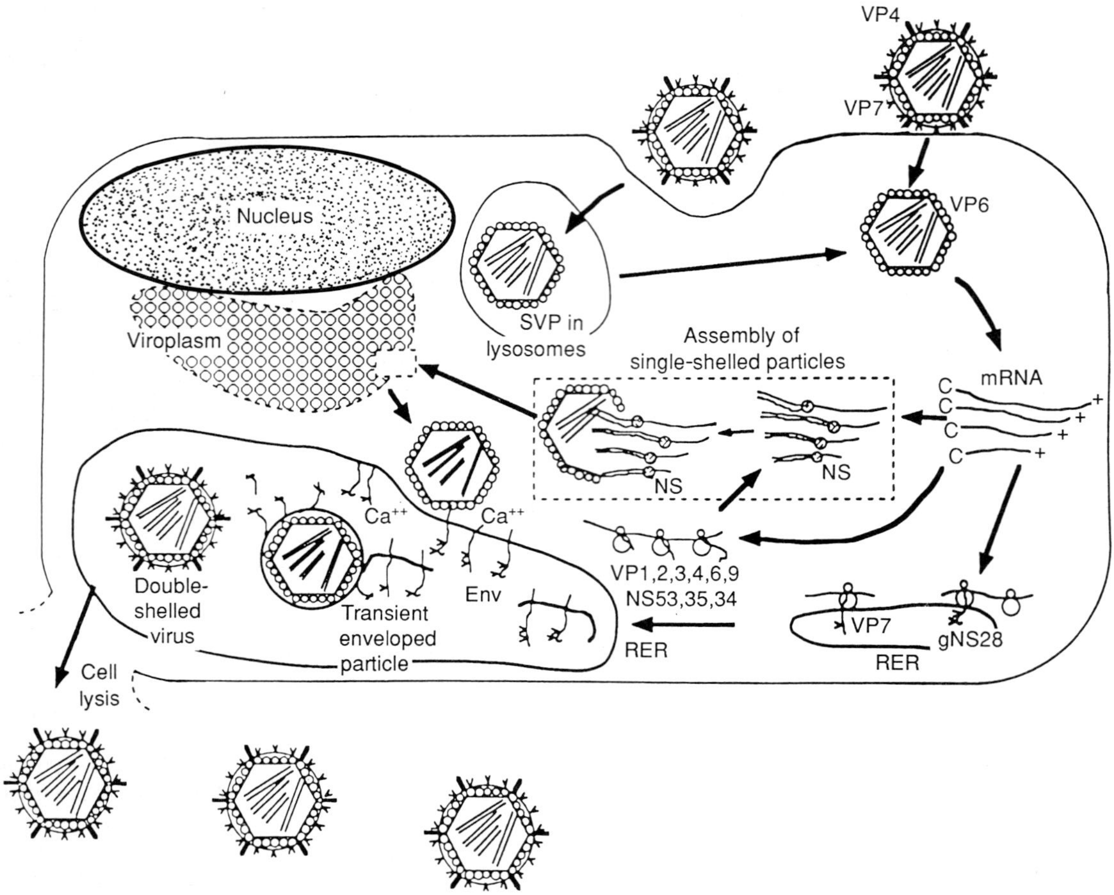

Figure 37–3. Overview of the rotavirus replication cycle. (Reproduced, with permission, from Estes MK: Rotaviruses and their replication. Pages 1329–1352 in: *Virology,* 2nd ed. Fields BN et al [editors]. Raven Press, 1990.)

viruses and are demonstrable by Nt tests. At least six serotypes have been identified among human rotaviruses, and at least three more serotypes exist among animal isolates. Some animal and human rotaviruses share serotype specificity. For example, monkey virus SA11 is very similar to human serotype 3. The gene-coding assignments responsible for the antigenic specificities of rotavirus proteins are shown in Figure 37–4.

The viruses usually associated with human gastroenteritis are classified as group A rotaviruses, but antigenically and genomically distinct rotaviruses have also caused diarrheal outbreaks.

Molecular epidemiologic studies have analyzed isolates based on differences in the migration of the 11 genome segments following electrophoresis of the RNA in polyacrylamide gels (Figure 37–5). Extensive genome heterogeneity has been demonstrated in numerous studies. These differences in electropherotypes cannot be used to predict serotypes; however, electropherotyping can be a useful epidemiologic tool to monitor viral transmission.

Animal Susceptibility

Rotaviruses have a wide host range. Most isolates have been recovered from newborn animals with diarrhea. Cross-species infections can occur in experimental inoculations, but it is not clear if they occur in nature. In experimental studies, human rotavirus can induce diarrheal illness in newborn colostrum-deprived animals (eg, piglets, calves). Homologous infections may have a wider age range. Swine rotavirus infects both newborn and weanling piglets. Newborns often exhibit subclinical infection due perhaps to the presence of maternal antibody, whereas overt disease is more common in weanling animals.

Propagation in Cell Culture

Rotaviruses are fastidious agents to culture. Most human rotaviruses can be cultivated if pretreated with the proteolytic enzyme trypsin and if low levels of trypsin are included in the tissue culture medium. This cleaves an outer capsid protein and facilitates uncoating.

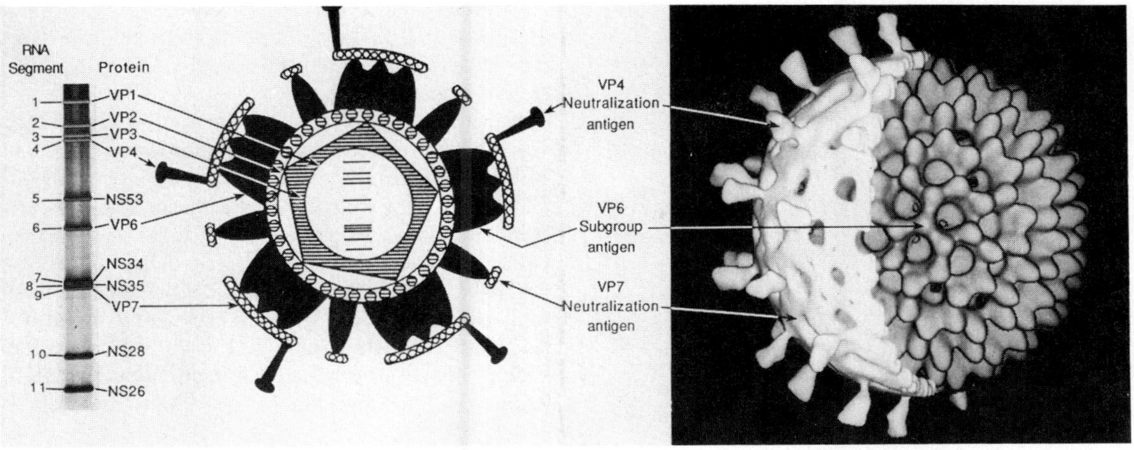

Figure 37–4. Gene-coding assignments for antigenic specificities of rotavirus proteins. Shown on the left are the genome RNA segments and the encoded protein products. In the center is a schematic representation of the rotavirus double-shelled particle with the location of the structural proteins indicated. The figure on the right shows the three-dimensional structure of a viral particle. A double-shelled particle is drawn on the left half; the structure of the core is represented on the right half. (Courtesy of MK Estes and BVV Prasad.)

Pathogenesis

Rotaviruses infect cells in the villi of the small intestine (gastric and colonic mucosa are spared). They multiply in the cytoplasm of enterocytes and damage their transport mechanisms. Damaged cells may slough into the lumen of the intestine and release large quantities of virus, which appear in the stool (up to 10^{10} particles per gram of feces). Viral excretion usually lasts 2–12 days in healthy patients but may be prolonged in those with poor nutrition. Diarrhea caused by rotaviruses may be due to impaired sodium and glucose absorption as damaged cells on villi are replaced by nonabsorbing immature crypt cells. It may take 3–8 weeks for normal function to be restored.

Clinical Findings & Laboratory Diagnosis

Rotaviruses cause the major portion of diarrheal illness in infants and children but not in adults (Table 37–2). There is an incubation period of 1–4 days. Typical symptoms include diarrhea, fever, abdominal pain, and vomiting, leading to dehydration.

In infants and children, severe loss of electrolytes and fluids may be fatal unless treated. Patients with milder cases have symptoms for 3–8 days and then recover completely. Asymptomatic infections, with seroconversion, occur.

Adult contacts may be infected, as evidenced by seroconversion, but they rarely exhibit symptoms, and virus is infrequently detected in their stools. A common source of infection is contact with pediatric cases. However, epidemics of severe disease have occurred in adults, especially in closed populations, as in a geriatric ward. Group B rotaviruses have been implicated in large outbreaks of severe gastroenteritis in adults in China (Table 37–2).

Laboratory diagnosis rests on demonstration of virus in stool collected early in the illness and on a rise in antibody titer. Virus in stool is demonstrated by immune electron microscopy, immunodiffusion, or ELISA. Dot hybridization using rotavirus-specific cDNA probes may prove convenient. It may be possible to type rotavirus nucleic acid from stool specimens by the polymerase chain reaction. Many serologic tests can be used to detect an antibody titer rise, particularly CF and ELISA.

Epidemiology & Immunity

Rotaviruses are the single most important worldwide cause of gastroenteritis in young children. Estimates range from 500 million to 1 billion for annual diarrheal episodes in children under 5 years of age in Africa, Asia, and Latin America, resulting in as many as 3.5 million deaths. Typically, 50–60% of cases of acute gastroenteritis of hospitalized children throughout the world are caused by rotaviruses.

Rotavirus infections usually predominate during the winter season. Symptomatic infections are most common in children between ages 6 months and 2 years, and transmission appears to be by the fecal-oral route. Nosocomial infections are frequent.

Rotaviruses are ubiquitous. By age 6 years, 60–90% of children have serum antibodies to one or more types. Both humans and animals can become infected even in the presence of antibodies. Local immune factors, such as secretory IgA or interferon, may be important in protection against rotavirus infection. Alternatively, reinfection in the presence of circulating

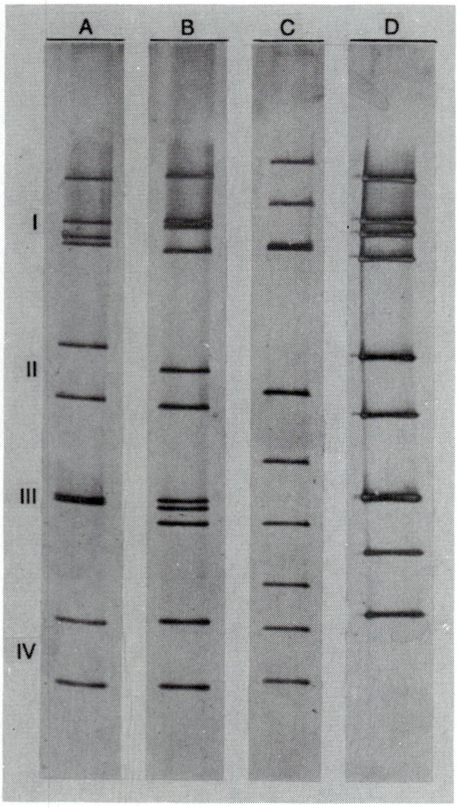

Figure 37–5. Electrophoretic profiles of rotavirus RNA segments. Viral RNAs were electrophoresed in 10% polyacrylamide gels and visualized by silver stain. Different rotavirus groups and RNA patterns are illustrated: a group A monkey virus (SA11; lane A), a group A human rotavirus isolated in Ohio in 1986 (lane B), a group B human adult diarrhea virus from Jinzhou, China, 1983 (lane C), and a group A rabbit virus that exhibits a "short" RNA pattern (lane D). Rotaviruses contain 11 genome RNA segments, but sometimes two or three segments migrate closely together and are difficult to separate. (Photograph provided by T Tanaka and MK Estes.)

antibody could reflect the presence of multiple serotypes of virus. Asymptomatic infections are common in infants before age 6 months, the time during which protective maternal antibody acquired passively by newborns should be present. Such neonatal infection does not prevent reinfection, but it may protect against the development of severe disease during reinfection. Rotavirus antibody has been detected in the mother's milk for up to 9 months postpartum.

Treatment & Control

Treatment of gastroenteritis is supportive, to correct the loss of water and electrolytes that may lead to dehydration, acidosis, shock, and death. Management consists of replacement of fluids and restoration of electrolyte balance either intravenously or orally, as feasible. The infrequent mortality from infantile diarrhea in developed countries is due to routine use of effective replacement therapy.

In view of the fecal-oral route of transmission, wastewater treatment and sanitation are significant control measures.

A live bovine rotavirus and a rhesus rotavirus are being evaluated as attenuated vaccines in humans. Other approaches toward vaccine development include the use of attenuated and cold-adapted human rotavirus mutants and of interspecies reassortant rotaviruses. Ultimately, an effective rotavirus vaccine should induce in very young infants protective antibodies to all the important serotypes of rotaviruses.

REOVIRUSES

The viruses of this genus, which have been studied most thoroughly by molecular biologists, are not known to cause human disease.

Classification & Antigenic Properties

Reoviruses are ubiquitous, with a very wide host range. Three distinct but related types of reovirus have been recovered from many species and are demonstrable by Nt and HI tests. All three types share a common complement-fixing antigen. Reoviruses contain a hemagglutinin for human O or bovine erythrocytes.

Epidemiology

Reoviruses cause many inapparent infections, because most people have serum antibodies by early adulthood. Antibodies are also present in other species.

All three types have been recovered from healthy children, from young children during outbreaks of minor febrile illness, from children with diarrhea or enteritis, and from chimpanzees with epidemic rhinitis.

Human volunteer studies have failed to demonstrate a clear cause-and-effect relationship of reoviruses to human illness. In inoculated volunteers, reovirus is recovered far more readily from feces than from the nose or throat. An association of reovirus type 3 with biliary atresia in infants has been suggested.

Pathogenesis

Reovirus has become an important model system for the study of the pathogenesis of viral infection at the molecular level. Defined recombinants from two reoviruses with differing pathogenic phenotypes are used to infect mice. Segregation analysis is then used to associate particular features of pathogenesis with specific viral genes and gene products. The pathogenic properties of reoviruses are primarily determined by the protein species ($\sigma 1$, $\mu 1C$, or $\sigma 3$) found on the outer

Table 37–2. Viruses associated with acute gastroenteritis in humans.[1]

Virus	Size (nm)	Epidemiology	Important as a Cause of Hospitalization
Rotavirus			
Group A	70	Single most important cause (viral or bacterial) of endemic severe diarrheal illness in infants and young children worldwide (in cooler months in temperate climates).	Yes
Group B	70	Outbreaks of diarrheal illness in adults and children in China.	No
Group C	70	Sporadic cases and occasional outbreaks of diarrheal illness in children.	No
Enteric adenovirus	70–80	Second most important viral agent of endemic diarrheal illness of infants and young children worldwide.	Yes
Norwalk virus and Norwalk-like viruses	27–32	Important cause of outbreaks of vomiting and diarrheal illness in older children and adults in families, communities, and institutions; frequently associated with ingestion of food.	No
Caliciviruses	28–40	Sporadic cases and occasional outbreaks of diarrheal illness in infants, young children, and the elderly.	No
Astroviruses	28	Sporadic cases and occasional outbreaks of diarrheal illness in infants, young children, and the elderly.	No

[1]Reproduced, with permission, from Kapikian AZ: Viral gastroenteritis. JAMA 1993;269:627.

capsid of the virion. The viral hemagglutinin ($\sigma 1$) is responsible for the receptor interactions that control cell and tissue tropisms; $\sigma 1$ is also the major determinant of the host humoral and cellular immune responses. The $\mu 1C$ protein determines the ability of the virus to replicate at the primary site of infection, the gastrointestinal tract, and subsequently undergo systemic spread; it also modulates the immune response to $\sigma 1$. The $\sigma 3$ protein is responsible for inhibiting the synthesis of host cell RNA and protein; thus, it controls the ability of reoviruses to kill and lyse cells. The picture which is emerging is that virion surface proteins play a critical role in pathogenesis. Studies also indicate that virulence is multigenically determined and represents the interactions of multiple viral and cellular genes and gene products.

ORBIVIRUSES

Orbiviruses are a genus within the reovirus family. They commonly infect insects, and many are transmitted by insects to vertebrates. About 100 serotypes are known. None of these viruses cause serious clinical disease in humans, but they may cause mild fevers. Serious animal pathogens include bluetongue virus of sheep and African horse sickness virus. Antibodies to orbiviruses are found in many vertebrates, including humans.

The genome consists of ten segments of double-stranded RNA, with a total molecular weight of 12×10^6. The replicative cycle is similar to that of reoviruses. Orbiviruses are sensitive to low pH, in contrast with the general stability of other reoviruses.

OTHER AGENTS OF VIRAL GASTROENTERITIS

In addition to rotaviruses and noncultivatable adenoviruses, a group of small, round enteric viruses has been associated with gastroenteritis in humans. These viruses are detected by electron microscopy and cannot be cultured (Figure 37–6). The best-studied are the Norwalk-like agents.

Norwalk Virus

The Norwalk agent has been definitely established as an important pathogen in epidemic gastroenteritis (Figure 37–1 and Table 37–2). It is most often associated with epidemic outbreaks of waterborne, foodborne, and shellfish-associated gastroenteritis. Community outbreaks can occur in any season. It is estimated that about 40% of outbreaks of acute, epidemic, nonbacterial gastroenteritis in the USA are caused by Norwalk virus and related agents, such as Hawaii and Snow Mountain viruses. There appear to be at least four serotypes of Norwalk-like viruses, based on human cross-challenge and immunoelectron microscopic studies.

Epidemic nonbacterial gastroenteritis is characterized by (1) absence of bacterial pathogens; (2) gastroenteritis with rapid onset and recovery and relatively mild systemic signs; and (3) an epidemiologic pattern of a highly communicable disease that spreads rapidly with no particular predilection in terms of age or geography. Various terms have been used in reports of different outbreaks (eg, epidemic viral gastroenteritis, viral diarrhea, winter vomiting disease), depending on the predominant clinical feature.

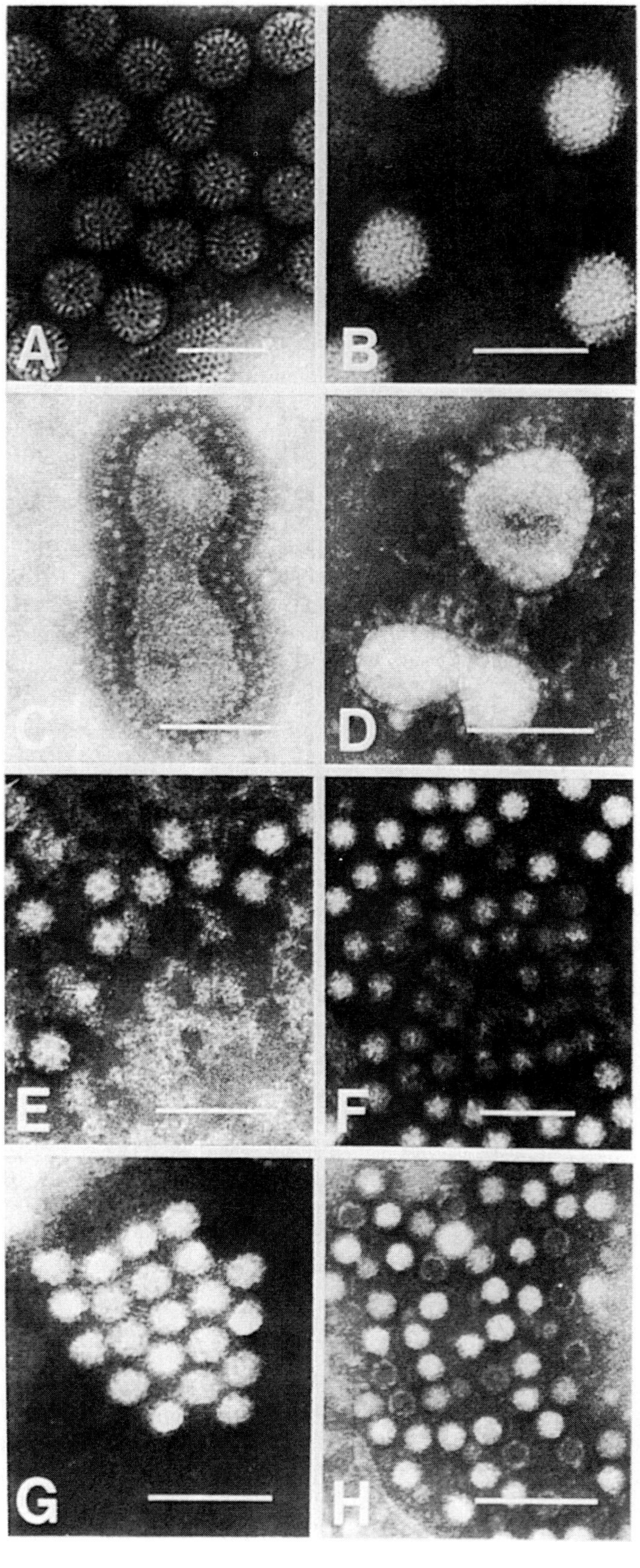

Figure 37–6. Electron micrographs of virus particles found in stools of patients with gastroenteritis. These viruses were visualized following negative staining. Specific viruses and the original magnifications of the micrographs are as follows. ***A:*** Rotavirus (185,000×). ***B:*** Enteric adenovirus (234,000×). ***C:*** Coronavirus (249,000×). ***D:*** Torovirus (coronavirus) (249,000×). ***E:*** Calicivirus (250,000×). ***F:*** Astrovirus (196,000×). ***G:*** Norwalk virus (calicivirus) (249,000×). ***H:*** Parvovirus (249,000×). The electron micrographs in panels C–H were originally provided by T Flewett; panel E was originally obtained from CR Madeley. Bars, 100 nm. (Reproduced, with permission, from Graham DY, Estes MK: Viral infections of the intestine. Pages 566–578 in: *Principles and Practice of Gastroenterology and Hepatology.* Gitnick G et al [editors]. Elsevier Science Publishing Co., 1988.)

Viral particles with a diameter of 27 nm were demonstrated by immune electron microscopy in stools from adults with acute gastroenteritis in a Norwalk, Ohio, outbreak and many subsequent outbreaks. There appear to be at least three serotypes. The Norwalk agent has not been grown in tissue culture, so it has not been extensively characterized biochemically. The Norwalk virus genome has been cloned and sequenced, and viral proteins have been synthesized using the baculovirus expression system in insect cells. The expressed proteins are being characterized. The Norwalk agent is now classified as a calicivirus. It replicates only in humans.

Viral gastroenteritis has an incubation period of 16–48 hours. Onset is rapid, and the clinical course is brief, lasting 24–48 hours; symptoms include diarrhea, nausea, vomiting, low-grade fever, abdominal cramps, headache, and malaise. Hospitalization is rarely required. No sequelae have been reported.

Volunteer experiments have clearly shown that the appearance of Norwalk virus coincides with clinical illness. Antibody develops during the illness and is usually protective against reinfection with the same agent, at least on a short-term basis. A radioimmunoassay blocking test and an immune adherence method can detect antibody to Norwalk-type viruses. Whereas rotavirus antibody develops early in childhood, Norwalk virus antibody is acquired later in life; more than 50% of adults have such antibody.

Treatment is symptomatic. Because of the infectious nature of the stools, care should be taken in their disposal.

Caliciviruses

Caliciviruses are similar to picornaviruses but are slightly larger (35–39 nm) and contain a single major structural protein. They exhibit a distinctive morphology in the electron microscope (Figure 37–6E). There appear to be several serotypes of human caliciviruses, in addition to Norwalk virus, that do not cross-react antigenically with known animal strains. Human caliciviruses seem to be relatively common causes of gastroenteritis in children, especially in Southeast Asia, Japan, and the United Kingdom.

Astroviruses

Astroviruses are about 30 nm in diameter and, like caliciviruses, exhibit a distinctive morphology in the electron microscope (Figure 37–6F). They have been seen in stools from infants and young children and from calves and lambs with diarrhea. Several serotypes are recognized. Astroviruses may be shed in extraordinarily large quantities in feces.

The presence of astrovirus has been associated with diarrhea in young children in day care centers in the USA (Table 37–2). Volunteer studies indicate that astroviruses may be only minimally pathogenic, failing to induce disease in many infected persons. The extent of their role in human gastroenteritis remains unclear.

Small Round Viruses

The final group of agents associated with acute nonbacterial gastroenteritis contains unclassified, small (20–30 nm), round, featureless particles devoid of clear surface structure. They have not been characterized biochemically, and their epidemiologic significance in sporadic cases of acute diarrhea in children is unknown. It has recently been suggested that a substantial number of unidentified "small round viruses" recovered from stools may be parvoviruses (Figure 37–6H).

REFERENCES

Bern C, Glass RI: Impact of diarrheal diseases worldwide. In: *Viral Infections of the Gastrointestinal Tract,* 2nd ed. Kapikian AZ (editor). Marcel Dekker, 1994.

Bern C et al: The magnitude of the global problem of diarrhoeal disease: a ten-year update. Bull WHO 1992;70:705.

Cukor G, Blacklow NR: Human viral gastroenteritis. Microbiol Rev 1984;48:157.

Dimitrov DH, Graham DY, Estes MK: Detection of rotaviruses by nucleic acid hybridization with cloned DNA of simian rotavirus SA11 genes. J Infect Dis 1985;152: 293.

Dolin R, Treanor JJ, Madore HP: Novel agents of viral enteritis in humans. J Infect Dis 1987;155:365.

Estes MK, Cohen J: Rotavirus gene structure and function. Microbiol Rev 1989;53:410.

Gouvea V et al: Polymerase chain reaction amplification and typing of rotavirus nucleic acid from stool specimens. J Clin Microbiol 1990;28:276.

Hrdy DB: Epidemiology of rotaviral infection in adults. Rev Infect Dis 1987;9:461.

Jiang X et al: Norwalk virus genome cloning and characterization. Science 1990;250:1580.

Kapikian AZ et al: Prospects for development of a rotavirus vaccine against rotavirus diarrhea in infants and young children. Rev Infect Dis 1989;11:S539.

Lew JF et al: Astrovirus and adenovirus associated with diarrhea in children in day care settings. J Infect Dis 1991; 164:673.

Nakata S et al: Humoral immunity in infants with gastroenteritis caused by human calicivirus. J Infect Dis 1985;152: 274.

Oliver AR, Phillips AD: An electron microscopical investigation of faecal small round viruses. J Med Virol 1988; 24:211.

Saif LJ, Theil KW (editors): *Viral Diarrheas of Man and Animals.* CRC Press, 1989.

38 Arthropod-Borne & Rodent-Borne Viral Diseases

The **arthropod-borne viruses,** or **arboviruses,** are a group of infectious agents that are transmitted by bloodsucking arthropods from one vertebrate host to another. They multiply in the tissues of the arthropod without evidence of disease or damage. The vector acquires a lifelong infection through the ingestion of blood from a viremic vertebrate. Some arboviruses are maintained in nature by transovarian transmission in arthropods.

The major arbovirus diseases worldwide are yellow fever, dengue, Japanese B encephalitis, St. Louis encephalitis, western equine encephalitis, eastern equine encephalitis, Russian spring-summer encephalitis, West Nile fever, and sandfly fever. In the USA the most important arboviral infections are western equine encephalitis, eastern equine encephalitis, St. Louis encephalitis, and California encephalitis.

Because of the importance of ecologic factors governing their transmission, **rodent-borne (robo) viral diseases** also are considered in this chapter. They are maintained in nature by direct intraspecies or interspecies transmission from rodent to rodent without participation of arthropod vectors. Viral infection is usually persistent. Transmission occurs through many routes by contact with body fluids or excretions.

Arboviruses and roboviruses represent ecologic groupings of viruses with diverse physical and chemical properties. They belong to several virus families.

Classification of Arboviruses & Roboviruses

Individual viruses were sometimes named after a disease (dengue, yellow fever) or after the geographical area where the virus was first isolated (St. Louis encephalitis, West Nile fever). Although arboviruses are found in all temperate and tropical zones, they are most prevalent in the tropical rain forest with its abundance of animals and arthropods.

There are more than 450 arboviruses and roboviruses; of these, about 100 are known pathogens for humans. They are classified according to their chemical and physical properties and their antigenic relationships. Arboviruses and roboviruses are placed among toga-, flavi-, bunya-, reo-, arena-, filo-, and rhabdovirus groups (Table 38–1, Figure 38–1).

Togaviruses: The alphavirus subgroup consists of 28 viruses that are 70 nm in diameter and possess an enveloped, positive-sense RNA genome. The envelope contains two glycoproteins and lipid.

Flaviviruses: The family consists of 65 viruses that are 40–50 nm in diameter and have an enveloped, positive-sense RNA. The envelope contains a single glycoprotein and lipid.

Both alphaviruses and flaviviruses replicate in the cytoplasm; alphaviruses mature by budding nucleocapsids through the plasma membrane, whereas flaviviruses mature through intracytoplasmic membranes (particularly the endoplasmic reticulum). Unlike alphaviruses, some flaviviruses may cause persistent infections, and many are transmitted between vertebrate hosts without intermediate arthropod vectors.

Bunyaviruses: More than 300 viruses, mostly arthropod-transmitted, are classified in this family. Spherical particles contain a single-stranded, negative-sense RNA genome that is segmented. They have a lipid-containing envelope and measure 90–100 nm. The nucleocapsids have helical symmetry and contain a major viral protein. The envelope has two glycoproteins in the lipid bilayer and surface projections (10 nm) of glycopeptides clustered to form hollow cylinders. Several produce mosquito-borne encephalitides of humans and animals, others hemorrhagic fevers. Some are transmitted by sandflies. A newly recognized disease in the USA, hantavirus pulmonary syndrome, is caused by a virus transmitted by deer mice.

Reoviruses: (See Chapter 37.) A few arboviruses are members of the genus *Orbivirus,* including African horse sickness and bluetongue viruses. Colorado tick fever is classified in the genus *Coltivirus.* Some infect birds, small mammals, and ticks.

Arenaviruses: (See Chapter 29.) Pleomorphic particles contain a segmented single negative-sense RNA genome, are surrounded by an envelope, and measure 50–300 nm. They contain granules believed to be ribosomes. Several hemorrhagic fever viruses are members of this group. Most have a rodent host in their natural cycle.

Filoviruses: Long, filamentous particles of varying length, 80 nm in diameter. Negative-sense RNA genome. Probably have a rodent host. Highly virulent in humans (Figure 38–1).

Rhabdoviruses: (See Chapter 42.) Several bullet-shaped arboviruses fall into this group (see Figure 42–1).

Table 38–1. Taxonomic status of some arboviruses and roboviruses.

Taxonomic Classification	Important Arbovirus and Robovirus Members	Virus Properties
Togaviridae Genus *Alphavirus*	Chikungunya, eastern equine encephalitis, Mayaro, O'Nyong-nyong, Ross River, Semliki Forest, Sindbis, and Venezuelan and western equine encephalitis viruses	Spherical, 70 nm in diameter. Genome: positive-sense, single-stranded RNA. Envelope. Three or four major structural polypeptides, one or two glycosylated. Replication: cytoplasm. Assembly: budding through host cell membranes.
Flaviviridae Genus *Flavivirus*	Brazilian encephalitis (Rocio virus), dengue, Japanese B encephalitis, Kyasanur Forest disease, louping ill, Murray Valley encephalitis, Omsk hemorrhagic fever, Powassan, Russian spring-summer encephalitis, St. Louis encephalitis, tick-borne encephalitis, West Nile fever, and yellow fever viruses	Spherical, 40 nm in diameter. Genome: positive-sense RNA. Envelope. Three or four structural polypeptides, one or two glycosylated. Replication: cytoplasm. Assembly: within endoplasmic reticulum.
Bunyaviridae Genus *Bunyavirus*	Anopheles A and B, California encephalitis, Guama, Simbu (Oropouche), and Turlock viruses	Spherical, 90–100 nm in diameter. Genome: triple-segmented, negative-sense, single-stranded RNA. Virion contains a transcriptase. Four major polypeptides. Envelope. Replication: cytoplasm. Assembly: budding on smooth membranes of the Golgi system.
Genus *Phlebovirus*	Sandfly (*Phlebotomus*) fever viruses and Rift Valley fever viruses	
Genus *Nairovirus*	Crimean-Congo hemorrhagic fever, Nairobi sheep disease, and Sakhalin viruses	
Genus *Hantavirus*	Hantaan virus (Korean hemorrhagic fever, hemorrhagic fever with renal syndrome, hantavirus pulmonary syndrome)	
Reoviridae Genus *Orbivirus*	African horse sickness and bluetongue viruses	Spherical, 70 nm in diameter. Genome: 10 segments of linear, double-stranded RNA.
Genus *Coltivirus*	Colorado tick fever virus	No envelope. Six to 10 structural polypeptides. Replication and assembly: cytoplasm.
Rhabdoviridae Genus *Vesiculovirus*	Hart Park, Kern Canyon, and vesicular stomatitis viruses	Bullet-shaped, about 75 nm in diameter × 180 nm in length. Genome: negative-sense, single-stranded RNA. Virion contains a transcriptase. Four major polypeptides, including a surface-projection glycoprotein. Envelope. Replication: cytoplasm. Assembly: budding from plasma and intracytoplasmic membranes.
Arenaviridae Genus *Arenavirus*	Junin, Lassa, Machupo, and Pichinde viruses	Spherical, about 120 nm in diameter. Genome: double-segmented, negative-sense, single-stranded RNA. Virion contains a transcriptase. Three major polypeptides. Envelope. Replication: cytoplasm. Assembly: incorporates ribosome-like particles and buds from plasma membrane.
Filoviridae	Marburg and Ebola viruses	Long filaments, 80 nm in diameter × varying length (> 1000 nm). Genome: negative-sense, single-stranded RNA. Five polypeptides. Envelope. Replication: cytoplasm. Assembly: budding from cell membrane.

HUMAN ARBOVIRAL INFECTIONS

About 100 arboviruses can infect humans, but not all cause overt disease. Those infecting humans are all believed to be zoonotic, with humans the accidental hosts who play no important role in the maintenance or transmission cycle of the virus. Exceptions are urban yellow fever and dengue. Some of the natural cycles are simple and involve infection of a nonhuman vertebrate host (mammal or bird) transmitted by a species of mosquito or tick (eg, jungle yellow fever, Colorado tick fever). Others, however, are quite complex. For example, many cases of central European diphasic meningoencephalitis occur following ingestion of raw milk from goats and cows infected by grazing in tick-infested pastures where a tick-rodent cycle is occurring.

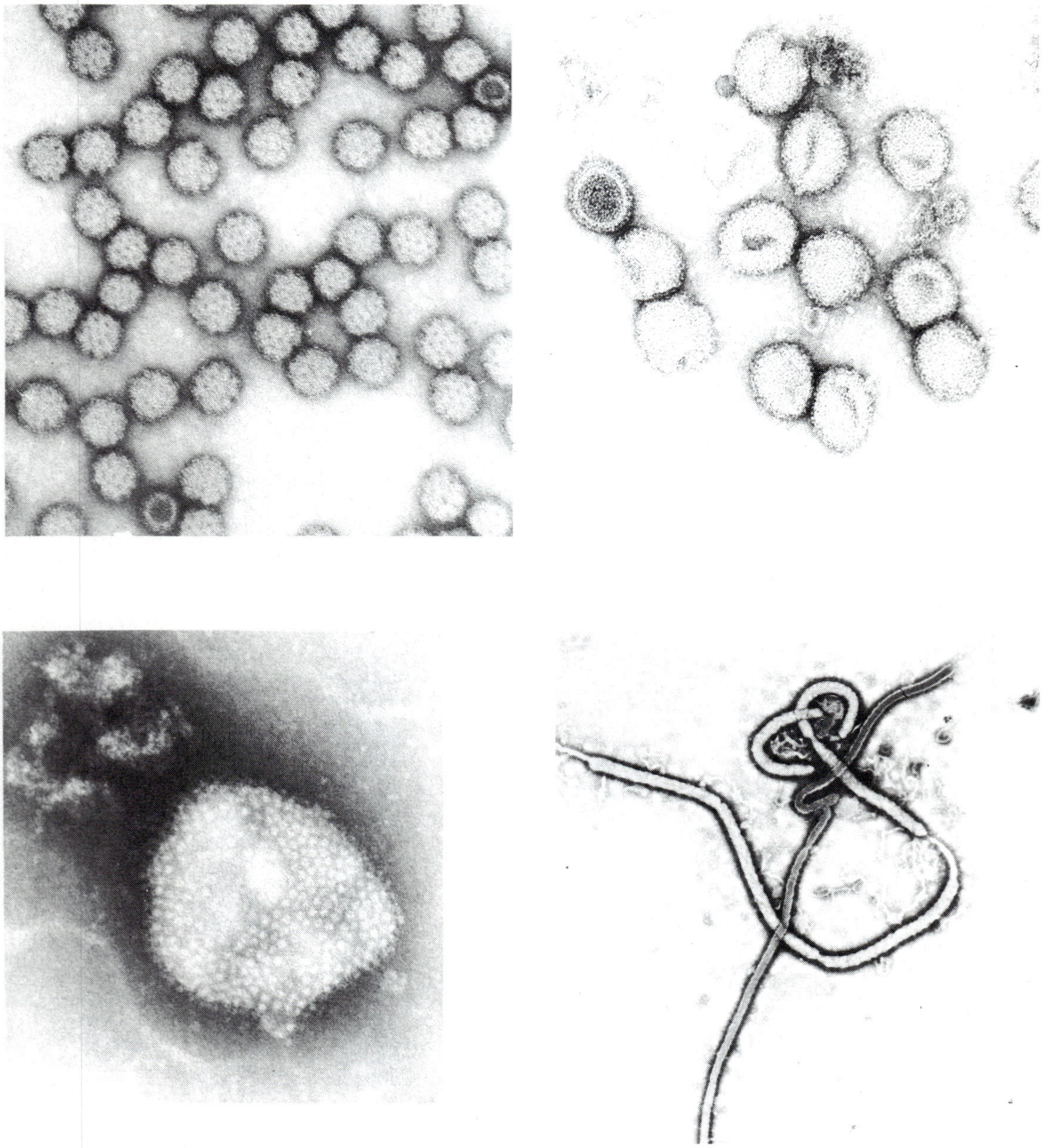

Figure 38–1. Electron micrographs of typical arboviruses and roboviruses. ***Upper left:*** An alphavirus, Semliki Forest virus (Togaviridae). ***Upper right:*** A representative member of Bunyaviridae, Uukuniemi virus. ***Lower left:*** An arenavirus, Tacaribe virus. ***Lower right:*** Ebola virus, Filoviridae. (Courtesy of FA Murphy and EL Palmer.)

Overview of Arbovirus Infections: Diseases produced by arboviruses may be divided into three clinical syndromes: (1) fevers of an undifferentiated type with or without a maculopapular rash and usually benign; (2) encephalitis, often with a high case-fatality rate; and (3) hemorrhagic fevers, also frequently severe and fatal. These categories are somewhat arbitrary, and some arboviruses may be associated with more than one syndrome, eg, dengue.

The intensity of viral multiplication and its predominant site of localization in tissues determine the clinical syndrome. Thus, individual arboviruses can produce a minor febrile illness in some patients and encephalitis or a hemorrhagic diathesis in others. However, in an epidemic situation, one of the syndromes usually predominates, permitting tentative diagnosis. Final diagnosis is based on further epidemiologic and serologic data.

After infection with an arbovirus, there is an incubation period during which viral multiplication takes place. This is followed by abrupt onset of clinical manifestations that are closely related to viral dissemination. Malaise, headache, nausea, vomiting, and myalgia accompany fever, which is an invariable symptom and sometimes the only one. The illness may terminate at this stage, recur with or without a rash, or reveal hemorrhagic manifestations secondary to vascular abnormalities. Frequently, the period of viremia is asymptomatic, with acute onset of encephalitis following localization of the virus in the central nervous system.

Encephalitis Overview: Encephalitis can be produced by many different viruses. Arbovirus encephalitis occurs in distinct geographic distributions and vector patterns (Table 38–2). Each continent tends to have its own arbovirus pattern, and names are usually suggestive, eg, Venezuelan equine encephalitis, Japanese B encephalitis, Murray Valley (Australia) encephalitis. All of the preceding are alpha- and flavivirus infections spread by mosquitoes with a distinct ecologic distribution. California encephalitis is caused by bunyaviruses. However, on a given continent there may be a shifting distribution depending on viral hosts and vectors in a given year.

Encephalitis or meningoencephalitis can also occur with viruses that involve tissues other than the central nervous system—measles, mumps, hepatitis, chickenpox, zoster, herpes simplex, and others. Some of these viruses replicate actively in the central nervous system, producing inflammation. At other times, the viral infection sets off an immunologic reaction that results in "postinfectious" encephalomyelitis, with a prominent demyelinating component.

In some parts of the world, epidemics of arbovirus infection have involved thousands of individuals with symptomatic infection; many more were asymptomatically infected. In the USA, the number of cases varies widely from year to year. In 1975, 4308 cases of encephalitis were reported, with 340 deaths. Cases occurred in almost every state. Of the entire number, 42% were due to St. Louis encephalitis, 7% to other arboviruses, 4% to mumps, 3% to enteroviruses, and 2% to herpesviruses; 40% could not be identified by laboratory means. In 1984 in the USA, arboviral infections of the central nervous system occurred in more than 100 persons. Thirty-three cases were caused by St. Louis encephalitis virus, 26 of them in California. Seventy-six cases were caused by California (La Crosse) encephalitis virus, five by eastern equine encephalitis virus, and two by western equine encephalitis virus. In 1987, only five cases of St. Louis encephalitis but 37 cases of western equine encephalitis were reported.

Table 38–2. Summary of major human arbovirus and rodent-borne virus infections that occur in the USA.

Diseases	Exposure	Distribution	Vectors	Infection: Case Ratio (Age Incidence)	Sequelae	Mortality Rate (%)
Western equine encephalitis (*Alphavirus*)	Rural	Pacific, Mountain, West Central, Southwest	*Culex tarsalis*	50:1 (under 5) 1000:1 (over 15)	+	3–7
Eastern equine encephalitis (*Alphavirus*)	Rural	Atlantic, southern coastal	*Aedes sollicitans* *Aedes vexans*	10:1 (infants) 50:1 (middle-aged) 20:1 (elderly)	+	50–70
Venezuelan equine encephalitis (*Alphavirus*)	Rural	South and Central America, southern USA	*Aedes* *Psorophora* *Culex*	25:1 (under 15) 1000:1 (over 15)	±	20–30 (children) < 10 (adults)
St. Louis encephalitis (*Flavivirus*)	Urban-rural	Widespread	*Culex pipiens* *Culex quinquefasciatus* *C tarsalis* *Culex nigrapalpus*	800:1 (under 9) 400:1 (9–59) 85:1 (over 60)	±	5–10 (under 65) 30 (over 65)
California encephalitis (La Crosse) (*Bunyavirus*)	Rural	North Central, Atlantic, South	*Aedes triseriatus*	Unknown ratio (most cases under 20)	Rare	Fatalities rare
Colorado tick fever (*Coltivirus*)	Rural	Pacific, Mountain	*Dermacentor andersoni*	Unknown ratio (all ages affected)	Rare	Fatalities rare
Hantavirus pulmonary syndrome (*Bunyavirus*)	Rural	Southwestern and western USA	*Peromyscus maniculatus*[1]	Unknown	Unknown	60

[1]Rodent reservoir, no vector.

TOGAVIRUS & FLAVIVIRUS ENCEPHALITIS

Characteristics of the Viruses

A. Properties: (See Table 38–1.) The viruses infect many cell lines, embryonated eggs, mice, birds, bats, mules, horses, and other animals.

In susceptible vertebrate hosts, primary viral multiplication occurs either in myeloid and lymphoid cells or in vascular endothelium. Multiplication in the central nervous system depends on the ability of the virus to pass the blood-brain barrier and to infect nerve cells. In natural infection of birds and mammals, an inapparent infection develops in a majority. However, for several days there is viremia, and arthropod vectors acquire the virus by sucking blood during this period—the first step in its dissemination to other hosts. These characteristics apply to the main flavi- and alphavirus infections in the western hemisphere, particularly St. Louis encephalitis, western equine encephalitis, eastern equine encephalitis, and Venezuelan equine encephalitis (Table 38–2). They also apply to Japanese B encephalitis, which occurs in the Far East.

B. Replication: The alphavirus RNA genome is positive-sense; it produces 42–50S and 26S mRNAs during transcription. The 42–50S mRNA translates precursor polyproteins, including nonstructural proteins, whereas the 26S mRNA encodes structural proteins. The proteins are elaborated by posttranslational cleavage. Sequence data indicate that western equine encephalitis virus is a genetic recombinant of eastern equine encephalitis and Sindbis viruses.

The flavivirus RNA genome also is positive-sense and produces a 40–45S mRNA during transcription. A precursor protein has not been identified, and it has been proposed that multiple initiation sites account for the multiple proteins.

C. Virus Assays: Viral multiplication can be measured by cytopathic changes, virus-specific immunofluorescence, or hemadsorption tests that detect the production of viral hemagglutinin in cell culture. Plaque counts can be done in most cultures. Arboviruses usually interfere with the replication of other arboviruses in coinfected cells. Arboviruses are susceptible to inhibition by interferon.

D. Antigenic Properties: Complement-fixing antigens and viral hemagglutinins may be prepared from infected brains of newborn mice (because of their low fat content). The hemagglutinins are part of the infectious viral particle and can agglutinate goose or newly hatched chick red blood cells. The erythrocyte-virus complex is still infective, but it can be neutralized by the addition of antibody.

Some of these viruses have an overlapping antigenicity, most readily demonstrated by cross-reactions in HI tests. Antigenic overlap is due to the presence of one or more cross-reactive antigens in addition to the strain-specific antigen. Thus, immune sera prepared for one strain will contain strain-specific as well as group-specific antibodies. An immune serum can be made more specific by adsorption with a heterologous virus of the same group. Such an adsorbed serum will react only with the homologous virus and is useful in the identification of newly isolated strains.

Pathogenesis & Pathology

Pathogenesis of encephalitis in humans has not been well studied, but the disease in experimental animals may afford a model for human disease. The equine encephalitides in horses are diphasic. In the first phase (minor illness), the virus multiplies in nonneural tissue and is present in the blood 3 days before the first signs of involvement of the central nervous system. In the second phase (major illness), the virus multiplies in the brain, cells are injured and destroyed, and encephalitis becomes clinically apparent. The two phases may overlap. It is not known whether in humans there is a period of primary viral multiplication in nonneural tissues with a secondary liberation of virus into the blood before its entry into the central nervous system. High concentrations of virus in brain tissue are necessary before the clinical disease becomes manifest.

The primary encephalitides are characterized by lesions in all parts of the central nervous system, including the basal structures of the brain, the cerebral cortex, and the spinal cord. Small hemorrhages with perivascular cuffing and meningeal infiltration—chiefly with mononuclear cells—are common. Nerve cell degeneration associated with neuronophagia occurs. Purkinje's cells of the cerebellum may be destroyed. There are also patches of encephalomalacia; acellular plaques of spongy appearance in which medullary fibers, dendrites, and axons are destroyed; and focal microglial proliferation. Thus, not only the neurons but also the cells of the supporting structure of the central nervous system are attacked.

Widespread neuronal degeneration occurs with all arbovirus-induced encephalitides.

Clinical Findings

Incubation periods of the encephalitides are between 4 and 21 days. There is a sudden onset with severe headache, chills and fever, nausea and vomiting, generalized pains, and malaise. Within 24–48 hours, marked drowsiness develops and the patient may become stuporous. Nuchal rigidity is common. Mental confusion, dysarthria, tremors, convulsions, and coma develop in severe cases. Fever lasts 4–10 days. The mortality rate in encephalitides varies (Table 38–2). With Japanese B encephalitis, the mortality rate in older age groups may be as high as 80%. Sequelae may include mental deterioration, personality changes, paralysis, aphasia, and cerebellar signs.

Abortive infections simulate aseptic meningitis or nonparalytic poliomyelitis. Inapparent infections are common.

In California, where both western equine encephalitis and St. Louis encephalitis are prevalent, western equine encephalitis has a predilection for children and infants. In the same area, St. Louis encephalitis rarely occurs in infants, even though both viruses are transmitted by the same arthropod vector *(Culex tarsalis).*

Laboratory Diagnosis

A. Recovery of Virus: The virus occurs in the blood only early in the infection, usually before the onset of symptoms. The virus is most often recovered from the brains of fatal cases by intracerebral inoculation of newborn mice, and then it should be identified by serologic tests with known antisera.

B. Serology: Neutralizing and hemagglutination-inhibiting antibodies are detectable within a few days after the onset of illness. Complement-fixing antibodies appear later. The neutralizing and the hemagglutination-inhibiting antibodies endure for many years. The complement-fixing antibody may be lost within 2–5 years.

The HI test with newly hatched chick erythrocytes is the simplest diagnostic test, but it primarily identifies the group rather than the specific causative virus.

It is necessary to establish a rise in specific antibodies during infection in order to make the diagnosis. The first sample of serum should be taken as soon after the onset as possible and the second sample 2–3 weeks later. The paired specimens must be run in the same serologic test.

The cross-reactivity that takes place within the alphavirus or flavivirus group must be considered in making the diagnosis. Thus, following a single infection by one member of the group, antibodies to other members may also appear. These group-specific antibodies are usually of lower titer than the type-specific antibody. Serologic diagnosis becomes difficult when an epidemic caused by one member of the serologic group occurs in an area where another group member is endemic, or when an infected individual has been infected previously by a closely related virus. Under these circumstances, a definite etiologic diagnosis may not be possible. Neutralizing, complement-fixing and hemagglutination-inhibiting antibodies have a decreasing degree of specificity for the causative viral type (in the order listed).

Immunity

Immunity is believed to be permanent after a single infection. In endemic areas, the population may build up immunity as a result of inapparent infections; the proportion of persons with antibodies to the local arthropod-borne virus increases with age.

Effective killed-virus vaccines have been developed to protect horses against eastern and western equine encephalitis. No effective vaccines for these diseases are currently available for humans.

An excellent attenuated live-virus vaccine for Venezuelan equine encephalitis is available for curtailing epidemics among horses and has been used experimentally in humans. A killed-virus vaccine for Japanese B encephalitis has been used in Japan and China.

Because of antigens common to several members within a group, the response to immunization or to infection with one of the viruses of a group may be modified by prior exposure to another member of the same group. In general, the homologous response is greater than a cross-reacting one. This mechanism may be important in conferring protection on a community against an epidemic of another related agent (eg, no Japanese B encephalitis in areas endemic for West Nile fever).

Treatment

There is no specific treatment. In experimental animals, hyperimmune serum is ineffective if given after the onset of disease. However, if given 1–2 days after the introduction of the virus but before signs of encephalitis are obvious, specific hyperimmune serum can prevent a fatal outcome of the infection.

Epidemiology

In severe epidemics caused by encephalitis viruses, the case rate is about 1/1000. St. Louis encephalitis is the most important arthropod-borne viral disease of humans in the USA, having caused about 10,000 cases and 1000 deaths since it was first recognized in 1933. In the large urban epidemic of St. Louis encephalitis that occurred in 1966 in Dallas (population 1 million), there were 545 reported cases and 145 (27%) laboratory-confirmed cases, with a case-fatality rate of 10%. All deaths were in persons age 45 years or older. The incidence of St. Louis encephalitis continues to vary each year in the USA; the largest epidemic (1815 cases) was recorded in 1975, and only five cases were reported in 1987.

In most years, western equine encephalitis transmission occurs at a low level in the rural West, where birds and *C tarsalis* mosquitoes are involved in the maintenance cycle of the virus. Infections of humans and equines rarely occur outside the maintenance cycle, as indicated by the few sporadically occurring cases. However, at intervals of 5–10 years (for reasons poorly understood), viral transmission in the maintenance cycle becomes intense, and humans and equines become infected at epidemic and epizootic levels. In 1987, 37 human and 32 equine cases were reported. Outbreaks have often affected wide areas of the western USA and Canada, where in 1941 more than 3400 human cases occurred.

A. Serologic Epidemiology: In highly endemic areas, almost the entire human population may become infected with the arbovirus, and most infections are asymptomatic. High infection-to-case ratios exist among specified age groups for many arbovirus infections (Table 38–2).

In the 1964 St. Louis encephalitis epidemic in Houston (712 reported cases), there was an inapparent infection rate of 8% in a random city survey, but in the epidemic area of the city the inapparent infection rate was 34%. The infection-to-case ratio remained about the same. It is obvious that the presence of infected mosquitoes is required before human infections can occur, although socioeconomic and cultural factors (air conditioning, screens, mosquito control) affect the degree of exposure of the population to these virus-carrying vectors.

In endemic areas of California, 11% of infants are born with maternal antibody to western equine encephalitis and 27% have St. Louis encephalitis maternal antibody. A direct relationship exists between the length of residence of the mother in the endemic area and the acquisition of antibody.

Japanese B encephalitis is the leading cause of viral encephalitis in Asia. About 50,000 cases occur annually in China, Japan, Korea, and the Indian subcontinent. Seroprevalence studies indicate nearly universal exposure to Japanese B encephalitis virus by adulthood.

B. Mosquito-Borne Encephalitis: Infection of humans occurs when a mosquito like *C tarsalis, Culex quinquefasciatus, Culex pipiens,* or *Culex tritaeniorhynchus* (Japan) or another arthropod bites first an infected animal and later a human.

The equine encephalitides, eastern, western, and Venezuelan, are transmitted by culicine mosquitoes to horses or humans from a mosquito-bird-mosquito cycle. Equines, like humans, are unessential hosts for the maintenance of the virus. An epizootic of encephalitis in horses should alert physicians to the possibility that an arbovirus epidemic in humans may be developing. Both eastern and Venezuelan equine encephalitis in horses are severe, with up to 90% of affected animals dying. Epizootic western equine encephalitis is less frequently fatal for horses. In addition, eastern equine encephalitis produces severe epizootics in certain domestic game birds. A mosquito-bird-mosquito cycle also occurs in St. Louis encephalitis and Japanese B encephalitis. Swine are an important host of Japanese B encephalitis. Mosquitoes remain infected for life (several weeks to months). Only the female feeds on blood and can feed and transmit the virus more than once. The cells of the mosquito's mid gut are the site of primary viral multiplication. This is followed by viremia and invasion of organs—chiefly salivary glands and nerve tissue, where secondary viral multiplication occurs. The arthropod remains healthy.

Infection of insectivorous bats with arboviruses produces a viremia that lasts 6–12 days without any illness or pathologic changes in the bat. While the viral concentration is high, the infected bat may infect mosquitoes that are then able to transmit the infection to wild birds and domestic fowl as well as to other bats.

C. Overwintering of Arboviruses: The epidemiology of the arthropod-borne encephalitides must account for the maintenance and dissemination of the viruses in nature in the absence of humans. Most infections with arboviruses occur in mammals or birds, with humans serving as accidental hosts. The virus is transmitted from animal to animal through the bite of an arthropod vector. Viruses have been isolated from mosquitoes and ticks, which serve as reservoirs of infection. In ticks, the viruses may pass from generation to generation by the transovarian route, and in such instances the tick acts as a true reservoir of the virus as well as its vector. In tropical climates, where mosquito populations are present throughout the year, arboviruses cycle continually between mosquitoes and reservoir animals.

In temperate climates, the virus may be reintroduced each year from the outside (eg, by birds migrating from tropical areas) or it may survive the winter in the local area. Three possible but unproved overwintering mechanisms are as follows: (1) hibernating mosquitoes at the time of their emergence may reinfect birds and thus reestablish a simple bird-mosquito-bird cycle; western equine encephalitis virus was isolated from adult mosquitoes collected as larvae from a California marsh, providing evidence for vertical transmission in mosquitoes in nature; (2) the virus may remain latent in winter within birds, mammals, or arthropods; and (3) cold-blooded vertebrates (snakes, turtles, lizards, alligators, frogs) may act as winter reservoirs. Garter snakes experimentally infected with western equine encephalitis virus can hibernate over the winter and circulate virus in high titers and for long periods the following spring. Normal mosquitoes can be infected by feeding on emerged snakes and can then transmit the virus. Virus has been found in the blood of wild snakes. Western equine encephalitis virus has also been isolated from winter collections of *C tarsalis* mosquitoes in the Rio Grande valley.

In nature, mosquitoes are closely associated with bats, both in summer and during the winter (in hibernation sites). Experimentally, mosquitoes have been shown to transmit virus to bats that could maintain a latent viral infection, with no detectable viremia, for over 3 months at 10 °C. When bats were returned to room temperature, viremia appeared after 3 days. The mosquito-bat-mosquito cycle may be a possible overwintering mechanism for some arboviruses.

Tick-Borne Encephalitis Complex

A. Russian Spring-Summer Encephalitis: This disease occurs chiefly in the early summer, particularly in humans exposed to the ticks *Ixodes persulcatus* and *Ixodes ricinus* in the uncleared forest. Ticks can become infected at any stage in their metamorphosis, and virus can be transmitted transovarially. The virus persists through the winter in hibernating ticks or in vertebrates such as hedgehogs or bats. Virus is secreted in the milk of infected goats for long periods, and infection may be transmitted to those who drink unpasteurized milk. Characteristics of the disease are involvement of the bulbar area or the cervical cord and the development of ascending paralysis or hemiparesis. The mortality rate is about 30%.

B. Louping Ill: This disease of sheep in Scotland and northern England is spread by the tick *I ricinus.* Humans are occasionally infected.

C. Tick-Borne Encephalitis (Central European or Diphasic Meningoencephalitis): This virus is antigenically related to Russian spring-summer encephalitis virus and louping ill virus. Typical cases have a diphasic course, the first phase being influenza-like and the second a meningoencephalitis with or without paralysis.

D. Kyasanur Forest Disease: This is an Indian hemorrhagic disease caused by a virus of the Russian spring-summer encephalitis complex. In addition to humans, langur *(Presbytis entellus)* and bonnet *(Macaca radiata)* monkeys are naturally infected in southern India.

E. Powassan Encephalitis: This tick-borne virus is the first member of the Russian spring-summer complex isolated in North America. Human infection is rare. Since 1959, when the original fatal case was reported from Canada, several additional cases have been confirmed in the northeastern portion of the USA.

Control

Biologic control of the natural vertebrate host is generally impractical, especially when the hosts are wild birds. The most effective method is arthropod control. Since the period of viremia in the vertebrate is of short duration (3–6 days for St. Louis encephalitis infections of birds), any suppression of the vector for this period should break the transmission cycle.

During urban St. Louis encephalitis outbreaks, public health authorities recommend that persons seek protection from the *Culex* vector by being indoors at dusk. This recommendation assumes that houses are adequately sealed against mosquitoes. Repairing window screens may be an effective protective measure in poor neighborhoods where the risk of urban St. Louis encephalitis is highest.

An inactivated vaccine for Japanese B encephalitis derived from infected mouse brain was licensed for use in the USA in 1992. The same vaccine has been licensed and used successfully in Japan since 1954. The vaccine is recommended for travelers to Asia who will be in endemic areas for extended periods of time. Other killed-virus vaccines are not available for arboviruses in the USA. Attenuated live encephalitis virus vaccines continue to be investigated. A live-virus vaccine was used successfully to halt the severe epidemic of Venezuelan equine encephalitis in horses in Texas in 1971.

VENEZUELAN EQUINE ENCEPHALITIS

Venezuelan equine encephalitis is a mosquito-borne viral disease that produces primarily an undifferentiated febrile illness in humans and encephalitis in equines. It is caused by a togavirus, subgroup alphavirus. There is a partial cross-immunity between Venezuelan equine and eastern equine encephalitis.

Clinical Findings

Over 50% of equines infected develop central nervous system symptoms after an incubation period of 24–72 hours, while the remainder have an undifferentiated febrile illness. Symptoms include high fever, depression, diarrhea, anorexia, and weight loss. In nonfatal cases, the fever subsides and convalescence is protracted. In fatal cases, fever persists, weakness ensues, and the horse loses balance and dies within 2–4 days.

The disease in humans is influenza-like in about 97% of patients who develop symptoms and consists of high fever, headache, and severe myalgia. Convalescence is often prolonged. Encephalitis occurs in about 3%. A mortality rate of 0.5% has been reported, usually in younger patients who develop neurologic signs. Leukopenia is common in both equines and humans.

Laboratory Diagnosis

The virus may be isolated from whole blood, serum, nasopharyngeal washings, many organs, and occasionally the cerebrospinal fluid during the acute phase of the illness. Isolations are made by intracerebral inoculation of suckling mice or in cell cultures. The antibody response is similar to that found in other arbovirus diseases. Neutralizing and hemagglutination-inhibiting antibodies appear 2–3 weeks after onset but fall within 2–5 years. Serologic tests, listed in order of specificity, include Nt, CF, and HI. Cross-reactions with other alphaviruses are extensive using the HI test, although homologous titers are higher than the heterologous antibodies.

Epidemiology

The natural cycle for Venezuelan equine encephalitis involves mammals and mosquitoes. Birds and bats are susceptible. Humans are tangentially involved.

First reported in Venezuela in 1936, the disease gradually appeared in Panama and Mexico. In 1971, a severe epidemic occurred along the Texas-Mexico border, with the death of several thousand horses and the occurrence of several hundred human cases. In Florida, Venezuelan equine encephalitis is enzootic in rodents. Serologic evidence indicates that much subclinical human infection with this agent occurs in Florida, but clinical central nervous system disease is rare.

Control

Because of the presence of virulent Venezuelan equine encephalitis in Mexican border states, immunization of all equines (including revaccination of previously vaccinated equines) with an attenuated live-virus vaccine and local and aerial spraying of mosquitoes were begun on a routine basis in 1972. So far, these measures have proved effective in limiting spread of the disease. Strict quarantine to prevent movement of equines into areas free of the disease is also necessary. The attenuated Venezuelan equine encephalitis vaccine has been used experimentally in humans but is not available for general use.

BUNYAVIRUS ENCEPHALITIS

The California encephalitis virus complex comprises 14 antigenically related bunyaviruses, including La Crosse virus.

Clinical Findings & Diagnosis

The onset of California encephalitis viral infection is abrupt, typically with a severe bifrontal headache, a fever of 38–40 °C, sometimes vomiting, lethargy, and convulsions. Less frequently, there is only aseptic meningitis.

Histopathologic changes include neuronal degeneration and patchy inflammation, with perivascular cuffing and edema in the cerebral cortex and meninges.

The prognosis is excellent, although convalescence may be prolonged. Fatalities and neurologic sequelae are rare.

Serologic confirmation by HI, CF, or Nt tests is done on acute and convalescent specimens.

Epidemiology

These viruses were originally found in California, but they occur mainly in the Mississippi and Ohio River valleys, with scattered cases elsewhere. From 30 to 160 cases occur annually between July and September in the USA, particularly in the young (ages 4–14 years).

These viruses are probably transmitted between various woodland mosquitoes, primarily *Aedes triseriatus,* and small mammals such as squirrels and rabbits. Human infection is tangential. Overwintering in diapause eggs of the mosquito vector has been demonstrated. The virus is transmitted transovarially, and adult mosquitoes that develop from infected eggs can transmit the virus by bite.

OROPOUCHE FEVER

Oropouche virus is a member of the Simbu serologic group of bunyaviruses. It is a major cause of human febrile illness in Brazil. Outbreaks are frequent in urban centers in the eastern Amazon region. At least 220,000 persons were involved in 1978–1981, when the greatest wave yet recorded affected 19 localities. Outside the Amazon region, human infection caused by Oropouche virus has been documented only in Trinidad.

Three types of clinical syndromes have been associated with Oropouche virus infection: febrile illness, febrile illness with rash, and meningitis or meningismus. Many patients become severely ill, some to the point of prostration. The disease may be confused with malaria or other febrile conditions. The incubation period varies from 4 to 8 days. Fever, chills, severe headache, myalgias, arthralgia, dizziness, and photophobia are the most common clinical manifestations. Virtually all patients are viremic during the first 2 days of illness, but only 23% are still viremic on the fifth day.

Most of those infected develop clinical disease. In outbreaks in large cities, the distribution of virus is markedly uneven, whereas in small villages the agent is spread throughout. This pattern correlates with the distribution of the insect *Culicoides paraensis,* which is the main vector of Oropouche virus.

All outbreaks have occurred during the rainy season, and in several localities their decline has coincided with the end of this period. In some places, viral activity has been detected for a period of 6 months.

Oropouche virus probably occurs in nature in two distinct cycles: a jungle cycle (with the vector still unknown), which is responsible for maintaining the virus in nature, where primates, sloths, and possibly certain species of wild birds are implicated as vertebrate hosts; and an urban cycle, during which humans may be infected and, once infected, probably serve as an amplifying host of the virus among hematophagous insects.

Two insect species have been implicated as viral vectors in urban settings: the ceratopogonid midge *C paraensis* and the mosquito *C quinquefasciatus.* Transmission studies using hamsters have demonstrated that *C paraensis* is the more efficient of the two vectors. Furthermore, *C paraensis* can transmit the virus from humans to hamsters, which emphasizes the insect's role as a vector.

Methods for control of *C paraensis* are needed to prevent or interrupt epidemics, particularly in view of the increasing activity of the virus in urban centers of the eastern Amazon region and the report of an epidemic in 1981 in the western part of the Amazon region, where the large city of Manaus was extensively affected. It is also possible that Oropouche fever may spread to other areas, since *C paraensis* is widely distributed throughout South America, Central America, Mexico, and the eastern USA.

WEST NILE FEVER

West Nile fever is an acute, mild, febrile disease with lymphadenopathy and rash that occurs in the Middle East, tropical or subtropical Africa, and southwest Asia. It is caused by a flavivirus.

Clinical Findings

The virus is introduced through the bite of a *Culex* mosquito and produces viremia and a generalized systemic infection characterized by lymphadenopathy, sometimes with an accompanying maculopapular rash. Transitory meningeal involvement may occur during the acute stage. The virus may produce fatal encephalitis in older people, who have a delayed (and low) antibody response.

Laboratory Diagnosis

Virus can be recovered from blood taken in the acute stage of the infection. On paired serum specimens, complement-fixing, hemagglutination-inhibiting and neutralizing antibody titer rises may be diagnostic. Neutralizing antibodies persist longer than complement-fixing antibodies. During convalescence, heterologous complement-fixing and neutralizing antibodies develop to Japanese B and St. Louis encephalitis. The heterologous response is shorter and of lower titer than the homologous response.

Immunity

Only one antigenic type exists, and immunity is presumably permanent. Maternal antibodies are transferred from mother to offspring and disappear during the first 6 months of life.

Epidemiology & Control

Although West Nile fever appeared to be limited to the Middle East, antibodies to the virus have also been found in Africa, India, and Korea. In nonimmune populations, subclinical or clinical infections are common. In Cairo, 70% of persons over age 4 years have antibodies. In 1984, the virus was reported to have been isolated from the brains of three children who died of viral encephalitis.

The disease is more common in summer and more prevalent in rural than urban areas. The virus has been isolated from *Culex* mosquitoes during epidemics, and experimentally infected mosquitoes can transmit the virus. Mosquito abatement appears to be a logical, if unproved, control measure.

YELLOW FEVER

Yellow fever is an acute, febrile, mosquito-borne illness. Severe cases are characterized by jaundice, proteinuria, and hemorrhage. Yellow fever has been recognized as a serious health threat for many years. There was a resurgence of cases in the late 1980s, despite the availability of a safe and effective vaccine.

Yellow fever virus is a flavivirus. It multiplies in many different types of animals and in mosquitoes. It grows in embryonated chicks and in cell cultures made from chick embryos. Strains freshly isolated from humans, monkeys, or mosquitoes are pantropic, ie, the virus invades many cell types. Fresh strains usually produce a severe (often fatal) infection with marked damage to the livers of monkeys after parenteral inoculation. After serial passage in the brains of monkeys or mice, such strains lose much of their viscerotropism; they cause encephalitis after intracerebral injection but only asymptomatic infection after subcutaneous injection. Cross-immunity exists between the pantropic and neurotropic strains of the virus.

During the serial passage of a pantropic strain of yellow fever virus through tissue cultures, the relatively avirulent 17D strain was recovered. This strain lost its capacity to induce a viscerotropic or neurotropic disease in monkeys and in humans and has been used as a vaccine for over 40 years.

Pathogenesis & Pathology

Our understanding of the pathogenesis of yellow fever is based on work with the experimental infection in monkeys. The virus enters through the skin and then spreads to the local lymph nodes, where it multiplies. From the lymph nodes, it enters the circulating blood and becomes localized in the liver, spleen, kidney, bone marrow, and lymph glands, where it may persist for days.

The lesions of yellow fever are due to the localization and propagation of the virus in a particular organ. Death may result from necrotic lesions in the liver and kidney. The most frequent site of hemorrhage is the mucosa at the pyloric end of the stomach.

Distribution of necrosis in the liver may be spotty but is most evident in the mid zones of the lobules. Hyaline necrosis may be restricted to the cytoplasm; the hyaline masses are eosinophilic (Councilman bodies). Intranuclear eosinophilic inclusion bodies are also present and are of diagnostic value. During recovery, parenchymatous cells are replaced, and the liver may be completely restored.

In the kidney, there is fatty degeneration of the tubular epithelium. Degenerative changes also occur in the spleen, lymph nodes, and heart. Intranuclear, acidophilic inclusion bodies may be present in the nerve and glial cells of the brain. Perivascular infiltrations with mononuclear cells also occur in the brain.

Clinical Findings

The incubation period is 3–6 days. At the onset, the patient has fever, chills, headache, and backache, followed by nausea and vomiting. A short period of remission often follows the prodrome. On about the fourth day, the period of intoxication begins with a slow pulse (90–100) relative to a high fever and moderate jaundice. In severe cases, marked proteinuria and hemorrhagic manifestations appear. The vomitus may be black with altered blood. Lymphopenia is present. When the disease progresses to the severe stage (black vomitus and jaundice), the mortality rate is high. On the other hand, the infection may be so mild as to go unrecognized. Regardless of severity, there are no sequelae; patients either die or recover completely.

Laboratory Diagnosis

A. Recovery of Virus: The virus may be recovered from the blood up to the fifth day of the disease by intracerebral inoculation of mice. Isolated virus is identified by neutralization with specific antiserum.

B. Serology: Neutralizing antibodies develop early (by the fifth day) even in severe and fatal cases. In patients who survive the infection, circulating antibodies endure for life.

Complement-fixing antibodies are rarely found after mild infection or vaccination with the attenuated, live 17D strain. In severe infections, they appear later than neutralizing antibodies and disappear more rapidly.

The serologic response in yellow fever may be of two types. In **primary infections** of yellow fever, specific hemagglutination-inhibiting antibodies appear first, followed rapidly by antibodies to other flaviviruses. The titers of homologous hemagglutination-inhibiting antibodies are usually higher than those of heterologous antibodies. Complement-fixing and neutralizing antibodies rise slowly and are usually specific.

In **secondary infections** where yellow fever occurs in a patient previously infected with another flavivirus, hemagglutination-inhibiting and complement-fixing antibodies appear rapidly and to high titers. There is no suggestion of specificity. The highest hemagglutination-inhibiting and complement-fixing antibody titers are usually heterologous. Accurate diagnosis even by Nt test may be impossible.

Histopathologic examination of the liver in fatal cases is useful in those regions where the disease is endemic.

Immunity

Subtle antigenic differences exist between yellow fever strains isolated in different locations and between pantropic and vaccine (17D) strains. Monoclonal antibodies have been derived that can distinguish virulent and avirulent viruses.

An infant born of an immune mother has antibodies at birth that are gradually lost during the first 6 months of life. Reacquisition of similar antibodies is dependent upon the individual's exposure to the virus under natural conditions or by vaccination.

Epidemiology

Two major epidemiologic cycles of yellow fever are recognized: (1) classic (or urban) epidemic yellow fever and (2) sylvan (or jungle) yellow fever. Urban yellow fever involves person-to-person transmission by domestic *Aedes* mosquitoes. In the western hemisphere and west Africa, this species is primarily *Aedes aegypti,* which breeds in the accumulations of water that accompany human settlement. Mosquitoes remain close to houses and become infected by biting a viremic individual. Urban yellow fever is perpetuated in areas where there is a constant influx of susceptible persons, cases of yellow fever, and *A aegypti.* With use of intensive measures for mosquito abatement, the incidence of urban yellow fever has been markedly reduced in South America, even though 200–400 cases are recognized annually, mainly in persons occupationally exposed in forested areas. The disease is probably underreported. In Africa, epidemics involving forest mosquito vectors affect tens of thousands of humans at intervals of a few years, but only a few cases are officially reported.

Jungle yellow fever is primarily a disease of monkeys. In South America and Africa, it is transmitted from monkey to monkey by arboreal mosquitoes (ie, *Haemagogus, Aedes*) that inhabit the moist forest canopy. The infection in animals may be severe or inapparent. Persons such as woodcutters, nut-pickers, or road-builders come in contact with these mosquitoes in the forest and become infected. Jungle yellow fever may also occur when an infected monkey visits a human habitation and is bitten by *A aegypti,* which then transmits the virus to a human.

The virus multiplies in mosquitoes, which remain infectious for life. After the mosquito ingests a virus-containing blood meal, an interval of 12–14 days is required for it to become infectious. This interval is called the **extrinsic incubation period.**

All age groups are susceptible, but the disease in infants is milder than that in older groups. Large numbers of inapparent infections occur. Yellow fever has never been reported in India or the Orient, even though the vector, *A aegypti,* is widely distributed there.

New outbreaks continue to occur. The majority occur in Africa. The most recent resurgence of yellow fever in Africa occurred in the late 1980s. Over 8000 cases with 2200 deaths were reported in 1988–1990; the actual incidence and the number of deaths were certainly much higher, as only a small percentage of yellow fever cases are actually reported. Epidemics usually occur in a typical emergence zone for yellow fever: humid and semihumid savanna adjoining a rain forest where the sylvatic cycle is maintained in a large monkey population.

Such outbreaks indicate that yellow fever is a zoonosis that is difficult to control and is capable of causing unpredictable epidemics in human populations. A gradual increase in yellow fever cases has recently been observed in South America: 50 cases were reported in 1983, 125 in 1985, and 552 cases with 449 deaths during 1988–1990. Reported cases were chiefly from Peru, Bolivia, Brazil, and Colombia.

Yellow fever in the Americas continues to present epidemiologic features typical of its jungle cycle: most cases are in males aged 15–45 years and engaged in agricultural or forestry activities.

Yellow fever continues to infect and kill thousands of persons worldwide because they have failed to be immunized (see below). Annually, yellow fever strikes 200,000 persons, of whom about 30,000 die.

Control

Vigorous mosquito abatement programs have virtually eliminated urban yellow fever. The last reported outbreak of yellow fever in the USA occurred in 1905.

However, with the speed of modern air travel, the threat of a yellow fever outbreak exists wherever *A aegypti* is present. Most countries insist upon proper mosquito control on airplanes and vaccination of all persons at least 10 days before arrival in or from an endemic zone. The yellow fever vaccination requirement for travelers entering the USA was eliminated in 1972.

In 1978, a yellow fever outbreak occurred in Trinidad. Eight human cases and a number of infected forest monkeys were detected. The outbreak was quickly stopped by a mass immunization campaign and *A aegypti* control measures.

An excellent attenuated live-virus vaccine is available in the 17D strain. Vaccine is prepared in eggs and dispensed as a dried powder. It is a live virus and must be kept cold. It is rehydrated just before use and injected subcutaneously by skin scarification or by jet injector. A single dose produces a good antibody response in over 95% of vaccinated persons that persists for at least 10 years. After vaccination, the virus multiplies and may be isolated from the blood before antibodies develop.

The virulent Asibi strain of yellow fever virus has been sequenced and its sequence compared to that of the 17D vaccine strain, which was derived from it. These two strains differ by more than 240 passages. The two RNA genomes (10,862 nucleotides long) differ at 68 nucleotide positions, resulting in a total of 32 amino acid differences. It should be possible to determine the specific genetic changes responsible for loss of virulence.

DENGUE (Breakbone Fever)

Dengue is a mosquito-borne infection characterized by fever, muscle and joint pain, lymphadenopathy, and rash. It is caused by a flavivirus. Dengue and yellow fever viruses are antigenically related, but this does not result in significant cross-immunity.

Pathogenesis & Pathology

Viremia is present at the onset of fever and may persist for 3 days. The histopathologic lesion is in small blood vessels, with endothelial swelling, perivascular edema, and infiltration with mononuclear cells.

Clinical Findings

The onset of fever may be sudden or there may be prodromal symptoms of malaise, chills, and headache. Pains soon develop, especially in the back, joints, muscles, and eyeballs. The temperature returns to normal after 5–6 days or may subside on about the third day and rise again about 5–8 days after onset ("saddle-back" form). A rash (maculopapular or scarlatiniform) may appear on the third or fourth day and last for 24–72 hours, fading with desquamation. Lymph nodes are frequently enlarged. Leukopenia with a relative lymphocytosis is a regular occurrence. Convalescence may take weeks, although complications and death are rare. Especially in young children, dengue may be a mild febrile illness lasting 1–3 days.

A more severe syndrome—dengue hemorrhagic fever—may occur in individuals (usually children) with passively acquired (as maternal antibody) or endogenously produced heterologous dengue antibody. Although initial symptoms simulate normal dengue, the patient's condition abruptly worsens and is associated with hypoproteinemia, thrombocytopenia, prolonged bleeding time, and elevated prothrombin time. Dengue shock syndrome, characterized by shock and hemoconcentration, may supervene. These altered manifestations of dengue have been observed, often in epidemic form, in the Philippines, Southeast Asia, and India—regions in which several dengue serotypes are regularly present; the mortality rate is 5–10%. In studies of the dengue diseases in Southeast Asia, where most cases of dengue hemorrhagic fever, with or without shock, occur, it was found that the acute vascular permeability syndrome occurred more frequently when dengue type 2 was the secondary infecting virus and the patient was a female aged 3 years or older. In 1981, more than 40 deaths from type 2 dengue occurred in Cuba as a result of hemorrhage and shock. That outbreak established that blacks are relatively resistant to the hemorrhagic fever–shock syndrome. The pathogenesis of the severe syndrome is not understood, but it seems to involve preexisting dengue antibody. It is postulated that virus-antibody complexes are formed within a few days of the second dengue infection and that they activate the complement system and lead to the disseminated intravascular coagulation seen in the hemorrhagic fever syndrome.

Laboratory Diagnosis

Isolation of the virus is difficult. Injection of early fresh serum into mice rarely produces disease, but the animals may subsequently be immune to challenge. Dengue viruses often grow in cell cultures.

Neutralizing and hemagglutination-inhibiting antibodies appear within 7 days of onset of dengue fever and complement-fixing antibodies somewhat later. Homotypic antibodies tend to reach higher titers than heterotypic ones.

Immunity

At least four antigenic types of the virus exist.

Reinfection with a virus of a different serotype 2–3 months after the primary attack may give rise to a short, mild illness without a rash. Mosquitoes feeding on these reinfected patients can transmit the disease.

Epidemiology

The known geographic distribution of dengue viruses today is India, Southeast Asia, China, Japan and the Pacific Islands, the Hawaiian and Caribbean Islands, Central and South America, Africa, and the Middle East. Dengue has occurred in the southern

USA (1934) and in Australia. Most subtropical and tropical regions around the world where *Aedes* vectors exist are endemic or potentially endemic areas. For example, more than 500,000 cases of dengue occurred in Colombia in 1972 following reinfestation of the Atlantic coastal areas by *A aegypti*. More than 100,000 cases occurred in 1981 in Cuba.

The infectious cycle is as follows:

$$\begin{array}{ccccccc} \textbf{\textit{Aedes}} & \rightarrow & \textbf{Human} & \rightarrow & \textbf{\textit{Aedes}} & \rightarrow & \textbf{Human} \\ & \nearrow & & \nearrow & & \nearrow & \\ \textbf{\textit{Aedes}} & \rightarrow & \textbf{Monkey} & \rightarrow & \textbf{\textit{Aedes}} & \rightarrow & \textbf{Monkey} \end{array}$$

A aegypti is a domestic mosquito; *Aedes albopictus* exists in the bush or jungle and may be responsible for maintaining the infection among monkeys.

In urban communities, dengue epidemics are explosive and involve appreciable portions of the population. They often start during the rainy season, when the vector mosquito, *A aegypti,* is abundant. The mosquito has a short flight range, and urban spread of dengue is frequently house-to-house. The mosquito breeds in tropical or semitropical climates in artificial water-holding receptacles around human habitation or in tree holes or plants close to human dwellings. It apparently prefers the blood of humans to that of other animals. Since *A aegypti* is also the vector of yellow fever, the outbreak of dengue in the Caribbean serves as a warning of even more serious epidemics. Epidemics can be controlled by aerial spraying to kill adult mosquitoes and by treatment of breeding sites to kill larvae.

A aegypti is the primary vector mosquito for dengue in the western hemisphere. The female acquires the virus by feeding upon a viremic human. Mosquitoes are infective after a period of 8–14 days (extrinsic incubation time). In humans, clinical disease begins 2–15 days after an infective mosquito bite. Once infective, a mosquito probably remains so for the remainder of her life (1–3 months or more). Dengue virus is not passed from one generation of mosquitoes to the next. In the tropics, mosquito breeding throughout the year maintains the disease.

Epidemics of dengue are usually observed when the virus is newly introduced into an area or if susceptible persons move into an endemic area. The endemic dengue in the Caribbean and Mexico is a constant threat to the USA, where *A aegypti* mosquitoes are prevalent in the summer months.

World War II was responsible for the spread of dengue from Southeast Asia to Japan and the Pacific Islands. In 1977, a dengue type 1 virus was isolated from mosquitoes and from patients in Jamaica, from where it spread to the Bahamas, Trinidad, Cuba, and the USA. This was the first time type 1 virus had been isolated in the western hemisphere.

In 1979, an epidemic of dengue type 4 broke out on Tahiti, the first known appearance of type 4 outside Southeast Asia. There were 6800 reported cases on the island (population 97,000). In 1981, dengue type 4 was first recognized in the western hemisphere, with the first cases in the French Antilles (contacts from French Polynesia) and then a spread to other islands, including Puerto Rico, Jamaica, Haiti, Trinidad, and St. Thomas. The virus has also been found on the mainland of Central America and South America.

Concurrent with the increased epidemic activity of dengue in the tropics, there has been an increase in the number of cases imported into the USA. Many of these cases continue to be imported into states where competent mosquito vectors are found, underscoring the need for effective surveillance, especially during periods of increased dengue activity in the tropics.

A albopictus, a mosquito of Asian origin, was discovered in Texas in 1985; by 1989 it had spread throughout the southeastern USA, where *A aegypti,* the principal vector of dengue virus, is prevalent. However, *A aegypti* cannot overwinter in northern states; this is in contrast to *A albopictus,* which can overwinter as far as 42 °N and in summer can extend much farther north, increasing the risk of epidemic dengue in the USA.

Control

Control depends upon antimosquito measures, eg, elimination of breeding places and the use of insecticides. A number of laboratories are now approaching dengue vaccines through molecular virology.

SANDFLY FEVER

Sandfly fever is a mild, insect-borne disease that occurs commonly in countries bordering the Mediterranean Sea and in Russia, Iran, Pakistan, India, Panama, Brazil, and Trinidad. The sandfly *Phlebotomus papatasii* is present in endemic areas between 20 and 45 degrees of latitude. Sandfly fever (also called *Phlebotomus* fever) is caused by a bunyavirus.

Clinical Findings

In humans, the bite of the sandfly results in small itching papules on the skin that persist for up to 5 days. The disease begins abruptly after an incubation period of 3–6 days. For 24 hours before and 24 hours after the onset of fever, the virus is found in the blood. Clinical features consist of headache, malaise, nausea, fever, conjunctival injection, photophobia, stiffness of the neck and back, abdominal pain, and leukopenia. All patients recover. There is no specific treatment. The pathology in humans is not known.

Laboratory Diagnosis

The diagnosis is usually made on clinical grounds. It may be confirmed by demonstrating a rise in antibody titer in paired serum specimens by Nt or HI tests.

Immunity

There are at least 20 separate antigenic types, but only five appear to cause human illness. Immunity is specific for each type and persists for at least 2 years.

Epidemiology

The disease is transmitted by the female sandfly, a midge only a few millimeters in size. In the tropics, the sandfly is prevalent all year; in cooler climates, only during the warm seasons. Transovarial transmission may occur.

The extrinsic incubation period in the sandfly is about 1 week. The insect feeds at night; during the day, it may be found in dark places (cracks in walls, caves, houses, and tree trunks). Eggs are laid a few days after a blood meal. About 5 weeks are required for the eggs to develop into winged insects. The adult lives only a few weeks in hot weather.

In endemic areas, infection is common in childhood. When nonimmune adults (eg, troops) arrive, large outbreaks can occur among the new arrivals and are occasionally mistaken for malaria.

Control

Sandflies are most common just above the ground. Because of their small size, they can pass through ordinary screens and mosquito nets. Their flight range is up to 200 yards. Prevention of disease in endemic areas relies on use of insect repellents during the night and residual insecticides in and around living quarters.

RIFT VALLEY FEVER

The agent of this disease, a bunyavirus of the phlebovirus subgroup, is pathogenic primarily for sheep and other domestic animals. Humans are secondarily infected during the course of epizootics in domesticated animals in Africa and the Middle East. Infection among laboratory workers is common.

Clinical features are similar to those of dengue: acute onset, fever, prostration, pain in the extremities and joints, and gastrointestinal distress. The temperature curve is like that of dengue and yellow fever (saddle back type). There is a marked leukopenia. The disease is short-lived, and recovery almost always is complete.

The virus can be isolated from human blood early in the disease. Complement-fixing, neutralizing, and hemagglutination-inhibiting antibodies develop and persist for years.

Rift Valley fever was believed to be relatively benign for humans until 1977, when it spread to Egypt. There it caused enormous losses of sheep and cattle, and thousands of human cases occurred, with 600 deaths. Although mosquitoes are known to transmit the virus in epizootics and epidemics, the reservoir of the virus in nature and the means of interepizootic maintenance are unknown. Vaccination of livestock with available killed-virus or attenuated live-virus vaccines should prevent transmission to both humans and animals. Movement of animals should be restricted when an epizootic is in progress. Rift Valley fever can be expected to spread from Africa to countries of the Mediterranean basin and southwest Asia.

COLORADO TICK FEVER

Colorado tick fever, also called mountain fever or tick fever, is a mild febrile disease, without rash, that is transmitted by a tick. It is caused by a coltivirus (Table 38–1). During the acute stage, the virus is present in the blood and can be isolated in cell culture or suckling mice. It appears to be antigenically distinct from other known viruses. The pathologic features of the disease in humans are unknown, since the disease is self-limited.

Clinical Findings

The incubation period is 4–6 days. The disease has a sudden onset with chilly sensations and myalgia. Symptoms include headache, deep ocular pain, muscle and joint pains, lumbar backache, and nausea and vomiting. The temperature is usually diphasic. After the first bout of 2 days, the patient may feel well. Symptoms and fever then reappear and last 3–4 more days.

Laboratory Diagnosis

The virus may be isolated from whole blood by inoculation of suckling mice. Viremia may persist for 2 weeks. Specific neutralizing and complement-fixing antibodies appear in the second week of illness and persist for years.

Immunity

Only one antigenic type is known. A single infection is believed to produce lasting immunity.

Epidemiology

Colorado tick fever is limited to areas where the wood tick *Dermacentor andersoni* is distributed, primarily Colorado, Oregon, Utah, Idaho, Montana, and Wyoming. Patients have been in a tick-infested area 4–5 days before onset of symptoms, and in many cases ticks are found attached to the patient, as their bite is painless. Cases occur chiefly in adult males, the group with greatest exposure to ticks.

D andersoni collected in nature can carry the virus. This tick is a true reservoir, and the virus is transmitted transovarially by the adult female. Natural infection occurs in rodents, which act as hosts for immature stages of the tick.

Control

The disease can be prevented by avoiding tick-infested areas and by using protective clothing or repellent chemicals. An experimental live-virus vaccine has been made.

RODENT-BORNE HEMORRHAGIC FEVERS

The zoonotic rodent-borne hemorrhagic fevers include Korean (Hantaan virus), South American (Junin and Machupo viruses), and Lassa fevers. Although the natural reservoir and mode of transmission of Marburg and Ebola viruses (African hemorrhagic fever) are not known, it is strongly suspected that they are harbored by rodents.

Common clinical features of the epidemic hemorrhagic fevers include fever; petechiae or purpura; gastrointestinal, nasal, and uterine bleeding; leukopenia; hypotension; shock; proteinuria; thrombocytopenia; and central nervous system signs, often ending in death.

In 1993 an outbreak of severe respiratory illness in the USA, now designated the hantavirus pulmonary syndrome, was found to be caused by a novel hantavirus. This agent is the first hantavirus recognized to cause disease in North America and the first to cause primarily an adult respiratory distress syndrome.

HEMORRHAGIC FEVER WITH RENAL SYNDROME (Hantaan Virus)

Hemorrhagic fever with renal syndrome is an acute viral infection that causes an interstitial nephritis that can lead to acute renal insufficiency and renal failure in the clinically severe forms of the disease that occur in Asia, particularly in Korea. Generalized hemorrhage and shock may occur, with a case-fatality rate of 10%. In a milder clinical form—nephropathia epidemica, which is prevalent in Scandinavia—the interstitial nephritis generally resolves without hemorrhagic complications, and fatalities are rare.

Hantaan virus is classified as a bunyavirus. More than 2000 cases of hemorrhagic fever with renal syndrome occurred among United Nations troops during the Korean war, but Hantaan virus was isolated only in 1976. The agent was recovered in Korea from *Apodemus agrarius,* a rodent previously shown by epidemiologic investigations to be associated with transmission of epidemic hemorrhagic fever. In the 1980s, hemorrhagic fever with renal syndrome caused by Hantaan virus has been recognized in different areas of France.

Hemorrhagic fever with renal syndrome is not restricted to rural areas where infected field and sylvatic rodents constitute the animal-host reservoir. Urban rats are now known to be persistently infected with Hantaan virus, and it has been suggested that rats on trading ships may have dispersed hantaviruses worldwide. Serosurveys indicated that rats in the USA also were infected with a Hantaan-related virus, and this virus has recently been isolated from a domestic rat, *Rattus norvegicus.* Infected laboratory rats were proved to be sources of Hantaan outbreaks in scientific institutes in Europe and Asia. Hantaan-related infections have not been detected in laboratory rats raised in the USA. However, Hantaan virus-related infections have occurred in persons whose occupations place them in contact with seropositive rats. For example, 6% of longshoremen in Baltimore had neutralizing antibody to Hantaan virus.

HANTAVIRUS PULMONARY SYNDROME

A newly recognized hantavirus was identified as the etiologic agent of an outbreak of severe respiratory distress that occurred in the southwestern USA in 1993. Since that time, cases have been identified from a wide geographic area in the USA.

Of 53 persons with confirmed cases of hantavirus pulmonary syndrome in 1993, 32 (60%) died. This case-fatality rate is substantially higher than that of other hantavirus infections. Patient ages ranged from 12 to 69 years, and males and females were equally affected. The disease is characterized by prodromal fever, myalgia, and other symptoms, including cough, headache, and nausea and vomiting, followed by rapidly progressive pulmonary edema. There are no signs of hemorrhage. The pathogenesis of the pulmonary findings is not known but may reflect an increased permeability of pulmonary capillaries. Hantaviral antigens were widespread in patients, being detected in the endothelium of lung, heart, kidney, pancreas, and skeletal muscle tissue.

The virus has been isolated; it is a new virus in the bunyavirus family, most closely related genetically to the Prospect Hill strain of hantavirus. The primary reservoir of the virus, the deer mouse *(Peromyscus maniculatus),* is widespread throughout the USA. Thirty percent of the mice tested in the southwestern USA were seropositive for hantaviral antibodies. It is presumed that human infections were acquired by inhalation of dust containing rodent excreta, as hantaviruses are shed in saliva, urine, and feces from infected rodents. Person-to-person transmission of hantaviruses is thought not to occur.

Current therapy for hantavirus pulmonary syndrome consists of maintenance of adequate oxygenation and support of hemodynamic functioning. Intravenous ribavirin is being investigated as possible therapy. Preventive measures are based on rodent control and avoidance of contact with rodents and rodent droppings.

AFRICAN HEMORRHAGIC FEVERS (Marburg & Ebola Viruses)

Marburg and Ebola viruses are members of the filovirus family (Figure 38–1). They cause acute diseases characterized by high fever, with bleeding into skin (petechiae, purpura) and from the nose, gastrointestinal tract, and genitourinary tract; thrombocytopenia; and marked toxicity, often leading to shock and death. Marburg virus disease was recognized in 1967 among laboratory workers exposed to tissues of African green monkeys *(Cercopithecus aethiops)* imported into Germany and Yugoslavia. Transmission from patients to medical personnel occurred, with high mortality rates.

There have been no cases since then in Europe or the USA, but antibody surveys have indicated that the virus is present in east Africa and causes infection in monkeys and humans.

Marburg virus has been isolated in guinea pigs and various cell culture systems. The viral particle contains RNA and has a cylindrical or filamentous shape by electron microscopy. It superficially resembles a rhabdovirus but has no antigenic relationship with any known virus. Experimentally inoculated monkeys developed a uniformly fatal disease resembling hemorrhagic fever in humans.

Treatment is directed at maintaining renal function and electrolyte balance and combating hemorrhage and shock. Transfusion of convalescent plasma may have some benefit. Extreme care is needed to prevent exposure of medical personnel to blood, saliva, and urine of patients.

In 1976, two severe epidemics of hemorrhagic fever occurred in Sudan and Zaire. The virus responsible, provisionally named Ebola virus after a river in Zaire, resembles Marburg virus morphologically but is antigenically distinct. The outbreaks involved more than 500 cases and at least 400 deaths due to clinical hemorrhagic fever. The illness was marked by a sudden onset of severe headache, fever, muscle pains, and prostration, quickly followed by profuse diarrhea and vomiting. In each outbreak, hospital staff became infected through close and prolonged contact with patients, their blood, or their excreta. In one hospital, 41 of 76 infected staff members died.

It is probable that Marburg and Ebola viruses have a reservoir host, perhaps a rodent, and become transmitted to humans only accidentally. Human infection, however, is highly communicable to human contacts. By means of rapid travel, such diseases may spread to distant nonendemic areas and present a risk.

Because the natural reservoirs of Marburg and Ebola viruses are still unknown, no control activities can be organized. Hospital spread has been a marked feature of both diseases, and management of patients therefore requires special attention. Patients should be nursed in medical units in the locality where the cases occur. A team trained in the techniques of barrier nursing and management of infectious patients should be available.

In late 1989, infections caused by a filovirus closely related to Ebola virus were detected in cynomolgus monkeys *(Macaca fascicularis)* imported into the USA from the Philippines and held in a private quarantine facility in Virginia. The infection spread to only a few of the 149 persons who came in contact with the infected monkeys or their tissues, but none of the workers became sick, indicating that the virus was not as virulent as Ebola virus. Personnel involved in the transit and care of nonhuman primates should be instructed about the potential hazards of handling such animals.

LASSA FEVER

The first recognized cases of this disease occurred in 1969 among Americans stationed in the Nigerian village of Lassa. Lassa virus is extremely virulent: the mortality rate was 36–67% in four documented epidemics in west Africa involving about 100 cases. In western and central Africa, the annual toll includes about 300,000 infections and 5000 deaths. Lassa virus is active in all western African countries situated between Senegal and Zaire. In Sierra Leone, Lassa fever accounts for 10% of all febrile patients admitted to hospitals and for almost 2% of the general mortality rate. In some areas, Lassa virus has infected about 50% of the population—more than malaria, which is generally believed to be the chief killer in Africa.

Lassa fever can involve almost all the organ systems, although symptoms may vary in the individual patient. The disease is characterized by very high fever, mouth ulcers, severe muscle aches, skin rash with hemorrhages, pneumonia, and heart and kidney damage. Benign, febrile cases do occur. The virus can be isolated from the patient's blood in Vero monkey cell cultures.

Lassa virus is an arenavirus (see Chapter 29). Four arenaviruses cause human disease—Lassa, lymphocytic choriomeningitis, Junin, and Machupo. They can be distinguished by immunofluorescent antibody tests.

Lassa virus seems to be transmitted by human-to-human contact and also to have a nonhuman cycle. A house rat *(Mastomys natalensis)* is the principal rodent reservoir of Lassa virus. When the virus spreads within a hospital, human contact is the mode of transmission. Meticulous barrier nursing procedures and universal precautions to avoid contact with virus-contaminated blood and body fluids can prevent transmission to hospital personnel.

Until 1986, the only available therapy for Lassa fever used hyperimmune serum from recovered patients. The antiviral drug ribavirin has since been shown to be an effective treatment, particularly if it is given early in the disease process.

A potential vaccine is under study. A vaccinia virus recombinant that expressed the nucleocapsid gene of Lassa virus was constructed. Guinea pigs immunized with the recombinant virus were protected against challenge with Lassa virus, whereas control animals showed the usual disease course, including pyrexia, anorexia, viremia, and death. It is of interest that the only part of the virus needed to mediate this protective immune response was the internal protein component.

SOUTH AMERICAN HEMORRHAGIC FEVERS (Junin & Machupo Viruses)

Junin hemorrhagic fever is a major public health problem in certain agricultural areas of Argentina; over 18,000 cases were reported between 1958 and 1980, with a mortality rate of 10–15% in untreated patients. A gradual increase in the endemic area of this hemorrhagic fever has been observed since 1958. The disease has a marked seasonal variation, and the infection occurs almost exclusively among workers in maize and wheat fields who are exposed to the reservoir rodent, *Calomys musculinus.*

Junin virus produces both humoral and cell-mediated immunodepression; deaths due to Junin hemorrhagic fever may be related to an inability to initiate a cell-mediated immune response. Administration of convalescent human plasma to patients during the first week of illness reduced the mortality rate from 15% to 1%. Were it not for the humoral immunodepression regularly induced by Junin virus and the related Machupo virus, the infection in humans would be no more than a brief, nonspecific illness.

The first outbreak of Machupo hemorrhagic fever was identified in Bolivia in 1962. It is estimated that 2000–3000 persons were affected by the disease, with a case-fatality rate of 20%. A small nosocomial outbreak involving six persons, five of whom died, was reported in 1971.

An effective rodent control program directed against infected *Calomys callosus,* the host of Machupo virus, was undertaken in Bolivia, and as a result no human cases of Machupo hemorrhagic fever have been recorded since 1974.

REFERENCES

Advisory Committee on Immunization Practices: Inactivated Japanese encephalitis virus vaccine. Morb Mortal Wkly Rep 1993;42(Suppl RR-1).

Brandt WE: Current approaches to the development of dengue vaccines and related aspects of the molecular biology of flaviviruses. J Infect Dis 1988;157:1105.

Brès PL: A century of progress in combating yellow fever. Bull WHO 1986;64:775.

Cosgrif TM (editor): International symposium on hemostatic impairment associated with hemorrhagic fever viruses. Rev Infect Dis 1989;11:S669.

Duchin JS et al: Hantavirus pulmonary syndrome: A clinical description of 17 patients with a newly recognized disease. N Engl J Med 1994;330:949.

Elliott RM: Molecular biology of the Bunyaviridae. J Gen Virol 1990;71:501.

Fulhorst CF et al: Natural vertical transmission of western equine encephalomyelitis virus in mosquitoes. Science 1994;263:676.

George S et al: Isolation of West Nile virus from the brains of children who had died of encephalitis. Bull WHO 1984;62:879.

Hahn CS et al: Western equine encephalitis virus is a recombinant virus. Proc Natl Acad Sci USA 1988;85:5997.

Halstead SB: The XXth century dengue pandemic: Need for surveillance and research. World Health Stat Q 1992;45: 292.

Holmes GP et al: Lassa fever in the United States: Investigation of a case and new guidelines for management. N Engl J Med 1990;323:1120.

Lanciotti RS et al: Molecular evolution and epidemiology of dengue-3 viruses. J Gen Virol 1994;75:65.

Lee HW, van der Groen G: Hemorrhagic fever with renal syndrome. Prog Med Virol 1989;36:62.

Levine B, Hardwick JM, Griffin DE: Persistence of alphaviruses in vertebrate hosts. Trends Microbiol 1994; 2:25.

Luby JP: St. Louis encephalitis. Epidemiol Rev 1979;1:55.

McCormick JB et al: Lassa fever: Effective therapy with ribavirin. N Engl J Med 1986;314:20.

Monath TP et al: Immunoglobulin M antibody capture enzyme-linked immunosorbent assay for diagnosis of St. Louis encephalitis. J Clin Microbiol 1984;20:784.

Nichol ST et al: Genetic identification of a hantavirus associated with an outbreak of acute respiratory illness. Science 1993;262:914.

Rice CM et al: Nucleotide sequence of yellow fever virus: Implications for flavivirus gene expression and evolution. Science 1985;229:726.

Sangkawibha N et al: Risk factors in dengue shock syndrome: A prospective epidemiologic study in Rayong, Thailand. 1. The 1980 outbreak. Am J Epidemiol 1984; 120:653.

Shope RE, Peters CJ, Davies FG: The spread of Rift Valley fever and approaches to its control. Bull WHO 1982;60: 299.

Theiler M, Downs WG: *The Arthropod-Borne Viruses of Vertebrates: An Account of the Rockefeller Foundation Virus Program, 1951–1970.* Yale Univ Press, 1973.

Tsai TF, Monath TP: Viral diseases in North America transmitted by arthropods or from vertebrate reservoirs. In: *Textbook of Pediatric Infectious Diseases,* 2nd ed. 2 vols. Feigin RD, Cherry JD (editors). Saunders, 1987.

Orthomyxoviruses (Influenza Viruses)

39

Respiratory illnesses are responsible for more than half of all acute illnesses each year in the USA. The **Orthomyxoviridae** (influenza viruses) are a major determinant of morbidity and mortality caused by respiratory disease, and outbreaks of infection sometimes occur in worldwide epidemics. Influenza has been responsible for millions of deaths worldwide during this century. The mutability and high frequency of genetic reassortment characteristic of orthomyxoviruses and resultant antigenic changes in the viral surface glycoproteins make influenza viruses formidable challenges for control efforts. Influenza type A is highly variable antigenically and is responsible for most cases of epidemic influenza. Influenza type B may exhibit antigenic changes and sometimes causes epidemics. Influenza type C is antigenically stable and causes only mild illness.

PROPERTIES OF ORTHOMYXOVIRUSES

All known orthomyxoviruses are influenza viruses. Three immunologic types are known, designated A, B, and C. Antigenic changes continually occur within the type A group of influenza viruses and to a lesser degree in the type B group, whereas type C appears to be antigenically stable. Influenza A strains are also known for pigs, horses, and birds. Some of the strains isolated from animals are antigenically similar to strains circulating in the human population.

The following descriptions are based on influenza virus type A, the best-characterized type (Table 39–1).

Distinction From Paramyxoviruses

The term "myxovirus" implies an affinity for mucins and originally denoted a large group of enveloped viruses able to attach to glycoprotein cell surface receptors. These viruses have now been separated into two distinct groups—the orthomyxoviruses and the paramyxoviruses—because of fundamental differences in their structures and their patterns of replication (Table 39–2). The orthomyxoviruses are considered here, and the paramyxoviruses are discussed in Chapter 40.

Structure & Composition

Influenza virus particles are usually spherical and about 100 nm in diameter, although virions may display great variation in size (Figure 39–1). Long filamentous forms up to several micrometers in length are commonly observed during early passages of new isolates.

The single-stranded RNA genomes of influenza A and B viruses occur as eight separate segments. Sizes and protein-coding assignments are known for all the segments (Table 39–3). Most of the segments code for a single protein. Because of the segmented nature of the genome, when a cell is coinfected by two different viruses of a given type, mixtures of parental gene segments may be assembled into progeny virions. This phenomenon, called **genetic reassortment,** may result in sudden changes in viral surface antigens—a property that explains the epidemiologic features of influenza and poses significant problems for vaccine development (described below).

Influenza virus particles contain seven different structural proteins. Three large proteins (PB1, PB2, and PA) are bound to the viral RNA and are responsible for RNA transcription and replication. The nucleoprotein (NP) associates with the viral RNA to form a structure 9 nm in diameter that assumes a helical configuration. The matrix (M) protein, which forms a shell underneath the viral lipid envelope, is important in particle morphogenesis and is a major component of the virion (about 40% of viral protein).

A lipid envelope derived from the cell surrounds the viral particle. Two virus-encoded glycoproteins, the hemagglutinin (HA) and the neuraminidase (NA), are inserted into the envelope and are exposed as spikes about 10 nm long on the surface of the particle. These two surface glycoproteins are the important antigens that determine antigenic variation of influenza viruses and host immunity. The HA represents about 25% of viral protein.

Influenza viruses are relatively hardy and may be stored at 0–4 °C for weeks without loss of viability. The virus loses infectivity more rapidly at −20 °C than at +4 °C. Ether and protein denaturants destroy infectivity. The hemagglutinin and internal antigens are more stable to inactivation than the infective virus; both infectivity and hemagglutination are

Table 39–1. Important properties of orthomyxoviruses.

Virion: Spherical, pleomorphic, 80–120 nm in diameter (helical nucleocapsid, 9 nm).
Composition: RNA (1%), protein (73%), lipid (20%), carbohydrate (6%).
Genome: Single-stranded RNA, segmented (8 molecules), negative-sense, total MW 5 million.
Proteins: Seven structural proteins.
Envelope: Contains viral hemagglutinin (HA) and neuraminidase (NA) proteins.
Replication: Nuclear transcription; capped 5′ termini of cellular RNA scavenged as primers; particles mature by budding from plasma membrane.
Outstanding characteristics: Genetic reassortment is common. Influenza viruses cause worldwide epidemics.

more resistant to inactivation at alkaline pH than at acid pH.

Classification & Nomenclature

Antigenic differences exhibited by two of the internal structural proteins, the NP and M proteins, are used to divide influenza viruses into types A, B, and C. These proteins possess no cross-reactivity among the three types. Antigenic variations in the surface glycoproteins, HA and NA, are used to subtype the viruses.

The standard nomenclature system for influenza virus isolates includes the following information: type, host of origin, geographic origin, strain number, and year of isolation. Antigenic descriptions of the HA and the NA are given in parentheses for type A. The host of origin is not indicated for human isolates, eg, A/Hong Kong/03/68(H3N2), but it is for others, eg, A/swine/Iowa/15/30(H1N1).

So far, 14 subtypes of HA (H1–H14) and nine subtypes of NA (N1–N9), in many different combinations, have been recovered from birds, animals, or humans. Three HA (H1–H3) and two NA (N1, N2) subtypes have been recovered from humans.

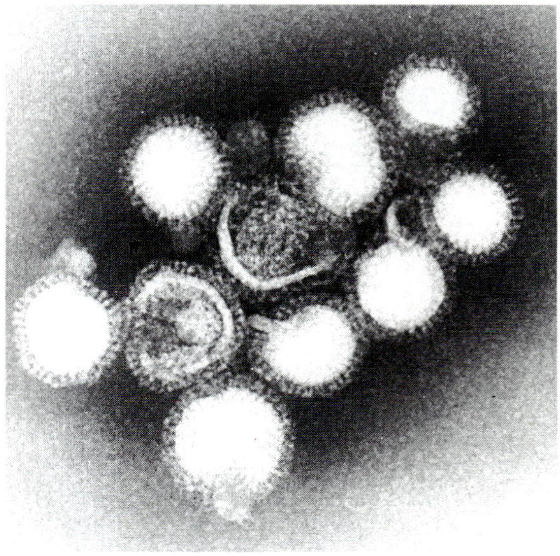

Figure 39–1. Influenza virus A/Hong Kong/1/68(H3N2). Note pleomorphic shapes and glycoprotein projections covering particle surfaces (315,000×). (FA Murphy and EL Palmer.)

Table 39–2. Differences between orthomyxoviruses and paramyxoviruses.

Property	Orthomyxoviruses	Paramyxoviruses
Diseases caused in humans	Influenza types A, B, and C	Parainfluenza 1–4 infections, respiratory syncytial disease, mumps, measles
Genome organization	Single-stranded RNA in eight pieces	Single-stranded RNA in single piece
Inner ribonucleoprotein helix	9 nm in diameter	18 nm in diameter
Transcription of viral RNA	Host cell nucleus	Host cell cytoplasm
Genetic reassortment	Frequent	Rare
Rate of antigenic change	High	Low

Structure & Function of the Hemagglutinin

The HA protein of influenza virus has been studied in great detail because of its biologic significance. It binds viral particles to susceptible cells and is the major antigen against which neutralizing (protective) antibodies are directed; variability in it is primarily responsible for the continual evolution of new strains and subsequent influenza epidemics. The HA derives its name from its ability to agglutinate erythrocytes under certain conditions.

The complete amino acid sequence for HA has been calculated from the sequence of cloned DNA copies of the HA gene, and the 3-dimensional structure of the protein has been revealed by x-ray crystallography. It is now possible to correlate functions of the HA molecule with its structure.

The primary sequence of HA contains 566 amino acids (Figure 39–2A). A short signal sequence at the amino terminus inserts the polypeptide into the endoplasmic reticulum; the signal is then removed. The HA protein is cleaved into two subunits, HA1 and HA2, that remain tightly associated by a disulfide bridge. A hydrophobic stretch near the carboxy terminus of HA2 anchors the HA molecule in the membrane, with a short hydrophilic tail extending into the cytoplasm. Oligosaccharide residues are added at several sites.

The HA molecule is folded into a complex structure (Figure 39–2B). Each linked HA1 and HA2 dimer

Table 39–3. Coding assignments of influenza virus A RNA segments.[1]

Genome Segment Number[2]	Encoded Polypeptide			
	Designation	Molecular Weight[3]	Approximate Number of Molecules per Virion	Function
1	PB2	96,000	30–60	RNA transcriptase components
2	PB1	87,000		
3	PA	85,000		
4	HA	≃75,000	500	Hemagglutinin; trimer; envelope glycoprotein; mediates virus attachment to cells
5	NP	56,000	1000	Associated with RNA and polymerase proteins; helical structure
6	NA	≃56,000	100	Neuraminidase; tetramer; envelope glycoprotein; enzyme
7	M_1	28,000	3000	Matrix protein; major component of virion; lines inside of envelope; involved in assembly
	M_2	15,000	0	Nonstructural; ion channel; from spliced mRNA
8	NS_1	26,000	0	Nonstructural; function unknown
	NS_2	14,000	0	Nonstructural; function unknown; from spliced mRNA

[1]Adapted from Lamb RA, Choppin PW: Annu Rev Biochem 1983;**52**:467.
[2]RNA segments are numbered in order of decreasing size.
[3]Estimated by gel electrophoresis. The molecular weights of the two glycoproteins, HA and NA, are for the glycosylated monomeric polypeptides.

forms an elongated stalk capped by a large globule. The base of the stalk anchors it in the membrane. Analysis of viral variants has identified five antigenic sites on the HA molecule that exhibit extensive mutations. These sites occur at regions exposed on the surface of the structure, are apparently not essential to the molecule's stability, and are involved in viral neutralization. Other regions of the HA molecule are conserved in all isolates that have been sequenced, presumably because they are necessary for the molecule to retain its structure and function.

The HA spike on the viral particle is a trimer, composed of three intertwined HA1 and HA2 dimers (Figure 39–2C). The trimerization imparts greater stability to the spike than could be achieved by an HA monomer. The cellular receptor binding site (viral attachment site) is located at the top of each large globule.

The cleavage that separates HA1 and HA2 is necessary for the viral particle to be infectious and occurs extracellularly by cellular proteases abundant in the respiratory tract environment. Viral particles with uncleaved HA can attach to cell receptors but are noninfectious. The amino terminus of HA2, generated by the cleavage event, is necessary for the viral envelope to fuse with the cell membrane, an essential step in the process of viral infection.

Structure & Function of the Neuraminidase

The antigenicity of NA, the other glycoprotein on the surface of influenza virus particles, is also important in determining the subtype of influenza virus isolates.

The complete sequence of NA is known. The spike on the viral particle is a tetramer, composed of four identical monomers (Figure 39–2D). A slender stalk is topped with a box-shaped head. There is a catalytic site for neuraminidase on the top of each head, so that each NA spike contains four active sites.

The NA functions at the end of the viral life cycle. It is a sialidase enzyme that removes sialic acid from glycoconjugates. It facilitates release of viral particles from infected cell surfaces during the budding process and helps prevent self-aggregation of virions by removing sialic acid residues from viral glycoproteins.

Antigenic Drift & Antigenic Shift

Influenza viruses are remarkable because of the frequent antigenic changes that occur in HA and NA. Antigenic variants of influenza virus have a selective advantage over the parental virus in the presence of antibody directed against the original strain. This phenomenon is responsible for the unique epidemiologic features of influenza. Other respiratory tract agents do not display significant antigenic variation.

The two surface antigens of influenza undergo antigenic variation independent of each other. Minor antigenic changes are termed **antigenic drift;** major antigenic changes in HA or NA, called **antigenic shift,** result in the appearance of a new subtype (Figure 39–3).

Antigenic drift is due to the accumulation of point mutations in the gene, resulting in amino acid changes

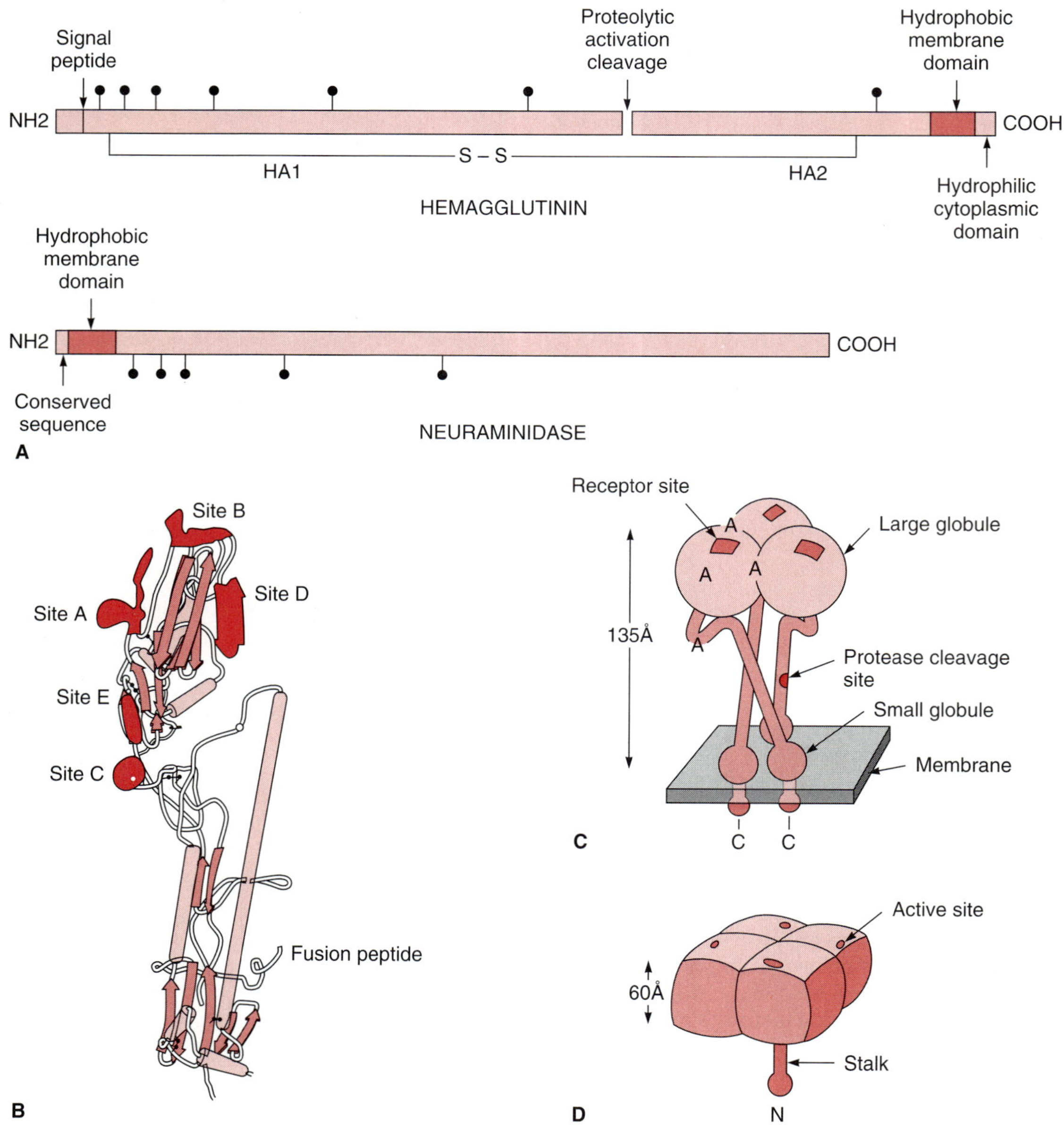

Figure 39–2. Influenza virus hemagglutinin and neuraminidase surface glycoproteins. ***(A)*** Primary structures of HA and NA polypeptides. The cleavage of HA into HA1 and HA2 is necessary for virus to be infectious. HA1 and HA2 remain linked by a disulfide bond (S–S). No posttranslational cleavage occurs with NA. Carbohydrate attachment sites (↓) are shown. The hydrophobic amino acids that anchor the proteins in the viral membrane are located near the C-terminus of HA and the N-terminus of NA. ***(B)*** Folding of the HA1 and HA2 polypeptides in an HA monomer. Five major antigenic sites (sites A–E) that undergo change are shown as shaded areas. The N-terminus of HA2 provides fusion activity (fusion peptide). ***(C)*** Structure of the HA trimer as it occurs on a viral particle or the surface of infected cells. Some of the sites involved in antigenic variation are shown (A). Carboxyterminal residues (C) protrude through the membrane. ***(D)*** Structure of the NA tetramer. Each NA molecule has an active site on its upper surface. The N-terminal region (N) of the polypeptides anchors the complex in the membrane. (Redrawn, with permission, from ***[A, B]*** Murphy BR, Webster RG: Influenza viruses, p 1179, and ***[C, D]*** Kingsbury DW: Orthomyxo- and paramyxoviruses and their replication, p 1157. In: *Virology.* Fields BN et al [editors]. Raven Press, 1985.)

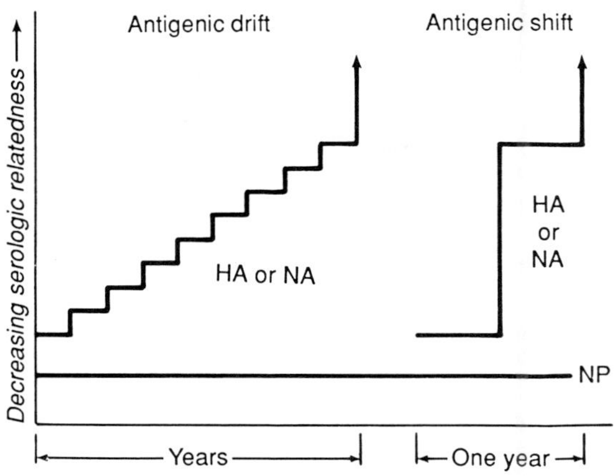

Figure 39–3. Principles of antigenic drift and antigenic shift that account for antigenic changes in the two surface glycoproteins (HA and NA) of influenza virus. Antigenic drift is a gradual change in antigenicity due to point mutations that affect major antigenic sites on the glycoprotein. Antigenic shift is an abrupt change due to genetic reassortment with an unrelated strain. Changes in HA and NA occur independently. Internal proteins of the virus, such as the nucleoprotein (NP), do not undergo such antigenic changes.

in the protein. Sequence changes can alter antigenic sites on the molecule such that a virion can escape recognition by the host's immune system. A variant must sustain two or more mutations before a new, epidemiologically significant strain emerges.

Antigenic shift reflects drastic changes in the sequence of a viral surface protein, changes too extreme to be explained by mutation. The segmented genomes of influenza viruses reassort readily in doubly infected cells. One probable mechanism for shift is genetic reassortment between human and nonhuman influenza viruses, especially those of avian origin. Influenza B and C viruses do not exhibit antigenic shift, perhaps because few related viruses exist in animals.

Influenza Virus Replication

A. Viral Attachment, Penetration, and Uncoating: The virus attaches to cell-surface sialic acid via the receptor site located on the top of the large globule of the HA. Influenza C binds to a different cell receptor from that of influenza A and B. Viral particles are then internalized within endosomes. The next step involves fusion between the viral envelope and cell membrane, triggering uncoating. The amino terminus of HA2, generated by proteolytic cleavage of the precursor HA polypeptide, is essential for this step. The low pH within the endosome is optimal for virus-mediated membrane fusion; it probably causes a conformational change in the HA structure to bring the HA2 "fusion peptide" in correct contact with the membrane. Viral nucleocapsids are then released into the cell cytoplasm.

B. Transcription and Translation: Transcription mechanisms used by orthomyxoviruses differ markedly from those of other RNA viruses in that cellular functions are more intimately involved. Viral transcription occurs in the nucleus. The virus-encoded polymerase, consisting of a complex of the three P proteins, is primarily responsible for transcription. However, its action must be primed by scavenged capped and methylated 5′ termini from cellular transcripts that are newly synthesized by cellular RNA polymerase II. This explains why influenza virus replication is inhibited by dactinomycin and α-amanitin, which block cellular transcription, whereas other RNA viruses (including paramyxoviruses) are not affected because they do not use cellular transcripts in viral RNA synthesis.

Six of the genome segments yield monocistronic mRNAs that are translated in the cytoplasm into six viral proteins. The other two transcripts undergo splicing, each yielding two mRNAs that are translated in different reading frames. The two glycoproteins, HA and NA, are synthesized and modified using the secretory pathway.

C. Viral RNA Replication: Viral genome replication is accomplished by the same virus-encoded polymerase proteins involved in transcription. The mechanisms that regulate the alternative transcription and replication roles of the same proteins are related to the abundance of one or more of the viral nucleocapsid proteins.

As with all other negative-strand viruses, templates for viral RNA synthesis (transcription or replication) remain coated with nucleoproteins. The only completely free RNAs are mRNAs.

The first step in genome replication is production of positive-strand complete copies of each segment. These antigenome copies differ from mRNAs at both termini; the 5′ ends are not capped, and the 3′ ends are neither truncated nor polyadenylated. These copies then serve as templates for synthesis of faithful copies of genomic RNAs.

There are common sequences at both ends of all viral RNA segments, which means that they can be recognized efficiently by the RNA-synthesizing machinery. It is not known how the appropriate segments become assembled within the nucleocapsids of progeny virions. Intermingling of genome segments derived from different parents in coinfected cells is presumably responsible for the high frequency of genetic reassortment typical of influenza viruses. Frequencies of reassortment as high as 40% have been observed.

D. Maturation: The virus matures by budding from the apical surface of the cell. Individual viral components arrive at the budding site by different routes. The nucleocapsids are assembled in the nucleus and move out to the cell surface. The glycoproteins, HA and NA, are synthesized in the endoplasmic reticulum, are modified and assembled into trimers and tetramers, respectively, and are inserted into the plasma membrane. The matrix (M_1) protein, synthesized in the cytoplasm, serves as a bridge, linking the nucleocapsid to the cytoplasmic ends of the glycoproteins. Progeny virions bud off the cell. During this sequence of events, the HA is cleaved into HA1 and HA2 if the host cell possesses the appropriate extracellular proteolytic enzyme. The NA removes terminal sialic acids from cellular and viral surface glycoproteins, thus facilitating release of viral particles from the cell and preventing their aggregation, so that each can act as a separate infectious unit. Otherwise, large clumps of particles would form because of the affinity of the HA binding site for sialic acid.

The viral multiplication cycle proceeds rapidly. New progeny viruses are produced within 8–10 hours.

Many (90% or more) of the particles produced are not infectious. Particles sometimes fail to encapsidate the complete complement of genome segments; frequently, one of the large RNA segments is missing. These noninfectious particles are capable of causing hemagglutination and can interfere with the replication of intact virus.

INFLUENZA VIRUS INFECTIONS IN HUMANS

Pathogenesis & Pathology

Influenza virus spreads from person to person by airborne droplets or by contact with contaminated hands or surfaces. A few cells of respiratory epithelium are infected if deposited viral particles avoid removal by the cough reflex and escape neutralization by any preexisting specific IgA antibodies or inactivation by nonspecific inhibitors in the mucous secretions. Progeny virions are soon produced and spread to adjacent cells, where the replicative cycle is repeated. Viral NA lowers the viscosity of the mucous film in the respiratory tract, laying bare the cellular surface receptors and promoting the spread of virus-containing fluid to lower portions of the tract. Within a short time, many cells in the respiratory tract are infected and eventually killed.

The incubation period from time of exposure to virus and the onset of illness varies from 1 to 4 days, depending partly upon the size of the viral dose and the immune status of the host. Viral shedding starts the day preceding onset of symptoms, peaks within 24 hours, remains elevated for 1–2 days, and then declines rapidly.

Interferon is detectable in respiratory secretions about 1 day after viral shedding begins. Influenza viruses are sensitive to the antiviral effects of interferon, and it is believed that the interferon response contributes to host recovery from infection. Specific antibody and cell-mediated responses cannot be detected for another 1–2 weeks.

Influenza infections cause cellular destruction and desquamation of superficial mucosa of the respiratory tract but do not affect the basal layer of epithelium. Complete reparation of cellular damage probably takes up to 1 month. Viral damage to the respiratory tract epithelium lowers its resistance to secondary bacterial invaders, especially staphylococci, streptococci, and *Haemophilus influenzae.*

Edema and mononuclear infiltrations in response to cell death and desquamation due to viral replication probably account for local symptoms. The prominent systemic symptoms associated with influenza are difficult to explain. Although they suggest viral spread, infectious virus is very rarely recovered from blood.

Clinical Findings

A. Uncomplicated Influenza: Symptoms of influenza usually appear abruptly and include chills, headache, and dry cough, followed closely by high fever, generalized muscular aches, malaise, and anorexia. The fever usually lasts 3 days, as do the systemic symptoms. Respiratory symptoms typically last another 3–4 days. The cough and weakness may persist for 1–3 weeks after major symptoms subside. Mild or asymptomatic infections may occur.

The symptoms described above may be induced by any strain of influenza A or B. In contrast, influenza C rarely (if ever) causes the influenza syndrome, effecting instead a common cold illness.

Clinical symptoms of influenza in children are similar to those in adults, although children may have higher fever and a higher incidence of gastrointestinal manifestations. Influenza A viruses are an important cause of croup in children under 1 year of age.

When influenza appears in epidemic form, clinical findings are consistent enough so that the disease can be diagnosed in most cases. Sporadic cases cannot be diagnosed on clinical grounds. Influenza C does not occur in epidemics.

B. Pneumonia: Serious complications usually occur only in the elderly and debilitated, especially those with underlying cardiopulmonary or other chronic disease. Pregnancy has appeared to be a risk factor for lethal complications in some epidemics.

The lethal impact of an influenza epidemic is reflected in the excess deaths due to pneumonia and cardiovascular and renal diseases.

Pneumonia complicating influenza infections can be viral, secondary bacterial, or a combination of the two. Increased mucous secretion helps carry agents into the lower respiratory tract. Influenza infection enhances susceptibility of patients to bacterial superinfection. This is attributed to loss of ciliary clearance, dysfunction of phagocytic cells, and provision of a rich bacterial growth medium by the alveolar exudate. Bacterial pathogens are most often *Staphylococcus aureus, Streptococcus pneumoniae,* and *H influenzae.*

Combined viral-bacterial pneumonia is approximately three times more common than primary influenza pneumonia. *S aureus* coinfection has been reported to have a fatality rate of up to 42%. Recent studies suggest a molecular basis for a synergistic effect between virus and bacteria. Some *S aureus* strains secrete a protease able to cleave the influenza HA, thereby allowing production of much higher titers of infectious virus in the lungs. Such viral activation would promote extensive spread of viral infection in the lungs.

C. Reye's Syndrome: Reye's syndrome is an acute encephalopathy of children and adolescents, usually between 2 and 16 years of age. Fatty degeneration of the liver is associated with the syndrome. The mortality rate is high (10–40%).

The cause of Reye's syndrome is unknown, but it is a recognized complication of influenza B, influenza A, and herpesvirus varicella-zoster infections. Epidemic cases of Reye's syndrome have been associated with outbreaks of influenza B infection.

There is a possible relationship between salicylate use and subsequent development of Reye's syndrome. Although a causal role has not been proved, it is advisable that children with flu-like symptoms not be given aspirin-containing compounds for fever.

Immunity

Antibodies against HA and NA are important in immunity to influenza, whereas antibodies against the other virus-encoded proteins are not protective. Resistance to initiation of infection is related to antibody against the HA, whereas decreased severity of disease and decreased ability to transmit virus to contacts are related to antibody directed against the NA. Antibodies against the ribonucleoprotein are type-specific and are useful in typing viral isolates (as influenza A or B).

Protection correlates with both serum antibodies and secretory IgA antibodies in nasal secretions. The local secretory antibody is probably most important in preventing infection. Antibody also modifies the course of illness. A person with low titers of antibody may be infected but will experience a mild form of disease.

The three types of influenza viruses are antigenically unrelated and therefore induce no cross-protection. When a viral type undergoes antigenic drift, a person with preexisting antibody to the original strain may suffer only mild infection with the new strain.

Serum antibodies persist for many months to years, whereas secretory antibodies are shorter-lived (usually only several months).

The role of cell-mediated immune responses in influenza is unclear. Presumably, cytotoxic T cells help recovery by lysing infected cells. Interestingly, the cytotoxic T lymphocyte response is cross-reactive (able to lyse cells infected with any strain of virus) rather than "strain-specific" and appears to be directed predominantly against the viral nucleoprotein rather than surface glycoproteins.

Laboratory Diagnosis

Clinical characteristics of viral respiratory infections can be produced by many different viruses. Consequently, diagnosis of influenza relies on isolation of the virus, identification of viral antigens in the patient's cells, or demonstration of a specific immunologic response by the patient.

A. Isolation and Identification of Virus: Nasal washings and throat swabs are the best specimens for viral isolation and should be obtained within 3 days of the onset of symptoms. The sample should be held at 4 °C until inoculation into cell culture, as freezing and thawing reduce the ability to recover virus. However, if storage time will exceed 5 days, the sample should be frozen at −70 °C. There is a greater loss of viral infectivity at freezing temperatures between 0 and −50 °C.

Classically, embryonated eggs and primary monkey kidney cells have been the isolation methods of choice for influenza viruses. More recently, continuous cell lines derived from canine kidney (MDCK) or rhesus monkey kidney (LLC-MK_2) have been preferred. Inoculated cell cultures are incubated in the absence of serum, which may contain nonspecific viral inhibitory factors, and in the presence of trypsin, which cleaves and activates the HA so that replicating virus will spread throughout the culture.

The culture fluid is examined for virus after 7 days by hemagglutination. If the results are negative, a passage is made into fresh cultures. This passage may be necessary, because primary viral isolates are often fastidious and grow slowly.

Viral isolates are identified by hemagglutination inhibition, a procedure that permits rapid determination of the influenza type and subtype. To do this, reference sera to currently prevalent strains must be used. Hemagglutination by the new isolate will be inhibited by antiserum to the homologous subtype. Alternatively, the phenomenon of hemadsorption may be used for early detection of viral growth in cell cultures. Positive hemadsorption results in red blood cells firmly attached as rosettes or chains to the cell culture sheets. The antigenic specificity of an isolate can be determined by blocking the hemadsorption reaction with specific reference antisera (hemadsorption inhibition).

If identification cannot be accomplished by hemagglutination inhibition, a type-specific test can be used to confirm that the isolate is influenza A or B. Type-specific tests include CF and immunofluorescence tests using antisera specific for the NP or M proteins.

It is possible to identify viral antigen directly in exfoliated cells in nasal aspirates using fluorescent antibodies. This test is rapid but must be rigorously controlled to give valid results. This approach is not as sensitive as viral isolation, does not provide full details about the viral strain, and does not yield an isolate that can be characterized. Rapid tests based on detection of influenza RNA in clinical specimens using nucleic acid hybridization are also possible.

B. Serology: Routine serodiagnostic tests in use are based on hemagglutination inhibition and complement fixation. ELISA and RIA will eventually replace these assays as purified antigens become more readily available. Paired acute and convalescent sera are necessary, because normal individuals usually have influenza antibodies. A fourfold or greater increase in titer must occur to indicate influenza infection. Human sera often contain nonspecific mucoprotein inhibitors that must be destroyed by treatment with RDE (receptor-destroying enzyme of *Vibrio cholerae* cultures), trypsin, or periodate before testing.

The HI test reveals the strain of virus responsible for infection only if the correct antigen is available for use. Complement fixation measures antibodies against NP and M proteins, indicating the type of influenza (A, B, or C) that caused the infection. Nt tests are the most sensitive and the best predictor of susceptibility to infection but are more unwieldy and time-consuming to perform than the other tests.

Complications may be encountered in attempting to identify the strain of infecting influenza virus by the patient's antibody response. For instance, the predominant antibodies elicited by a currently circulating strain of virus may be directed against the first strain of influenza experienced years earlier, a phenomenon called "original antigenic sin."

Epidemiology

The three types of influenza vary markedly in their epidemiologic patterns. Influenza C is least significant; it causes mild, sporadic respiratory disease but not epidemic influenza. Influenza B sometimes causes epidemics, but influenza type A can sweep across continents and around the world in massive epidemics called pandemics.

The incidence of influenza peaks during the winter. In the USA, influenza epidemics usually occur from January through April. There is no evidence that influenza establishes latent infections, so a continuous person-to-person chain of transmission must exist for viral survival. Maintenance of the agent between epidemics is not clearly established, but some viral activity can be detected in large population centers throughout each year, indicating that the virus remains endemic in the population and causes a few subclinical or minor infections.

Periodic outbreaks appear because of antigenic changes in one or both surface glycoproteins of the virus, which result in a relatively more susceptible population. When the number of susceptible persons in a population reaches a sufficient level, the new strain of virus causes an epidemic. The change may be gradual (hence the term "antigenic drift"), due to point mutations reflected in alterations at major antigenic sites on the glycoprotein (see Figure 39–3), or drastic and abrupt (hence the term "antigenic shift"), owing to genetic reassortment during coinfection with an unrelated strain.

All three types of influenza virus exhibit antigenic drift. However, only influenza A undergoes antigenic shift, perhaps because types B and C are restricted to humans, whereas related influenza A viruses circulate in animal and bird populations. These animal strains are believed to account for antigenic shift, by genetic reassortment of the glycoprotein genes.

Avian influenza ranges from highly lethal infections in chickens and turkeys to inapparent infections. The possibility that influenza viruses are transmitted between birds and mammals, including humans, would seem unlikely if transfer were to be solely by the respiratory route. However, influenza viruses of ducks multiply in cells lining the intestinal tract and are shed in high concentrations into water, where they remain viable for days or weeks. It is possible that avian influenza is a waterborne infection, moving from wild to domestic birds and even to humans.

Influenza outbreaks occur in waves, although there is no regular periodicity in the occurrence of epidemics. The experience in any given year will reflect the interplay between extent of antigenic drift of the predominant virus and waning immunity in the population. The period between epidemic waves of influenza A tends to be 2–3 years; the interepidemic period for type B is longer (3–6 years).

Every 10–40 years, when a new subtype of influenza A appears, a pandemic results. This happened in 1918 (H1N1), 1957 (H2N2), and 1968 (H3N2). The H1N1 subtype reemerged in 1977 and has continued to cocirculate with H3N2 since then. It is interesting that the HA of the 1968 pandemic virus (A/Hong Kong/68[H3N2]) was barely distinguishable from that of isolates from ducks and horses (A/duck/Ukraine/63 [H3N8] and A/equine/Miami/63[H3N8]), lending credence to the explanation of genetic reassortment with influenza viruses from animals as the basis for antigenic shift. Furthermore, the last three major shifts in influenza A originated in China, where much of the population is rural and in close contact with pigs and ducks.

School-age children are the predominant vectors of influenza transmission. Crowding in schools favors the aerosol transmission of virus, and children take the virus home to the family. The economic impact of influenza A outbreaks is significant, due to the morbidity associated with infections. Economic costs have been estimated at $1–3 billion, depending on the size of the epidemic.

Surveillance for influenza outbreaks is more extensive than for any other disease in order to identify the early appearance of new strains, with the aim of preparing vaccines against them before an epidemic occurs. That surveillance also extends into animal populations, especially birds, pigs, and horses. Isolation of a virus with an altered hemagglutinin in the late spring during a mini-epidemic signals a possible epidemic the following winter. This warning sign, termed a "herald wave," has been observed to precede influenza A and B epidemics.

Human influenza virus was first isolated in 1933 using ferrets. The subtypes that circulated prior to that time have been deduced using retrospective seroepidemiology (seroarcheology). This technique is based on screening hemagglutination-inhibition titers against numerous HA subtypes of virus with sera from many individuals in different age groups.

In early life, the range of the influenza antibody spectrum is narrow, but it becomes progressively broader in later years. Antibodies (and immunity) acquired from initial infections in childhood are of limited range and reflect dominant antigens of the prevailing strains. Later exposures to viruses of related but differing antigenic composition result in an antibody spectrum broadening toward a larger number of common antigens of influenza viruses. Exposures later in life to antigenically related strains result in progressive reinforcement of the primary antibody. The highest antibody levels in a particular age group therefore reflect dominant antigens of the virus responsible for childhood infections of the group. Thus, a serologic recapitulation of past infection with influenza viruses of different antigenic makeup can be obtained by studying age distribution of influenza antibodies in normal populations.

This approach suggests that the epidemic of 1890 was probably caused by an H2N8 subtype and the epidemic of 1900 by an H3N8 virus. The catastrophic pandemic of 1918–1919 (Spanish flu) was apparently caused by the abrupt appearance of the H1N1 subtype, the swine-like influenza. (More than 20 million people died during this pandemic, mainly from complicating bacterial pneumonias.) Subsequent antigenic shifts have been documented by viral isolations; for example, H2N2 (Asian flu) appeared in 1957 and was replaced in 1968 by the H3N2 subtype (Hong Kong flu). The H1N1 strain reappeared in 1977 (Russian flu), supporting the belief that human strains recirculate. However, it failed to spread in spite of a lack of immunity in most persons under age 50 years, and no epidemic materialized.

Prevention & Treatment by Drugs

Amantadine hydrochloride and one of its analogues, rimantadine, are antiviral drugs for systemic use in the prevention of influenza A. The drugs block uncoating of influenza A virus in the host cell and prevent viral replication. They are ineffective against influenza B and C viruses. Amantadine and rimantadine reportedly induce protection from influenza illness in about 70% of recipients. However, the drugs appear ineffective in protecting household contacts from influenza; drug-resistant mutants of virus develop and spread. Amantadine is relatively nontoxic but may produce central nervous system stimulation with dizziness and insomnia, particularly in the elderly. It should be considered for individuals who are at high risk (eg, those with chronic diseases) if they have not been vaccinated yearly or if a new influenza A strain is epidemic, as well as for hospital personnel who might spread infection. Amantadine may also modify the severity of influenza A if administration is begun within 24–48 hours after onset of illness.

Aspirin helps reduce headache, fever, and myalgias of the influenza syndrome. However, aspirin should not be given to those under 16 years of age because of its possible association with Reye's syndrome.

There is no specific therapy for complications other than pneumonia (including Reye's syndrome).

Prevention & Control

Inactivated viral vaccines are the primary means of prevention of influenza in the USA. However, certain characteristics of influenza viruses, described above, make prevention and control of the disease by immunization especially difficult. Existing vaccines are continually being rendered obsolete as the viruses undergo antigenic drift and shift. Surveillance programs by government agencies and the World Health Organization constantly monitor subtypes of influenza circulating around the world to promptly detect the appearance and spread of new strains.

Several other problems are worthy of mention. Protection is at best about 70% for a year following immunization and may be much lower. Inactivated viral vaccines do not generate local IgA or cell-mediated immune responses. Vaccination is also complicated by the phenomenon of original antigenic sin (ie, annual immunizations may predominantly boost antibody levels directed against irrelevant strains to which the person had once been exposed).

A. Preparation of Inactivated Viral Vaccines: Federal bodies and the World Health Organization make recommendations each year about which strains should be included in the vaccine. The vaccine is usually a cocktail containing both a type A and a type B virus of the strains isolated in the previous winter's outbreaks. Two A types are sometimes included in addition to the B type when both A types circulated widely the previous winter and scientists are not able to predict with confidence which strain might be most important in the succeeding flu season. Such a trivalent vaccine has been used for several years. The three viral strains incorporated into the 1994–1995 vaccine contain H3N2, H1N1, and B antigens.

Selected seed strains are grown in embryonated eggs, the substrate used for vaccine production. Sometimes the natural isolates grow too poorly in eggs to permit vaccine production, in which case a reassortant virus is made in the laboratory. The reassortant virus, which carries the genes for the surface antigens of the desired vaccine with the replication genes from an egg-adapted laboratory virus, is then used for vaccine production.

Virus is harvested from the egg allantoic fluid, purified, concentrated by zonal centrifugation, and inactivated with formalin. The quantity of HA is standardized in each vaccine dose (approximately 15 μg of antigen), but the quantity of NA is not standardized, as it is more labile under purification and storage conditions. Each dose of vaccine contains the equivalent of about 10^{10} viral particles.

B. Use of Influenza Vaccines: The only contraindication to vaccination is a history of allergy to egg protein. Since vaccine strains are grown in eggs, some egg protein antigens are present in the vaccine. Individuals who are allergic to eggs may develop symptoms and signs of hypersensitivity.

Annual influenza vaccination is currently recommended for high-risk groups (ie, individuals at increased risk of dying from pulmonary complications associated with influenza infection, including those with either chronic heart or lung disease or metabolic or renal disorders; residents of nursing homes; medical personnel who have extensive contact with high-risk patients; and, finally, those 65 years of age and older).

The vaccine is safe but has a protective efficacy of only about 70%. Whatever immunity results from an inactivated viral vaccine appears to be of short duration—probably 1–3 years against the homologous

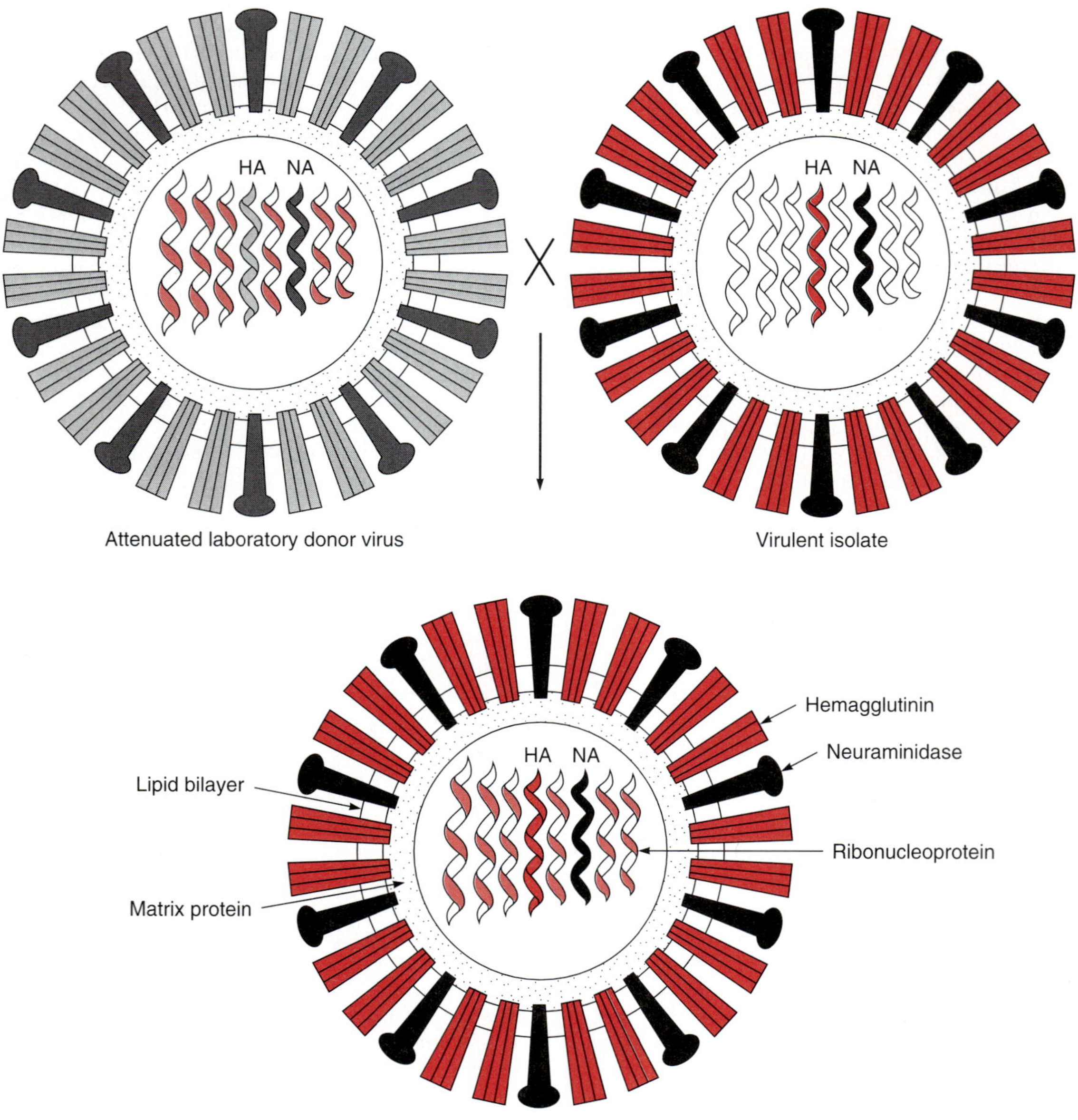

Figure 39–4. Principle of using genetic reassortment to construct an attenuated live vaccine virus. Cells are coinfected with an attenuated laboratory donor virus and a virulent wild-type influenza virus isolate. The desired reassortant vaccine virus will contain the HA and NA genes from the wild-type virulent virus and other viral genes that confer attenuation from the attenuated donor virus.

virus. As noted above, killed-virus vaccines, unfortunately, do not induce secretory IgA antibodies in the respiratory tract.

The vaccine may produce mild local side effects in about 25% of vaccinees and systemic effects, including fever, in about 1%. Guillain-Barré syndrome, an ascending paralysis, was statistically associated with the **swine influenza** vaccination program of 1976. The syndrome occurred in one in 100,000 vaccinees, 5% of whom died. However, no such increased risk of contracting Guillain-Barré syndrome has been associated with any previous or subsequent standard influenza vaccines.

C. New Approaches to Better Influenza Vaccines: Modern technologies offer new strategies for producing inactivated vaccines against influenza. Cloned DNA copies of the HA gene can be used to express the protein in bacteria or yeast. Purified HA could then be used as a vaccine. Secondly, oligopeptides that correspond to the sequence of crucial functional domains on the HA molecule could be synthesized in vitro and used as immunogens. These approaches have not yet resulted in practical influenza vaccines.

Researchers are trying to develop a reliable live-virus vaccine. Current inactivated viral vaccines do not provide complete protection and fail to induce local immunity, which is especially important in resistance to respiratory pathogens. A live-virus vaccine must be attenuated so as not to induce the disease it is designed to prevent. In view of the constantly changing face of influenza viruses in nature and the extensive laboratory efforts required to attenuate a virulent virus, the only feasible strategy is to devise a way to transfer defined attenuating genes from an attenuated master donor virus to each new epidemic or pandemic isolate. The principle of using genetic reassortment to construct attenuated live vaccine viruses is shown in Figure 39–4.

Several approaches to vaccine preparation are being evaluated. A cold-adapted donor virus, able to grow at 25 °C but not at 37 °C, the temperature of the lower respiratory tract, should replicate somewhat in the nasopharynx, which has a cooler temperature (33 °C). A variation of this approach is the use of an avian influenza donor virus that is restricted in its ability to replicate in primate cells. The stability of the attenuation phenotype in any such vaccine virus reassortant would have to be proved.

REFERENCES

Carson JL, Collier AM, Hu SS: Acquired ciliary defects in nasal epithelium of children with acute viral upper respiratory infections. N Engl J Med 1985;312:463.

Douglas RG Jr: Prophylaxis and treatment of influenza. N Engl J Med 1990;322:443.

Edwards KM et al: A randomized controlled trial of cold-adapted and inactivated vaccines for the prevention of influenza A disease. J Infect Dis 1994;169:68.

Frank AL et al: Influenza B virus infections in the community and the family: The epidemics of 1976–1977 and 1979–1980 in Houston, Texas. Am J Epidemiol 1983; 118:313.

Lamb RA, Choppin PW: The gene structure and replication of influenza virus. Annu Rev Biochem 1983;52:467.

Langmuir AD et al: An epidemiologic and clinical evaluation of Guillain-Barré syndrome reported in association with the administration of swine influenza vaccines. Am J Epidemiol 1984;119:841.

Palese P, Young JF: Variation of influenza A, B, and C viruses. Science 1982;215:1468.

Riddiough MA, Sisk JE, Bell JC: Influenza vaccination: Cost-effectiveness and public policy. JAMA 1983;249: 3189.

Tashiro M et al: Role of *Staphylococcus* protease in the development of influenza pneumonia. Nature 1987;325:536.

Webster RG et al: Influenza–A model of an emerging virus disease. Intervirology 1993;35:16.

Webster RG et al: Molecular mechanisms of variation in influenza viruses. Nature 1982;296:115.

Weis W et al: Structure of the influenza virus haemagglutinin complexed with its receptor, sialic acid. Nature 1988; 333:426.

Yewdell JW et al: Influenza A virus nucleoprotein is a major target antigen for cross-reactive anti-influenza A virus cytotoxic T lymphocytes. Proc Natl Acad Sci USA 1985; 82:1785.

40 Paramyxoviruses & Rubella Virus

The paramyxoviruses include the most important agents of respiratory infections of infants and young children (respiratory syncytial virus and the parainfluenza viruses) as well as the causative agents of two of the most common contagious diseases of childhood (mumps and measles). The World Health Organization estimates that acute respiratory infections are responsible for the deaths of 4 million children annually under 5 years of age. Worldwide, such infections account for 20–40% of children's admissions to hospitals. Paramyxoviruses are the major respiratory pathogens in this age group.

All members of the **Paramyxoviridae** family initiate infection via the respiratory tract. Replication of the respiratory pathogens is limited to the respiratory epithelia, whereas measles and mumps become disseminated throughout the body and produce generalized disease.

Rubella virus, though classified as a togavirus because of its chemical and physical properties (see Chapter 29), can be considered with the paramyxoviruses on an epidemiologic basis.

PROPERTIES OF PARAMYXOVIRUSES

The differences between paramyxoviruses and orthomyxoviruses are described in Chapter 39 and summarized in Table 39–2. Major properties of paramyxoviruses are shown in Table 40–1.

Structure & Composition

The morphology of **Paramyxoviridae** resembles that of influenza viruses, but paramyxoviruses are larger (150–300 nm in diameter) and much more pleomorphic, with particles ranging in size from 100 to 700 nm. A typical particle is shown in Figure 40–1. The envelope of paramyxoviruses seems to be fragile, making viral particles labile to storage conditions and prone to distortion in electron micrographs.

The viral genome is linear, single-stranded RNA with a molecular weight of $5–7 \times 10^6$ (about 15,000 nucleotides). In contrast to the genome of orthomyxoviruses, it is not segmented, and this negates any opportunity for frequent reassortment. All members of the paramyxovirus group are antigenically stable.

The six structural proteins of the paramyxoviruses are generally analogous to those of the influenza viruses. Three proteins are complexed with the viral RNA—the nucleoprotein (NP or N) that forms the helical nucleocapsid (18 nm in diameter) and represents the major internal protein and two large proteins (designated P and L), which are probably involved in the viral polymerase activity that functions in transcription and RNA replication. Three proteins participate in the formation of the viral envelope. A matrix (M) protein underlies the viral envelope; it has an affinity for both the NP and the viral surface glycoproteins and is important in virion assembly.

The nucleocapsid is surrounded by a lipid envelope that is studded with 10-nm spikes of two different trans-membrane glycoproteins. The activities of these surface glycoproteins distinguish the three genera of the **Paramyxoviridae** family (Table 40–2; see Classification, below). The larger glycoprotein (HN or H) may possess both hemagglutinin and neuraminidase activities and is responsible for host cell attachment. It is assembled as a tetramer in the mature virion. The other glycoprotein (F) mediates membrane fusion and hemolysin activities.

A diagram of a paramyxovirus particle is shown in Figure 40–2.

Classification

The **Paramyxoviridae** family is divided into three genera (Table 40–2). Most of the members are mono-

Table 40–1. Important properties of paramyxoviruses.

Virion: Spherical, pleomorphic, 150–300 nm in diameter (helical nucleocapsid, 18 nm).
Composition: RNA (1%), protein (73%), lipid (20%), carbohydrate (6%).
Genome: Single-stranded RNA, linear, nonsegmented, negative-sense, MW 5–7 million (~15,000 nucleotides).
Proteins: Six structural proteins.
Envelope: Contains viral hemagglutinin (HN) glycoprotein (which sometimes carries neuraminidase activity) and fusion (F) glycoprotein; very fragile.
Replication: Cytoplasm; particles bud from plasma membrane.
Outstanding characteristics: Antigenically stable; particles are labile yet highly infectious.

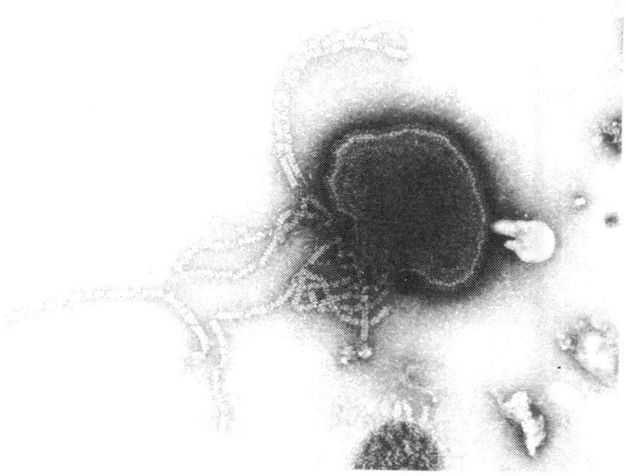

Figure 40–1. Ultrastructure of parainfluenza virus type 1. The virion is partially disrupted, showing the nucleocapsid. Surface projections are visible along the edge of the particle. (FA Murphy and EL Palmer.)

typic (ie, they consist of a single serotype); all are antigenically stable.

The *Paramyxovirus* genus contains the four serotypes of human parainfluenza viruses as well as mumps virus. Early names for parainfluenza viruses were "hemadsorption agent 2" for type 1, "croup-associated" virus for type 2, and "hemadsorption agent 1" for type 3. Some animal viruses are related to the human strains. Sendai virus of mice, which was the first parainfluenza virus isolated and is now recognized as a common infection in mouse colonies, is a subtype of human type 1 virus. SV5, a common contaminant of primary monkey cells, is a subtype of type 2, whereas shipping fever virus of cattle and sheep, SF4, is a subtype of type 3. Newcastle disease virus, the prototype avian parainfluenza virus, is also related to the human viruses.

All members of the *Paramyxovirus* genus share common antigenic determinants. Although the viruses can be distinguished antigenically using well-defined reagents, hyperimmunization stimulates cross-reactive

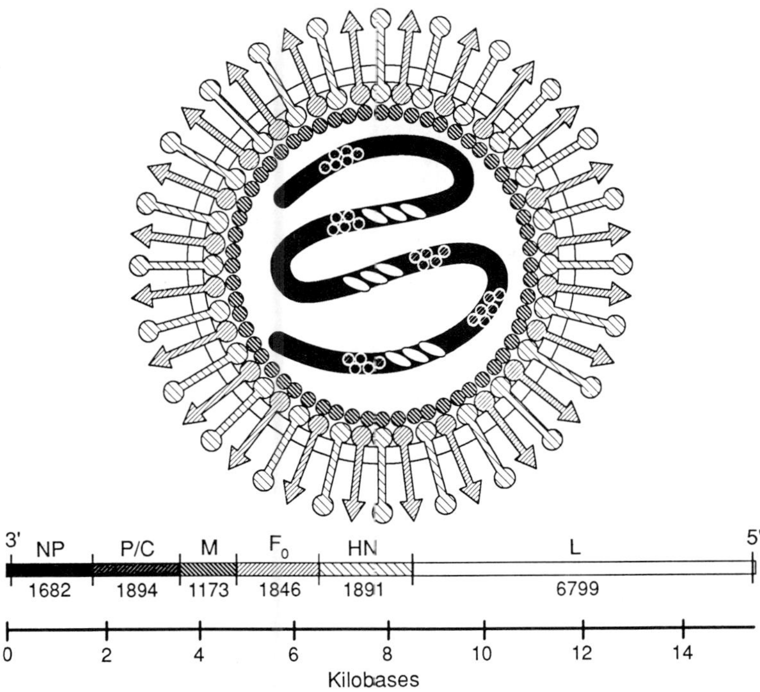

Figure 40–2. Diagram of a typical paramyxovirus particle. The genetic map of the virion RNA of Sendai virus is drawn beneath the particle. Vertical marks on the map are the sites of gene boundaries. The number beneath each gene is its length in bases. Genes and the encoded polypeptides are correlated by similar shadings. The internal viral nucleocapsid (black spiral) contains the negative-strand viral genomic RNA complexed with the nucleocapsid protein, NP. Also present internally are nucleocapsid proteins, L (white ovals) and P (densely shaded circles). The lipid bilayer of the viral envelope (outer white circle) is cell-derived; it is penetrated by molecules of the viral attachment glycoprotein, HN (light shading, rounded tips), and the fusion protein, F (darker shading, pointed tips). Cytoplasmic domains of the glycoproteins are anchored by the nonglycosylated envelope protein, M (shaded circles). The shapes of the different viral proteins are schematic; actual structures have not been defined. (Reproduced, with permission, from Kingsbury DW: Paramyxoviridae and their replication. Pages 945–962 in: *Virology,* 2nd ed. Fields BN et al [editors]. Raven Press, 1990.)

Table 40–2. Characteristics of genera in the family Paramyxoviridae.

Property	Genus			
	Paramyxovirus		***Morbillivirus***	***Pneumovirus***
Human viruses	Parainfluenza 1–4	Mumps	Measles (rubeola)	Respiratory syncytial virus
Serotypes	4	1	1	1
Diameter of nucleocapsid (nm)	18	18	18	13
Membrane fusion (F protein)	+	+	+	+
Hemolysin[1]	+	+	+	0
Hemagglutinin	+[2]	+[2]	+[3]	0
Hemadsorption	+	+	+	0
Neuraminidase	+[2]	+[2]	0	0
Inclusions[4]	C	C	N,C	C

[1]Hemolysin activity carried by F glycoprotein.
[2]Hemagglutination and neuraminidase activities carried by HN glycoprotein.
[3]Hemagglutination of monkey erythrocytes only, by H glycoprotein that lacks neuraminidase activity.
[4]C, cytoplasm; N, nucleus.

antibodies that react with all four parainfluenza viruses, mumps virus, and Newcastle disease virus. Such heterotypic antibody responses, which include antibodies directed against both internal and surface proteins of the virus, are commonly observed in older people. This phenomenon makes it difficult to determine by serodiagnosis the most likely infecting type. All members of the *Paramyxovirus* genus possess hemagglutinating and neuraminidase activities, both carried by the HN glycoprotein, as well as membrane fusion and hemolysin properties, both functions of the F protein.

The *Morbillivirus* genus contains measles virus (rubeola) of humans, as well as canine distemper virus and rinderpest virus of cattle. These three viruses are antigenically related but do not cross-react with members of the other two genera. The F protein seems to be highly conserved among morbilliviruses, whereas the H proteins display more variability. Measles virus has a hemagglutinin (that agglutinates only monkey erythrocytes) but lacks neuraminidase activity. In contrast to the other paramyxoviruses, whose cytopathic effects are limited to the cytoplasm of cells, measles virus induces formation of intranuclear inclusions as well.

Respiratory syncytial virus and pneumonia virus of mice constitute the *Pneumovirus* genus. They are immunologically unrelated to agents in the other genera. Their nucleocapsid is smaller (13 nm in diameter). The larger surface glycoprotein of pneumoviruses lacks hemagglutinating and neuraminidase activities characteristic of parainfluenza viruses, so it is designated the G protein. The F protein of respiratory syncytial virus exhibits membrane fusion activity but no hemolysin activity.

Structure & Function of the Fusion Protein

The fusion (F) protein is a key factor in infection and pathogenesis by paramyxoviruses. It mediates fusion of the viral envelope with the plasma membrane of the host cell, an essential step in initiation of infection. It also is responsible for cell-to-cell fusion, which permits direct viral spread. The latter phenomenon causes formation of large syncytia (giant cells), which are characteristic of paramyxovirus infections (hence the name respiratory syncytial virus).

Synthesis and processing of the F glycoprotein bear several resemblances to those of the influenza virus hemagglutinin. The F protein is synthesized as an inactive precursor, F_0. To acquire biologic activity, the precursor must be cleaved by an extracellular protease, generating two subunits, F_1 and F_2, which remain joined by a disulfide bond. This cleavage results in a new hydrophobic amino terminus (on F_1) that can cause membrane fusion. Cleavage must occur to activate the fusion and hemolytic functions; otherwise, the viral particle is not infectious. Production of an appropriate protease able to cleave the F_0 precursor is a major determinant of host-cell permissiveness in vitro and probably of host range and tissue tropism in vivo.

The sequence of the hydrophobic amino terminus of the F_1 cleavage product is highly conserved among paramyxoviruses and shares homology with the influenza virus HA_2 N-terminus. Synthetic oligopeptides analogous to the N-terminus of F_1 inhibit viral replication in vitro (by an unknown mechanism) and are being considered as potential antiviral agents.

The F protein readily causes cell fusion at neutral pH, in contrast to the low pH requirement for influenza virus HA_2-mediated cell fusion. That is why inactivated Sendai virus is a popular choice as a fusion factor for cell hybrid formation, an important tool in somatic cell genetics.

If suitable extracellular proteases are present, F_0 molecules on the cell surface will be cleaved. The activated F_1 protein can then cause contiguous cell surfaces to fuse. This process permits replicating virus to spread from one cell to the next and thereby evade any circulating antibodies. If paramyxovirus vaccines are to be effective, they must elicit antibodies against both the F protein and the HN antigen; otherwise, the host cannot prevent direct cell-to-cell viral spread. It has been suggested that this accounts for the failure of inactivated paramyxovirus vaccines tested in the past.

Paramyxovirus Replication

A. Virus Attachment, Penetration, and Uncoating: Paramyxoviruses attach to host cells via the hemagglutinin glycoprotein (HN or H protein). In the case of measles virus, the receptor appears to be the membrane CD46 molecule. Next, the virion envelope fuses with the cell membrane by the action of the F_1 cleavage product. If the F_0 precursor is not cleaved, it has no fusion activity; virion penetration does not occur, and the viral particle is unable to initiate infection (Figure 40–3). Fusion by F_1 occurs at the neutral pH of the extracellular environment, allowing release of the viral nucleocapsid directly into the cell. Thus, paramyxoviruses are able to bypass internalization through endosomes (required for entry of influenza viruses, as HA_2-mediated fusion occurs only at the low pH found in endosomes).

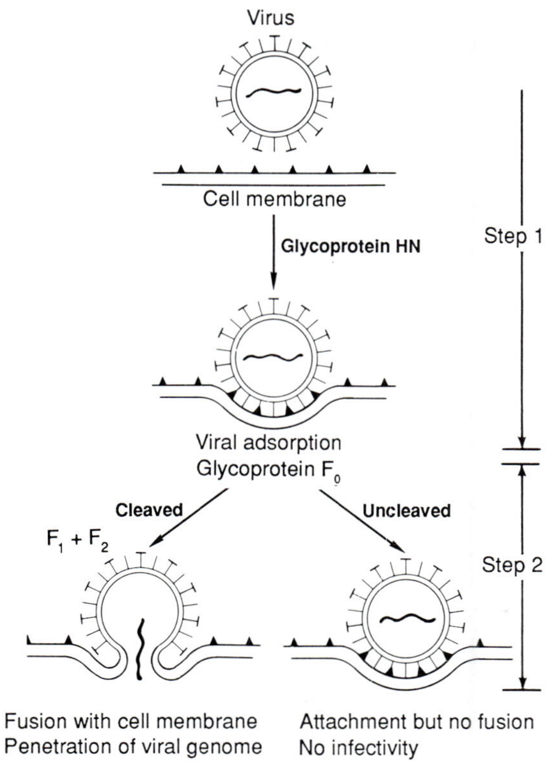

Figure 40–3. Initiation of infection. Adsorption of paramyxovirus to receptors on the cell membrane is mediated by the HN glycoprotein. Penetration of the cell by the virus by means of fusion of viral and cell membranes is mediated by the F_0 glycoprotein, which must be cleaved into two subunits, F_1 and F_2, to be active. If the F_0 protein is not cleaved, the virus will attach but will not fuse with the cell membrane, and the viral genome does not penetrate the cell. (After PW Choppin and A Scheid.)

B. Transcription, Translation, and RNA Replication: Paramyxoviruses contain a nonsegmented, negative-strand RNA genome. Messenger RNA transcripts are made in the cell cytoplasm by the viral RNA polymerase. There is no need for exogenous primers and therefore no dependence on cell nuclear functions. The mRNAs are much smaller than genomic size; each represents a single gene. Transcriptional regulatory sequences at gene boundaries signal transcriptional start and termination. The position of a gene relative to the 3′ end of the genome correlates with transcription efficiency. The most abundant class of transcripts in an infected cell is from the NP gene, located nearest the 3′ end of the genome, whereas the least abundant is from the L gene, located at the 5′ end (Figure 40–2).

Viral proteins are synthesized in the cytoplasm, and the quantity of each gene product corresponds to the level of mRNA transcripts from that gene. Viral glycoproteins are synthesized and glycosylated in the secretory pathway.

The viral polymerase protein complex (P and L proteins) is also responsible for viral genome replication. For successful synthesis of a positive-strand antigenome intermediate template, the polymerase complex must disregard the termination signals interspersed at gene boundaries. Full-length progeny genomes are then copied from the antigenome template.

The nonsegmented genome of paramyxoviruses negates the possibility of gene segment reshuffling so important to the natural history of influenza viruses. The HN and F surface proteins of paramyxoviruses exhibit minimal antigenic variation over long periods of time. It is surprising that they do not undergo antigenic drift as a result of mutations introduced during replication, as RNA polymerases tend to be error-prone. One possible explanation is that nearly all the amino acids in the primary structures of paramyxovirus glycoproteins may be involved in structural or functional roles, leaving little opportunity for substitutions that would not markedly diminish the viability of the virus.

C. Maturation: The virus matures by budding from the cell surface. Progeny nucleocapsids form in the cytoplasm and migrate to the cell surface. They are attracted to sites on the membrane that are studded with viral HN and F_0 glycoprotein spikes. The M protein is essential for particle formation, probably serving to link the viral envelope to the nucleocapsid. During budding, most host proteins are excluded from the membrane.

The neuraminidase activity of the HN protein of parainfluenza viruses and mumps virus presumably functions similarly to the NA protein of influenza virus to prevent self-aggregation of viral particles. Other paramyxoviruses do not possess neuraminidase activity (Table 40–2).

If appropriate host cell proteases are present, F_0 proteins in the plasma membrane will be activated by cleavage. Activated fusion protein will then cause fusion of adjacent cell membranes, resulting in formation of large syncytia (Figure 40–4).

D. Fate of the Cell: Syncytium formation is a common response to paramyxovirus infection. Acidophilic cytoplasmic inclusions are regularly formed (Figure 40–4). Inclusions are believed to reflect sites of viral synthesis and have been found to contain recognizable nucleocapsids and viral proteins. Measles virus also produces intranuclear inclusions (Figure 40–4), though it is not known if the cell nucleus plays any role in measles virus multiplication.

Paramyxoviruses usually have minimal effects on host cell metabolism (unless extensive cell fusion occurs). Persistent noncytocidal infections readily develop and can be traced to many different mechanisms (eg, lack of synthesis of a viral protein, presence of antibody or interferon, nonpermissive nature of cell type). The clinical importance of this property may explain the serious complication of measles infection, subacute sclerosing panencephalitis (see pp 472 and 473).

PARAINFLUENZA VIRUS INFECTIONS

Parainfluenza viruses are ubiquitous and cause common respiratory illnesses in persons of all ages. They are major pathogens of severe respiratory tract disease in infants and young children; only respiratory syncytial virus causes more cases of serious respiratory disease in children. Of the four serotypes of parainfluenza viruses able to infect humans, only the first three are associated with severe disease.

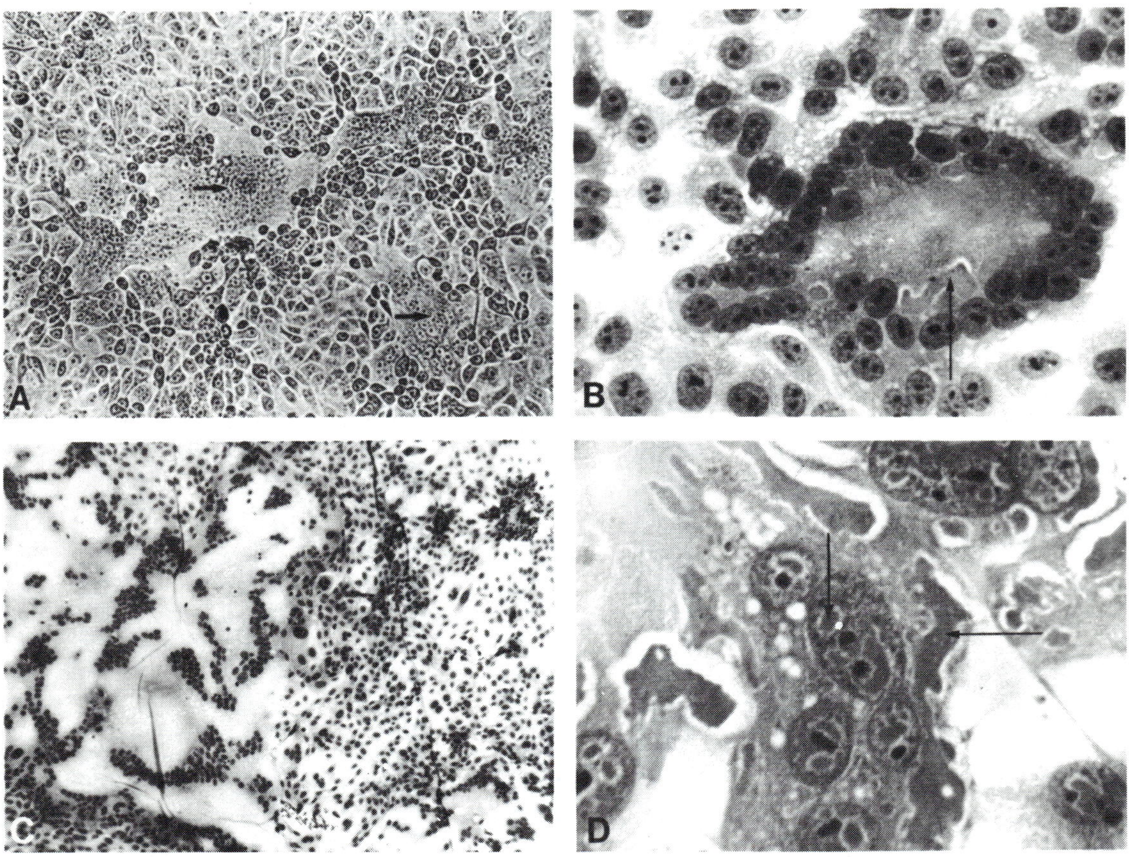

Figure 40–4. Syncytial formation induced by paramyxoviruses. ***(A)*** Respiratory syncytial virus in MA104 cells (unstained, 100×). Syncytia (arrows) result from fusion of plasma membranes; nuclei are accumulated in the center. ***(B)*** Respiratory syncytial virus in HEp-2 cells (H&E stain, 400×). Syncytium contains many nuclei and acidophilic cytoplasmic inclusions (arrow). ***(C)*** Measles virus in human kidney cells (H&E stain, 30×). Huge syncytium contains hundreds of nuclei. ***(D)*** Measles virus in human kidney cells (H&E stain, 400×). Multinucleated giant cell contains acidophilic nuclear inclusions (vertical arrow) and cytoplasmic inclusions (horizontal arrow). (Courtesy of I. Jack; reproduced from White DO, Fenner FJ: *Medical Virology,* 3rd ed. Academic Press, 1986.)

Pathogenesis & Pathology

Parainfluenza viruses are transmitted by direct person-to-person contact or by large-droplet aerosols. Replication appears to be limited to respiratory epithelia. Viremia, if it occurs at all, is uncommon. The infection may involve only the nose and throat, resulting in a harmless "common cold" syndrome. Infection may be more extensive and, especially with types 1 and 2, involve the larynx and upper trachea, resulting in croup (laryngotracheobronchitis). Croup is characterized by respiratory obstruction due to swelling of the larynx and related structures. The infection may spread deeper to the lower trachea and bronchi, culminating in pneumonia or bronchiolitis (or both), especially with type 3. More than one-half of initial infections with parainfluenza virus types 1–3 result in febrile illness. It is estimated that about 25% of primary type 1 infections produce bronchitis, but only 2–3% develop into croup.

Factors that determine the severity of parainfluenza virus disease are unclear but include both viral and host properties, such as susceptibility of the F_0 protein to cleavage by different proteases, production of an appropriate protease by host cells, immune status of the patient, and airway hyperreactivity.

The presence of host cell proteases able to cleave and activate the fusion protein of an infecting parainfluenza virus enables that virus to replicate well and disseminate throughout the respiratory tract.

Primary infections tend to be the most severe and generally occur during the first 5 years of life. Reinfections are common but usually cause only mild, nonfebrile, upper respiratory infections. Antibodies from previous infections do not confer absolute protection against reinfection but do modify the course of ensuing illnesses.

It has been suggested but not proved that rapid and abundant production of virus-specific IgE antibodies which mediate histamine release in the trachea may contribute to production of croup symptoms.

The incubation period in pediatric infections is unknown, but in adult volunteers it ranges from 2 to 6 days. Viral shedding continues for about 1 week, although prolonged shedding has been observed occasionally.

Clinical Findings

The relative importance of parainfluenza viruses as a cause of respiratory diseases in different age groups is indicated in Table 30–3.

Primary infections in young children usually result in rhinitis and pharyngitis, often with fever and some bronchitis. However, children with primary infections caused by parainfluenza virus type 1, 2, or 3 may have serious illness, ranging from laryngotracheitis and croup (particularly with types 1 and 2) to bronchiolitis and pneumonia (particularly with type 3). The severe illness associated with type 3 occurs mainly in infants under the age of 6 months; croup or laryngotracheobronchitis is more likely to occur in older children.

Parainfluenza virus type 4 does not cause serious disease, even on first infection.

Newcastle disease virus is an avian paramyxovirus that produces pneumoencephalitis in young chickens and "influenza" in older birds. In humans, it may produce inflammation of the conjunctiva. Recovery is complete in 10–14 days. Infection in humans is an occupational disease limited to laboratory workers handling infected birds.

Immunity

Virtually all infants have maternal antibodies to parainfluenza viruses in serum, yet such antibodies do not prevent infection or disease. Reinfection of older children and adults also occurs in the presence of antibodies arising from an earlier infection. However, those antibodies modify the disease, since such reinfections usually present simply as nonfebrile upper respiratory infections (colds).

Natural infection stimulates appearance of IgA antibody in nasal secretions and concomitant resistance to reinfection. The secretory IgA antibodies are most important for providing protection against reinfection but unfortunately disappear within a few months. Reinfections are thus common even in adults.

As successive reinfections occur, the antibody response becomes broader because of shared antigenic determinants among parainfluenza viruses and mumps virus. This makes it difficult to diagnose the specific paramyxovirus associated with a given infection using serologic assays.

The relative importance of serum antibodies to HN and F viral surface proteins in determining resistance is unknown. The F antibodies are probably more important, as they both neutralize virus infectivity and prevent cell-to-cell spread by cell fusion; HN antibodies only neutralize infectivity.

Infants produce local IgA antibodies that do not neutralize virus well, and they tend to exhibit poor F antibody responses. The combination of these two factors probably explains the frequent reinfections with parainfluenza viruses that occur during early childhood.

The importance of interferon in recovery from parainfluenza virus infections is unknown. About one-third of young patients have been reported to develop a detectable interferon response.

Laboratory Diagnosis

The immune response to the initial parainfluenza virus infection in life is type-specific. However, with repeated infections the response gets broader and broader, and cross-reactions extend even to mumps virus. Heterotypic responses make specific diagnosis by serologic testing extremely difficult; definitive diagnosis relies on viral isolation from appropriate specimens.

A. Isolation and Identification of Virus: Throat and nasal swabs and nasal washes are good specimens for viral isolation. Primary human and monkey kidney cells are the most sensitive for isolation of parainfluenza viruses. However, such cells are difficult to obtain, and monkey cells may be contaminated with an adventitious simian paramyxovirus, SV5. A continuous monkey kidney cell line, LLC-MK_2, is a suitable alternative, provided trypsin is included in the culture medium to cleave and activate the viral F glycoprotein. Prompt inoculation of samples into cell cultures is important for successful viral isolation, as viral infectivity drops rapidly if clinical specimens are stored.

Parainfluenza viruses grow slowly and produce very little cytopathic effect. To detect the presence of virus, hemadsorption using guinea pig erythrocytes is performed. Depending on the amount of virus, 10 days or more of incubation may be necessary before the cultures become hemadsorption-positive.

Isolates may be typed by immunofluorescence or hemadsorption inhibition of infected monolayers or by hemagglutination inhibition using virus from the cell culture media.

Direct identification of viral antigens in specimens is possible. Antigens may be detected in exfoliated nasopharyngeal cells by immunofluorescence or ELISA. These methods are rapid but less sensitive than viral isolation and must be carefully controlled. Highly specific immune reagents are essential if specific serotype identification is desired.

B. Serology: Serodiagnosis should be based on paired sera. Antibody responses can be measured using Nt, HI, ELISA, or CF tests. A fourfold rise in titer is indicative of infection with a parainfluenza virus. However, because of the problem of shared antigens, it is impossible to be confident of the specific virus type involved. Even the Nt test does not provide total specificity with this group of viruses.

Epidemiology

Parainfluenza viruses are second only to respiratory syncytial virus as a cause of lower respiratory tract disease in young children. Parainfluenza viruses are widely distributed geographically. Type 3 is most prevalent. It is estimated that half of all children are infected during the first year of life; 95% have antibodies to type 3 by age 6 years.

Type 3 is endemic, with some increase during the spring, whereas types 1 and 2 tend to cause epidemics during the fall or winter, frequently on a 2-year cycle.

Types 1 and 2 cause croup in infants. In one study, 20% of patients with croup in a pediatric practice yielded parainfluenza virus type 1. Type 3 is a frequent cause of pneumonia and bronchiolitis in infants under 6 months of age. Reinfections are common throughout childhood and in adults and result in mild upper respiratory tract illnesses.

Parainfluenza viruses are usually introduced into a group by preschool children and then spread readily from person to person. Type 3 virus especially will generally infect all susceptible individuals in a semiclosed population, such as a family or a nursery, within a short time. Parainfluenza viruses are troublesome causes of infection in pediatric wards in hospitals. Other high-risk situations include day-care centers and schools.

Treatment & Prevention

The antiviral drug ribavirin shows promise of being beneficial when delivered by small-particle aerosol, as in the treatment of respiratory syncytial virus infections.

Experimental killed-virus vaccines have been found to induce serum antibodies but are not protective against infection. This is not surprising, as inactivated vaccines are poor inducers of local immunity, and secretory IgA is of major importance in resistance to parainfluenza virus infections.

There are currently no immediate candidates for a live-virus vaccine.

RESPIRATORY SYNCYTIAL VIRUS INFECTIONS

Respiratory syncytial virus is the most important cause of lower respiratory tract illness in infants and young children, usually outranking all other microbial pathogens as the cause of bronchiolitis and pneumonia in infants under 1 year of age. Respiratory syncytial virus accounts for about half of cases of bronchiolitis and one-fourth of pneumonias in infants. It is estimated to cause about 4500 deaths per year in the USA.

Pathogenesis & Pathology

Respiratory syncytial virus is transmitted via large droplets, so spread can occur by contact with contaminated hands or surfaces. Viral replication occurs initially in epithelial cells of the nasopharynx. Virus may spread into the lower respiratory tract, probably carried there by secretions. Although virus can spread from cell to cell, it is doubtful that this is the major mode of dissemination in vivo. Viremia has not been detected.

The incubation period between exposure and onset of illness is 4–5 days. Viral shedding may persist for 1–3 weeks.

An intact immune system seems to be important to clear an infection, as patients with impaired cell-mediated immunity may become persistently infected with respiratory syncytial virus and shed virus for months. Spread outside the respiratory epithelium (kidney, liver, myocardium) has been noted in several fatal infections in individuals who lacked cell-mediated immunity.

Although the airways of very young infants are narrow and more readily obstructed by inflammation and edema, it is not known why only a subset of young babies develops severe respiratory syncytial virus disease.

Possible involvement of the immune response in the pathogenesis of some respiratory syncytial virus respiratory symptoms, especially bronchiolitis, has been the subject of much speculation for many years. In the late 1960s, an experimental formalin-inactivated respiratory syncytial virus vaccine was tested. Recipients developed high titers of serum antibodies. But when immunized children encountered a subsequent infection with wild-type respiratory syncytial virus, they suffered significantly more severe lower respiratory tract illness than did children from the control group. Thus, respiratory syncytial disease was felt to be the result of an immunopathologic process mediated by maternal antibodies. However, it appears from more recent studies that serum antibody does not participate in the pathogenesis of respiratory syncytial virus-induced disease. It is possible, though, that an immediate hypersensitivity to virus-IgE interactions may be involved. Nasal secretions of children experiencing severe reactions to the virus contain histamine and also anti-respiratory syncytial virus IgE.

At autopsy, the lungs of infants who have died of respiratory syncytial virus infection show extensive bronchopneumonia accompanied by sloughing of bronchiolar epithelium and infiltration by monocytes and other immunologic cells. There is abundant mucus secretion. These processes result in obstruction of small bronchioles.

Clinical Findings

Most respiratory syncytial virus infections are symptomatic. The spectrum of respiratory illness ranges from the common cold in adults, through febrile bronchitis in infants and older children and pneumonia in infants, to bronchiolitis in very young babies.

In 25–40% of primary respiratory syncytial virus infections, the lower respiratory tract is involved. The child may wheeze. Almost 1% of babies develop disease severe enough to require hospitalization.

Progression of symptoms may be very rapid, culminating in death. With availability of modern pediatric intensive care, the mortality rate in normal infants is low (about 1% of hospitalized patients). But if a respiratory syncytial virus infection is superimposed on preexisting disease, such as congenital heart disease, the mortality rate may be as high as 35%.

The role of respiratory syncytial virus in the sudden infant death syndrome is not clear. Virus has been detected in the lungs of children who die suddenly and unexpectedly. It is likely that a subset of such sudden deaths can be attributed to respiratory syncytial virus.

Children who suffered from respiratory syncytial virus bronchiolitis and pneumonia as infants and apparently recovered completely often exhibit abnormal pulmonary function for many years. However, no cause and effect relationship has been shown between respiratory syncytial virus infections and long-term abnormalities. It may be that certain individuals have some underlying physiologic traits that predispose them to both severe respiratory syncytial virus infections and chronic pulmonary abnormalities.

Respiratory syncytial virus is an important etiologic agent of otitis media: About one-third of children with respiratory syncytial virus illness develop middle-ear infections.

Reinfection is common in both children and adults. Although reinfections in all ages tend to be symptomatic, the illness is usually limited to the upper respiratory tract, resembling a cold.

Respiratory syncytial virus may cause pneumonia in the elderly.

Immunity

High levels of neutralizing antibody that is maternally transmitted and present during the first 2 months of life are believed to be critical in protective immunity. Severe respiratory syncytial disease begins to occur in infants at 2–4 months of age, when maternal antibody levels are falling. The natural rate of decrease is about 50% each month; thus, the antibody titer soon falls below the protective level. Healthy 1-month-old infants have antibody titers up to four times higher than those of age-matched infants with respiratory syncytial virus bronchiolitis or pneumonia.

Respiratory syncytial virus is not an effective inducer of interferon, in contrast to influenza and parainfluenza virus infections, in which interferon levels are high and correlate with disappearance of virus.

Both serum and secretory antibodies are made in response to respiratory syncytial virus infection. However, the role of the immune response in viral infection is unclear. It is probable that secretory IgA in nasal secretions is involved in protection against reinfection and that cellular immunity is important in recovery from infection. There is evidence of a role for serum antibody in protection as well. It is apparent that immunity is only partially effective and is often overcome under natural conditions; reinfections are common, but the severity of ensuing disease is lessened.

Laboratory Diagnosis

A rise in serum antibody is a reasonably reliable indication of respiratory syncytial virus infection in adults, but isolation of virus or detection of viral antigen in respiratory secretions is the procedure of choice. Respiratory syncytial virus differs from other paramyxoviruses in that it does not have a hemagglutinin; therefore, diagnostic methods cannot use hemagglutination or hemadsorption assays.

A. Isolation and Identification of Virus: A nasopharyngeal swab or a nasal wash is a good source of virus. Respiratory syncytial virus is extremely labile. Samples should be inoculated into cell cultures immediately; freezing of clinical specimens may result in complete loss of infectivity.

Human heteroploid cell lines HeLa and HEp-2 are the most sensitive for viral isolation. Cultured cells may lose sensitivity to respiratory syncytial virus, so it is important that cell lines be monitored regularly to ensure that they retain susceptibility to the virus.

The presence of respiratory syncytial virus can usually be recognized by development of giant cells and syncytia in inoculated cultures. It may take as long as 10 days for cytopathic effects to appear. Definitive diagnosis can be established by detecting viral antigen in infected cells using a defined antiserum and the immunofluorescence test.

Direct identification of viral antigens in clinical samples is rapid and sensitive. Immunofluorescence on exfoliated cells or ELISA on nasopharyngeal secretions may be used. These tests are simplified because currently only one serotype of respiratory syncytial virus is recognized.

Detection of respiratory syncytial virus is strong evidence that the virus is involved in a current illness, because it is almost never found in healthy people.

B. Serology: Serum antibodies can be assayed in a variety of ways—immunofluorescence, ELISA, CF, and Nt tests are all used. Measurable amounts of antibody are frequently encountered in acute-phase serum samples, but this does not preclude a significant rise in titer during a current infection.

Measurements of serum antibody are important for epidemiologic studies but play only a small role in clinical decision making.

Epidemiology

Respiratory syncytial virus is distributed worldwide and is recognized as the major pediatric respiratory tract pathogen. Serious bronchiolitis or pneumonia is most apt to occur in infants between the ages of 6 weeks and 6 months, with peak incidence at 2 months. Respiratory syncytial virus is the most common cause of viral pneumonia in children under age 5 years but may also cause pneumonia in the elderly or in immunocompromised persons. The virus can be isolated from about 40% of infants under age 6 months suffering from bronchiolitis and from about 25% with pneumonitis, but it is almost never isolated from healthy infants. Respiratory syncytial virus infection in older infants and children results in milder respiratory tract infection than in those under age 6 months.

Reinfection occurs frequently (in spite of the presence of specific antibodies), but resulting symptoms are those of a mild upper respiratory infection (a cold). In families with an identified case of respiratory syncytial infection, virus spread to siblings and adults is common.

Respiratory syncytial virus spreads extensively in children every year during the winter season. Outbreaks tend to peak in February or March in the northern hemisphere. In tropical areas, respiratory syncytial virus epidemics may coincide with rainy seasons.

Respiratory syncytial virus causes nosocomial infections in nurseries and on pediatric hospital wards. Transmission occurs primarily via the hands of staff members. Hospital staff members and parents of infants with respiratory syncytial virus disease often develop colds with fever or pharyngitis (or both).

Treatment

Treatment of serious respiratory syncytial virus infections depends primarily on supportive care (eg, removal of secretions, administration of oxygen).

The antiviral drug ribavirin, administered in a continuous aerosol for 3–6 days, has been found to be clinically beneficial to hospitalized infants. In addition, viral shedding was decreased. When administered as an aerosol, the drug has little or no systemic toxicity.

It was reported in 1993 that administration of immune globulin with a high titer of antibodies against respiratory syncytial virus was an effective means of preventing serious infections in infants and children. The immune globulin was given as monthly intravenous infusions.

Prevention & Control

Much research effort has been devoted to attempts to develop a respiratory syncytial virus vaccine. As noted above, problems with a formalin-inactivated vaccine necessitated abandonment of that approach. To date, attempts to develop an attenuated live-virus vaccine have not been successful.

Respiratory syncytial virus poses special problems for vaccine development. The target group, newborns, would have to be immunized soon after birth to afford protection at the time of greatest risk of serious respiratory syncytial virus infection. Eliciting a protective immune response at this early age, in the presence of maternal antibody, continues to be an elusive goal.

MUMPS VIRUS INFECTIONS

Mumps is an acute contagious disease characterized by nonsuppurative enlargement of one or both parotid glands. Other organs that may also be involved include the pancreas, testes, and ovaries as well as the central nervous system. More than one-third of all mumps infections are asymptomatic.

Pathogenesis & Pathology

Humans are the only natural hosts for mumps virus. Transmission is from person to person by large droplets. Primary replication occurs in nasal or upper respiratory tract epithelial cells. Viremia then disseminates the virus to the salivary glands and other major organ systems. Involvement of the parotid gland is not an obligatory step in the infectious process.

The incubation period is typically about 18 days but may range from 7 to 25 days. Virus is shed in the saliva from as long as 6 days before to 1 week after the onset of salivary gland swelling. About one-third of infected individuals do not exhibit obvious symptoms (inapparent infections) but are equally capable of transmitting infection. It is difficult to control transmission of mumps because of the variable incubation periods, the presence of virus in saliva before clinical symptoms develop, and the large number of asymptomatic but infectious cases.

The testes and ovaries may be affected, especially after puberty. Twenty percent of males over age 13 years who are infected with mumps virus develop orchitis (often unilateral). Because of the lack of elasticity of the tunica albuginea, which does not allow the inflamed testis to swell, the complication is extremely painful. Atrophy of the testis may occur as a result of pressure necrosis, but only rarely does sterility result.

Virus frequently infects the kidneys. As a result, virus can be detected in the urine of most patients. Viruria may persist for up to 14 days after the onset of clinical symptoms. The central nervous system is also commonly infected and may be involved in the absence of parotitis. Mumps is a systemic viral disease with a propensity to replicate in epithelial cells in various visceral organs. Parotitis is only one manifestation of viral infection.

Little tissue damage is associated with uncomplicated mumps. The ducts of the parotid glands show desquamation of the epithelium and the presence of polymorphonuclear cells in the lumina. Interstitial edema and lymphocytic infiltration occur. With severe orchitis, the testis is congested and punctate hemorrhage, as well as degeneration of germinal epithelial cells, occurs. Central nervous system lesions may vary from perivascular edema to inflammatory reaction, glial reaction, hemorrhage, or demyelination.

Clinical Findings

The clinical features of mumps reflect the pathogenesis of the infection. At least one-third of all mumps infections are subclinical. The most characteristic feature of symptomatic cases is swelling of the salivary glands, which occurs in about 95% of patients.

A prodromal period of malaise and anorexia is followed by rapid enlargement of parotid glands as well as other salivary glands. Swelling may be confined to one parotid gland, or one gland may enlarge several days before the other. Gland enlargement is associated with pain, especially when acid substances are consumed. Salivary adenitis is commonly accompanied by low-grade fever and lasts for approximately 1 week.

Mumps accounts for 10–15% of cases of aseptic meningitis observed in the USA and is more common among males than females. Meningoencephalitis usually occurs 5–7 days after inflammation of the salivary glands, but it may occur simultaneously or in the absence of parotitis and is usually self-limited. Cases of mumps meningitis and meningoencephalitis usually resolve without sequelae, although unilateral deafness has been observed. The mortality rate from mumps encephalitis is about 1%.

Rare complications of mumps include (1) a self-limited polyarthritis that resolves without residual deformity; (2) pancreatitis, usually mild but rarely severe (it has been suggested that diabetes mellitus may occasionally follow); (3) nephritis; (4) thyroiditis; and (5) unilateral nerve deafness (hearing loss is complete and permanent). Mumps may be a possible causative agent in the production of aqueductal stenosis and hydrocephalus in children.

Immunity

Immunity is permanent after a single infection. There is only one antigenic type of mumps virus, and it does not exhibit significant antigenic variation.

Antibodies to the HN glycoprotein (V antigen), the F glycoprotein, and the internal nucleocapsid protein (S antigen) develop in serum following natural infection. Antibodies to S antigen appear earliest (3–7 days after onset of clinical symptoms) but are transient and are usually gone within 6 months. Antibodies to V antigen develop more slowly (about 4 weeks after onset) but persist for years.

Antibodies against the HN antigen correlate well with immunity. Even subclinical infections are thought to generate lifelong immunity.

A cell-mediated immune response also develops. Its role in recovery and protection is unknown. Interferon is induced early in mumps infection, with unknown consequences.

Passive immunity is transferred from mother to offspring; thus, it is rare to see mumps in infants under age 6 months.

Laboratory Diagnosis

Laboratory studies are not usually required to establish the diagnosis of typical cases. However, mumps can sometimes be confused with enlargement of the parotids due to suppuration, drug sensitivity, tumors, etc. In cases without parotitis (particularly in aseptic meningitis), the laboratory can be helpful in establishing the diagnosis.

A. Isolation and Identification of Virus: The most appropriate clinical samples for viral isolation are saliva, cerebrospinal fluid, and urine collected within a few days after onset of illness. Virus can be recovered from the urine for up to 2 weeks.

Monkey kidney cells are preferred for viral isolation. Samples should be inoculated shortly after collection, as mumps virus is thermolabile. Cytopathic effects typical of mumps virus consist of cell rounding and giant cell formation. However, not all primary isolates show characteristic syncytial formation, so the hemadsorption test is used to demonstrate the presence of a hemadsorbing agent. The test is done 1 and 2 weeks after cell inoculation, whether or not cytopathic effect is evident.

An isolate can be confirmed as mumps virus by hemadsorption inhibition using mumps-specific antiserum. It is important that the antiserum not cross-react with parainfluenza viruses.

For more rapid diagnosis, immunofluorescence using mumps-specific antiserum can detect mumps virus antigens as early as 2–3 days after inoculation of cell cultures.

B. Serology: Antibody rise can be detected using paired sera: a fourfold or greater rise in antibody titer is evidence of mumps infection. The CF or HI test is commonly used. Problems can be encountered with cross-reactive antibodies induced by parainfluenza viruses, however. Recently described ELISA procedures are more sensitive, and heterotypic antibodies do not seem to interfere.

ELISA is useful because it can be designed to detect either mumps-specific IgM antibody or mumps-specific IgG antibody. Mumps IgM is uniformly present early in the illness and seldom lasts longer than 60 days. Therefore, demonstration of mumps-specific IgM in serum drawn early in illness strongly suggests recent infection. Heterotypic antibodies induced by parainfluenza virus infections do not cross-react in the mumps IgM ELISA.

A CF test on a single serum sample obtained soon after onset of illness may also provide a presumptive diagnosis. Antibodies to the nucleocapsid protein (S antigen) develop within a few days after onset and sometimes reach a high titer before antibodies to the HN glycoprotein (V antigen) can be detected. In early convalescence, both S and V antibodies are present at high levels. Subsequently, S antibodies disappear, leaving V antibodies as a marker of previous infection for several years.

Epidemiology

Mumps occurs endemically worldwide. Cases appear throughout the year. Outbreaks occur where crowding favors dissemination of the virus. Mumps is primarily an infection of children. The disease reaches its highest incidence in children aged 5–15 years, but epidemics may occur in army camps. In children under 5 years of age, mumps may commonly cause upper respiratory tract infection without parotitis.

Mumps is quite contagious; most susceptible individuals in a household will acquire infection from an infected member. The virus is transmitted by direct contact, airborne droplets, or fomites contaminated with saliva or urine. The period of communicability is from about 6 days before to about 1 week after the onset of symptoms. However, closer contact is necessary for transmission of mumps than for transmission of measles or varicella.

About one-third of infections with mumps virus are inapparent. During the course of inapparent infection, the patient can transmit the virus to others. Individuals with subclinical mumps acquire immunity.

The overall mortality rate for mumps is low (1–3.8 deaths per 10,000 cases in the USA). The ratio of encephalitis to reported mumps cases varies widely, averaging about 2.6:1000; and 1–2% of encephalitis cases are fatal.

The incidence of mumps and associated complications have declined markedly since introduction of the live-virus vaccine.

Treatment

Mumps immune globulin does not prevent infection when administered to an exposed susceptible person and is of no value for decreasing the incidence of orchitis even when given immediately after parotitis is first noted.

Prevention & Control

Immunization with attenuated live mumps virus vaccine is the best approach to reducing mumps-associated morbidity and mortality rates. Attempts to minimize viral spread during an outbreak by using isolation procedures are futile because of the high incidence of asymptomatic cases and the degree of viral shedding before clinical symptoms appear.

An effective attenuated live-virus vaccine made in chick embryo cell culture is available. It produces a subclinical, noncommunicable infection.

The vaccine is recommended for children over age 1 year and for adolescents and adults who have not had mumps parotitis. It is contraindicated in pregnancy and in patients who are allergic to egg protein or neomycin. A single dose of the vaccine given subcutaneously produces detectable antibodies in 95% of vaccinees, and antibody persists for at least 10 years.

Mumps vaccine is available in monovalent form (mumps only) or in combinations with rubella (MR) or measles and rubella (MMR) live-virus vaccines. Combination live-virus vaccines produce antibodies to each of the viruses in about 95% of vaccinees.

In 1967, the year mumps vaccine was licensed, there were about 200,000 mumps cases (and 900 patients with encephalitis) in the USA. After 18 years of vaccine use, the number of mumps cases in 1985 was less than 3000, with fewer than 20 cases of encephalitis. This represents a fall in the incidence of mumps from prevaccine levels of 50–250 cases per 100,000 population to a current low of about 1.2 per 100,000. Further declines in the incidence of mumps are expected, as more children entering school are required to provide proof of mumps vaccination.

MEASLES (RUBEOLA) VIRUS INFECTIONS

Measles is an acute, highly infectious disease characterized by a maculopapular rash, fever, and respiratory symptoms. Complications are common and may be quite serious. The introduction of an effective live-virus vaccine has dramatically reduced the incidence of this disease in the USA, but measles is still a leading cause of death of young children in many developing countries. It is of concern that a significant percentage of preschool children in the USA are susceptible to measles because they have not been vaccinated.

Pathogenesis & Pathology

Humans are the only natural hosts for measles virus, although numerous other species, including monkeys, dogs, and mice, can be experimentally infected.

The pathogenesis of measles (Figure 40–5) is assumed to be similar to that of mousepox, another generalized skin disease (see Figure 30–3).

The virus gains access to the human body via the respiratory tract, where it multiplies locally; the infection then spreads to the regional lymphoid tissue, where further multiplication occurs. Primary viremia disseminates the virus, which then replicates in the reticuloendothelial system. Finally, a secondary viremia seeds the epithelial surfaces of the body, including the skin, respiratory tract, and conjunctiva, where focal replication occurs. Measles can replicate in certain lymphocytes, which aids in dissemination throughout the body. Multinucleated giant cells with intranuclear inclusions are seen in lymphoid tissues throughout the body (lymph nodes, tonsils, appendix).

The events described above occur during the incubation period, which typically lasts 9–11 days but may be prolonged for up to 3 weeks in older people. Onset of illness is usually abrupt and characterized by coryza, cough, conjunctivitis, fever, and Koplik's spots in the mouth. Koplik's spots—pathognomonic for measles—are small, bluish-white ulcerations on the buccal mucosa, opposite the lower molars. These spots contain giant cells, viral antigens, and recognizable viral nucleocapsids.

During the prodromal phase, which lasts 2–4 days, virus is present in tears, nasal and throat secretions, urine, and blood. The characteristic maculopapular rash appears about day 14 just as circulating antibodies become detectable, the viremia disappears, and the fever falls. The rash develops as a result of interaction

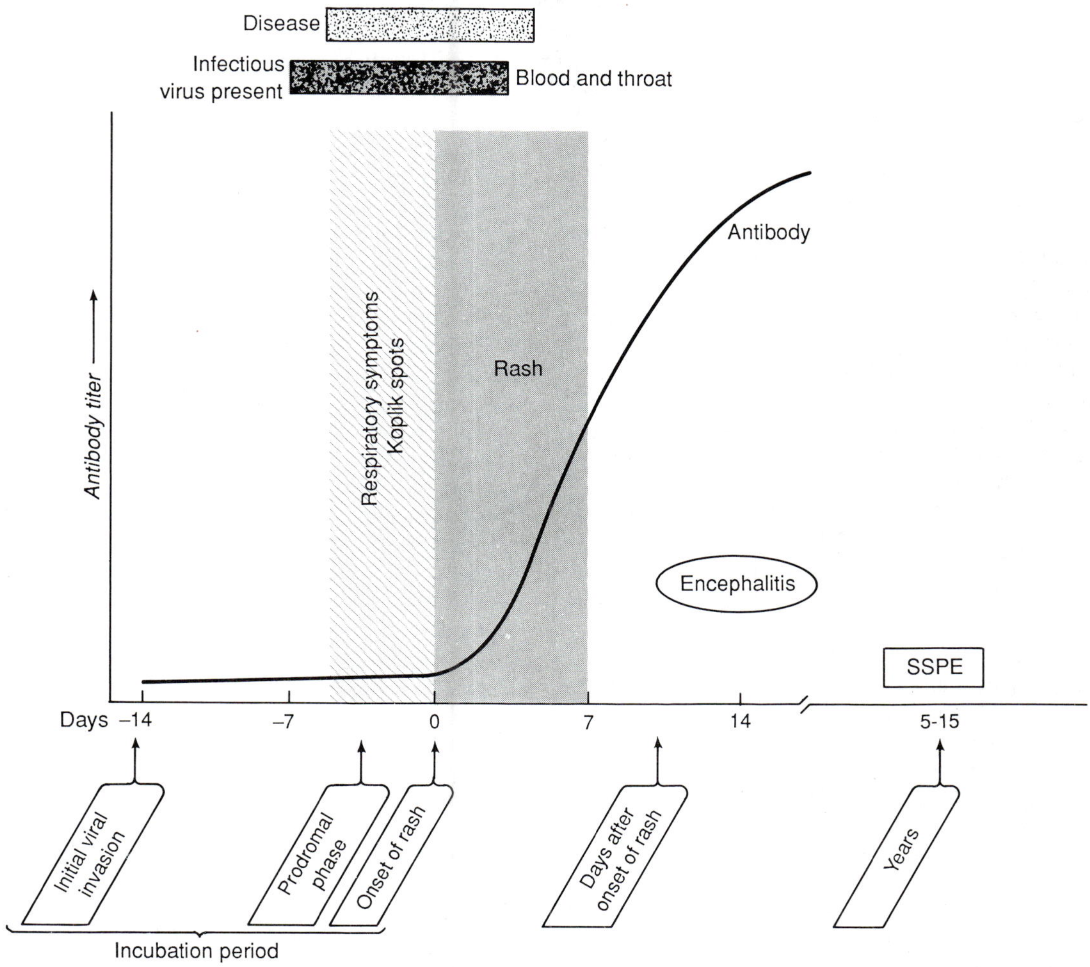

Figure 40–5. Natural history of measles infection. Encephalitis occurs in about one of every 1000 cases of measles. Subacute sclerosing panencephalitis (SSPE) is a late, rare complication that develops in about one of 1 million cases.

of immune T cells with virus-infected cells in the small blood vessels and lasts about 1 week. (In patients with defective cell-mediated immunity, no rash develops.)

Involvement of the central nervous system is common in measles. Symptomatic encephalitis develops in about 1:1000 cases. Because infectious virus is rarely recovered from the brain, it has been suggested that an autoimmune reaction is the mechanism responsible for this complication.

In contrast, acute progressive infectious encephalitis may develop in patients with defective cell-mediated immunity. Actively replicating virus is present in the brain in this usually fatal form of disease.

A rare late complication of measles is subacute sclerosing panencephalitis. This fatal disease develops years after the initial measles infection and is caused by virus that remains in the body after acute measles infection. Large amounts of measles antigens are present within inclusion bodies in infected brain cells, but no viral particles mature. Viral replication is defective owing to lack of production of one or more viral gene products, often the matrix protein. It is not known what mechanisms are responsible for selection of the pathogenic defective virus.

The presence of latent intracellular measles virus in the brain cells of patients with subacute sclerosing panencephalitis suggests a failure of the immune system to clear the viral infection. Expression of viral antigens on the cell surface is modulated by the addition of measles antibody to cells infected with measles virus. By expressing fewer viral antigens on the surface, cells may avoid being killed by antibody- or cell-mediated cytotoxic reactions yet may retain viral genetic information. Whether this process plays a role in the persistent infections found in patients with subacute sclerosing panencephalitis is unknown.

Children who were immunized with inactivated measles vaccine and then exposed to natural measles virus, may experience a syndrome called atypical measles. The inactivation procedure employed in vaccine production destroyed the immunogenicity of the viral F protein; although vaccinees developed a good antibody response to the H protein, in the absence of F antibody infection could be initiated and virus could spread from cell to cell by fusion. These conditions would be appropriate for immune pathologic reactions that might mediate atypical measles. Killed measles virus vaccine is no longer used.

Clinical Findings

After an incubation period of 9–11 days, measles is typically a 7- to 11-day illness (with a prodromal phase of 2–4 days followed by an eruptive phase of 5–7 days).

The prodromal phase is characterized by fever, sneezing, coughing, running nose, redness of the eyes, Koplik's spots, and lymphopenia. The conjunctivitis is commonly associated with photophobia. The fever and cough persist until the rash appears and then subside within 1–2 days. The rash, which starts on the head and then spreads progressively to the chest, the trunk, and down the limbs, appears as light pink, discrete maculopapules that coalesce to form blotches, becoming brownish in 5–10 days. The fading rash resolves with desquamation. Symptoms are most marked when the rash is at its peak but subside rapidly thereafter.

Atypical measles, now seen occasionally in young adults who received killed measles virus vaccine as children, is characterized by high fever, pneumonitis, edema of the extremities, and an unusual rash (raised papules, wheals, and tiny hemorrhages in the skin) located predominantly on the extremities. Koplik's spots are not present. Atypical measles may be confused with Rocky Mountain spotted fever.

Modified measles occurs in infants with residual maternal antibody. The incubation period is prolonged, prodromal symptoms are diminished, Koplik's spots are usually absent, and rash is mild.

Secondary bacterial infections, most often involving β-hemolytic streptococci, are common in measles. The most common complication is otitis media. Lower respiratory tract infections follow in about 15% of measles cases and may be serious; pulmonary complications account for more than 90% of measles-related deaths.

A different form of disease, giant cell pneumonia, may occur as a complication in children with immune deficiencies and is believed to be due to unchecked viral replication. As the name implies, extensive cell fusion is seen in lung tissue. It is usually fatal.

Complications involving the central nervous system are the most feared. About 50% of children with regular measles register electroencephalographic changes. Acute encephalitis occurs in about 1:1000 cases. There is no apparent correlation between the severity of the measles and the appearance of neurologic complications. The cause of measles encephalitis is unknown. Symptoms referable to the brain usually appear a few days after the rash, often after it has faded. There is a second bout of fever, with drowsiness or convulsions and pleocytosis of the cerebrospinal fluid. Survivors may show permanent mental changes (psychosis or personality change) or physical disabilities (particularly seizure disorders). The mortality rate in encephalitis associated with measles is about 15%, and 25% of survivors show sequelae.

Immunologically deficient children may develop acute progressive infectious encephalitis, as well as giant cell pneumonia, due to active viral replication.

Subacute sclerosing panencephalitis is a rare late complication of measles infection, with an incidence between 1:300,000 and 1:1 million cases. The disease begins insidiously 5–15 years after a case of measles; it is characterized by progressive mental deterioration, involuntary movements, muscular rigidity, and coma. It is invariably fatal. Patients with subacute sclerosing panencephalitis exhibit high titers of measles antibody in cerebrospinal fluid and serum and defective measles virus in brain cells. With the widespread use of measles vaccine, subacute sclerosing panencephalitis has become less common (and may someday be eliminated).

Immunity

There is only one antigenic type of measles virus. Infection confers lifelong immunity. Most so-called second attacks represent errors in diagnosis of either the initial or the second illness.

The presence of humoral antibodies indicates immunity. However, cellular immunity must also be relevant to protection: patients with immunoglobulin deficiencies recover from measles and resist reinfection, whereas patients with cellular immune deficiencies do very poorly when they acquire measles infections.

Laboratory Diagnosis

Typical measles is reliably diagnosed on clinical grounds; laboratory diagnosis may be necessary in cases of modified or atypical measles. Serologic diagnoses are preferred with measles because viral isolation methods are inefficient and slow.

A. Isolation and Identification of Virus: Nasopharyngeal swabs and blood samples taken from a patient 2–3 days before the onset of symptoms up to 1 day after the appearance of rash (essentially during the febrile period of measles) are appropriate sources for viral isolation. Monkey or human kidney cells or human amnion cells are optimal for isolation attempts. Measles virus grows slowly; typical cytopathic effects (multinucleated giant cells containing both intranuclear and intracytoplasmic inclusion bodies) take 7–10 days to develop. Hemadsorption or immunofluorescence assays can be used to confirm measles antigens in the inoculated cultures.

B. Serology: Serologic confirmation of measles infection depends on a fourfold rise in antibody titer between acute- and convalescent-phase sera or on demonstration of measles-specific IgM antibody in a single serum specimen drawn between 1 and 2 weeks after the onset of rash. HI, CF, and Nt tests all may be used to measure measles antibodies, though HI is the most practical method.

Measles and canine distemper virus are antigenically related, with the F protein being the most highly conserved. Measles patients develop antibodies that cross-react with canine distemper virus—and, similarly, dogs develop antibodies that fix complement with measles antigen after infection with distemper virus.

The major part of the immune response is directed against the NP protein. Only in cases of atypical measles is a pronounced response to the M protein observed. Patients with subacute sclerosing panencephalitis display an exaggerated antibody response, with titers 10- to 100-fold higher than those seen in typical convalescent sera. The hyperimmune response in subacute sclerosing panencephalitis often does not include antibodies to the M protein.

Epidemiology

The key epidemiologic features of measles are as follows: the virus is highly contagious, there is a single serotype, there is no animal reservoir, inapparent infections are rare, and infection confers lifelong immunity. Prevalence and age incidence of measles are related to population density, economic and environmental factors, and use of an effective live-virus vaccine.

Transmission occurs predominantly via the respiratory route. A continuous supply of susceptible individuals is required for the virus to persist in a community. A population size approaching 500,000 is necessary to sustain measles as an endemic disease; in smaller communities, the virus disappears until it is reintroduced from the outside after a critical number of nonimmune persons accumulates.

Measles is endemic throughout the world. In general, epidemics recur regularly every 2–3 years. A population's state of immunity is the determining factor; the disease will flare up when there is an accumulation of susceptible children. The severity of an epidemic is a function of the number of susceptible individuals. Finally, the more widely dispersed the population, the lower the rate of spread and the longer-lasting the epidemic.

When the disease is introduced into isolated communities where it has not been endemic, an epidemic builds rapidly and attack rates are almost 100%. All age groups develop clinical measles. A classic example of this phenomenon occurred in 1846 when measles was introduced into the Faroe Islands; only people over age 60 years, who had been alive during the last epidemic, escaped the disease. In places where the disease strikes rarely, its consequences are often disastrous and the mortality rate may be as high as 25%.

Measles rarely causes death in healthy people in developed countries. However, in malnourished children in developing countries where adequate medical care is unavailable, measles is a leading cause of infant mortality.

In industrialized countries, measles occurs in 5- to 10-year-old children, whereas in developing countries it commonly infects children under 5 years of age.

Measles cases occur throughout the year in temperate climates. Epidemics tend to occur in late winter and early spring. In the USA, peak activity is in March and April.

Treatment

There are no available antiviral drugs effective against measles or its complications. Bacterial superinfections should be treated with antibiotics. Various antiviral agents and interferon have been given to patients with subacute sclerosing panencephalitis, without obvious benefit.

Measles may be prevented or modified by administering antibody early in the incubation period. Passive immunization is indicated for neonates, susceptible pregnant women, and immunosuppressed patients. If mild disease occurs, immunity ensues. With a large dose of immune globulin administered promptly, the disease may be prevented, but the individual will remain susceptible to infection at a later date. Antibodies given more than 6 days after exposure are not likely to influence the course of the disease.

Prevention & Control

A highly effective, safe, attenuated live measles virus vaccine is available. It has reduced indigenous measles in the USA from prevaccine levels of more than 500,000 cases annually to about 3000 cases in 1988. Before measles vaccine was developed, the rate of measles deaths per year was 400, but death from measles is now rare.

The vaccine is more than 95% effective. However, measles has not been eliminated, because of failure to vaccinate some children before they reach school age and because of cases of vaccine failure. The failures may be attributed to vaccine inactivation or administration to infants with residual maternal antibody. In 1989, a substantial number of measles cases occurred on college campuses, coupled with several large outbreaks among unvaccinated children under school age.

These outbreaks prompted new recommendations for measles vaccination: (1) Each child should receive two doses of measles vaccine, the first at 15 months of age and the second just before entering school. Both doses should preferably be given as combined measles-mumps-rubella (MMR) vaccine. (2) If the child lives in a high-risk area, the first dose should be administered at 12 months of age. (3) Colleges should require any entering student to receive two doses of vaccine at least 1 month apart or to provide evidence of immunity. (4) Individuals given live-virus vaccine along with immune globulin (routinely done from 1963 through the middle 1970s) should be considered unvaccinated and should receive two doses of vaccine. (5) Other persons vaccinated according to earlier recommendations (live-virus vaccine before first birthday or the killed-virus vaccine given from 1963 to 1967) should also be considered unvaccinated and should receive two doses of vaccine.

Mild clinical reactions (fever or mild rash) will occur in 10–15% of vaccinees, but there is little or no virus excretion and no transmission. Antibody titers tend to be lower than after natural infection, but immunity lasts at least 18 years and is probably lifelong.

There are few contraindications to the use of the vaccine. The World Health Organization recommends that all children be vaccinated except when their general condition calls for hospitalization. Although there is no evidence of fetal infection or teratogenicity by the vaccine virus, it is prudent to exempt pregnant women from vaccination. In addition, vaccination is not recommended in persons with febrile illnesses or egg allergies or in persons with immune defects. The attenuated vaccine virus can cause giant cell pneumonia in immunodeficient patients.

Special problems are associated with the use of live-virus vaccine in developing countries. Storage and transport of the labile vaccine are difficult. Furthermore, the vaccine must be given early in life to prevent the disease, with its attendant high mortality rates, in children under 1 year of age. An aerosolized form of the measles vaccine has been tested for vaccination in the first few months of life in the presence of maternal antibody. It may prove particularly useful.

The use of killed measles virus vaccine was discontinued by 1970, as certain vaccinees became sensitized and developed severe atypical measles when infected with wild virus.

GUILLAIN-BARRÉ SYNDROME

Guillain-Barré syndrome is an inflammatory and demyelinating disorder of the nervous system. It is a rare sequela of acute viral infections, especially measles, rubella, varicella-zoster, or mumps. It can also follow vaccination, especially with vaccinia virus or some types of influenza virus vaccine. In 1976, swine influenza virus vaccine inoculation of humans was followed by Guillain-Barré syndrome five times more often than occurred in matched individuals who had not been given this vaccine. Very rarely, this syndrome has followed infections by enteroviruses and cytomegalovirus.

Symptoms may range from minor neuropathy with paresthesia or weakness to rapidly progressive ascending paralysis and occasional death. Treatment is symptomatic.

RUBELLA (GERMAN MEASLES) VIRUS INFECTIONS

Rubella (German measles, or 3-day measles) is an acute febrile illness characterized by a rash and posterior auricular and suboccipital lymphadenopathy that affects children and young adults. It is the mildest of common viral exanthems. However, infection during early pregnancy may result in serious abnormalities of the fetus, including congenital malformations and mental retardation. The consequences of rubella in utero are referred to as the congenital rubella syndrome.

Classification

Rubella virus, a member of the **Togaviridae** family, is the sole member of the *Rubivirus* genus. Although its morphologic features and physicochemical properties place it in the togavirus group, rubella is not transmitted by arthropods.

Togavirus structure and replication are described in Chapter 38.

1. POSTNATAL RUBELLA

For clarity in presentation, postnatal rubella and congenital rubella infections will be described separately.

Pathogenesis & Pathology

Infection occurs through the mucosa of the upper respiratory tract. Little is known about events that occur during the 2- to 3-week incubation period. Initial viral replication probably occurs in the respiratory tract, followed by multiplication in the cervical lymph nodes. Viremia develops after 5–7 days and lasts until the appearance of antibody on about day 13–15. The development of antibody coincides with the appearance of the rash, suggesting an immunologic basis for the rash. After the rash appears, the virus remains detectable only in the nasopharynx, where it may persist for several weeks (Figure 40–6). In about 25% of cases, primary infection is subclinical.

Clinical Findings

Rubella usually begins with malaise, low-grade fever, and a morbilliform rash appearing on the same day. Less often, systemic symptoms may precede the rash by 1 or 2 days, or the rash and lymphadenopathy may occur without systemic symptoms. The rash starts on the face, extends over the trunk and extremities, and rarely lasts more than 3 days. No feature of the rash is pathognomonic for rubella. Posterior auricular and suboccipital lymphadenopathy are present.

Transient arthralgia and arthritis are commonly seen in women. Despite certain similarities, rubella arthritis is not etiologically related to rheumatoid arthritis. Rare complications include thrombocytopenic purpura and encephalitis.

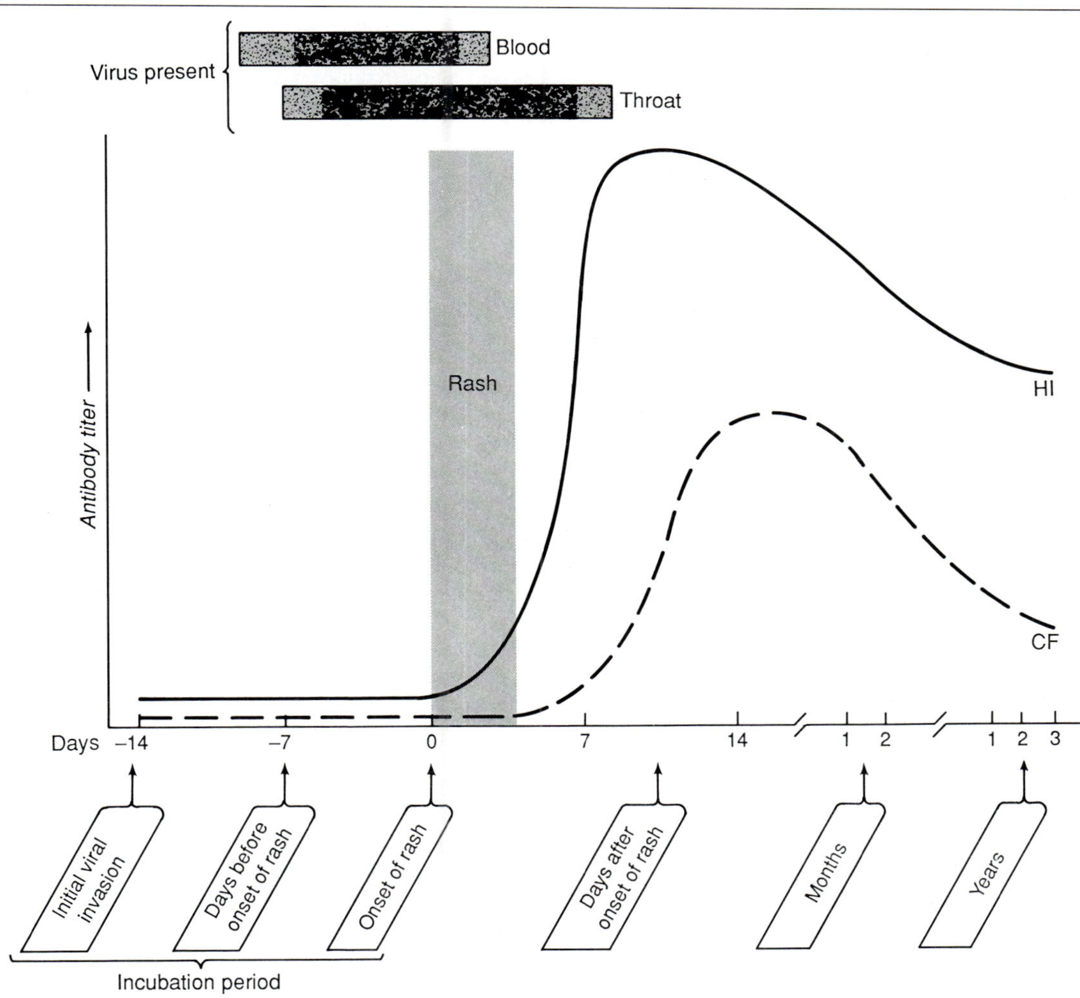

Figure 40–6. Natural history of primary rubella infection: virus production and antibody responses.

Unless an epidemic occurs the disease is difficult to diagnose clinically, since the rash caused by other viruses (eg, enteroviruses) is similar.

Immunity

Rubella antibodies appear in the serum of patients as the rash fades and the antibody titer rises rapidly over the next 1–3 weeks. Much of the initial antibody consists of IgM antibodies, which generally do not persist beyond 6 weeks after the illness. IgM rubella antibodies found in a single serum sample obtained 2 weeks after the rash give evidence of recent rubella infection. IgG rubella antibodies usually persist for life.

One attack of the disease confers lifelong immunity, as only one antigenic type of the virus exists. A history of "rubella" is not a reliable index of immunity. Immune mothers transfer antibodies to their offspring, who are then protected for 4–6 months.

Laboratory Diagnosis

Clinical diagnosis of rubella is unreliable because many viral infections produce symptoms similar to those of rubella. Certain diagnosis rests on specific laboratory studies (isolation of virus or evidence of seroconversion).

A. Isolation and Identification of Virus: Viral isolation is seldom attempted for routine diagnosis because recovery methods are time-consuming (sometimes taking several weeks) and insensitive.

Nasopharyngeal or throat swabs taken within 3–4 days after symptoms appear are the best source of rubella virus. Various tissue culture cell lines of monkey (BSC-1, Vero) or rabbit (RK-13, SIRC) origin, as well as primary African green monkey kidney cultures, may be used. Rubella produces a rather inconspicuous cytopathic effect in most of the cell lines, whereas its presence in primary cells must be detected indirectly by its ability to interfere with replication of an unrelated challenge enterovirus. Perhaps the most sensitive method for recovery of rubella virus from clinical specimens entails the interference technique in primary monkey kidney cells with coxsackievirus A9 as the challenge virus.

Absolute identification of an isolate requires specific neutralization with reference rubella antibody.

B. Serology: The HI test is the standard serologic test for rubella. However, serum must be pretreated to remove nonspecific inhibitors before testing. CF tests are of limited usefulness. Complement-fixing antigens have not yet been correlated with specific viral proteins. ELISA tests developed recently are not only comparable in sensitivity to older tests but advantageous in that serum pretreatment is not required and they can be adapted to detect specific IgM.

Detection of IgG is evidence of immunity, as there is only one serotype of rubella virus. To accurately confirm a recent rubella infection (critically important in the case of a pregnant woman), either a rise in antibody titer must be demonstrated between two serum samples taken at least 10 days apart or rubella-specific IgM must be detected in a single specimen.

Accurate serologic testing for rubella antibodies is so important that various diagnostic kits are now commercially available. Most individuals are unable to assess their rubella immunity status reliably, because subclinical infections are common and rashes induced by other viruses may be mistaken for rubella.

Epidemiology

Rubella is worldwide in distribution. Infection occurs throughout the year with a peak incidence in the spring. Epidemics occur every 6–10 years, with explosive pandemics every 20–25 years. Infection is transmitted by the respiratory route, but—for reasons that are not understood—rubella is not as contagious as measles. The use of rubella vaccine has eliminated epidemic rubella in the USA.

Treatment

Rubella is a mild, self-limited illness, and no specific treatment is given.

Laboratory-proved rubella in the first 3–4 months of pregnancy is almost uniformly associated with fetal infection; therapeutic abortion is the only means of avoiding the risk of malformed infants in such cases.

Immune globulin USP injected into the mother does not protect the fetus against rubella infection, because it is usually not given early enough to prevent viremia. However, in cases in which infection occurs early in pregnancy and termination of pregnancy will not be considered, immune globulin should be administered on the slim chance that it might be helpful.

Prevention & Control

Attenuated live rubella vaccines have been available since 1969. The original one (HPV77) was prepared in duck embryo cells; it was replaced in 1979 by a second vaccine, RA27/3, grown in human diploid cells. It produces much higher antibody titers and a more enduring and solid immunity than does HPV77, and there is evidence that it is highly effective in preventing subclinical superinfection with wild virus. It may also produce IgA antibody in the respiratory tract and thus interfere with infection by wild virus. This vaccine is available as a single antigen or combined with measles and mumps vaccine.

The vaccine virus multiplies in the body and is shed in small amounts, but it does not spread to contacts. Vaccinated children pose no threat to mothers who are susceptible and pregnant. In contrast, nonimmunized children can bring home wild virus and spread it to susceptible family contacts. The vaccine induces immunity in at least 95% of recipients, and that immunity endures for at least 10 years.

The vaccine is safe and causes few side effects in children. There may be mild fever, lymphadenopathy, and a fleeting rash but no permanent residual effects. In adults, the only significant side effect is arthralgia. In postpubertal females, the vaccine produces self-limited arthralgia and arthritis in about one-third of vaccinees.

In the USA, control of rubella is being attempted by routine vaccination of children aged 1–12 years and selective immunization of adolescents and women of childbearing age. Before vaccine became available in 1969, about 70,000 cases were being reported annually. Vaccination decreased the incidence of rubella to only 220 cases in 1988, a decrease of more than 99%. However, the decrease occurred primarily in children; in persons 15 years of age and older, only a small decrease in incidence occurred.

Since the introduction of vaccine, scattered outbreaks of rubella still occur, chiefly among nonvaccinated adolescents in high school and college. The changing age incidence of rubella since introduction of vaccine is similar to the changing epidemiologic pattern with measles (see above).

Rubella vaccine virus can cross the placenta and infect the fetus. However, it is not teratogenic. More than 200 infants have been born to susceptible mothers inadvertently vaccinated with rubella virus vaccine during pregnancy; none had congenital rubella syndrome. Therefore, accidental immunization during pregnancy is not an indication for termination. Nevertheless, it is still prudent to avoid vaccination during pregnancy, and nonpregnant women vaccinees should be advised to delay conception for at least 3 months.

It has been suggested that, because immunity may wane in individuals vaccinated as children, pregnant women may be at risk of infection. Therefore, vaccination of prepubertal girls and women in the immediate postpartum period has been proposed. It may be wise for all pregnant women to undergo a serum antibody test for rubella and, if found to be susceptible, receive a vaccination immediately after delivery.

The 1989 recommendations for a routine two-dose measles vaccination schedule encouraged the use of the combined measles-mumps-rubella vaccine for both doses. Although rubella vaccine failure has not been a major problem, the use of measles-mumps-rubella as recommended should provide an additional safeguard against the potential serious consequences of vaccine failure (ie, congenital rubella syndrome).

2. CONGENITAL RUBELLA SYNDROME

Pathogenesis & Pathology

Maternal viremia associated with rubella infection during pregnancy may result in infection of the placenta and fetus. Only a limited number of fetal cells become infected. Although the virus does not destroy the cells, the growth rate of infected cells is reduced, resulting in fewer numbers of cells in affected organs at birth. The infection may lead to deranged and hypoplastic organ development, resulting in structural anomalies in the newborn.

Timing of the fetal infection determines the extent of teratogenic effect. In general, the earlier in pregnancy infection occurs, the greater the damage to the fetus. Infection during the first trimester of pregnancy is most critical. Infection in the first month of pregnancy results in abnormalities in the infant in about 50% of cases, whereas detectable defects are found in about 20% of infants who acquired the disease during the second month of gestation and in about 4% of infants infected during the third month. Birth defects are uncommon if maternal infection occurs after the 18th week of pregnancy.

Inapparent maternal infections can produce these anomalies as well. Rubella infection can also result in fetal death and spontaneous abortion.

Intrauterine infection with rubella is associated with chronic persistence of the virus in the newborn. At birth, virus is easily detectable in pharyngeal secretions, multiple organs, cerebrospinal fluid, urine, and rectal swabs. Viral excretion may last for 12–18 months after birth, but the level of shedding gradually decreases with age.

Clinical Findings

Rubella virus has been isolated from many different organs and cell types from infants infected in utero, and rubella-induced damage is similarly widespread.

Clinical features of congenital rubella syndrome may be grouped into three broad categories: (1) transient effects in infants, (2) permanent manifestations that may be apparent at birth or become recognized during the first year, and (3) developmental abnormalities that appear and progress during childhood and adolescence.

The most common permanent defects are congenital heart disease (patent ductus arteriosus, pulmonary and aortic stenosis, pulmonary valvular stenosis, and ventricular or atrial septal defect), total or partial blindness (cataracts, glaucoma, chorioretinitis), and neurosensory deafness. Infants may also display transient symptoms of growth retardation, failure to thrive, hepatosplenomegaly, thrombocytopenic purpura, anemia, osteitis, and meningoencephalitis.

Central nervous system involvement is more global. The most common developmental manifestation of congenital rubella is moderate to profound mental retardation. Problems with balance and motor skills develop in preschool children. Psychiatric disorders and behavioral manifestations may occur in preschool and school-age children. The encephalitic manifestations of congenital rubella syndrome are persistent and diverse, with 9- to 12-year-old children displaying significant learning deficits, poor balance, muscle weakness, and deficits in tactile perception.

There is a 20% mortality rate among congenitally virus-infected infants symptomatic at birth. Surprisingly, some virus-infected infants appear normal at birth but manifest abnormalities later. Severely affected infants may require institutionalization.

Progressive rubella panencephalitis, a rare complication that develops in the second decade of life in children with congenital rubella, is a severe neurologic deterioration that inevitably progresses to death. It seems to be associated with chronic rubella virus infection; patients have high titers of rubella antibodies, and virus has been isolated from brain tissue by cocultivation techniques. The mechanism of rubella virus involvement in the pathogenesis of progressive rubella panencephalitis is unknown.

Immunity

Normally, maternal rubella antibody in the form of IgG is transferred to infants and is gradually lost over a period of 6 months. In infants infected in utero, persistence of rubella virus causes a rising titer of rubella-specific IgM and a rise in the specific IgG level that persists long after the fall in maternal IgG.

Laboratory Diagnosis

Infants infected in utero shed large amounts of virus in pharyngeal secretions and other body fluids for up to 18 months of age. Virus has been recovered from many tissues tested postmortem.

Demonstration of rubella antibodies of the IgM class in infants is diagnostic of congenital rubella. IgM antibodies do not cross the placenta, so their presence indicates that they must have been synthesized by the infant in utero. Children with congenital rubella exhibit impaired cell-mediated immunity specific for rubella virus.

Epidemiology

In the rubella epidemic of 1964, more than 20,000 infants were born with severe manifestations of congenital rubella. Mortality rates vary, depending on the timing of maternal infection and the particular congenital defects.

Congenitally infected infants who shed virus can transmit rubella to susceptible contacts, such as the nurses and physicians caring for them. Persons at risk should therefore avoid contact with these babies.

Treatment

There is no specific treatment for congenital rubella. Many abnormalities can be corrected by surgery or may respond to medical therapy. Specific lesions are managed clinically without regard to the fact that they resulted from rubella virus infection.

Prevention & Control

The primary impetus for the development of a rubella vaccine was to prevent congenital rubella, and it is being brought under control. In the USA, the incidence has declined from a high of almost 30,000 cases in 1964 (in the prevaccine period) to only three cases in 1987. To eliminate rubella and the congenital rubella syndrome, it is necessary to immunize women of childbearing age as well as all school-age children. In addition to the recommendations set forth above, it is advised that women be vaccinated as part of routine medical and gynecologic care (particularly during visits to family-planning clinics) and that proof of immunity (positive serologic tests or documented rubella vaccination) be required for women entering college and for female hospital personnel who might come in contact with rubella patients or pregnant women.

REFERENCES

Amler RW et al: Imported measles in the United States. JAMA 1982;248:2129.

Anderson LJ et al: Antigenic characterization of respiratory syncytial virus strains with monoclonal antibodies. J Infect Dis 1985;151:626.

Black NA et al: Post-partum rubella immunisation: A controlled trial of two vaccines. Lancet 1983;2:990.

Briss PA et al: Sustained transmission of mumps in a highly vaccinated population: Assessment of primary vaccine failure and waning vaccine-induced immunity. J Infect Dis 1994;169:77.

Carrigan DR, Kabacoff CM: Nonproductive, cell-associated virus exists before the appearance of antiviral antibodies in experimental measles encephalitis. Virology 1987;156:185.

Centers for Disease Control: Measles prevention: Recommendations of the Immunization Practices Advisory Committee (ACIP). Morb Mortal Wkly Rep 1989;38 (No. S–9):1.

Groothuis JR et al: Prophylactic administration of respiratory syncytial virus immune globulin to high-risk infants and young children. N Engl J Med 1993;329:1524.

Hall CB et al: Aerosolized ribavirin treatment of infants with respiratory syncytial viral infection: A randomized double-blind study. N Engl J Med 1983;308:1443.

Hinman AR et al: Elimination of indigenous measles from the United States. Rev Infect Dis 1983;5:538.

Johnson RT: The pathogenesis of acute viral encephalitis and postinfectious encephalomyelitis. J Infect Dis 1987;155:359.

Lamb RA: Paramyxovirus fusion: A hypothesis for changes. Virology 1993;197:1.

Leclair JM et al: Prevention of nosocomial respiratory syncytial virus infections through compliance with glove and gown isolation precautions. N Engl J Med 1987;317:329.

Orenstein WA et al: The opportunity and obligation to eliminate rubella from the United States. JAMA 1984;251:1988.

Remington PL et al: Airborne transmission of measles in a physician's office. JAMA 1985;253:1574.

Serdula MK et al: Serological response to rubella revaccination. JAMA 1984;251:1974.

Coronaviruses

41

Coronaviruses are large, enveloped RNA viruses. The human coronaviruses cause common colds and have been implicated in gastroenteritis in infants. Animal coronaviruses cause diseases of economic importance in domestic animals. Coronaviruses of lower animals establish persistent infections in their natural hosts. The human viruses are difficult to culture and therefore are poorly characterized.

PROPERTIES OF CORONAVIRUSES

Important properties of the coronaviruses are listed in Table 41–1.

Structure & Composition

Coronaviruses are enveloped, 80- to 160-nm particles that contain an unsegmented genome of single-stranded RNA (27–30 kb; MW 5–6 $\times 10^6$), the largest genome among RNA viruses. The helical nucleocapsid is 9–11 nm in diameter. There are 20-nm-long club- or petal-shaped projections that are widely spaced on the outer surface of the envelope, resembling a solar corona (Figure 41–1). The viral structural proteins include a 50–60K phosphorylated nucleocapsid protein, a 20–30K (E1) glycoprotein that serves as a matrix protein embedded in the envelope lipid bilayer and interacting with the nucleocapsid, and the E2 (180–200K) glycoprotein that makes up the petal-shaped peplomers. Some viruses contain a third glycoprotein (E3; 120–140 K) that causes hemagglutination and has acetylesterase activity.

Classification

There seem to be two antigenic groups of human coronaviruses, represented by strains 229E and OC43. There are two additional distinct antigenic groups when animal coronaviruses are included, one of which contains the well-studied avian infectious bronchitis virus. There appears to be significant antigenic heterogeneity among viral strains within a major antigenic group (ie, 229E-like). Cross-reactions occur between some human and some animal strains. Some strains have hemagglutinins.

The toroviruses represent a separate genus in the **Coronaviridae** family. The toroviruses are widespread in ungulates and appear to be associated with diarrheas.

Coronavirus Replication

Because human coronaviruses do not grow well in cell culture, details of viral replication have come from studies with mouse hepatitis virus, which is closely related to human strain OC43.

The virus attaches to receptors on target cells by the glycoprotein spikes on the viral envelope (either by E2 or by E3). Human and mouse coronaviruses utilize unrelated receptors. The receptor for human coronavirus is aminopeptidase N, whereas multiple isoforms of the carcinoembryonic antigen-related glycoprotein family serve as receptors for mouse coronavirus. The particle is then internalized, probably by absorptive endocytosis. The E2 glycoprotein may cause fusion of the viral envelope with the cell membrane.

The first event after uncoating is the synthesis of a virus-specific RNA-dependent RNA polymerase that transcribes a full-length complementary (minus-strand) RNA. This serves as the template for a nested set of 5–7 subgenomic mRNAs. These overlapping molecules have common 3′ ends, with each mRNA containing one additional gene at the 5′ end. Only the 5′ terminal gene sequence of each mRNA is translated. Each subgenomic mRNA contains at its 5′ end a leader sequence of about 70 bases that is also found at the 5′ end of the genomic RNA. Full-length genomic RNA copies are also transcribed off the complementary RNA. Coronaviruses undergo a high frequency of recombination during replication; this is unusual for an RNA virus with a nonsegmented genome and may ac-

Table 41–1. Important properties of coronaviruses.

Virion: Spherical, 80–160 nm in diameter, helical nucleocapsid.
Genome: Single-stranded RNA, linear, nonsegmented, positive-sense, 27–30 kb, MW 5–6 million, capped and polyadenylated, infectious.
Proteins: Two glycoproteins and one phosphoprotein. Some viruses contain a third glycoprotein (hemagglutinin esterase).
Envelope: Contains large, widely spaced, club- or petal-shaped spikes.
Replication: Cytoplasm; particles mature by budding into endoplasmic reticulum and Golgi.
Outstanding characteristics: Caue colds; display high frequency of recombination; difficult to grow in cell culture.

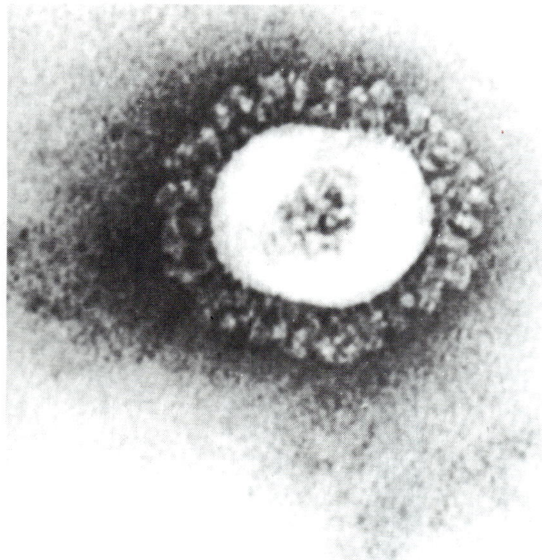

Figure 41–1. Human coronavirus OC43. Note the characteristic large, widely spaced spikes that form a "corona" around the virion (297,000×). (Courtesy of FA Murphy and EL Palmer.)

count for the observed antigenic variation. As each subgenomic mRNA is translated into a single polypeptide, polyprotein precursors are not common in coronavirus infections. It may be that genomic RNA encodes a large polyprotein that gets processed to yield the viral RNA polymerase.

Newly synthesized genomic RNA molecules interact in the cytoplasm with the nucleocapsid protein to form helical nucleocapsids. The nucleocapsids bud through membranes of the rough endoplasmic reticulum and the Golgi apparatus in areas that contain the viral glycoproteins. Mature virions may then be transported in vesicles to the cell periphery for exit or may wait until the cell dies to be released. Virions are not formed by budding at the plasma membrane. Large numbers of particles may be seen on the exterior of infected cells and are presumably adsorbed to it after virion release. Some coronaviruses establish persistent infections of cells rather than being cytocidal.

CORONAVIRUS INFECTIONS IN HUMANS

Pathogenesis

Coronaviruses tend to be highly species-specific. Little is known about the pathogenesis of coronavirus disease in humans. Most of the known animal coronaviruses display a tropism for epithelial cells of the respiratory or gastrointestinal tract. Coronavirus infections in humans usually remain limited to the upper respiratory tract. Coronavirus infection of tracheal organ cultures in vitro results in a slow, patchy destruction of ciliated epithelial cells and the loss of beating cilia. This destructive effect may be related to disease development in vivo. Rat and chicken coronavirus diseases are two animal models for respiratory infection.

There are several animal models for enteric coronaviruses. Disease occurs in young animals and is marked by epithelial cell destruction and loss of absorptive capacity.

Clinical Findings

A. Respiratory Disease: The human coronaviruses produce "colds," usually afebrile, in adults. The symptoms are similar to those produced by rhinoviruses, typified by nasal discharge and malaise. The incubation period is from 2 to 5 days, and symptoms usually last about 1 week. The lower respiratory tract is seldom involved, although pneumonia in military recruits has been attributed to coronavirus infection. Asthmatic children may suffer wheezing attacks, and chronic pulmonary disease in adults may exacerbate respiratory symptoms.

B. Gastrointestinal Disease: Coronavirus-like particles have been observed by electron microscopy in feces from both normal controls and patients with enteritis. It has not been proved that the particles are actually coronaviruses or that they cause disease in humans. However, such human viruses may exist; several animal coronaviruses are known that cause acute gastrointestinal infections.

C. Neurologic Disease: Some animal coronaviruses cause nervous system disease in animals. However, there is currently no evidence that coronaviruses are involved in human neurologic disease.

Immunity

As with other respiratory viruses, immunity develops but is not absolute. Secretory IgA is probably important, but this has not been proved. Immunity against the surface projection antigen is probably most important for protection. Resistance to reinfection may last several years, but reinfections with similar strains are common.

Laboratory Diagnosis

A. Isolation and Identification of Virus: Isolation of coronaviruses in cell culture has been difficult. Research laboratories may attempt viral isolation using organ cultures of human embryonic trachea.

B. Direct Examination: Coronavirus antigens in cells in respiratory secretions may be detected using the ELISA test if a high-quality antiserum is available. Enteric coronaviruses can be detected by examination of stool samples by electron microscopy.

C. Serology: Because of the difficulty of viral isolation, serodiagnosis using acute and convalescent sera is the only practical means of confirming coronavirus infections. CF, ELISA, and hemagglutination tests may be used. Serologic diagnosis of infections with strain 229E is possible using a passive hemagglutination test in which red cells coated with coronavirus antigen are agglutinated by antibody-containing sera.

Epidemiology

The coronaviruses are a major cause of respiratory illness in adults during some winter months when the incidence of colds is high but the isolation of rhinoviruses or other respiratory viruses is low.

Antibodies to respiratory coronaviruses appear in early childhood, increase in prevalence with age, and are found in more than 90% of adults. Different methods vary in ability to measure antibody; ELISA is probably the most sensitive and broadly reactive test available.

It is estimated that coronaviruses cause 15–30% of all colds. They have been found worldwide.

Very little is known about the epidemiology of enteric coronavirus infections.

REFERENCES

Lai MMC: Coronavirus: Organization, replication and expression of genome. Annu Rev Microbiol 1990;44:303.

Mortensen ML et al: Coronaviruslike particles in human gastrointestinal disease: Epidemiologic, clinical, and laboratory observations. Am J Dis Child 1985;139:928.

Siddell SG, Wege H, ter Meulen V: The biology of coronaviruses. J Gen Virol 1983;64:761.

Snijder EJ, Horzinek MC: Toroviruses: Replication, evolution and comparison with other members of the corona-virus-like superfamily. J Gen Virol 1993;74:2305.

Yeager CL et al: Human aminopeptidase N is a receptor for human coronavirus HCV-229E. Nature 1992;357:420.

42 Rabies & Slow Virus Infections

Many different viruses can invade the central nervous system and cause disease. This chapter considers rabies, a viral encephalitis feared since antiquity, and slow virus infections, rare neurodegenerative disorders that are caused either by typical viruses or by unconventional agents.

RABIES

Rabies is an acute infection of the central nervous system that is almost always fatal. The virus is usually transmitted to humans from the bite of a rabid animal. Although the number of human cases is small, rabies is a major public health problem because it is widespread among animal reservoirs.

Properties of the Virus

A. Structure: Rabies virus is a rhabdovirus with morphologic and biochemical properties in common with vesicular stomatitis virus of cattle and several animal, plant, and insect viruses (Table 42–1). The rhabdoviruses are rod- or bullet-shaped particles measuring 75 × 180 nm (Figure 42–1). The particles are surrounded by a membranous envelope with protruding spikes, 10 nm long, that are composed of a single glycoprotein. Inside the envelope is a ribonucleocapsid. The genome is single-stranded, negative-sense RNA (12 kb; MW 4.6×10^6) that is not infectious and does not serve as a messenger. Virions contain an RNA-dependent RNA polymerase.

B. Reactions to Physical and Chemical Agents: Rabies virus survives storage at 4 °C for weeks but is inactivated by CO_2. On dry ice, therefore, it must be stored in glass-sealed vials. Rabies virus is killed rapidly by exposure to ultraviolet radiation or sunlight, by heat (1 hour at 50 °C), by lipid solvents (ether, 0.1% sodium deoxycholate), by trypsin, by detergents, and by extremes of pH.

C. Virus Replication: The replication of rabies virus is similar to that of the most studied rhabdovirus, vesicular stomatitis virus. Rabies virus attaches to cells via its glycoprotein spikes; the nicotinic acetylcholine receptor may serve as a cellular receptor for rabies virus. The single-stranded RNA genome is transcribed by the virion-associated RNA polymerase to five mRNA species. These monocistronic mRNAs code for the five virion proteins. The genome is a template for a replicative intermediate responsible for the generation of progeny RNA. The genomic RNA associates with the viral transcriptase, phosphoprotein, and nucleoprotein. After encapsidation, the bullet-shaped particles acquire an envelope by budding through the plasma membrane. The viral matrix protein forms a layer on the inner side of the envelope, whereas the viral glycoprotein is on the outer layer and forms the spikes.

D. Animal Susceptibility and Growth of Virus: Rabies virus has a wide host range. All warm-blooded animals, including humans, can be infected. Susceptibility varies among mammalian species, ranging from most (foxes, coyotes, wolves) to least (opossums) susceptible; those with intermediate susceptibility include skunks, raccoons, and bats (Table 42–2). The virus is widely distributed in infected animals, especially in the nervous system, saliva, urine, lymph, milk, and blood. Recovery from infection is rare except in certain bats, where the virus has become peculiarly adapted to the salivary glands. Vampire bats may transmit the virus for months without themselves ever showing any signs of disease.

When freshly isolated in the laboratory, the strains are referred to as street virus. Such strains show long and variable incubation periods (usually 21–60 days in dogs) and regularly produce intracytoplasmic inclusion bodies. Serial brain-to-brain passage in rabbits yields a "fixed" virus that no longer multiplies in extraneural tissues. This fixed virus multiplies rapidly, and the incubation period is shortened to 4–6 days. Inclusion bodies are found only with difficulty.

E. Antigenic Properties: There is a single serotype for rabies virus. However, there are strain differences among viruses isolated from different species (raccoons, foxes, skunks, canines, bats) in different geographic areas. These viral strains can be distinguished by epitopes in the nucleoprotein and glycoprotein recognized by monoclonal antibodies as well as by specific nucleotide sequences. There are at least five antigenic variants found in terrestrial animals and eight other variants found in bats in the USA.

Avirulent mutants of rabies virus have been selected using certain monoclonal antibodies against the viral

Table 42–1. Important properties of rhabdoviruses.

Virion	Bullet-shaped, 75 nm in diameter × 180 nm in length
Composition	RNA (4%), protein (67%), lipid (26%), carbohydrate (3%)
Genome	Single-stranded RNA, linear, non-segmented, negative-sense, MW 4.6 million, 12 kb
Proteins	One envelope glycoprotein
Envelope	Present
Replication	Cytoplasm; virions bud from plasma membrane
Outstanding characteristics	Wide array of viruses with broad host ranges; group includes the deadly rabies virus

glycoprotein. A substitution at amino acid position 333 of the glycoprotein results in loss of virulence, indicating some essential role for that site of the protein in disease pathogenesis.

Purified spikes containing the viral glycoprotein elicit neutralizing antibody in animals. Antiserum prepared against the purified nucleocapsid is used in diagnostic immunofluorescence for rabies.

Pathogenesis & Pathology

Rabies virus multiplies in muscle or connective tissue at the site of inoculation and then enters peripheral nerves at neuromuscular junctions and spreads up the nerves to the central nervous system. It multiplies there and may then spread through peripheral nerves to the salivary glands and other tissues. Rabies virus has not been isolated from the blood of infected persons.

Susceptibility to infection and the incubation period may depend on the host's genetic background, the viral strain involved, the concentration of viral receptors on host cells, the amount of inoculum, the severity of lacerations, and the distance the virus has to travel from its point of entry to the central nervous system. There is a higher attack rate and shorter incubation period in persons bitten on the face or head.

Hyperemia and nerve cell destruction occur throughout the brain, especially in the cerebral cortex, cerebellum, hippocampus, and dorsal spinal ganglia. Demyelinization occurs in the white matter, and degeneration of axons and myelin sheaths is common. In the spinal cord, the posterior horns are most severely involved, with neuronophagia and cellular infiltrates.

Rabies virus produces a specific eosinophilic cytoplasmic inclusion, the Negri body, in infected nerve cells. The presence of such inclusions is pathognomonic of rabies but is not observed in at least 20% of cases. Therefore, the absence of Negri bodies does not rule out rabies as a diagnosis.

Rabies virus multiplies outside the central nervous system and may produce cellular infiltrates and necrosis in salivary and other glands, in the cornea, and elsewhere.

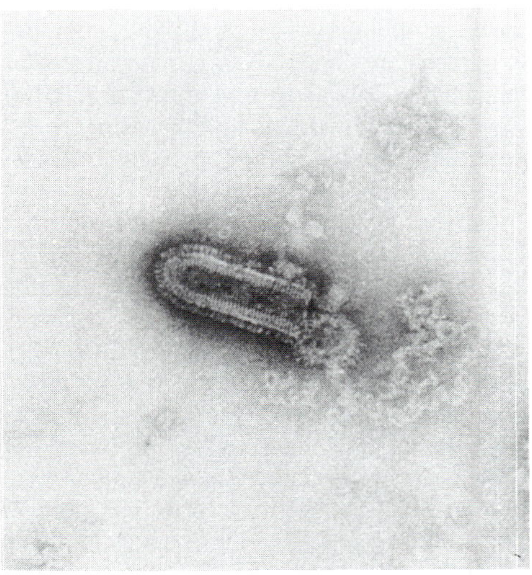

Figure 42–1. Electron micrograph of bullet-shaped particle typical of the rhabdovirus family (100,000×). Shown here is vesicular stomatitis virus negatively stained with potassium phosphotungstate. (RM McCombs, M Benyesh-Melnick, and JP Brunschwig.)

Clinical Findings

Rabies is primarily a disease of animals and is spread to humans by bites of rabid animals or by contact with saliva from rabid animals. The disease is an acute, fulminant, fatal encephalitis. The incubation period in humans typically varies from 2 to 16 weeks but may be as short as 10 days or as long as a year. It is usually shorter in children than in adults. The clinical spectrum can be divided into four phases: a short prodromal phase, a sensory phase, a period of excitement, and a paralytic or depressive phase. The prodrome, lasting 2–4 days, may show any of the following: malaise, anorexia, headache, nausea and vomiting, sore throat, and fever. Usually there is an abnormal sensation around the site of infection. The patient may

Table 42–2. Animal susceptibility to rabies.[1]

Susceptibility of Species			
Very High	**High**	**Moderate**	**Low**
Foxes Coyotes Jackals Wolves Cotton rats	Hamsters Skunks Raccoons Cats Bats Rabbits Cattle	Dogs Sheep Goats Horses Nonhuman primates	Opossums

[1]Modified from Baer GM, Bellini WJ, Fishbein DB: Rhabdoviruses. In: *Fields Virology,* vol. 1. Fields BN et al (editors). Raven Press, 1990.

show increasing nervousness and apprehension. General sympathetic overactivity is observed, including lacrimation, pupillary dilatation, and increased salivation and perspiration. Hallucinations, muscle spasms, and combativeness may appear. The act of swallowing precipitates a spasm of the throat muscles; a patient may allow saliva to drool from the mouth simply to avoid swallowing and the associated painful spasms. (Because of the patient's apparent fear of water, the disease has been known as hydrophobia since ancient days.) This phase is followed by convulsive seizures or coma and death, usually 3–5 days after onset. The major cause of death is respiratory paralysis. Progressive paralytic symptoms may develop before death. Recovery and survival is extremely rare.

The usual incubation period in dogs ranges from 3 to 8 weeks, but it may be as short as 10 days. Clinically, the disease in dogs is divided into three phases: prodromal, excitative, and paralytic. The prodromal phase is characterized by fever and a sudden change in the temperament of the animal. The excitative phase lasts 3–7 days, during which the dog shows symptoms of irritability, restlessness, nervousness, and exaggerated response to sudden light and sound stimuli. At this stage the animal is most dangerous because of its tendency to bite. The animal has difficulty in swallowing, suffers from convulsive seizures, and enters into a paralytic stage with paralysis of the whole body, coma, and death. Sometimes the animal goes into the paralytic stage without passing through the excitative stage.

Laboratory Diagnosis

A. Microscopy: Tissues infected with rabies virus are currently identified most rapidly and accurately by means of direct immunofluorescence using antirabies hamster serum. (See Chapter 47.) Impression preparations of brain or cornea tissue are often used.

A definitive pathologic diagnosis of rabies is based on the finding of Negri bodies in the brain or the spinal cord. Negri bodies are found in impression preparations or histologic sections. They are sharply demarcated, more or less spherical, and 2–10 μm in diameter, and they have a distinctive internal structure with basophilic granules in an eosinophilic matrix. Several may be found in the cytoplasm of large neurons. Negri bodies contain rabies virus antigens and can be demonstrated by immunofluorescence. Both Negri bodies and rabies antigen can usually be found in animals or humans suffering from rabies or dead from the infection, but they are rarely found in bats.

B. Viral Isolation: Available tissue (or saliva) is inoculated intracerebrally into suckling mice. Infection in mice results in flaccid paralysis of legs, encephalitis, and death. The central nervous system of the inoculated animal is examined for Negri bodies and rabies antigen. In specialized laboratories, hamster and mouse cell lines can be inoculated for rapid (2–4 day) growth of rabies virus; this is much faster than virus isolation in mice. An isolated virus is identified by Nt tests with specific antiserum.

C. Serology: Antibodies to rabies can be detected by immunofluorescence, CF, or Nt tests. Such antibodies may develop in infected persons or animals during progression of the disease.

D. Animal Observation: All animals considered "rabid or suspected rabid" (Table 42–3) should be sacrificed immediately for laboratory examination of tissues. Other animals, if available, should be held for observation for 10 days. If they show any signs of encephalitis, rabies, or unusual behavior, they should be killed humanely and the tissues examined in the laboratory. On the other hand, if they appear normal after 10 days, decisions must be made on an individual basis in consultation with public health officials.

Immunity & Prevention

Only one antigenic type of rabies virus is known. More than 99% of infections in humans and mammals who develop symptoms end fatally. Survival after proved rabies infection is extremely rare. It is therefore essential that individuals at high risk receive preventive immunization, that the nature and risk of any exposure be evaluated, and that individuals be given postexposure prophylaxis if their exposure is believed to have been dangerous (Table 42–3). Because treatment is of no benefit after the onset of disease, it is important that postexposure treatment be initiated promptly.

A. Pathophysiology of Rabies Prevention by Vaccine: Presumably the virus must be amplified in muscle near the site of inoculation until the concentration of virus is sufficient to accomplish infection of the central nervous system. If immunogenic vaccine or antibody can be administered promptly, virus replication can be depressed and virus can be prevented from invading the central nervous system. The action of passively administered antibody is to neutralize some of the inoculated virus and lower the concentration of virus in the body, providing additional time for a vaccine to stimulate active antibody production to prevent entry into the central nervous system.

B. Types of Vaccines: All vaccines for human use contain only inactivated rabies virus. Two vaccines are available in the USA, although a number of others are in use in other countries.

1. Human diploid cell vaccine (HDCV)–To obtain a rabies virus suspension free from nervous system and foreign proteins, rabies virus was adapted to growth in the WI-38 human normal fibroblast cell line. The rabies virus preparation is concentrated by ultrafiltration and inactivated with β-propiolactone. This material is sufficiently antigenic that only five doses of HDCV (Table 42–4) need to be given to obtain a substantial antibody response in most recipients. Local reactions (erythema, itching, swelling at the injection site) occur in 30–70% of recipients, and mild systemic reactions (headache, nausea, myalgia, dizziness) occur in about one-fifth of recipients. No serious anaphylac-

Table 42–3. Rabies postexposure prophylaxis guide.[1]

The following recommendations are only a guide. In applying them, take into account the animal species involved, the circumstances of the bite or other exposure, the vaccination status of the animal, and the presence of rabies in the region. ***Note:*** Local or state public health officials should be consulted if questions arise about the need for rabies prophylaxis.

Animal Type	Evaluation of Animal	Treatment of Exposed Person[2]
Domestic		
Dogs and cats	Healthy and available for 10 days of observation	None, unless animal develops symptoms of rabies[3]
	Rabid or suspected rabid	HRIG[4] and HDCV or RVA[5] immediately
	Unknown (escaped)	Consult public health officials. If treatment is indicated, give HRIG[4] and HDCV or RVA.
Wild		
Skunks, raccoons, bats, foxes, coyotes, and other carnivores	Regard as rabid unless geographic area is known to be free of rabies or until animal is proved negative for rabies by laboratory tests.[6]	HRIG[4] and HDCV or RVA[5] immediately
Other		
Livestock, rodents, and lagomorphs (rabbits and hares)	Consider individually. Local and state public health officials should be consulted about the need for rabies prophylaxis. Bites of squirrels, hamsters, guinea pigs, gerbils, chipmunks, rats, mice, other rodents, rabbits, and hares almost never require antirabies prophylaxis.	

[1]Modified from Morbid Mortal Wkly Rep 1991;40(RR-3).
[2]*All bites and wounds should immediately be thoroughly cleansed with soap and water.* If antirabies treatment is indicated, both human rabies immune globulin (HRIG) and human diploid cell rabies vaccine (HDCV) or rabies vaccine, adsorbed (RVA) should be given as soon as possible, *regardless* of the interval from exposure.
[3]During the usual holding period of 10 days, begin treatment with HRIG and vaccine at first sign of rabies in a dog or cat that has bitten someone. The symptomatic animal should be killed immediately and tested.
[4]If HRIG is not available, use antirabies serum, equine. Do not use more than the recommended dosage.
[5]Local reactions to vaccines are common and do not contraindicate continuing treatment. Discontinue vaccine if fluorescent antibody tests of the animal are negative.
[6]The animal should be killed and tested as soon as possible. Holding for observation is not recommended.

tic, neuroparalytic, or encephalitic reactions have been reported. This vaccine has been used in the USA since 1980.

2. Rabies vaccine, adsorbed (RVA)–A vaccine made in a diploid cell line derived from fetal rhesus monkey lung cells was licensed in the USA in 1988. This vaccine virus is inactivated with β-propiolactone and concentrated by adsorption to aluminum phosphate. The HDCV and RVA vaccines are equally efficacious and safe.

3. Nerve tissue vaccine–This is made from infected sheep, goat, or mouse brains and is used in many parts of the world including Asia, Africa, and South America. It causes sensitization to nerve tissue and results in postvaccinal encephalitis (an allergic disease) with substantial frequency (0.05%). It has not been used in the USA for several decades. Estimates of its efficacy in persons bitten by rabid animals vary from 5% to 50%.

4. Duck embryo vaccine–This was developed to minimize the problem of postvaccinal encephalitis. The rabies virus is grown in embryonated duck eggs, but the head is removed before the vaccine is prepared so as to remove nervous tissue and avoid allergic en-

Table 42–4. Rabies immunization regimens.[1]

Preexposure: Preexposure rabies prophylaxis for persons with special risks of exposure to rabies, such as animal care and control personnel, selected laboratory workers, and veterinarians, consists of immunization with either human diploid cell rabies vaccine (HDCV) or rabies vaccine adsorbed (RVA) according to the following schedule:

Type of Vaccination	Dose	Route of Administration	Regimen
Primary	1.0 mL	IM (deltoid area)	Days 0, 7, and 21 or 28
Booster[2]	1.0 mL	IM (deltoid area)	Day 0

Postexposure: Postexposure rabies prophylaxis for persons exposed to rabies consists of the immediate, thorough cleansing of all wounds with soap and water, administration of rabies immune globulin, and, for persons not previously vaccinated,[3] the initiation of either HDCV or RVA according to the following schedule: 1.0 mL IM (deltoid area) on days 0, 3, 7, 14, and 28.

[1]Modified from Morbid Mortal Wkly Rep 1991;40(RR-3).
[2]Administration of booster dose of vaccine depends on exposure risk category of individual.
[3]The postexposure regimen is greatly modified for someone with previously demonstrated rabies antibody.

cephalitis. It produces local reactions regularly and systemic reactions (fever, malaise, myalgia) in one-third of recipients. Neuroparalytic ($<0.001\%$) and anaphylactic ($<1\%$) reactions are infrequent, but the antigenicity of the vaccine is low. Consequently, many (16–25) doses have to be given to obtain a satisfactory postexposure antibody response. This vaccine was used in the USA in the past but is no longer used.

5. Live attenuated viruses–Live attenuated viruses adapted to growth in chick embryos (eg, Flury strain) are used for animals but *not* for humans. Occasionally, such vaccines can cause death from rabies in injected cats or dogs. Rabies viruses grown in various animal cell cultures have also been used as vaccines for domestic animals.

An experimental recombinant viral vaccine consisting of vaccinia virus carrying the rabies surface glycoprotein gene has successfully immunized animals following oral administration. This vaccine may prove valuable in the immunization of both wildlife reservoir species and domestic animals.

C. Types of Rabies Antibody:

1. Rabies immune globulin, human (HRIG)–is a gamma globulin prepared by cold ethanol fractionation from the plasma of hyperimmunized humans. The neutralizing antibody content is standardized to 150 IU/mL. The dose is 20 IU/kg, half given around the bite wound and the other half intramuscularly.

2. Antirabies serum, equine–is concentrated serum from horses hyperimmunized with rabies virus. It has been used in countries where HRIG is not available.

D. Choice of Rabies Immunizing Products: This is an application of the risk/benefit ratio, as far as known for each product. Human diploid cell vaccine has the greatest efficacy among known vaccines in stimulating antibody production, and few adverse effects are associated with it. There are fewer reactions to human rabies immune globulin (especially rare serum sickness, anaphylaxis) than to equine antirabies serum.

E. Preexposure Prophylaxis: This is indicated for persons at high risk of contact with rabies virus (research and diagnostic laboratory workers, spelunkers) or with rabid animals (veterinarians, animal control and wildlife workers, travelers to certain foreign areas). The goal is to attain an antibody level presumed to be protective by means of vaccine administration prior to any exposure. Current recommended immunization schedules are shown in Table 42–4.

F. Postexposure Prophylaxis: Since 1960, 0–5 cases of human rabies have occurred in the USA per year, but every year 20,000–30,000 persons receive some treatment for possible bite-wound exposure. *All* bites should be thoroughly cleaned with soap and water immediately, and tetanus prophylaxis should be considered. The decision to administer rabies antibody, rabies vaccine, or both, depends on (1) the nature of the biting animal (species, state of health, domestic or wild) and its vaccination status; (2) the availability of the animal for laboratory examination (*all* bites by wild animals and bats require rabies immune globulin and vaccine); (3) the existence of rabies in the area; (4) the manner of attack (provoked or unprovoked); (5) the severity of bite and contamination by saliva of the animal; and (6) advice from local public health officials (Table 42–3). Schedules for postexposure prophylaxis involving the administration of rabies immune globulin and vaccine are shown in the 1991 recommendations for the USA (Table 42–4). Different materials and schedules may be proposed in other parts of the world depending on availability of products and local experience.

Epidemiology

Rabies exists in two epizootic forms—urban (dogs and cats) and sylvatic (wildlife). Worldwide, about 15,000 cases of human rabies are estimated to occur each year, most of them in developing countries, eg, India, Southeast Asia, the Philippines, and South America. In these countries, where canine rabies is still endemic, most human cases develop from the bite of rabid dogs. Perhaps 1 million persons are given postexposure prophylaxis annually.

In the USA, Canada, and western Europe, where canine rabies has been controlled, dogs are responsible for very few cases. Rather, human rabies develops from bites of wild animals (especially skunks, foxes, and bats) or occurs in travelers bitten by dogs elsewhere in the world. In Latin America, rabies is transmitted especially by vampire bats that normally suck the blood of cattle (and may cause outbreaks among them) but may also bite humans. The increase in wildlife rabies in the USA and some other developed countries presents a far greater risk to humans than do dogs or cats. Wild animals trapped and sold as pets can be the source of human exposure.

From 1980–1993, 18 human rabies cases were diagnosed in the USA. Using molecular markers, seven of the nine cases known to have acquired rabies in the USA were proved to have bat-associated virus. All eight patients with imported rabies had dog-associated strains.

Raccoons have become an important reservoir for rabies in the eastern USA and now account for over half of all reported cases of animal rabies. It is believed that raccoon rabies was introduced into the mid-Atlantic region in the 1970s, when infected raccoons were transported there from the southeastern USA to replenish hunting stocks.

In 1981, over 7000 laboratory-confirmed cases of animal rabies were reported in the USA and its territories. Seven kinds of animals accounted for 97% of those cases: skunks (62%), bats (12%), raccoons (7%), cattle (6%), cats (4%), dogs (3%), and foxes (3%). Of these, 85% of cases occurred in wild animals and 15% in domestic animals. Approximately 95,000 animals were tested, giving a positive detection rate of 8%. In 1986, the USA reported about 5500 cases of animal rabies; wild animals accounted for 91% of all cases. The same year, Canada reported almost 4000 cases, the majority (80%) of which also occurred in wild animals. In contrast, most cases reported in Mexico in 1986 involved domestic and farm animals as principal hosts (97% of about 10,000 cases).

Bats present a special problem because they may carry rabies virus while they appear to be healthy, excrete it in saliva, and transmit it to other animals, including other bats, and to humans. South American vampire bats may transmit rabies to insectivorous bats living in caves. The latter, in turn, may transmit rabies to fruit-eating bats that visit such caves and migrate elsewhere. Bat caves may contain aerosols of rabies virus and present a risk to spelunkers. Migrating fruit-eating bats exist in all 48 contiguous states of the USA, in Canada, and in Latin America. They are a source of infection for many animals and humans. It has been speculated that bat rabies may be important in the initiation of terrestrial enzootics in new regions. *All* persons bitten by bats must receive postexposure rabies prophylaxis.

Human-to-human rabies infection is very rare. The only documented cases involve rabies transmitted by corneal transplants—the corneas came from donors who died with undiagnosed central nervous system diseases, and the recipients died from rabies 50–80 days later. Theoretically, rabies could originate from the saliva of a patient who has rabies and exposes attending personnel, but such transmission has never been documented.

Control

Historically, several key events have contributed to the control of human rabies: the development of a human rabies vaccine (1885), the discovery of the diagnostic Negri body (1903), the use of rabies vaccines for dogs (1940s), the addition of rabies immune globulin to human postexposure vaccination treatments (1954), the growth of rabies virus in cultured cells (1958), and the development of diagnostic fluorescent antibody tests (1959).

Preexposure vaccination is desirable for all persons who are at high risk of contact with rabid animals (Table 42–4). This applies particularly to veterinarians, animal care personnel, certain laboratory workers, and spelunkers. Persons traveling to developing countries where rabies control programs for domestic animals are not optimal should be offered preexposure prophylaxis if they plan to stay for more than 30 days. Persons on long-term international assignments in rabies-endemic areas who are at risk of inapparent exposure to rabies or a delay in postexposure prophylaxis should be advised to have a booster every 2 years or to have their serum tested for rabies-neutralizing antibody every 2 years and, if their titer is inadequate, have a booster. It should be emphasized that preexposure prophylaxis does not eliminate the need for prompt postexposure prophylaxis if an exposure to rabies occurs.

Rabies should be considered in any case of encephalitis or myelitis of unknown etiology, even in the absence of an exposure history, particularly in a person who has lived or traveled outside the USA.

Isolated countries, eg, Great Britain, that have no indigenous rabies in wild animals can establish quarantine procedures. Dogs and other pets to be imported are quarantined for 6–12 months. In countries where dog rabies exists, stray animals should be destroyed and vaccination of pet dogs and cats should be mandatory. In countries where wildlife rabies exists and where contact between domestic animals, pets, and wildlife is inevitable, all domestic animals and pets should be vaccinated and the incidence of rabies in wild animals should be continually ascertained.

Large-scale field tests of orally absorbed vaccines have proved effective at controlling rabies in foxes in parts of Europe. Such approaches may help control rabies in wildlife in certain regions of North America.

Dogs and cats that appear healthy but have made an unprovoked attack upon and bitten a person should be quarantined and observed for at least 10 days.

ASEPTIC MENINGITIS

This syndrome is characterized by acute onset, fever, headache, and stiff neck. There is pleocytosis of the spinal fluid, consisting largely of mononuclear cells. The fluid is bacteria-free, with a normal glucose content and often a slightly elevated protein content.

Etiology

Aseptic meningitis may be caused by a variety of agents: (1) primarily neurotropic viruses (poliovirus, lymphocytic choriomeningitis virus, and arthropod-borne encephalitis viruses); (2) viruses not primarily neurotropic (enteroviruses, mumps virus, herpes simplex virus, varicella-zoster virus, Epstein-Barr virus, hepatitis A virus, and measles virus); (3) spirochetes (*Treponema pallidum* and leptospirae); (4) bacteria, as in silent brain abscess and inadequately treated bacterial meningitis; and (5) mycoplasmas or chlamydiae.

Diagnosis

The diagnosis of aseptic viral meningitis is made by exclusion of bacterial causes of the symptom complex. Specific etiologic causes of aseptic meningitis can usually be determined only by isolation of the agent or the demonstration of a rise in specific antibodies. However, epidemiologic features have diagnostic value. (See discussions of specific agents in appropriate chapters.)

Laboratory Findings

The peripheral white count is usually normal, but in lymphocytic choriomeningitis, eosinophilia may appear a few days after onset. There is pleocytosis of the cerebrospinal fluid; polymorphonuclear cells often predominate during the first 24 hours, but a shift to lymphocytes usually occurs thereafter. The range is 100–800 cells or more, sometimes reaching 3000 cells in lymphocytic choriomeningitis. Protein levels of the spinal fluid are often elevated, but the glucose level is within normal limits.

LYMPHOCYTIC CHORIOMENINGITIS

Lymphocytic choriomeningitis is an acute disease with aseptic meningitis or a mild systemic influenza-like illness. Occasionally there is a severe encephalomyelitis or a fatal systemic disease. The incubation period is usually 18–21 days but may be as short as 1–3 days. The mild systemic form is rarely recognized clinically. There may be fever, malaise, generalized muscle aches and pains, weakness, sore throat, and cough. The fever lasts for 3–14 days.

Lymphocytic choriomeningitis is caused by an RNA-containing arenavirus (see Chapter 38).

Diagnosis

Specific diagnosis can be made by the isolation of virus from spinal fluid or blood during the acute phase and by tests demonstrating a rise in antibody titer between acute and convalescent serum specimens. Complement-fixing antibodies rise to diagnostic levels in 3–4 weeks, then fall gradually and reach normal levels after several months. Neutralizing antibodies appear later and reach diagnostic levels 7–8 weeks after onset; they may persist for 4–5 years.

Laboratory Findings

In the prodromal period (or mild systemic form), leukopenia with relative lymphocytosis is frequently present. In the meningitic form, there is pleocytosis in the spinal fluid (100–3000 cells/μL), with a predominance of lymphocytes. The glucose level is normal, and the protein level is slightly elevated.

Epidemiology & Control

The disease is endemic in mice and other animals (dogs, monkeys, guinea pigs) and is occasionally transmitted to humans. One large epidemic in the USA was caused by infected pet hamsters. There is no evidence of person-to-person spread.

Infected gray house mice, probably the most common source of human infection, excrete the virus in urine and feces. The virus may be harbored by mice throughout their lives, and females transmit it to their offspring, which in turn become healthy carriers. Mice inoculated as adults develop a rapidly fatal generalized infection. In contrast, congenitally or neonatally infected mice do not become acutely ill, but 10–12 months later many develop a fatal debilitating disease involving the central nervous system. The animals exhibit chronic glomerulonephritis and hypergammaglobulinemia; the glomerular lesions are due to deposition of antigen-antibody complexes, and the infection in mice is considered an immune complex disease. The mode of transmission from mice to humans is uncertain. Mice and their droppings should be controlled.

SLOW & UNCONVENTIONAL VIRUS DISEASES

Some chronic degenerative diseases of the central nervous system in humans are caused by "slow" or chronic, persistent viral infections. Among these are subacute sclerosing panencephalitis and progressive multifocal leukoencephalopathy. Other diseases, such as kuru and Creutzfeldt-Jakob disease, appear to be caused by unconventional transmissible agents (Table 42–5).

Several animal viruses and unconventional agents produce chronic infections of the central nervous system that result in progressive degenerative changes. These animal infections serve as models for similar disorders of humans and include visna of sheep in Iceland, scrapie of sheep in Great Britain, and transmissible mink encephalopathy. The progressive neurologic diseases produced by these agents may have incubation periods of up to 5 years before clinical manifestations of the infections become evident (Table 42–5).

Slow Virus Infections

A. Visna: Visna and **progressive pneumonia (maedi) viruses** are closely related agents that cause slow infections in sheep. These viruses are classified as retroviruses (subfamily Lentivirinae) because of structural similarities (see Chapter 43), although they are not tumorigenic. The viruses that cause acquired immunodeficiency syndrome are more closely related to visna virus than to the oncogenic retroviruses (see Chapter 44).

Visna virus infects all the organs of the body of the infected sheep; however, pathologic changes are confined primarily to the brain, lungs, and reticuloendothelial system. Inflammatory lesions develop in the central nervous system soon after infection, but there is usually a long incubation period (months to years) before observable neurologic symptoms appear. Disease progression can be either rapid (weeks) or slow (years).

Virus can be recovered for the life of the animal, but viral expression is restricted in vivo so that only minimal amounts of infectious virus are present in the infected host. Once recovered in culture, the virus is cytolytic and kills infected cells.

Antigenic variation occurs during the long-term persistent infections. Many mutations occur in the structural gene that codes for viral envelope glycoproteins. However, the role antigenic drift might play in the pathogenesis of disease is unknown.

Infected animals develop antibodies to the virus; these can be detected in the cerebrospinal fluid as well as in the serum of sick animals. Some animals develop neutralizing antibodies, whereas in other animals the antibodies appear to be nonneutralizing.

B. Subacute Sclerosing Panencephalitis: This is a rare disease of teenagers and young adults, with slowly progressive demyelination in the central nervous system ending in death. In electron microscopic studies of involved brain cells, structures are visible that resemble the nucleocapsid of paramyxoviruses. Defective measles virus has been recovered from brain material from patients with subacute sclerosing panencephalitis by cocultivation of brain cells with susceptible cells. Such isolates are mutated in one or more viral proteins, often the internal membrane or M viral protein that plays a role in viral assembly at the cell membrane. Patients with subacute sclerosing panencephalitis have high titers of antimeasles antibody in both serum and cerebrospinal fluid. However, antibody to the M protein is frequently lacking. The lack of M protein would explain one characteristic of the disease: persistence of infection but no production of mature infectious virus.

It is possible that subacute sclerosing panencephalitis represents a tolerant infection with defective cell-mediated responses in which latent measles virus persists for years. This may be the result of an immunologic dysfunction of the host, of a change in the virus so that some antigens are missing or are not expressed while the viral genetic information persists in host cells, or of both features. Experimentally, persistent infection with measles virus can be established in cell culture where some viral antigens are not expressed on the host cell surface, and such cells are not killed by lymphocytes (see Chapter 40).

A progressive panencephalitis has also been reported in patients with **congenital rubella.** The neurologic illness developed in the second decade and consisted of spasticity, ataxia, seizures, and progressive decline in intellectual ability.

C. Progressive Multifocal Leukoencephalopathy: Papovaviruses (see Chapter 43) have been isolated from brain tissue of patients with progressive multifocal leukoencephalopathy, a rare central nervous system complication found in patients suffering from chronic leukemia, Hodgkin's disease, or lymphosarcoma or in others receiving immunosuppressants. Demyelination in the central nervous system of patients with progressive multifocal leukoencephalopathy (usually immunosuppressed individuals) results from oligodendrocyte infection by papovaviruses.

The virus isolated, designated JC virus, is antigenically and biologically distinct from known papovaviruses. A related papovavirus, BK virus, has been isolated from the urine of renal transplant patients receiving immunosuppressive therapy but is not known to induce disease. JC and BK viruses are antigenically related to each other and to SV40. The human papovaviruses BK and JC commonly infect humans; antibodies to them are found in 70–80% of human sera. Antibody specific to SV40 occurs in about 3% of human sera.

In hamsters, the JC isolate induces brain tumors that resemble glioblastomas and medulloblastomas but without demyelination. BK virus lacks this oncogenicity but can transform hamster cells in culture.

Spongiform Encephalopathies of Humans & Animals

Degenerative central nervous system diseases—**kuru, Creutzfeldt-Jakob disease,** and the **Gerstmann-Sträussler-Scheinker syndrome** of humans, **scrapie** of sheep, **transmissible encephalopathy** of mink, and **bovine spongiform encephalopathy** of cattle and dairy cows—have similar pathologic features. These diseases are described as subacute spongiform viral encephalopathies. The causative agents do not appear to be conventional viruses; infectivity is associated with proteinaceous material devoid of detectable amounts of nucleic acid. The term prion has been proposed to designate this novel class of agents.

These agents are unusually resistant to standard means of inactivation. They are resistant to treatment with formaldehyde, β-propiolactone, ethanol, proteases, deoxycholate, and ionizing radiation. However, they are sensitive to phenol (90%), household bleach, ether, acetone, urea (6 mol/L), strong detergents (10% sodium dodecyl sulfate), iodine disinfectants, and autoclaving.

A. Characteristics of Diseases: There are several distinguishing hallmarks of diseases caused by these unconventional agents. The diseases are confined to the nervous system and exhibit reactive astrocytosis. Neurons may be vacuolated, or amyloid plaques may be present, or both. Long incubation periods (months to decades) precede the onset of clinical illness and are followed by chronic progressive pathology (weeks to years). The diseases are always fatal, with no known cases of remissions or recoveries. The host shows no inflammatory response and no immune response (the agents do not appear to be antigenic), no production of interferon is elicited, and there is no effect on host B or T cell function. Finally, immunosuppression of the host has no effect on pathogenesis of the disease.

B. Scrapie: Scrapie, which behaves like a recessive genetic trait in sheep, shows marked differences in susceptibility of different breeds. Susceptibility to experimentally transmitted scrapie ranges from zero to over 80% in sheep, whereas goats are almost 100% susceptible. Scrapie has also been transmitted to laboratory monkeys. The transmission of scrapie to mice and hamsters, in which the incubation period is greatly reduced, has facilitated study of the disease.

Infectivity can be recovered from lymphoid tissues early in infection, but high titers of the agent are found only in the brain, spinal cord, and eye (which are also the only places where pathologic changes are observed). Maximal titers of infectivity are reached in the brain long before neurologic symptoms appear. A feature of the disease is the development of amyloid plaques in the central nervous system of infected animals. These areas represent extracellular accumulations of protein; they stain with Congo red.

A protein designated PrP (MW 27,000–30,000) has been purified from scrapie-infected brain. It copurifies with scrapie infectivity, aggregates, and behaves like amyloid. Preparations containing only PrP and no detectable nucleic acid have been found to be infectious. PrP is encoded by a cellular gene (on chromosome 20 in humans). Transcripts from this gene are found in many normal tissues and in similar levels in normal and infected brains. The level of PrP, however, is elevated in infected brains as it becomes resistant to degradation. Genetic susceptibility to scrapie infection is associated with point mutations in the PrP gene. Mice genetically altered to be devoid of PrP are resistant to scrapie. It is still uncertain whether this protein represents the essential structural element of the infectious agent or a pathologic product that accumulates as a result of the disease.

C. Transmissible Mink Encephalopathy: This disease is caused by an agent that induces clinical disease and neurologic lesions in the gray matter of the brain similar to those of scrapie. It also has a long incubation period in mink that are naturally infected—presumably by the oral route. Transmissible mink encephalopathy probably represents a strain of sheep scrapie acquired when mink on mink ranches were fed scrapie-infected sheep carcasses.

D. Kuru: Two human spongiform encephalopathies are caused by "slow viruses," producing lesions similar to those of scrapie and transmissible mink encephalopathy. These are kuru and Creutzfeldt-Jakob disease. Brain material from patients who died from either disease can produce similar diseases when injected into chimpanzees, and the serial passage of diseased chimpanzee brain into healthy chimpanzees or rodents transfers the illness.

Kuru occurs only in the eastern highlands of New Guinea. The disease consists of relentless progressive cerebellar ataxia, tremors, dysarthria, and emotional lability without significant dementia. It occurs more frequently in women than in men, which coincides with the customs surrounding cannibalism. The remains of dead relatives were handled and eaten primarily by women and children. Since cannibalism has been outlawed, the incidence of the disease has decreased, and it is now felt that this was the primary mode of transmission of the agent.

E. Creutzfeldt-Jakob Disease: Creutzfeldt-Jakob disease (subacute presenile dementia) develops gradually, with progressive dementia, myoclonic fasciculations, ataxia, and somnolence, and leads to death in 8–12 months. The histologic lesions resemble those of kuru and scrapie, including the presence of amyloid plaques. (Gerstmann-Sträussler-Scheinker syndrome is a variant of familial Creutzfeldt-Jakob disease with a more protracted clinical course.) Creutzfeldt-Jakob disease occurs with a frequency of approximately one case per million population per year in the USA and Europe. Most cases occur sporadically and involve patients over 50 years of age. The estimated incidence is less than 1 case per 200 million for persons under 30 years of age. Creutzfeldt-Jakob disease has been transmitted accidentally by contaminated growth hormone preparations from human cadaver pituitary glands, by a corneal transplant, and by cadaveric human dura mater grafts used for surgical repair of head injury. It appears that recipients of contaminated dura mater grafts remain at risk of developing Creutzfeldt-Jakob disease for at least 8 years following receipt of grafts. Both kuru and Creutzfeldt-Jakob disease fail to show cerebrospinal fluid pleocytosis or abnormalities in sedimentation rate, blood chemistry, or body temperature.

A protein very similar to the scrapie PrP has been purified from brain tissue infected with Creutzfeldt-Jakob disease. It has been speculated that the agent of Creutzfeldt-Jakob disease was derived originally from scrapie-infected sheep and transmitted to humans by ingestion of poorly cooked sheep brains or eyeballs.

F. Alzheimer's Disease: There are some neuropathologic similarities between Creutzfeldt-Jakob disease and Alzheimer's disease, including the appearance of amyloid plaques. However, attempts to transmit disease to primates or rodents using brain samples from patients with Alzheimer's disease have been unsuccessful to date. The amyloid material in the brains of Alzheimer's patients is distinct from that containing PrP protein in brain tissue infected with scrapie or Creutzfeldt-Jakob disease.

REFERENCES

Banerjee AK, Barik S: Gene expression of vesicular stomatitis virus genome RNA. Virology 1992;188:417.

Blancou J et al: Oral vaccination of the fox against rabies using a live recombinant vaccinia virus. Nature 1986; 322:373.

Bockman JM et al: Creutzfeldt-Jakob disease prion proteins in human brains. N Engl J Med 1985;312:73.

Brochier B et al: Large-scale eradication of rabies using recombinant vaccinia-rabies vaccine. Nature 1991;354:520.

Büeler H et al: Mice devoid of PrP are resistant to scrapie. Cell 1993;73:1339.

Chatigny MA, Prusiner SB: Biohazards of investigations on the transmissible spongiform encephalopathies. Rev Infect Dis 1980;2:713.

Dietzschold B et al: Characterization of an antigenic determinant of the glycoprotein that correlates with pathogenicity of rabies virus. Proc Natl Acad Sci USA 1983; 80:70.

Fishbein DB, Robinson LE: Rabies. N Engl J Med 1993; 329:1632.

Flamand A et al: Avirulent mutants of rabies virus and their use as live vaccine. Trends Microbiol 1993;1:317.

Haase AT et al: Natural history of restricted synthesis and expression of measles virus genes in subacute sclerosing panencephalitis. Proc Natl Acad Sci USA 1985;82:3020.

Hunter N: Genetic control of scrapie incidence in sheep and its relevance for bovine spongiform encephalopathy in cattle. Rev Med Virol 1993;3:195.

Immunization Practices Advisory Committee: Rabies prevention—United States, 1991. Morb Mortal Wkly Rep 1991;40(RR-3).

Johnson RT: The contribution of virologic research to clinical neurology. N Engl J Med 1982;307:660.

Manuelidis L, Manuelidis EE: Creutzfeldt-Jakob disease and dementias. Microbial Pathogenesis 1989;7:157.

National Association of State Public Health Veterinarians: Compendium of animal rabies control, 1993. MMWR Morb Mortal Wkly Rep 199 1993;42(RR-3).

Wechsler SL, Meissner HC: Measles and SSPE viruses: Similarities and differences. Prog Med Virol 1982;28:65.

43 Tumor Viruses & Oncogenes

Viruses are now known to be etiologic factors in the development of several types of human tumors, including two of great significance worldwide—cervical cancer and liver cancer. The viruses that have been strongly associated epidemiologically with human cancers are listed in Table 43–1. They include human papillomaviruses, Epstein-Barr virus, hepatitis B virus, and a human retrovirus. Many viruses can cause tumors in animals, either as a consequence of natural infection or after experimental inoculation.

Animal viruses are studied to learn how a limited amount of genetic information (one or a few viral genes) can so profoundly alter the growth behavior of cells, ultimately converting a normal cell into a neoplastic one. Such studies will reveal insights into growth regulation in normal cells as well. Tumor viruses are agents that can produce tumors when they infect appropriate animals. Many studies are done using cultured animal cells rather than intact animals, because it is possible to analyze events at cellular and subcellular levels. In such cultured cells, tumor viruses can cause "transformation." However, animal studies are essential to study many of the steps in carcinogenesis, including complex host responses to tumor formation.

Studies with RNA tumor viruses revealed the involvement of cellular oncogenes in neoplasia; DNA tumor viruses implicated a role for cellular tumor suppressor genes. These discoveries revolutionized thinking in the 1980s about the molecular mechanisms of carcinogenesis.

GENERAL FEATURES OF VIRAL CARCINOGENESIS

Multistep Carcinogenesis

Carcinogenesis is a multistep process, ie, multiple genetic changes must occur to convert a normal cell into a malignant one. Intermediate stages have been identified in various systems and designated using terms such as "immortalization," "hyperplasia," and "preneoplastic." A long time is usually required for the appearance of tumors. The natural history of spontaneously occurring human and animal cancers suggests a multistep process of cellular evolution, probably involving repeated selection of rare cells with some selective growth advantage. The number of mutations underlying this process is estimated to range from three to eight. Some viral genes, eg, *myc* and polyoma large T antigen, can immortalize primary cells so that they will grow continuously in culture but not exhibit properties of complete transformation. Viral proteins may inactivate one or more tumor suppressor proteins so that cellular growth regulation is lost. An appropriate combination of different oncogenes (eg, *myc* and *ras*) can accomplish morphologic transformation of primary cells. Such observations suggest that multiple cellular oncogenes and tumor suppressor genes are involved in the evolution of tumors.

In most systems, it appears that a tumor virus acts as a cofactor, providing only some of the steps required to generate malignant cells.

Cellular transformation may be defined as a stable, heritable change in the growth control of cells in culture. No set of characteristics invariably distinguishes transformed cells from their normal counterparts. In practice, transformation is recognized by the cells' permanent acquisition of some growth property not exhibited by the parental cell type. The most prominent changes associated with transformed cells include: (1) Alterations in cell growth patterns: Growth to higher cell density, increased rate of growth, decreased requirement for serum growth factors, decreased cell adhesion to a substrate, enhanced ability to grow in semisolid medium (anchorage independence), and loss of "contact inhibition." The latter property means that transformed cells are no longer inhibited by contact with other cells, as normal cells are, but tend to pile up to form a "focus." Induction of foci can provide the basis for a quantitative assay for certain tumor viruses. (2) Alterations in cell surface: Increased rate of transport of cell nutrients, increased secretion of proteases or protease activators, increased agglutinability by plant lectins, and changes in composition of glycoproteins and glycolipids, sometimes including the presence of virus-encoded proteins. (3) Alterations in intracellular components and biochemical processes: Increased metabolic rate; increased glycolysis; altered levels of cyclic nucleotides; activation or repression of certain cellular genes; presence of viral DNA, mRNA, and viral coded proteins;

Table 43–1. Association of viruses with human cancers.

Virus Family	Virus	Human Cancer
Papovaviridae	Human papillomaviruses	Genital tumors (cervical, vulvar, penile cancers) Squamous cell carcinoma
Herpesviridae	EB virus	Nasopharyngeal carcinoma African Burkitt's lymphoma B-cell lymphoma
	Herpes simplex type 2	Cervical carcinoma?
Hepadnaviridae	Hepatitis B virus	Hepatocellular carcinoma
Retroviridae	HTL virus	Adult T cell leukemia

and changes in cell cytoskeleton, often resulting in a more rounded cell shape. (4) Tumorigenicity: Production of tumors when transformed cells are injected into appropriate test animals, especially immunologically deficient animals. Many transformed cells exhibit changes in growth behavior in vitro but are not transplantable in vivo. No in vitro growth characteristic can successfully predict tumorigenicity.

Types of Tumor Viruses

Like other viruses, tumor viruses are classified among different virus families according to the nucleic acid of their genome and the biophysical characteristics of their virions. All known tumor viruses either have a DNA genome or generate a DNA provirus after infection of cells. DNA tumor viruses are classified among the papova-, adeno-, herpes-, hepadna-, and poxvirus groups.

All RNA tumor viruses belong to the retrovirus family. Retroviruses carry an RNA-directed polymerase (reverse transcriptase) that constructs a DNA copy of the RNA genome of the virus. The DNA copy (provirus) becomes integrated into the DNA of the infected host cell, and it is from this integrated DNA copy that all proteins of the virus are translated. Among widely studied RNA tumor viruses are those causing avian sarcomas, avian leukoses, mouse leukemias, mouse sarcomas, mouse mammary tumors, feline leukemias, and human T cell leukemia.

RNA tumor viruses are of two general types with respect to tumor induction. The highly oncogenic (direct-transforming) viruses carry an oncogene of cellular origin (described below). The weakly oncogenic (slowly transforming) viruses do not contain an oncogene and induce leukemias after long incubation periods by indirect mechanisms (see below).

Interactions of Tumor Viruses With Host Cells

Host cells are either permissive or nonpermissive for replication of a given virus. Permissive cells support viral growth and production of progeny virus; nonpermissive cells do not. Especially with the DNA viruses, permissive cells are not transformed unless the viral replicative cycle that normally results in death of the host cell is blocked in some way; nonpermissive cells may be transformed. Cells that are permissive for one virus may be nonpermissive for another.

DNA tumor viruses replicate in certain cells of their natural host but rarely, if ever, produce tumors in those hosts. Conversely, DNA tumor viruses are usually unable to replicate in heterologous host cells but can, on occasion, transform them. An example is simian virus SV40, a virus that naturally infects rhesus monkeys. The virus replicates in monkey kidney cells but does not transform them. SV40 cannot replicate in cells of rodent origin but is able to transform them at low efficiency. These two types of virus-host interaction are illustrated in Figure 43–1. However, it must be noted that the DNA tumor viruses associated with human cancers are all human viruses. Fortunately, most infections by them do not result in tumors (see below).

RNA tumor viruses usually cause cancers in their natural hosts. They can both replicate in and transform homologous cells, because viral replication is not cytolytic. Certain viruses may be able to transform heterologous cells as well, usually in the absence of viral replication. Thus, RNA tumor viruses differ from DNA tumor viruses in that the former can transform both permissive and nonpermissive cells. A characteristic property of RNA tumor viruses is that they are not lethal for the cells in which they replicate (Figure 43–2). Cells infected with leukemia viruses exhibit no morphologic or cytopathic changes and continue to grow normally, whereas cells infected with sarcoma viruses undergo morphologic changes and grow like tumor cells.

Not all cells from the natural host species are susceptible to viral replication or transformation or both. Most tumor viruses exhibit marked tissue specificity, a property that probably reflects the variable presence of surface receptors for the virus or intracellular factors necessary for viral gene expression.

A. Integration of Tumor Virus Nucleic Acid Into a Host Cell: The stable genetic change from a normal to a neoplastic cell is attributed to the integration of certain viral genes into the host cell genome. With DNA tumor viruses, a portion of the DNA of the viral genome becomes integrated into the host cell chromosome (Figure 43–3). With RNA tumor viruses, viral RNA serves as a template for the synthesis of viral DNA (through the agency of a virus-encoded reverse transcriptase), and that DNA copy of the viral RNA is integrated into the host cell DNA (Figure 43–3). Generally, very few copies (perhaps one) of the viral genome are integrated in a transformed cell.

B. Recovery of Viral Genes and Transforming Genes From Tumor Cells: Transformed cells usually do not produce virus. Cells transformed by DNA tumor viruses never do, and those transformed by RNA

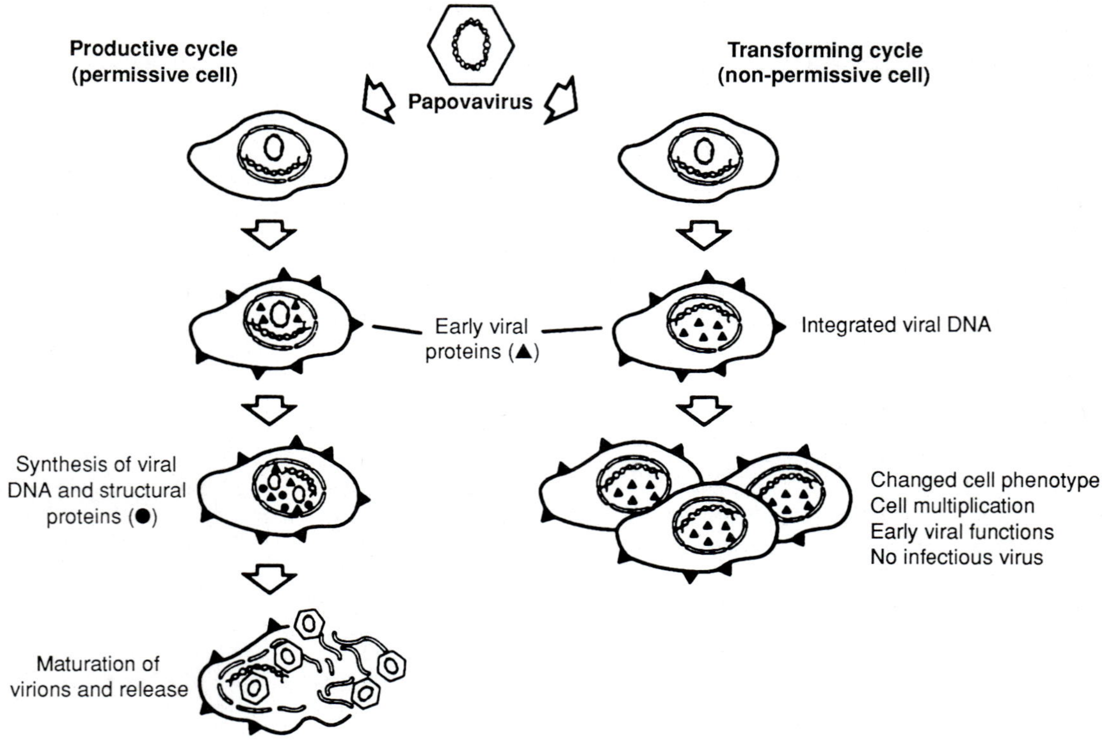

Figure 43–1. Schematic comparison of two types of interaction between a DNA tumor virus (papovavirus) and a host cell. The productive cycle that results in the synthesis of progeny virions is diagrammed on the left. The transforming cycle that is characterized by partial viral gene expression and cellular phenotypic changes is represented on the right. (After M Benyesh-Melnick and J Butel.)

tumor viruses may not. Recombinant DNA techniques can be used to recover virus-specific sequences regardless of whether a complete viral genome is present.

Cellular DNA can be extracted from tumor cells and inoculated onto a normal recipient cell line in the presence of a chemical facilitator that promotes ingestion of the DNA. This technique is called **transfection**. The transfected cells are observed for morphologic changes, eg, focus formation, as evidence of transforming activity expressed by the applied tumor cell DNA. The cellular sequences carrying the transforming activity can then be recovered using molecular cloning techniques. This approach has identified additional cellular oncogenes not carried by any known RNA tumor viruses.

C. Mechanisms of Cell Transformation by Viruses: Tumor viruses mediate changes in cell behavior by means of a limited amount of genetic information. There are two general patterns by which this is accomplished: (1) the tumor virus introduces a new "transforming gene" into the cell (Figure 43–3), or (2) the virus induces or alters the expression of a preexisting cellular gene. The result in either case is that the cell loses control of normal regulation of growth processes.

RNA TUMOR VIRUSES (Retroviruses)

RNA tumor viruses are classified as **retroviruses** because they contain an RNA-directed DNA poly-

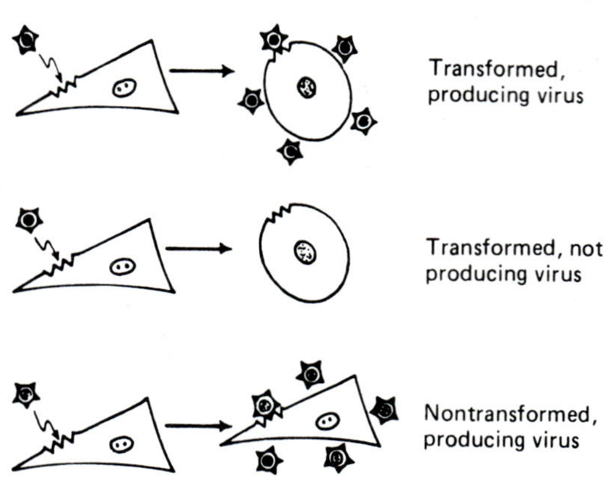

Figure 43–2. Schematic representation of the responses of fibroblasts to infection by retroviruses. (Courtesy of R Weiss.)

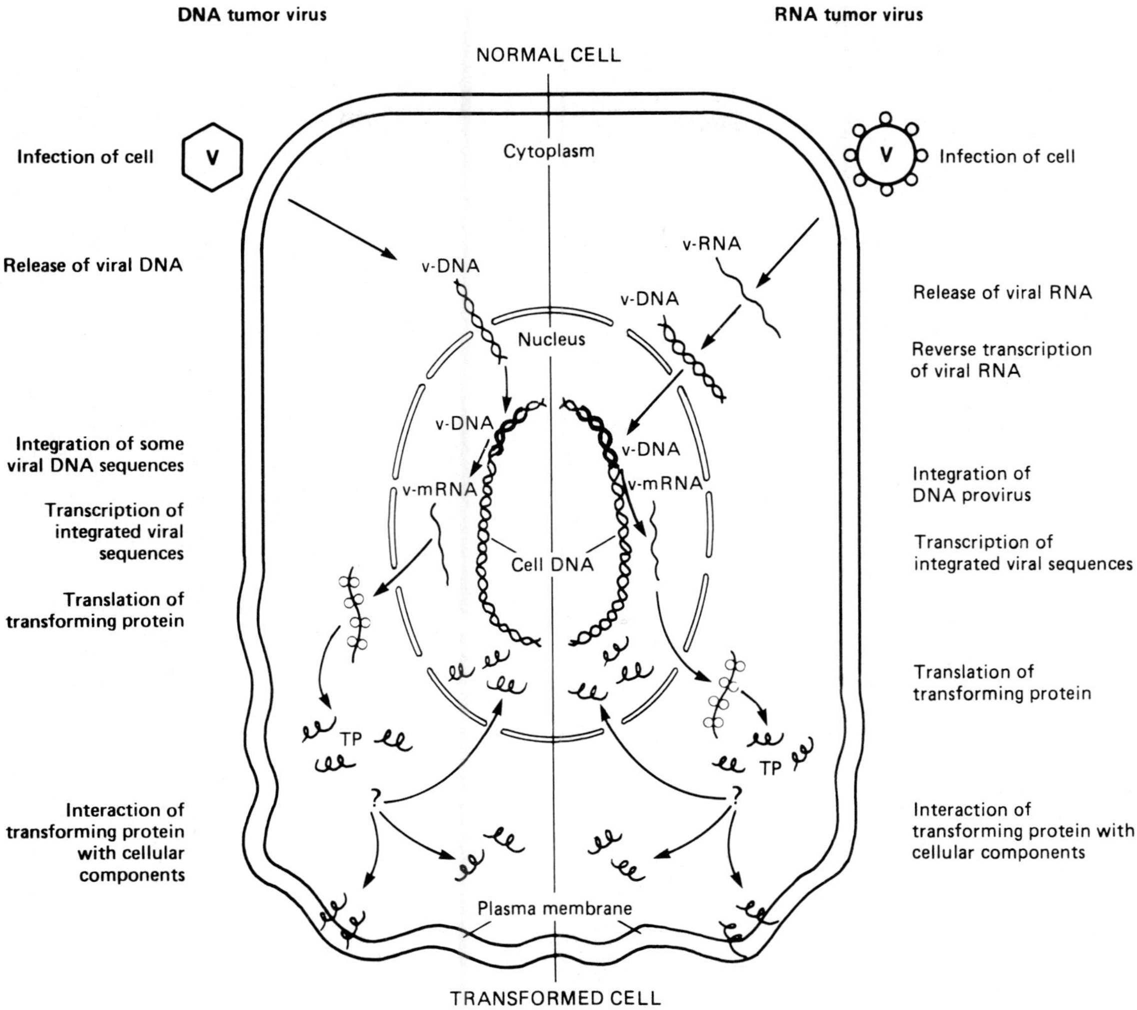

Figure 43–3. Molecular mechanism of cell transformation by tumor viruses carrying a transforming gene. Transformation by a DNA tumor virus is summarized on the left and transformation by an RNA tumor virus on the right. Viral nucleic acid (v-DNA, v-RNA) is released after infection of a normal cell by a virus (V) and, in the case of RNA tumor viruses, a DNA copy is reverse transcribed from the viral genomic RNA. Viral DNA is then integrated into a host cell chromosome. Messenger RNA (v-mRNA) is transcribed from the integrated viral sequences, transported to the cytoplasm, and translated on polyribosomes. The transforming protein (TP) product is then transported to appropriate locations within the cell to interact with cellular components, eg, the plasma membrane, the cytoplasm, the nucleus, or all of these. Some virus-specific transforming proteins appear to localize in only one cellular compartment, whereas others are found in more than one location. Cell regulatory processes are altered by the transforming protein with the result that the cell is transformed. Known viral transforming proteins differ structurally and functionally. The transforming genes carried by RNA tumor viruses are derived from cellular genes; no known cellular homologues exist for the DNA tumor virus transforming genes. A variation of the illustrated process of transformation occurs with some viruses (eg, leukemia viruses) that do not carry a transforming gene; the integrated viral DNA induces or alters the expression of a cellular gene that affects growth control.

merase (reverse transcriptase). RNA tumor viruses mainly cause tumors of the reticuloendothelial and hematopoietic systems (leukemias, lymphomas) or of connective tissue (sarcomas).

Important properties of the retroviruses are listed in Table 43–2.

Structure & Composition

The retrovirus genome consists of two identical subunits of single-stranded, positive-sense RNA, each 5–8 kb in size. Viral particles contain an RNA-directed DNA polymerase (reverse transcriptase), essential for viral replication.

Table 43–2. Important properties of retroviruses.

Virion: Spherical, 80–110 nm in diameter, helical nucleoprotein within icosahedral capsid.
Composition: RNA (1%), protein (about 65%), lipid (about 30%), carbohydrate (about 4%).
Genome: Single-stranded RNA, linear, positive-sense, 5–8 kb, diploid, total MW 3–6 million; may be defective; may carry oncogene.
Proteins: Reverse transcriptase enzyme contained inside virions.
Envelope: Present.
Replication: Reverse transcriptase makes DNA copy from genomic RNA; DNA (provirus) integrates into cellular chromosome; provirus is template for viral RNA.
Maturation: Virions bud from plasma membrane.
Outstanding characteristics: Infections do not kill cells; may transduce cellular oncogenes, may activate expression of cell genes. Proviruses remain permanently associated with cells and are frequently not expressed. Many members are tumor viruses.

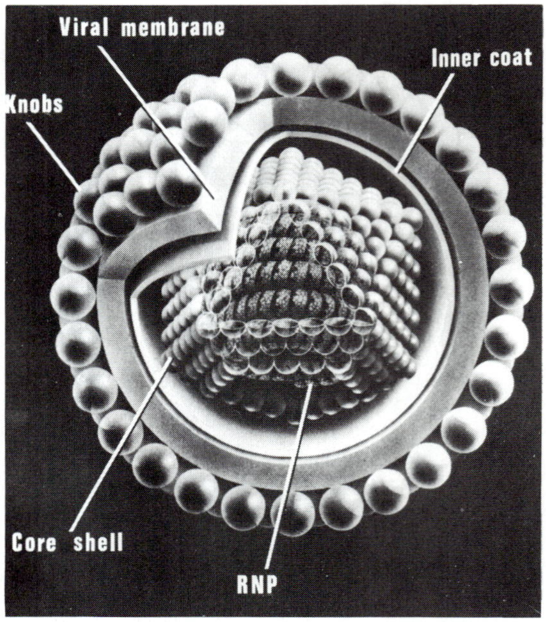

Figure 43–4. Three-dimensional model of a retrovirus. Removal of the front triangle of the icosahedral core shell allows the ribonucleoprotein (RNP) to be seen. Knobs + viral membrane + inner coat = viral envelope. Core shell + RNP = core. (Reproduced, with permission, from Frank H et al: Z Naturforsch 1978;33:124.)

Retrovirus particles have an icosahedral core that contains the ribonucleoprotein, surrounded by an outer membrane (envelope) containing glycoprotein and lipid. Two types of antigens are found in retroviruses: type-specific or subgroup-specific antigens associated with the glycoproteins in the viral envelope, which are encoded by the *env* gene; and group-specific antigens associated with the virion core, which are encoded by the *gag* gene. Cross-reactions do not occur between the envelope antigens of retroviruses from different species. A model of a retrovirus particle is shown in Figure 43–4.

Three morphologic classes of extracellular retrovirus particles, as well as an intracellular form, are known. They reflect slightly different processes of morphogenesis by different retroviruses. Examples of each are shown in Figure 43–5.

A type particles occur only intracellularly and appear to be noninfectious. Intracytoplasmic A type particles, 75 nm in diameter, are precursors of extracellular B type viruses, whereas intracisternal A type particles, 60–90 nm in diameter, are unknown entities that are not a stage in a viral life cycle. B type viruses are 100–130 nm in diameter and contain an eccentric nucleoid. The prototype of this group is the mouse mammary tumor virus, which occurs in "high mammary cancer" strains of inbred mice and is found in particularly large amounts in lactating mammary tissue and milk. It is readily transferred to suckling mice, in whom the incidence of subsequent development of adenocarcinoma of the breast is high. The C type viruses represent the largest group of retroviruses; some authors use the term "C type particle" to refer to typical retroviruses. The particles are 90–110 nm in diameter, and the electron-dense nucleoids are centrally located. The C type viruses may exist as exogenous or endogenous entities (see below). The lentiviruses are also C type viruses. Finally, the D type retroviruses are poorly characterized. The particles are 100–120 nm in diameter, contain an eccentric nucleoid, and exhibit surface spikes shorter than those on B type particles.

Classification

A. Subfamilies: The retrovirus family is divided into three subfamilies: Oncovirinae (which contains all the tumor viruses), Spumavirinae (which contains viruses able to cause "foamy" degeneration of inoculated cells but which are not associated with any known disease process), and Lentivirinae (which encompasses agents able to cause chronic infections with slowly progressive neurologic impairment, including the human immunodeficiency virus; see Chapter 44).

Further classification of tumor viruses within the Oncovirinae subfamily is very complicated. The members can be grouped in various ways. As described above, retroviruses may be grouped morphologically (B, C, and D type oncoviruses); the vast majority of isolates display C type characteristics.

B. Host of Origin: Retroviruses have been isolated from virtually all vertebrate species. Most viruses of a given type are isolated from a single species, although natural infections across species barriers may occur. Group-specific antigenic determinants on the major internal (core) protein are shared by viruses from the same host species. All mammalian viruses are more closely related to one another than to those from avian species.

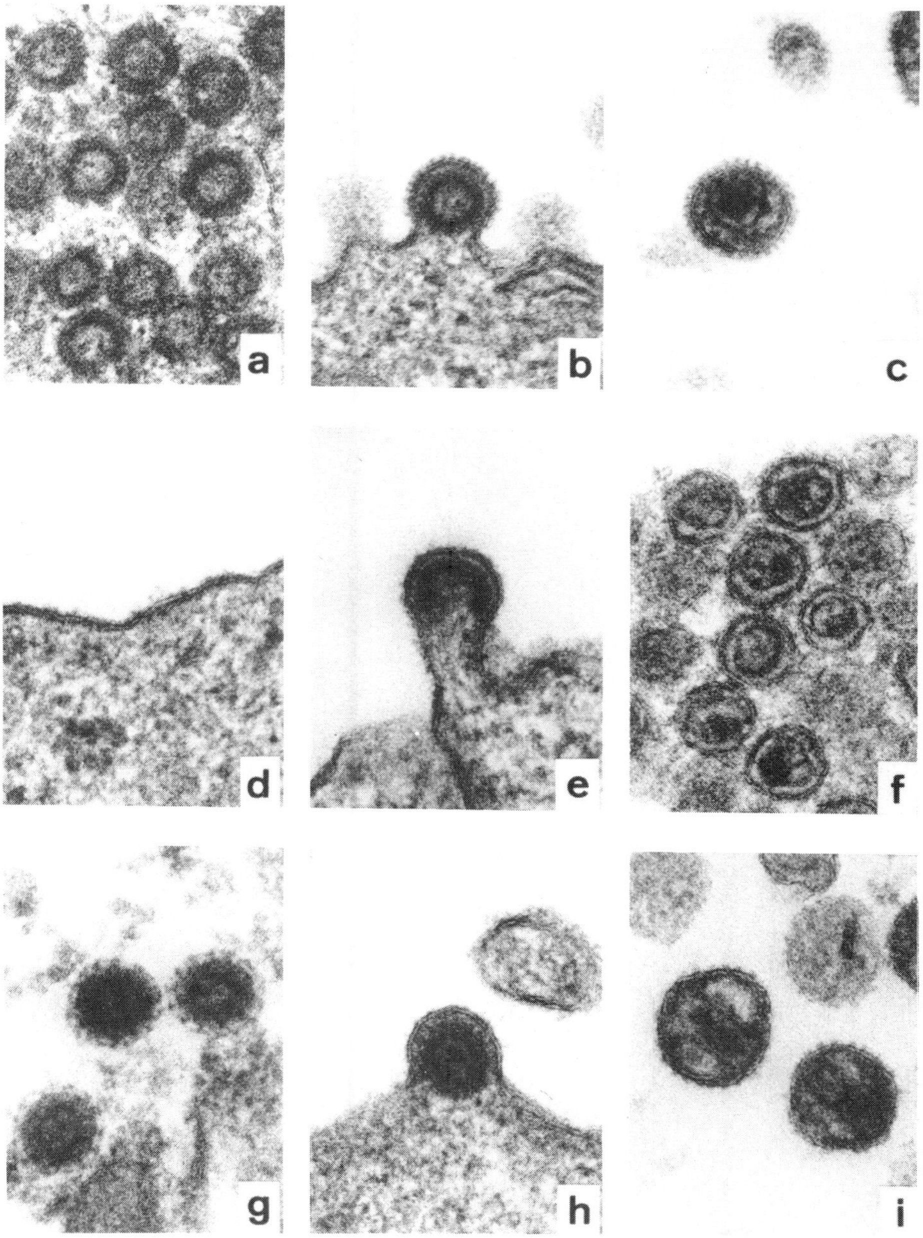

Figure 43–5. Comparative morphology of type A, B, C, and D retroviruses. ***a:*** Intracytoplasmic A type particles (representing immature precursor of budding B type virus). ***b:*** Budding B type virus. ***c:*** Mature, extracellular B type virus. ***d:*** Lack of morphologically recognizable intracytoplasmic form for C type virus. ***e:*** Budding C type virus. ***f:*** Mature, extracellular C type virus. ***g:*** Intracytoplasmic A type particle (representing immature precursor form of D type virus). ***h:*** Budding D type virus. ***i:*** Mature, extracellular D type virus. All micrographs are approximately × 87,000. Thin sections were double-stained with uranyl acetate and lead citrate. (Courtesy of D Fine and M Gonda.)

The RNA tumor viruses most widely studied experimentally are the sarcoma viruses of birds and mice and the leukemia viruses of mice, cats, birds, and humans. Representative examples are listed in Table 43–3.

C. Exogenous or Endogenous: Exogenous retroviruses are spread horizontally and behave as typical infectious agents. They initiate infection and transformation only after contact. In contrast to endogenous viruses, which are found in all cells of all in-

Table 43–3. Representative RNA-containing tumor viruses (retroviruses).

Virus	Abbreviations Used	Host of Origin	Natural Tumors (Host of Origin)	Persistence of Infectious Virus in Tumor	Carry Cellular Oncogene(s)	In Vitro Cell Transformation	Morphology (Particle Type)
Avian complex				Sometimes, but not always. Usually no for sarcoma viruses.			
Leukemia	ALV	Chicken	Yes		No	No	C
Sarcoma	ASV		Yes		Yes	Yes	
Murine complex							
Leukemia	MLV	Mouse	Yes		No	No	C
Sarcoma	MSV		No		Yes	Yes	
Murine mammary tumor	MMTV	Mouse	Yes		No	No	B
Feline complex							
Leukemia	FeLV	Cat	Yes		No	No	C
Sarcoma	FeSV		Yes		Yes	Yes	
Primate							
Human T-cell lymphotropic	HTLV	Human	Yes		No	No	C
Woolly monkey, sarcoma	SSV-1	Monkey	Yes		Yes	Yes	C
Gibbon, leukemia	GALV	Ape	Yes		No	No	C
Monkey, mammary carcinoma (Mason-Pfizer)	M-PMV	Monkey	?		No	No	D

dividuals of a given species, gene sequences of exogenous viruses are found only in infected cells. The pathogenic retroviruses all appear to be exogenous viruses.

Retroviruses may also be transmitted vertically through the germ line. Viral genetic information that is a constant part of the genetic constitution of an organism is designated as "endogenous." An integrated retroviral provirus behaves like a cluster of cellular genes and is subject to regulatory control by the cell. This cellular control usually results in partial or complete repression of viral gene expression. Its location in the cellular genome and the presence of appropriate cellular transcription factors determine to a great extent if (and when) viral expression will be activated. It is not uncommon for normal cells to maintain the endogenous viral infection in a quiescent form for extended periods of time.

Many vertebrates possess multiple copies of endogenous RNA viral sequences. The endogenous viral sequences are of no apparent benefit to the animal, and the reasons for retention and conservation of the sequences are not known. However, it has recently been discovered that endogenous proviruses of mammary tumor virus carried by inbred strains of mice express superantigen activities that influence the T cell repertoires of the animals. The proto-oncogene sequences present in all normal cells (see below) are not located in the cellular chromosome adjacent to any endogenous viral sequences.

Endogenous viruses are usually not pathogenic for their host animals. They do not produce any disease and cannot transform cells in culture. Even when activated, they are less oncogenic for their hosts than exogenous viruses. (There are examples of disease caused by replication of endogenous viruses in inbred strains of mice.)

One method to detect the presence of heritable viral genes in normal cells is to "activate" viral expression in tissue culture by exposure of cells to radiation, chemical carcinogens, or metabolic inhibitors. More commonly, endogenous viral sequences are detected and characterized at the molecular level by using nucleic acid hybridization techniques.

Important features of endogenous viruses can be summarized as follows: (1) DNA copies of RNA tumor virus genomes are covalently linked to cellular DNA and are present in all somatic and germ cells in the host; (2) endogenous viral genomes are transmitted genetically from parent to offspring; (3) the integrated state subjects the endogenous viral genomes to host genetic control; and (4) the endogenous virus may be induced to replicate either spontaneously or by treatment with extrinsic (chemical) factors.

D. Host Range: The presence or absence of an appropriate cell surface receptor is a major determinant of the host range of a retrovirus. Infection is initiated by an interaction between the viral envelope glycoprotein and a cell surface receptor. **Ecotropic** viruses infect and replicate only in cells from animals of the original host species. **Amphotropic** viruses exhibit a broad host range (able to infect cells not only of the natural host but of heterologous species as well) because they recognize a receptor that is widely distributed. **Xenotropic** viruses can replicate in some heterologous (foreign) cells but not in cells of the natural host. Many endogenous viruses have xenotropic host ranges.

E. Genetic Content: Retroviruses have a simple genetic content, but there is some variation in the number and type of genes contained. The genetic makeup of a virus influences its biologic properties. Genomic structure is a useful way of categorizing RNA tumor viruses (Figure 43–6).

The standard leukemia viruses contain three genes required for viral replication: *gag,* which encodes the core proteins (*g*roup-specific *a*nti*g*ens); *pol,* which encodes the reverse transcriptase enzyme (*pol*ymerase); and *env,* which encodes the glycoproteins that form projections on the *env*elope of the particle. The gene order in all retroviruses is 5′-*gag-pol-env*-3′.

Until 1988, the cleaved retrovirus proteins, products of the three common genes, were designated by the letter "p" followed by an approximate molecular weight. This system became cumbersome because different retrovirus species of proteins with different functions may have similar molecular weights and, conversely, proteins of similar functions may have different molecular weights. A unified nomenclature for proteins common to all retroviruses has now been proposed, based on an increased understanding of viral functions. The new nomenclature uses only two letters and reflects a known biologic function, location in virions, or enzymatic activity (Table 43–4). For example, the avian sarcoma and leukosis virus (ASLV) p15 protease would be referred to as the ASLV PR, or the murine leukemia virus (MuLV) p10 nucleocapsid protein would be referred to as the MuLV NC.

Some viruses, exemplified by the human retroviruses, contain a fourth gene, designated *tax* or *tat,* downstream from the *env* gene. It is a *t*rans*act*ivating regulatory gene that encodes a nonstructural protein that alters the transcription or translational efficiency of other viral genes. The lentiviruses, including human immunodeficiency virus, have a more complex genome and contain several additional accessory genes (see Chapter 44).

Retroviruses with either of these two genomic structures will be replication-competent (in appropriate cells). Because they lack a transforming (*onc*) gene, they cannot transform cells in tissue culture. However, they may have the ability to transform precursor cells in blood-forming tissues in vivo.

The directly transforming retroviruses carry an *onc* gene. The transforming genes carried by various RNA tumor viruses represent cellular genes that have been appropriated by those viruses at some time in the distant past and incorporated into their genomes (Figure 43–7). The avian sarcoma virus is one of the most intensively studied agents; its transforming gene is designated *src* (pronounced "sark"). This and other cellular oncogenes, as well as their normal cellular proto-oncogene predecessors, are described below.

Such viruses are highly oncogenic in appropriate host animals and can transform cells in culture. With very few exceptions, the addition of the cellular DNA results in the loss of portions of the viral genome (Figure 43–6). Consequently, the acute leukemia and sarcoma viruses are replication-defective; progeny virus is produced only in the presence of helper viruses. The helper viruses are generally other retroviruses (leukemia viruses), which may recombine in various ways with the defective viruses. These defective transforming retroviruses have been the source of most of the recognized cellular oncogenes. The most notable exception to the defective nature of sarcoma viruses is the famous Rous (avian) sarcoma virus in which the cellular *src* gene was inserted such that the necessary replication genes were not interrupted.

F. Oncogenic Potential: The retroviruses that contain oncogenes are highly oncogenic. They are sometimes referred to as "acute transforming" agents because they induce tumors in vivo after very short latent periods and rapidly induce morphologic transformation of cells in vitro. The known highly oncogenic retroviruses can induce a variety of tumor types (sarcomas, carcinomas, leukemias). However, a given virus usually displays a marked tissue tropism. The viruses that do not carry an oncogene have a much lower oncogenic potential. Disease (usually of blood cells) appears after a long latent period (ie, "slow transforming"); cultured cells are not transformed.

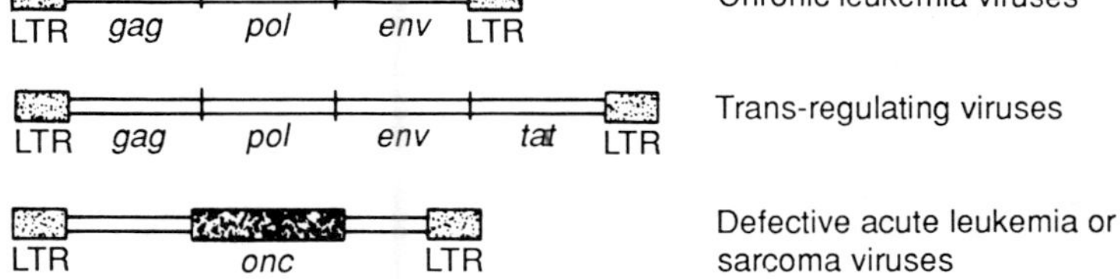

Figure 43–6. Provirus genomic structures of different categories of retroviruses. Standard leukemia viruses contain three genes required for replication: *gag, pol,* and *env.* Transregulating viruses, such as human immunodeficiency virus, contain a fourth gene, *tat* (called *tax* in HTLV-I). [The lentiviruses contain several accessory genes in addition to *tat* (see Chapter 44).] The directly transforming viruses carry a cellular gene, *onc,* usually acquired at the expense of portions of the viral genome, producing a transforming virus that is replication defective.

Table 43–4. New nomenclature for proteins common to all retroviruses.

Name of Protein[1]	Acronym	Previous Designations Based on Molecular Weight[2]
Matrix	MA	p10–p19
(Unnamed)	?	p10–p21
Capsid	CA	p24–p30
Nucleocapsid	NC	p7–p15
Protease	PR	p12–p15
Reverse transcriptase	RT	p66–p80
Integration	IN	p32–p46
Surface	SU	gp46–gp120
Transmembrane	TM	p15E–gp45

[1]Order of proteins 5′ to 3′ on the viral genome, from top to bottom of list.

[2]Includes examples from avian, murine, bovine, equine, simian, and human retroviruses.

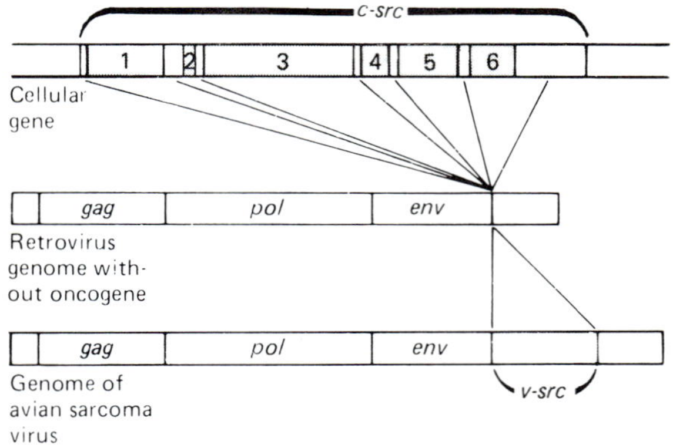

Figure 43–7. Split cellular gene c-*src (top)* consists of exons (light gray) and introns (dark gray). The cellular gene was somehow picked up by a preexisting retrovirus; the introns were eliminated and the exons, spliced together, were inserted into the viral genome *(middle)* to complete the avian sarcoma virus genome *(bottom).* In addition to *src,* the genes are *gag* (which encodes the protein of the viral capsid), *pol* (which encodes reverse transcriptase), and *env* (which encodes glycoprotein spikes of the viral envelope). Other retrovirus oncogenes are thought to have similar origins but represent different cellular genes. Usually the incorporation of cellular DNA is accompanied by the deletion of some of the viral genome, resulting in a replication-defective, transforming retrovirus. (After Bishop JM: Sci Am [March] 1982;246:80.)

Mechanisms of tumorigenesis by the weakly oncogenic leukemia viruses are considered below.

Briefly, neoplastic transformation by retroviruses is the result of a cellular gene that is normally expressed at low, carefully regulated levels becoming activated and expressed constitutively. In the case of the acute transforming viruses, a cellular gene has been inserted by recombination into the viral genome and is expressed as a viral gene under the control of the viral promoter. In the case of the leukemia viruses, the viral promoter or enhancer element is inserted adjacent to or near the cellular gene in the cellular chromosome.

Replication of Retroviruses

After viral particles have adsorbed to and penetrated host cells, the viral RNA serves as the template for the synthesis of viral DNA through the action of the viral enzyme reverse transcriptase. By a complex process, sequences from both ends of the viral RNA get duplicated, forming the long terminal repeat located at each end of the viral DNA (Figure 43–8). Long terminal repeats are present only in viral DNA. The newly formed viral DNA becomes integrated into the host cell DNA as a provirus. The structure of the provirus is constant, but its integration into the host cell genome can occur at different sites. The very precise orientation of the provirus after integration is achieved by specific sequences at the ends of both long terminal repeats.

Progeny viral genomes may then be transcribed from the provirus DNA into viral RNA. The U3 sequence in the long terminal repeat contains both a promoter and an enhancer. The enhancer may help confer tissue specificity on viral expression. The proviral DNA is transcribed by the host enzyme, RNA polymerase II. Full-length transcripts (capped, polyadenylated) may serve as genomic RNA for encapsidation in progeny virions. Some transcripts are spliced, and the subgenomic mRNAs are translated to produce viral precursor proteins that get modified and cleaved to form the final protein products.

If the virus happens to contain a transforming gene, the oncogene plays no role in replication. This is in marked contrast to the DNA tumor viruses in which the transforming genes are also essential viral replication genes.

Viral particles mature and emerge from infected host cells by budding from cytoplasmic membranes (Figure 43–9).

A salient feature of retroviruses is that they are not cytolytic, ie, they do not kill the cells in which they replicate. Furthermore, the provirus remains integrated within the cellular DNA for the life of the cell. There is currently no known way to cure a cell of a chronic retrovirus infection. There is probably a better chance of developing a means of altering viral expression than of eliminating a provirus from a cell.

Human Retroviruses

A human T cell lymphotropic retrovirus, HTLV-I, has been established as the causative agent of certain cutaneous T cell lymphomas of adults that express large quantities of interleukin-2 membrane receptors, as well as a nervous system degenerative disorder

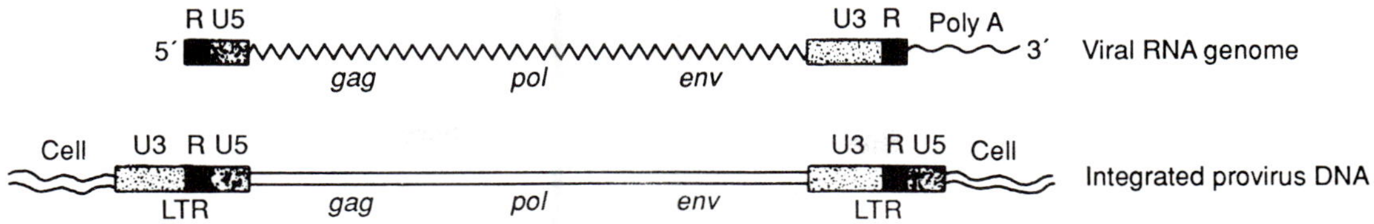

Figure 43–8. Comparison of structures of retrovirus RNA genome and integrated provirus DNA. A viral particle contains two identical copies of the single-stranded RNA genome. The 5′ terminus is capped, and the 3′ terminus is polyadenylated. A short sequence, R, is repeated at both ends; unique sequences are located near the 5′ (U5) and 3′ (U3) ends. U3 contains promoter and enhancer sequences. The integrated provirus DNA is flanked at each end by the long terminal repeat (LTR) structure generated during synthesis of the DNA copy by reverse transcription. Each long terminal repeat contains U3, R, and U5 sequences. The long terminal repeats and coding regions of the retrovirus genome are not drawn to scale.

called tropical spastic paraparesis. Two related human viruses, HTLV-II and HTLV-V, have been isolated but have not been conclusively associated with a specific disease.

The human lymphotropic viruses have a marked affinity for mature T cells. HTLV-I is expressed at very low levels in infected individuals, and its initial discovery in 1978 hinged on the use of T cell growth factor (interleukin-2) to amplify populations of malignant T cells in vitro, coupled with the use of sensitive molecular techniques to assay for virus-specific markers (DNA or protein). It appears that the viral promoter-enhancer sequences in the long terminal repeat

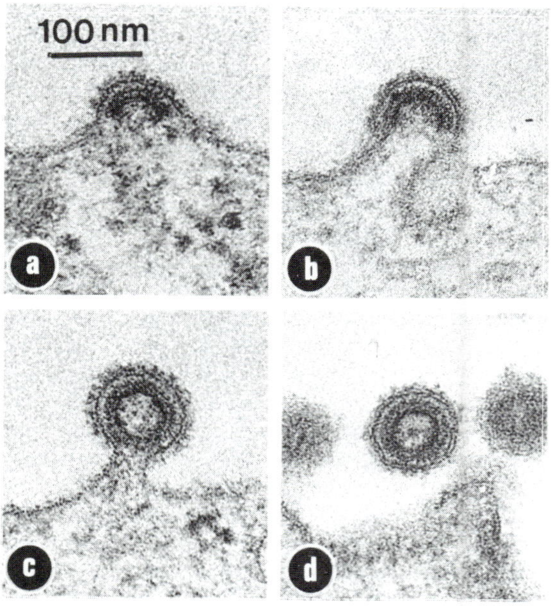

Figure 43–9. Sequential stages of the budding process of replicating retroviruses. Pictured is the Friend strain of murine leukemia virus. A core containing viral RNA acquires an envelope by budding through the cellular plasma membrane at a site containing viral glycoproteins. (Courtesy of H Frank.)

may be responsive to signals associated with the activation and proliferation of T cells. If so, the replication of the viruses may be linked to the replication of the host cells, a strategy that would ensure efficient propagation of the virus.

The human retroviruses are transregulating (Figure 43–6). They carry a gene, *tax,* the product of which alters the expression of other viral genes. Transactivating regulatory genes are believed to be necessary for viral replication in vivo and may contribute to oncogenesis by also modulating cellular genes that regulate growth. In fact, transgenic mice carrying the HTLV-I *tax* gene under the control of the HTLV-I regulatory region developed mesenchymal tumors, showing that a transactivating gene may be oncogenic. It is possible to transmit HTLV from donor cells to recipient cord blood or bone marrow cells by cocultivation experiments; transformed immortalized recipient cell lines of T cell origin will emerge. The fact that proviral sequences are found in the DNA of neoplastic T cells but not in normal human cells establishes that the virus is an exogenous agent.

The virus is distributed worldwide, with clusters of HTLV-associated disease in certain geographic areas (southern Japan, Melanesia, the Caribbean basin, the southern USA, and areas in South America and Africa). Although less than 1% of people worldwide have HTLV-I antibody, more than 10% of the population in endemic areas will be seropositive, and antibody may be found in 50% of relatives of virus-positive leukemia patients.

Transmission of HTLV-I seems to involve cell-associated virus. Mother-to-child transmission via breast feeding is an important mode. Efficiency of transmission from infected mother to child is estimated at 15–25%. Blood transfusion is an effective means of transmission, so retrovirus infections in apparently healthy blood donors must be considered. HTLV-I can be transmitted by sharing blood-contaminated needles (drug abusers) and by sexual intercourse.

Seroepidemiology has linked infection with HTLV-I to a syndrome called HTLV-I-associated myelopathy–tropical spastic paraparesis (HAM/TSP). The primary clinical feature is development of progressive weakness of the legs and lower body. The patient's mental faculties remain intact. HAM/TSP is described as being of the same magnitude and importance in the tropics as multiple sclerosis is in western countries. HAM/TSP patients display some immunologic features commonly seen in autoimmune diseases, and it has been proposed that infection by HTLV-I may trigger autoimmune abnormalities that cause the HAM/TSP symptoms.

A distantly related subfamily of human retroviruses has been established as the cause of acquired immunodeficiency syndrome (AIDS; see Chapter 44). The viruses are cytolytic and nontransforming and are classified as lentiviruses.

CELLULAR ONCOGENES

Oncogene is the general term given to genes that cause cancer. "Friendly" versions of these transforming genes are present in normal cells and have been designated proto-oncogenes.

Classification of Oncogenes

The discovery of cellular oncogenes came from studies with acutely transforming retroviruses. Surprisingly, it was found that normal cells contained highly related (but not identical) copies of various retrovirus transforming genes; cellular sequences had been captured and incorporated into the retrovirus genomes. Transduction of the cellular genes was probably an accident, reflecting the way the retroviruses replicate. The presence of the cellular sequences is of no benefit to the virus, and each particular "hybrid" virus probably would have perished with the death of the host animal had not an industrious tumor virologist isolated it from the tumor. About 20 different cellular oncogenes have been identified by virtue of their presence in retrovirus isolates. There are at least an equal number of other known cellular oncogenes that have not been segregated into retrovirus vectors. Gene transfer techniques have been successful in recovering such novel oncogenes from tumors of nonviral origin.

Cellular proto-oncogenes represent highly conserved sequences found in cells of species ranging from fruit flies to humans. This suggests that their functions are essential to normal activities of cells.

Cellular oncogenes can be broadly grouped on the basis of presumed function and predominant properties (Table 43–5). They are structurally and functionally heterogeneous entities. The picture emerging is that oncogenes represent individual components of complicated pathways responsible for regulating cell proliferation, division, and differentiation. Incorrect expression of any component might interrupt that regulation, resulting in uncontrolled growth of cells (cancer). Examples exist of tyrosine-specific protein kinases (eg, *src*), growth factors (*sis* is similar to human platelet-derived growth factor, a potent mitogen for cells of connective tissue origin), mutated growth factor receptors (*erb*-B is a truncated epidermal growth factor receptor), GTP-binding proteins (Ha-*ras*), and nuclear transcription factors (*myc, jun*).

Mechanisms of Oncogene Activation

The molecular mechanisms believed to be responsible for activating a benign proto-oncogene and converting it into a cancer gene vary. The following examples all involve genetic damage. All might cause malfunction of the proto-oncogene or its protein product. The gene may get overexpressed and a dosage effect of the overproduced oncogene product may be important in cellular growth changes. These mechanisms might result in constitutive activity (loss of normal regulation), so that the gene is expressed at the wrong time during the cell cycle or in inappropriate tissue types. Mutations might alter the carefully regulated interaction of a proto-oncogene protein with other proteins or nucleic acids.

A. Transduction by a Retrovirus: As described above, recombination between retroviral and cellular genes can introduce a cellular gene into the viral genome, where it can be replicated and transmitted like a viral gene. This is the most potent way of activating a cellular proto-oncogene into a cancer gene. The captured cell gene invariably ends up mutated in some way (point mutations, deletions, substitutions), plus the transduced gene is then expressed abundantly under the control of strong viral signals.

B. Insertional Mutagenesis: Overexpression of a proto-oncogene may occur as a result of a newly provided strong transcriptional promoter or "enhancer" sequences. Insertion of a retroviral promoter adjacent to a cellular oncogene may result in enhanced expression of that gene. A model of "promoter-insertion oncogenesis" by a leukemia virus is illustrated in Figure 43–10. This was first shown to occur in chicken lymphomas induced by avian leukosis virus; the c-*myc* gene was activated. More commonly, expression of the cellular gene may be increased through the action of nearby viral "enhancer" sequences. Insertional mutagenesis may also result in synthesis of truncated gene products.

C. Translocation: A chromosomal translocation that removes a proto-oncogene from its normal regulatory sequences and juxtaposes it near a strong promoter (such as used in immunoglobulin production) may activate expression of the oncogene. Translocations may be mutagenic as well, by deleting portions of the gene. Thus, translocations can affect either the expression of the proto-oncogene or the function of the gene product. Cancer cytogenetics studies have established that many human neoplasms have characteristic chromosomal abnormalities. It turns out that the location of proto-oncogenes (~20) is strongly associated with these cancer-specific breakpoints. The character-

Table 43–5. Representative cellular oncogenes.

General Class	Name of Oncogene	Origin: Prototype Retrovirus	Origin: Host Species[1]	Protein Product: Property	Protein Product: Subcellular Location
Nonreceptor protein tyrosine kinases	*src*	Rous sarcoma virus	Chicken	Tyrosine kinase	Plasma membrane
	abl	Abelson murine leukemia virus	Mouse		Plasma membrane, cytoplasm
	fes	ST feline sarcoma virus	Cat		Plasma membrane, cytoplasm
Receptor protein tyrosine kinases	*fms*	McDonough feline sarcoma virus	Cat	Related to colony-stimulating factor (CSF-1) receptor	Plasma membrane, endoplasmic reticulum
	erb-B	Avian erythroblastosis virus	Chicken	Epidermal growth factor receptor (truncated)	Plasma membrane, endoplasmic reticulum
	neu	None	Rat (neuroglioblastomas)	Related to epidermal growth factor receptor	Plasma membrane
Serine/threonine protein kinase	*mos*	Moloney murine sarcoma virus	Mouse		Cytoplasm
Growth factors	*sis*	Simian sarcoma virus	Woolly monkey	Platelet-derived growth factor-like	Cytoplasm, secreted
	int-2	None	Mouse	Related to fibroblast growth factor	
Membrane-associated G proteins	Ha-*ras*	Harvey murine sarcoma virus	Rat	Guanosine diphosphate-triphosphate binding; guanosine triphosphatase	Plasma membrane
	Ki-*ras*	Kirsten murine sarcoma virus			
	N-*ras*	None	Human (neuroblastomas)		
Nuclear transcription factors	*myb*	Avian myeloblastosis virus	Chicken	DNA binding	Nucleus
	myc	MC29 myelocytomatosis virus			
	fos	FBJ osteosarcoma virus	Mouse	Part of AP-1 transcription factor	
	jun	Avian sarcoma virus-17	Chicken	DNA binding; part of AP-1 transcription factor	
	erb-A	Avian erythroblastosis virus	Chicken	Mutant thyroxine (T_4) receptor	Cytoplasm, nucleus

[1]Proto-oncogene sequences are conserved among many species; column indicates initial recovery of oncogene.

istic 8:14 chromosomal translocation in Burkitt's lymphoma joins c-*myc* to immunoglobulin genes. Such translocations that activate oncogenes are probably early events in tumor development.

D. Gene Amplification: An increase in copy number often results in an increased amount of gene product. Oncogene sequences are amplified in some tumors. Amplification of the HER-2/*neu* oncogene occurs relatively frequently in human breast cancer and appears to correlate with disease relapse and shortened survival. It is likely that gene amplification is related to later steps in neoplastic progression, rather than initiation of transformation.

E. Mutation: There may be alterations in the structure of a proto-oncogene protein product due to point mutations or deletions in the gene. Such alterations might change the function of the protein (eg, substrate specificity of an enzymatic activity, binding specificity of a transcription factor). Specific point mutations resulting in substitutions of specific amino acids have been correlated with oncogenic activation of c-*ras*.

Role of Oncogenes in Human Cancer

Tumor development, in both humans and animals, is a complicated process. As many as eight indepen-

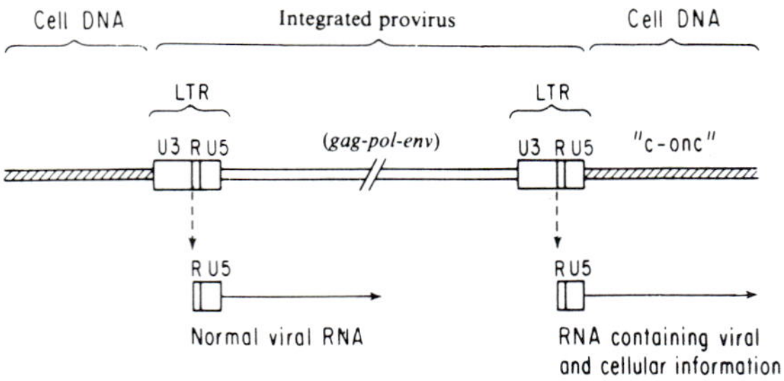

Figure 43–10. Structure and transcriptional products of an integrated leukemia virus provirus. The integrated provirus is flanked by sequences termed long terminal repeats (LTRs). Synthesis of normal viral RNA (genomic RNA and mRNAs) initiates within the left long terminal repeat. Initiation within the right long terminal repeat would generate a molecule containing viral 5′ sequences plus cellular information encoded in the adjacent cellular DNA. If, as shown, the provirus integrated upstream from a potentially oncogenic cellular gene (designated c-*onc*), initiation within the right long terminal repeat could cause elevated expression of the c-*onc* gene. (Courtesy of Hayward et al: Nature 1981;290:475.)

dent steps may be required for a malignant cell to emerge. Oncogene activations are believed to represent some of those steps, acting in collaboration with the inactivation of tumor suppressor genes. The best-characterized system is colon cancer and the genetic changes that contribute to its development. At least eight different genetic alterations have been identified in colon cancers, including alterations in tumor suppressor genes (eg, p53, DCC), oncogenes (eg, K-*ras*), and DNA repair genes. Some of these changes have been identified in families with hereditary risks of developing colon cancer. Changes in some of the genes seem to correlate with discrete intermediate stages in cancer development.

TUMOR SUPPRESSOR GENES

A newly recognized class of human cancer genes is involved in tumor development. These are the negative regulators of cell growth, variously called "tumor suppressor genes," "growth suppressor genes," or "anti-oncogenes." The **inactivation** or functional loss of both alleles of such a gene is required for tumor formation—in contrast to the **activation** that occurs with cellular oncogenes. The prototype of this inhibitory class of genes is the retinoblastoma (Rb) gene. The Rb protein appears to inhibit entry of cells into S phase by binding to key transcription factors. The function of normal Rb protein is regulated by phosphorylation. The loss of Rb gene function is causally related to the development of retinoblastoma, a rare ocular tumor of children, and appears to be involved in the development of several common human malignant tumors, including those of lung and bladder.

Another recognized tumor suppressor gene is the p53 gene. It can also block cell cycle progression; p53 acts as a transcription factor and regulates the synthesis of a protein that inhibits the function of certain cell cycle kinases. Experiments using homologous recombination to inactivate the p53 gene in mice showed that mice with no functional p53 developed normally but were prone to the appearance of spontaneous tumors. p53 appears to be altered in at least 50% of human tumors.

Specific chromosome deletions, detected by cytogenetic and molecular studies of restriction fragment length polymorphisms of cellular DNA, are often associated with human cancers; such chromosomal changes are suspected to reflect loss of tumor suppressor genes. It is thought that inactivation of tumor suppressor genes is as important in cancer development as activation of oncogenes. The transforming proteins of several DNA tumor viruses interact with the products of cellular tumor suppressor genes, and it is presumed that such protein-protein interactions are functionally important in tumor induction by those viruses.

DNA TUMOR VIRUSES

Fundamental differences exist between the oncogenes of DNA and RNA tumor viruses. The transforming genes carried by DNA tumor viruses encode functions required for viral replication and do not have normal homologues in cells. In contrast, retroviruses carry transduced cellular oncogenes that have no role in viral replication. Presumably, the DNA virus transforming proteins complex with normal cell proteins and alter their function. To understand the mechanism of action of DNA virus transforming proteins, it is important to identify the cellular targets with which they interact. Two such cellular proteins have been identified as the products of tumor suppressor genes (Rb, p53).

Five families of DNA-containing viruses contain members capable of tumor induction or cell transformation. Representative examples are shown in Table 43–6. A brief description of each of these families, with particular reference to oncogenesis, is given below.

Papovaviruses

Important properties of papovaviruses are given in Table 43–7.

A. Structure and Composition: These are small viruses (diameter 45–55 nm) that possess a circular genome of double-stranded DNA (MW $3–5 \times 10^6$; 5–8 kb pairs) enclosed within a nonenveloped capsid exhibiting icosahedral symmetry (Figures 43–11 and 43–12). Cellular histones are used to condense viral DNA inside viral particles.

Table 43–6. Representative DNA-containing tumor viruses.

Virus	Host of Origin	Natural Tumors (Host of Origin)	Persistence of Infectious Virus in Tumor	Encode Transforming Protein(s)	In Vitro Cell Transformation	Virion	
						Size (nm)	Structure
Papovaviruses							
Polyoma	Mouse	No			Yes		
SV40	Monkey	No	No		Yes		
BK, JC	Human	No		Yes	Yes	45–55	Icosahedral symmetry
Papilloma							
Human	Human	Yes					
Rabbit	Rabbit	Yes	Yes, but not always		No		
Bovine	Cow	Yes			Yes		
Adenoviruses							
Human (several types)	Human	No	No	Yes	Yes	70–90	Icosahedral symmetry
Simian (some)	Monkey	No					
Herpesviruses							
Human							
Herpes simplex type 2	Human				Yes		
EB virus	Human	Yes		Yes	Yes		
Cytomegalovirus	Human		No		Yes	100	Icosahedral symmetry
Monkey	Monkey	No					
Avian (Marek)	Chicken	Yes					
Frog (Lucké)	Frog	Yes					
Hepadnaviruses							
Human hepatitis B	Human	Yes	No	No	No	42	Complex
Woodchuck hepatitis	Woodchuck	Yes			No		
Poxviruses							
Molluscum contagiosum	Human	Yes			No		
Yaba	Monkey	Yes	Yes			230 × 400	Complex symmetry
Fibroma-myxoma	Rabbit, deer	Yes					

B. Classification: The **Papovaviridae** family contains two genera, *Polyomavirus* and *Papillomavirus.* The latter are slightly larger, possess a larger genome, and are more important to human disease. The genome organization of member viruses differs significantly between the two genera. Properties of these two subgroups are compared in Table 43–8.

There is widespread diversity among papillomaviruses. Since neutralization tests cannot be done as there is no in vitro infectivity assay, papillomavirus isolates are classified using molecular criteria. Virus "types" share less than 50% DNA homology. More than 70 distinct human papillomavirus (HPV) types have been recovered.

C. Polyomaviruses: SV40 and polyoma viruses are the best-characterized DNA-containing tumor viruses, since they contain a limited amount of genetic information (6 or 7 genes). The papovavirus genome contains "early" and "late" regions, as illustrated for SV40 (Figure 43–13). The late region consists of genes that code for the synthesis of coat proteins; they are not expressed in transformed cells. The early region is expressed soon after infection of cells; it contains genes that code for early proteins, eg, the SV40 tumor (T) antigen, which is necessary for the replication of viral DNA in permissive cells. The polyoma virus genome encodes three early proteins (small, middle, and large T antigens). One or two of the T antigens are required for the transformation of cells. (Even with

Table 43–7. Important properties of papovaviruses.

Virion: Icosahedral, 45–55 nm in diameter.
Composition: DNA (10%), protein (90%).
Genome: Double-stranded DNA, circular, MW 3–5 million, 5–8 kbp.
Proteins: Three structural proteins; cellular histones condense DNA in virion.
Envelope: None.
Replication: Nucleus.
Outstanding characteristics: Stimulate cell DNA synthesis. Polyomaviruses are important model tumor viruses; papillomaviruses are significant causes of human disease. Viral oncoproteins interact with cellular tumor suppressor proteins.

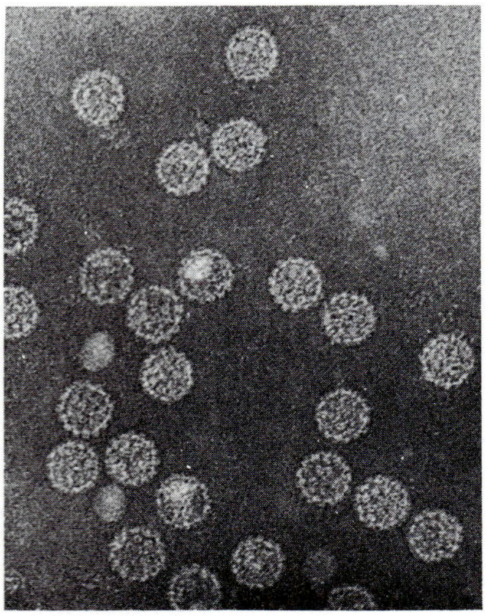

Figure 43–11. Papovavirus SV40. Purified preparation negatively stained with phosphotungstate (150,000×). (S McGregor and H Mayor.)

the larger DNA viruses such as adenoviruses, only two or three viral genes are involved in cell transformation.) The transforming proteins must be continuously synthesized for cells to stay transformed.

The polyoma large T antigen is found in the nucleus of transformed cells; the middle T antigen is associated with the cell membrane, where it complexes with the normal c-*src* protein and activates its tyrosine kinase activity. Most of the SV40 large T antigen is in the cell nucleus, but small amounts are localized in the plasma membrane, where it is a target for cytotoxic T cells involved in tumor rejection reactions. SV40 T antigen does not interact with the c-*src* protein but rather is found tightly complexed with cellular tumor suppressor gene products, p53 and Rb (Table 43–9). Presumably, these interactions of T antigen with cellular proteins are important in the transformation process.

Polyoma virus causes many different types of tumors following injection into newborn mice. Tumors do not develop as a result of natural infection among young mice. Polyoma virus replicates in mouse cells and transforms certain heterologous (eg, hamster) cells. SV40 replicates in cells of the natural host (monkey); it causes tumors in experimentally inoculated newborn hamsters and transforms various rodent cells. Tumor induction in the natural host—the rhesus monkey—has not been observed. SV40 contaminated early lots of live poliovirus vaccines that had been grown in monkey cells. Although many persons, including newborns, accidentally received such SV40-contaminated vaccines, these individuals have been

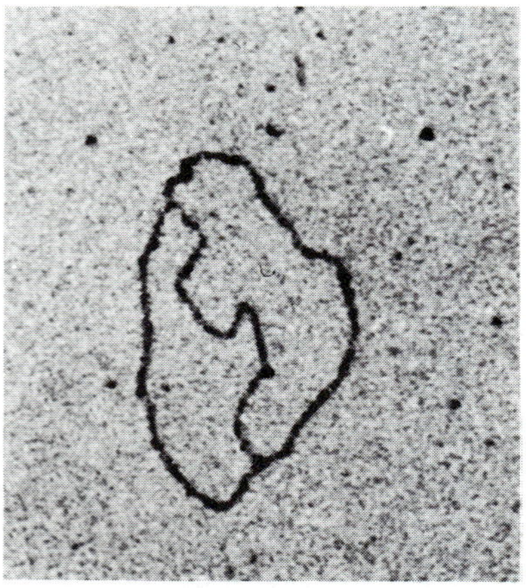

Figure 43–12. Circular double-stranded DNA genome of papovavirus SV40. This molecule is in the process of replicating. (From N Salzman et al.)

Table 43–8. Comparison of properties of polyomaviruses and papillomaviruses.

Characteristic	Genus: *Polyomavirus*	Genus: *Papillomavirus*
Virion		
Capsid structure	Icosahedral, no envelope	Icosahedral, no envelope
Size (diameter)	45 nm	55 nm
Genome		
Type, structure of nucleic acid	Circular, double-stranded DNA	Circular, double-stranded DNA
Size: MW, no. of base pairs	3×10^6; 5×10^3	5×10^6; 8×10^3
Coding information	On both strands	On one strand
Oncogenic potential		
Tumors in natural hosts	No	Yes
Result of natural infection	Usually inapparent	Benign tumor (wart)
Target tissue	Internal organs	Surface epithelia
Transform cells in vitro	Yes	Rarely
Genome in transformed cells	Integrated	Not integrated in warts; integrated in carcinomas
Individual members		
Viruses infecting humans	BK and JC viruses	Human papillomaviruses, >70 types
Most significant human illness	Progressive multifocal leukoencephalopathy	Skin warts, genital warts, laryngeal papillomas, cervical carcinoma
Important animal isolates	Polyoma virus (mouse), SV40 (monkey)	Papillomaviruses from cows and rabbits

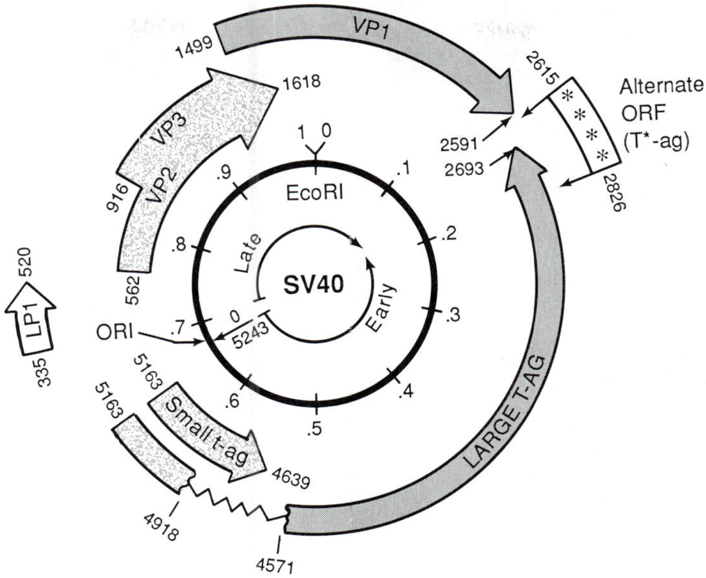

Figure 43–13. Genetic map of the papovavirus SV40. The thick circle represents the circular SV40 DNA genome. The unique *Eco*RI site is shown at map unit 0/1. Nucleotide numbers begin and end at the origin (ori) of viral DNA replication (0/5243). Boxed arrows indicate the open reading frames that encode the viral proteins. Arrowheads point in the direction of transcription; the beginning and end of each open reading frame is indicated by nucleotide numbers. Various shadings depict different reading frames used for different viral polypeptides. Note that large T antigen (T-ag) is coded by two noncontiguous segments on the genome. The alternative open reading frame (ORF) that could be used for a unique carboxy terminus of the putative third tumor antigen, T*-ag, is indicated. The genome is divided into "early" and "late" regions that are expressed before and after the onset of viral DNA replication, respectively. Only the early region is expressed in transformed cells. (Reproduced, with permission, from Butel JS, Jarvis DL: Biochim Biophys Acta 1986;865:171.)

followed for over 25 years, and no SV40-related tumors have been reported.

The human papovaviruses (BK and JC) have been isolated from immunocompromised patients. BK virus is not known to cause human disease, but JC virus is regularly isolated from brains of patients with progressive multifocal leukoencephalopathy. The two viruses are antigenically distinct, but both induce a T antigen that is related to SV40 T antigen. BK and JC viruses are widely distributed in human populations, as evidenced by the presence of specific antibody in 70–80% of adult sera. Infection usually occurs during early childhood. Both viruses may persist in the kidneys of healthy individuals after primary infection and may reactivate when the host's immune response is impaired, eg, by renal transplantation, or during pregnancy. These human viruses can transform rodent cells and induce tumors in newborn hamsters. However, they have not been associated with any human tumors.

D. Papillomaviruses: The papillomaviruses are slightly larger in diameter (55 nm) than the polyomaviruses (45 nm) and contain a larger genome (MW 5×10^6 versus 3×10^6). The organization of the papillomavirus genome is more complex (Figure 43–14).

Papillomaviruses are highly tropic for epithelial cells of the skin and mucous membranes. Viral nucleic acid can be found in basal stem cells, but late gene expression (capsid proteins) is restricted to the uppermost layer of differentiated keratinocytes (Figure 43–15). Stages in the viral replicative cycle are probably dependent on specific factors that are present in sequential differentiated states of epithelial cells. Molecular and biologic studies with the papillomaviruses have progressed slowly, because they have not been propagated in vitro in cell culture. This difficulty in culturing is probably a reflection of the strong depen-

Table 43–9. Interactions between DNA tumor virus oncoproteins and cellular tumor suppressor proteins.

Virus	Viral Oncoproteins	Complex Formation With Cellular Protein: Rb[1]	p53[2]
Papovavirus SV40	Large T-antigen	T-antigen	T-antigen
Human papillomavirus	E6, E7	E7	E6
Adenovirus	E1A, E1B	E1A	E1B

[1]Rb = M_r 105,000 phosphoprotein, product of the retinoblastoma gene.
[2]p53 = M_r 53,000 phosphoprotein, product of the p53 gene.

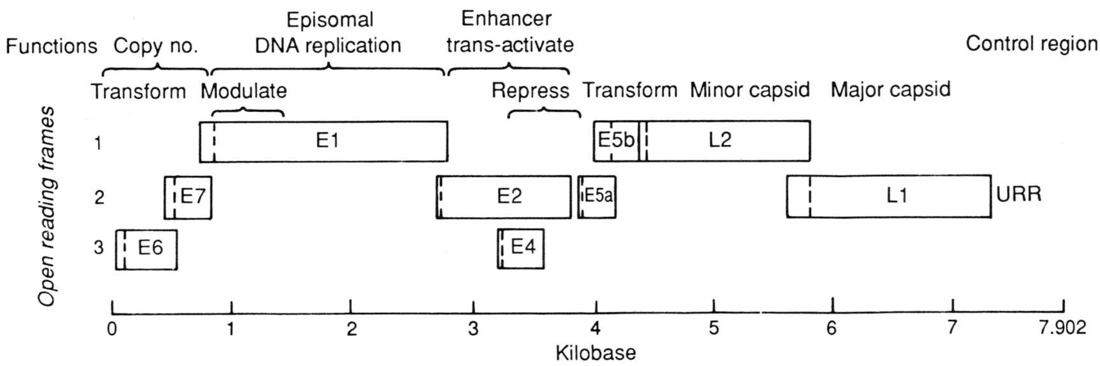

Figure 43–14. Map of the human papillomavirus genome (HPV-6, 7902 base pairs). The papillomavirus genome is circular but is shown linearized in the upstream regulatory region (URR). The upstream regulatory region contains the origin of replication and enhancer and promoter sequences. Early (E1–E7) and late (L1, L2) open reading frames and their functions are shown. All the open reading frames are on the same strand of viral DNA. Biologic functions are extrapolated from studies with the bovine papillomavirus. The organization of the papillomavirus genome is much more complex than that of SV40 (compare with Figure 43–13). (Reproduced, with permission, from Broker TR: Structure and genetic expression of papillomaviruses. Obstet Gynecol Clin North Am 1987;14:329.)

dence of viral replication on the differentiated state of the host cell.

Papillomaviruses are biologically distinguished from the related polyomaviruses by their dependence on the differentiated state of host cells for viral replication, the induction of tumors in natural hosts, the presence of viral particles in some tumor tissues, and the maintenance of viral DNA as episomal copies in some transformed cells.

Papillomaviruses cause several different kinds of

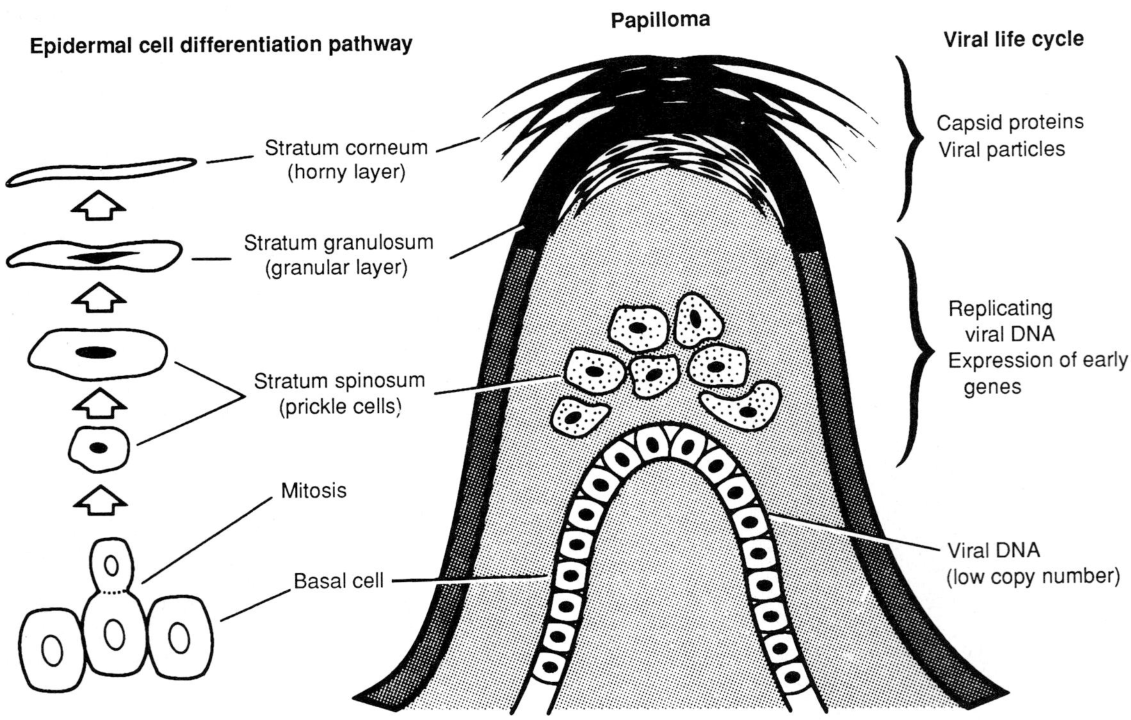

Figure 43–15. Schematic representation of a skin wart (papilloma). The papillomavirus life cycle is tied to epithelial cell differentiation. The terminal differentiation pathway of epidermal cells is shown on the left. Events in the virus life cycle are noted on the right. Late events in viral replication (capsid protein synthesis and virion morphogenesis) occur only in terminally differentiated cells. (Reproduced, with permission, from Butel JS: Papovaviruses. In: *Medical Microbiology,* 2nd ed. Albrecht T, Baron S [editors]. Churchill Livingstone, 1990.)

warts in humans, including skin warts, plantar warts, flat warts, genital condylomas, and laryngeal papillomas (Table 43–10). HPV-associated sexually transmitted genital lesions are becoming more common. More importantly, there is strong evidence that links HPV infection with premalignant and malignant disease of the vulva, cervix, penis, and anus.

The multiple types of human papillomavirus isolates are preferentially associated with certain clinical lesions, although distribution patterns are not absolute. Clinicians believe there is a spectrum of HPV-related disease that ranges from genital condylomas through grades of dysplasia to invasive cancer. Cervical cancer is the second most frequent cancer in women worldwide (~500,000 new cases annually) and is a major cause of cancer deaths in developing countries.

The majority of cervical, penile, and vulvar cancers carry HPV DNA. Most frequently, HPV-16 or HPV-18 is found, although some cancers contain DNA from HPV type 11, 31, 33, or 35. HeLa cells, a widely used tissue culture cell line derived many years ago from a cervical carcinoma, have been found to contain HPV-18 DNA.

It is likely that cofactors are involved in the progression of high-risk HPV lesions to carcinomas. Suspected cofactors include tobacco smoke and coinfection with herpes simplex virus.

Laryngeal papillomas in children are caused by HPV-6 and HPV-11. The infection is probably acquired during passage through the birth canal of a mother with genital warts. While laryngeal papillomas are rare, the growths may obstruct the larynx and must be removed repeatedly by surgical means. Viral DNA can be detected in normal tissues of the larynx of patients in remission. This latent infection may serve as a source of new lesions. Interferon has been used to treat laryngeal papillomas with some success.

Based on relative occurrence of DNA in certain cancers, HPV types 16 and 18 are considered to be high cancer risk, type 31 is classified as intermediate risk, and types 6 and 11 are viewed as low risk. Many HPV types are considered benign. For this reason, it will become important to be able to diagnose the specific HPV type associated with a clinical lesion.

Integrated copies of viral DNA are present in cancer cells, although HPV DNA is generally not integrated (episomal) in noncancerous cells or premalignant lesions. Viral early proteins E6 and E7 are synthesized in cancer tissue. These are HPV transforming proteins, and they have been found able to complex with cellular proteins Rb and p53 (Table 43–9).

The behavior of HPV lesions is influenced by immunologic factors. Cell-mediated immunity is probably important. Warts tend to disappear spontaneously with time, whereas immunosuppressed patients experience an increased incidence of warts and of intraepithelial neoplasia of the vulva and cervix as well. The role of the immune response in protection against infection and in the regression of papillomavirus lesions needs to be better understood before the feasibility of vaccine development can be assessed.

Table 43–10. Association of human papillomaviruses with clinical lesions.[1]

Human Papillomavirus Type	Clinical Lesion	Suspected Oncogenic Potential
1	Plantar warts	Benign
2	Common warts	Benign
3, 10, 28	Flat warts, epidermodysplasia verruciformis	Rarely malignant
5, 8	Epidermodysplasia verruciformis in patients with cell-mediated immune deficiency	30% progress to malignancy
6, 11	Anogenital condylomas; laryngeal papillomas; dysplasias and intraepithelial neoplasias, grades I and II	Low
7	Hand warts of meat and animal handlers	Benign
9, 12, 14, 15, 17, 19–25, 36, 40	Epidermodysplasia verruciformis	Some progress to carcinomas (eg, HPV-12, 17, 20)
13, 32	Oral focal epithelial hyperplasia (Heck's disease)	Possible progression to carcinoma
16, 18, 31, 33, 35, 39	High-grade dysplasias and carcinomas of genital mucosa; laryngeal and esophageal carcinomas; Bowen's disease	High correlation with genital and oral carcinomas
26, 27, 29	Cutaneous warts	?
30, 40	Laryngeal carcinoma	Malignant
37	Keratoacanthoma	Benign
41, 42	Genital warts	Benign

[1]Modified, with permission, from Broker TR: Structure and genetic expression of papillomaviruses. *Obstet Gynecol Clin North Am* 1987;14:329.

Adenoviruses (See Chapter 32.)

The adenoviruses comprise a large group of agents widely distributed in nature. They are medium-sized, nonenveloped viruses containing a linear genome of double-stranded DNA (MW 20–25 × 10^6). Replication is species-specific, occurring in cells of the natural hosts. Adenoviruses commonly infect humans, causing mild acute illnesses, mainly of the respiratory and intestinal tracts.

Adenoviruses can transform rodent cells and induce the synthesis of virus-specific early antigens that localize in both the nucleus and the cytoplasm of transformed cells. The E1A early proteins complex with the cellular Rb protein as well as with several other unidentified cellular proteins. Another early protein, E1B, binds the cellular p53 protein (Table 43–9). The adenoviruses are important models for studying the molecular mechanisms by which DNA tumor viruses usurp cellular growth control processes. Different serotypes of adenoviruses manifest varying degrees of oncogenicity in newborn hamsters. No association of adenoviruses with human neoplasms has been found.

Herpesviruses (See Chapter 33.)

These large viruses (diameter 100–200 nm) contain a linear genome of double-stranded DNA (MW 100×10^6) and have a capsid with icosahedral symmetry surrounded by an outer lipid-containing envelope. Herpesviruses typically cause acute infections followed by latency and eventual recurrence in each host, including humans.

Some herpesviruses (herpes simplex virus types 1 and 2 and cytomegalovirus) can transform cells in culture but at a very low frequency. Transformed hamster cells produce tumors when injected into hamsters.

Some herpesviruses are associated with tumors in lower animals. Marek's disease is a highly contagious lymphoproliferative disease of chickens that can be prevented by vaccination with an attenuated strain of Marek's disease virus. The prevention of cancer by vaccination in this case establishes the virus as the causative agent and suggests the possibility of a similar approach to prevention of some human tumors if a virus is identified as a causative agent. Other examples of herpesvirus-induced tumors in animals include lymphomas of certain types of monkeys and adenocarcinomas of frogs. The simian viruses cause inapparent infections in their natural hosts but induce malignant T cell lymphomas when transmitted to other species of monkeys. The diseases induced by Marek's disease virus and the monkey viruses may be good models for human Burkitt's lymphoma, which is caused by Epstein-Barr virus. The kidney tumors induced by the frog virus, in contrast, are reminiscent of nasopharyngeal carcinoma (related to Epstein-Barr virus), because epithelial cells are transformed rather than lymphocytes.

In humans, herpesviruses have been linked epidemiologically to a few specific types of tumors. Carcinoma of the cervix shows an association with herpes simplex virus type 2, although that association is not as strong as for HPV and cervical cancer. No specific herpesvirus transforming gene has yet been identified. It is possible that herpesvirus-induced oncogenesis involves insertional mutagenesis rather than transformation mediated by a viral transforming protein.

Epstein-Barr (EB) herpesvirus causes acute infectious mononucleosis when it infects B lymphocytes of susceptible humans. In a few immunodeficient children, such EB virus infections have progressed to a B cell lymphoma. One tragic case of severe combined immunodeficiency demonstrated that EB virus can cause B cell lymphoma. A 12-year-old child kept in a gnotobiotic environment since birth received a bone marrow transplant and died 124 days later of multiple B cell proliferations proved to be due to EB virus.

EB virus has been linked to Burkitt's lymphoma, a tumor most commonly found in children in central Africa, and to nasopharyngeal carcinoma, the incidence of which is higher in Chinese male populations in Southeast Asia than elsewhere. Cells from these two types of tumors usually contain EB viral DNA (both integrated and episomal forms) and viral antigens. Normal human lymphocytes have a limited life span in vitro, but EB virus can transform such lymphocytes into lymphoblast cell lines that grow indefinitely in culture. All cells that carry EB virus genomes express virus-specific nuclear antigens (called EBNAs) regardless of whether mature virus is released.

The confounding attributes of herpesviruses (ubiquitous, establish lifelong persistent infections) make their association with tumor cells difficult to interpret. Because of their low efficiencies of transformation in vitro and the difficulties in defining a transforming gene (except for EB virus), it is likely that herpesvirus effects represent only one step in a complex sequence leading to neoplasia. EB virus appears to be one cofactor in the pathogenesis of Burkitt's lymphoma. A characteristic chromosomal translocation that activates the c-*myc* proto-oncogene may play a role in that cancer. The c-*myc* gene is transposed from the distal end of chromosome 8 to a position near an immunoglobulin gene (usually on chromosome 14). The transcriptional activity regulating immunoglobulin synthesis results in enhanced expression of the translocated c-*myc* gene. The striking geographic distribution of Burkitt's lymphoma and nasopharyngeal carcinoma suggests that either a genetic predisposition or an environmental cofactor is involved in those cancers. The etiologic role of EB virus in either tumor probably will not be verified until an EB virus vaccine can be shown to protect against cancer development.

Poxviruses (See Chapter 34.)

Poxviruses are large, brick-shaped viruses with a linear genome of double-stranded DNA (MW $130–240 \times 10^6$). Yaba virus produces benign tumors (histiocytomas) in its natural host, monkeys. Shope fibroma virus produces fibromas in some rabbits and is able to alter cells in culture. Molluscum contagiosum virus produces small benign growths in humans. Very little is known about the nature of these proliferative diseases, but the poxvirus-encoded growth factor that is related to epidermal growth factor and to transforming growth factor may be involved.

Hepatitis B Virus (See Chapter 35.)

Hepatitis B virus, the prototype member of the **Hepadnaviridae** family, is characterized by 42-nm spherical virions with a circular genome of double-stranded

DNA (MW 1.6 × 10^6). One strand of the DNA is incomplete and variable in length. Studies of the virus are hampered because it has not been grown in cell culture.

In addition to causing hepatitis, hepatitis B virus is a risk factor in the development of liver cancer in humans. Epidemiologic and laboratory studies have proved persistent infection with hepatitis B virus to be an important cause of chronic liver disease and have strongly implicated the virus in the development of hepatocellular carcinoma (Figure 43–16). Tumor cells

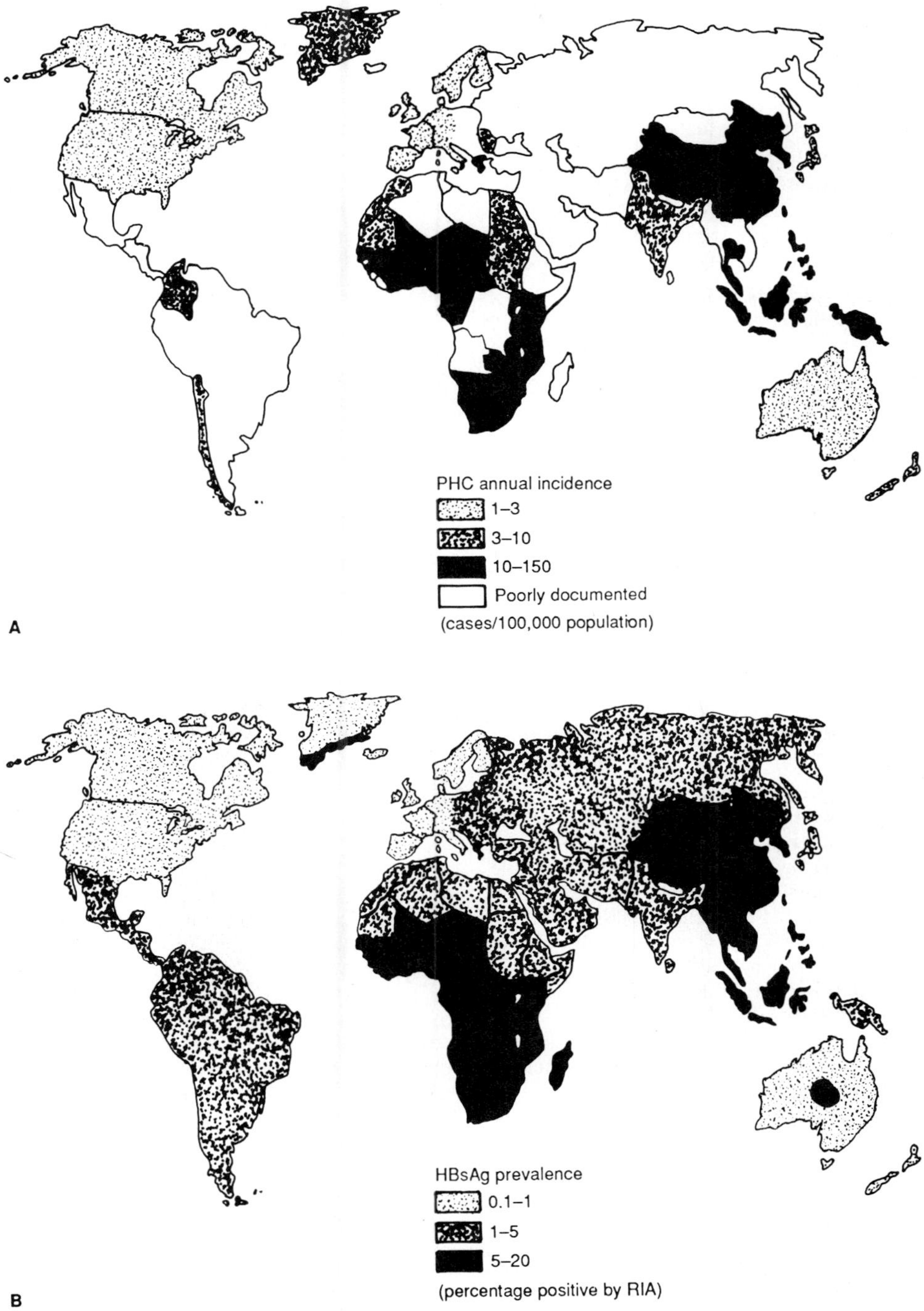

Figure 43–16. Maps showing world distributions of primary hepatocellular carcinoma (panel A) and HBsAg carrier rate (panel B). Note that high liver cancer rates correspond to areas with high hepatitis B virus carrier rates. (Reproduced, with permission, from Maupas P, Melnick JL: Hepatitis B infection and primary liver cancer. Prog Med Virol 1981;27:1.)

obtained from patients who are hepatitis B carriers often contain integrated hepatitis B virus DNA. The precise mechanism of oncogenesis remains obscure. As hepatitis B virus does not carry an oncogene, the virus probably is involved indirectly, perhaps by an insertional mutagenesis or transactivating mechanism. The advent of an effective hepatitis B vaccine for the prevention of primary infection raises the possibility of prevention of hepatocellular carcinoma, particularly in areas of the world where infection with hepatitis B virus is hyperendemic (eg, Africa, China, Southeast Asia). Because of the long latent period before cancer development, however, the effects of vaccination will not be apparent for at least 20 years.

Woodchucks are an excellent model for hepatitis B virus infections of humans. A similar virus, woodchuck hepatitis virus, establishes chronic infections in both newborn and adult woodchucks, many of which develop hepatocellular carcinomas within a 3-year period. This animal model will permit genetic studies of viral involvement in tumorigenesis, as well as facilitate the development of antiviral drugs.

VIRUSES & HUMAN CANCER

It is now clear that viruses are involved in the genesis of a few specific human tumors. Proving a causal relationship between a virus and a given type of cancer is, in general, very difficult. Obviously, controlled human transmission studies cannot be done to fulfill Koch's postulates.

If a virus is the etiologic agent of a specific cancer, it should be found at some stage in tumor development in every case of that type of cancer. Only if the continued expression of a viral function is necessary for maintenance of transformation will viral genes necessarily persist in every tumor cell. If the virus provides an early step in multistep carcinogenesis, the viral genome may be lost as the tumor progresses to more altered stages (perhaps mediated by the activation of cellular oncogenes). Conversely, a virus may be found associated frequently with a tumor but be there simply as a passenger because of an affinity for the cell type.

Tumor viruses are usually not replicating in transformed cells, so it is necessary to search for viral nucleic acids or proteins in cells to detect virus presence. As viral structural proteins are frequently not expressed, virus-encoded nonstructural proteins are more common markers of virus presence.

Tumor induction in laboratory animals and transformation of cultured cells are good circumstantial lines of evidence that a virus is tumorigenic, and those systems can provide models for molecular analyses of the transformation process. However, they do not constitute proof that the virus causes a particular human cancer.

The most definitive proof of a causal relationship will depend on intervention methods designed to prevent infection by the virus. Such an approach should be effective in reducing the occurrence of the cancer, even if the virus is only one of multiple cofactors.

REFERENCES

Bishop JM: The molecular genetics of cancer. Science 1987; 235:305.

Broker TR: Structure and genetic expression of papillomaviruses. Obstet Gynecol Clin North Am 1987;14:329.

Butel JS, Jarvis DL: The plasma-membrane-associated form of SV40 large tumor antigen: Biochemical and biological properties. Biochim Biophys Acta 1986;865:171.

de Villiers EM: Heterogeneity of the human papillomavirus group. J Virol 1989;63:4898.

Donehower LA et al: Mice deficient for p53 are developmentally normal but susceptible to spontaneous tumours. Nature 1992;356:215.

Finlay CA, Hinds PW, Levine AJ: The p53 proto-oncogene can act as a suppressor of transformation. Cell 1989;57: 1083.

Gallo RC: The first human retrovirus. Sci Am (Dec) 1986;255:88.

Genital human papillomavirus infections and cancer: Memorandum from a WHO meeting. Bull WHO 1987;65:817.

Hardy WD Jr: Biology of feline retroviruses. In: *Retrovirus Biology and Human Disease.* Gallo RC, Wong-Staal F (editors). Marcel Dekker, 1990.

Heldin CH, Westermark B: Growth factors: Mechanism of action and relation to oncogenes. Cell 1984;37:9.

Levine AJ: The tumor suppressor genes. Annu Rev Biochem 1993;62:623.

Macnab JC: Herpes simplex virus and human cytomegalovirus: Their role in morphological transformation and genital cancers. J Gen Virol 1987;68:2525.

Moran E: Interaction of adenoviral proteins with pRB and p53. FASEB J 1993;7:880.

Nevins JR: E2F: A link between the Rb tumor suppressor protein and viral oncoproteins. Science 1992;258:424.

Ring CJA: The B cell-immortalizing functions of Epstein–Barr virus. J Gen Virol 1994;75:1.

Schiffman MH et al: Epidemiologic evidence showing that human papillomavirus infection causes most cervical intraepithelial neoplasia. J Natl Cancer Inst 1993; 85:958.

Shearer WT et al: Epstein-Barr virus-associated B-cell proliferations of diverse clonal origins after bone marrow transplantation in a 12-year-old patient with severe combined immunodeficiency. N Engl J Med 1985;312:1151.

Slagle BL, Becker SA, Butel JS: Hepatitis viruses and liver cancer. In: *Viruses and Cancer.* Minson A, Neil J, McCrae M (editors). Cambridge Univ Press, 1994.

Stanbridge EJ: Identifying tumor suppressor genes in human colorectal cancer. Science 1990;247:12.

Tooze J (editor): *The Molecular Biology of Tumor Viruses,* 2nd ed. *DNA Tumor Viruses,* 1981; *RNA Tumor Viruses,* 1982. Cold Spring Harbor Laboratory.

Varmus H, Bishop JM (editors): Biochemical mechanisms of oncogene activity: Proteins encoded by oncogenes. Cancer Surv 1986;5:153.

Weinberg RA: Oncogenes, antioncogenes, and the molecular basis of multi-step carcinogenesis. Cancer Res 1989; 9:3713.

Whyte P, Williamson NM, Harlow E: Cellular targets for transformation by the adenovirus E1A proteins. Cell 1989;56:67.

Yoshida M: HTLV-1 Tax: Regulation of gene expression and disease. Trends Microbiol 1993;1:131.

44 AIDS & Lentiviruses

Human immunodeficiency virus (HIV), a nononcogenic retrovirus, is the primary etiologic agent of acquired immunodeficiency syndrome (AIDS). The illness was first described in 1981, and the virus was isolated by the end of 1983. Since then, AIDS has become a worldwide epidemic, expanding in scope and magnitude as HIV infections have affected different populations and geographic regions. Millions are now infected worldwide; once infected, individuals remain infected for life. Within a decade, the vast majority of HIV-infected individuals develop fatal opportunistic infections as a result of HIV-induced deficiencies in the immune system. AIDS promises to be a major health problem worldwide into the next century.

PROPERTIES OF LENTIVIRUSES

Important properties of lentiviruses, a special subfamily of retroviruses, are summarized in Table 44–1.

Structure & Composition

It is a tribute to modern molecular virology that only 4 years from the time an unusual disease syndrome (AIDS) was first recognized in 1981, the causative agent was isolated and identified and the genomes of a number of isolates were sequenced.

HIV is a retrovirus, a member of the **Lentivirinae** subfamily, and exhibits many of the physicochemical features typical of the family (see Chapter 43). The unique morphologic characteristic of HIV is a cylindrical nucleoid in the mature virion (Figure 44–1). The diagnostic bar-shaped nucleoid is visible in electron micrographs in those extracellular particles that happen to be sectioned at the appropriate angle.

The RNA genome of lentiviruses is more complex than that of transforming retroviruses (Figure 44–2). The virus contains the three genes required for a replicating retrovirus—*gag, pol,* and *env* (see Chapter 43). Six additional genes regulate viral expression and are important in disease pathogenesis in vivo. Although these auxiliary genes show little sequence homology among lentiviruses, their functions are conserved. The lack of sequence identity among these genes may help explain the marked species specificity exhibited by lentiviruses. One early phase replication protein, the tat protein, functions in "transactivation," whereby a viral gene product is involved in transcriptional activation of other viral genes. Transactivation in HIV is highly efficient and may account, in part, for the virulent nature of HIV infections. The rev protein is required for the expression of viral structural proteins. Rev facilitates the export of unspliced viral transcripts from the nucleus; structural proteins are translated from unspliced mRNAs during the late phase of viral replication. The precise functions of most of the viral regulatory genes have not yet been determined, as only *tat* and *rev* appear necessary for replication in cultured cells. Strikingly, a strain of simian virus with the *nef* gene deleted has been found to lose its virulence in monkeys and to induce immunity to challenge with pathogenic strains of simian immunodeficiency virus (SIV). Only the primate lentiviruses possess a *nef* gene.

The many different isolates of HIV are not identical but appear to comprise a spectrum of related viruses. The regions of greatest divergence among different isolates are localized to the *env* gene, which codes for the viral envelope proteins. Divergent populations of viral genomes are found in an infected individual. Another lentivirus, visna virus, typically undergoes pro-

Table 44–1. Important properties of lentiviruses (nononcogenic, cytocidal retroviruses).

Virion: Spherical, 100–140 nm in diameter, cylindrical core.
Genome: Single-stranded RNA, linear, positive-sense, 9–10 kb, diploid; genome more complex than that of oncogenic retroviruses, contains at least six additional replication genes.
Proteins: Envelope glycoprotein undergoes antigenic variation; reverse transcriptase enzyme contained inside virions.
Envelope: Present.
Replication: Reverse transcriptase makes DNA copy from genomic RNA; provirus DNA is template for viral RNA. Genetic variability is common.
Maturation: Particles bud from plasma membrane.
Outstanding characteristics: Members are nononcogenic and may be cytocidal. Infect cells of the immune system. Proviruses remain permanently associated with cells. Viral expression is restricted in vivo; cause slowly progressive, chronic diseases. Replication is highly species-specific. Group includes the causative agents of AIDS.

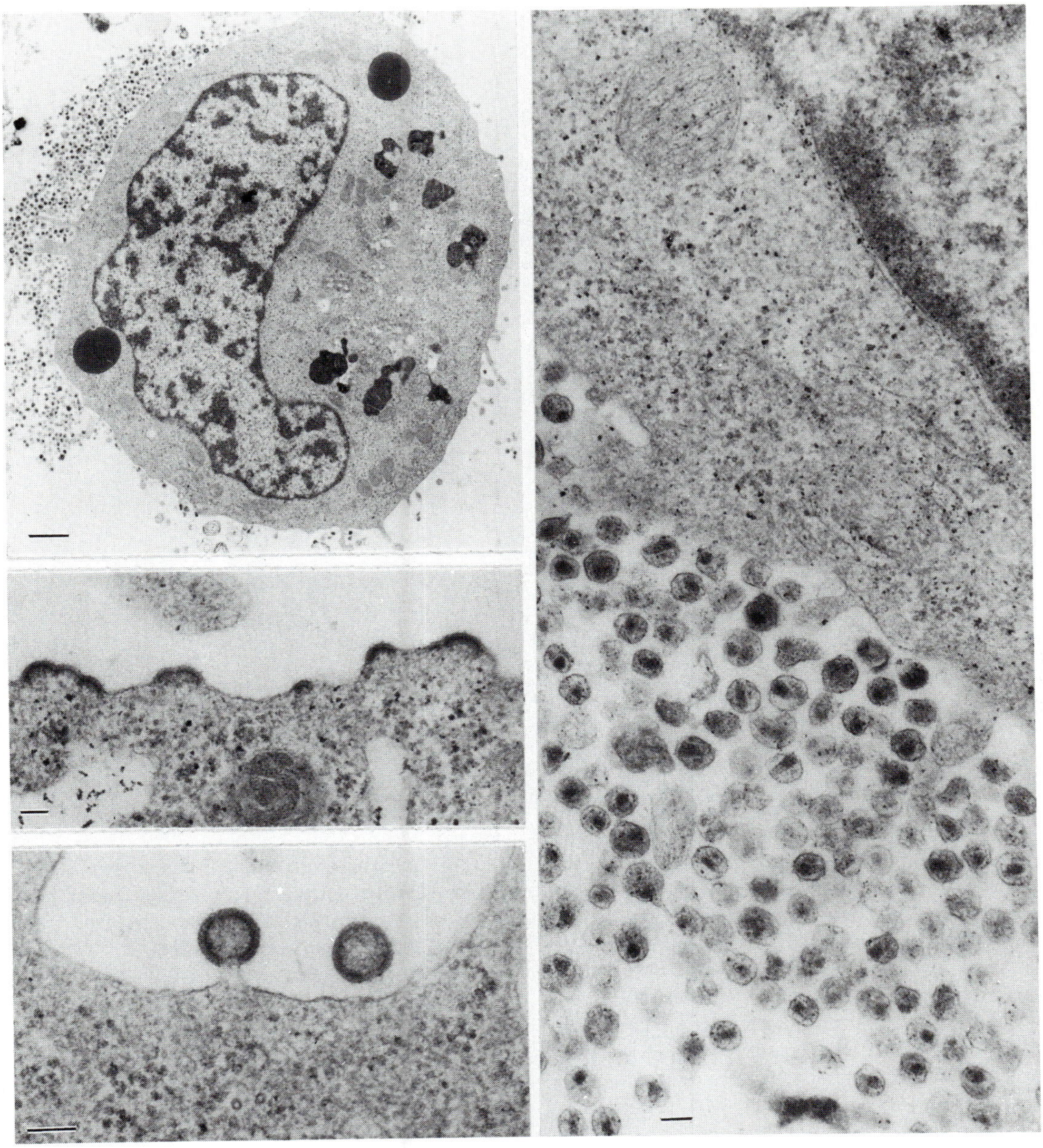

Figure 44–1. Electron micrographs of HIV-infected lymphocytes, showing a large accumulation of freshly produced virus at the cell surface (**upper left,** 5660×, bar = 1000 nm; and **right,** 46,450×, bar = 100 nm); newly formed virus budding from cytoplasmic membrane (**middle left,** 49,000×, bar = 100 nm); two virions about to be cast off from cell surface (**lower left,** 75,140×, bar = 100 nm).

gressive antigenic variation in reaction to the host's immune response during persistent infection. The divergence in the envelope of HIV complicates efforts to develop an effective vaccine for AIDS.

Lentiviruses are completely exogenous viruses; in contrast to the transforming retroviruses, the lentiviral genome does not contain any conserved cellular genes (see Chapter 43). Individuals become infected by the introduction of virus from outside sources and not by the activation of silent sequences contained in cellular DNA.

Classification

Lentiviruses have been isolated from many species (Table 44–2). The human AIDS viruses are not homogeneous, but most are variants of HIV-1. A second

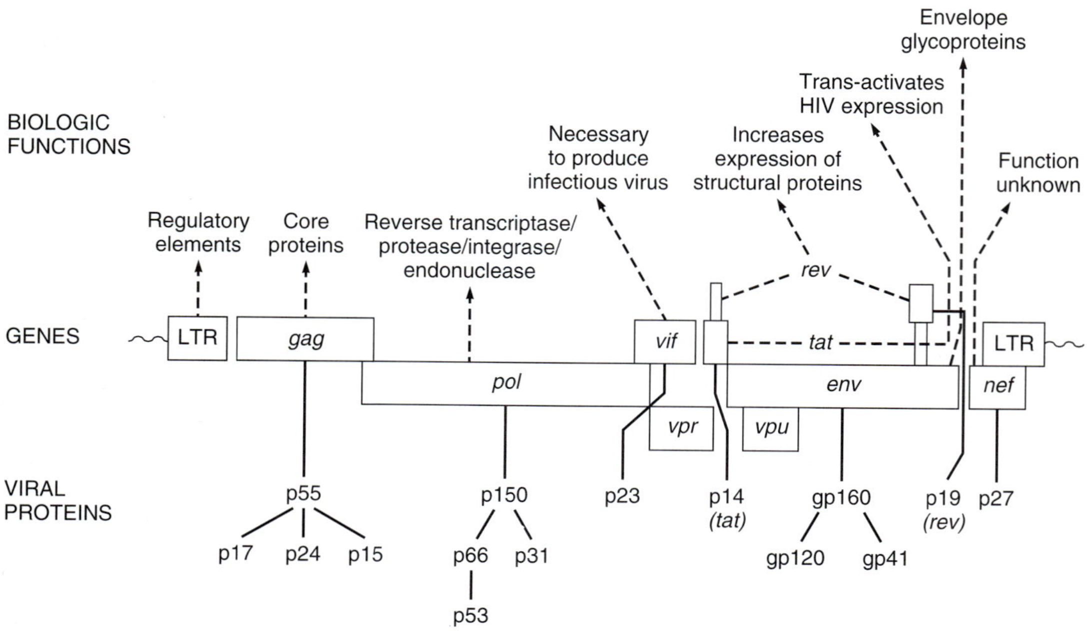

Figure 44–2. HIV-1 genome structure. The recognized viral genes, protein products, and their biologic functions are illustrated. The DNA provirus form of the viral genome is shown.

virus, HIV-2, seems to be prevalent only in West Africa and is much less virulent. Only about 40% of the sequences of HIV-1 and HIV-2 are identical.

Numerous retrovirus isolates have been obtained from nonhuman primate species. SIV from sooty mangabeys (a type of monkey in west Africa) and HIV-2 are similar enough that they are now considered to be variants of the same virus. The chimpanzee isolates are more closely related to HIV-1 than any of the simian isolates. The SIVs from African green monkeys and mandrills form a discrete group equidistant to HIV-1 and HIV-2. Captured adult monkeys of African species commonly have serologic evidence of SIV infection.

The organization of the genomes of primate lentiviruses (human and simian) is very similar. One difference is that HIV-1 and the chimpanzee virus carry a *vpu* gene, whereas HIV-2 and most SIVs have a *vpx* gene. The sequences of the *gag* and *pol* genes are highly conserved. There is significant divergence among the envelope glycoprotein genes; the sequences of the trans-membrane protein portion are more conserved than the external glycoprotein sequences (the protein component exposed on the exterior of the viral particle). Antigenic cross-reactivity between HIV-1 and SIV is most pronounced for the viral core antigens and less evident for the envelope antigens.

The SIVs appear to be nonpathogenic in their host species of origin (African green monkey, sooty mangabey); these species are known to be infected in their natural habitats. In contrast, rhesus monkeys are not infected naturally in the wild in Asia but are susceptible to induction of simian AIDS by various SIV isolates. The virus first recovered from captive rhesus monkeys is the sooty mangabey/HIV-2 strain.

It is an increasingly popular theory that HIV in humans originated from infections by simian viruses, probably in rural Africa. The sooty mangabey SIV is presumably the predecessor of HIV-2. No clear progenitor has been identified for HIV-1, but the closest nonhuman virus found to date is from a chimpanzee. HIV-1 will replicate in experimentally inoculated chimpanzees but not in any species of monkey.

The nonprimate lentiviruses include a number of viruses that establish persistent infections affecting various animal species. These viruses cause chronic debilitating diseases and sometimes immunodeficiency. The prototype agent, visna virus (also called maedi virus), causes neurologic symptoms or pneumonia in sheep in Iceland. Other viruses cause infectious anemia in horses and arthritis and encephalitis in goats. Feline and bovine lentiviruses may cause an immunodeficiency. Nonprimate lentiviruses are not known to infect any primates, including humans.

Disinfection & Inactivation

HIV is completely inactivated ($\geq 10^5$ units of infectivity) by treatment for 10 minutes at room temperature with any of the following: 10% household bleach, 50% ethanol, 35% isopropanol, 1% Nonidet P40, 0.5% Lysol, 0.5% paraformaldehyde, or 0.3% hydrogen peroxide. The virus is also inactivated by extremes

Table 44–2. Representative members of the lentivirus subfamily.

Origin of Isolates	Virus	Disease(s)
Human	HIV-1 HIV-2	AIDS
Nonhuman primates		
Macaques rhesus cynomolgus	SIV	Simian AIDS[1]
African green monkey	SIV	
Sooty mangabey	SIV	
Mandrill	SIV	
Chimpanzee	SIV	
Nonprimate		
Cat	Feline immunodeficiency virus	Feline AIDS
Cow	Bovine immunodeficiency virus	
Sheep	Visna/maedi	Lung/CNS
Horse	Equine infectious anemia	Anemia
Goat	Caprine arthritis/ encephalitis	Arthritis/ encephalitis

[1]Disease not caused in host of origin by SIVs; requires transmission to a different species of monkey (rhesus are most susceptible to disease). The Asian macaques (rhesus) show no evidence of SIV infection in the wild; SIVs were probably accidentally introduced to macaques in captivity. Nonprimate lentiviruses cause disease in species of origin.

in pH (pH 1.0 and 13.0). Virus is rapidly inactivated (<1 minute) by exposure to undiluted household bleach.

The virus is not inactivated by 2.5% Tween-20. Although paraformaldehyde inactivates virus free in solution, it is not known if it penetrates tissues sufficiently to inactivate all virus that might be present in cultured cells or tissue specimens.

HIV is readily inactivated in liquids or 10% serum by heating at 56 °C for 10 minutes, but dried proteinaceous material affords marked protection. Lyophilized blood products would need to be heated at 68 °C for 72 hours to ensure inactivation of contaminating virus.

Lessons From Animal Lentivirus Systems

Insights into the biologic characteristics of lentivirus infections have been gained from experimental infections, particularly sheep with visna virus. Virus is always present in the host but at very low levels, and it may take years for disease to occur. Lentiviruses differ from other retroviruses in that they can infect nondividing, terminally differentiated cells. However, those cells must be activated before viral replication ensues and progeny virus is produced. Virus is cell-associated in monocytes and macrophages, but only about one cell per million is infected. Monocytes carry the virus around the body in a form that the immune system cannot recognize, seeding other tissues. Viral isolation requires cocultivation of white blood cells with susceptible cells. Visna virus can also be isolated from other tissues. Once virus is recovered in tissue culture, it grows well and is cytolytic; it is never transforming.

Virus is present for the life of the sheep. Infected animals usually make antibodies, but they do not clear the infection. New antigenic variants periodically arise in infected hosts, but it is not known if this variation is important in the progression of disease. Most mutations occur in envelope glycoproteins. Clinical symptoms may develop at any time from 3 months to 8 years after infection.

Viral replication is restricted in vivo at the level of transcription. An unusual feature of lentiviruses is that in addition to an integrated provirus, multiple copies of viral DNA are often found free in the cytoplasm of infected cells. Restriction of viral expression probably accounts for the slow progression of infection and may explain why infected cells escape destruction by host immune surveillance mechanisms.

Simian lentiviruses share molecular and biologic characteristics with HIV and cause an AIDS-like disease in selected nonhuman primates. The SIV model is important for understanding disease pathogenesis and developing vaccine and treatment strategies. The nonprimate models—particularly the feline and bovine lentiviruses—are useful for studying induction of protective immunity and for screening potential antiviral agents.

Chimpanzees can be infected with HIV-1, and they exhibit a humoral immune response similar to that seen in humans. Neutralizing antibodies and cell-mediated immunity have been detected. However, chimpanzees do not develop clinical features of AIDS, so they cannot be used to study disease pathogenesis.

HIV INFECTIONS IN HUMANS

Pathogenesis & Pathology

A. Overview of Course of HIV Infection: The typical course of HIV infection spans about a decade (Figure 44–3). Stages include the primary infection, dissemination of virus to lymphoid organs, clinical latency, induction of HIV expression, clinical disease, and death. The duration between primary infection and progression to clinical disease averages about 10 years. Death usually occurs within 2 years after the onset of clinical symptoms.

Following primary infection, viral replication occurs and viremia is detectable for about 8–12 weeks. Virus is widely disseminated throughout the body during this time, and the lymphoid organs become seeded. An acute mononucleosis-like syndrome may develop

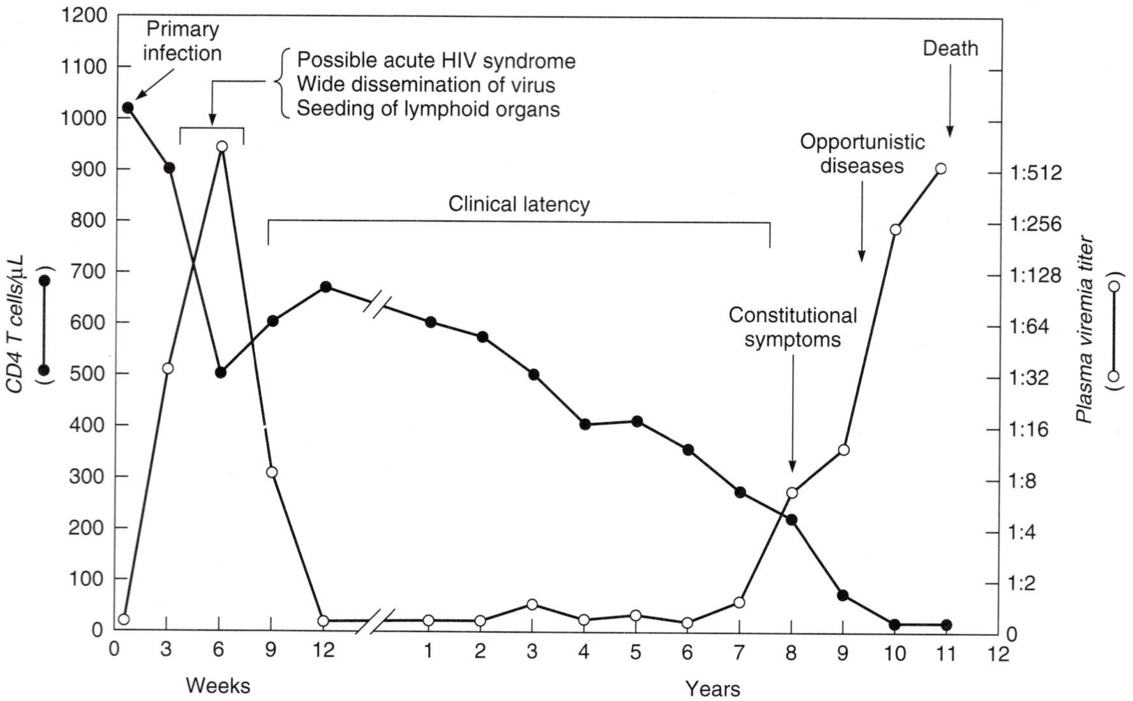

Figure 44–3. Typical course of HIV infection. During the early period after primary infection, there is widespread dissemination of virus and a sharp decrease in the number of CD4 T cells in peripheral blood. An immune response to HIV ensues, with a decrease in detectable viremia followed by a prolonged period of clinical latency. The CD4 T cell count continues to decrease during the following years until it reaches a critical level below which there is a substantial risk of opportunistic diseases. (Reproduced, with permission, from Pantaleo G, Graziosi C, Fauci AS: The immunopathogenesis of human immunodeficiency virus infection. N Engl J Med 1993;328:327.)

in many patients (50–75%) 3–6 weeks after primary infection. There is a significant drop in numbers of circulating CD4 T cells at this early time. An immune response to HIV occurs 1 week to 3 months after infection, plasma viremia drops, and levels of CD4 cells rebound. However, the immune response is unable to clear the infection completely, and HIV-infected cells persist in the lymph nodes.

This period of clinical latency may last for as long as 10 years. Although very few infected cells are in the peripheral blood ($1{:}10^3$–$1{:}10^4$), it is not a time of true latency as virus-expressing cells are present in lymphoid organs and the immune system gradually deteriorates, manifested by a decline in circulating CD4 cells.

Eventually, the patient will develop constitutional symptoms and clinically apparent disease, such as opportunistic infections or neoplasms. Virus is readily detectable during the advanced stages of infection. HIV found in patients with late-stage disease is usually much more virulent and cytopathic than the strains of virus found early in infection. Often, a shift from monocyte- or macrophage-tropic strains of HIV-1 to lymphocyte-tropic variants accompanies progression to AIDS.

B. CD4 T Lymphocyte Depletion: The cardinal feature of HIV infection is the depletion of T helper-inducer lymphocytes—the result of the tropism of HIV for this population of lymphocytes, which express the CD4 phenotypic marker on their surface. The CD4 molecule is the major receptor for HIV; it has a high affinity for the viral envelope. Infection can be blocked by monoclonal antibodies to CD4 and by recombinant soluble CD4. Certain subsets of monocytes and macrophages also express the CD4 molecule, and these cells can bind and be infected by HIV.

The progressive decline in circulating CD4 T cells during the asymptomatic phase of HIV infection cannot be explained solely by direct cytopathogenicity of the virus, as there are low levels of HIV-infected cells in the peripheral blood at that time. Indirect mechanisms that may contribute to cell loss include cell fusion, mediated by HIV gp120 molecules on the surface of an infected T cell binding to CD4 molecules on uninfected cells, resulting in large multinucleated cells (syncytia). Uninfected CD4 T cells might bind free gp120 released from other cells and then be killed by cellular cytotoxicity responses. Complexes of gp120 and antibody can bind to CD4 molecules; this may induce anergy and make the cells unresponsive to appropriate signals. Disruption of normal cell control pathways may induce apoptosis (programmed cell death).

The consequences of CD4 T cell dysfunction caused by HIV infection are devastating because the CD4 T lymphocyte plays a critical role in the human immune response. It is responsible directly or indirectly for induction of a wide array of lymphoid and nonlymphoid cell functions. These effects include activation of macrophages; induction of functions of cytotoxic T cells, natural killer cells, and B cells; and secretion of a variety of soluble factors that induce growth and differentiation of lymphoid cells and affect hematopoietic cells.

C. B Cells: Individuals with AIDS also exhibit abnormal B cell function as manifested by polyclonal activation, hypergammaglobulinemia, circulating immune complexes, and autoantibodies. B cells from HIV-infected patients may spontaneously secrete high levels of cytokines. The polyclonal hyperactivity of the B cell limb of the immune response may be due to other factors, such as increased incidence of infections with Epstein-Barr (EB) virus and cytomegalovirus, both of which are polyclonal B cell activators. Despite the heightened responsiveness of the B cell repertoire of these individuals, there is a deficient antibody response to new antigens. Although certain T cell-dependent B cell responses may be abnormal as a result of defects in the helper function of the CD4 T cell, other defective responses result from abnormalities at the B cell level. One such defective response is an inability to mount an adequate immunoglobulin M (IgM) response to antigenic challenge; this often results in a fatal illness in infants and children infected with HIV who have not been previously exposed to various pathogenic bacterial organisms and must rely on an initial IgM response for adequate host defenses. Adult patients also manifest increased susceptibility to various pyogenic bacteria.

D. Monocytes and Macrophages: Monocytes and macrophages may play a major role in the dissemination and pathogenesis of HIV infection. These phagocytic cells can engulf the virus. Certain subsets of monocytes express the CD4 surface antigen and therefore bind to the envelope of HIV. However, HIV does not induce a cytopathic effect in monocytes. In the brain, the major cell type infected with HIV appears to be the monocyte-macrophage, and this may have important consequences for the development of neuropsychiatric manifestations associated with HIV infection. Infected pulmonary alveolar macrophages may play a role in the interstitial pneumonitis seen in certain patients with AIDS.

The infectivity of monocytes with HIV suggests that the monocyte serves as a major reservoir for HIV in the body. Unlike the CD4 T lymphocyte, the monocyte is relatively refractory to the cytopathic effects of HIV, so that the virus can not only survive in this cell but can be transported to various organs in the body (such as the lungs and brain). The noncytopathic, restricted replication of HIV in monocytes is reminiscent of infection with other lentiviruses (such as visna virus of sheep) against which effective immune surveillance does not develop. Persistence of HIV in human monocytes may in part explain the inability of an HIV-specific immune response to completely clear the body of virus.

E. Lymphoid Organs: It is now established that lymphoid organs play a central role in HIV infection (Figure 44–4). It is in the lymphoid organs that specific immune responses are generated. Lymphocytes in the peripheral blood represent only about 2% of the total lymphocyte pool, the remainder being located chiefly in lymphoid organs. The network of follicular dendritic cells in the germinal centers of lymph nodes traps antigens and stimulates an immune response. During the stage of clinical latency when minimal levels of HIV-infected cells are in the blood, HIV is sequestered and actively replicating in lymphoid tissues. The microenvironment of the lymph node is ideal for the establishment and spread of HIV infection. Cytokines are released, activating a large pool of CD4 T cells that are highly susceptible to HIV infection. It is now estimated that the viral burden in lymphoid tissue during early-stage disease is several orders of magnitude higher than in the peripheral blood. As the late stages of HIV disease progress, the architecture of the lymph nodes becomes disrupted. This degeneration and loss of virus-trapping function may allow release of virus into the circulation, accounting for the typical rise in viremia.

F. Neural Cells: Neurologic abnormalities are common in AIDS and occur to varying degrees in 40–90% of patients. These include HIV encephalopathy, myelopathy, peripheral neuropathies, and, most serious, AIDS dementia complex. Both direct and indirect pathogenic mechanisms might explain the neuropsychiatric manifestations of HIV infection. The predominant cell type in the brain that is infected with HIV is the monocyte-macrophage. Virus may enter the brain through infected monocytes and release cytokines that are toxic to neurons as well as chemotactic factors that lead to infiltration of the brain with inflammatory cells. HIV has been found in neurons, oligodendrocytes, and astrocytes. Galactosylceramide, a common nervous system glycolipid, is an alternative receptor for gp120 and may mediate HIV entry into glial cells. Viral products, such as gp120, may be involved in tissue damage without actual infection of all cells. It is speculated that gp120 may activate macrophages, microglia, and astrocytes and cause the release of cytokines and neurotoxins that injure neighboring neuronal cells.

G. Viral Coinfections: Activation signals are required for the establishment of a productive HIV infection. In the HIV-infected individual, a wide range of in vivo antigenic stimuli seem to serve as cellular activators. Other concomitant viral infections—

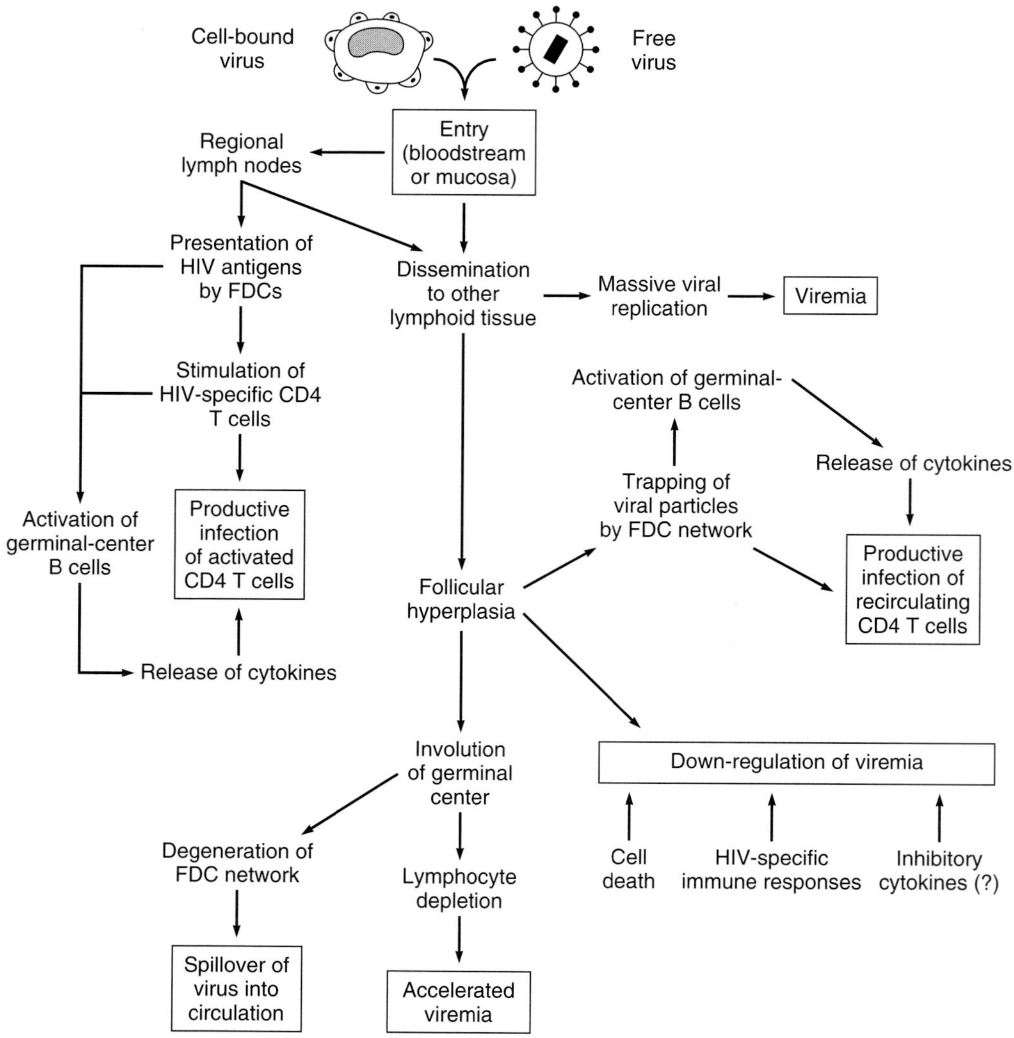

Figure 44–4. The complex roles of lymphoid organs in the pathogenesis of HIV disease. Lymphoid tissues are reservoirs of HIV during the asymptomatic phase of clinical latency. The virus is sequestered and actively replicating in these sites. (FDC, follicular dendritic cell.) (Reproduced, with permission, from Pantaleo G, Graziosi C, Fauci AS: The immunopathogenesis of human immunodeficiency virus infection. N Engl J Med 1993;328:327.)

EB virus, cytomegalovirus, herpes simplex virus, or hepatitis B virus—induce HIV expression and may serve as cofactors of AIDS. There is a high prevalence of cytomegalovirus infection in HIV-positive individuals.

HIV-antibody complexes can infect cells in vitro by means of receptors for the Fc portion of immunoglobulins. Infection by HIV-antibody complexes, mediated by the receptors for Fc, is independent of CD4. Infection of cells by human herpesviruses, such as cytomegalovirus and herpes simplex virus, can induce the expression of these receptors. This might permit HIV to infect a wider range of cell types. Once HIV enters cytomegalovirus-infected cells by means of the receptor for Fc, its replication could be enhanced by cytomegalovirus transactivating factors.

Clinical Findings

AIDS is characterized by a pronounced suppression of the immune system and the development of unusual neoplasms (especially Kaposi's sarcoma) or a wide variety of severe opportunistic infections. The more serious symptoms in adults are often preceded by a prodrome ("diarrhea and dwindling") that can include fatigue, malaise, weight loss, fever, shortness of breath, chronic diarrhea, white patches on the tongue (hairy leukoplakia, oral candidiasis), and lymphadenopathy. Disease symptoms in the gastrointestinal tract from the esophagus to the colon are a major cause of debility. The period between primary infection with HIV and the first appearance of clinical disease is usually long in adults, averaging about 10 years. Death occurs about 2 years later.

A. Pediatric AIDS: The situation is different in infected neonates as compared with HIV-infected adults. Pediatric AIDS—acquired from mothers in high-risk groups—usually presents with clinical symptoms by 2 years of age; death follows in another 2 years. The neonate is particularly susceptible to the devastating effects of HIV because the immune system has not developed at the time of primary infection. Clinical findings may include lymphoid interstitial pneumonitis, pneumonia, severe oral candidiasis, encephalopathy, wasting, generalized lymphadenopathy, bacterial sepsis, hepatosplenomegaly, diarrhea, and failure to thrive. Children with perinatally acquired HIV-1 infection have a very poor prognosis. A high rate of disease progression occurs in the first few years of life.

B. Neurologic Disease: Neurologic dysfunction occurs frequently in HIV-infected persons. Forty to 90 percent of patients have neurologic symptoms, and many are found during autopsy to have neuropathologic abnormalities. Associated neurologic diseases include toxoplasmosis, cryptococcosis, and primary lymphoma of the central nervous system. Several distinct neurologic syndromes frequently occur, including subacute encephalitis, vacuolar myelopathy, aseptic meningitis, peripheral neuropathy, and myopathy. AIDS dementia complex, the most common neurologic syndrome, occurs as a late manifestation of HIV infection and is characterized by poor memory, inability to concentrate, apathy, and psychomotor retardation. Focal motor abnormalities and behavioral changes may also occur. Symptoms usually progress rapidly. Cerebrospinal fluid analyses and radiographic examinations generally show nonspecific changes. HIV infection is thought to have both direct and indirect effects on the brain in the pathogenesis of these dysfunctions.

Pediatric AIDS patients also display neurologic abnormalities. These include seizure disorders, progressive loss of behavioral developmental milestones, encephalopathy, and attention deficit disorders. HIV encephalopathy may occur in as many as 12% of children, usually in concert with profound immune deficiency. Bacterial pathogens predominate in pediatric AIDS as the most common cause of meningitis.

C. Opportunistic Infections: The predominant causes of morbidity and mortality among patients with late-stage HIV infection are opportunistic infections, ie, severe infections induced by agents that rarely cause serious disease in immune-competent individuals. As treatments are developed for some common opportunistic pathogens and management of AIDS patients permits longer survivals, the spectrum of opportunistic infections changes.

The most common opportunistic infections in AIDS patients include the following:

(1) Protozoa—*Toxoplasma gondii, Isospora belli, Cryptosporidium.*

(2) Fungi—*Candida albicans, Cryptococcus neoformans, Coccidioides immitis, Histoplasma capsulatum, Pneumocystis carinii* (formerly classified as a protozoan).

(3) Bacteria—*Mycobacterium avium-intracellulare, Mycobacterium tuberculosis, Listeria monocytogenes, Nocardia asteroides, Salmonella, Streptococcus.*

(4) Viruses—Cytomegalovirus, herpes simplex virus, varicella-zoster virus, adenovirus, JC human papovavirus, hepatitis B virus.

Coinfection with DNA viruses can lead to enhanced expression of HIV in cells in vitro. These findings suggest that infection with other viruses in HIV-infected patients has the potential to activate HIV in vivo and accelerate disease progression. Herpesvirus infections are common in AIDS patients. Cytomegalovirus retinitis is the most common severe ocular complication of AIDS.

D. Cancer: AIDS patients exhibit a marked predisposition to the development of cancer, another consequence of immune suppression. Proven types of AIDS-associated cancers are non-Hodgkin's lymphoma and Kaposi's sarcoma. Other cancers that also appear more often in HIV-infected people are anogenital cancers and Hodgkin's lymphoma. The lymphomas are polyclonal B cell malignancies; many are classified as Burkitt's lymphoma, and EB viral DNA is found in the majority of those. Burkitt's lymphoma occurs 1000 times more commonly in AIDS patients than in the general population. Kaposi's sarcoma is a vascular tumor thought to be of endothelial origin that appears in skin, mucous membranes, lymph nodes, and visceral organs. Before this type of malignancy was observed in AIDS patients, it was considered to be a very rare cancer that occurred infrequently in older men of Mediterranean origin and with a higher frequency in children and young adults in equatorial Africa. Kaposi's sarcoma is now 20,000 times more common in AIDS patients than in the general population, although for reasons that are not understood, it is found more often in homosexual men than in other categories of patients. The cause of the cancer is unclear. The anogenital cancers may arise as a result of coinfections with human papillomaviruses. Hairy oral leukoplakia, although not a frank tumor, is a lesion on the tongue caused by the replication of EB virus in epithelial cells.

Immunity

Antibodies to a number of viral antigens develop soon after infection (Table 44–3), but the response pattern against specific viral antigens changes over time as patients progress to AIDS. Antibodies to the enve-

Table 44–3. Major gene products of HIV that are useful in diagnosis of infection.

Gene Product[1]	Description
gp160[2]	Precursor of envelope glycoproteins
gp120[2]	Outer envelope glycoprotein of virion
p66	Reverse transcriptase in polymerase gene product
p55	Precursor of core proteins
p53	Reverse transcriptase in polymerase gene product
gp41[2]	Trans-membrane envelope glycoprotein
p31	Endonuclease component of polymerase gene product
p24[2]	Nucleocapsid core protein of virion
p17	Matrix core protein of virion

[1]Number refers to the approximate molecular weight of the protein in kilodaltons.
[2]Antibodies to these viral proteins are the most commonly detected.

lope glycoproteins (gp41, gp120, gp160) are maintained, but those directed against the core protein (p24) decline. The decline of anti-p24 may herald the beginning of clinical signs and other immunologic markers of progression (Figure 44–5).

Neutralizing antibodies can be measured in vitro by means of inhibiting HIV infection of susceptible lymphocyte cell lines. Viral infection is quantified by (1) reverse transcriptase assay, which measures the enzyme activity of released HIV particles; (2) indirect immunofluorescence assay, which measures the percentage of infected cells; and (3) cell fusion assay, which measures the capability of the virus to produce cell fusion and subsequent cell death. Relatively low neutralizing activity is present in the sera of both asymptomatic seropositive individuals and patients with AIDS. Higher titers of anti-p24 are found in persons who remain asymptomatic, but neutralizing antibody levels are no different from those in patients whose disease progresses. The roles of cytotoxic T lymphocytes, NK cells, and lymphokine-activated cells are all under study.

A sustained protective immunity against HIV may not be readily achievable, because HIV is very mutable. Infected patients usually contain a "swarm" of viral variants. A problem confronting AIDS vaccine research is that the correlates of protective immunity are not known, including the relative importance of humoral and cell-mediated immune responses.

Laboratory Diagnosis

A. Isolation and Identification of Virus: The polymerase chain reaction can be used to detect HIV DNA and RNA in test samples.

HIV can be cultured from lymphocytes in peripheral blood. The numbers of circulating infected cells vary with the stage of disease (Figure 44–3). Higher titers of virus are found in the plasma and in peripheral blood cells of patients with AIDS, as compared with asymptomatic individuals. The magnitude of plasma viremia appears to be a better correlate of the clinical stage of HIV infection than the presence of any antibodies (Figure 44–5).

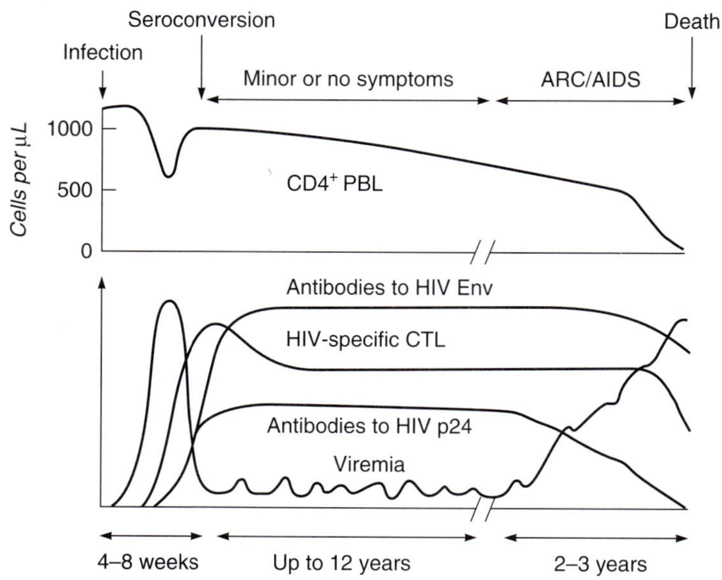

Figure 44–5. Pattern of HIV antibody responses related to the course of HIV infection. (ARC, AIDS-related complex; PBL, peripheral blood lymphocytes; CTL, cytotoxic T lymphocytes.) (Reproduced, with permission, from Weiss RA: How does HIV cause AIDS? Science 1993;260:1273.)

HIV can be grown in lymphocyte cultures containing abundant CD4-reactive target cells. Primary isolates of HIV grow very slowly compared with laboratory-adapted strains. Primary cells must be stimulated with a mitogen, eg, phytohemagglutinin, and supplemented with interleukin-2 (IL-2). Viral growth is detected by the appearance of a magnesium-dependent reverse transcriptase about 7–14 days after infection together with a pronounced cytopathic effect. Virus-specific antigens also develop in the cultures and are measured by enzyme immunoassay, indirect immunofluorescence, or radioimmunoprecipitation methods. Because viral expression is restricted in most cells in vivo, T cells from infected persons must be cultured in vitro before they will yield positive assays for viral antigen. A persistent HIV antigenemia is associated with a poor clinical diagnosis.

Early diagnosis of HIV infection in infants born to infected mothers is difficult. The presence of maternal antibodies makes serologic tests uninformative. Testing for p24 antigen at birth identifies only a small proportion (<10%) of infected infants. Viral culture of peripheral blood can correctly identify about half of infected newborns. There are also problems of false-negative rates using polymerase chain reaction technology on neonate samples, presumably reflecting a low virus load near the time of delivery. These assays can diagnose the majority of HIV-infected infants by 6 months of age.

B. Serology: Test kits are commercially available for measuring antibodies by enzyme-linked immunosorbent assay (ELISA). In almost 100% of persons with positive antibody tests, HIV can be recovered from cultured lymphocytes. When ELISA-based antibody tests are used for screening populations with a low prevalence of HIV infections, a positive test in a serum sample must be confirmed by a repeat test before the serum donor is notified. If the repeat ELISA test is negative, the specimen should be tested by another method. Alternative tests have included immunofluorescence and radioimmunoprecipitation assays, but the most extensive experience has been with the Western blot technique, in which antibodies to HIV proteins of specific molecular weights can be detected. The major gene products of HIV, detected in various diagnostic tests, are listed in Table 44–3. Antibodies to viral core protein p24 or envelope glycoproteins gp41, gp120, or gp160 are most commonly detected. It has been reported that a few individuals who have recently been vaccinated for influenza show a transient false-positive ELISA for HIV antibody.

The majority of individuals seroconvert within 2 months after viral exposure. HIV infection for longer than 6 months without a detectable antibody response is very uncommon.

Epidemiology

A. Worldwide Spread of AIDS: AIDS was first recognized in the USA in 1981 as a new disease entity in homosexual men. Thirteen years later, AIDS had become a worldwide epidemic that continues to expand. The World Health Organization estimated that by mid 1993 more than 13 million people worldwide had become infected with HIV, the majority by heterosexual contact (Figure 44–6). An estimated 1 million children had been infected perinatally. By 1994, over 4 million HIV-infected adults had developed full-blown AIDS, and most of those had died.

Based on 1993 data, sub-Saharan Africa had the highest number of HIV infections. In certain high-prevalence cities in Africa, as many as one of every three adults was infected with the virus. However, in-

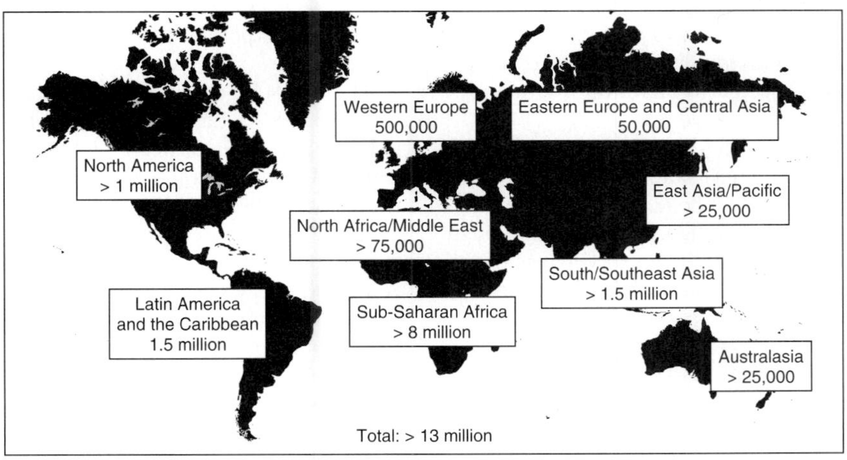

Figure 44–6. Estimated distribution of cumulative HIV infections in adults, by continent or region, as of mid 1993. Data from the World Health Organization. (Reproduced, with permission, from Merson MH: Slowing the spread of HIV: Agenda for the 1990s. Science 1993;260:1266.)

fections were spreading most rapidly in southern and southeastern Asia.

The World Health Organization has estimated that 30–40 million people will be infected with HIV by the end of the century, with 90% of all new infections occurring in developing countries. In those countries, AIDS is overwhelmingly a heterosexually transmitted disease, and there are about equal numbers of male and female cases.

It is hypothesized that the rapid dissemination of HIV globally was fostered by massive migration of rural inhabitants to urban centers, coupled with international movement of infected individuals as a consequence of civil disturbances, tourism, and business travels.

B. USA: The face of the AIDS epidemic changed in the USA between 1981 and 1994. At first, most of the cases occurred in homosexual men. Then the disease was identified in injecting drug users. By 1994, about 1 million people were infected with HIV, and 400,000 AIDS cases had been reported (of whom over one-half had died). There were 104,400 new AIDS cases in 1993 alone, and AIDS had become the number one cause of death among young men aged 25–44 years (19.9% of all deaths). This reflected a death rate of 52.8 per 100,000 for the general population, 136.0 per 100,000 for black men, and 42.1 per 100,000 for white men. HIV infection ranked as the fourth leading cause of death (7.3%) for women in this age group, with a similar overrepresentation in the black population. The largest proportionate increases of AIDS cases in the 1990s occurred among women, blacks and Hispanics, and persons exposed to HIV through heterosexual contacts. Most heterosexually acquired AIDS cases were attributed to sexual contact with an injecting drug user or a partner with HIV infection (about 9% of reported AIDS cases in 1993). Of these cases, 65% occurred in women, 50% of whom were black and 24% Hispanic.

Pediatric AIDS increased as the number of HIV-infected women increased. It was estimated that 1800 newborns acquired the virus in 1991 in the USA. Infants can become infected in utero, during the birth process, or through breast feeding.

The annual incidence of AIDS for persons who had received blood transfusions before screening of donated blood or persons with hemophilia who received tainted clotting factors declined in the 1990s, though such cases continued to be diagnosed because of the long interval between infection with HIV and onset of AIDS; they represented a very small fraction of all AIDS cases.

C. Routes of Transmission: HIV is transmitted during sexual contact, through parenteral exposure to contaminated blood or blood products, and from mother to child during the perinatal period. The presence of other sexually transmitted diseases, such as syphilis, gonorrhea, or chancroid, increases the risk of sexual HIV transmission as much as a hundredfold. Presumably, the inflammation and sores facilitate the transfer of HIV-infected cells. Asymptomatic virus-positive individuals can transmit the virus. Since the first description of AIDS, promiscuous homosexual activity has been recognized as a major risk factor for acquisition of the disease. The risk increases in proportion to the number of sexual encounters with different partners.

Transfusion of infectious blood or blood products is an effective route for viral transmission. For example, over 90% of hemophiliac recipients of contaminated clotting factor concentrates in the USA (before HIV was detected) developed antibodies to HIV. Users of illicit drugs are commonly infected through the use of contaminated needles.

Careful testing is necessary to ensure a safe blood supply. Furthermore, the World Health Organization has reported that voluntary nonremunerated blood donation is far safer than paid donations. Donor recruitment is important because even with testing, the risk of transmission of HIV by blood transfusions exists during the "window" between the time a donor is infected and the time detectable antibodies develop.

Health care workers have been infected by HIV following a needlestick with contaminated blood. The numbers of infections are relatively few in comparison with the number of needlesticks that have occurred involving contaminated blood.

The routes of transmission (blood, sex, and birth) described above account for almost all HIV infections, but there has been considerable concern that in rare circumstances other types of transmission may occur, particularly through contact with saliva, other "casual" contact with HIV-infected persons, or insect vectors. There is no evidence of virus transmission under these casual conditions.

HIV has been recovered from saliva, but the isolation rate is very much lower than that from blood. Many health care workers have been followed, and none have become infected after parenteral or mucous membrane exposure to the saliva of HIV-infected persons.

The risk of HIV transmission through "casual" contact has been evaluated in family members of both children and adults with HIV infection. The only documented cases of transmission by contact have occurred where there was repeated exposure to the blood or other body secretions or excretions of the HIV-infected person. HIV is not easily transmitted by this route; the risk has been estimated to be less than 0.1% for a single mucous membrane exposure to HIV-infected blood and even lower for skin exposure. Persons providing home nursing care for HIV-infected patients should take precautions to reduce exposures to blood and body fluids. The potential risk of transmission in other social settings, such as schools and offices, is even lower than in such household settings.

HIV can survive for several hours to days in insects fed blood with high concentrations of HIV or injected with HIV-contaminated blood. However, HIV does not replicate in insects or insect cell lines, and epidemiologic studies show no pattern of HIV infection consistent with transmission by insect vectors.

Prevention, Treatment, & Control

A. Vaccines Against HIV: Various approaches toward developing a vaccine are being investigated (Table 44–4). Viral vaccines are typically preventive, ie, given to uninfected individuals to prevent either infection or disease. Consideration is also being given to the possibility of therapeutic HIV vaccines, whereby HIV-infected individuals would be treated to boost anti-HIV immune responses, decrease the numbers of virus-infected cells, or delay the onset of AIDS. Vaccine development is difficult because HIV mutates rapidly, is not expressed in many cells that are infected, and is not completely cleared by the host immune response after primary infection. HIV isolates show a marked variation, especially in the envelope antigens—variability that probably promotes the emergence of neutralization-resistant mutants (Figure 44–7). Most troubling, the correlates of protective immunity are not known, so it is unclear what immune responses a vaccine should elicit. Furthermore, very little is known about the nature of mucosal immunity required for protection from infection by HIV-positive cells at mucosal surfaces.

Table 44–4. Candidate vaccines against AIDS.

General Vaccine Approach	Possible Specific Approaches
Whole virus vaccines	Live attenuated virus (HIV) Killed whole virus (HIV) Defective virus (HIV)
Subunit vaccines (monovalent or multivalent)	Based on: gp160 (gp120 plus gp41) gp120 gp41 As expressed in: bacteria, animal cells As part of: vaccinia envelope adenovirus capsid protein herpesvirus outer membrane bacterial outer membrane protein As synthetic epitopes of the envelope glycoproteins
Target cell protection	Antibodies to the viral attachment protein Antibodies to the CD4 receptor Genetically engineered viral attachment protein Genetically engineered CD4 receptor protein Anti-idiotype antibody equivalent to the viral attachment protein Anti-idiotype antibody equivalent to the CD4 receptor Intracellular immunization (gene therapy) to induce resistance in cells
Antigen presentation options	Immunostimulatory complexes Attached to bacterial vectors Added with T cell growth factors Nonspecific immunostimulants

Because of the difficulty of ensuring safety against possible vector-induced disease, vaccines based on attenuated or inactivated HIV or on simian isolates are viewed with apprehension. Recombinant viral proteins—especially those of the envelope glycoproteins—seem to be more likely candidates, whether delivered with adjuvants or with heterologous viral vectors. An effective subunit vaccine will have to be able to induce antibodies against natural isolates of HIV, as well as the laboratory strain used for its production.

Novel methods are under investigation. For example, a soluble form of CD4 has been made by recombinant DNA techniques and is being studied as a viral blocking agent. As CD4 is the HIV receptor on cells, soluble CD4 may inhibit HIV from infecting cells; may block gp120-mediated events, such as cell fusions; and may serve as a targeting signal to direct cytotoxic agents (eg, CD4-ricin) to HIV-infected cells. A modification of the soluble CD4 approach involves a molecular fusion of the gp120-binding domain of CD4 with the Fc domain of immunoglobulin to form a new molecule termed a CD4 immunoadhesion. This extends the plasma half-life of the CD4 immunoadhesion, improving the possibility of therapeutic application.

Gene therapy approaches are being developed that are designed to achieve "intracellular immunization," ie, genetically alter target cells to make them resistant to HIV. One strategy aims to express an altered form of an HIV replication protein that interferes with wild-type function, disrupting viral replication and thereby protecting the engineered CD4 T cells. Another concept uses ribozymes—RNA molecules that enzymatically cut targeted RNA into fragments—to block HIV replication in cells.

A large hurdle for vaccine development is the lack of an appropriate animal model for HIV. Chimpanzees are the only animals that are susceptible to HIV. Not only is the supply scarce, but chimpanzees develop only viremia and antibodies; they do not develop immunodeficiency. The SIV-macaque model of simian AIDS does develop disease and may prove more useful for vaccine development studies. However, very little is known about the immunology of macaques, so it will be difficult to extrapolate results to humans.

B. Antiviral Drugs: Four antiviral drugs are currently approved for treatment of HIV infections. All are nucleoside inhibitors of the viral enzyme reverse transcriptase. They are zidovudine (AZT), didanosine (ddI), zalcitabine (ddC), and stavudine (d4T). These drugs slow the progression of disease and have enabled patients to live longer and enjoy improved quality of life. However, none of the drugs appear to prevent the onset of AIDS, and all have toxic side-effects. Drug-resistant mutants of HIV emerge in most patients; the viral reverse transcriptase is highly error-

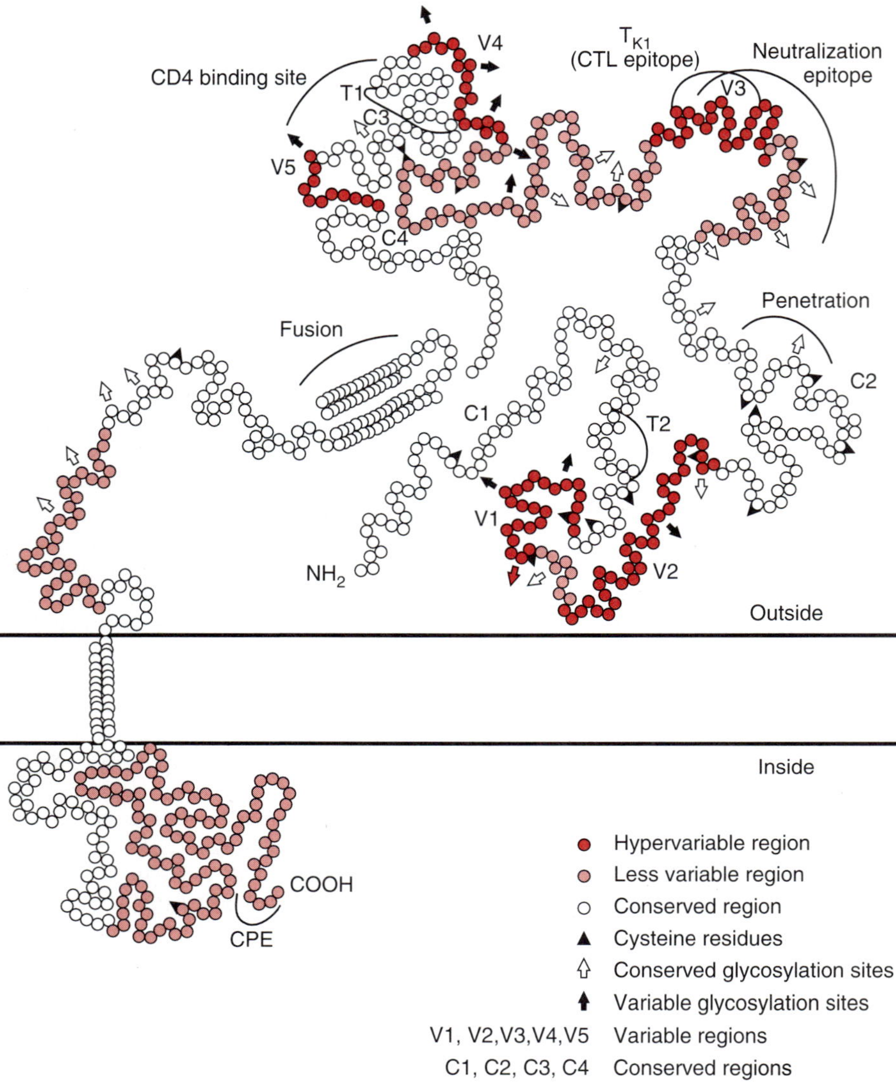

Figure 44–7. Structure of HIV envelope proteins. gp120 is on the outside of the cell, gp41 is a transmembrane protein. Functional domains are shown (CD4 binding, neutralization, penetration, fusion). Hypervariable regions are shown as closed circles and labeled V1–V5; conserved regions are denoted as open circles and labeled C1–C4. (CTL, cytotoxic T lymphocyte.) (Reproduced, with permission, from Gallo RC: Human retroviruses: A decade of discovery and link with human disease. J Infect Dis 1991;164:235.)

prone, and resistant mutants are selected in the presence of long-term antiviral chemotherapy. The molecular basis of resistance is associated with changes in several specific codons in the viral reverse transcriptase gene. Drugs are being developed that target other steps in the viral life cycle. However, it is a concern that HIV drug resistance will continue to be an obstacle to the development of effective antivirals.

AZT has been found to significantly reduce the transmission of HIV from mother to infant. AZT therapy during pregnancy and after birth reduced the risk of perinatal transmission from 25% to 8%.

C. Control Measures: Without control by drugs or vaccines, the only way to avoid epidemic spread of HIV is to maintain a lifestyle that minimizes or eliminates the high-risk factors discussed above. No cases have been documented to result from such common exposures as sneezing, coughing, sharing meals, or other casual contacts.

Because HIV may be transmitted in blood, all donor blood should be tested for antibody and, when such tests become commercially available, for virus or for viral antigens. Properly conducted antibody tests appear to detect almost all HIV-1 and HIV-2 carriers.

Since the introduction of widespread screening of blood donors for viral exposure and the rejection of contaminated blood, transmission by blood transfusion has virtually disappeared.

Public health authorities have recommended that persons reported to have an HIV infection be provided the following information and advice:

1. Available data indicate that almost all persons will remain infected for life and will develop the disease.

2. Although asymptomatic, such individuals may transmit HIV to others. Regular medical evaluation and follow-up are advised.

3. Infected persons should refrain from donating blood, plasma, body organs, other tissues, or sperm.

4. There is a risk of infecting others by sexual intercourse (vaginal or anal), by oral-genital contact, or by sharing of needles. The consistent and proper use of condoms can reduce transmission of the virus, though prevention is not absolute.

5. Toothbrushes, razors, and other implements that could become contaminated with blood should not be shared.

6. Seropositive women or women with seropositive sexual partners are themselves at increased risk of acquiring AIDS. If they become pregnant, their offspring also are at high risk of acquiring AIDS.

7. After accidents that result in bleeding, contaminated surfaces should be cleaned with household bleach freshly diluted 1:10 in water.

8. Devices that have punctured the skin, eg, hypodermic and acupuncture needles, should be steam-sterilized by autoclaving before reuse or should be safely discarded. Dental instruments should be heat-sterilized between patients. Whenever possible, disposable needles and equipment should be used.

9. When seeking medical or dental care for intercurrent illness, infected persons should inform those responsible for their care that they are seropositive, so that appropriate evaluation can be undertaken and precautions taken to prevent transmission to others.

10. Testing for HIV antibody should be offered to persons who may have been infected as a result of their contact with seropositive individuals (eg, sexual partners, persons with whom needles have been shared, infants born to seropositive mothers).

11. Most persons with a positive test for HIV do not need to consider a change in employment unless their work involves significant potential for exposing others to their blood or other body fluids. There is no evidence of viral transmission by food handling.

12. Seropositive persons in the health care professions who perform invasive procedures or have skin lesions should take precautions similar to those recommended for hepatitis B carriers to protect patients from the risk of infection.

13. Children with positive tests should be allowed to attend school, since casual person-to-person contact of schoolchildren poses no risk. However, a more restricted environment is advisable for preschool children or children who lack control of their body secretions, display biting behavior, or have oozing lesions.

D. Health Education: Without a vaccine or treatment, the prevention of cases of AIDS relies on the success of education projects involving behavioral changes. The health education messages for the general public have been summarized as follows:

1. Any sexual intercourse (outside of mutually monogamous HIV antibody-negative relationships) should be protected by a condom.

2. Do not share unsterile needles or syringes.

3. All women who have been potentially exposed should seek HIV antibody testing before becoming pregnant and, if the test is positive, should consider avoiding pregnancy. HIV seropositivity in pregnant women can be considered grounds for termination of pregnancy if the woman so wishes.

REFERENCES

Blumberg BM et al: Human immunodeficiency virus type 1 *nef* quasispecies in pathological tissue. J Virol 1992;66:5256.

Bozzette SA et al: A cross-sectional comparison of persons with syncytium- and non-syncytium-inducing human immunodeficiency virus. J Infect Dis 1993;168:1374.

Brady HJM et al: CD4 cell surface downregulation in HIV-1 Nef transgenic mice is a consequence of intracellular sequestration. EMBO J 1993;12:4923.

Cameron PU et al: Dendritic cells exposed to human immunodeficiency virus type-1 transmit a vigorous cytopathic infection to CD4+ T cells. Science 1992;257:383.

Centers for Disease Control: Agent summary statement for human immunodeficiency virus and report on laboratory-acquired infection with human immunodeficiency virus. Morb Mortal Wkly Rep 1988;37(Suppl S-4).

Centers for Disease Control: Interpretation and use of the western blot assay for serodiagnosis of human immunodeficiency virus type 1 infections. Morb Mortal Wkly Rep 1989;38(Suppl S-7).

Centers for Disease Control: Public Health Service statement on management of occupational exposure to human immunodeficiency virus, including considerations regarding zidovudine postexposure use. Morb Mortal Wkly Rep 1990;39(RR-1).

Centers for Disease Control: Testing for antibodies to human immunodeficiency virus type 2 in the United States. Morb Mortal Wkly Rep 1992;41(RR-12).

Centers for Disease Control: Zidovudine for the prevention

of HIV transmission from mother to infant. Morb Mortal Wkly Rep 1994;43:285.

Clements JE, Payne SL: Molecular basis of the pathobiology of lentiviruses. Virus Res 1994;32:97.

Cook DG et al: Binding of human immunodeficiency virus type 1 (HIV-1) gp120 to galactosylceramide (GalCer): Relationship to the V3 loop. Virology 1994;201:206.

Daniel MD et al: Protective effects of a live attenuated SIV vaccine with a deletion in the *nef* gene. Science 1992;258: 1938.

Fineberg HV: Education to prevent AIDS: Prospects and obstacles. Science 1988;239:592.

Hanson CG, Shearer WT: Pediatric HIV infection and AIDS. In: *Textbook of Pediatric Infectious Diseases,* 3rd ed. Feigin RD, Cherry JD (editors). Saunders, 1992.

Haynes BF: Scientific and social issues of human immunodeficiency virus vaccine development. Science 1993;260: 1279.

Johnston MI, Hoth DF: Present status and future prospects for HIV therapies. Science 1993;260:1286.

Kohlstaedt LA et al: Crystal structure at 3.5 Å resolution of HIV-1 reverse transcriptase complexed with an inhibitor. Science 1992;256:1783.

Levine AM: AIDS-related malignancies: The emerging epidemic. J Natl Cancer Inst 1993;85:1382.

McNearney T et al: Relationship of human immunodeficiency virus type 1 sequence heterogeneity to stage of disease. Proc Natl Acad Sci USA 1992;89:10247.

Merson MH: Slowing the spread of HIV: Agenda for the 1990s. Science 1993;260:1266.

Pantaleo G, Graziosi C, Fauci AS: The immunopathogenesis of human immunodeficiency virus infection. N Engl J Med 1993;328:327.

Quinn TC: Population migration and the spread of types 1 and 2 human immunodeficiency viruses. Proc Natl Acad Sci USA 1994;91:2407.

Richman KM, Rickman LS: The potential for transmission of human immunodeficiency virus through human bites. J Acq Immune Def Syndr 1993;6:402.

Scott GB et al: Survival in children with perinatally acquired human immunodeficiency virus type 1 infection. N Engl J Med 1989;321:1791.

Talbott R et al: Mapping the determinants of human immunodeficiency virus 2 for infectivity, replication efficiency, and cytopathicity. Proc Natl Acad Sci USA 1993;90: 4226.

Wainberg MA et al: Clinical correlates and molecular basis of HIV drug resistance. J Acq Immune Def Syndr 1993;6 (Suppl 1):S36.

Medical Mycology

45

*Jeffrey C. Edman, MD**

There are thousands of known species of yeasts and molds, but only about 100 of them cause disease in humans or animals (many others cause disease in plants). Only the dermatophytes and *Candida* species are commonly transmitted from one human to another.

For convenience, human mycotic infections may be grouped into superficial, cutaneous, subcutaneous, and deep (or systemic) mycoses (Table 45–1). Infections with fungi that cause superficial, cutaneous, or subcutaneous infections of skin, hair, and nails may be chronic and resistant to treatment but rarely affect the general health of the patient. The deep mycoses are caused by pathogenic fungi or by opportunistic fungi infecting immunosuppressed patients. Deep fungal infections may produce systemic involvement and are sometimes fatal. The actinomycetes are not fungi but filamentous branching bacteria. However, since they produce diseases that clinically resemble fungal infections, they are included in this chapter.

Deep mycoses are caused by organisms that live free in nature in the soil or on decaying organic material and are frequently limited to certain geographic areas. In such areas, many people acquire the fungal infection, but the majority develop only minor symptoms or none at all; only a small minority of infections progress to full-blown serious or fatal disease. The host's cell-mediated immune reactions are of paramount importance in determining the outcome of such infections.

Pathogenic fungi generally produce no toxins. In the host, they regularly induce hypersensitivity to their

*Associate Professor of Laboratory Medicine, University of California, San Francisco.

GLOSSARY

Conidia: Propagative forms produced by asexual reproduction. Some fungi form both large (macroconidia) and small conidia (microconidia).

- **Arthroconidia (arthrospores):** Structures resulting from fragmentation of a hypha into individual cells (eg, in Coccidioides immitis; Figure 45–15).
- **Blastoconidia (blastospores):** Simple structures that develop by budding, with subsequent separation of the bud from the parent cell (eg, in yeasts; Figure 45–1).
- **Chlamydoconidia (chlamydospores):** Terminal or intercalary cells in a hypha that enlarge and develop thick walls. These structures are resistant to unfavorable environmental conditions and germinate when conditions become more favorable for vegetative growth (Figure 45–2).

Dimorphic: Fungi that have two forms, hyphae and yeasts, that develop under different growth conditions (eg, Histoplasma capsulatum, which forms hyphae in nature and yeasts when infecting humans).

Hyphae: Long filaments or strands of cells. Hyphae that do not have cross-walls are called "aseptate"; those with cross-walls are "septate." Vegetative hyphae grow under the surface of agar and absorb nutrients. Aerial hyphae grow above the surface of agar and support reproductive structures.

Imperfect fungi ("fungi imperfecti"): Fungi with no recognized or existing sexual stage of reproduction

Molds: Hyphae.

Mycelia: Hyphae or mats of hyphae.

Perfect fungi: Those that have a sexual reproductive stage

Spore: Reproductive structure. (See also Conidia, which are reproductive structures formed asexually.) The following types of spores are formed by sexual reproduction:

- **Ascospores:** Following meiosis, four to eight spores form within a specialized cell called an ascus (Figure 45–1).
- **Basidiospores:** Following meiosis, four spores usually form on the surface of a specialized cells called a basidium.
- **Zygospores:** In certain zygomycetes, the tips of approximating hyphae fuse, meiosis occurs, and large, thick-walled zygospores develop.

Yeasts: Single oval to round fungal cells that bud (form blastoconidia) to reproduce

Table 45–1. The major fungal infections and causative organisms.

Type of Infection	Causative Organism	Disease
Superficial	*Malassezia furfur*	Pityriasis versicolor
Cutaneous	*Trichophyton, Epidemophyton,* and *Microsporum* species *Candida albicans*	Dermatophytosis (ringworm of skin, scalp, nails). Candidiasis of skin, oral candidiasis (thrush) of mucous membranes
Subcutaneous	*Sporothrix schenkii*	Sporotrichosis
Deep	*Blastomyces dermatitidis* *Coccoidioides immitis* *Histoplasma capsulatum* *Paracoccidioides brasiliensis*	Blastomycosis Coccidioidomycosis Histoplasmosis Paracoccidioidomycosis
Deep opportunistic	*Aspergillus fumigatus* and other *Aspergillus* species *Candida albicans* and other *Candida* species *Cryptococcus neoformans* *Mucor* and *Rhizopus* species	Aspergillosis Candidiasis Cryptococcosis Zygomycosis

chemical constituents. In systemic mycoses, the typical tissue reaction is a chronic granuloma with varying degrees of necrosis and abscess formation.

CLASSIFICATION OF FUNGI

The comparative position of fungi in the overall classification of microorganisms is discussed in Chapter 1.

The fungi are classified on the basis of their mode of **sexual reproduction;** however, the sexual stages can be difficult to induce and are rarely observed in clinical specimens. Most fungi reproduce by forming **conidia** through mitosis **(asexual reproduction),** during which the chromosome number remains the same. The descriptions of species deal principally with various asexual structures, and the fungi are identified on the basis of the morphologic characteristics of the hyphae, yeasts, and conidia, which may form on specialized **conidiophores,** on the sides or ends of nonspecialized hyphae, or from a hyphal cell. Specialized names have been given to each developmental form of conidia. (See Figures 45–1 to 45–9.) Some pathogenic and many nonpathogenic fungi respond to environmental stimuli and can exhibit different morphologic forms **(dimorphism).** Demonstration of the two phases can be a key diagnostic criteria. Reactivity in biochemical tests is used to identify yeasts and some other fungi. Because the sexual stages of fungi are so seldom seen and because identification is based on asexual stages, the organisms will often have two formal names (eg, *Filobasidiella neoformans* and *Cryptococcus neoformans* for the sexual and asexual stages, respectively). The names of the asexual stages are used commonly.

The fungi are classified as follows:

Ascomycotina (the ascomyces): Sexual fusion results in a sac, or ascus, containing the meiotic products as four or eight spores (ascospores). Asexual spores (conidia) are borne externally at the tips of hyphae. ***Examples:*** *Trichophyton (Arthroderma), Microsporum (Nannizzia), Blastomyces (Ajellomyces).*

Basidiomycotina (the basidiomyces): Sexual fusion results in formation of a club-shaped organ called a basidium, on the surface of which are borne the four meiotic products (basidiospores). Asexual spores (conidia) are borne externally at the tips of hyphae. ***Example:*** *Cryptococcus neoformans (Filobasidiella neoformans).*

Deuteromycotina (the imperfect fungi): This is not a true phylogenetic group but rather an artificial class into which are temporarily placed all forms in which the sexual process has not yet been observed. Most of the members of the group resemble ascomyces morphologically. ***Examples:*** *Epidermophyton, Sporothrix, Candida* species.

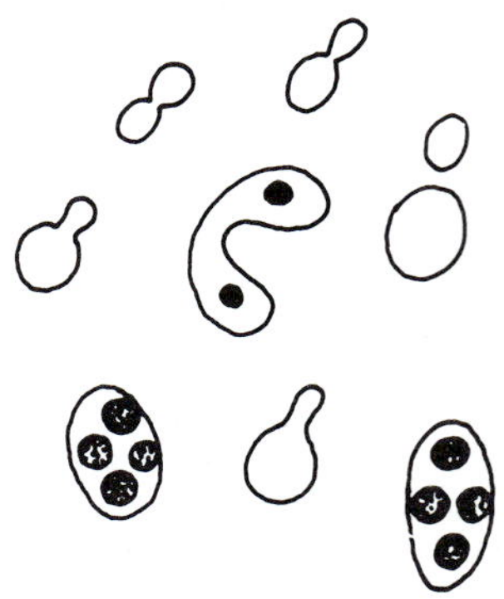

Figure 45–1. *Saccharomyces.* Budding blastoconidia (blastospores). Conjugating blastoconidia. Ascus containing ascospores.

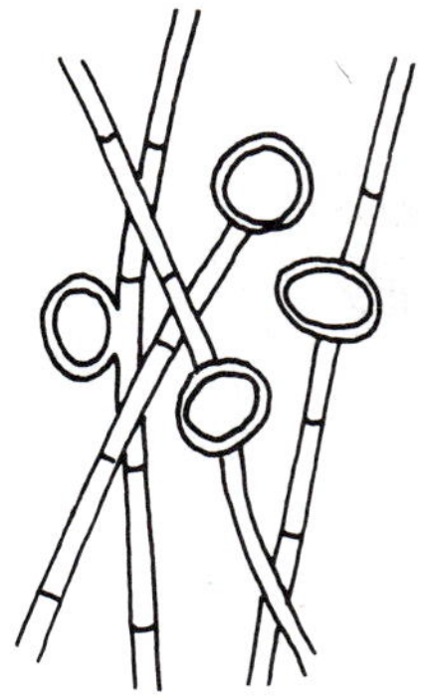

Figure 45–2. Terminal and intercalary chlamydoconidia (chlamydospores).

Zygomycotina (the phycomyces): Mycelium usually nonseptate; asexual spores produced in indefinite numbers within a structure called a sporangium. Sexual fusion results in formation of a resting, thick-walled cell termed a zygospore. ***Example:*** *Rhizopus nigrans* (opportunistic pathogens only).

GROWTH & ISOLATION OF FUNGI

Most fungi occur in nature and grow readily on simple sources of nitrogen and carbohydrate. Traditionally, Sabouraud's agar, which contains glucose and beef extract (pH 5.0), has been used because it does not readily support the growth of bacteria. The morphologic characteristics of fungi used for identification have also been defined for growth on Sabouraud's agar. The specimens used for isolation of fungi and other media used to isolate them are discussed in Chapter 48.

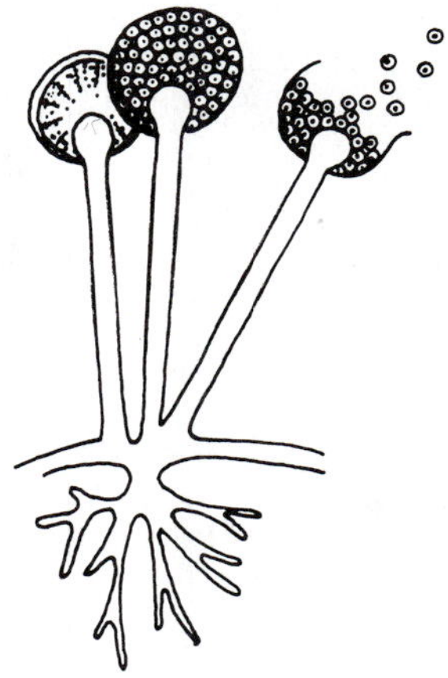

Figure 45–4. *Rhizopus.* Developing sporangioconidia (sporangiospores). Sporangioconidia released. Rhizoid.

SUPERFICIAL MYCOSES

TINEA VERSICOLOR (Pityriasis Versicolor)

Tinea versicolor is a common mild superficial infection that appears to be the result of overgrowth of *Malassezia furfur,* a yeast-like fungus that is a member of the normal skin flora. Growth within the skin (stratum corneum) of clusters of spherical, thick-walled budding cells and short, bent hyphae of *Malassezia furfur* usually causes no pathologic signs other than fine to brawny scales. Lesions appear prin-

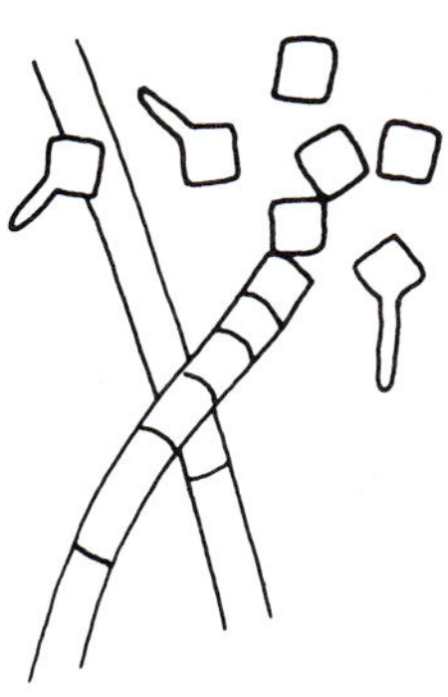

Figure 45–3. *Geotrichum.* Arthroconidia (arthrospore) formation. Germinating arthroconidia.

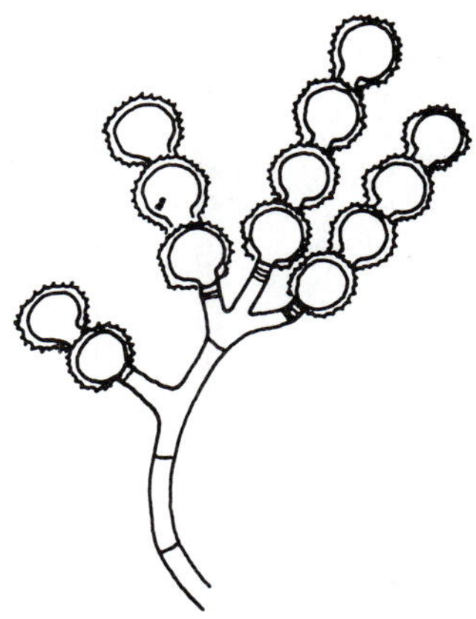

Figure 45–5. *Scopulariopsis.* Conidiophore shows spore scars. Terminal conidium is oldest.

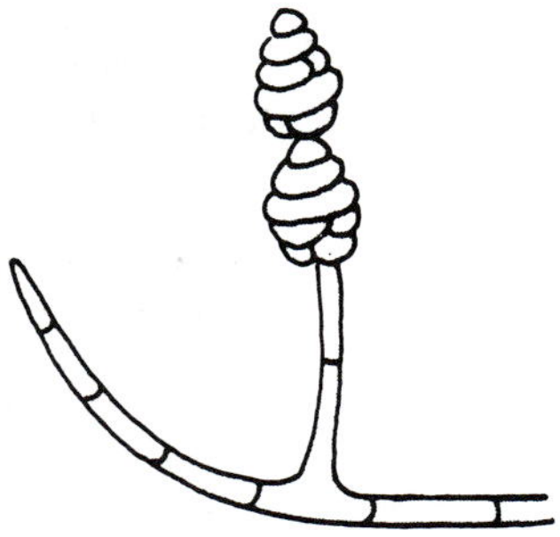

Figure 45–6. *Alternaria.* Black, multicellular conidia in chains. Terminal conidium is youngest.

cipally on the chest, back, abdomen, neck, and upper arms. The lesions range from depigmented to brownish-red and are of only cosmetic importance. Rarely, *Malassezia furfur* causes fungemia in association with intravenous lipid therapy.

Treatment consists of 1% selenium sulfide applied every other day for 15 minutes and then washed off. Treatment of catheter-associated *Malassezia furfur* fungemia consists of removing the offending catheter.

TINEA NIGRA

Light brown to blackish macular areas appear most commonly on the palmar or plantar stratum corneum. These are filled with brownish, branched, septate hyphae and budding cells of *Exophiala werneckii.* No scaling or other reaction develops. Treatment consists of topical undecylenic acid or antifungal azole.

PIEDRA

Hard black nodules (black piedra) are formed around the scalp hair by *Piedraia hortae.* Softer, white to light brown nodules (white piedra) caused by *Trichosporon beigelii* form on axillary, pubic, beard, and scalp hair. Treatment for both forms consists of removal of hair and application of a topical antifungal. Relapse is common.

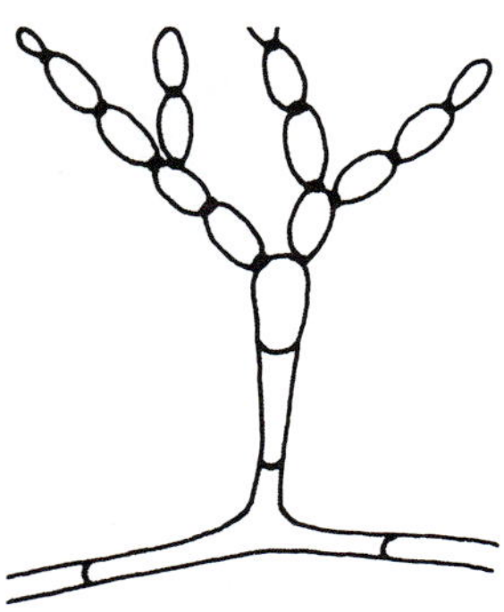

Figure 45–7. *Cladosporium.* Chains of conidia. Terminal conidium is youngest and has budded from subterminal conidium.

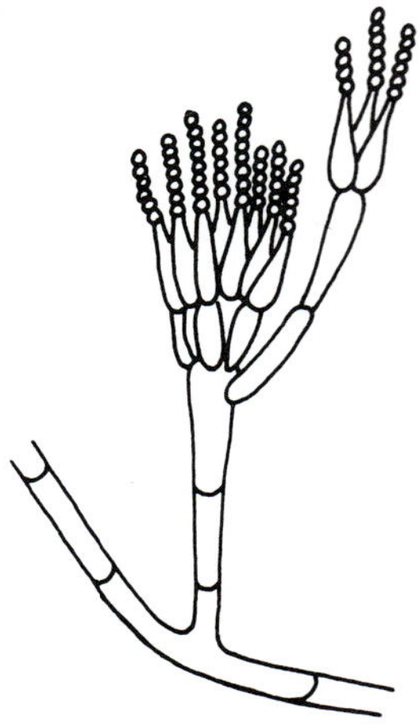

Figure 45–8. *Penicillium.* Conidia form within a phialide. Terminal conidium is oldest.

CUTANEOUS MYCOSES

The cutaneous mycoses are caused by fungi that invade only superficial keratinized tissue (skin, hair, and

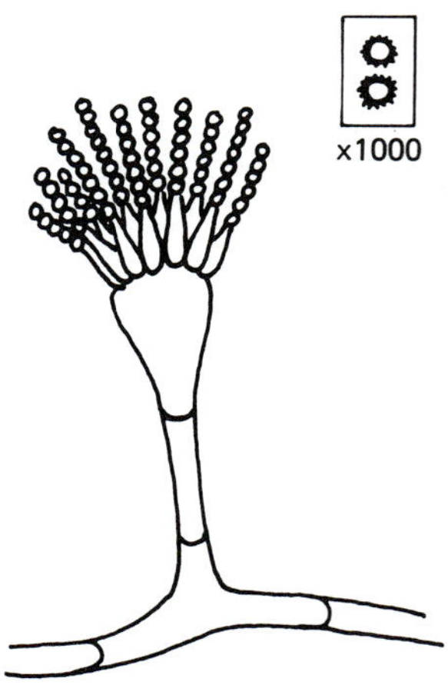

Figure 45–9. *Aspergillus fumigatus.* Phialides form on top of swollen vesicle. Terminal conidium is oldest. Mature conidia have rough walls.

nails) and not the deeper tissues. The most important of these are the dermatophytes, a group of closely related fungi classified into three genera: *Epidermophyton, Microsporum,* and *Trichophyton.* In nonviable keratinized tissue, these form only hyphae and arthroconidia. In culture, they develop characteristic colonies and conidia by means of which they can be divided into species. Sexual spores of some species have been found. All dermatophytes with a demonstrable sexual state belong to a single genus *Arthroderma.* Some species are found only in soil and never produce infection. Other soil species may produce disease in humans. Others have evolved to complete parasitism, are communicable, and are not found in soil.

Most dermatophytes are worldwide in distribution, but some species show a higher incidence in certain regions than in others (eg, *Trichophyton schoenleinii* in the Mediterranean, *Trichophyton rubrum* in tropical climates). Many domestic and other animals have infections caused by dermatophytes and may transmit them to humans (eg, *Microsporum canis* from cats and dogs).

Morphology & Identification

Representative colonies form on Sabouraud's agar at room temperature. Conidia formation may be observed by means of slide cultures.

A. *Trichophyton:* Microconidia are the predominant spore form. Smooth-walled, pencil-shaped macroconidia with blunt ends are rarer. Each species varies in colony morphology and pigmentation. Conidia formation may also vary according to the species under observation (Figure 45–10). The medium on which the fungi grow greatly influences these characteristics. The use of different nutritional media is sometimes necessary in order to differentiate among the species.

In culture, colonies of *Trichophyton mentagrophytes* range from granular to powdery, and they usually display abundant grape-like clusters of subspherical microconidia on terminal branches. Some cottony strains develop only rare teardrop-shaped microconidia along the sides of the hyphae. Coiled hyphae are frequent. *T rubrum* usually has some teardrop-shaped microconidia along the sides of the hyphae; in some strains, these may be abundant. Colonies often develop a red color on the reverse side. The larger microconidia of *Trichophyton tonsurans* are usually numerous and clavate and may be borne on short branches. Colonies are usually powdery.

B. *Microsporum:* Macroconidia are the predominant conidial form (Figure 45–11). They are large, rough-walled, multicellular, and spindle-shaped, and they form on the ends of hyphae. Microconidia are not used as a means of differentiating species. *Microsporum* species usually infect skin and hair but rarely the nails.

M canis forms numerous thick-walled, 8- to 15-celled macroconidia that frequently have curved or hooked spiny tips. A yellow-orange pigment usually develops on the reverse side of the colony. Infected hairs fluoresce a bright green under Wood's light. *Microsporum gypseum* has abundant thinner-walled, four- to six-celled macroconidia in buff to brownish-colored colonies. *Microsporum audouini* rarely forms conidia in the colony, but many thick-walled chlamydoconidia may be present. This fungus grows poorly on sterile rice grains, whereas other *Microsporum* species show rapid growth. Infected hairs fluoresce.

C. *Epidermophyton floccosum:* In this monotypic genus, only one- to five-celled, club-shaped macroconidia (Figure 45–11) are formed in the greenish-yellow colony, which mutates readily to form a sterile white overgrowth. This fungus invades skin and nails but never hair.

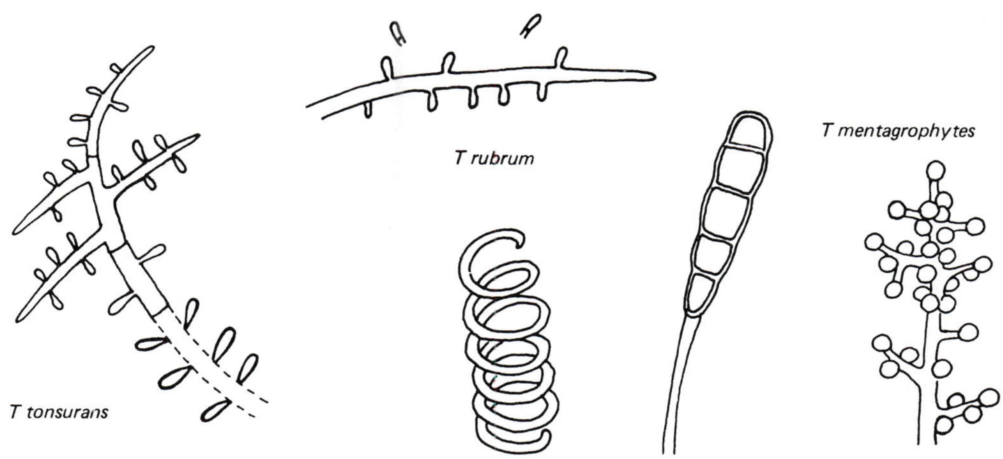

Figure 45–10. *Trichophyton* species. Microconidia and typical macroconidium.

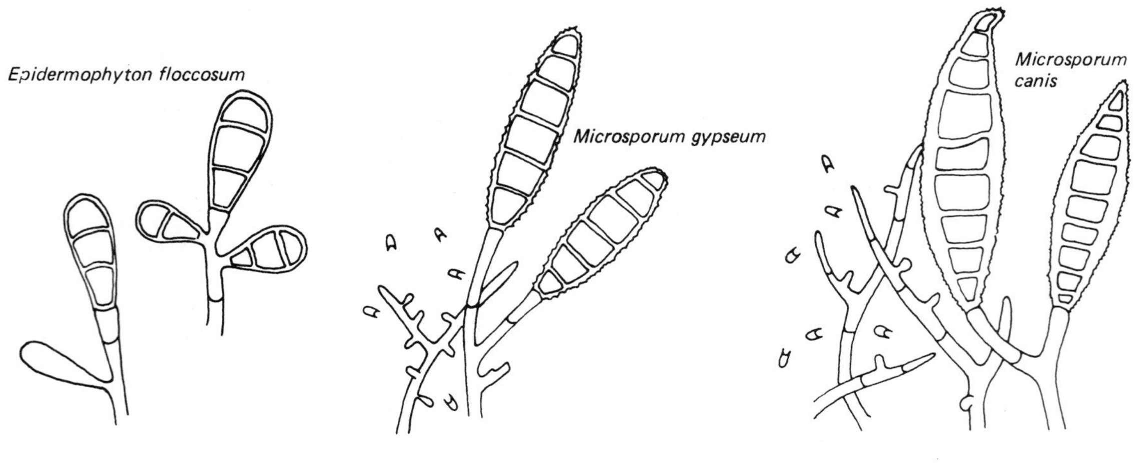

Figure 45–11. Macroconidia and microconidia.

Antigenic Structure

Trichophytin, a crude extract from dermatophytes, produces a positive tuberculin-like response in most adults. A galactomannan peptide is the reactive component. The carbohydrate portion is related to an immediate response, whereas the peptide moiety is associated with the delayed response and is believed also to be associated with immunity. Patients without the delayed type reaction or with an immediate type reaction are more susceptible to chronic dermatophytosis. Resistance to infection, both partial and local, may be acquired after the primary infection. This resistance varies in duration and degree depending on the host, site, and species of fungus causing the infection.

Clinical Findings (Table 45–2)

A. Tinea Pedis (Athlete's Foot): This is the most prevalent of all dermatophytoses. The toe webs are infected with a *Trichophyton* species or with *E floccosum.* Initially, there is itching between the toes and the development of small vesicles that rupture and discharge a thin fluid. The skin of the toe webs becomes macerated and peels, whereupon cracks appear that are prone to secondary bacterial infection. When secondary infection does occur, lymphangitis and lymphadenitis develop. When the fungal infection becomes chronic, peeling and cracking of the skin are the principal manifestations. Nail infection (tinea unguium, onychomycosis) follows prolonged tinea pedis. Nails become yellow, brittle, thickened, or crumbling.

In the course of dermatophytosis, the individual may become hypersensitive to constituents or products of the fungus and may develop allergic manifestations, called dermatophytids (usually vesicles), elsewhere on the body (most often on the hands). The trichophytin skin test is markedly positive in such persons.

B. Tinea Corporis, Tinea Cruris (Ringworm): Dermatophytosis of the nonhairy skin of the body commonly gives rise to the annular lesions of ringworm, with a clearing, scaly center surrounded by a red advancing border that often contains vesicles. *E floccosum, T rubrum,* and *T mentagrophytes* are the most common isolates.

Dermatophytes grow only within dead, keratinized tissue. Fungal metabolic products diffuse through the malpighian layer to cause erythema, vesicle formation, and pruritus. The role of antibody activity is not understood. As hyphae age and break up into arthrospores, the cells containing them are shed, which partly accounts for the central clearing of the "ringworm" lesion. Active hyphal growth is into the peripheral "ring" of uninfected stratum corneum. Continuing growth downward into the newly forming stratum corneum of the thicker plantar and palmar surfaces accounts for the persistent infections at those sites.

C. Tinea Capitis (Ringworm of the Scalp): *Microsporum* infection occurs in childhood and usually heals spontaneously by puberty. Untreated *Trichophyton* infections may persist into adulthood. Infection begins on the skin of the scalp, with subsequent growth of the dermatophyte down the keratinized wall of the hair follicle. Infection of the hair takes place just above the hair root. The fungus continues to grow downward on the upward-growing hair shaft. *Microsporum* species grow primarily as a sheath around the hair (ectothrix), whereas *Trichophyton* species vary in their growth patterns. Some invade the hair shaft (endothrix), making it so fragile that it breaks off within or at the surface of the hair follicle (black-dot ringworm). In infections with other species, the hair breaks a short distance above the scalp, leaving short stubs in a balding, usually circular patch. Redness, edema, scaling, and vesicle formation may be seen. In some patients, a pronounced inflammation called kerion may occur around the area of infection and may even resemble pyogenic infection. *T schoenleinii* forms cup-like crusts (scutula) around infected follicles.

Table 45–2. Some clinical features of dermatophyte infection.

Skin Disease	Location of Lesions	Clinical Appearance	Fungi Most Frequently Responsible
Tinea corporis (ringworm)	Nonhairy, smooth skin.	Circular patches with advancing red, vesiculated border and central scaling. Pruritic.	*Microsporum canis, Trichophyton mentagrophytes*
Tinea pedis[1] (athlete's foot)	Interdigital spaces on feet of persons wearing shoes.	Acute: itching, red vesicular. Chronic: itching, scaling, fissures.	*Trichophyton rubrum, T mentagrophytes, Epidermophyton floccosum*
Tinea cruris (jock itch)	Groin.	Erythematous scaling lesion in intertriginous area. Pruritic.	*T rubrum, T mentagrophytes, E floccosum*
Tinea capitis	Scalp hair. Endothrix: fungus inside hair shaft. Ectothrix: fungus on surface of hair.	Circular bald patches with short hair stubs or broken hair within hair follicles. Kerion rare. *Microsporum*-infected hairs fluoresce.	*M canis, Trichophyton tonsurans*
Tinea barbae	Beard hair.	Edematous, erythematous lesion.	*T rubrum, T mentagrophytes*
Tinea unguium (onychomycosis)	Nail.	Nails thickened or crumbling distally; discolored; lusterless. Usually associated with tinea pedis.	*T rubrum, T mentagrophytes, E floccosum*
Dermatophytid (id reaction)	Usually sides and flexor aspects of fingers. Palm. Any site on body.	Pruritic vesicular to bullous lesions. Most commonly associated with tinea pedis.	No fungi present in lesion. May become secondarily infected with bacteria.

[1]May be associated with lesions of hands and nails (onychomycosis).

Infection with *Trichophyton* species may involve the bearded region of humans (tinea barbae); the highly inflammatory reaction they cause closely resembles pyogenic infections of that area. Rarely, dermatophytes not only colonize a human but produce systemic infection, eg, infective endocarditis. This occurs only in immunocompromised persons.

Diagnostic Laboratory Tests

A. Specimens: Specimens consist of scrapings from both the skin and the nails plus hairs plucked from involved areas. *Microsporum*-infected hairs fluoresce under Wood's light in a darkened room.

B. Microscopic Examination: Specimens are placed on a slide in a drop of 10–20% potassium hydroxide, covered with a coverslip, and examined immediately and then again after 20 minutes. In skin or nails, branching hyphae or chains of arthrospores are seen (Figure 45–12). In hairs, *Microsporum* species form dense sheaths of spores in a mosaic pattern around the hair; *Trichophyton* species form parallel rows of spores outside (ectothrix) or inside (endothrix) the hair shaft.

C. Culture: All final identification of dermatophytes rests on cultures. Specimens are inoculated onto Sabouraud's agar slants containing cycloheximide and chloramphenicol to suppress mold and bacterial growth, incubated for 1–3 weeks at room temperature, and further examined in slide cultures if necessary. Species determination is made on the basis of colonial morphology, microscopic examination, and in some cases biochemical tests.

Treatment

Therapy consists of thorough removal of infected and dead epithelial structures and application of a topical antifungal chemical. Overtreatment often causes dermatophytids. Attempts must be made to prevent reinfection. In widespread involvement, oral administration of griseofulvin for 1–4 weeks has been effective. Nail infections require months of griseofulvin treatment and sometimes surgical removal of the nail. Relapse of nail infections is common.

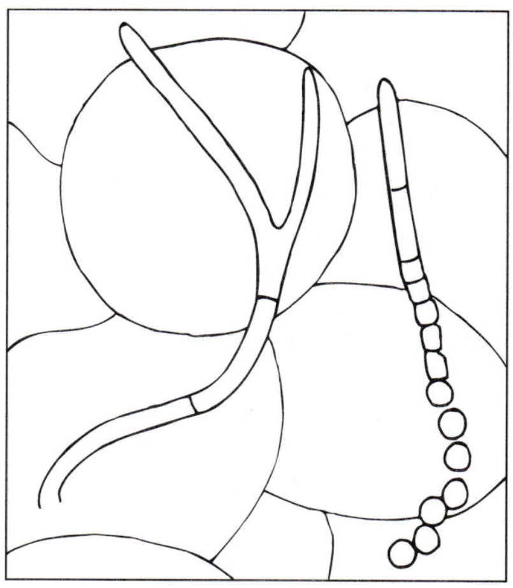

Figure 45–12. Dermatophyte in potassium hydroxide mount of skin or nail scraping. Branching hyphae. Arthroconidia formation.

A. Scalp Infections: In scalp infections, hairs can be plucked manually, clipped, or otherwise epilated. Griseofulvin may be given for 1–2 weeks. Frequent shampoos and miconazole cream or other antifungal agents may be effective if used for weeks.

B. Body Infections: Use miconazole cream, undecylenic acid cream, salicylic acid, or benzoic acid.

C. Foot Infections:

1. Acute phase–Soak in potassium permanganate 1:5000 until the acute inflammation subsides; then apply antifungal chemicals as described above.

2. Chronic phase–Apply antifungal chemicals as creams at night (as powders during the day) as outlined above. Higher concentrations may be tolerated.

Epidemiology & Control

Infection arises from contact of uninfected skin or hair with infected skin scales or hair stubs. Hyphae then grow into the stratum corneum. Sporadic cases of ringworm infection are acquired from cats or dogs *(M canis).* Epidemics of tinea capitis have been traced to the use of shared barbershop clippers, transfer of infected hairs on headrests in common carriers, and person-to-person contact. Control depends on cleanliness, sterilization of instruments (using hot mineral oil), effective treatment of cases, and reduced contact with infectious materials.

Athlete's foot is found only in people who wear shoes. Infection spreads through the use of common showers and dressing rooms, where infected desquamated skin serves as a source of infection. No really effective control measures are available other than proper hygiene and the use of talc to keep interdigital spaces dry. In many persons, chronic athlete's foot is asymptomatic and becomes activated only in excessive heat or moisture or with unsuitable footwear. Open-toed shoes or sandals are best for general wear.

SUBCUTANEOUS MYCOSES

The fungi that cause subcutaneous mycoses grow in soil or on decaying vegetation. They must be introduced into subcutaneous tissue in order to produce disease. In general, lesions spread slowly from the area of implantation. Extension via lymphatics draining the lesion is slow except in sporotrichosis. Each of these fungi has developed a unique morphologic form as a pathogen, except for *Basidiobolus haptosporus* and *Entomophthora coronata,* zygomycetes that grow as branching hyphae within subcutaneous lesions.

SPOROTHRIX SCHENCKII

Sporothrix schenckii is a dimorphic fungus that lives on plants or wood and causes **sporotrichosis,** a chronic granulomatous infection, when traumatically introduced into the skin. There is often a characteristic spread along lymphatics draining the area.

Morphology & Identification

The organisms are rarely seen in pus and tissues from human infections. They may appear as small, round to cigar-shaped, gram-positive budding cells. In cultures at room temperature on Sabouraud's agar, cream-colored to black, folded, leathery colonies develop within 3–5 days. (Pigment formation of different strains of *S schenckii* is variable.) Simple, ovoid conidia are borne in clusters at the tips of long, slender conidiophores (resembling a daisy; see Figure 45–13) as well as along the sides of the thin hyphae. Culture at 37 °C produces spherical to ovoid budding cells.

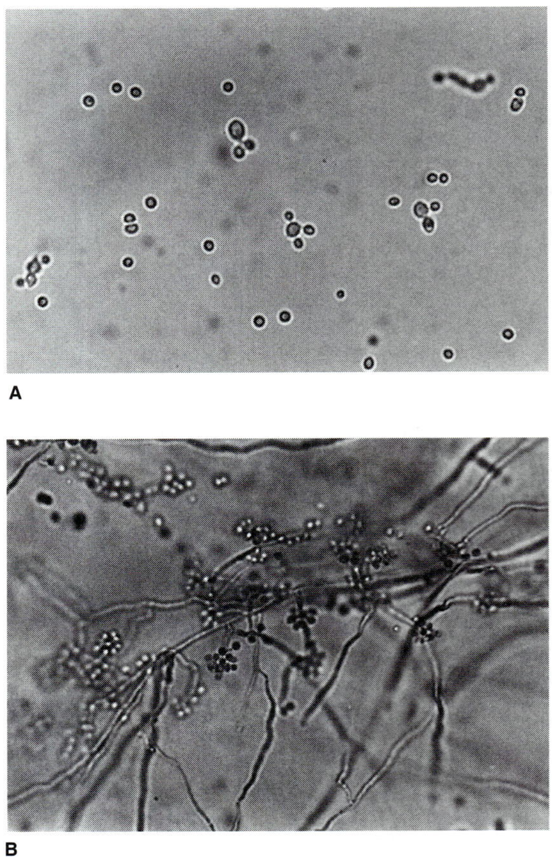

Figure 45–13. *Sporothrix schenckii.* ***A:*** Blastoconidia (blastospores) seen in tissue or 37 °C culture. ***B:*** Conidia formation in 20 °C culture.

Antigenic Structure

Heat-killed saline suspensions of cultures (or carbohydrate fractions from them) give positive delayed skin tests in infected humans or animals. A variety of antibodies are found in infected patients and sometimes also in normal individuals.

Pathogenesis & Clinical Findings

The fungus is introduced into the skin by trauma. The location of the initial lesion is usually on the extremities but can be found anywhere (children often present with facial lesions). A local lesion develops as a pustule, abscess, or ulcer, and the lymphatics leading from it become thickened and cord-like. Multiple subcutaneous nodules and abscesses occur along the lymphatics. Usually there is little systemic illness associated with these lesions, but dissemination of the infection—especially to joints—sometimes occurs, especially in debilitated patients. Rarely, primary infection in humans occurs through the lung. A variety of animals (rats, dogs, mules, and horses) are naturally infected.

Histologically, the lesions show both chronic inflammation and granulomas that undergo necrosis.

Yeast forms in tissue stain with Gomori methenamine silver and other fungal stains (though often not seen). Organisms can also be identified by specific immunofluorescence. In some endemic areas (South Africa and Japan), an eosinophilic antigen-antibody complex ("asteroid body") may be seen in hematoxylin-eosin stains.

Diagnostic Laboratory Tests

A. Specimens: Specimens consist of pus or biopsy from lesions.

B. Microscopic Examination: In human lesions, organisms are seen infrequently, whereas budding cells are abundant in laboratory infections of mice.

C. Culture: On Sabouraud's agar, typical colonies with clusters of conidia are diagnostic. They should convert to yeast morphology during incubation at 37 °C.

D. Serology: Agglutination of yeast cell suspensions or of latex particles coated with antigen occurs in high titer with sera of infected patients but is not diagnostic.

Treatment

In a majority of cases, the infection is self-limited though chronic. Potassium iodide administered orally for weeks has some therapeutic benefit in the cutaneous-lymphatic form. In systemic involvement, amphotericin B is given intravenously. Oral ketoconazole may be beneficial.

Epidemiology & Control

S schenckii occurs worldwide in nature on plants (particularly sphagnum moss in the USA), thorns, and decaying wood; in soil; and on infected animals. Occupational exposure of gardeners, nursery workers, miners, and others in contact with plants and wood accounts for most cases. Prevention of trauma in these occupations is effective, since the organism must be introduced subcutaneously in order to cause disease.

CHROMOBLASTOMYCOSIS (Chromomycosis)

Chromoblastomycosis is a slowly progressive granulomatous infection of skin caused by several species of black molds. *Phialophora verrucosa, Fonsecaea pedrosoi, Rhinocladiella aquaspersa,* and *Cladosporium carrionii* have been isolated most frequently.

Morphology & Identification

In exudates and tissues, these fungi produce dark brown, thick-walled, rounded cells 5–15 μm in diameter that divide by septation. Septation in different planes with delayed separation may give rise to a cluster of four to eight cells, the so-called "sclerotic bodies" (Figure 45–14). Cells within superficial crusts of pus may germinate into brown, branching hyphae. Colonies vary in pigmentation from olive-gray to brown to black. The surface is generally velvety over a black, dense mat of mycelium.

A. *P verrucosa:* Conidia are primarily produced by vase-shaped phialides.

B. *F pedrosoi:* Most conidia form in short branching chains with the terminal cell budding to form a new conidium. Conidia may also form without chains directly on the top and sides of a conidiophore. Phialides are rare.

C. *Rhinocladiella aquaspersa:* Short branched chains of elliptical conidia are formed on conidiophore tips.

D. *C carrionii:* Only long, branching chains of conidia form on elongated conidiophores.

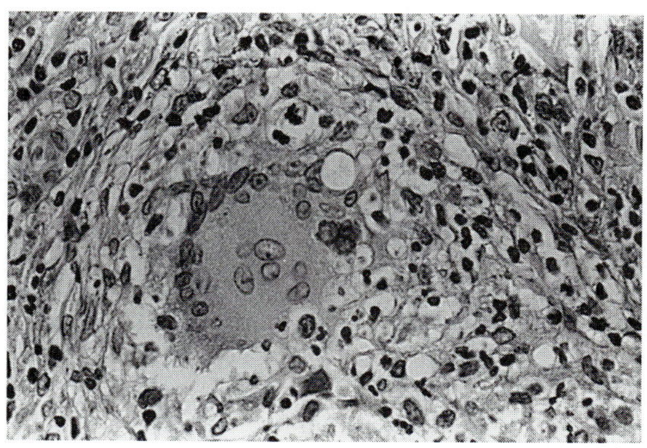

Figure 45–14. Chromomycosis. Pigmented fungal cells seen in giant cell.

Pathogenesis & Clinical Findings

The fungi are introduced by trauma into the skin, often of the legs or feet. Slowly—over months or years—wart-like growths extend along the lymphatics of the affected area. Cauliflower-like nodules with crusting abscesses eventually cover the area. Small ulcerations or "black dots" of hemopurulent material are present on the warty surface. Rarely, elephantiasis may result from secondary infection, obstruction, and fibrosis of lymph channels. Dissemination to other parts of the body is very rare, though satellite lesions can occur due either to local lymphatic spread or to autoinoculation.

Histologically, the lesions are granulomas; within leukocytes or giant cells, the dark brown, round fungus cells may be seen.

Diagnostic Laboratory Tests

A. Specimens: Specimens consist of scrapings or biopsy from lesions.

B. Microscopic Examination: Scrapings are placed in 10% potassium hydroxide and examined microscopically for dark, round fungus cells. Detection of the sclerotic bodies is diagnostic. Tissue sections show granulomas and organisms.

C. Culture: Specimens should be cultured on Sabouraud's agar so that the characteristic conidial structures and arrangement described above may be detected. Pathogenic species are distinguished from similar saprophytic black molds by the inability of the former to digest gelatin.

Treatment

Surgical excision with wide margins is the therapy of choice for small lesions. Chemotherapy with flucytosine or itraconazole may be efficacious for larger lesions. Local applied heat is also beneficial. Relapse is common.

Epidemiology

Chromoblastomycosis occurs mainly in the tropics. The fungi are saprophytic in nature, probably occurring on vegetation and in soil. The disease occurs chiefly on the legs of barefoot farm workers, presumably following traumatic introduction of the fungus. The disease is not communicable. Wearing shoes and protecting the legs probably would prevent infection.

PHAEOHYPHOMYCOSIS

Phaeohyphomycosis, broadly defined, is that group of clinical syndromes caused by dematiaceous (dark-walled) fungi that do not conveniently fit into other clinical or taxonomic groupings. Over 100 fungal species have been associated with the phaeohyphomycosis group of clinical entities. In tissue, these fungi vary from yeast-like bodies to long hyphae and combinations of multiple forms.

MYCETOMA

Mycetoma is a localized, swollen lesion with granules that are compact colonies of the causative agent draining from sinuses. It is caused by a variety of fungi and aerobic actinomycetes (filamentous bacteria). The term **actinomycetoma** is used to distinguish those cases caused by actinomycetes. Mycetoma develops when these soil organisms are implanted by trauma into subcutaneous tissue. The term **maduromycosis** or **Madura foot** is often used to denote those infections caused by fungi, but the clinical disease resembles actinomycetoma, though therapy is different. Mycetoma occurs worldwide but chiefly in people who do not wear shoes. Mycetomas are rarely seen outside of the tropics and are particularly prevalent in India, Africa, and Latin America.

Morphology & Identification

White, yellow, red, or black granules are extruded in pus. The granules due to fungi consist of intertwined, septate hyphae (3–5 μm), and, depending on the species, they may have larger, thick-walled cells at the periphery. The actinomycete granule consists only of filamentous hyphae (1 μm in diameter). There are distinct geographic differences in the distribution of causative agents of mycetoma. *Pseudallescheria boydii* is among the more common fungal causes of mycetoma. The gray colony produces abundant ovoid conidia and occasionally ascospores within brown cleistothecia. *P boydii* may also cause opportunistic disease of the lungs and other organs in compromised hosts. Other fungi causing mycetoma are *Madurella* species, *Phialophora* species, *Exophiala,* and *Acremonium* species. Each has its own characteristic colonial and microscopic morphology.

The most common causes of actinomycetoma are *Nocardia brasiliensis, Streptomyces somaleliensis,* and *Actinomadura madurae. N brasiliensis* may be acid-fast. These and other pathogenic actinomycetes are differentiated by biochemical tests and chromatographic analysis of cell wall components.

Pathogenesis & Clinical Findings

After one of the causative microorganisms has been introduced into the subcutaneous tissue (usually the foot, hand, or back) by trauma, abscesses form that may extend through muscle and even into bone, eventually draining through chronic sinuses. The organism can be seen as a compact granule in the pus. Untreated lesions persist for years and extend deeper and peripherally, causing deformity and loss of function.

Histologically, the lesions resemble those of actinomycosis, with prominent abscess formation, granulation tissue, necrotic foci, and fibrosis. Within the abscess, the granule may be surrounded by an eosinophilic matrix of host material and immune complexes.

Very rarely, *P boydii* disseminates in an immunocompromised host or produces infection of a foreign body (eg, a cardiac pacemaker).

Diagnostic Laboratory Tests

Some granules have characteristic morphologic characteristics as well as a characteristic color that aids in identification when cultures cannot be made. The diagnosis of mycetoma should never be made unless granules are seen.

Treatment

Actinomycetomas respond well to various combinations of streptomycin, trimethoprim-sulfamethoxazole, and dapsone if therapy is begun early, before extensive deformity has occurred. Surgical drainage assists in healing. There is no established therapy for fungal mycetoma, though prolonged treatment with oral ketoconazole or itraconazole may be beneficial. Surgical excision of early lesions may prevent spread.

Epidemiology & Control

The organisms producing mycetoma occur in soil and on vegetation. Barefoot farm laborers are therefore commonly exposed. Properly cleaning wounds and wearing shoes are reasonable control measures.

DEEP MYCOSES (Systemic Mycoses)

The deep mycoses are caused by soil fungi. Infection is acquired by inhalation, and most infections are asymptomatic. In symptomatic disease, dissemination of infection may occur to any organ, though each fungus shows some predilection for certain anatomic sites. These fungi appear to cause disease in specific persons, in whom disseminated, often fatal infection may develop. The genetic features that predispose to disseminated disease are not clearly understood. All of these fungi are dimorphic in that they have a unique morphologic adaptation to existence in tissue or to growth at 37 °C. A summary of the deep mycoses is given in Table 45–3.

COCCIDIOIDES IMMITIS

Coccidioides immitis is a soil fungus that causes **coccidioidomycosis.** The infection is endemic in some arid regions of the southwestern USA and Latin America. Infection is usually self-limited; dissemination is rare but may be fatal.

Morphology & Identification

In histologic sections of tissue, in pus, or in sputum, *Coccidioides* appears as a spherule 15–60 μm in diameter, with a thick, doubly refractile wall (Figure 45–15). Endospores form within the spherule and fill it. Upon rupture of the wall, they are released into surrounding tissue, where they enlarge to form new spherules.

When grown on bacteriologic media or on Sabouraud's agar, a white to tan cottony colony develops. The aerial hyphae form alternating arthroconidia (arthrospores) and empty cells. Hyphae fragment easily and release the conidia. The arthroconidia are light, float in air, and are highly infectious. When they are inoculated into animals or inhaled by humans, these infectious conidia develop into tissue spherules. Spherules can also be produced in the laboratory by cultivation of *Coccidioides* using specialized methods.

Antigenic Structure

Coccidioidin is a sterile filtrate from broth in which *Coccidioides* mycelium has been grown. Spherulin is a sterile filtrate from broth in which spherules have been grown. These materials give positive skin tests (in dilutions up to 1:10,000) in infected persons and serve as antigens in immunodiffusion (precipitin), latex agglutination, complement fixation (CF), and

Table 45–3. Summary of the deep mycoses.

Disease	Organism	Dimorphism (20 °C → 37 °C)	Distribution	Manifestations	Comments
Coccidioidomycosis (Valley fever, desert rheumatism)	*Coccidioides immitis*	Hyphae → Spherule	Southwestern USA, Mexico	Pulmonary, meningeal, osteomyelitis	Increased disease in pregnancy, AIDS, Filipino, African-American, Mexican
Histoplasmosis	*Histoplasma capsulatum*	Hyphae → Yeast	Ohio and Mississippi River Valleys	Pulmonary, reticulo-endothelial system	Increased disease in AIDS
Blastomycosis (North American blastomycosis)	*Blastomyces dermatitidis*	Hyphae → Yeast	Northern midwest USA and Canada	Skin	
Paracoccidioidomycosis (South American blastomycosis)	*Paracoccidioides brasiliensis*	Hyphae → Yeast	Central and South America	Skin, reticuloendothelial system	

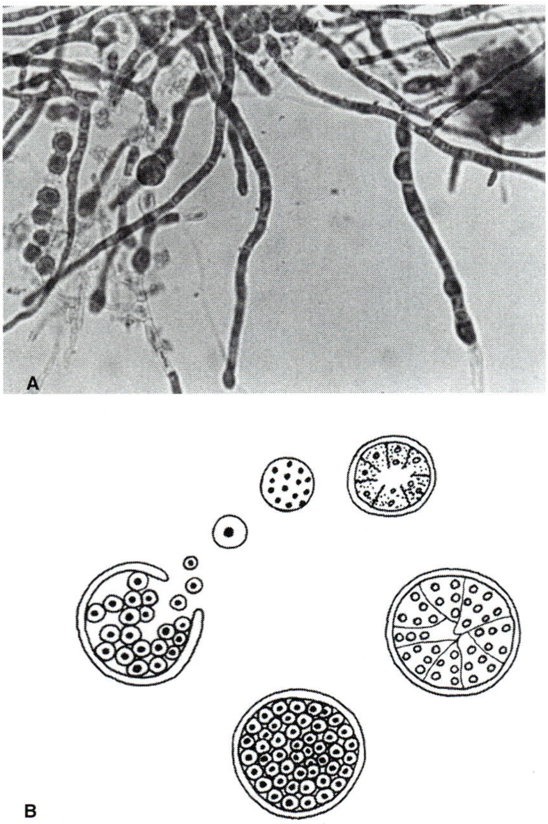

Figure 45–15. *Coccidioides immitis. **A:*** In soil. Arthroconidia (arthrospore) formation and germination. ***B:*** In tissue. Spherule formation with endospores.

other tests. In low dilutions (1:10), these antigens cross-react with antigens of other fungi *(Histoplasma, Paracoccidioides)*. Some antisera give highly specific immunofluorescence tests with spherules in tissue.

Pathogenesis & Clinical Findings

Infection is acquired through the inhalation of airborne arthroconidia. Two-thirds of persons with primary infections are completely asymptomatic, and infection may be evident only by the development of precipitating antibodies and a positive skin test in 2–3 weeks. In the remainder, primary coccidioidal disease may occur, manifested as an influenza-like illness with fever, malaise, cough, arthralgia, and headache. About 15% of individuals in the latter category develop hypersensitivity reactions 1–2 weeks later in the form of rash, erythema nodosum, or erythema multiforme. This symptom complex is called **valley fever** or desert rheumatism and is self-limited. Some radiologic changes occur in the lungs in more than half of cases, taking the form of infiltrates, pneumonia, pleural effusions, or hilar adenopathy. Pulmonary residua occur in about 5%, usually in the form of solitary nodules or thin-walled cavities. The latter may heal or may become chronic.

In fewer than 1% of persons who have been infected with *Coccidioides* does the disease progress to the disseminated, often lethal form. This occurs much more frequently in some races (eg, Filipinos, African-Americans, Mexicans) and possibly in pregnant women. The immunologic basis for racial susceptibility is not understood; general lowering of cell-mediated reactions may be responsible. In addition, the elevated levels of estradiol and progesterone in pregnancy can enhance the growth of *Coccidioides.* Spontaneous dissemination, if it occurs, usually develops within 1 year after initial infection, either by direct extension of a lesion or by hematogenous spread; cutaneous, joint, meningeal, and bone lesions are common. Dissemination suggests some defect in the individual's ability to localize and control *Coccidioides* infection. Disease resulting from massive exposure (usually occupational) also has an increased tendency to disseminate. Most persons can be considered immune to reinfection after their skin tests have become positive. However, if such individuals become immunocompromised by drugs or disease (eg, AIDS), dissemination can occur many years after primary *Coccidioides* infection (reactivation disease). Coccidioidomycosis in AIDS patients often presents with a rapidly fatal diffuse reticulonodular pneumonitis. Because of the radiologic overlap between this disease and *Pneumocystis* pneumonia (see below) and the different therapies for these two entities, it is important to be aware of the possibility of coccidioidal pneumonia in AIDS patients. Blood cultures are often positive for *Coccidioides.*

Disseminated coccidioidomycosis is comparable to tuberculosis in that lesions develop in many organs, bones, and the central nervous system. Histologically, these are typical granulomas with giant cells and interspersed suppuration. Histologic diagnosis depends on detection of typical spherules filled with endospores. The clinical course often includes remissions and exacerbations.

Diagnostic Laboratory Tests

A. Specimens: Specimens consist of sputum, pus, spinal fluid, tissue biopsy samples for culture, and blood for serologic testing.

B. Microscopic Examination: Materials should be examined fresh (after centrifuging, if necessary) for typical spherules.

C. Cultures: Cultures can be grown on blood agar at 37 °C and on Sabouraud's agar at 20 °C. ***Note:*** Extreme caution must be used, since arthrospores from cultures are highly infectious.

D. Animal Inoculation: Mice injected intraperitoneally develop progressive lesions from which *Coccidioides* can be grown.

E. Serology: IgM and IgG precipitating antibodies to coccidioidin develop within 2–4 weeks after infection and can be detected readily by immunodiffusion and latex agglutination tests. These titers decline within a few months. CF antibodies rise at about the same time and persist in lower titer for 6–8 months but are sometimes undetectable in self-limited infection. By contrast, if dissemination occurs, the CF antibody titer continues to rise. Such high CF titers are a poor prognostic sign. Their fall during treatment suggests improvement. In coccidioidal meningitis, the CF antibody titer may be high in cerebrospinal fluid and low in serum.

Patients with active disease or recent infection usually have high levels of IgE and circulating immune complexes. However, IgE levels do not permit differentiation of active pulmonary coccidioidomycosis from general dissemination.

F. Skin Test: (See Antigenic Structure, above.) The coccidioidin skin test reaches maximum induration (>5 mm in diameter) between 24 and 48 hours after injection of 0.1 mL of 1:100 dilution. It is often negative in disseminated disease. Cross-reactions with other fungi occur at a dilution of 1:10. Spherulin is more sensitive than and as specific as coccidioidin in detecting reactors. Reactions to skin tests tend to diminish in size and intensity years after primary infection in persons residing in endemic areas, but skin testing exerts a "booster" effect.

Immunity

Following recovery from primary infection with *Coccidioides,* there is usually immunity to reinfection.

Treatment

In most persons, symptomatic primary infection is self-limited and requires only supportive treatment. However, in patients with immunosuppression or disease resulting from massive exposure, amphotericin B followed by several months of oral azole therapy may be indicated. In disseminated coccidioidomycosis (not involving the meninges), intravenous amphotericin B for months may result in remission. Oral azole therapy with ketoconazole, fluconazole, or itraconazole for disseminated disease does not show significantly greater efficacy than amphotericin B. However, their decreased toxicities and ease of administration make the azoles attractive alternatives. Surgical resection of pulmonary cavities is sometimes necessary and often curative. In coccidioidal meningitis, intrathecal amphotericin B must also be given when used as single agent therapy, but the long-term results are often poor. Promising results have been obtained with oral fluconazole or itraconazole therapy for coccidioidal meningitis, but therapy must be maintained for many months to achieve symptomatic improvement. Relapse after cessation of antifungal therapy is common.

Epidemiology & Control

The endemic area of *Coccidioides* in the USA includes the arid regions ("lower sonoran life zone") of the southwestern states, particularly the San Joaquin and Sacramento Valleys of California, areas around Tucson and Phoenix in Arizona, and western Texas. *Coccidioides* also occurs in some arid areas of Central and South America. In these areas, the fungus is found in the soil and in rodents, and many humans have been infected, as shown by positive skin tests. The infection rate is highest during the dry months of summer and autumn, when dust is most prevalent. A high incidence of infection and disease may follow dust storms. During an epidemic of coccidioidomycosis in the San Joaquin Valley of California in 1991–1993, the rate of coccidioidomycosis increased more than tenfold. Increased precipitation in the spring months of these years has been suggested as an environmental stimulus.

The disease is not communicable from person to person, and there is no evidence that infected rodents contribute to its spread. A certain amount of control can be achieved by reducing dust, paving roads and airfields, planting grass or crops, and using oil sprays.

HISTOPLASMA CAPSULATUM

Histoplasma capsulatum is a dimorphic soil fungus occurring primarily in the United States. It causes **histoplasmosis,** an intracellular mycosis of the reticuloendothelial system. The ascomycetous, sexual stage of the fungus is called *Ajellomyces capsulatus.*

Morphology & Identification

Histoplasma forms oval, uninucleate budding cells measuring 2–4 μm in phagocytic cells and on glucose-cysteine blood agar slants or in tissue culture incubated at 37 °C (Figure 45–16). The bud arises at the smaller end of the yeast on a narrow bud base. On Sabouraud's agar incubated at room temperature, white to tan, cottony colonies develop, with either large (8–14 μm), thick-walled, spherical conidia that usually have finger-like projections (tuberculate conidia) or small (2–4 μm) microconidia, or both (Figure 45–17).

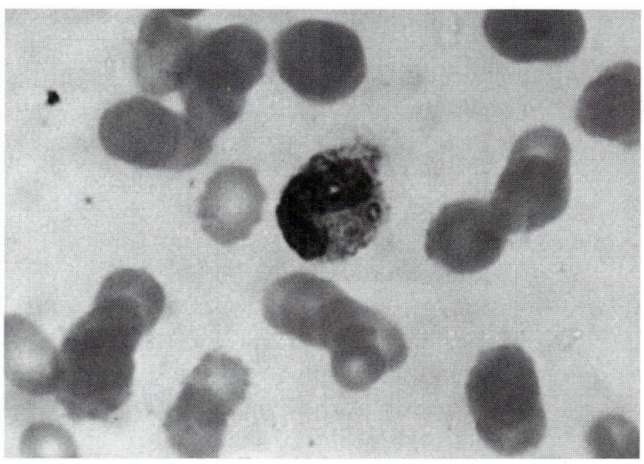

Figure 45–16. *Histoplasma capsulatum.* Macrophage containing blastoconidia (blastospores).

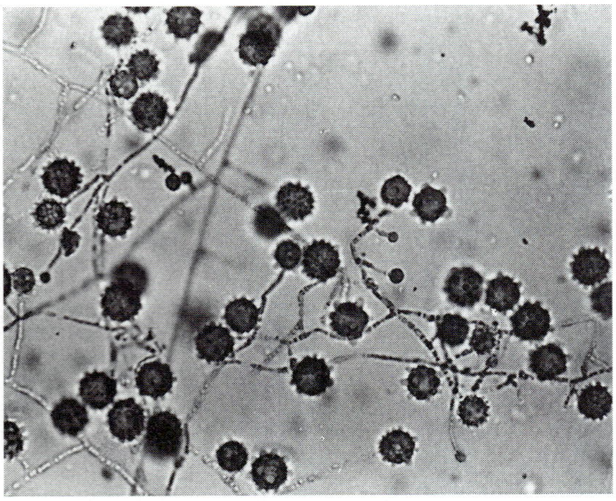

Figure 45–17. *Histoplasma capsulatum.* Macro and microconidia in culture at 20 °C.

Antigenic Structure

After initial infection with *Histoplasma,* persons have positive responses to skin tests with histoplasmin, a filtrate of broth in which *Histoplasma* has been grown. The reaction is delayed and tuberculin-like. Polysaccharides with precipitating and CF activity can be isolated from the yeast phase or mycelium. Cross-reactions with blastomycin are significant.

Pathogenesis & Clinical Findings

Infection with *Histoplasma* occurs via the respiratory tract. Inhaled conidia are engulfed by alveolar macrophages and eventually develop into budding cells. Although organisms are soon spread throughout the body, more than 99% of infections are asymptomatic. In the remainder, a self-limited flu-like syndrome with fever, chills, myalgias, headaches, and nonproductive cough is typical. These symptoms resolve spontaneously with no therapy. The small inflammatory or granulomatous foci in the lungs and spleen heal with calcification. If infection is the result of heavy exposure (usually do to disturbance or contact with contaminated soil), then symptomatic acute histoplasmosis can occur in up to 100% of exposed individuals. Chronic cavitary histoplasmosis occurs most often in men. Severe, disseminated histoplasmosis develops in a small minority of infected individ-uals, particularly infants, the elderly, and immunosuppressed individuals (including AIDS). The reticuloendothelial system is particularly involved, with lymphadenopathy, enlarged spleen and liver, high fever, anemia, and a high mortality rate in the absence of antifungal therapy. Ulcers of the nose, mouth, tongue, and intestine can occur. In such individuals, the histologic lesion shows focal areas of necrosis in small granulomas in many organs. Phagocytic cells (mononuclear or polymorphonuclear leukocytes of the blood, fixed reticuloendothelial cells of liver, spleen, and bone marrow) contain the small, oval yeast cells.

Many animals, including dogs and rodents, are spontaneously infected in endemic areas. Many laboratory animals can be infected with cultures.

Diagnostic Laboratory Tests

A. Specimens: Specimens consist of sputum, urine, scrapings from lesions, or buffy coat blood cells for culture; biopsies from bone marrow, skin, or lymph nodes for histologic study; and blood for serologic testing. Bone marrow culture has the highest yield in disseminated disease.

B. Microscopic Examination: The small, ovoid cells may be detected intracellularly in histologic sections stained with Gomori methenamine silver or in Giemsa-stained smears of bone marrow or blood. Specific immunofluorescence tests can identify *Histoplasma* cells in sections or smears.

C. Culture: Specimens are cultured at 37 °C on glucose-cysteine blood agar and on Sabouraud's agar at room temperature. Cultures must be kept for 3 weeks or more. Injection of organisms into mice may yield *Histoplasma* in lesions of spleen and liver upon culture.

D. Serology: Latex agglutination, precipitation, and immunodiffusion tests become positive within 2–5 weeks after infection. CF titers rise later in the disease; they fall to very low levels if the disease is inactive. With progressive disease, the CF test remains positive in high titer (1:32 or more). CF antibody cross-reacts with other fungal antigens. In immunodiffusion tests, two precipitin bands can be diagnostic: one (H) often connotes active histoplasmosis; the other (M) may arise from repeated skin testing or past contact.

E. Skin Test: The histoplasmin skin test (1:100) becomes positive soon after infection and remains positive for years. It may be negative in disseminated progressive disease. Repeated skin testing stimulates serum antibodies and thus interferes with serologic diagnosis.

Immunity

Following initial infection with *Histoplasma,* most persons appear to develop some degree of immunity. Immunosuppression may lead to dissemination. Although reactivation of quiescent histoplasmosis does occur, most disseminated disease appears to be the result of primary or repeat infection.

Treatment

Supportive therapy and rest enable most persons with symptomatic primary pulmonary histoplasmosis to recover. In disseminated disease, systemic treatment with amphotericin B is often curative, though prolonged treatment and monitoring for relapse are necessary. Patients with AIDS typically relapse despite therapy that would be curative in patients without AIDS. Therefore, maintenance therapy with oral ketoconazole or weekly amphotericin B is required. Ketoconazole can be of benefit for mild to moderate infection.

Epidemiology & Control

Histoplasmosis occurs at highest incidence in the United States. In the USA, areas endemic for *Histoplasma* include the central and eastern states and in particular the Ohio River Valley and portions of the Mississippi River Valley. The fungus has been recovered from the soil where human or animal outbreaks of infection have occurred. *Histoplasma* grows abundantly in soil mixed with bird feces (eg, starling roosts, chicken houses) or bat guano (caves). Exposure in such places may result in massive infection (eg, cave disease). Birds are not infected or carriers of the fungus; their excrement merely provides optimal culture conditions for growth.

In endemic areas, small infective inocula are spread by dust. A large proportion of inhabitants apparently become infected early in life but without symptoms. They develop positive histoplasmin skin tests and occasionally have miliary calcifications in the lungs. In the USA, midwestern cities have experienced large urban outbreaks of histoplasmosis following windstorms carrying dust. Clinical histoplasmosis infection in such outbreaks occurred somewhat more frequently in black than in white residents. The disease is not communicable from person to person. Spraying of formaldehyde on infected soil may destroy *Histoplasma.*

HISTOPLASMA CAPSULATUM VAR *DUBOISII*

Histoplasma capsulatum var *duboisii* is a variant of *H capsulatum* and is the cause of African histoplasmosis. The disease differs from classic histoplasmosis in that there is very little if any lung involvement. There are suppurative and granulomatous lesions of the cutaneous and subcutaneous tissues and bone. Pathologically, there are many large yeasts found within giant cells.

BLASTOMYCES DERMATITIDIS

Blastomyces dermatitidis is a dimorphic fungus that grows in mammalian tissues as a budding cell and in culture at 20 °C as a mold (Figure 45–18). It causes **blastomycosis,** a chronic granulomatous disease which until recently was recognized only in Canada, the USA, and Mexico and was referred to as **North American blastomycosis.** Indigenous cases have now been reported in Central and South America, Africa, the Middle East, Poland, and India, indicating a worldwide distribution. Nonetheless, it is associated with specific geographic locales. For example, North American disease is never seen in the Far West or New England.

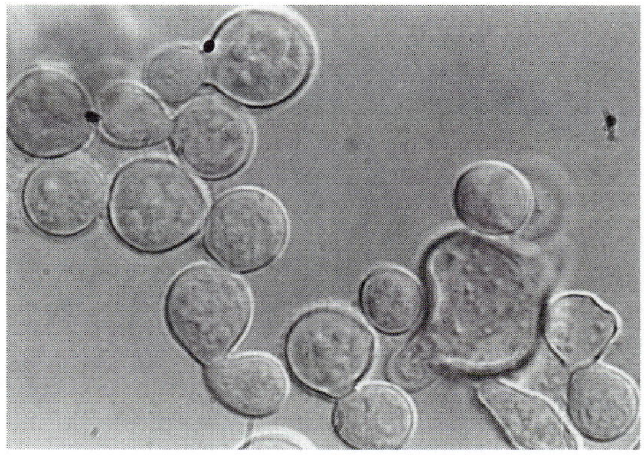

A

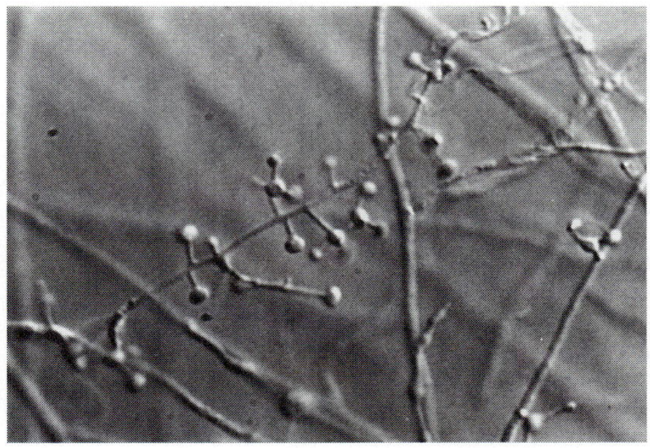

B

Figure 45–18. *Blastomyces dermatitidis.* ***A:*** In tissue or culture at 37 °C. ***B:*** In culture at 20 °C on Sabouraud's agar.

The ascomycetous sexual stage is called *Ajellomyces dermatitidis.*

Morphology & Identification

In tissue, pus, or exudates, *Blastomyces* appears as a round, multinucleate, budding cell (8–15 μm) with a doubly refractile wall. Each cell usually has only one bud with a broad base. Colonies on blood agar at 37 °C are wrinkled, waxy, and soft, and the cells are morphologically similar to those in the tissue stage, though short hyphal segments may also be present. When cells are grown on Sabouraud's agar at room temperature, a white or brownish colony develops, with branching hyphae bearing round or ovoid conidia 2–10 μm in diameter on slender terminal or lateral conidiophores.

Antigenic Structure

Extracts of culture filtrates of *Blastomyces* contain **blastomycin,** probably a mixture of antigens. Blastomycin as a skin test gives positive delayed reactions in less than 50% of patients and lacks specificity. Cross-reactions with histoplasmin are common. Positive skin tests rapidly revert to negative in repeat testing, making epidemiologic surveys impossible. In CF tests, blastomycin is an unreliable antigen, giving cross-reactions with other fungal infections but also reacting to high titer in persons with widespread blastomycosis. Specific animal sera permit the demonstration of budding *Blastomyces* cells in tissues by means of immunofluorescence.

Pathogenesis & Clinical Findings

Human infection probably occurs most commonly via the respiratory tract. Mild and self-limited cases are recognized infrequently, but this may be due to the lack of an adequate skin or serologic test for subclinical or resolved primary infection. The most common clinical presentation is a pulmonary infiltrate in association with a variety of constitutional symptoms indistinguishable from other acute lower respiratory infections (fever, malaise, night sweats, cough, myalgias). Patients can also present with a chronic pneumonia. Histologic examination reveals a distinct "pyogranulomatous" reaction with neutrophils and noncaseating granulomas. When dissemination occurs, skin lesions on exposed surfaces are most common. They may evolve into ulcerated verrucous granulomas with an advancing border and central scarring. The border is filled with microabscesses and has a sharp, sloping edge. Lesions of bone, prostate, epididymis, and testis occur; other sites are less frequently involved. Unlike the other systemic mycoses, there does not appear to be an increased incidence of blastomycosis in the immunosuppressed (including AIDS).

Diagnostic Laboratory Tests

A. Specimens: Specimens consist of sputum, pus, exudates, urine, and biopsies from lesions.

B. Microscopic Examination: Wet mounts of specimens may show broadly attached buds on thick-walled cells. These may also be apparent in histologic sections and are most helpful in diagnosis.

C. Culture: Initial growth is best on Sabouraud's or enriched blood agar at 30 °C; cellular morphology is most typical at 37 °C.

D. Animal Inoculation: Massive doses of blastoconidia cultures injected intravenously or intraperitoneally into mice, guinea pigs, or rabbits are fatal in 5–20 days.

E. Serology: Blastoconidia antigens may give positive results in CF and immunodiffusion tests. A titer rise in successive sera may have diagnostic significance, but cross-reactions with other fungal antigens and false-positives are common. Results of serologic tests contribute little to diagnosis.

Treatment

Prior to the introduction of amphotericin B in 1956, blastomycosis carried a grave prognosis. Intravenous amphotericin B is curative in the majority of patients with pulmonary and disseminated disease. Relapse is rare. Ketoconazole and itraconazole for 6 months have both been shown to be efficacious in the treatment of blastomycosis, and treatment failure can usually be attributed to noncompliance. The decreased toxicities and oral route of administration make these agents the drugs of choice for blastomycosis, although amphotericin B is still used for the control of rapidly progressive or life-threatening disease.

Epidemiology

Blastomycosis is a relatively common finding in dogs and some other animals in endemic areas. Increases in the canine form may presage human outbreaks. Blastomycosis is not communicable from animals or humans. It is assumed that both animals and humans are infected by inhaling conidia from *Blastomyces* growing in soil. Unlike *Histoplasma,* direct isolation from the environment has rarely been successful even in point-source outbreaks. Successful isolation has been reported in association with rotting wood and beaver dams with high contents of organic matter.

PARACOCCIDIOIDES BRASILIENSIS

Paracoccidioides brasiliensis (Blastomyces brasiliensis) is a dimorphic fungus that causes **paracoccidioidomycosis,** the predominant systemic mycosis in Latin America.

Morphology & Identification

P brasiliensis resembles *B dermatitidis.* The principal difference is that in tissue and in culture at 37 °C, *P brasiliensis* forms thick-walled yeast cells (10–60 μm in tissue) that characteristically have multiple buds (Figure 45–19). At room temperature, cultures are slow-growing, mycelial with small conidia.

Pathogenesis & Clinical Findings

The infected organism is inhaled, and early lesions occur in the lung. Dissemination occurs later, primar-

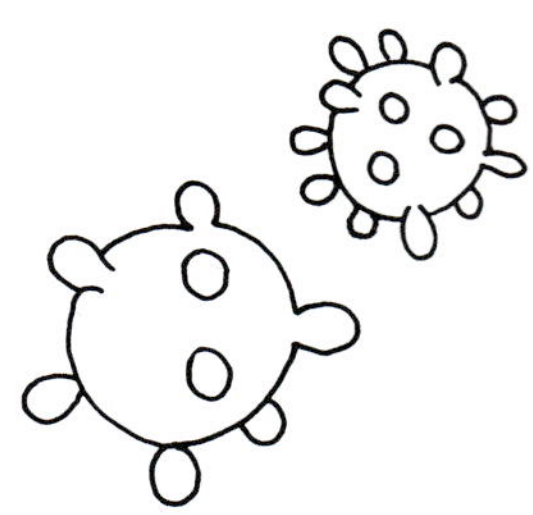

Figure 45–19. *Paracoccidioides brasiliensis.* In tissue or culture at 37 °C; multiple budding.

ily to the spleen, liver, mucous membranes, and skin. Asymptomatic lung infections may be followed by dissemination (sometimes years to decades), with frequent and severe oral mucous membrane lesions. Lymph node enlargement or gastrointestinal disturbances may be the presenting symptom. Histologically, there is either a granuloma with central caseation or microabscess formation. Organisms are frequently seen in giant cells or in pus and are always characterized by their multiple budding.

Skin tests can be performed using **paracoccidioidin,** a sterile filtrate of old broth cultures of the organism or extracts of the yeast phase. Some cross-reactions may occur with histoplasmin and blastomycin.

Diagnostic Laboratory Tests

In sputum, exudates, pus, or other material from lesions, the organism is often seen microscopically. Cultures on Sabouraud's or yeast extract agar are incubated at room temperature. Serologic testing is most useful for diagnosis. Paracoccidioidin is used as an antigen in such tests. The sera of healthy persons living in endemic areas fail to react in CF or precipitin tests. A significant serum antibody titer denotes tissue involvement with the disease, and CF titers of 1:2048 or more occur in active disease. In immunodiffusion tests, two well-defined precipitin lines are said to be diagnostic of paracoccidioidomycosis. In such persons, the skin test is also positive, but it is not diagnostic.

Treatment

In paracoccidioidomycosis of mild or moderate severity, oral administration of sulfonamides may produce striking remissions. Ketoconazole is effective in the management of cases that fail to respond to sulfonamides and of more severe paracoccidioidomycosis. Amphotericin B is currently a drug of last resort.

Epidemiology

Paracoccidioidomycosis occurs mainly in rural areas of Latin America, particularly among farmers. The disease manifestations are much more frequent in males than in females, but infection occurs equally in both sexes. The fungus has been isolated from soil. The disease is not communicable.

OPPORTUNISTIC MYCOSES

Fungi that usually do not induce disease may do so in persons who have altered host defense mechanisms. Such opportunists may infect any or all organs of the body. The underlying predisposing condition may allow only certain opportunistic fungi or actinomycetes to infect the host. Often several organisms infect a severely immunocompromised patient. *Candida* and other yeasts may be acquired from an endogenous source. Conidia of other fungi are commonly found in the air. Additional opportunists are *Fusarium, Penicillium, Geotrichum, Paecilomyces, Scopulariopsis,* and a number of black molds. Disease caused by known pathogenic fungi is often accelerated by impaired host defense mechanisms.

CANDIDA & RELATED YEASTS

Candida albicans is an oval, budding yeast that produces pseudohyphae both in culture and in tissues and exudates. It is a member of the normal flora of the mucous membranes in the respiratory, gastrointestinal, and female genital tracts. In such locations, it may gain dominance and be associated with pathologic conditions. Sometimes it produces progressive systemic disease in debilitated or immunosuppressed patients, particularly if cell-mediated immunity is impaired. *Candida* may produce bloodstream invasion, thrombophlebitis, endocarditis, or infection of the eyes and virtually any organ or tissue when introduced intravenously (tubing, needles, hyperalimentation, narcotics abuse, etc).

Morphology & Identification

In smears of exudates, *Candida* appears as a gram-positive, oval, budding yeast, 2–3 × 4–6 μm, gram-positive, elongated budding cells in chains **(pseudohyphae)** (Figure 45–20), or true hyphae. On Sabouraud's agar incubated at room temperature, soft, cream-colored colonies with a yeasty odor develop. The surface growth consists of oval budding cells. The submerged growth consists of **pseudomycelium.** This is composed of pseudohyphae that form blastoconidia at the nodes and sometimes chlamydoconidia terminally. *C albicans* ferments glucose and maltose, producing both acid and gas, and does not attack lactose. These carbohydrate fermentations, together with colonial and morphologic characteristics, differentiate *C albicans* from the other species of *Candida. C albicans* is much more common than any other *Candida* species in causing symptomatic infections; other *Candida* species that occasionally cause disease include *Candida parapsilosis, Candida tropicalis,* and *Torulopsis glabrata.* Other *Candida* species that live in soil and at times occur in normal human flora and are rarely implicated in human disease include *Candida kefyr, Candida krusei,* and *Candida guilliermondii.* Only the budding cells of 24-hour-old cultures of *C albicans*—and not of other species—will form germ tubes in 2–3 hours when placed in serum at 37 °C. The species *Candida stellatoidea* is a sucrose-negative variant of *Candida albicans* and *Candida pseudotropicalis* is a synonym for *Candida kefyr.*

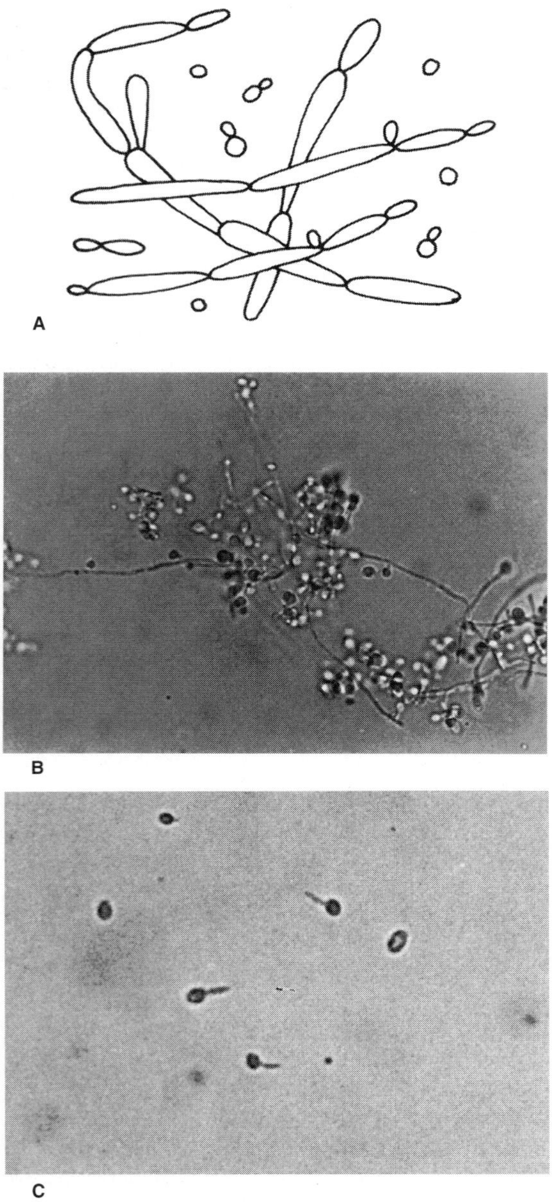

Figure 45–20. *Candida albicans. **A:*** Blastoconidia (blastospores) and pseudohyphae in exudate. ***B:*** Blastoconidia, pseudohyphae, and chlamydoconidia (chlamydospores) in culture at 20 °C. ***C:*** Young culture forms germ tubes when placed in serum for 3 hours at 37 °C.

Antigenic Structure

Agglutination tests with absorbed sera show that *C albicans* strains fall into two large serologic groups, A and B. Group A includes *C tropicalis. Candida* extracts for serologic and skin tests appear to consist of mixtures of antigens. Antibodies can be detected by precipitation, immunodiffusion, counterimmunoelectrophoresis, latex agglutination, and other tests, but the detection of circulating antibodies is not clinically useful for diagnosing disease due to *Candida.* In disseminated candidiasis, there are often circulating mannan antigens of *Candida,* and precipitating antibodies to nonmannan antigens can sometimes be detected. Virtually all normal human sera will contain IgG antibodies directed against *Candida mannan.*

Pathogenesis & Pathology

Upon intravenous injection into mice or rabbits, dense suspensions of *C albicans* result in widespread abscesses, particularly in the kidney, and death in less than 1 week.

Histologically, the various skin lesions in humans show inflammatory changes. Some resemble abscess formation; others resemble chronic granuloma. Large numbers of *Candida* are sometimes found in the intestinal tract following administration of oral antibiotics, eg, tetracyclines, but this usually causes no symptoms. *Candida* may be carried by the bloodstream to many organs, including the meninges, but usually cannot establish itself and cause miliary abscess formation except in a grossly debilitated host. Dissemination and sepsis may occur in patients with compromised cellular immunity, eg, those undergoing cancer chemotherapy or those with lymphoma, AIDS, or other conditions.

Clinical Findings

Among the principal predisposing factors to *Candida* infection are the following: diabetes mellitus, general debility, immunodeficiency, indwelling urinary or intravenous catheters, intravenous opioid abuse, administration of antimicrobials (which alter the normal bacterial flora), and corticosteroids.

A. Mouth: Infection of the mouth (thrush) occurs—mainly in infants and in AIDS patients—on the buccal mucous membranes and appears as white adherent patches consisting largely of pseudomycelium and desquamated epithelium, with only minimal erosion of the membrane. Growth of *Candida* in the mouth is enhanced by corticosteroids, antibiotics, high levels of glucose, and immunodeficiency.

B. Female Genitalia: Vulvovaginitis resembles thrush but produces irritation, intense itching, and discharge. Loss of an acid pH in the vagina predisposes to candidal vulvovaginitis. Acid pH is normally maintained by the bacterial flora in the vagina. Diabetes, pregnancy, progesterone, and antibiotic therapy predispose to disease.

C. Skin: Infection of the skin occurs principally in moist, warm parts of the body, such as the axilla, intergluteal folds, groin, or inframammary folds; it is most common in obese and diabetic individuals. The infected areas become red and weeping and may develop vesicles.

Candida infection of the interdigital webs of the hands is seen most frequently following repeated prolonged immersion in water; it is most common in homemakers, cooks, and vegetable and fish handlers.

D. Nails: Painful, reddened swelling of the nail fold, resembling a pyogenic paronychia, may lead to thickening and transverse grooving of the nails and eventually loss of the nail.

E. Lungs and Other Organs: *Candida* infection may be a secondary invader of lungs, kidneys, and other organs where a preexisting disease is present (eg, tuberculosis or cancer). In uncontrolled leukemia and in immunosuppressed or surgical patients, candidal lesions may occur in many organs. *Candida* endocarditis (often due to *C parapsilosis*) occurs particularly in narcotics addicts or on prosthetic valves. Candiduria sometimes develops after urinary catheterization, but it tends to subside spontaneously.

F. Chronic Mucocutaneous Candidiasis: This disorder is a sign of deficiency of cellular immunity in children.

Diagnostic Laboratory Tests

A. Specimens: Specimens consist of swabs and scrapings from surface lesions, sputum, exudates, and material from removed intravenous catheters.

B. Microscopic Examination: Sputum, exudates, thrombi, etc, may be examined in Gram-stained smears for pseudohyphae and budding cells. Skin or nail scrapings are first placed in a drop of 10% potassium hydroxide.

C. Culture: All specimens are cultured on Sabouraud's agar at room temperature and at 37 °C; typical colonies are examined for cells and budding pseudomycelia. Chlamydoconidia production by *C albicans* on cornmeal-polysorbate 80 agar is an important differential test.

D. Serology: A carbohydrate extract of group A *Candida* gives positive precipitin reactions with sera of 50% of normal persons and 70% of persons with mucocutaneous candidiasis. In systemic candidiasis, a rise in the titer of antibodies to *Candida* may be detected by various tests, but serologic testing for candidiasis has no proved clinical utility.

E. Skin Test: A *Candida* skin test is almost universally positive in normal adults. It is therefore used as an indicator of competent cellular immunity.

Immunity

Animals can be immunized actively and are then resistant to disseminated candidiasis. Human sera often contain IgG antibody that clumps *Candida* in vitro and may be candidacidal. The basis of resistance to candidiasis is complex and incompletely understood.

Treatment

Orally administered nystatin is not absorbed, remains in the gut, and has no effect on systemic *Candida* infections. Ketoconazole has produced striking therapeutic response in some systemic *Candida* infections, especially in mucocutaneous candidiasis. Amphotericin B intravenously is the widely accepted effective treatment for most forms of deep candidiasis. Amphotericin B can be given in conjunction with flucytosine orally for enhanced effect in disseminated candidiasis. In *Candida* vulvovaginitis, ketoconazole maintenance therapy may be required.

Mucocutaneous candidiasis occurs mainly in immunodeficient children and occasionally responds to the administration of transfer factor obtained from persons with active cell-mediated reactions to *Candida.* Ketoconazole therapy is the drug of choice for long-term control of chronic mucocutaneous candidiasis.

Local lesions are best treated by removing the cause, ie, avoiding moisture; keeping affected areas cool, powdered, and dry; and withdrawing antibiotics. There is no evidence to support vaccine therapy. Various chemicals have been employed topically with more or less success, eg, 1% gentian violet for thrush and parahydroxybenzoic acid esters, sodium propionate, candicidin, or 2% miconazole for vaginitis. Nystatin suppresses intestinal and vaginal candidiasis.

Epidemiology & Control

The most important preventive measure is to avoid interfering with the normal balance of microbial flora and with normal host defenses. *Candida* infection is not communicable, since virtually all persons normally harbor the organism.

CRYPTOCOCCUS NEOFORMANS

Cryptococcus neoformans is a yeast characterized by a thick carbohydrate capsule both in culture and in tissue fluids. It occurs widely in nature and is found in very large numbers in dry pigeon feces. Human disease is usually associated with immunosuppression or malignancy but occasionally is seen in apparently normal hosts.

Morphology & Identification

In spinal fluid or tissue, *Cryptococcus* is round or ovoid, 4–12 μm in diameter, often budding, and surrounded by a thick capsule (Figure 45–21). On Sabouraud's agar at room temperature, the cream-colored colonies are shiny and mucoid. Cultures do not ferment carbohydrates but assimilate glucose, maltose, sucrose, and galactose (but not lactose). Urea is hydrolyzed. In contrast to nonpathogenic cryptococci, *Cryptococcus* grows well at 37 °C on most laboratory media provided they do not contain cycloheximide. Mating of serotypes A and D or B and C gives rise to mycelia and basidiospores of *Filobasidiella neoformans* var *neoformans* or *Filobasidiella neoformans* var *gatti.*

Antigenic Structure

Four serologic types of capsular polysaccharides–A, B, C, and D—have been identified. The capsular anti-

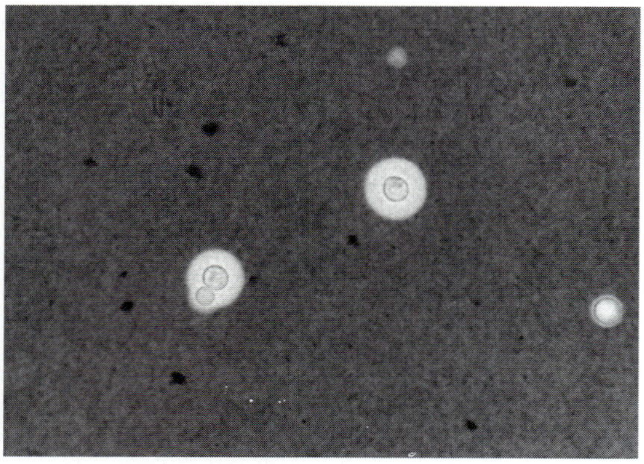

Figure 45–21. *Cryptococcus neoformans.* India ink preparation of spinal fluid.

gen may be dissolved in spinal fluid, serum, or urine and can be detected with specific antisera to the carbohydrate by latex agglutination (particles coated with antibody) and other tests. The detection of cryptococcal capsular antigen is diagnostically reliable. Several serologic tests also can detect antipolysaccharide antibodies. The presence of these antibodies does not denote increased resistance to recurrence.

Pathogenesis

Infection in humans occurs via the respiratory tract and is either asymptomatic or associated with nonspecific pulmonary signs and symptoms. Very massive inhalation of cells may result in progressive systemic disease in a normal person. Usually, however, cryptococcosis is an opportunistic infection. In immunodeficient or immunosuppressed persons, the pulmonary infection may disseminate systemically and establish itself in the central nervous system and other organs.

Histologically, the reaction varies from mild inflammation to formation of typical granulomas.

Clinical Findings

Infection with *Cryptococcus* may remain subclinical. The commonest clinical manifestation is a slowly developing chronic meningitis with spontaneous remissions and exacerbations. The meningitis may resemble a brain tumor, brain abscess, degenerative central nervous system disease, or any mycobacterial or fungal meningitis. Cerebrospinal fluid pressure and protein content may be greatly increased and the cell count elevated, whereas the sugar content is normal or low. In addition, there may be lesions of skin, lungs, or other organs.

The course of cryptococcal meningitis may fluctuate over long periods, but ultimately all untreated cases are fatal. The disease is particularly common in immunocompromised persons, eg, AIDS patients. It is not transmitted from person to person.

Diagnostic Laboratory Tests

A. Specimens: Specimens consist of spinal fluid, exudates, sputum, urine, and serum.

B. Microscopic Examination: Specimens are examined in wet mount, both directly and after mixing with India ink (which makes the large capsule stand out around the budding cell). Immunofluorescent stain is applied to dried smears. Filtration of cerebrospinal fluid through Millipore filters may reveal the organism.

C. Culture: Growth is rapid at 20–37 °C on Sabouraud's agar and other laboratory media provided they do not contain cycloheximide. Urea is hydrolyzed. *Cryptococcus* colonies produce a diagnostic brown pigment on bird seed (Niger seed) media.

D. Serology: Tests for cryptococcal polysaccharide capsular antigen can be performed on cerebrospinal fluid and serum. Latex slide agglutination for cryptococcal antigen in either cerebrospinal fluid or serum are positive in 90% of patients with cryptococcal meningitis. With effective treatment, the antigen titer drops.

Treatment

Combination therapy of amphotericin B and flucytosine has been considered the treatment of choice for cryptococcal meningitis, although the benefit of the added flucytosine remains controversial. Fluconazole penetrates the cerebrospinal fluid well and may become the preferred therapy for cryptococcal meningitis. Ketoconazole does not benefit patients with cryptococcal meningitis. Although amphotericin B (with or without flucytosine) is curative in most patients with cryptococcal meningitis, AIDS patients with cryptococcosis will almost always relapse when amphotericin B is withdrawn. For AIDS patients, long-term suppressive therapy with oral fluconazole is required.

Epidemiology & Control

Bird droppings (particularly pigeons) containing *Cryptococcus* are the major source of infection for animals and humans. The organism grows luxuriantly in pigeon excreta, but the birds are not infected. One method of control is reduction of the pigeon population and site decontamination with alkali. Serologic studies indicate that most individuals have been exposed to *Cryptococcus* and presumably had subclinical infections.

ASPERGILLOSIS

Broadly defined, **aspergillosis** is a group of mycoses with diverse causes and pathogenesis. *Aspergillus fumigatus* is a ubiquitous mold found on decaying vegetation. It may colonize and then invade tissues in a traumatized cornea or in burns, wounds, or the external ear (otitis externa). It and other *As-*

pergillus species become opportunistic invaders in immunodeficient persons (eg, in patients with chronic granulomatous disease—but not in AIDS patients) or individuals with anatomic abnormalities of the respiratory tract (pulmonary aspergillosis). Various species of *Aspergillus* produce aflatoxins in foods.

In tissues, exudates, or sputum, *Aspergillus* species occur as filamentous, septate structures that usually branch dichotomously. Cultures on Sabouraud's agar incubated at 37–40 °C grow as gray-green colonies with a central dome of conidiophores. The latter support characteristic radiating chains of conidia (Figure 45–9). Extracts of cultures, particularly carbohydrates, are used as antigens in various serologic tests. Different forms of aspergillosis produce different serologic results, and rising antibody titers are of limited diagnostic help.

Pulmonary aspergillosis may occur in distinct forms. One is a "fungus ball" growing in a preexisting cavity (eg, tuberculous cavity, paranasal sinus, bronchiectasis) in which the *Aspergillus* does not invade tissue. Aspergillomas of the lung do not respond to antifungal therapy and are best managed by conservative measures unless massive hemoptysis is seen, in which case surgical resection is indicated and often curative. Paranasal aspergillomas respond to surgical resection. Aspergillomas may result in significant antibody responses to *Aspergillus* antigens.

A second form is an invasive pulmonary aspergillosis with *Aspergillus* spreading in the lung, giving rise to necrotizing pneumonia, hemoptysis, and secondary dissemination to other organs. This occurs mainly in immunodeficient or immunosuppressed persons and requires active antifungal drug therapy with amphotericin B. (Flucytosine is sometimes added, but its benefits are controversial.)

A third form is allergic bronchopulmonary aspergillosis, with asthma, eosinophilia, high serum IgE, and only minimal tissue invasion but abnormal bronchograms. *Aspergillus* antibodies may be demonstrable but have little diagnostic value. It has been claimed that the demonstration of galactomannan antigens in the circulating blood is evidence for invasive aspergillosis. Corticosteroids are beneficial for symptomatic relief.

Diagnosis of aspergillosis rests most securely on demonstration of hyphal fragments in tissue biopsies by methenamine-silver stain. Treatment of invasive aspergillosis in immunosuppressed patients is only marginally successful. The same applies to the rare postsurgical *Aspergillus* endophthalmitis that usually leads to rapid loss of the infected eye.

Other fungi that may invade tissues in an immunosuppressed host and produce hyphae that resemble *Aspergillus* species include *Pseudallescheria, Fusarium,* and *Curvularia.* These may produce disease states resembling the several forms of aspergillosis.

MUCORMYCOSIS (Zygomycosis, Phycomycosis)

Saprophytic zygomycetes of the order Mucorales (eg, *Mucor, Rhizopus* [Figure 45–4]) occasionally infect a specific group of compromised hosts. Patients suffering from diabetes mellitus (particularly with acidosis), extensive burns, leukemia, lymphoma, chronic illness, immunosuppression, and dialysis patients treated with deferoxamine are the most commonly infected with mucormycosis. *Rhizopus, Mucor,* and other species invade and proliferate in the walls of blood vessels, producing thrombosis. This most commonly occurs as rhinocerebral mucormycosis wherein the organism invades via the palate or nasal or paranasal sinus mucous membranes. Rapid extension into retro-orbital regions, other sinuses, regional and internal carotid arteries, and the brain is typical. Ischemic necrosis ensues, with massive tissue destruction. Less commonly, pulmonary, gastrointestinal, and disseminated mucormycosis occur and are also characterized by rapid tissue destruction.

Despite their rapid growth and simple nutritional requirements, the organisms are rarely cultured during life but are seen in histologic preparations of tissues as broad, nonseptate, irregular hyphae in thrombosed vessels or sinuses with surrounding leukocytic and giant cell responses.

In mucormycosis diagnosed during life, intensive therapy of the underlying disorder accompanied by systemic amphotericin B therapy and aggressive surgical debridement of infected tissue has resulted in remissions and occasional cure.

PNEUMOCYSTIS CARINII

Pneumocystis carinii until recently was thought to be a protozoan; however, on the basis of molecular biologic studies, is now recognized as a fungus with a close relationship to Ascomycotina. It is widely distributed in mammalian species (rats, mice, dogs, cats, ferrets, rabbits) but in the absence of immunosuppression rarely causes disease. Until the AIDS epidemic, human disease was confined to interstitial plasma cell pneumonitis in malnourished infants and immunosuppressed patients (corticosteroid therapy, antineoplastic therapy, and transplant recipients). Prior to the introduction of effective chemoprophylactic regimens, it was the leading cause of death among AIDS patients. Chemoprophylaxis has resulted in a dramatic decrease in the incidence of pneumocystis disease but has appeared to "chase" *Pneumocystis* out of lungs and into organs where *Pneumocystis* was heretofore rarely or never seen (spleen, lymph nodes, bone marrow).

Morphology & Identification

Pneumocystis occurs in two morphologically distinct forms, the so-called "trophozoites" and "cysts." The cyst form is the presumed sexual state, and intermediate forms may be seen. Trophozoites are small 2–6 μm, with irregular borders and a single nucleus. Cyst forms are large and contain four to eight nuclei. The cyst form stains with silver stain, toluidine blue, and calcofluor. As seen in most clinical specimens, the trophozoite and cyst forms are present in a tightly adherent mass of intermingled organisms that probable reflects their mode of growth in the host.

Antigenic Structure

Pneumocystis contains a surface glycoprotein of 90–120 kDa that can be detected by analysis of sera from acutely ill and normal individuals. Other minor antigens are also present. There is little or no cross-reaction between *Pneumocystis* found in human infections and those from animal infections.

Pathogenesis & Clinical Findings

Pneumocystis carinii is an extracellular pathogen. In the lung, growth is limited to the surfactant layer above alveolar epithelium. In non-AIDS patients, infiltration of the alveolar spaces with plasma cells leads to the so-called "interstitial plasma cell pneumonitis." Plasma cells are absent in AIDS-related pneumocystis pneumonia. Blockage of the gas-exchange interface results in cyanosis. Decreases in Po_2 are typically out of proportion to the radiologic findings.

Diagnostic Laboratory Tests

A. Specimens: Bronchoalveolar lavage or lung biopsy is usually necessary to make a diagnosis of pneumocystis pneumonia. Induced sputum can be used in some AIDS patients.

B. Microscopic Examination: Specimens can be stained for detection of either the "cyst" or "trophozoite" forms. Giemsa staining is rapid and reveals the clumps of the small trophozoite, but the procedure requires patience and a practiced eye. Toluidine blue, methenamine silver, or calcofluor staining will demonstrate the large cyst forms readily, though caution must be exercised to avoid misidentification of yeasts with *Pneumocystis* cysts. A specific monoclonal antibody is available for direct fluorescent examination of specimens.

C. Culture: While there are reports of maintaining viable organisms in coculture with tissue culture cells, there are no methods for the continuous in vitro culture of *Pneumocystis.* Cultivation is never used for diagnosis.

D. Animal Inoculation: While animal-to-animal transfer may be possible, there is no evidence that *Pneumocystis* from human infections can be transferred to any animal model.

E. Serology: While not clinically useful, serology has been used to establish the prevalence of infection (see below).

Immunity

In the absence of immunosuppression, *Pneumocystis* does not cause disease. Serologic evidence suggests that most individuals are infected in early childhood, and the organism has a worldwide distribution. Cell-mediated immunity presumably plays a dominant role in the resistance to disease, as AIDS patients often have significant antibody titers and *Pneumocystis* pneumonia is not usually seen until the CD4 lymphocyte count drops below 400/μL.

Treatment

Treatment can be divided into acute therapy and chemoprophylaxis. The same agents can be used for either. Trimethoprim-sulfamethoxazole, trimethoprim-dapsone, or pentamidine can be used. For acute therapy, parenteral therapy is necessary for rapid control. Prophylaxis can be achieved with oral trimethoprim-sulfamethoxazole or inhaled pentamidine.

Epidemiology & Control

The mode of infection is unknown. While some studies suggest acquisition via an airborne route, conclusive evidence is lacking. Horizontal transmission may be possible. No natural reservoir has been demonstrated, and it may be that *Pneumocystis* is an obligate parasite that is part of the normal human flora. Control of disease in susceptible patients can be achieved through chemoprophylaxis.

ACTINOMYCETES

The actinomycetes are a heterogeneous group of filamentous bacteria related to corynebacteria and mycobacteria and superficially resembling fungi. Characteristically, they grow as gram-positive, branching organisms that tend to fragment into bacteria-like pieces. Some actinomycetes are acid-fast. Most are free-living, particularly in soil. The anaerobic species are part of the normal flora of the mouth. Some of the aerobic species found in soil *(Nocardia, Streptomyces)* may cause disease in humans and animals.

ACTINOMYCOSIS

Actinomycosis is a chronic suppurative disease that spreads by direct extension, forms draining sinus tracts, and is caused by *Actinomyces israelii* and related anaerobic filamentous bacteria, including *Arachnia* species. These form part of the normal flora of the oral cavity, and it is not clear what transforms carriage of the organisms into invasive disease. When they invade tissues, *Actinomyces* species are often associated with other oral bacteria. *Actinomyces bovis* causes "lumpy jaw" in cattle.

Morphology & Identification

In tissue, *Actinomyces* species occur as branching filaments surrounded by suppurating, fibrosing inflammation. The typical finding is a "sulfur granule" in pus (Figure 45–22). It consists of a colony of gram-positive mycelial filaments surrounded by eosinophilic "clubs." The latter may be antigen-antibody complexes.

A. Typical Organisms: When a sulfur granule in pus is washed and crushed, it reveals a tangled mass of filaments that readily breaks up into coccoid or bacillary forms that are gram-positive and non-acid-fast and show characteristic V or Y branching.

B. Culture: "Sulfur granules" or other pus-containing *Actinomyces* can be washed and inoculated into thioglycolate liquid medium, streaked onto brain-heart infusion agar, and incubated anaerobically at 37 °C. In thioglycolate, *A israelii* grows as fluffy balls near the bottom of the tube, whereas *A bovis* produces general turbidity. On solid media, *A israelii* produces small "spidery" colonies in 2–3 days that in 10 days become white, heaped-up, irregular—or sometimes smooth—larger colonies. Other species may have different colony forms.

C. Growth Characteristics: Of the three species most commonly responsible for actinomycosis, *A israelii* does not hydrolyze starch but ferments xylose and mannitol, whereas *A bovis* hydrolyzes starch but does not ferment these sugars. *Arachnia propionica* yields large amounts of propionic acid. Most *Actinomyces* species are nonhemolytic, nonproteolytic, and catalase-negative.

Antigenic Structure

Gel diffusion methods or immunofluorescence can differentiate *A israelii* from other actinomycete species and from other filamentous anaerobes that may produce granules in tissues. Species-specific antigens (mainly polysaccharides from the cell wall) occur in acetone extracts of culture supernate. There are at least two serotypes of *A israelii.*

Pathogenesis & Pathology

Typical *A israelii* can be found on teeth and in tonsillar crypts of most normal persons. It is likely that trauma (eg, tooth extraction), pyogenic or necrotizing bacterial infection, or aspiration precipitates clinical actinomycosis.

The typical lesion consists of an abscess with central necrosis, surrounded by granulation tissue and fibrous tissue; the pus often contains "sulfur granules" and may drain to the outside through sinuses. Histologically, the lesions are not typical unless sulfur granules can be found or *Actinomyces* cultured. In early lesions, a mixed bacterial flora is often seen.

Clinical Findings

The characteristic appearance of actinomycosis is a hard, red, relatively nontender swelling that usually develops slowly. It becomes fluctuant, points to a surface, and eventually drains, forming a chronic sinus tract with little tendency to heal. Lesions extend by contiguity. Dissemination via the bloodstream is very rare.

In about half of cases of actinomycosis, the initial lesion is cervicofacial, involving the face, neck, tongue, or mandible. Dental procedures or maxillofacial injuries are typical precipitating events. About one-fifth of cases show predominant involvement of lungs (thoracic actinomycosis), with abscesses or empyema. In a similar number, the primary lesion is in the cecum, appendix, or pelvic organs and may develop multiple draining fistulas (abdominal actinomycosis). Most patients with abdominal actinomycosis have a recent history of surgery, penetrating trauma, or intestinal perforation. Pelvic actinomycosis has occurred particularly in women wearing intrauterine contraceptive devices (IUDs). Rarely, central nervous

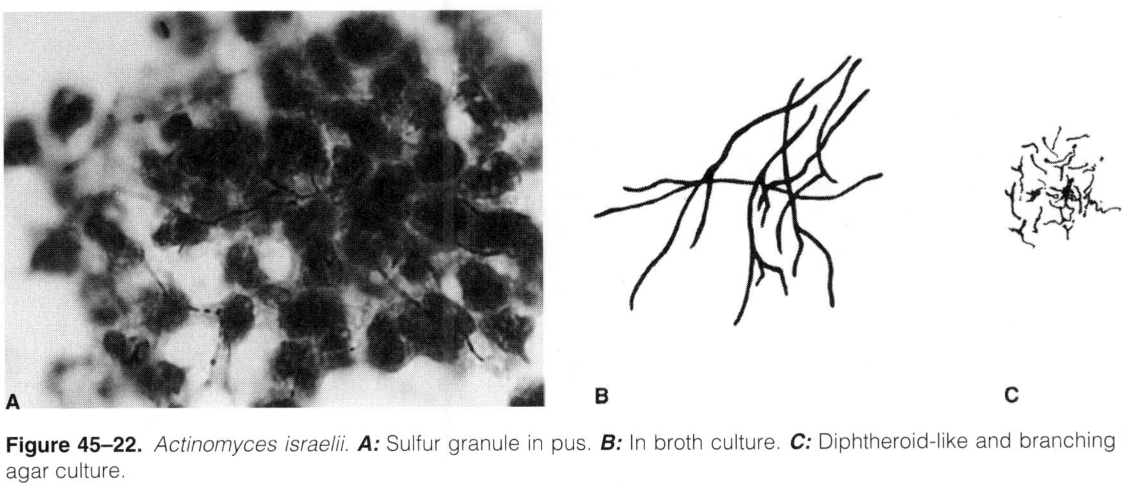

Figure 45–22. *Actinomyces israelii.* ***A:*** Sulfur granule in pus. ***B:*** In broth culture. ***C:*** Diphtheroid-like and branching in agar culture.

system and musculoskeletal actinomycosis is reported. *A israelii, A propionica,* and other species may cause similar disease.

Diagnostic Laboratory Tests

Animal inoculation, skin tests, and serologic tests are not useful.

A. Specimens: Specimens consist of pus from lesions, sinus tracts, or fistulas and sputum or tissue biopsy material.

B. Microscopic Examination: Every effort must be made to find "sulfur granules." These are rinsed, crushed, examined, and cultured. The appearance in wet mount of the central mycelium and peripheral clubs is characteristic (Figure 45–22). If no granules are found, stained smears of gram-positive branching rods and filaments are suggestive.

C. Culture: Material inoculated into thioglycolate medium and streaked onto brain-heart infusion blood agar plates must be incubated anaerobically for at least 2 weeks. The cultures are examined intermittently for characteristic morphologic features.

Immunity

Actinomyces organisms are part of the normal body flora. It is uncertain whether antibodies or cell-mediated reactions are produced until tissue invasion occurs. Eosinophilic clubs are not present on granules found in tonsillar crypts; these eosinophilic reactions in tissue granules may denote an antigen-antibody complex.

Treatment

Prolonged administration of penicillin is effective in many cases. Clindamycin or erythromycin are effective in penicillin-allergic patients. However, drugs may penetrate the abscesses poorly, and some of the tissue destruction may be irreversible. Surgical drainage and surgical removal are accepted forms of treatment.

Epidemiology

Because of the many free-living actinomycetes and the occurrence of "lumpy jaw" in cattle, it was at one time believed that actinomycosis in humans was acquired from grasses, straws, etc, which acted by traumatizing the mucous membranes and introducing the causative organism. However, it is now established that potentially pathogenic *A israelii* is a common inhabitant of mucous membranes in the mouth, so that no introduction from the outside need be postulated. The disease is not communicable from one person to another.

Most isolates from human sources are *A israelii;* most isolates from bovine sources are *A bovis.*

NOCARDIOSIS

Nocardia species and *Streptomyces* species are aerobic actinomycetes that occur in soil. *N asteroides* is the main cause of nocardiosis, an opportunistic human pulmonary disease that may spread to other parts of the body. *N brasiliensis* and *N caviae* are infrequent causes of nocardiosis. These organisms may also produce mycetoma (see above under Subcutaneous Mycoses).

Morphology & Identification

N asteroides has thin, gram-positive, branching filaments that may fragment into bacillary or coccoid forms. Many isolates are acid-fast when decolorized with 1% sulfuric acid ("partial acid-fastness"). Bacillary and filamentous forms may be seen in tissue exudates or in pus. Granules similar to those in actinomycosis or mycetoma are never seen, though filamentous clusters and colonies may occur. *Streptomyces* organisms are not acid-fast and do not fragment into bacillary forms.

Nocardia species grow aerobically on many simple media. Growth is variable and slow. Colonies are waxy, with pigmentation varying from yellow to orange or red. White aerial hyphae may form over the surface of the colony. Sporulation occurs by fragmentation into arthrospores. *N asteroides* will not grow in gelatin media and is unable to digest casein or ferment carbohydrates. *N brasiliensis* gives positive results in these tests and often produces β-lactamase. All nocardiae are urease-positive. Chromatographic identification of cell wall constituents is used to differentiate species.

Antigenic Structure

Filtrates from *Nocardia* grown in broth can serve as antigen in various serologic tests. Antibodies occur in disease, but false-positive reactions occur in mycobacterial infections. Nocardiae and mycobacteria evidently share antigens.

Pathogenesis & Clinical Findings

Nocardiosis begins as a pulmonary infection that may be subclinical or produce pneumonia. It can easily be confused with tuberculosis and pulmonary malignancy. The localized lesion may remain chronic as an enlarging abscess, sinus tract, or cavity. There is a predilection for brain abscess formation by hematogenous spread. Kidney lesions may also develop and extend through the cortex to the medulla. Disease caused by these organisms is most commonly seen in patients immunosuppressed by disease (eg, leukemia, lymphoma, AIDS) or drugs.

Diagnostic Laboratory Tests

A. Specimens: Specimens consist of sputum, pus, spinal fluid, and biopsy material. Serologic tests are unreliable at present. Sonicated extracts of *Nocardia* species may give precipitin lines with sera of infected persons in immunodiffusion tests.

B. Microscopic Examination: Gram-stained smears show coccal and bacillary forms or tangled masses of branching rods. Some strains are partially acid-fast.

C. Culture: *Nocardia* species grow on most laboratory media but may be inhibited by the presence of antibacterial antibiotics in the media. Guinea pigs, mice, and rabbits are susceptible to experimental infection.

D. Tissue Sections: Nocardiae are stained by methenamine-silver stain.

Treatment

The sulfonamides are the drugs of choice; trimethoprim-sulfamethoxazole may be slightly better, and minocycline is also effective. Amikacin and third-generation cephalosporins also show significant in vitro activity and may be useful either alone or in combination with trimethoprim-sulfamethoxazole. Surgical drainage or resection may be required. Treatment of the underlying disorder should be attempted.

Epidemiology

Potentially pathogenic nocardiae are ubiquitous in soil and probably enter the body by the respiratory route or through breaks in the skin. Infections in dogs, other pets, and farm animals are fairly common. Mastitis in dairy cattle is at times widespread. Nocardiosis is not transmitted from person to person.

HYPERSENSITIVITY TO FUNGI

In the course of many fungal infections, delayed type hypersensitivity develops to one or more antigens of the fungus. This is true whether the organism grows as a saprophyte (see section on *Aspergillus*) or as an invasive opportunist and whether it grows on surfaces, in cavities, or in tissues. Inhalation of actinomycetes or molds growing in the environment may cause allergic pneumonitis (see Chapter 8). Hypersensitivity evidenced by positive skin tests with fungal extracts may be helpful in diagnosis, but such skin tests are often negative in persons with disseminated systemic involvement. The return of a positive skin test reaction may be a sign of effective chemotherapy and of improved prognosis.

MYCOTOXINS

Many fungi produce poisonous substances called mycotoxins that can cause acute or chronic intoxication and damage. The mycotoxins are not directly related to the invasion or disease caused by fungi but represent intoxications. Ingestion of poisonous mushrooms (eg, *Amanita phalloides*) may cause severe or fatal damage to the liver and kidney. Chronic damage or neoplasms may be induced in animals or humans following ingestion of small quantities of toxin on contaminated food (eg, **aflatoxin** from *Aspergillus flavus*). Derivatives of fungal products (eg, LSD) may cause profound mental derangement.

ANTIFUNGAL CHEMOTHERAPY

In stark contrast to the ever-expanding armamentarium of antibacterial agents is the limited number of clinically useful antifungal agents. The reasons for this discrepancy lie in the close relation between the pathogenic fungi and their mammalian hosts. Many biochemical pathways that provide useful targets for antibacterial agents are simply lacking in fungi, and pathways that could be targets are shared by the mammalian host. For these reasons, many compounds that show significant in vitro antifungal activity cannot be used therapeutically because of host toxicity. The primary target of antifungal chemotherapeutic agents is the fungal membrane. Most fungi contain ergosterol as the principal membrane sterol. Humans do not synthesize ergosterol and utilize cholesterol as the predominant membrane sterol. With the exceptions of griseofulvin and flucytosine (which have very narrow indications), antifungal agents act by either binding ergosterol (amphotericin B) or inhibiting ergosterol biosynthesis (antifungal azoles).

AMPHOTERICIN B

Description

Amphotericin B is a complex antibiotic polyene produced by a *Streptomyces* species and has negligible antibacterial properties. It strongly inhibits the growth of several pathogenic fungi in vitro and in vivo. Amphotericin B binds to sterols on the fungal cell membranes and disturbs their function.

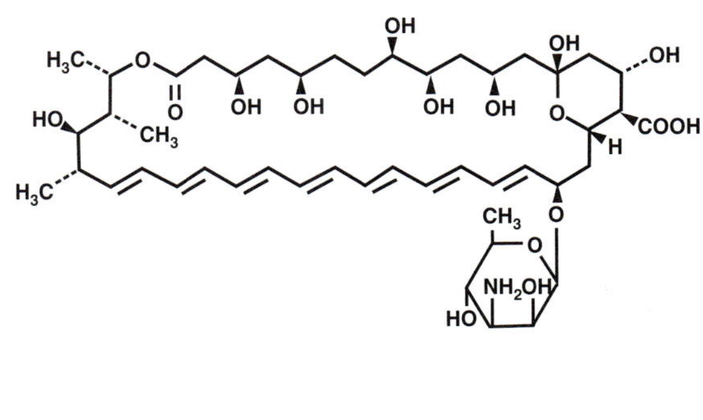

Mechanism of Action

Amphotericin B is given intravenously as micelles with sodium deoxycholate dissolved in dextrose solution. Though the drug is widely distributed in tissues, it penetrates poorly to the cerebrospinal fluid. Upon encountering a fungal cell, amphotericin B firmly binds to ergosterol in the cell membrane. This interaction results in changes in membrane fluidity and perhaps the introduction of "amphotericin pore." Small molecules and ions are lost from the fungal cell, eventually resulting in cell death. Mammalian cells are relatively resistant to these actions because they lack ergosterol. Amphotericin binds weakly to the cholesterol in mammalian cell membranes, and this interaction probably accounts for its toxic side effects.

Indications

Amphotericin B is a broad-spectrum antifungal agent with demonstrated efficacy against most of the major systemic mycoses, including, but not limited to, coccidioidomycosis, blastomycosis, histoplasmosis, sporotrichosis, cryptococcosis, mucormycosis, and candidiasis. The response of the particular infection is dependent on the rapid institution of amphotericin B, the site of the infection, the immune status of the patient, and the inherent sensitivity of the pathogen. For fungal meningitis due to *Coccidioides* (but not *Cryptococcus*), intrathecal administration is necessary. Intra-articular therapy is useful in fungal joint infections. Combination therapy with flucytosine is probably beneficial in infections due to *Candida* and *Cryptococcus*. It is of note that infections caused by *Pseudallescheria boydii* appear to be refractory to amphotericin B.

Side Effects

Acute reactions that usually accompany the intravenous administration of amphotericin B include fever, chills, dyspnea, and hypotension. These effects can usually be alleviated by prior or concomitant administration of hydrocortisone or acetaminophen. Tolerance to the acute side effect develops during therapy.

Chronic side effects are usually the result of nephrotoxicity. Azotemia is almost always seen with amphotericin B therapy, and serum creatinine and ion levels must be closely monitored. Hypokalemia, anemia, renal tubular acidosis, headache, nausea, and vomiting are also frequently observed. While some of the nephrotoxicity is reversible, permanent reduction in glomerular and renal tubular function does occur. This damage can be correlated with the total dose of amphotericin B given.

FLUCYTOSINE

Description

Flucytosine (5-fluorocytosine) is a fluorinated derivative of cytosine. It is an oral antifungal compound that is primarily used in conjunction with amphotericin B for infections caused by *Candida* and *Cryptococcus*. It penetrates well into all tissues, including cerebrospinal fluid.

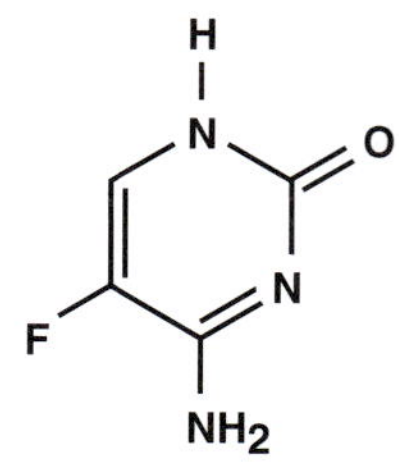

Flucytosine

Mechanism of Action

Susceptible fungi are capable of accumulating flucytosine via a membrane-bound permease. Flucytosine is then converted to fluorouracil by cytosine deaminase. Fluorouracil is a potent inhibitor of thymidylate synthetase, and this inhibition results in cell death. Mammalian cells lack cytosine deaminase and are therefore protected from the toxic effects of fluorouracil. Unfortunately, resistant mutants rapidly emerge, limiting the utility of flucytosine.

Indications

Flucytosine is primarily used in conjunction with amphotericin B for treatment of *Candida* and *Cryptococcus* infections. Flucytosine acts synergistically with amphotericin B in vitro against these organisms, and clinical trials suggest a beneficial effect of the combination, particularly in cryptococcal meningitis. The combination has also been shown to delay or eliminate the appearance of flucytosine-resistant mutants.

Side Effects

While flucytosine itself probably has little toxicity for mammalian cells and is relatively well tolerated, its conversion to fluorouracil results in a highly toxic compound that is probably responsible for the major side effects of this agent. Prolonged administration of flucytosine results in bone marrow suppression, hair loss, and abnormal liver function. The conversion of flucytosine to fluorouracil by enteric bacteria may cause colitis. Patients with AIDS may be more susceptible to bone marrow suppression by flucytosine, and serum levels should be closely monitored.

ANTIFUNGAL AZOLES (Figure 45–23)

Description

The antifungal imidazole (ketoconazole) and triazoles (fluconazole and itraconazole) are orally active agents useful in therapy in a wide range of systemic and localized fungal infections. The indications for their use are still being evaluated, but it is likely that

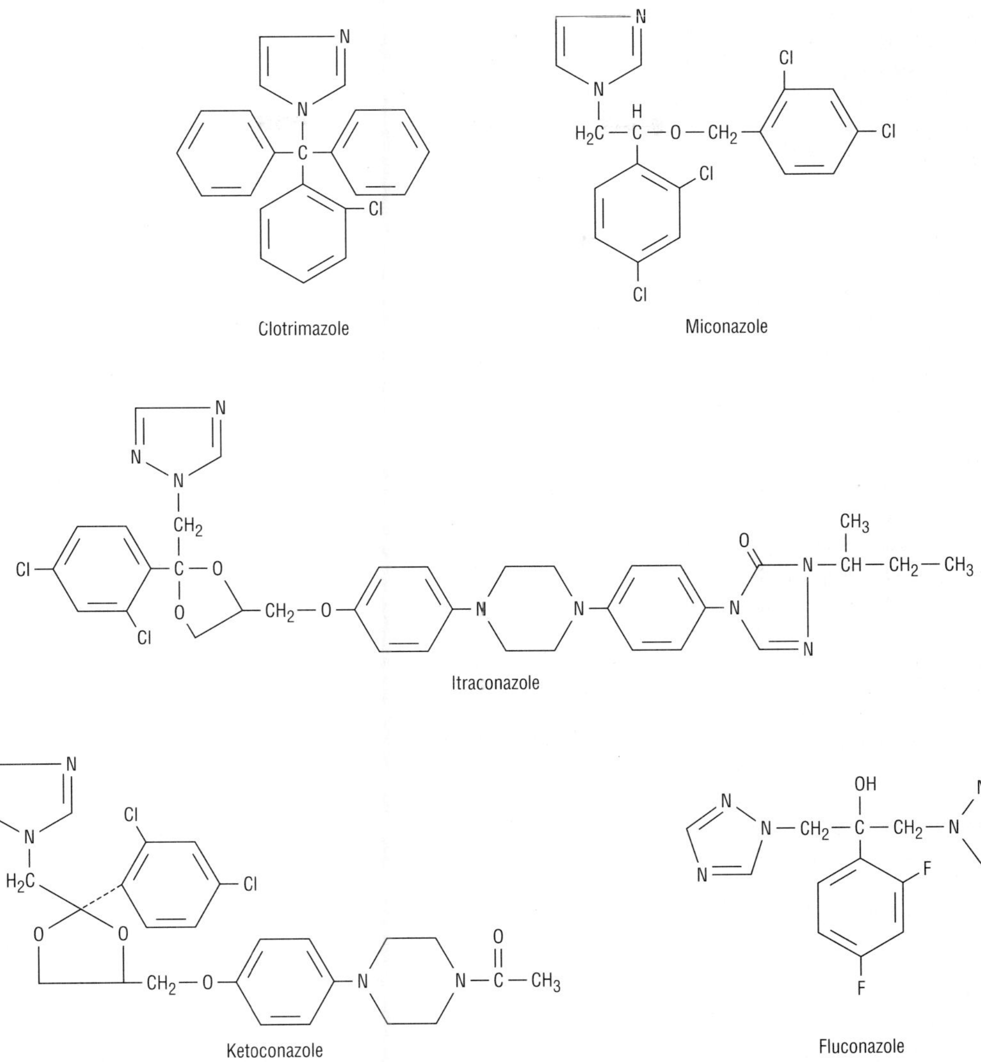

Figure 45–23. Structural formulas of the antifungal azoles. (Reproduced, with permission, from Katzung BG [editor]: *Basic and Clinical Pharmacology,* 6th ed. Appleton & Lange, 1995.)

they will supplant amphotericin B in many fungal infections because they can be administered orally and with less toxicity. Other imidazoles (miconazole and clotrimazole) which are too toxic for systemic administration are useful as topical agents and are discussed with the topical agents below.

Mechanism of Action

All antifungal azoles act by inhibition of fungal ergosterol biosynthesis. This inhibition is achieved by drug binding and interference with the function of the heme group in cytochrome P450 oxidases. The fungal P450 oxidase that is most sensitive to inhibition is 14-lanosterol demethylase. Other P450 enzymes (including mammalian enzymes involved in steroidogenesis) can be inhibited at higher concentrations. The blockage of ergosterol production leads to alterations in fungal membrane structure and function.

Indications

As noted above, the indications for the use of antifungal azoles will broaden as the results of long-term studies become available. Accepted indications for the use of antifungal azoles is listed below.

Ketoconazole is useful in the treatment of chronic mucocutaneous candidiasis and in extrameningeal chronic forms of blastomycosis, coccidioidomycosis, paracoccidioidomycosis, and histoplasmosis.

Fluconazole is unique among the antifungal azoles currently available in its ability to penetrate to the cerebrospinal fluid. This property and its demonstrated clinical efficacy make fluconazole an attractive alternative to amphotericin B in the treatment of cryptococcal and coccidioidal meningitis. In AIDS patients with cryptococcal meningitis, lifelong fluconazole maintenance therapy can prevent relapse. Oropharyngeal candidiasis in AIDS patients and candidemia in immunocompetent patients can also be treated with fluconazole.

Itraconazole indications overlap somewhat with those for fluconazole but may have activity against aspergillosis also. Although large-scale clinical trials have not been completed, animal models and case reports suggest that itraconazole may be useful in the treatment of invasive aspergillosis, which generally responds poorly to amphotericin B. Itraconazole has demonstrated efficacy in the primary and maintenance therapy of histoplasmosis in AIDS patients, histoplasmosis in immunocompetent patients, extrameningeal coccidioidomycosis, sporotrichosis, and blastomycosis.

Mucormycosis does not respond to antifungal azole therapy, and amphotericin B (in conjunction with surgical debridement) should be used for these infections.

Side Effects

The adverse effects of the antifungal azoles are primarily related to their ability to inhibit mammalian cytochrome P450 enzymes. Ketoconazole is the most toxic in this regard and will at therapeutic doses inhibit the synthesis of testosterone and cortisol. These inhibitions lead to gynecomastia, decreased libido, impotence, menstrual irregularity, and occasionally adrenal insufficiency. Fluconazole and itraconazole at recommended therapeutic doses do not show significant impairment of mammalian steroidogenesis, but this may change if increased dosages are used for the treatment of recalcitrant infections. All the antifungal azoles can cause both asymptomatic elevations in liver function tests and rare cases of hepatitis.

Since antifungal azoles interact with P450 enzymes that are also responsible for drug metabolism, some important drug interactions can occur. Increased antifungal azole concentrations can be seen when isoniazid, phenytoin, or rifampin is used. Antifungal azole therapy can also lead to higher than expected serum levels of cyclosporine, phenytoin, oral hypoglycemics, anticoagulants, digoxin, and probably many others. Serum monitoring of both drugs may be necessary to achieve a proper therapeutic ranges.

GRISEOFULVIN

Description

Griseofulvin is an orally administered antibiotic obtained from certain *Penicillium* species. It has no effect on bacteria or fungi producing systemic mycoses but suppresses certain dermatophytes.

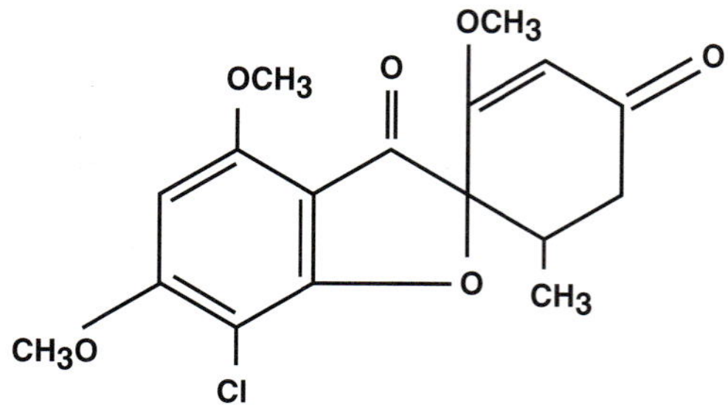

Griseofulvin

Mechanism of Action

After oral administration, griseofulvin is distributed throughout the body. The drug accumulates in the epidermis and other keratinized tissues (hair and nails). Keratin is the major nutritional source for dermatophytes, and the degradation of griseofulvin-impregnated keratin by these fungi results in the ingestion of the drug. Within the organism, griseofulvin is thought to interact with microtubules and disrupt mitotic spindle function, resulting in growth inhibition.

Indications

Griseofulvin is clinically useful for the treatment of dermatophyte infections of the skin, hair, and nails caused by *Trichophyton, Epidermophyton,* and *Microsporum* species. It has no effect on superficial or systemic candidiasis or any other systemic mycosis. Oral therapy for weeks to months is usually required.

Side Effects

Griseofulvin is generally well-tolerated. The most common side effect is headache, which usually resolves without discontinuation of the drug. Less frequently observed are gastrointestinal disturbances, drowsiness, and hepatotoxicity.

TOPICAL ANTIFUNGAL AGENTS

Nystatin

Nystatin is a polyene antibiotic structurally related to amphotericin B and probably shares a common mode of action. It can be useful in treatment of local candidal infections of the mouth and vagina. Nystatin may also suppress subclinical esophageal candidiasis and gastrointestinal overgrowth of *Candida.* No systemic absorption occurs, and there are no side effects.

Tolnaftate & Naftifine

Tolnaftate and naftifine are topical antifungal agents used in the treatment of tinea pedis, tinea cruris, tinea corporis, and tinea versicolor. Infections due to *Candida* are relatively resistant to these agents. Over-the-counter formulations are available as creams, powders, and sprays.

Clotrimazole, Miconazole, & Other Azoles

A variety of antifungal azoles which are too toxic for systemic use are available for topical uses. Clotrimazole and miconazole are the most widely used and are available in over-the-counter formulations. Ecoconazole, butoconazole, tioconazole, and terconazole are also available. There are no documented differences in efficacy or tolerance between any of these agents.

Topical antifungal azoles have a broad spectrum of activity. Tinea pedis, tinea corporis, tinea cruris, tinea versicolor, and cutaneous candidiasis respond well to local application of creams or powders. Vulvovaginal candidiasis can be treated with vaginal suppositories or creams. Clotrimazole is also available as an oral troche for treatment of oral and esophageal thrush in immunocompetent patients.

Other Topical Antifungal Agents

Undecylenic acid is available in many formulations for the over-the-counter treatment of tinea pedis and tinea cruris. Although it is effective and well-tolerated, antifungal azoles, naftifine, and tolnaftate are more effective. Haloprogin and ciclopirox are topical agents commonly used in dermatophyte infections.

REFERENCES

General

Kwon-Chung KJ, Bennett JE: *Medical Mycology,* Lea & Febiger, 1992.

Rippon JW: *Medical Mycology: The Pathogenic Fungi and the Pathogenic Actinomycetes,* 3rd ed. Saunders, 1988.

Actinomycosis

Burden P: Actinomycosis. J Infect 1989;19:95.

Schaal KP, Lee H-J: Actinomycete infections in humans: A review. Gene 1992;115:201.

Weese WC, Smith IM: Study of 57 cases of actinomycosis over a 36-year period. Arch Intern Med 1975;135: 1562.

Aspergillosis

Levitz SM: Aspergillosis. Infect Dis Clin North Am 1989; 3:1.

Rinaldi MG: Invasive aspergillosis. Rev Infect Dis 1983; 5:1061.

Blastomycosis

Bradsher RW: Blastomycosis. Clin Infect Dis 1992;14: S82.

Sarosi GA, Davies SF: Blastomycosis. Am Rev Respir Dis 1979;120:911.

Candidiasis

Crislip MA, Edwards JE: Candidiasis. Infect Dis Clin North Am 1989;3:103.

Saral R: *Candida* and *Aspergillus* infections in immunocompromised patients: An overview. Rev Infect Dis 1991;13:487.

Chromoblastomycosis

Fader RC, McGinnis MR: Infections caused by dematiaceous fungi: Chromoblastomycosis and phaeohyphomycosis. Infect Dis Clin North Am 1988;2:925.

Coccidioidomycosis

Ampel NM et al: Coccidioidomycosis: Clinical update. Rev Infect Dis 1989;11:897.

Einstein HE, Johnson RH: Coccidioidomycosis: New aspects of epidemiology and therapy. Clin Infect Dis 1993;16:349.

Galgiani JN: Coccidioidomycosis: Changes in clinical expression, serological diagnosis and therapeutic options. Clin Infect Dis 1992;14:S100.

Galgiani JN: Coccidioidomycosis. West J Med 1993;159: 153.

Cryptococcosis

Bulmer GS: Twenty-five years with *Cryptococcus neoformans.* Mycopathologia 1990;109:111.

Ellis DH, Pfeiffer TJ: Ecology, life cycle, and infectious propagule of *Cryptococcus neoformans.* Lancet 1990;336:923.

Kwon-Chung KJ et al: Recent advances in biology and immunology of *Cryptococcus neoformans.* J Med Vet Mycol 1992;30(Suppl 1):133.

Dermatophytes

Klotz SA: *Malassezia furfur.* Infect Dis Clin North Am 1989;3:53.

Macura AB: Dermatophyte infections. Int J Dermatol 1993;32:313.

Histoplasmosis

Sarosi GA, Johnson PC: Disseminated histoplasmosis in patients infected with human immunodeficiency virus. Clin Infect Dis 1992;14:S60.

Wheat LJ: Histoplasmosis. Infect Dis Clin North Am 1988;2:841.

Mucormycosis

Boelaert JR et al: Deferoxamine therapy and mucormycosis in dialysis patients: Report of an international registry. Am J Kidney Dis 1991;18:660.

Ingram CW et al: Disseminated zygomycosis: Report of four cases and review. Rev Infect Dis 1989;11:741.

Rinaldi MG: Zygomycosis. Infect Dis Clin North Am 1989;3:19.

Mycetoma

McGinnis MR, Fader RC: Mycetoma: A contemporary concept. Infect Dis Clin North Am 1988;2:939.

Mycotoxins

Berry CL: The pathology of mycotoxins. J Pathol 1988;154:301.

Klein AS et al: *Amanita* poisoning: Treatment and the role of liver transplantation. Am J Med 1989;86:187.

Krogh P: The role of mycotoxins in disease of animals and man. Soc Appl Bacteriol Symp Ser 1989;18:99S.

Nocardia

Beaman BL et al: Nocardia and nocardiosis. J Med Vet Mycol 1992;30(Suppl 1):317.

Curry WA: Human nocardiosis: A clinical review with selected case reports. Arch Intern Med 1980;140:818.

Smego RA Jr, Gallis HA: The clinical spectrum of *Nocardia brasiliensis* infection in the United States. Rev Infect Dis 1984;6:164.

Paracoccidioidomycosis

Brummer E et al: Paracoccidioidomycosis: An update. Clin Microbiol Rev 1993;6:89.

Restrepo A et al: The gamut of paracoccidioidomycosis. Am J Med 1976;61:33.

Pneumocystis carinii

Lipschik GY, Masur H: *Pneumocystis carinii* pneumonia (PCP). Prog Clin Parasitol 1991;2:27.

Masur H: Prevention and treatment of pneumocystis pneumonia. N Eng J Med 1992;327:1853.

Smulian AG, Walzer PD: The biology of *Pneumocystis carinii.* Crit Rev Microbiol 1992;18:191.

Sporotrichosis

Belknap, BS: Sporotrichosis. Dermatol Clin 1989;7:193.

Pluss JL, Opal SM: Pulmonary sporotrichosis: Review of outcome and treatment. Medicine 1986;65:143.

Antifungal Chemotherapy

Como JA, Dismukes WE: Oral azole drugs as systemic antifungal therapy. N Engl J Med 1993;330:263.

Odds FC: Itraconazole: A new oral antifungal agent with a very broad spectrum of activity in superficial and systemic mycoses. J Dermatol Sci 1993;5:65.

Warnock DW: Amphotericin B: An introduction. J Antimicrob Chemother 1991;28(Suppl B):27.

Medical Parasitology 46

*Donald Heyneman, PhD**

Although all of the medically significant microorganisms considered in this chapter are parasitic in their human hosts, the biomedical discipline of **parasitology** has traditionally been concerned only with the parasitic protozoa, helminths, and arthropods. This chapter offers a brief survey of the protozoan and helminthic parasites of medical importance. The text is supplemented by tabular materials and illustrations.† The books and articles listed at the end of the chapter are recommended for reference.

CLASSIFICATION OF PARASITES

The parasites of humans in the kingdom **Protozoa** are now classified under three phyla: **Sarcomastigophora** (containing the flagellates and amebas); **Apicomplexa** (containing the sporozoans); and **Ciliophora** (containing the ciliates). Within these great assemblages are found the important human parasites.

(1) Mastigophora, the flagellates, have one or more whip-like flagella and, in some cases, an undulating membrane (eg, trypanosomes). These include intestinal and genitourinary flagellates *(Giardia, Trichomonas, Dientamoeba, Chilomastix)* and blood and tissue flagellates *(Trypanosoma, Leishmania).*

(2) Sarcodina are typically ameboid and are represented in humans by species of *Entamoeba, Endolimax, Iodamoeba, Naegleria,* and *Acanthamoeba.*

(3) Sporozoa undergo a complex life cycle with alternating sexual and asexual reproductive phases, usually involving two different hosts (eg, arthropod and vertebrate, as in the blood forms). The subclass **Coccidia** contains the human parasites *Isospora, Toxoplasma,* and others. One of these, *Cryptosporidium,* has been implicated as a cause of intractable diarrhea among the immunosuppressed. Among the **Haemosporina** (blood sporozoans) are the malarial parasites (*Plasmodium* species) and the subclass *Piroplasmia,* which includes *Babesia* species. *Pneumocystis* has recently been shown to be a member of the Fungi rather than the Protozoa. It is another opportunistic parasite of immunosuppressed individuals.

(4) Ciliophora are complex protozoa bearing cilia distributed in rows or patches, with two kinds of nuclei in each individual. *Balantidium coli,* a giant intestinal ciliate of humans and pigs, is the only human parasite representative of this group.

The parasitic worms, or helminths, of human beings belong to two phyla:

(1) Platyhelminthes (flatworms) lack a true body cavity (celom) and are characteristically flat in dorsoventral section. All medically important species belong to the classes **Cestoda** (tapeworms) and **Trematoda** (flukes). The tapeworms of humans are band-like and segmented; the flukes are typically leaf-shaped, and the schistosomes narrow and elongate. The important tissue and intestinal cestodes of humans belong to the genera *Diphyllobothrium, Spirometra, Taenia, Echinococcus, Hymenolepis,* and *Dipylidium.* Medically important trematode genera include *Schistosoma, Paragonimus, Clonorchis, Opisthorchis, Heterophyes, Metagonimus, Fasciolopsis,* and *Fasciola.*

(2) Nemathelminthes (worm-like, separate-sexed, unsegmented roundworms) include many parasitic species that infect humans.

These are listed in Table 46–4 together with the other parasitic helminths. An essential procedure in diagnosis of many helminthic infections is microscopic recognition of ova or larvae in feces, urine, blood, or tissues. Illustrations of diagnostically important stages are found in appropriate sections of the text; important characteristics of microfilariae are listed in Table 46–5.

*Professor of Parasitology Emeritus, Department of Epidemiology and International Health, University of California, San Francisco; and Chairman, Emeritus, University of California, Berkeley–University of California, San Francisco, Joint Medical Program.

†The illustrations in this chapter are by P.H. Vercammen-Grandjean, DSc.

INTESTINAL FLAGELLATES

GIARDIA LAMBLIA

Giardia lamblia, a flagellate, is the only common protozoan found in the duodenum and jejunum of humans. It is the cause of giardiasis.

Giardia duodenalis is another name commonly ascribed to the parasite that causes human giardiasis; the term *Giardia intestinalis* is frequently used in Europe and *Lamblia intestinalis* in the former USSR. Much of the confusion is due to merging of species names now that human giardiasis is recognized as a zoonosis and species based on supposed single-host parasitism have been synonymized (see Epidemiology). Pending further taxonomic clarification, the name of the species first described, *G lamblia,* will be retained.

Morphology & Identification

A. Typical Organisms: The trophozoite of *G lamblia* is a heart-shaped, symmetric organism 10–20 μm in length (Figure 46–1). There are four pairs of flagella, two nuclei with prominent central karyosomes, and two axostyles (supporting rod-like organelles). A large concave sucking disk in the anterior portion occupies much of the ventral surface. The swaying or dancing motion of *Giardia* trophozoites in fresh preparations is unmistakable. As the parasites pass into the colon, they typically encyst. Cysts are found in the stool—often in enormous numbers. They are thick-walled, highly resistant, 8–14 μm in length, and ellipsoid and contain two nuclei as immature, four as mature cysts.

B. Culture: Cultivation, though possible, is not diagnostically useful.

Pathogenesis & Clinical Findings

G lamblia is usually only weakly pathogenic for humans. Cysts may be found in large numbers in the stools of entirely asymptomatic persons. In some persons, however, large numbers of parasites attached to the bowel wall may cause irritation and low-grade inflammation of the duodenal or jejunal mucosa, with consequent acute or chronic diarrhea associated with crypt hypertrophy, villous atrophy or flattening, and epithelial cell damage. The stools may be watery, semisolid, greasy, bulky, and foul-smelling at various times during the course of the infection. Malaise, weakness, weight loss, abdominal cramps, distention, and flatulence can occur. Children are more liable to clinical giardiasis than adults. Immunosuppressed individuals are especially liable to massive infection with severe clinical manifestations. Symptoms may continue for long periods.

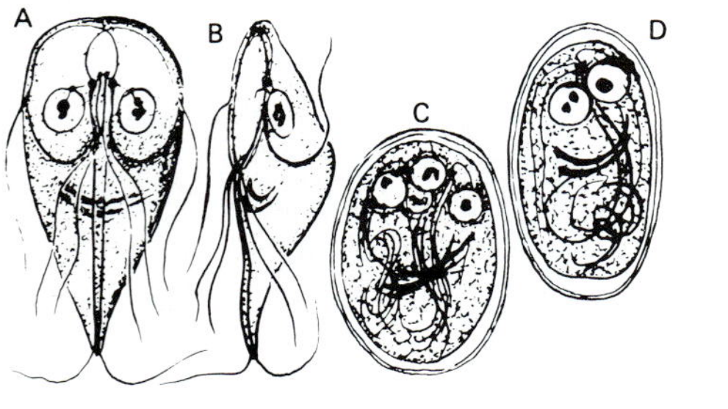

Figure 46–1. *Giardia lamblia. **A:*** "Face" and ***B:*** "profile" of vegetative forms; ***C*** and ***D:*** cysts (binucleate ***[D]*** and quadrinucleate stages). 2000×.

Diagnostic Laboratory Tests

Diagnosis depends upon finding the distinctive cysts in formed stools, or cysts and trophozoites in liquid stools. Development of a stool enzyme-linked immunosorbent assay (ELISA) has been shown to be both a specific and sensitive rapid diagnostic tool (Seradyn Color Vue–Giardia; LMD Laboratories). Examination of the duodenal contents may be necessary to establish the diagnosis, as cyst production may be sporadic and not found in the stool by an ovum and parasite fecal smear examination. Duodenal aspiration or use of the duodenal capsule technique (Entero-Test) may therefore be superior to fecal examination for diagnosis. A series of three or more stool examinations on alternate days is recommended.

Treatment

Metronidazole (Flagyl) will clear over 90% of *G lamblia* infections. Oral quinacrine hydrochloride (Atabrine) and furazolidone (Furoxone) are alternatives. Tinidazole (Fasigyn), used for 1-day treatment, is widely and effectively used but is not available in the USA. Paromomycin (Humatin) may be useful in pregnancy.

Treatment may be repeated if necessary. Only symptomatic patients require treatment.

Epidemiology

G lamblia occurs worldwide. Humans are infected by ingestion of fecally contaminated water or food containing *Giardia* cysts or by direct fecal contamination, as may occur in day-care centers for children, refugee camps, or jails. Epidemic outbreaks have been reported at ski resorts in the USA where overloading of sewage facilities or contamination of the water supply has resulted in sudden outbreaks of giardiasis. Cysts can survive in water for up to 3 months. Outbreaks among campers in wilderness areas suggest that humans may be infected with various animal *Giardia* harbored by rodents, deer, cattle, sheep, horses, or household pets. This suggests that human infection can also be a zoonosis and that *G lamblia* has a broad spectrum of hosts, contrary to earlier views. Extensive variation occurs in the *Giardia* complex, and though species definitions are still unresolved, it is clear that a great number of distinct and probably variable clones exist.

TRICHOMONAS

The trichomonads are flagellate protozoa with 3–5 anterior flagella, other organelles, and an undulating membrane. *Trichomonas vaginalis* causes the most common form of trichomoniasis in humans.

Morphology & Identification

A. Typical Organisms: *T vaginalis* is pear-shaped, with a short undulating membrane lined with a flagellum and four anterior flagella (Figure 46–2). It measures about 10 × 7 μm, though its length may vary from 5 to 30 μm and its width from 2 to 14 μm. The organism moves with a characteristic wobbling and rotating motion. The nonpathogenic trichomonads, *Trichomonas hominis* (Figure 46–3) and *Trichomonas tenax,* cannot readily be distinguished from *T vaginalis* when alive. For all practical purposes, trichomonads found in the mouth are *T tenax;* in the intestine, *T hominis;* and in the genitourinary tract (both sexes), *T vaginalis.*

B. Culture: *T vaginalis* may be cultivated in many solid and fluid cell-free media, in tissue cultures, and in chick embryo. Simplified trypticase serum is usually used for semen cultures.

C. Growth Requirements: *T vaginalis* grows best at 35–37 °C under anaerobic conditions, less well aerobically. The optimal pH for growth in vitro (5.5–6.0) suggests why vaginal trichomoniasis is more severe in women with higher than normal vaginal pH.

Pathogenesis, Pathology, & Clinical Findings

T hominis and *T tenax* are generally considered to be harmless commensals. *T vaginalis* is capable of causing low-grade inflammation. The intensity of infection, the pH and physiologic status of the vaginal and other genitourinary tract surfaces, and the accompanying bacterial flora are among the factors affecting pathogenicity. The organisms do not survive at normal vaginal acidity of pH 3.8–4.4.

In females, the infection is normally limited to vulva, vagina, and cervix; it does not usually extend to the uterus. The mucosal surfaces may be tender, inflamed, eroded, and covered with a frothy yellow or cream-colored discharge. In males, the prostate, seminal vesicles, and urethra may be infected. Signs and symptoms in females, in addition to profuse vaginal discharge, include local tenderness, vulval pruritus, and burning. About 10% of infected males have a thin, white urethral discharge.

Diagnostic Laboratory Tests

A. Specimens and Microscopic Examination: Vaginal or urethral secretions or discharge should be examined microscopically in a drop of saline for characteristic motile trichomonads. Dried smears may be stained with hematoxylin or other stains for later study.

B. Culture: Culture of vaginal or urethral discharge, of prostatic secretion, or of a semen specimen may reveal organisms when direct examination is negative.

Immunity

Infection confers no apparent immunity, although over time reinfections appear to cause less severe symptoms in women, suggesting that some resistance may develop.

Treatment

Successful treatment of vaginal infection requires destruction of the trichomonads, for which topical and systemic metronidazole (Flagyl) is best. Tinidazole (Fasigyn) and ornidazole (Tiberal) are equally effective, with fewer side effects, but are not available in the USA. The patient's sexual partner should be examined and treated simultaneously. Postmenopausal patients may require treatment with estrogens to improve the condition of the vaginal epithelium. Prostatic infection can be cured with certainty only by systemic treatment with metronidazole or one of the above-mentioned nitroimidazoles.

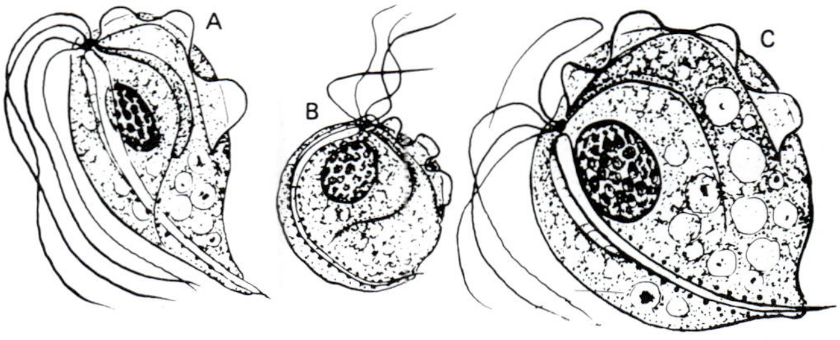

Figure 46–2. *Trichomonas vaginalis* (found in vaginal and prostatic secretions). ***A:*** Normal trophozoite; ***B:*** round form after division; ***C:*** common form seen in stained preparation. Note that the undulating membrane extends only two-thirds of the way down the parasite, not the full length, as in the other trichomonads of humans. Cysts not found. 2000×.

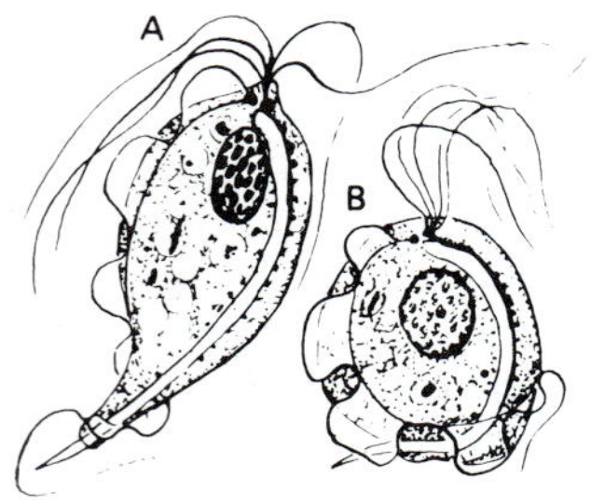

Figure 46–3. *Trichomonas hominis.* ***A:*** normal and ***B:*** round forms of trophozoites, probably a staining artifact. Cysts not found. 2000×.

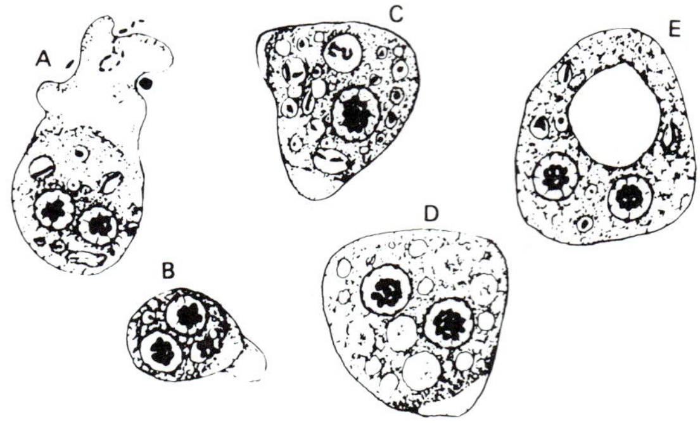

Figure 46–4. *Dientamoeba fragilis.* Trophozoites (cysts not found). ***A:*** active, ***B:*** small, ***C:*** mononuclear, ***D*** and ***E:*** resting. 2000×.

Epidemiology & Control

T vaginalis is a common parasite of both males and females. Infection rates vary greatly but may be quite high (40% or higher). Transmission is by sexual intercourse, but contaminated towels, douche equipment, examination instruments, and other objects may be responsible for some new infections. Infants may be infected during birth. Most infections, in both sexes, are asymptomatic or mild. Control of *T vaginalis* infections always requires simultaneous treatment of both sexual partners. Mechanical protection (condom) should be used during intercourse until the infection is eradicated in both partners.

OTHER INTESTINAL FLAGELLATES

Dientamoeba fragilis

Long classified with the amebas, this occasionally pathogenic organism is now recognized as an ameboflagellate in the same order as *Trichomonas.* In its ameba stage it measures 4–18 μm, has one or two nuclei, and is often bilobate or bean-shaped (Figure 46–4). It is commonly found in the human colon along with the true amebas, but it contains a flagellate structure (the parabasal body) near the nuclei and, like *Trichomonas,* lacks a cyst stage. *Dientamoeba fragilis* is a parasite of humans but has been found in apes, monkeys, and sheep as well. It is mildly pathogenic in about 25% of infected individuals, who may experience abdominal pain and flatulence, diarrhea, vomiting, weakness, and weight loss similar to giardiasis. Treatment is as for *Entamoeba histolytica* infection. Morphologic distinction from intestinal amebas is included in the section on amebiasis.

Chilomastix mesnili

This parasite can be confused with *Trichomonas* in the laboratory. It is found throughout the world. The trophozoite is pear-shaped and resembles *Trichomonas,* but the spiral motion of the trophozoite is unlike that of *Trichomonas.* The cyst is lemon-shaped, uninucleate, and 7–10 μm long (Figure 46–5).

THE HEMOFLAGELLATES

The hemoflagellates of humans include the genera *Trypanosoma* and *Leishmania.* There are two distinct types of human trypanosomes: (1) African, which causes sleeping sickness and is transmitted by tsetse flies *(Glossina): Trypanosoma brucei rhodesiense* and *Trypanosoma brucei gambiense;* and (2) American, which causes Chagas' disease and is transmitted by conenose bugs (*Triatoma,* etc): *Trypanosoma (Schizotrypanum) cruzi.* The genus *Leishmania,* divided into a number of species infecting humans, causes cutaneous (Oriental sore), mucocutaneous (espundia), and visceral (kala-azar) leishmaniasis. All of these infections are transmitted by sandflies (*Phlebotomus, Lutzomyia,* and *Psychodopygus*).

The genus *Trypanosoma* appears in the blood as trypomastigotes, with elongated bodies supporting a longitudinal lateral undulating membrane and a flagellum that borders the free edge of the membrane and emerges at the anterior end as a whip-like extension. The kinetoplast is a darkly staining body lying immediately adjacent to the tiny node (blepharoplast) from which the flagellum arises. Other developmental forms among the hemoflagellates include (1) a leish-

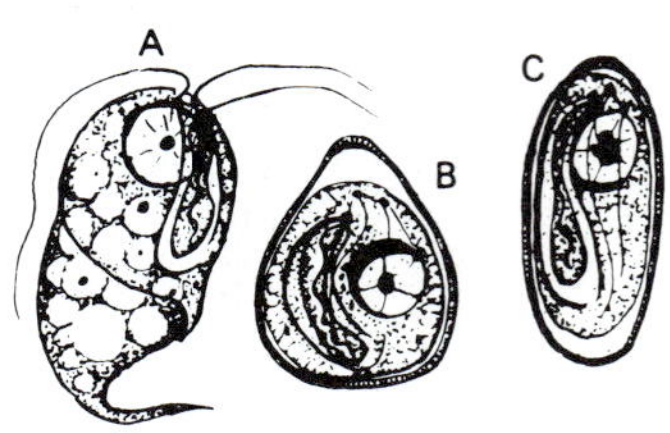

Figure 46–5. *Chilomastix mesnili.* ***A:*** Trophozoite; ***B*** and ***C:*** cysts. 2000×.

manial rounded intracellular stage, the amastigote; (2) a flagellated extracellular stage, the promastigote, a lanceolate form without an undulating membrane, with a kinetoplast at the anterior end; and (3) an epimastigote, a more elongated extracellular stage with a short undulating membrane and a kinetoplast placed more posteriorly, near the nucleus.

In *Leishmania* life cycles, only the amastigote and promastigote are found, the latter being restricted to the insect vector. In *T cruzi,* all three developmental stages may occur in humans, and trypomastigote and epimastigote in the vector. In African trypanosomes, the latter two flagellated stages also occur in the tsetse fly vector, but only the trypomastigote in humans.

LEISHMANIA

The genus *Leishmania,* widely distributed in nature, has a number of species that are nearly identical morphologically. Differentiation is not possible morphologically and therefore is based on a number of biochemical and epidemiologic criteria: electrophoretic mobility profile of a battery of isoenzymes (zymodeme pattern); excretory factor serotyping; kinetoplast DNA restriction analysis (schizodemes); lectin conjugation patterns on the parasite surface; use of monoclonal probes to detect specific antigens; promastigote growth patterns in vitro in the presence of antisera; developmental characteristics of promastigotes in the specific sandfly vector; vectors, reservoir hosts, and other epidemiologic factors. Clinical characteristics of the disease produced are traditional differentiating characteristics, but many exceptions are now recognized (see below). Visceral leishmaniasis results from infection with members of the *Leishmania donovani* complex, which includes many different species or subspecies. The New World forms are all carried by sandflies of the genera *Lutzomyia* and *Psychodopygus;* Old World leishmanias are transmitted by sandflies of the genus *Phlebotomus.* The different leishmanias present a range of clinical and epidemiologic characteristics that, for convenience only, are combined under three clinical groupings: (1) visceral leishmaniasis (kala-azar), (2) cutaneous leishmaniasis (Oriental sore, Baghdad boil, wet cutaneous sore, dry cutaneous sore, chiclero ulcer, uta, and other names), and (3) mucocutaneous or naso-oral leishmaniasis (espundia). However, some species can induce several disease syndromes (eg, visceral leishmaniasis from one of the agents of cutaneous leishmaniasis or cutaneous leishmaniasis from the agent of visceral leishmaniasis). Similarly, the same clinical condition can be caused by different agents.

Morphology & Identification

A. Typical Organism: (Figure 46–6.) Only the nonflagellated amastigote (Leishman-Donovan [LD] body) occurs in mammals. The sandfly transmits the infective promastigotes by bite. The promastigotes rapidly change to amastigotes after phagocytosis by macrophages, then multiply, filling the cytoplasm of the macrophages. The infected cells burst, the released parasites are again phagocytosed, and the process is repeated, producing a cutaneous lesion or visceral infection depending upon the species of parasite and the host response. The amastigotes are oval, 2–6 × 1–3 μm, with a laterally placed oval vesicular nucleus and a dark-staining, rod-like kinetoplast.

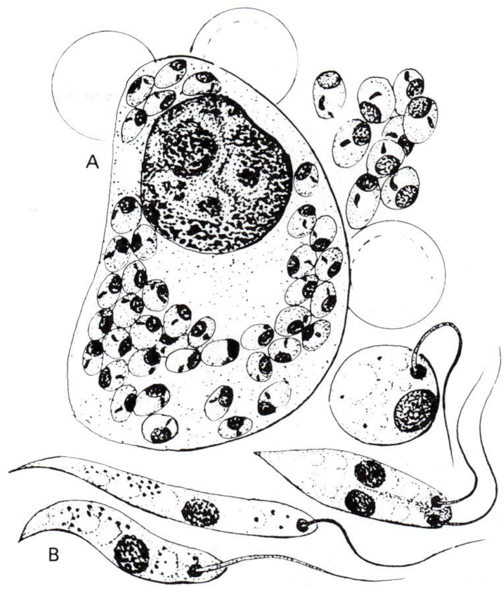

Figure 46–6. *Leishmania donovani.* ***A:*** Large reticuloendothelial cell of spleen with amastigotes. ***B:*** Promastigote as seen in sandfly gut or in culture. ***C:*** Dividing form. 2000×. (Simple double circles represent the size of red cells.)

B. Culture and Growth Characteristics: In NNN or Tobie's medium, only the promastigotes are found. *L donovani* usually grows slowly, the promastigotes forming tangled clumps in the fluid. *Leishmania tropica* grows more quickly, promastigotes forming small rosettes attached by their flagella in the fluid, while *Leishmania braziliensis* may produce a wax-like surface with fewer, smaller promastigotes. In contrast, *Leishmania mexicana* produces rapid growth of large organisms in simple blood agar medium. In tissue cultures, intracellular amastigotes may occur in addition to the extracellular promastigotes.

C. Variations: There are strain differences in virulence, tissue tropism, and biologic and epidemiologic characteristics, as well as the serologic and biochemical criteria previously noted. The New World species (or subspecies) of cutaneous and mucocutaneous leishmaniasis have been placed within the *L mexicana* and *L braziliensis* complexes, respectively, and the agents of visceral leishmaniasis have been placed within the *L donovani* complex as geographically distinct species (or subspecies).

Pathogenesis, Pathology, & Clinical Findings

L donovani, which causes kala-azar, spreads from the site of inoculation to multiply in reticuloendothelial cells, especially macrophages in spleen, liver, lymph nodes, and bone marrow. This is accompanied by marked hyperplasia of the spleen. Progressive emaciation is accompanied by growing weakness. There is irregular fever, sometimes hectic. Untreated cases with symptoms of kala-azar usually are fatal. Some forms, especially in India, develop a postcure florid cutaneous resurgence, with abundant parasites in cutaneous vesicles, 1–2 years later (post-kala-azar dermal leishmanoid).

L tropica, L major, L mexicana, L braziliensis and other dermotropic forms induce a dermal lesion at the site of inoculation by the sandfly: cutaneous leishmaniasis, Oriental sore, Delhi boil, etc. Mucous membranes are rarely involved. The dermal layers are first affected, with cellular infiltration and proliferation of amastigotes intracellularly and spreading extracellularly, until the infection penetrates the epidermis and causes ulceration. Satellite lesions may be found (hypersensitivity or recidivans type of cutaneous leishmaniasis) that contain few or no parasites, do not readily respond to treatment, and induce a strongly granulomatous scarring reaction. In Venezuela, a cutaneous disseminating form, caused by *Leishmania mexicana pifanoi,* is known. In Ethiopia, a form known as *Leishmania aethiopica* causes a similar nonulcerating, blistering, spreading cutaneous leishmaniasis. Both forms are typically anergic and nonreactive to skin test antigen and contain large numbers of parasites in the dermal blisters.

Leishmania braziliensis braziliensis causes mucocutaneous or nasopharyngeal leishmaniasis in Amazonian South America. It is known by many local names. The lesions are slow-growing but extensive (sometimes 5–10 cm). From these sites, migration appears to occur rapidly to the nasopharyngeal or palatine mucosal surfaces, where no further growth may take place for years. After months to over 20 years, relentless erosion may develop, destroying the nasal septum and surrounding regions in an often intractable, fungating, polypoid course. In such instances, death occurs from asphyxiation due to blockage of the trachea, starvation, or respiratory infection. This is the classic clinical picture of espundia, most commonly found in the Amazon basin. At high altitudes in Peru, the clinical features (uta) resemble those of Oriental sore. *Leishmania braziliensis guyanensis* infection frequently spreads along lymphatic routes, where it appears as a linear chain of nonulcerating lesions. *L mexicana* infection is more typically confined to a single, indolent, ulcerative lesion that heals in about 1 year, leaving a characteristic depressed circular scar. In Mexico and Guatemala, the ears are frequently involved (chiclero ulcer), usually with a cartilage-attacking infection without ulceration and with few parasites.

Diagnostic Laboratory Tests

A. Specimens: Lymph node aspirates, scrapings, and biopsies from the margin of the lesion, not the center, are important in the cutaneous forms; lymph node aspirates, blood, and spleen, liver, or bone marrow puncture are important in kala-azar. Purulent discharges are of no value for diagnosis, although nasal scrapings may be useful. An enzyme-linked immunosorbent assay (ELISA) technique using a 70-kDa antigen has been studied as a rapid and accurate field-applied tool to detect visceral leishmaniasis (in place of splenic aspiration or the direct agglutination test [DAT], which remains positive for some years after cure, a disadvantage for current diagnosis).

B. Microscopic Examination: Giemsa-stained smears and sections may show amastigotes, especially in material from kala-azar and under the rolled edges of cutaneous sores.

C. Culture: NNN medium is the medium most generally used. A diphasic rabbit blood agar culture, Tobie's medium, at about 26–28 °C, is especially suitable. Blood culture is satisfactory for *L donovani* and *L braziliensis.* Lymph node aspirates are suitable for all forms; and tissue aspirates, biopsy material, scrapings, or small biopsies from the edges of ulcers are useful for the cutaneous forms and often for kala-azar also. However, only promastigotes can be cultivated in the absence of living cells.

D. Serology: The formol-gel (aldehyde) test of Napier is a nonspecific test that detects an elevated serum globulin level in kala-azar. The IHA (indirect hemagglutination antibody) test or the IFA (indirect fluorescent antibody) test may be useful, but they lack sufficient sensitivity and may cross-react with *T cruzi.* The ELISA (enzyme-linked immunosorbent assay) test is more promising. A skin test (Montenegro test) is epidemiologically important in indicating past exposure to any of the leishmanias.

Immunity

Recovery from cutaneous leishmaniasis confers a solid and permanent immunity, although it usually is species-specific and may be strain-specific as well. Natural resistance varies greatly among individuals and with age and sex. Vaccination with a living inoculum from a recently isolated culture significantly reduces the incidence of Oriental sore.

Immunity to kala-azar may develop but varies with the time of treatment and condition of the patient.

Treatment

Single lesions may be cleaned, curetted, treated with antibiotics if secondarily infected, and then covered and left to heal. For larger or nonhealing forms, pentavalent antimony sodium gluconate (Pentostam,

Solustibosan) is the drug of choice. Pentamidine isethionate (Lomidine) is useful for kala-azar resistant to antimony sodium gluconate. Cycloguanil pamoate in oil (Camolar) and amphotericin B (Fungizone) can be used for espundia, which is frequently quite unresponsive to treatment. Local heat with hot water compresses (39–42 °C) applied directly 20–30 min/d for 12–30 days or by exposure to ultraviolet or infrared radiation for 20 min/d may be effective against the nonresponsive recidivans form of *L tropica* infection.

Epidemiology, Prevention & Control

Kala-azar, caused by *L donovani,* is found focally in most tropical and subtropical countries. Its local distribution is related to the prevalence of specific sandfly vectors. In the Mediterranean littoral and in middle Asia and South America, domestic and wild canids are reservoirs, and in the Sudan, various wild carnivores and rodents are reservoirs of endemic kala-azar. No animal reservoirs have been found for the forms from India and Kenya. Control is aimed at destroying breeding places and dogs, where appropriate, and protecting people from sandfly bites. Oriental sore occurs mostly in the Mediterranean region, North Africa, and the Middle and Near East. The "wet" type, caused by *L major,* is rural, and burrowing rodents are the main reservoir; the "dry" type, caused by *L tropica,* is urban, and humans are presumably the only reservoir. For *L braziliensis,* there are a number of wild but apparently no domestic animal reservoirs. Sandfly vectors are involved in all forms.

TRYPANOSOMA

Hemoflagellates of the genus *Trypanosoma* occur in the blood of mammals as mature elongated trypomastigotes. A multiplying epimastigote stage precedes the formation of infective trypomastigotes in the intermediate host (an insect vector) in all species of trypanosomes that infect humans. Trypanosomiasis is expressed as African sleeping sickness; Chagas' disease of southern USA, Mexico, and Central and South America; and asymptomatic trypanosomiasis in Central and South America.

The parent form in Africa is *Trypanosoma brucei brucei,* which causes nagana in livestock and game animals; the two human forms are *T brucei rhodesiense* and *T brucei gambiense.* The three forms are indistinguishable morphologically but differ biochemically, ecologically, and epidemiologically.

Morphology & Identification

A. Typical Organisms: (Figures 46–7 and 46–8.) African *T b gambiense* and *T b rhodesiense* vary in size and shape of the body and length of the flagellum (usually 15–30 μm) but are essentially indistinguishable. A "stumpy" short form is infective to the insect host and possesses a full battery of enzymes for energy metabolism. The elongated form requires host metabolic assistance and is specialized for rapid multiplication in the richly nutritious vertebrate bloodstream. The same forms are seen in blood as in lymph node aspirates.

The blood forms of American *T cruzi* are present during the early acute stage and at intervals thereafter in smaller numbers. They are typical trypomastigotes, varying about a mean of 20 μm, frequently curved in a C shape when fixed and stained. A large, rounded terminal kinetosome in stained preparations is characteristic. The tissue forms, which are most common in heart muscle, liver, and brain, develop from amastigotes that multiply to form an intracellular colony after invasion of the host cell or phagocytosis of the parasite. *Trypanosoma rangeli* of South and Central America infects humans without causing disease and must therefore be carefully distinguished from the pathogenic species (Table 46–1).

B. Culture: *T cruzi* and *T rangeli* are readily cultivated (3–6 weeks) in the epimastigote form in fluid or diphasic media. Diagnosis of patients in the early, blood-borne phase of infection can be aided by using the multiplying powers of parasites in laboratory-reared, clean vector insects (kissing, conenose, or triatomine bugs) that have been allowed to feed on patients (see Xenodiagnosis, below).

C. Variation: There are variations in morphology (see above), virulence, and antigenic constitution. The African trypanosomes of the *T brucei* complex are remarkable in that they undergo development of a series of genetically controlled glycoprotein antigenic coats (variant surface glycoproteins, or VSGs). Successive

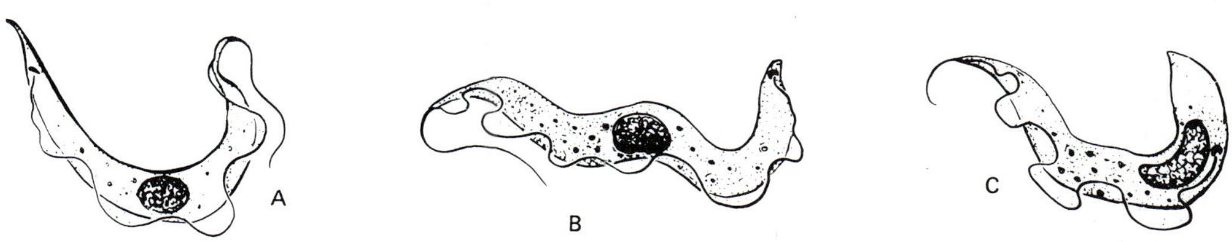

Figure 46–7. *Trypanosoma brucei gambiense* (or *Trypanosoma brucei rhodesiense,* indistinguishable in practice). ***A, B:*** Trypomastigotes in blood; ***C:*** epimastigote (intermediate type; kinetoplast not yet anterior to nucleus); found in tsetse fly, *Glossina* species. 1700×.

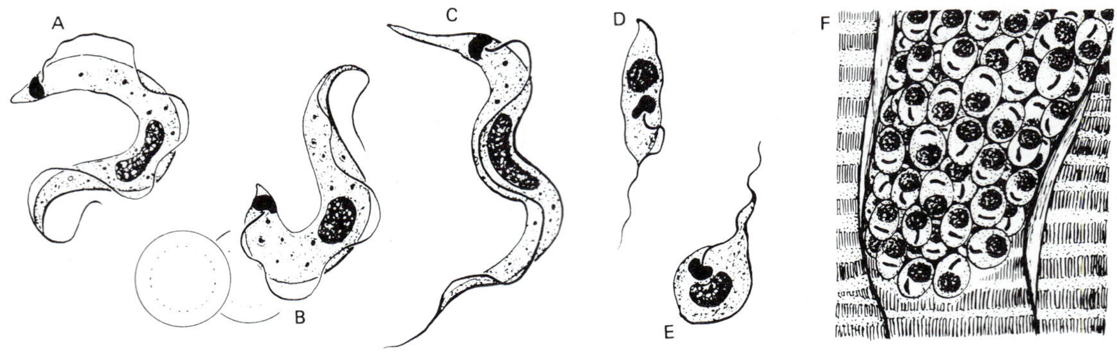

Figure 46–8. *Trypanosoma cruzi.* ***A, B, C:*** Trypomastigotes in blood; ***D, E:*** epimastigote (with short anterior undulating membrane); ***F:*** amastigote colony in heart muscle. 1700×.

waves of parasites in the host bloodstream are each covered with a distinct coat, one of an apparently unlimited number. This process is due to genetically induced changes in the development of the surface glycoprotein coat; it is viewed as a means of continuously escaping the host's antibody response by producing different antigenic membranes. Each population is reduced but is promptly replaced with another antigenic type before the preceding one is eliminated. Each trypanosome is thought to possess about 1000 VSG genes, an example of mosaic gene formation.

Pathogenesis, Pathology, & Clinical Findings

Infective trypanosomes of *T b gambiense* and *T b rhodesiense* are introduced through the bite of the tsetse fly and multiply at the site of inoculation to cause variable induration and swelling (the primary lesion), which may progress to form a trypanosomal chancre. They spread to lymph nodes, to the bloodstream, and, in terminal stages, to the central nervous system, where they produce the typical sleeping sickness syndrome: lassitude, inability to eat, tissue wasting, unconsciousness, and death.

Table 46–1. Differentiation of *T cruzi* and *T rangeli.*

	T cruzi	*T rangeli*
Blood forms Size	20 μm	Over 30 μm
Shape	Often C-shaped in fixed preparations	Rarely C-shaped
Posterior kinetoplast	Terminal, large	Distinctly subterminal, small
Developmental stages in tissues	Amastigote to epimastigote	Not found (only trypomastigotes)
Triatomine bugs In salivary gland or proboscis (or both)	Always absent	Usually present
In hindgut or feces	Present	Present

Infective forms of *T cruzi* do not pass to humans by triatomine bug bites (which is the mode of entry of the nonpathogenic *T rangeli*); rather, they are introduced when infected bug feces are rubbed into the conjunctiva, the bite site, or a break in the skin. At the site of *T cruzi* entry, there may be a subcutaneous inflammatory nodule or chagoma. Chagas' disease is common in infants. Unilateral swelling of the eyelids (Romaña's sign) is characteristic at onset, especially in children. The primary lesion is accompanied by fever, acute regional lymphadenitis, and dissemination to blood and tissues. The parasites can usually be detected within 1–2 weeks as trypomastigotes in the blood. Subsequent development depends upon the organs and tissues affected and on the nature of multiplication and release of toxins.

The African forms multiply extracellularly as trypomastigotes in the blood as well as in lymphoid tissues. *T cruzi* multiplies mostly within reticuloendothelial cells, going through a cycle starting with large agglomerations of amastigotes. In both African and American forms, multiplication in the tissues is punctuated by phases of parasitemia with later destruction by the host of the blood forms, accompanied by bouts of intermittent fever gradually decreasing in intensity. Parasitemia is more common in *T b rhodesiense* and is intermittent and scant with *T cruzi.*

The release of toxins explains much of the systemic and local reactions. The organs most seriously affected are the central nervous system and heart muscle. Interstitial myocarditis is the most common serious element in Chagas' disease. Other organs affected are the liver, spleen, and bone marrow, especially with chronic *T cruzi* infection. Invasion or toxic destruction of nerve plexuses in the alimentary tract walls leads to megaesophagus and megacolon, especially in Brazilian Chagas' disease. Megaesophagus and megacolon are absent in Colombian, Venezuelan, and Central American Chagas' disease. Central nervous system involvement is most characteristic of African trypanosomiasis. *T b rhodesiense* appears in the cerebrospinal fluid in about 1 month and *T b gambiense* in several months, but both are present in small numbers. *T b gambiense* infection is chronic and leads to progressive diffuse meningoencephalitis, with death from the sleeping syndrome usually following in 1–2 years. The more rapidly fatal *T b rhodesiense* produces somnolence and coma only during the final weeks of a terminal infection. All three trypanosomes are transmissible through the placenta, and congenital infections occur in hyperendemic areas.

Diagnostic Laboratory Tests

A. Specimens: Blood, preferably collected when the patient's temperature rises; cerebrospinal fluid; lymph node or primary lesion aspirates; or specimens obtained by iliac crest, sternal bone marrow, or spleen puncture are used.

B. Microscopic Examination: Fresh blood (or aspirated tissue in saline) is kept warm and examined immediately for the actively motile trypanosomes. Thick films may be stained with Giemsa's stain. Thin films stained with Giemsa's stain are necessary for confirmation. Centrifugation may be necessary. Tissue smears must be stained for identification of the pretrypanosomal stages. Centrifuged cerebrospinal fluid should be similarly examined; there is seldom more than one trypanosome per milliliter. The most reliable tests are smears of blood for *T b rhodesiense,* of lymph gland puncture specimens for *T b gambiense,* and of cerebrospinal fluid for *T b rhodesiense* and advanced *T b gambiense.*

C. Culture: Any specimens may be inoculated into Tobie's, Wenyon's semisolid, NNN, or other media for culture of *T cruzi* or *T rangeli.* The organisms are grown at 22–24 °C and subcultured every 1–2 weeks. Centrifuged material is examined microscopically for trypanosomes. Culture of the African forms is unsatisfactory.

D. Animal Inoculation: *T cruzi* and *T rangeli* may be detected by inoculating blood intraperitoneally into mice (when available, pups and kittens are animals of first choice). *T b rhodesiense* is often detectable and *T b gambiense* sometimes detectable by this procedure. Trypanosomes appear in the blood in a few days after successful inoculation.

E. Serology: A positive IHA, IFA, or CF (Machado's) test provides confirmatory support in *T cruzi* infection. Recently developed ELISAs using recombinant antigens now provide a highly specific and sensitive serodiagnostic tool for detection of *T cruzi.* These tests are especially useful for blood bank screening. African forms cause IFA reactions after about 12 days of infection. This is especially useful for *T b gambiense* diagnosis. A card test for direct agglutination is valuable for field use or for rural medical stations, using lyophilized trypanosome antigen.

F. Xenodiagnosis: This is the method of choice in suspected Chagas' disease if other examinations are negative, especially during the early phase of disease onset. *Because laboratory infection with* T cruzi *is a distinct hazard, the test should be performed only by workers trained in the procedure.* About six clean laboratory-reared triatomine bugs are fed on the patient, and their droppings are examined in 7–10 days for the various developmental forms. Defecation follows shortly after a fresh meal or may be forced by gently probing the bug's anus and then squeezing its abdomen. Xenodiagnosis is impracticable for the African forms.

Differential Diagnosis

T b rhodesiense and *T b gambiense* are morphologically identical but may be distinguished by their geographic distribution, vector species, and clinical disease in humans. The presence of specific IgM in the cerebrospinal fluid is considered pathognomonic for the encephalitic stage of African trypanosomiasis. The differentiation of *T cruzi* from *T rangeli* (Table 46–1) is important. A laboratory-based procedure has been described that differentiates the two species based on total parasite DNA digestant electrophoresed on agarose gels which are then stained with ethidium bromide.

Immunity

Humans show some individual variation in natural resistance to trypanosomes. Strain-specific CF and protecting antibodies can be detected in the plasma, and these presumably lead to the disappearance of blood forms. Each relapse of African trypanosomiasis is due to a strain serologically distinct from the preceding one. Apart from such relapses, Africans free from symptoms may still have trypanosomes in the blood.

Treatment

There is no effective drug treatment for American trypanosomiasis, although nifurtimox (Bayer 2502) plus gamma interferon may shorten the acute phase and may temporarily relieve some patients with trypomastigotes still present in the blood. Benznidazole (Rochagan) is a recently tested alternative drug. African trypanosomiasis is treated principally with suramin sodium (Germanin) or pentamidine isethionate (Lomidine). Late disease with central nervous system involvement requires melarsoprol (Mel B), as well as suramin or tryparsamide. A promising new drug is eflornithine (difluoromethylornithine; DFMO; [Ornidyl], which works against both the blood and central nervous system phases of *T b gambiense* infection and the hemolymphatic stage of *T b rhodesiense.*

Epidemiology, Prevention, & Control

African trypanosomiasis is restricted to recognized tsetse fly belts. *T b gambiense,* transmitted by the streamside tsetse *Glossina palpalis* and several other humid forest tsetse vectors, extends from west to central Africa and produces a relatively chronic infection with progressive central nervous system involvement. *T b rhodesiense,* transmitted by the woodland-savanna *Glossina morsitans, Glossina pallidipes,* and *Glossina fuscipes,* occur in the east and southeast savannahs of Africa, with foci west of Lake Victoria. It causes a smaller number of cases but is more virulent. Bushbuck and other antelopes may serve as reservoirs of *T b rhodesiense,* whereas humans are the principal reservoir of *T b gambiense.* Control depends upon searching for and then isolating and treating patients with the disease; controlling movement of people in and out of fly belts; using insecticides in vehicles; and instituting fly control, principally with aerial insecticides and by altering habitats. Contact with reservoir animals is difficult to control, and insect repellent is of little value against tsetse bites.

Chemoprophylaxis, eg, with suramin sodium, is difficult and short-lived.

American trypanosomiasis (Chagas' disease) is especially important in Central and South America, although infection of animals extends much more widely—eg, to Maryland and southern California. A few autochthonous human cases have been reported in Texas and southern California. Certain triatomine bugs become as domiciliated as bedbugs, and infection may be brought in by rats, opossums, or armadillos—which may spread the infection to domestic animals such as dogs and cats. Since no effective treatment is known, it is particularly important to control the vectors with residual insecticides and habitat destruction and to avoid contact with animal reservoirs. Chagas' disease occurs largely among people in poor economic circumstances. An estimated 20–25 million persons harbor the parasite, and many of these sustain heart damage, with the result that their ability to work and their life expectancy are sharply reduced.

INTESTINAL AMEBAS

ENTAMOEBA HISTOLYTICA

Entamoeba histolytica is a common parasite in the large intestine of humans, certain other primates, and some other animals. Many cases are asymptomatic except in humans or among animals living under stress (eg, zoo-held primates).

Morphology & Identification

A. Typical Organisms: Three stages are encountered: the active ameba, the inactive cyst, and the intermediate precyst. The ameboid trophozoite is the only form present in tissues. It is also found in fluid feces during amebic dysentery. Its size is 15–30 μm. The cytoplasm is granular and may contain red cells (pathognomonic) but ordinarily contains no bacteria. Iron-hematoxylin or Wheatley's trichrome staining shows the nuclear membrane to be lined by fine, regular granules of chromatin. Movement of trophozoites in fresh material is brisk and unidirectional. Pseudopodia are finger-like and broad.

Cysts are present only in the lumen of the colon and in mushy or formed feces. Subspherical cysts of pathogenic amebas range from 10 to 20 μm. Smaller cysts, from 10 μm ranging down to 3.5 μm, are considered nonpathogenic *Entamoeba hartmanni.* The cyst wall, 0.5 μm thick, is hyaline. The initial uninucleate cyst may contain a glycogen vacuole and chromatoidal bodies with characteristic rounded ends (in contrast to splinter chromatoidals in developing cysts of *Entamoeba coli*). Nuclear division within the cyst produces the final quadrinucleate cyst, during which time the chromatoid bodies and glycogen vacuoles disappear. Diagnosis in most cases rests on the characteristics of the cyst, since trophozoites usually appear only in diarrheic feces in active cases and survive for only a few hours, though they may be excellently preserved in polyvinyl alcohol (PVA) fixative. Stools may contain cysts with 1–4 nuclei depending on their degree of maturation.

B. Culture: Trophozoites are readily studied in cultures; both encystation and excystation can be controlled.

C. Growth Requirements: Growth is most vigorous in various rich complex media or cell culture under partial anaerobiosis 37 °C and pH 7.0—with a mixed flora or at least a single coexisting species.

D. Variation: Variations in cyst size are due to nutritional differences or to the presence of the small nonpathogenic form, *E hartmanni.* The invasive or pathogenic form is now considered enzymatically distinct from the more common lumen-dwelling nonpathogenic form, given an older name, *E dispar,* with the name *E histolytica* reserved for the pathogenic form. However, the transmutability of the nonpathogenic to the pathogenic form remains controversial.

Pathogenesis, Pathology, & Clinical Findings

The trophozoites multiply by binary fission. The trophozoite emerges from the ingested cyst (metacyst) after activation of the excystation process in the stomach and duodenum. The metacyst divides rapidly, producing four amebulae (one for each cyst nucleus), each of which divides again to produce eight small trophozoites per infective cyst. These pass to the cecum and produce a population of lumen-dwelling trophozoites. Disease results (in about 10% of infections) when the trophozoites invade the intestinal epithelium. Mucosal invasion by amebas with the aid of proteolytic enzymes occurs through the crypts of Lieberkühn, forming discrete ulcers with a pinhead-sized center and raised edges, from which mucus, necrotic cells, and amebas pass. Pathologic changes are always induced by trophozoites: *E histolytica* cysts are not produced in tissues. The mucosal surface between ulcers typically is normal. Amebas multiply and accumulate above the muscularis mucosae, often spreading laterally. Healing may occur spontaneously with little tissue erosion if regeneration proceeds more rapidly than destruction, or the amebic trophozoites may break through the muscularis into the submucosa. Rapid lateral spread of the multiplying amebas follows, undermining the mucosa and producing the characteristic "flask-shaped" ulcer of primary amebiasis: a small point of entry, leading via a narrow neck through the mucosa into an expanded necrotic area in the submucosa. Bacterial invasion usually does not occur at this time, cellular reaction is limited, and damage is by lytic necrosis. Subsequent spread may coalesce colonies of amebas, undermining large areas of the mucosal surface. Trophozoites may penetrate the muscular coats and occasionally the serosa, leading to perforation into the peritoneal cavity. Subsequent enlargement of the necrotic area produces gross changes in the ulcer, which may develop shaggy overhanging edges, secondary bacterial invasion, and accumulation of neutrophilic leukocytes. Secondary intestinal lesions may develop as extensions from the primary lesion (usually in the cecum, appendix, or nearby portion of the ascending colon). The organisms may travel to the ileocecal valve and terminal ileum, producing a chronic infection. The sigmoid colon and rectum are favored sites for these later lesions. An amebic inflammatory or granulomatous tumor-like mass (ameboma) may form on the intestinal wall.

Factors that determine invasion of amebas include the following: the number of amebas ingested, the pathogenic capacity of the parasite strain or one of several enzymatically distinguishable xymodemes (which range from mild or noninvasive forms, as commonly found among homosexual men, to fully invasive virulent strains), host factors such as gut motility and immune competence, and the presence of suitable enteric bacteria that enhance amebic growth. Most infected persons are not diseased but harbor only lumen-dwelling amebas that form cysts passed in the feces. Trophozoites, especially with red cells in the cytoplasm, found in liquid or semiformed stools are pathognomonic. Formed stools usually contain cysts only, while patients with active disease and liquid stools (flecked with blood and mucus strands containing numerous amebas) usually pass trophozoites only. Symptoms vary greatly depending upon the site and intensity of lesions. Extreme abdominal tenderness, fulminating dysentery, dehydration, and incapacitation occur in serious disease. In less acute disease, onset of symptoms is usually gradual, and episodes of diarrhea, abdominal cramps, nausea and vomiting, and an urgent desire to defecate. More frequently, there will be weeks of cramps and general discomfort, loss of appetite, and weight loss with general malaise. Symptoms may develop within 4 days of exposure, may occur up to a year later, or may never occur. However, a change in host resistance or malnutrition (especially protein deficiency) may predispose asymptomatic carriers to develop the full syndrome.

Extraintestinal infection is metastatic and rarely occurs by direct extension from the bowel. By far the most common form is amebic hepatitis or liver abscess (4% or more of clinical infections), which is assumed to be due to microemboli, including trophozoites carried through the portal circulation. It is assumed that hepatic microembolism with trophozoites is a common accompaniment of bowel lesions but that these diffuse focal lesions rarely progress. A true amebic abscess is progressive, nonsuppurative (unless secondarily infected), and destructive without compression and formation of a wall. The contents are necrotic and bacteriologically sterile, active amebas being confined to the walls. A characteristic "anchovy paste" is produced in the abscess and seen on surgical drainage. More than half of patients with amebic liver abscess give no history of intestinal infection, and only one-eighth of them pass cysts in their stools. Rarely, amebic abscesses also occur elsewhere (eg, lung, brain, spleen, or draining through the body wall). Any organ or tissue in contact with active trophozoites may become a site of invasion and abscess.

Diagnostic Laboratory Tests

A. Specimens:

1. Fluid feces–

a. Fresh and warm for immediate examination for trophozoites.

b. Preserved in polyvinyl alcohol (PVA) fixative or Merthiolate-iodine-formalin (MIF) fixative for mailing to a diagnostic laboratory (in a waterproofed or double mailing tube, the inner one of metal).

c. After a saline purge (or high enema after saline purge) for cysts and trophozoites.

2. Formed feces for cysts.

3. Scrapings and biopsies obtained through a sigmoidoscope.

4. Liver abscess aspirates collected from the edge of the abscess, not the necrotic center. Viscous aspirates should be treated with a liquefying enzyme such as streptodornase, then cultured or examined microscopically (see Beaver, Jung, and Cupp reference, p 592).

5. Blood for serologic tests and cell counts.

B. Microscopic Examination: If possible, always examine fresh warm feces for trophozoites if the patient is symptomatic and has diarrheic stools. Otherwise, stain smears with trichrome or iron-hematoxylin stain. The stools in amebic dysentery can usually be distinguished from those in bacillary dysentery: the former contain much fecal debris, small amounts of blood with strings of nontenacious mucus and degenerated red cells, few polymorphonuclear cells or macrophages, scattered Charcot-Leyden crystals, and trophozoites. Although considerable experience is required to distinguish *E histolytica* from commensal amebas (see below), it is necessary to do so because misdiagnosis often leads to unnecessary treatment, overtreatment, or a failure to treat.

Differentiation of *E histolytica* (H) and *Entamoeba coli* (C), the most common other intestinal ameba, can be made in stained smears as follows:

1. Trophozoites–The cytoplasm in H is glassy and contains only red cells and spherical vacuoles. The cytoplasm in C is granular, with many bacterial and other inclusions and ellipsoid vacuoles. The nucleus of H has a very small central endosome and fine regular chromatin granules lining the periphery; the nucleus of C has a larger, eccentric endosome, and the peripheral chromatin is more coarsely beaded and less evenly distributed around the nuclear membrane. Moribund trophozoites and precysts of H and C are usually indistinguishable.

2. Cysts–Glycogen vacuoles disappear during successive divisions. Nuclei resemble those of the trophozoites. Rare cysts of H and C may have eight and 16 nuclei, respectively. Cysts of H in many preparations contain many uninucleate early cysts; these are rarely seen with C. Binucleate developing cysts of C often show the nuclei pushed against the cell wall by the large central glycogen vacuole. Chromatoidal bodies in early cysts of H are blunt-ended bars; those of C are splinter-like and often occur in clusters.

C. Culture: Diagnostic cultures are made in a layer of fluid overlying a solid nutrient base in partial anaerobiosis. Dobell's diphasic and Cleveland-Collier media are most often used.

D. Serology: The CF test is not always satisfactory, because a good and highly specific antigen is not available. Serologic testing is primarily for extraintestinal amebiasis, when stools are often negative. Serodiagnosis, most commonly by IHA test, is considered sensitive and specific. Serologic testing in intestinal infections is less reliable except in cases in which considerable tissue invasion has occurred. Commercially available preparations employ the latex agglutination technique (Serameba); Ouchterlony double diffusion (ParaTek); and counterelectrophoresis (Amoebogen). Positive responses to several tests are of value in supporting a tentative diagnosis in doubtful cases of extraintestinal amebiasis. The ENZYMEBA test is based on the finding of histolysain (the major cysteine protease of the virulent form) in the intestine plus circulating antibodies to histolysain after tissue invasion. The test is a solid-phase enzyme immunoassay to detect histolysain in stools. This test is especially helpful in cases where cysts or trophozoites are not found microscopically. Another test to distinguish pathogenic from nonpathogenic strains *(E dispar)* in a stool specimen is an ELISA that uses monoclonal antibodies against the galactose adhesin, a pathogen-specific epitope of *E histolytica.*

Treatment

Asymptomatic (cyst-passing) amebiasis can be treated with iodoquinol (Yodoxin); *or* diloxanide furoate (Furamide); *or* paromomycin (Humatin).

Metronidazole (Flagyl) is probably a drug of choice for symptomatic amebiasis even though it is mutagenic in bacteria. For mild to moderate intestinal disease, give metronidazole *or* tinidazole (Fasigyn) (an excellent drug of low toxicity but not available in the USA). For severe intestinal disease (amebic dysentery), give the regimen described above *or* dehydroemetine (or emetine). For hepatic or other extraintestinal involvement *or* for ameboma, give metronidazole *or* tinidazole *or* dehydroemetine (*or* emetine) followed by chloroquine phosphate.

Epidemiology, Prevention, & Control

Cysts are usually ingested through contaminated water. In the tropics, contaminated vegetables and food are also important cyst sources; flies have been incriminated in areas of fecal pollution. Asymptomatic cyst passers are the main source of contamination and may be responsible for severe epidemic outbreaks where sewage leaks into the water supply or breakdown of sanitary discipline occurs (as in mental, geriatric, prison, or children's institutions). A high-carbohydrate, low-protein diet favors the development of amebic dysentery both in experimental animals and in known human cases. Control measures consist of improving environmental and food sanitation. Treatment of carriers is controversial, although it is agreed that they should be barred from food handling. The danger of transformation from an asymptomatic lumen infection to an invasive tissue disease as well as possible environmental contamination should be considered in the treatment decision for an asymptomatic cyst passer. No fully satisfactory and safe drug is yet available for chemoprophylaxis, and the mix of drugs required for therapy attests to the problems of treating amebiasis.

OTHER INTESTINAL AMEBAS (Figure 46–9)

Entamoeba histolytica must be distinguished from four other ameba-like organisms that are also intestinal parasites of humans: (1) *Entamoeba coli,* which is very common; (2) *D fragilis,* the only intestinal parasite other than *E histolytica* that has been suspected of causing diarrhea and dyspepsia, but not by invasion (this flagellate considered on p 335 is included here for diagnostic convenience); (3) *Iodamoeba bütschlii;* and (4) *Endolimax nana.* To facilitate detection, cysts should be concentrated by zinc sulfate flotation or a similar technique. Unstained, trichrome- or iron-hematoxylin stained, and iodine-stained preparations should be searched systematically. Mixed infections

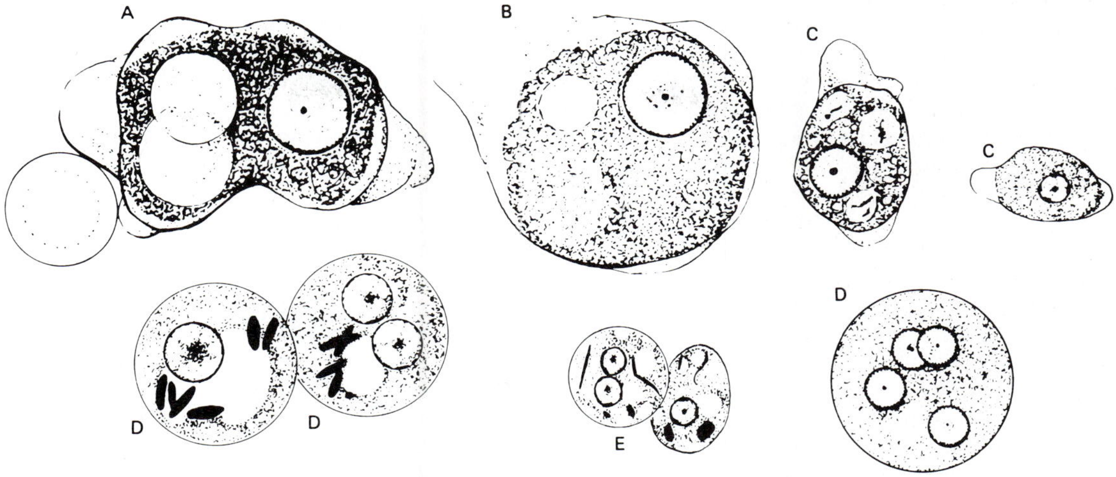

Entamoeba histolytica. A, B: Trophozoite (vegetative form) with ingested red cells in *A; C: Entamoeba hartmanni* trophozoite with food vacuoles, not red cells; *D:* cysts with 1, 2, and 4 nuclei and chromatoid bodies; *E: E hartmanni* binucleate cyst (left), uninucleate precyst (right).

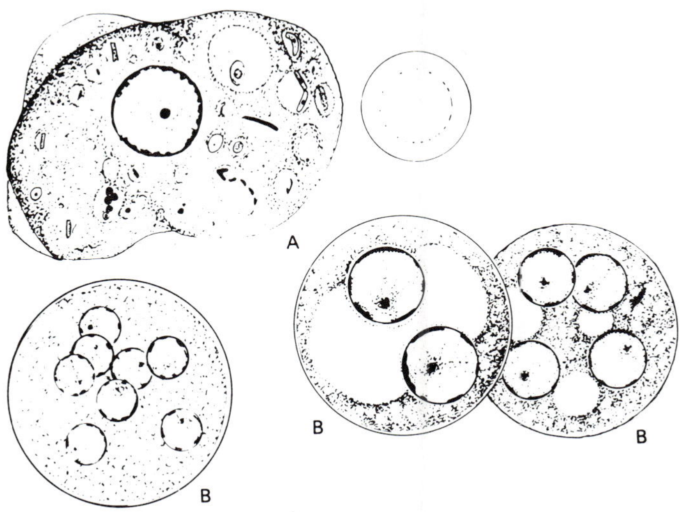

Entamoeba coli. A: Trophozoite with vacuoles and inclusions; *B:* cysts with 2, 4, and 8 nuclei, the latter being mature.

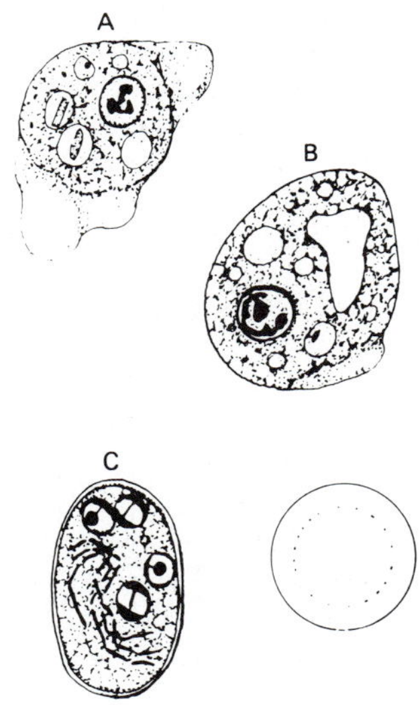

Endolimax nana. A: Trophozoite; *B:* precystic form; *C:* binucleate cyst.

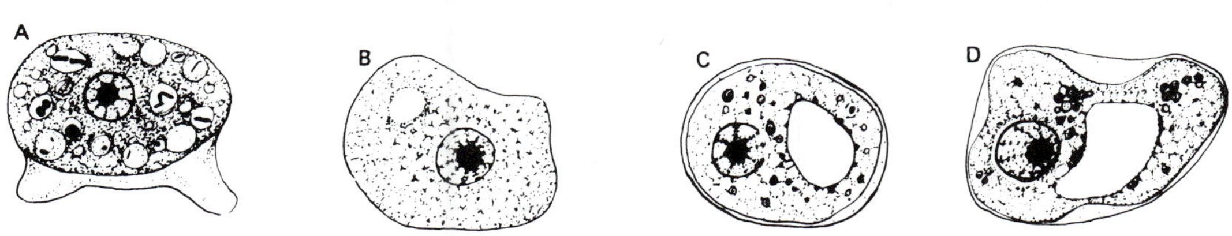

*Iodamoeba bütschlii. A:*Trophozoite; *B:* precystic form; *C* and *D:* cysts showing large glycogen vacuole (unstained in iron-hematoxylin preparation). Note variable shape of cysts.

Figure 46–9. Intestinal amebas. 2000×. (Simple double circles represent the size of red cells.)

may occur. Polyvinyl alcohol (PVA) fixation is especially valuable for preservation of trophozoites. The presence of nonpathogenic amebas is strongly indicative of poor sanitation or of accidental fecal contamination—both warnings of possible exposure to pathogenic *E histolytica*—or a possible pre-AIDS immunodeficient state.

BALANTIDIUM COLI

Balantidium coli, the cause of balantidiasis or balantidial dysentery, is the largest intestinal protozoan of humans. Morphologically similar ciliate parasites are found in swine and lower primates.

Morphology & Identification

A. Typical Organisms: (Figure 46–10.) The trophozoite is a ciliated, oval organism, 60 × 45 μm or larger. Its motion is a characteristic combination of steady progression and rotation around the long axis. The cell wall is lined with spiral rows of cilia. The cytoplasm surrounds two contractile vacuoles, food particles and vacuoles, and two nuclei—a large, kidney-shaped macronucleus and a much smaller, spherical micronucleus. When the organism encysts, it secretes a double-layered wall. The macronucleus, contractile vacuoles, and portions of the ciliated cell wall may be visible in the cyst, which ranges from 46–65 μm in diameter.

B. Culture: These organisms may be cultivated in many media used for cultivation of intestinal amebas.

Pathogenesis, Pathology, & Clinical Findings

When cysts are ingested by the new host, the cyst walls dissolve and the released trophozoites descend to the colon, where they feed on bacteria and fecal debris, multiply, and form cysts that pass in the feces. Most infections are apparently harmless. However, rarely, the trophozoites invade the mucosa and submucosa of the large bowel and terminal ileum. As they multiply, abscesses and irregular ulcerations with overhanging margins are formed. The number of lesions formed depends upon intensity of infection and degree of individual host susceptibility. Chronic recurrent diarrhea, alternating with constipation, is the most common clinical manifestation, but there may be bloody mu-

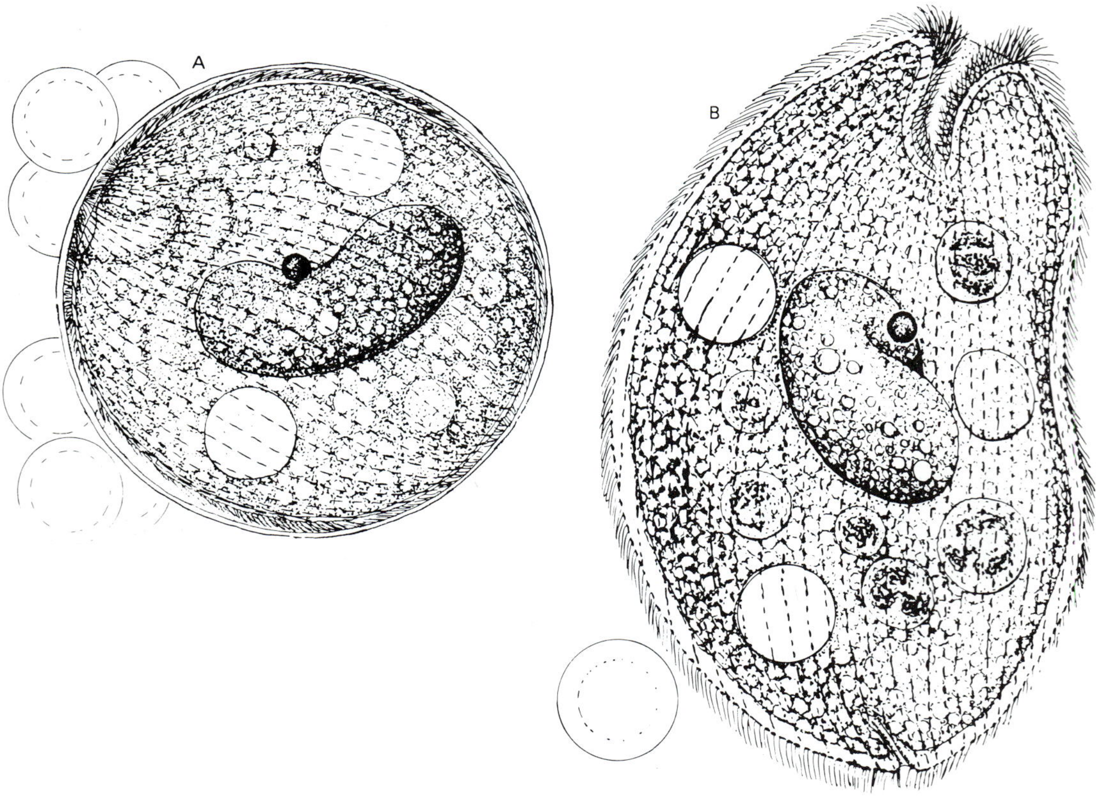

Figure 46–10. *Balantidium coli. **A:*** Cyst; ***B:*** trophozoite. 2000×. (Simple double circles represent the size of red cells.)

coid stools, tenesmus, and colic. Extreme cases may mimic severe intestinal amebiasis, and some have been fatal.

Diagnostic Laboratory Tests

The diagnosis of balantidial infection, whether symptomatic or not, depends upon laboratory detection of trophozoites in liquid stools or, more rarely, of cysts in formed stools. Sigmoidoscopy may be useful for obtaining material directly from ulcerations for examination. Culturing is rarely necessary.

Immunity

Humans appear to have a high natural resistance to balantidial infection. Factors underlying individual susceptibility are not known.

Treatment

A course of oxytetracycline may be followed by iodoquinol or metronidazole if necessary.

Epidemiology

B coli is found in humans throughout the world, particularly in the tropics, but it is a rare infection. Only a few hundred cases have been recorded. Infection results from ingestion of viable cysts previously passed in the stools by humans and possibly by swine. The strain found in swine was noninfective in volunteers. Outbreaks have been reported in crowded encampments, jails, or mental institutions.

FREE-LIVING AMEBAS

Primary amebic meningoencephalitis occurs in Europe and North America from amebic invasion of the brain. The free-living soil amebas *Naegleria fowleri, Acanthamoeba castellani,* and possibly species of *Hartmanella* have been implicated. Most cases have developed in children who were swimming and diving in warm, soil-contaminated pools, either indoors or—usually—outdoors. The amebas, primarily *N fowleri,* apparently enter via the nose and the cribriform plate of the ethmoid, passing directly into brain tissue, where they rapidly form nests of amebas that cause extensive hemorrhage and damage, chiefly in the basilar portions of the cerebrum and the cerebellum. In most cases, death ensued in less than a week. Entry of *Acanthamoeba* into the central nervous system from skin ulcers or traumatic penetration, such as keratitis from puncture of the corneal surface or ulceration from contaminated saline used with contact lenses, has also been reported. Diagnosis is by microscopic examination of the cerebrospinal fluid, which contains the trophozoites and red cells but no bacteria. Amebas can be readily cultured on nonnutrient agar plates seeded with *Escherichia coli.* These soil amebas are distinguished by a large, distinct nucleus; by the presence of contractile vacuoles and mitochondria (absent in *Entamoeba*); and by cysts that have a single nucleus and lack glycogen or chromatoidal bodies. *Acanthamoeba* may encyst in invaded tissues, whereas *Naegleria* does not. Treatment with amphotericin B has been successful in a few cases, chiefly when diagnosis can be made quickly.

BLOOD SPOROZOANS

THE PLASMODIA

The sporozoa of the genus *Plasmodium* are pigment-producing ameboid intracellular parasites of vertebrates, with one habitat in red cells and another in cells of other tissues. Transmission to humans is by the bloodsucking bite of female *Anopheles* mosquitoes of various species.

Morphology & Identification

A. Typical Organisms: Four species of plasmodia typically infect humans: *Plasmodium vivax, Plasmodium ovale, Plasmodium malariae,* and *Plasmodium falciparum.* The morphology and certain other characteristics of these species are summarized in Tables 46–2 and 46–3 and illustrated in Figure 46–11.

B. Culture: Human malaria parasites have been successfully cultivated in fluid media containing serum, erythrocytes, inorganic salts, and various growth factors and amino acids. Continuous cultivation of the erythrocytic phase undergoing schizogony (asexual multiple division) has been achieved and is of critical importance in vaccine development.

C. Growth Characteristics: In host red cells, the parasites convert hemoglobin to globin and hematin; the latter becomes modified into the characteristic malarial pigment. Globin is split by proteolytic enzymes and digested. Oxygen, dextrose, lactose, and erythrocytic protein are also utilized.

D. Variation: Variations of strains exist within each of the four species that infect humans. Variations have been detected in morphology, pathogenicity, enzyme characteristics, resistance to drug therapy, infectivity for mosquitoes, and other characteristics.

Pathogenesis, Pathology, & Clinical Findings

Human infection results from the bite of an infected female *Anopheles* mosquito, in which the **sporozoites,** resulting from the sexual or sporogonic cycle of de-

Table 46–2. Some characteristic features of the malaria parasites of humans (Romanowsky-stained preparations).

	P vivax (Benign Tertian Malaria)	P malariae (Quartan Malaria)	P falciparum (Malignant Tertian Malaria)	P ovale (Ovale Malaria)
Parasitized red cells	Enlarged, pale. Fine stippling (Schüffner's dots). Primarily invades reticulocytes, young red cells.	Not enlarged. No stippling (except with special stains). Primarily invades older red cells.	Not enlarged. Coarse stippling (Maurer's clefts). Invades all red cells regardless of age.[1]	Enlarged, pale. Schüffner's dots conspicuous. Cells often oval, fimbriated, or crenated.
Level of usual maximum parasitemia	Up to 30,000/μL of blood.	Fewer than 10,000/μL.	Max exceed 200,000/μL; commonly 50,000/μL.	Fewer than 10,000/μL.
Ring stage trophozoites	Large rings (1/3–1/2 red cell diameter). Usually one chromatin granule; ring delicate.	Large rings (1/3 red cell diameter). Usually one chromatin granule; ring thick.	Small rings (1/5 red cell diameter). Often 2 granules; multiple infections common; ring delicate, may adhere to red cells.	Large rings (1/3 red cell diameter). Usually one chromatin granule; ring thick.
Pigment in developing trophozoites	Fine; light brown; scattered.	Coarse; dark brown; scattered clumps; abundant.	Coarse; black; few clumps.	Coarse; dark yellow-brown; scattered.
Older trophozoites	Very pleomorphic.	Occasional band forms.	Compact and rounded.[1]	Compact and rounded.
Mature schizonts (segmenters)	More than 12 merozoites (14–24).	Fewer than 12 large merozoites (6–12). Often in rosette.	Usually more than 12 merozoites (8–32). Very rare in peripheral blood.[1]	Fewer than 12 large merozoites (6–12). Often in rosette.
Gametocytes	Round or oval.	Round or oval.	Crescentic.	Round or oval.
Distribution in peripheral blood	All forms.	All forms.	Only rings and crescents (gametocytes).[1]	All forms.

[1]Ordinarily, only ring stages or gametocytes are seen in peripheral blood infected with *P falciparum;* post-ring stages make red cells sticky, and they tend to be retained in deep capillary beds except in overwhelming, usually fatal infections.

velopment in the mosquito are injected into the human bloodstream. The sporozoites rapidly (usually within 1 hour) enter parenchymal cells of the liver, where the first stage of development in humans takes place (exoerythrocytic phase of the life cycle). Subsequently, numerous asexual progeny, the merozoites, rupture and leave the liver cells, enter the bloodstream, and invade erythrocytes. Parasites in the red cells multiply in a species-characteristic fashion, breaking out of their host cells synchronously. This is the **erythrocytic cycle,** with successive broods of merozoites appearing at 48-hour intervals (*P vivax, P ovale,* and *P falciparum*) or every 72 hours *(P malariae).* The incubation period includes the exoerythrocytic cycles (usually 2) and at least one or two erythrocytic cycles. For *P vivax* and *P falciparum,* this period is usually 10–15 days, but it may be weeks or months. The incubation period of *P malariae* averages about 28 days. There is no return of merozoites from red blood cells to liver cells. Without treatment, falciparum infection ordinarily will terminate spontaneously in less than 1 year unless it ends fatally. The other three species continue to multiply in liver cells long after the initial bloodstream invasion, or there may be *delayed* multiplication in the liver. These exoerythrocytic cycles coexist with erythrocytic cycles and may persist as nongrowing resting forms, or **hypnozoites,** after the parasites have disappeared from the peripheral blood. Resurgence of an erythrocytic infection **(relapse)** occurs when merozoites from the liver break out, are not phagocytosed

Table 46–3. Time factors of the various plasmodia in relation to cycles.

	Length of Sexual Cycle (in mosquito at 27°C)	Prepatent Period[1] (in humans) (preerythrocytic cycle)	Length of Asexual Cycle (in humans)
P vivax (tertian or vivax malaria)	8–9 days	8 days	48 hours
P malariae (quartan or malariae malaria)	15–20 days	15–16 days	72 hours
P falciparum (malignant tertian or falciparum malaria)	9–10 days	5–7 days	36–48 hours
P ovale (ovale malaria)	14 days	9 days	48 hours

[1]Preerythrocytic period only. Full incubation period before clinical malaria usually includes prepatent period (which ends 48 hours after infection of the erythrocytes) plus 2 or 3 erythrocytic schizogonic cycles and may extend over a much longer time.

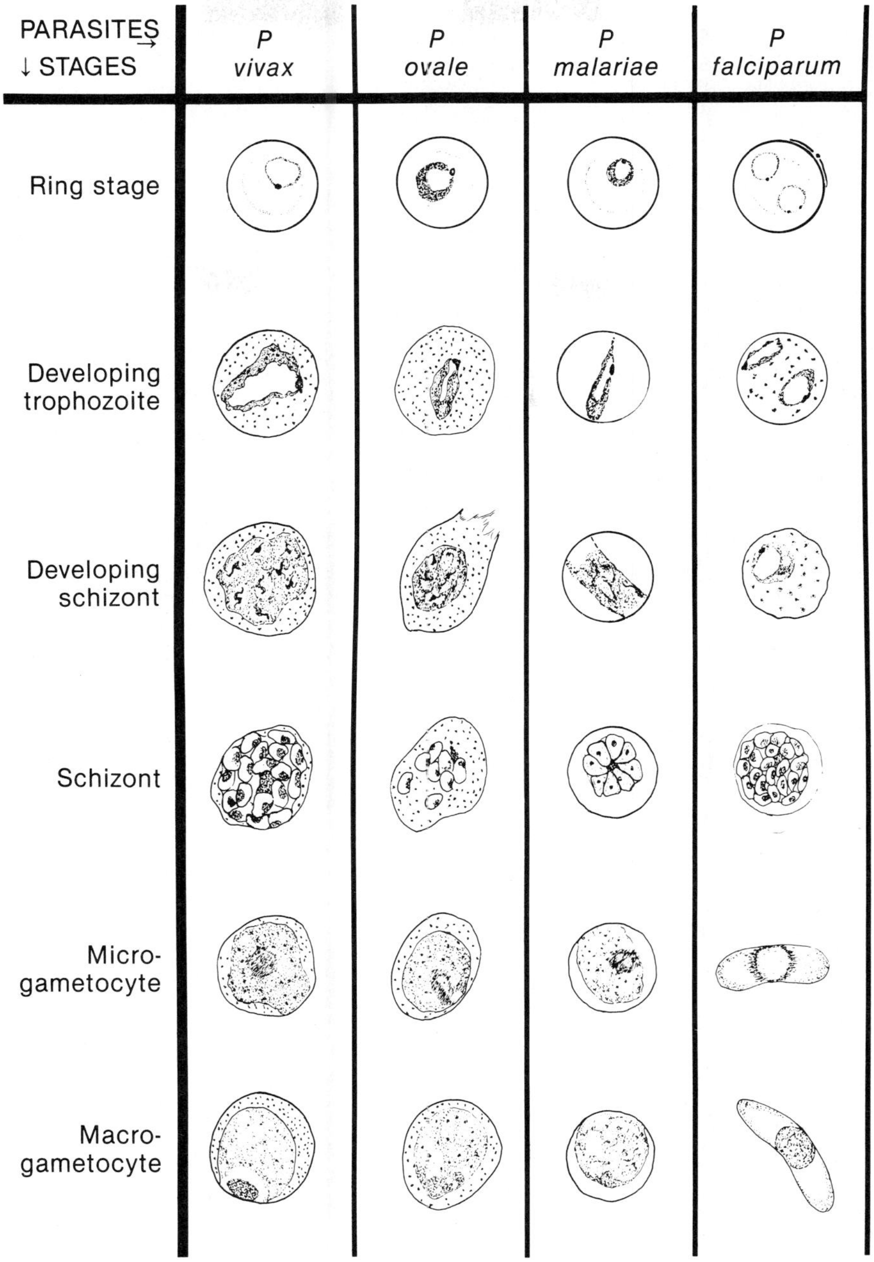

Figure 46–11. Morphologic characteristics of developmental stages of malarial parasites in the red blood cell. Note cytoplasmic Schüffner's dots and enlarged host cells in *P vivax* and *P ovale* infections, the band-shaped trophozoite often seen in *P malariae* infection, and the small, often multiply-infecting rings and the sausage-shaped gametocytes in *P falciparum* infections. Rings and gametocytes only are typically seen in peripheral blood smears from patients with *P falciparum* infections. (Reproduced, with permission, from Goldsmith R, Heyneman D: *Tropical Medicine and Parasitology.* Appleton & Lange, 1989.)

in the bloodstream, and succeed in reestablishing a red cell infection (clinical malaria). Without treatment, *P vivax* and *P ovale* infections may persist as periodic relapses for up to 5 years. *P malariae* infections lasting 40 years have been reported; they are thought to be cryptic erythrocytic rather than exoerythrocytic infections and are therefore termed **recrudescences.**

During the erythrocytic cycles, certain merozoites enter red cells and become differentiated as male or female gametocytes. The sexual cycle therefore begins in the vertebrate host, but then for its continuation into the sporogonic phase, the gametocytes must be taken up and ingested by bloodsucking female *Anopheles* as outlined in Figure 46–12.

P vivax, P malariae, and *P ovale* parasitemias are relatively low-grade, primarily because the parasites favor either young or old red cells but not both; *P falciparum* invades red cells of all ages, including the erythropoietic stem cells in bone marrow, so parasitemia may be very high. *P falciparum* also causes parasitized red cells to produce numerous projecting knobs that adhere to the endothelial lining of blood vessels, with resulting obstruction, thrombosis, and local ischemia. *P falciparum* infections are therefore far more serious than the others, with a much higher rate of severe and frequently fatal complications (cerebral malaria, malarial hyperpyrexia, gastrointestinal disorders, algid malaria, blackwater fever). Consequently, correct and prompt diagnosis of falciparum malaria is imperative and may be lifesaving. *P malariae* has been implicated in a nephrotic syndrome in children—"quartan nephrosis"—with a peak incidence at about age 5 years.

Periodic paroxysms of malaria are closely related to events in the bloodstream. An initial chill, lasting from 15 minutes to 1 hour, begins as a synchronously dividing generation of parasites rupture their host red cells and escape into the blood. Nausea, vomiting, and headache are common at this time. The succeeding febrile stage, lasting several hours, is characterized by a spiking fever that may reach 40 °C or more. During this stage, the parasites presumably invade new red cells. The third, or sweating, stage concludes the episode. The fever subsides, and the patient falls asleep and later awakes feeling relatively well. In the early stages of infection, the cycles are frequently asynchronous and the fever pattern irregular; later, paroxysms may recur at regular 48- or 72-hour intervals, although *P falciparum* pyrexia may last 8 hours or longer and may exceed 41 °C. As the disease progresses, splenomegaly and, to a lesser extent, hepatomegaly appear. A normocytic anemia also develops, particularly in *P falciparum* infections.

Diagnostic Laboratory Tests

A. Specimens and Microscopic Examination: The thick blood film stained with Giemsa's stain is the mainstay of malaria diagnosis. This preparation concentrates the parasites and permits detection even of mild infections. Examination of thin blood films stained with Giemsa's stain is necessary for species differentiation. A promising antigen-capture test (potentially a valuable tool for field use) to detect a trophozoite-derived protein in the blood (*Para*Sight-F

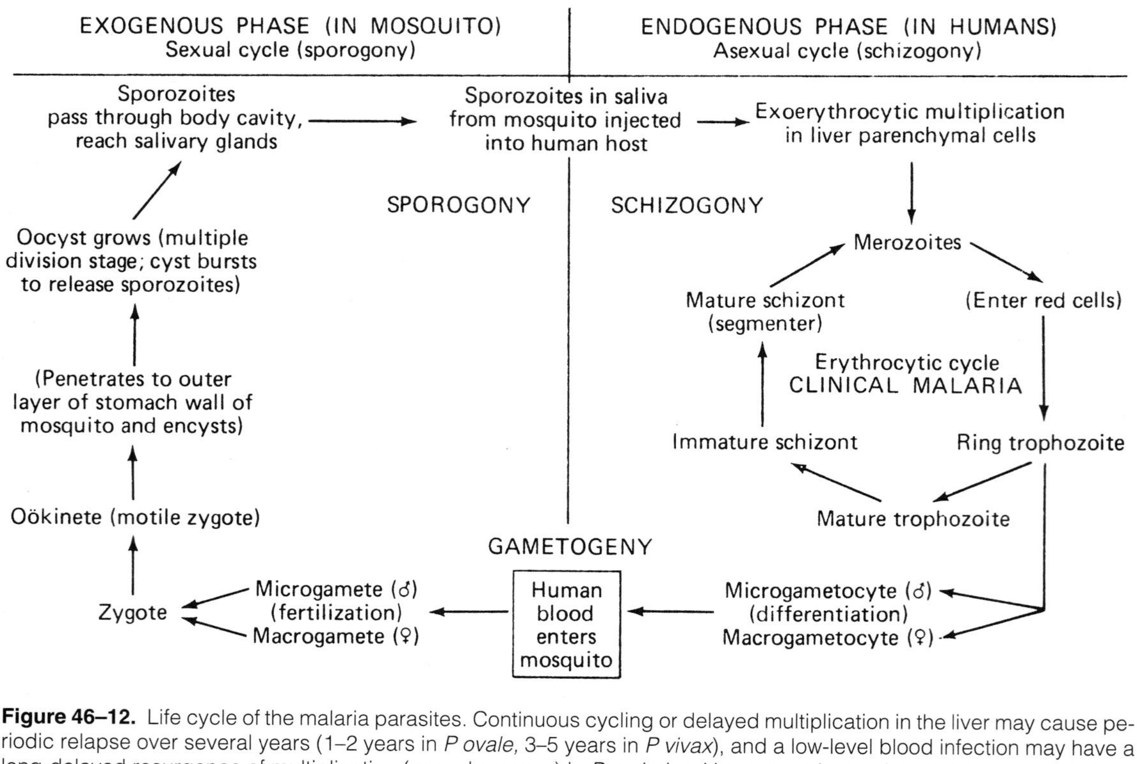

Figure 46–12. Life cycle of the malaria parasites. Continuous cycling or delayed multiplication in the liver may cause periodic relapse over several years (1–2 years in *P ovale,* 3–5 years in *P vivax*), and a low-level blood infection may have a long-delayed resurgence of multiplication (recrudescence) in *P malariae.* However, relapse does not occur with *P falciparum,* though a long prepatent period may occur (perhaps drug-suppressed), resulting in initial symptoms appearing up to 6 months or more after exposure.

test) can be used for rapid diagnosis without need of microscopic examination.

B. Other Laboratory Findings: Normocytic anemia of variable severity may be detected. During the paroxysms there may be transient leukocytosis; subsequently, leukopenia develops, with a relative increase in large mononuclear cells. Liver function tests may give abnormal results during attacks but revert to normal with treatment or spontaneous recovery. The presence of protein and casts in the urine of children with *P malariae* is suggestive of quartan nephrosis. In severe *P falciparum* infections, renal damage may cause oliguria and the appearance of casts, protein, and red cells in the urine.

Immunity

The mechanisms of immunity in malaria are still not clearly understood. An acquired strain-specific immunity has been observed that appears to depend upon the presence of a low-level parasitemia that somehow inhibits new infections or maintains the infection at a nonsymptomatic level. This so-called **premunition,** or **concomitant immunity,** is soon lost after the parasites disappear from the blood. Exoerythrocytic forms in the liver cannot alone support premunition, and they elicit no host inflammatory response. Hence, superinfection of the liver by homologous strains can continue to occur. Natural genetically determined partial immunity to malaria occurs in some populations, notably in Africa, where sickle cell disease, glucose-6-phosphate dehydrogenase deficiency, and thalassemia provide some protection against lethal levels of falciparum infection. Most blacks in West Africa, where malaria is endemic, are totally resistant to *P vivax* malaria because they lack the Duffy antigen (FyFy), which acts as a receptor for *P vivax;* in its absence, *P vivax* cannot invade erythrocytes. *P ovale* frequently replaces *P vivax* in this region.

The gene responsible for the sporozoite coating antigen has been identified and cloned using monoclonal antibody and hybridoma techniques. An antisporozoite vaccine has been developed; its initial testing in humans was not successful, however. A synthetic tripeptide vaccine, SPf66, developed by Patarroyo and colleagues, has been tested in Colombia and found to be partially effective (<50%). A complete prophylactic vaccine would have to be active against both sporozoites and merozoites of the target species, with an antigametocyticidic effect to curb transmission; this is some years in the future.

Treatment & Prevention

Chloroquine (Aralen) is the drug of choice for treatment of all susceptible forms of malaria during the acute attack; 1.5 g of chloroquine (base) is given over a 3-day period or 1.8 g over 4 days. In cases of falciparum malaria coma (cerebral or algid malaria), parenteral quinine dihydrochloride (no longer available in the USA) or quinidine gluconate should be used until oral therapy is possible. *P vivax* strains resistant to chloroquine have recently been reported, but chloroquine is still the drug of choice for all malarias except chloroquine-resistant falciparum infection. Primaquine, an 8-aminoquinoline, eliminates the exoerythrocytic forms in the liver (potentially relapsing malaria), permitting a so-called radical cure. Falciparum malaria does not remain in the liver after its erythrocytic phase, so a cure of the clinical form is a radical cure. Primaquine therapy should follow treatment for clinical malaria. Individuals deficient in glucose-6-phosphate dehydrogenase, frequently blacks or persons originally from the eastern Mediterranean, should be given a longer low-level course of primaquine (or none), owing to the possibility of hemolytic anemia. Primaquine also has gametocyticidal activity against *P falciparum* after a single dose (for adults) of 45 mg base.

Drug-resistant strains of *P falciparum* (multiply resistant in some areas, particularly Southeast Asia) are now found in all endemic tropical regions except the Arabian peninsula, Central America, and the Caribbean region. These resistant strains should be treated with quinine sulfate plus pyrimethamine-sulfadoxine (Fansidar), with quinine plus tetracycline, or with quinine plus clindamycin. Mefloquine (Lariam) and halofantrine (Halfan) are recommended alternative drugs for treatment of chloroquine-resistant *P falciparum* malaria.

Malarial coma should be treated with parenteral quinine or quinidine as for nonchloroquine-resistant cerebral malaria.

Suppressive prophylaxis can be achieved with chloroquine phosphate or amodiaquine except in chloroquine-resistant falciparum areas. Mefloquine is now the chemoprophylactic drug of choice in areas of chloroquine resistance. Doxycycline, taken daily, can be used in areas of multiple drug resistance of *P falciparum,* such as in Thailand near its western border with Myomar (Burma) and its eastern border with Cambodia, though mefloquine has been shown to be an effective suppressant among pregnant women in the Thai-Burma border area. Alternatively, chloroquine can be taken for prophylaxis and pyrimethamine-sulfadoxine withheld for presumptive treatment (as a single dose of 3 tablets) in case of a malarial breakthrough. In Africa south of the Sahara, an additional regimen of proguanil (Paludrine) is recommended. An alternative chemoprophylactic regimen consists of giving doxycycline daily. (For contraindications in pregnancy and other special considerations, see MacLeod, 1992). *No drug regimen can ensure prevention of malaria.* Travelers should avoid mosquito bites, use diethyltoluamide (deet) repellent, and sleep under a mosquito net impregnated with pyrethrin (RID).

In pregnancy, continued prophylaxis with chloroquine (not pyrimethamine or a sulfonamide) is essential because of the danger of transplacental transmission of malarial agents to the fetus.

Epidemiology & Control

Malaria today is generally limited to the tropics and subtropics, although outbreaks in Turkey attest to the capacity of this disease to reappear in areas cleared of the agent. Malaria in the temperate zones is relatively uncommon, although severe epidemic outbreaks may occur when the largely nonimmune populations of these areas are exposed; it is usually unstable and relatively easy to control or eradicate. Tropical malaria is usually more stable, difficult to control, and far harder to eradicate. In the tropics, malaria generally disappears at altitudes above 6000 feet. *P vivax* and *P falciparum,* the most common species, are found throughout the malaria belt. *P malariae* is also broadly distributed but considerably less common. *P ovale* is rare except in west Africa, where it seems to replace *P vivax.* All forms of malaria can be transmitted transplacentally or by blood transfusion or by needles shared among addicts when one is infected. Such cases do not develop a liver or exoerythrocytic infection; thus, relapse does not occur. Natural infection (other than transplacental transmission) takes place only through the bite of an infected female *Anopheles* mosquito.

Malaria control depends upon elimination of mosquito breeding places, personal protection against mosquitoes (screens, pyrethrin-treated netting, repellents), suppressive drug therapy for exposed persons, and adequate treatment of cases and carriers. Eradication requires prevention of biting contact between *Anopheles* mosquitoes and humans long enough to prevent transmission, with elimination of all active cases by treatment and by spontaneous cure. The results of massive efforts in highly endemic tropical areas have been unsuccessful. Many costly eradication projects undertaken between 1955 and 1970 have been replaced with control programs specifically geared to the mosquito vector ecology and malaria epidemiology of each area. These programs must be continued as permanent public health responsibilities.

BABESIA MICROTI

Babesia species are widespread animal parasites, causing infectious jaundice of dogs and Texas cattle fever (redwater fever). Babesiosis, a red cell-infecting tick-borne piroplasmosis caused by *Babesia microti,* is a human disease reported in increasing numbers from Massachusetts, the primary focus being Nantucket Island. A case of babesiosis in a splenectomized soldier that was reported from California was attributed to *B gibsoni.* However, recent outbreaks have been in healthy individuals with no record of splenectomy, corticosteroid therapy, or recurrent infection. The great majority of infections in immunologically intact individuals are asymptomatic, but in affected persons the illness develops 7–10 days after the tick bite and is characterized by malaise, anorexia, nausea, fatigue, fever, sweats, myalgia, arthralgia, and depression. *Babesia* may be mistaken in humans for *P falciparum* in its ring form in red cells, though its "Maltese cross" form in the red cell without pigment is diagnostic. Human babesiosis is more severe in the elderly than in the young. Splenectomized individuals may develop progressive hemolytic anemia, jaundice, and renal insufficiency with prolonged parasitemia. Chloroquine provides clinical relief but is not curative. Good clinical results follow treatment with clindamycin and quinine.

OTHER SPOROZOANS

ISOSPORA

Isospora belli, a sporozoan of the human intestine, causes coccidiosis in humans. Numerous species of intestinal sporozoa or coccidia occur in other animals and cause some of the most economically important diseases of domestic mammals and fowl. *I belli* is one of the few coccidia that multiply sexually in the human intestine—ie, in which humans are the definitive host.

Morphology & Identification

A. Typical Organisms: Only the elongated ovoid oocysts are known for *I belli.* Intestinal biopsies of patients with chronic isosporosis demonstrated both asexual schizogonic and oocyst-producing sexual phases. The oocyst of *I belli* is 25–33 × 12–16 μm and often has an asymmetric cyst wall.

B. Culture: These parasites have not been cultivated.

Pathogenesis & Clinical Findings

I belli inhabits the small intestine. Signs and symptoms of coccidiosis apparently are due to the invasion and multiplication of the parasites in the intestinal mucosa. Oocysts are shed into the intestinal lumen and passed in the stools. Infections may be silent or symptomatic. About 1 week after ingestion of viable cysts, a low-grade fever, lassitude, and malaise may appear, followed soon by mild diarrhea and vague abdominal pain. The infection is usually self-limited after 1–2 weeks, but diarrhea, weight loss, and fever may last for 6 weeks to 6 months. Symptomatic coccidiosis is more common in children than in adults. Chronic infections occur in poorly nourished people living under unsanitary conditions where continued reinfection is more likely, and in immunosuppressed persons.

Diagnostic Laboratory Tests

Diagnosis rests upon detection of oocysts in fresh stool specimens. Stool concentration techniques are usually necessary.

Immunity

Immunity to the coccidia following active infection is well documented in animals, although data from human infection are lacking. The many coccidia species are notably host-specific.

Treatment

Treatment of mild cases consists of bed rest and a bland diet for a few days. Treatment for more severe and chronic cases is with trimethoprim-sulfamethoxazole. Patients allergic to sulfonamides (eg, some AIDS patients) may respond to daily pyrimethamine. Immunosuppressed patients may have to be treated continuously.

Epidemiology

Human coccidiosis results from ingestion of cysts. It is usually sporadic and most common in the tropics and subtropics, although it occurs elsewhere, including the USA.

SARCOCYSTIS

Sarcocystis species are coccidia with a biphasic life cycle: an intestinal (sexual) stage in gut mucosal cells of carnivores, and an encysted tissue (asexual) stage in muscle or other cells of herbivores or other prey animals. Humans apparently serve as both intermediate and final hosts depending on the species of *Sarcocystis.* Human volunteers fed raw beef and pork with *Sarcocystis* cysts later passed *Isospora*-like oocysts in their stools; similar results have been obtained with dogs and cats. Human sarcocystosis develops from ingestion of undercooked beef *(S bovihumanis)* and pork *(S suihumanis).*

Morphology & Identification

In the muscles, the parasites develop in elongated sarcocysts that range from less than 0.1 mm to several centimeters long. When the infective zoites (bradyzoites) are freed from a sarcocyst in the gut of a definitive host, they invade the cells of the intestinal mucosa and enter a sexual stage to produce the oocysts, which typically separate into two sporocysts, each containing four infective sporozoites. The sporocysts are later discharged in the host's feces. When ingested by an intermediate host, the oocysts open in the gut, each releasing four sporozoites. The sporozoites penetrate the gut wall, pass to tissue sites, and invade host cells, where each sporozoite develops into a new sarcocyst with numerous bradyzoites.

Pathogenesis & Clinical Findings

Heavy *Sarcocystis* infections may be fatal in some animals (eg, mice, sheep, swine). Extracts of the parasite contain sarcocystin, a toxin that is probably responsible for the pathogenic effects. It is not clear that the parasite is pathogenic for humans. Fleeting subcutaneous swellings, eosinophilia, and heart failure have, however, been attributed to *Sarcocystis.* Sarcocysts have been found in the human heart, larynx, and tongue as well as in skeletal muscles of the extremities, called *"S lindemanni,"* probably an invalid group designation.

Diagnostic Laboratory Tests

The infection ordinarily causes no symptoms or signs in humans, though severe symptoms presumably would develop in immunosuppressed persons. A reliable CF test has been developed for detection of suspected infections.

Treatment

There is no known effective treatment.

Epidemiology

Intestinal infections in humans result from ingestion of raw or poorly cooked infected lamb, beef, or other meats.

CRYPTOSPORIDIUM

Cryptosporidium species can infect the intestine in immunocompromised persons (eg, those with AIDS) and cause severe intractable diarrhea. The organisms are coccidia related to *Isospora.* They have long been known as parasites of rodents, fowl, rhesus monkeys, and cattle and other herbivores and have probably been an unrecognized cause of self-limited, mild gastroenteritis and diarrhea in humans.

Morphology & Identification

The parasites are minute (2–5 μm) intracellular spheres found in great numbers just under the outer mucosal lining of the stomach or intestine. The mature trophozoite (schizont) divides into eight arc-shaped merozoites, which are released from the parent cell to begin a new cycle. Oocysts measuring 4–5 μm and containing four sporozoites may be seen, but no sporocysts have been demonstrated. Oocysts passed into feces are presumed to be the infective agents.

Pathology & Clinical Findings

Cryptosporidium inhabits the brush border, just within the outer limiting membrane of mucosal epithelial cells of the gastrointestinal tract, especially the surface of villi of the lower small bowel. The prominent clinical feature of cryptosporidiosis is diarrhea, which is mild and self-limited (1–2 weeks) in normal persons but may be severe and prolonged in immunocompromised or very young or old individuals.

Diagnostic Laboratory Tests

Diagnosis depends on detection of oocysts in fresh stool samples. Stool concentration techniques using a modified acid-fast stain are usually necessary (Garcia and Bruckner, 1993).

Treatment

Treatment is unnecessary for patients with normal immunity. For those receiving immunosuppressant drugs, cessation of immunosuppressants may be indicated; for those with AIDS or congenital immunodeficiency, only supportive therapy is available. Spiramycin (Rovamycine) may temporarily be effective.

Epidemiology & Control

Cryptosporidiosis is acquired from infected animal or human feces or from feces-contaminated food or water. Mild cases are common in farm workers. For those at high risk (immunosuppressed and very young or old persons), avoidance of animal feces and careful attention to sanitation are required. The organisms are widespread and probably infect asymptomatically a significant proportion of the human population. Occasional outbreaks, such as the one that occurred in Milwaukee in early 1993, affecting 370,000 people, can result from inadequate protection, treatment, or filtration of water supplies for large urban centers.

TOXOPLASMA GONDII

Toxoplasma gondii is a coccidian protozoan of worldwide distribution that infects a wide range of animals and birds but does not appear to cause disease in them. The normal final hosts are strictly the cat and its relatives in the family Felidae, the only hosts in which the oocyst-producing sexual stage of *Toxoplasma* can occur. Organisms (either sporozoites from oocysts or bradyzoites from tissue cysts) invade the mucosal cells of the cat's small intestine, where they form schizonts or gametocytes. After sexual fusion of the gametes, oocysts develop, exit from the host cell into the gut lumen, and pass out via the feces. These infective, resistant oocysts resemble those of *Isospora.* Within each oocyst, two sporocysts form, and in about 48 hours, four sporozoites form within each sporocyst. The oocyst with its eight sporozoites, when ingested, can either repeat its sexual cycle in a cat or—if ingested by certain birds or by a rodent or other mammal, including humans—can establish an infection in which it reproduces asexually. In the latter case, the oocyst opens in the animal's duodenum and releases the eight sporozoites, which pass through the gut wall, circulate in the body, and invade various cells, where they form trophozoites, multiply, break out, and spread the infection to lymph nodes and other organs. These rapidly multiplying crescentic cells (tachyzoites) initiate the acute stage of disease. Subsequently, they penetrate nerve cells, especially of the brain and eye, where they multiply slowly (as bradyzoites) to form quiescent tissue cysts, initiating the chronic stage of disease. The tissue cysts (formerly called pseudocysts) are infective when ingested by cats (resulting in the intestinal sexual stage followed by oocyst production) or other animals (resulting in production of more tissue cysts).

The organism in humans produces either congenital or postnatal toxoplasmosis. Congenital infection, which develops only when nonimmune mothers are infected during pregnancy, is usually of great severity; postnatal toxoplasmosis is usually much less severe. Most human infections are asymptomatic. However, fulminating fatal infections may develop in patients with AIDS, presumably by alteration of a chronic infection to an acute one. Varying degrees of disease may occur in immunosuppressed individuals, resulting in retinitis or chorioretinitis, encephalitis, pneumonitis, or various other conditions.

Morphology & Identification

A. Typical Organisms: (Figure 46–13.) The trophozoites are boat-shaped, thin-walled cells that are 4–7 × 2–4 μm within tissue cells and somewhat larger outside them. They stain lightly with Giemsa's stain; fixed cells often appear crescentic. Packed intracellular aggregates are occasionally seen. True cysts are found in the brain or certain other tissues. These cysts contain many thousands of spore-like bradyzoites, which can initiate a new infection in a mammal ingesting the cyst-bearing tissue.

B. Culture: T gondii may be cultured only in the presence of living cells, in cell culture or eggs. Typical intracellular and extracellular organisms may be seen.

C. Growth Requirements: Optimal growth is at about 37–39 °C in living cells.

D. Variations: There is considerable strain variation in infectivity and virulence, possibly related to the degree of adaptation to a particular host. All of these forms are thought to comprise a single species, *T gondii.*

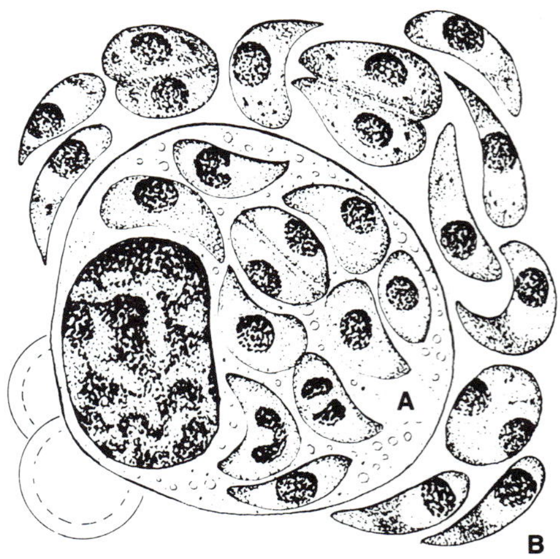

Figure 46–13. *Toxoplasma gondii.* ***A:*** Trophozoites in large mononuclear cell; ***B:*** free in blood. Not found within red cells but parasitize many other cell types, particularly reticuloendothelial cells. Cyst not shown. 2000×.

Pathogenesis, Pathology, & Clinical Findings

The tachyzoite directly destroys cells and has a predilection for parenchymal cells and those of the reticuloendothelial system. Humans are relatively resistant, but a low-grade lymph node infection resembling infectious mononucleosis may occur. When a tissue cyst ruptures, releasing numerous bradyzoites, a local hypersensitivity reaction may cause inflammation, blockage of blood vessels, and cell death near the damaged cyst. Congenital infection leads to stillbirths, chorioretinitis, intracerebral calcifications, psychomotor disturbances, and hydrocephaly or microcephaly. In these cases, the mother was infected for the first time during pregnancy. Prenatal toxoplasmosis is a major cause of blindness and other congenital defects. Infection during the first trimester generally results in stillbirth or major central nervous system anomalies. Second- and third-trimester infections induce less severe neurologic damage, though they are far more common. Clinical manifestations of these infections may be delayed until long after birth, even beyond childhood. Neurologic problems or learning difficulties may be caused by the long-delayed effects of late prenatal toxoplasmosis.

Diagnostic Laboratory Tests

A. Specimens: Blood (buffy coat of heparinized sample), sputum, bone marrow, cerebrospinal fluid, and exudates; lymph node, tonsillar, and striated muscle biopsy material; and ventricular fluid (in neonatal infections) may be required.

B. Microscopic Examination: Smears and sections stained with Giemsa's or other special stains, such as the periodic acid-Schiff technique, may show the organisms. The densely packed cysts, chiefly in the brain or other parts of the central nervous system, suggest chronic infection.

C. Animal Inoculation: This is commonly used for definitive diagnosis. A variety of specimens are inoculated intraperitoneally into groups of mice that are free from infection. If no deaths occur, the mice are observed for about 6 weeks, and tail or heart blood is then tested for specific antibody. The diagnosis is confirmed by demonstration of cysts in the brains of the inoculated mice.

D. Serology: The Sabin-Feldman dye test depends upon the appearance in 2–3 weeks of antibodies that will render the membrane of laboratory-cultured living *T gondii* impermeable to alkaline methylene blue, so that organisms are unstained in the presence of positive serum. It is being replaced by the IHA latex, IFA, and ELISA tests. None of these tests expose technologists to the danger of living organisms, as is required for the dye tests. A CF test may be positive (1:8 titer) as early as 1 month after infection, but it is valueless in many chronic infections. The IFA and IHA tests are routinely used for diagnostic purposes. Frenkel's intracutaneous test is useful for epidemiologic surveys. See Goldsmith and Heyneman (1989) for further information.

Immunity

Some acquired immunity may develop in the course of infection. Antibody titers in mothers, as detected in either blood or milk, tend to fall within a few months. Yet, the fact that prenatal infection is limited to infants born of mothers who were first exposed during their pregnancy strongly suggests that the presence of circulating antibodies is at least partially protective. Immune deficiency diseases (eg, AIDS), immunosuppressant drugs, or changes in host resistance may cause chronic infection with *Toxoplasma* to become a fulminating, acute toxoplasmosis.

Treatment

Acute infections can be treated with a combination of pyrimethamine and sulfadiazine or trisulfapyrimidines. Alternative drug include spiramycin, clindamycin, trimethoprim-sulfamethoxazole, and various other sulfonamide drugs. For use in pregnancy, spiramycin (Rovamycine) is recommended, continued until delivery.

Epidemiology, Prevention, & Control

Transplacental infection of the fetus has long been recognized. Domestic cats have been incriminated in the transmission of the parasite to humans; the infection is transmitted by an *Isospora*-like oocyst found only in the feces of cats and related animals. Rodents play a role in transmission, since they harbor in their tissues infective cysts that may be ingested by cats. Avoidance of human contact with cat feces is clearly important in control, particularly for pregnant women with negative serologic tests. Since oocysts usually take 48 hours to become infective, daily changing of cat litter (and its safe disposal) can prevent transmission. However, pregnant women should avoid all contact with cats, particularly kittens. An equally important source of human exposure is raw or undercooked meat, in which infective tissue cysts are frequently found. Humans (and other mammals) can become infected either from oocysts in cat feces or from tissue cysts in raw or undercooked meat.

MICROSPORIDA

Microsporida belongs to the protozoan phylum Microspora, a unique assemblage of intracellular parasites characterized by a unicellular spore containing a coiled spring-like tubular polar filament through which the sporoplasm is forcibly discharged into a host cell. The invading parasite grows into a spherical or oblong schizont, with two to eight or more nuclei which become separate merozoites, followed by a complex series of sexual and asexual divisions leading to more spore production. Identification of species and genera is based upon electron microscopic morphology of the spore, nuclei, and coiled polar filament. A modified trichrome-blue stain was used successfully to detect microsporidia in urine, stool, and nasopharyngeal specimens. All classes of vertebrates—especially fish—and many invertebrate groups—especially insects—are infected in essentially all tissues.

Transmission is chiefly by ingestion of spores in food or water. Transplacental transmission is common. Few cases were known among humans until intestinal, ophthalmic, and systemic infections were observed among AIDS patients. Microsporida is now increasingly recognized as a group of opportunistic parasites, probably widespread, abundant, and nonpathogenic in immunologically intact persons but a continuing threat to the immunocompromised. They often occur along with *Cryptosporidium* in AIDS patients.

The following microsporidial infections have been found among immunosuppressed individuals (mostly AIDS patients) (Pol et al, 1993; Ortega et al, 1993).

Ocular Infection

A. *Encephalitozoon hellum:* Treatment is with fumagillin (Fumidil-B) eyedrops; possibly itraconazole.

B. *Nosema corneum:* No treatment is effective; keratoplasty may be successful.

Intestinal Infection

A. *Enterocytozoon bineusi:* Treatment is with octreotide (Sandostatin) or albendazole (Zentel).

B. *Septata intestinalis:* (Also in gall bladder and kidney.) Treatment is with albendazole (Zentel).

Disseminated Infection

Encephalitozoon hellum, Nosema connori, Encephalitozoon cuniculi, Pleistophora species. No treatment established.

HELMINTHS*

Table 46–4 shows the principal diseases that are caused by helminths. Eggs may be detected in feces (or urine, with *Schistosoma haematobium;* occasionally *Schistosoma mansoni,* especially with dual infections; and sometimes *Schistosoma japonicum*), preferably after concentration by zinc sulfate centrifugal sedimentation or other techniques (especially for operculated and schistosome eggs; see Garcia and Bruckner, 1993). Eggs of *Enterobius* may be collected directly from the anal margins with cellulose tape on the end of a spatula.

*Eggs in feces are shown in Figures 46–14, 46–15, and 46–16; microfilariae in blood and tissues are characterized in Table 46–5.

THE NEMATODES (Figure 46–14)

Members of the phylum Nemathelminthes, class Nematoda, are a richly varied and highly successful group, consisting of enormous numbers of small worms that occupy essentially every habitat in which multicellular organisms can survive—terrestrial, marine, and freshwater. However, they are best known (though no more biologically significant) in the parasitic realm. Nematodes infect nearly every species of plant and are abundant in every class of vertebrate hosts. Insects as well as other invertebrates are heavily parasitized. In vertebrate hosts, nematodes parasitize a variety of tissues and organs and usually reach a far larger size than do their free-living relatives.

Nematodes can parasitize either intermediate or final hosts. In intermediate hosts, worms in the juvenile, larval, or developmental stages are found, whereas in final (or definitive) hosts, worms occur in the adult or sexually reproductive stage. In some instances, the same host serves in both capacities, as with the many mammalian hosts of *Trichinella,* the agent of trichinosis. Prehistoric humans that were cannibalized or consumed by predatory mammals could have served as both intermediate and final hosts, but today trichinosis cannot be transmitted by humans (ie, humans are dead-end hosts for *Trichinella*).

Characteristics of nematodes that adapt the group to a parasitic existence include a resistant noncellular cuticle that is shed four times during ontogeny; longitudinal muscles that permit a probing, penetrating movement; a complete digestive system that is well-adapted for active ingestion of the host's gut contents, cells, blood, or cellular breakdown products; and a highly developed separate-sexed reproductive system. Eggs and the four larval stages are well-suited for survival in the external environment or in various intermediate hosts. Consequently, various complex life cycle patterns have evolved among nematodes, as is well illustrated by those found in humans. A dozen nematode species are significant human parasites (Table 46–4, nematodes marked with N). An additional dozen or more nematode species are occasional, zoonotic human parasites (ie, animal parasites able to infect humans), most of which are unable to complete their life cycles in humans. Examples are the agents of angiostrongyliasis, anisakiasis, dirofilariasis, gnathosto-

Table 46–4. Diseases due to helminths.

C = cestode (tapeworm) N = nematode (roundworm) T = trematode (fluke)

Disease and Parasite	Location in Host	Mode of Transmission	Geographic Distribution	Treatment of Choice
Angiostrongyliasis; eosinophilic meningoencephalitis *Angiostrongylus cantonensis* (larval) (N), rat lungworm	Larvae in meninges.	Eating raw shrimps, prawns; raw garden slugs; aquatic and land snails; infested lettuce.	Local in Pacific, especially southwest.	Mebendazole (experimental).
Angiostrongyliasis; intestinal angiostrongyliasis *Angiostrongylus costaricensis* (N), cotton rat arterial worm	Larval stages in bowel wall, especially appendix; also regional lymph nodes in mesenteric arteries.	Ingestion of infected snails, slugs, contaminated salad vegetables.	Central America, Brazil.	Surgical excision, thiabendazole (experimental).
Anisakiasis *Anisakis, Phocanema,* other related genera (larval) (N)	Larvae in stomach or intestinal wall, rarely penetrate.	Eating raw or pickled marine fish.	Around Pacific basin (Japan, California, Hawaii) among people who eat raw fish.	Surgical excision, usually short-lived.
Ascariasis *Ascaris lumbricoides* (N), common roundworm	Small intestine; larvae through lungs.	Eating viable eggs from feces-contaminated soil or food.	Worldwide, very common.	Pyrantel pamoate, mebendazole, albendazole.
Capillariasis *Capillaria philippinensis* (N)	Small intestine (mucosa).	Undercooked marine fish.	Philippines, Thailand.	Mebendazole, albendazole, thiabendazole.
Clonorchiasis *Clonorchis sinensis* (T), Chinese liver fluke	Liver (bile ducts).	Uncooked freshwater fish.	China, Korea, Indochina, Japan, Taiwan.	Praziquantel.
Cysticercosis (bladder worm) *Taenia solium* (larval) (C)	Subcutaneous; eye, meninges, brain, etc.	Ingestion of eggs or regurgitation of gravid proglottid from lower GI tract.	Worldwide.	Surgical excision, albendazole, praziquantel.
Dracunculiasis *Dracunculus medinensis* (N), Guinea worm	Subcutaneous; usually leg, foot	Drinking water with *Cyclops.*	Africa, Arabia to Pakistan; locally elsewhere in Asia.	Mechanical or surgical extraction, metronidazole, thiabendazole.
Echinococcosis, hydatidosis *Echinococcus granulosus* (larval) (C), unilocular hydatid cyst	Liver, lung, brain, peritoneum, long bones, kidney.	Contact with dogs, foxes, other canids; eggs from feces.	Worldwide but local; sheep-raising areas.	Surgical aspiration and excision, albendazole, praziquantel (experimental).
Echinococcus multilocularis (larval) (C), alveolar (multilocular) hydatid cysts	Liver.	Fox fur trappers—from contact with fecal matter in fur.	Northern temperate areas with fox-vole cycle.	
Echinostomiasis *Echinostoma ilocanum* (T)	Small intestine.	Freshwater snails.	SE Asia.	Praziquantel.

(*continued*)

Table 46–4. Diseases due to helminths. (*Continued*)

C = cestode (tapeworm) N = nematode (roundworm) T = trematode (fluke)

Disease and Parasite	Location in Host	Mode of Transmission	Geographic Distribution	Treatment of Choice
Enterobiasis *Enterobius vermicularis* (N), pinworm	Cecum, colon (lumen).	Anal-oral; self-contamination and internal reinfection.	Worldwide.	Pyrantel pamoate, mebendazole, albendazole.
Fascioliasis *Fasciola hepatica* (T), sheep liver fluke	Liver (bile ducts, after migration through parenchyma).	Watercress, aquatic vegetation.	Worldwide, especially sheep-raising areas.	Bithionol.
Fasciolopsiasis *Fasciolopsis buski* (T), giant intestinal fluke	Small intestine.	Aquatic vegetation.	E and SE Asia.	Praziquantel, niclosamide.
Filariasis *Wuchereria bancrofti, Brugia malayi* (N), human filarial worms	Lymph nodes; microfilariae in blood.	Bite of mosquitoes; several species.	Tropical and subtropical, very local but widespread.	Diethylcarbamazine, ivermectin (experimental).
Filariasis, occult *Dirofilaria* species (N), heartworm	Lungs (larvae).	Infected mosquitoes.	India, SE Asia.	Diethylcarbamazine, mebendazole, or not treated.
Gnathostomiasis *Gnathostoma spinigerum* (N) rat stomach worm	Subcutaneous, migratory.	Uncooked fish.	E and SE Asia.	Surgical excision, mebendazole.
Heterophyiasis *Heterophyes heterophyes* (T), intestinal fish fluke of humans	Small intestine.	Uncooked fish (mullet).	China, Korea, Japan, Taiwan; Israel; Egypt.	Praziquantel.
Hookworms *Ancylostoma duodenale, Necator americanus* (N)	Small intestine; larvae through lungs.	Through skin, infected soil, from drinking contaminated water (*Ancylostoma*).	Worldwide tropics and North America (*Necator*); temperature zones (*Ancylostoma*).	Mebendazole, pyrantel pamoate, albendazole.
Larva migrans: Cutaneous, creeping eruption *Ancylostoma braziliense* and other domestic animal hookworms (N)	Subcutaneous, migrating larvae.	Contact with soil contaminated by dog or cat feces.	Worldwide.	Thiabendazole, albendazole.
Visceral *Toxocara* species (N), cat and dog roundworms	Liver, lung, eye, brain, other viscera; migrating larvae.	Ingesting soil contaminated by dog or cat feces.	Worldwide.	Thiabendazole, diethylcarbamazine, mebendazole, ivermectin (experimental), albendazole (experimental).
Loiasis *Loa loa* (N)	Subcutaneous, migratory; surface of eye. Microfilariae in blood.	Bite of deer flies, *Chrysops.*	Equatorial Africa.	Surgical removal, diethylcarbamazine, or not treated.

Mansonelliasis *Mansonella ozzardi* (N), (nonpathogenic) Ozzard's filaria	Body cavities, microfilariae in blood.	Bite of gnat *Culicoides.*	Argentina, N coast of S America; Caribbean Islands; Panama, Yucatan.	Invermectin (experimental) or not . treated.
Mansonella perstans (N) (*Dipetalonema perstans*) (nonpathogenic?)	Peritoneal and other cavities; microfilariae in blood.	Bite of gnat *Culicoides.*	Equatorial Africa; N coast of S America, Argentina, Panama, Trinidad.	Mebendazole or not treated.
Metagonimiasis *Metagonimus yokogawai* (T), intestinal fish fluke of humans	Small intestine.	Uncooked fish.	As for *Heterophyes* plus former USSR, Balkans, Spain.	Praziquantel.
Onchocerciasis *Onchocerca volvulus* (N), nodular or binding worm	Subcutaneous; microfilariae in skin, eyes.	Bite of black fly *Simulium.*	Equatorial Africa; C and S America.	Surgery, ivermectin.
Opisthorchiasis *Opisthorchis felineus, Opisthorchis viverrini* (T), Asian liver flukes	Liver (bile duct).	Uncooked fish.	E Europe, former USSR; Thailand.	Praziquantel.
Paragonimiasis *Paragonimus westermani* (T), lung fluke (several species)	Lung (paired worms in cyst), brain, other sites.	Raw crabs and other freshwater crustaceans.	E and S Asia; central Africa; S America; animals in N America.	Praziquantel, bithionol.
Schistosomiasis *Schistosoma haematobium* (T), schistosomes or bilharzia worms, blood flukes; vesicular blood fluke	Venous vessels of urinary bladder, large intestine; liver.	Cercariae (larvae) penetrate skin in snail-infested water.	Africa, widely; Madagascar; Arabia to Lebanon.	Praziquantel, metrifonate.
Schistosoma japonicum (T), Japanese blood fluke	Venous vessels of intestine; liver.	Cercariae (larvae) penetrate skin in snail-infested water.	China, Philippines, Japan; potentially Taiwan.	Praziquantel.
Schistosoma mansoni (T), Manson's blood fluke	Venous vessels of colon, rectum; liver.	Cercariae (larvae) penetrate skin in snail-infested water.	Africa to Near East; parts of S America; Caribbean tropics and subtropics.	Praziquantel, oxamniquine.
Schistosoma mekongi (T), Mekong blood fluke	Venous vessels of intestine; liver.	Cercariae (larvae) penetrate skin in snail-infested water.	Mekong delta of Thailand (Khong Island).	Praziquantel.
Sparganosis *Spirometra mansonoides; Spirometra erinacei* (larvae) (C); pseudophyllidean larva or sparganum from frogs, snakes, some birds and mammals (adult worms in felids or canids)	Intraorbital wound, other wounds or contusions if used as poultice; subtaneous tissues if from ingestion of procercoid or sparganum.	Native poultices such as infected raw frog flesh; drinking water with infected copepods; ingestion of raw frogs, tadpoles, snakes.	Orient; occasionally other countries, including N and S America.	Surgical removal.
Stronglyoidiasis *Strongyloides stercoralis* (N), threadworm	Duodenum, jejunum; larvae through skin, lungs.	Through skin and (rarely) by internal autoreinfection.	Worldwide.	Thiabendazole, albendazole (experimental), ivermectin (experimental).

(*continued*)

Table 46–4. Diseases due to helminths. (*Continued*)

C = cestode (tapeworm) N = nematode (roundworm) T = trematode (fluke)

Disease and Parasite	Location in Host	Mode of Transmission	Geographic Distribution	Treatment of Choice
Tapeworm disease (see also Cysticercosis, Hydatidosis, Echinococcosis, Sparganosis); taeniasis *Diphyllobothrium latum* (C), broad fish tapeworm	Small intestine.	Uncooked freshwater fish.	Alaska, E Canada, Great Lakes area, NW Florida; parts of S America; N Europe; E Mediterranean, Asiatic USSR, Japan; Australia.	Praziquantel, niclosamide.
Dipylidium caninum (C), dog tapeworm	Small intestine.	Ingestion of crushed fleas, lice from pets.	Worldwide.	Praziquantel, niclosamide.
Hymenolepis diminuta (C), rat tapeworm	Small intestine.	Indirectly from rats, mice via infected insects.	Worldwide.	Praziquantel, niclosamide.
Hymenolepis nana (C), dwarf tapeworm	Small intestine.	Anal-oral transfer of eggs or infestion of infected insects; internal reinfection.	Worldwide.	Praziquantel, niclosamide.
Taenia saginata (C), beef tapeworm	Small intestine.	Uncooked beef.	Worldwide.	Praziquantel, niclosamide.
Taenia solium (C), pork tapeworm (see also Cysticercosis)	Small intestine.	Uncooked pork.	Worldwide.	Praziquantel, niclosamide.
Trichinosis *Trichinella spiralis* (N), trichina worm	Larvae in striated muscle (coiled within enlarged fiber cell).	Uncooked pork.	Worldwide.	Mebendazole (plus steroids for severe infection).
Trichostrongyliasis *Trichostrongylus* species (N)	Small intestine.	Ingestion of infective third stage from feces-contaminated food or soil; contact with herbivore feces.	E Europe, former USSR, Iran.	Pyrantel pamoate, thiabendazole.
Trichuriasis *Trichuris trichiura* (N), whipworm	Cecum; colon.	Ingestion of eggs from feces-contaminated soil.	Worldwide.	Mebendazole, albendazole.

Table 46–5. Microfilariae.

Filariid	Disease	Distribution	Vectors	Microfilariae		
				Sheath	Tail Nuclei	Periodicity[1]
Wuchereria bancrofti	Bancroftian and Malayan filariasis: lymphangitis, hydrocele, elephantiasis	Worldwide 41 N to 28 S	Culicidae (mosquitoes)	+	Not to tip	Nocturnal or nonperiodic
Brugia malayi		Oriental region to Japan	Culicidae (mosquitoes)	+	Two distinct	Nocturnal or subperiodic
Loa loa	Loiasis; Calabar swellings; conjunctival worms	Western and central Africa	*Chrysops,* deer fly, mango fly	+	Extend to tip	Diurnal
Onchocerca volvulus	Onchocerciasis: skin nodules, blindness, dermatitis, hanging groin	Africa, Central and South America	*Simulium,* buffalo gnat, black fly	–	Not to tip	Nonperiodic in skin fluids
Mansonella (Dipetalonema) perstans	Mansonelliasis or dipetalonemiasis (minor disturbances)	Africa and South America	*Culicoides,* biting midge	–	Extend to tip	Nocturnal or diurnal or nonperiodic
Mansonella streptocerca	Usually nonpathogenic	Western and central Africa	*Culicoides,* biting midge	–	Extend to tip	In skin only, nonperiodic
Mansonella ozzardi	Ozzard's mansonelliasis (benign), occasionally hydrocele	Central and South America	*Culicoides,* biting midge	–	Not to tip	Nonperiodic

[1]Microfilariae are found in peripheral blood (in blood smear) only at night (nocturnal periodicity), largely at night or during crepuscular hours (subperiodicity), largely during daylight hours (diurnal periodicity), or without clear distinction (nonperiodic). Periodicity appears to be correlated with the bloodsucking habits of the chief vector insect in the particular area of transmission of the filaria.

miasis, and cutaneous and visceral larva migrans (Table 46–4).

Typically, nematode parasites of humans infect enormous numbers of hosts. More than 1 billion persons are hosts for *Ascaris lumbricoides,* the giant roundworm of humans; 600–800 million have hookworm (*Ancylostoma duodenale* or *Necator americanus*); hundreds of millions are infected with filarial worms (chiefly *Wuchereria bancrofti*); and equal numbers have pinworm *(Enterobius vermicularis).*

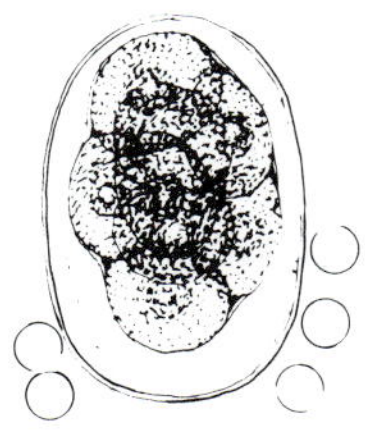

Ancylostoma duodenale or *Necator americanus.* Note shape, thin shell, 4- to 8-cell stage.

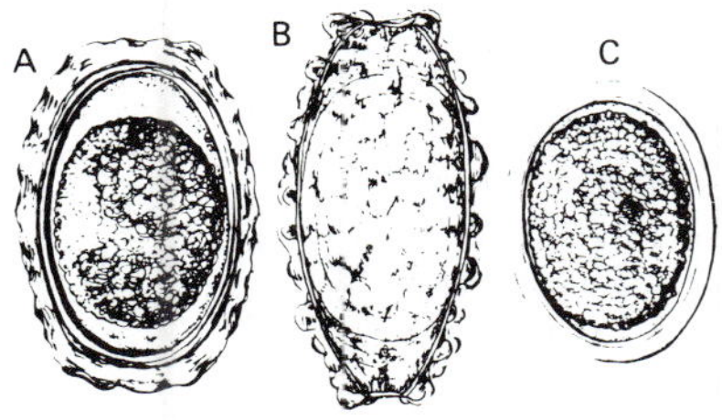

Ascaris lumbricoides. A: Fertilized unembryonated ovum; *B:* unfertilized ovum; *C:* fertilized decorticated ovum. Note heavy protective tuberculated shell in A.

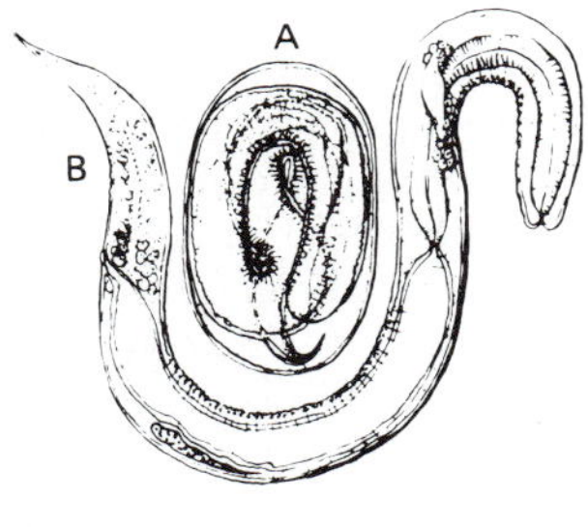

Strongyloides stercoralis. A: Embryonated ovum (rare in feces); *B:* rhabditiform larva (usually seen in feces).

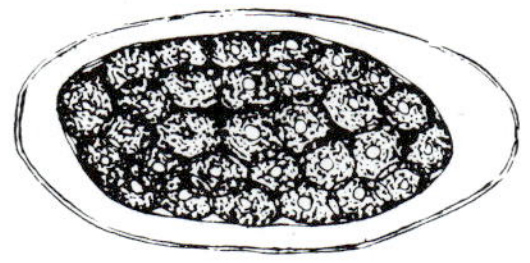

Trichostrongylus orientalis. Unembryonated ovum. (Rare in humans except in specific areas, eg, Iran.)

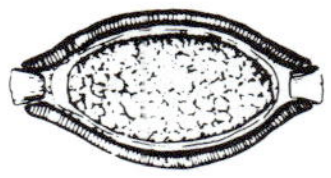

Trichuris trichiura. Unembryonated double-plug ovum.

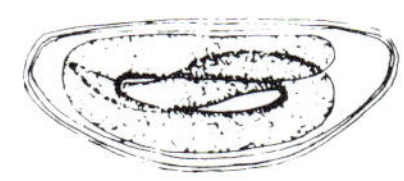

Enterobius vermicularis. Embryonated ovum. Note flattening on one side, thin shell. Deposited on perianal skin.

Figure 46–14. Ova of nematodes. 400×. (Simple circles represent the size of red cells.)

Infection patterns vary widely. Human intestinal nematodes infect via food-borne, water-borne, and soil-borne routes. *Ascaris* and *Trichuris trichiura* (whipworm) infect by eggs that are strongly resistant to desiccation and other environmental factors; hookworms and *Strongyloides stercoralis* (the small roundworm of humans) infect by skin-penetrating, third-stage infective larvae; *Trichinella spiralis* (trichina worm) infect by undercooked meat, usually pork, containing the encysted larvae. The pinworm is unique among human nematodes in that the eggs are viable shortly after being laid directly on the perianal skin by the gravid female. The viable eggs can then be scratched from the pruritic skin surface and accidentally ingested or passed on fingers, clothing, or fecal flecks to others, chiefly children. Consequently, they are mainly urban parasites, in contrast with the other intestinal nematodes, which are passed as eggs or larvae in stool or sewage to the soil and which must undergo varying periods of development before they are infective to humans. They therefore are parasites largely in rural areas. The trichina worm, *Trichinella,* is infective only as encysted larvae in cyst-bearing meat.

Of the tissue-infecting filarial nematodes, *W bancrofti* and *Brugia malayi* are transmitted by mosquitoes; *Loa loa,* the rarely pathogenic eyeworm, by deerflies of the genus *Chrysops; Onchocerca volvulus,* feared agent of river blindness, by blackflies of the genus *Simulium;* and the relatively nonpathogenic filariae of the genus *Mansonella* by various biting gnats or midges of the genus *Culicoides.* Onchocerciasis is a major cause of blindness, especially in western and central Africa. Major control efforts by WHO and supporting agencies have made significant inroads in the prevalence of this disease in West Africa. The distantly related guinea worm *Dracunculus medinensis* has an aquatic cycle via copepods ("water fleas"—an abundant group of aquatic microcrustaceans), which ingest larvae released from skin blisters that burst when immersed in cold water, spewing forth great numbers of larvae. Infected copepods, when drunk inadvertently in water, transmit developed infective guinea worm larvae to humans. In about 1 year, they mature and mate. The females then travel to the skin—usually of the lower leg—where they induce blisters to form; the blisters are again filled with larvae ready to infect copepods. *D medinensis* induces a broad range of pathologic changes depending on the site of adult infection and host response to the parasites' presence or to the worm's removal. Disease caused by guinea worms is a result of secondary infections. These infections may be due to sepsis at the point of emergence of the anterior end of the worm and its larvae from cutaneous blisters. Killed adult worms (or pieces of them) in the skin may also initiate severe infection, leading to gangrene or anaphylaxis. These worms are important causes of debility and economic loss in Africa, where control efforts directed toward eradication are under way.

Intestinal parasites, which are usually well adjusted to the human host (attested to by the vast number of hosts infected), are relatively well tolerated except when present in large numbers (in which case young children are particularly vulnerable). In children, ascariasis and trichuriasis have been shown to cause malnutrition and growth retardation owing to their great number and frequency of reinfection—a major health concern for undernourished populations. This is also true with hookworms, whose bloodsucking can cause severe anemia; with *Strongyloides,* which can overwhelm an immunosuppressed or vulnerable host by its capacity to undergo internal reinfection within humans; and with *Trichinella,* which also multiplies within the host (but to the encysted larval stage only) and may induce a fatal toxic reaction following a heavy initial infection. Fortunately, a strong immune reaction prevents recurrence of severe trichinosis.

The pathologic features of the tissue-infecting nematodes are closely tied to the host response. Elephantiasis, a morbid gross enlargement of limbs, breasts, and genitalia, is an immunopathologic response to long-continued filarial infection by *Wuchereria* or *Brugia.* Lesser enlargement of these tissues, accompanied by severe lymphangina, lymphadenitis, and lymphedema, is a far more common earlier indication of these infections. It is the microfilariae of *Onchocerca* that cause the most severe damage: migrating embryos in the interstitial fluids of the skin and subdermal tissues (*not* the bloodstream) cause changes in skin pigment and loss of elastic fibers, leading to "hanging groin," other skin changes, and severe pruritus, sometimes intractable and intolerable. Far more serious is the blindness that affects millions, mainly in Africa (primarily men). Visual loss develops over many years from an accumulation of microfilariae in the vitreous humor, since the microfilariae are not blood-borne and can concentrate and remain in the fluids of the eye. Visual clouding, photophobia, and ultimate retinal damage result in incurable blindness. The reason for the sex difference in prevalence of onchocercal blindness is unknown.

Treatment of intestinal worms is usually successful using mebendazole (Vermox), pyrantel pamoate (Antiminth), and other drugs (see Table 46–4). Thiabendazole (Mintezol) and, in severe cases, steroids are used—with modest success—against trichinosis. Diethylcarbamazine (Hetrazan) has been used to kill circulating filarial microfilariae, but immunologic toxic reactions may be severe. Ivermectin (Mectizan) is extremely effective in the treatment of early onchocerciasis and may prove effective against the other filariae as well.

THE TREMATODES (Figure 46–15)

The class Trematoda of the phylum Platyhelminthes (flatworms) are soft-bodied syncytial worms, com-

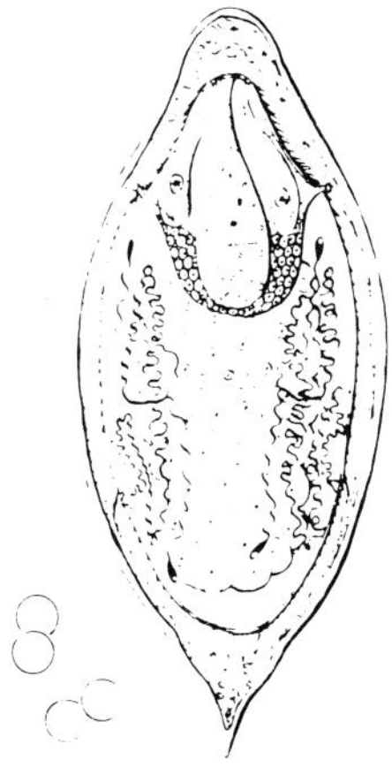

Schistosoma haematobium. Terminally spined embryonated ovum (containing miracidium).

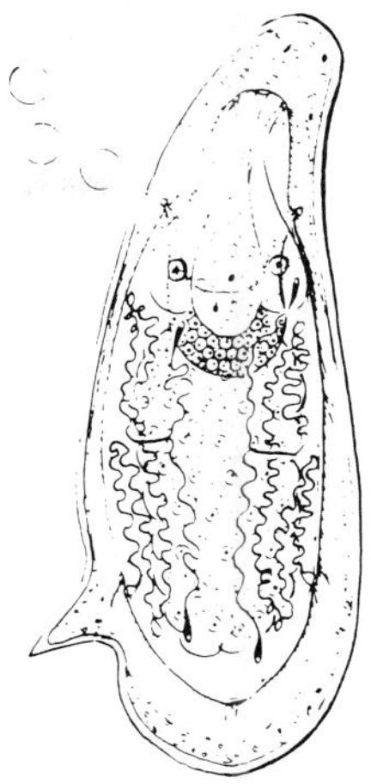

Schistosoma mansoni. Laterally spined embryonated ovum (containing miracidium).

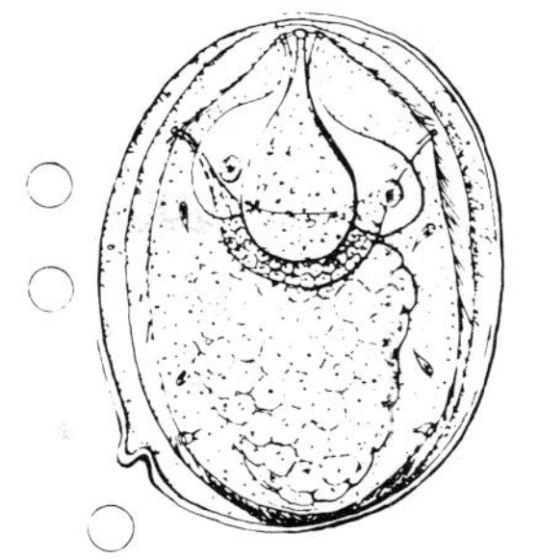

Schistosoma japonicum. Embryonated ovum with small lateral spine, often not visible.

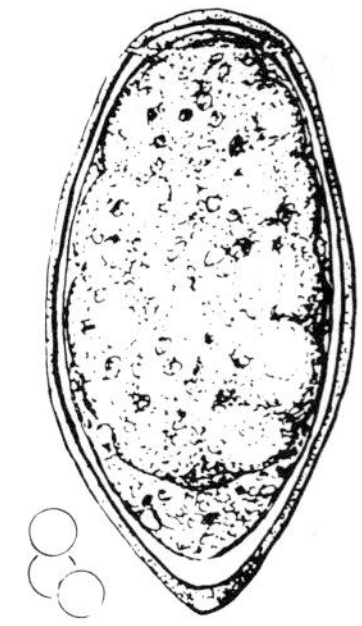

Paragonimus westermani. Unembryonated operculated ovum.

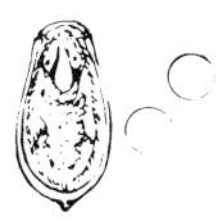

Clonorchis sinensis. Small operculated and embryonated ovum.

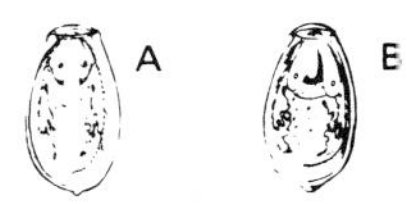

A: Heterophyes heterophyes or *B: Metagonimus yokogawai.* Minute embryonated operculated ova.

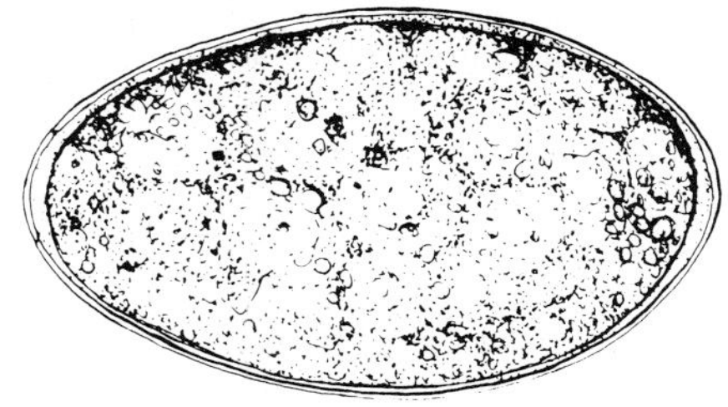

Fasciola hepatica or *Fasciolopsis buski.* Unembryonated operculated ovum.

Figure 46–15. Ova of trematodes as seen in feces. 400×. (Simple circles represent the size of red cells.)

monly called flukes, that are typically flattened and leaf-shaped or elongated with a pair of suckers and a bipartite gut ending blindly with no anus. Flukes possess both circular and longitudinal muscles; they lack the cuticle characteristic of nematodes and instead have a cellular epithelium. A complex reproductive system fills most of the worm's body.

Morphology, life cycles, and infection sites differ markedly among the many species, but the clearest distinction is between the hermaphroditic ("typical") flukes and the separate-sexed schistosomes. The latter are diecious with strong sexual dimorphism; they lack an encysted stage or a second intermediate host. Instead, schistosomes cause infection by penetrating the skin rather than by being ingested with an intermediate or transport host. Schistosomes are morphologically and immunologically specialized to reside in the vascular system of their human—and other—final hosts. In contrast, all other flukes of humans are monoecious and encyst in a second intermediate host or on a transfer medium (such as vegetation) in order to reach the human. There the sexually mature adult nonschistosome flukes develop in the intestine, liver, or lung.

All trematodes undergo a complex asexual reproductive phase through several distinct generations of larval stages in a snail, their first intermediate host. The life cycle of human trematodes is typically initiated by eggs passed to fresh water via body wastes. The eggs develop, hatch, and release a ciliated, snail-seeking first larval form, the **miracidium.** Some flukes, such as the fish-borne *Clonorchis sinensis, Opisthorchis felineus, Opisthorchis viverrini,* and *Heterophyes heterophyes,* have eggs small enough to be eaten by the snail host. Hatching and development within the snail follow. The snail host is usually highly specific to the fluke species, sometimes being limited to a particular strain of the host in a given geographic area. A series of larval generations soon fills most of the snail viscera by a germline process of internal budding within each larva. The miracidium sheds its ciliated coat to form a **sporocyst,** which buds internally to form a group of **rediae,** which then leave and migrate to the snail digestive organ or gonad and produce one or more additional generations of rediae. Ultimately the final larval stage is formed—the **cercaria.** These swarm out of the snail each day and swim with a rapid thrashing of the tail to locate and encyst in a second intermediate host or on vegetation, the sequence being constant for each species. In contrast, the distinctive schistosomes pass through only two generations, both sporocysts, without rediae. The last sporocyst generation of schistosomes forms numerous fork-tailed cercariae that are able to hang from the water surface by the flanges of their terminally forked tails. This ability increases their opportunity to seek and invade the skin of a human or other vertebrate final host. The encysted or **metacercaria** stage found in all other fluke life cycles of humans is thus entirely omitted.

Within these remarkable general patterns of development, each fluke species follows its own unique genetically programmed pattern. *Fasciolopsis buski,* the giant intestinal fluke of humans in China, India, and Southeast Asia, encysts on vegetation, such as the water chestnut *(Eleocharis)* or red caltrop *(Trapa).* The metacercariae are ingested with uncooked vegetation and then excyst and mature in the intestine. These intestinal flukes develop in humans but more commonly in pigs.

Fasciola hepatica, the sheep liver fluke, similarly encysts on aquatic vegetation and may be inadvertently eaten by humans, or cysts may wash off grasses or other vegetation on which metacercariae are usually found and be ingested with drinking water. Adult flukes, rare in humans but abundant in sheep, cattle, and other herbivores, penetrate the gut and then the liver from the body cavity, maturing in the bile ducts.

The human lung fluke *Paragonimus westermani* produces great numbers of cercariae in the infected host snail; these larvae leave the snail and crawl over the aquatic substrate, aided by a short, nonswimming adhesive tail. The larvae seek and penetrate a crustacean second intermediate host, such as a crayfish or freshwater crab. When infected host tissues are eaten raw (often as crushed crab, filtered to produce a liquid salad dressing), metacercariae excyst in the human gut, and young worms migrate to the lungs, where they usually pair and become encapsulated in lung tissue. Eggs are laid, work their way out of the capsule, and are carried by air ducts to the mouth to be expectorated or swallowed and returned to the freshwater environment in feces.

The remaining common flukes of humans are encysted in various freshwater fish. Cysts are digested free in the human duodenum. The minute fish fluke *H heterophyes* remains in the intestine. The mechanical damage to the mucosa it may cause is limited to cases of exceptionally heavy infections. Human liver flukes—*C sinensis* (Chinese liver fluke), *O felineus* (cat liver fluke), and *O viverrini* (civet liver fluke)—are found encysted in a great variety of freshwater fish and infect many humans in East Asia (where all fish-borne flukes are found) and in eastern Europe (where *Heterophyes* and *O felineus* are found). Humans are infected by eating raw, smoked, or pickled fish. Young worms excysted from metacercariae in digested fish flesh pass into the liver through the common bile duct and mature in the bile ducts or remain in the gut (in the case of *Heterophyes*). Heavy infection, especially with *Clonorchis,* can produce cachexia and other severe manifestations. Epigastric pain, edema, and diarrhea are most frequently found.

Treatment has been greatly enhanced by availability of praziquantel (Biltricide), which is now the drug of choice for treatment of all fluke infections except *Fasciola,* for which bithionol (Bitin) is still preferred.

THE CESTODES (Figure 46–16)

The cestodes, or tapeworms, are an example of extreme adaptation to the parasitic life-style. Their ribbon-like chain of segments **(strobila),** each segment bearing a complete male and female system, is capable of prodigious reproductive output. There is no mouth and no trace of an alimentary system. Instead, glucose or other simple predigested nutrients are absorbed directly from the host gut through millions of submicroscopic hair-like extensions, or **microtriches,** which interdigitate with the host's microvilli (brush border). An efficient, highly muscular anterior holdfast organ **(scolex)**—consisting of suckers and, with some species, anterior rings of muscle-controlled spines—maintains the worm's position in the gut or permits it to move freely in the small intestine. All stages of tapeworms are parasitic. The adult is usually found in the intestine, whereas larvae develop in the

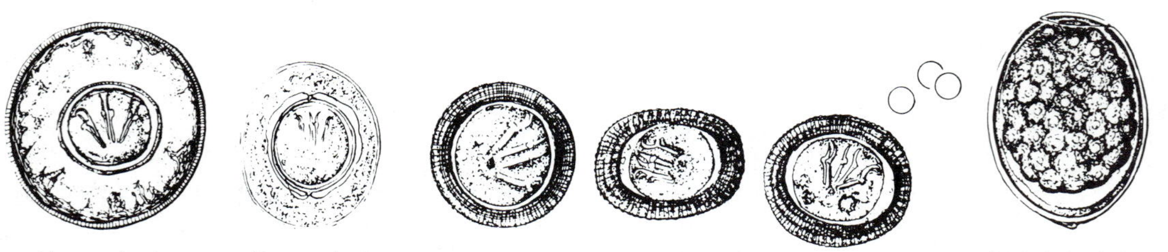

Figure 46–16. Ova of cestodes. Eggs of *Taenia* species are microscopically indistinguishable. 400×. (Simple circles represent the size of red cells.)

tissues of various intermediate hosts, either vertebrate or invertebrate.

In one striking exception, *Hymenolepis nana,* the dwarf tapeworm of humans, the eggs can short-circuit the usual development phase in an insect and infect humans directly from eggs passed in feces of other humans. In this abbreviated (or **direct**) cycle, ingested eggs hatch in the intestine. Each egg releases a 6-hooked microscopic embryo (**hexacanth,** or **oncosphere**), which penetrates a villus. There it forms into the same larva (**cysticercoid**) that usually develops in an insect. After 4 days, the larvae break out of the villi, return to the gut lumen, attach, and mature into small adult worms in the same human host. All other members of this large genus must use an arthropod intermediate host for development of the cysticercoid.

Three groups of tapeworms infect humans: (1) the *Taenia* group, giant adult tapeworms (3–10 m in length), and *Echinococcus* and its relatives, minute tapeworms of dogs and other carnivores, for which humans and many herbivores serve as intermediate hosts for the large larval form (**hydatid cyst**) but never as hosts of the intestinal adult worms; (2) the *Hymenolepis* group, referred to above, and related forms, such as the double-pored tapeworm of dogs, *Dipylidium caninum,* that develop in insects; and (3) the broad fish tapeworm *Diphyllobothrium latum,* which follows an aquatic, copepod-to-fish-to-human developmental pathway.

The first group is noteworthy for another exceptional variant. Adults of *Taenia solium,* the pork tapeworm, develop in the human gut. "Measly pork," containing bladder-like larvae (**cysticerci**) the size of rice grains, is digested in the human intestine to release these larval worms, which develop to adult worms in 3 months. Egg-filled segments then break off and pass out with human feces. These eggs, consumed in water contaminated with human feces, can hatch in the human gut as well as in swine, the normal intermediate host. In both, the hatched egg releases a typical tapeworm embryo, the 6-hooked hexacanth (oncosphere), which can then invade the gut wall and migrate to various tissues such as muscles or the brain, producing cysticercosis. The beef tapeworm *Taenia saginata* appears only able to develop in humans as an adult worm derived from the cysticercus developed in beef. Eggs from the ensuing adult worm develop only in cattle or other herbivores and cannot cause human cysticercosis.

Echinococcus is a genus of minute, 3-segmented tapeworms found in the intestine of dogs and other carnivores. The eggs leave these hosts and infect grazing animals. In the herbivore gut, the eggs hatch and release hexacanths, which penetrate the gut and pass to various tissues, especially liver and other viscera, muscle, and brain. Here larvae grow into huge, fluid-filled cysts in which thousands of future scoleces form. These large hydatid cysts are infective to dogs that feed on the viscera of a diseased sheep or cow. The condition that develops in a sheep can afflict humans as well: hydatid disease, or hydatidosis, occasionally results in the development of a cyst containing many liters of fluid. Humans are infected only from dog feces. Echinococcus eggs are inadvertently ingested with bits of fecal matter, often adhering to the fur. The dog, in turn, can acquire the infection only from an infected herbivore. Several species of *Echinococcus* infect humans, but only the hydatid stage can develop, never the adult intestinal worms.

Of the members of the second group, *H nana* is probably the most common tapeworm of humans, owing to its direct life cycle permitting human-to-human transmission. The **indirect** pathway of *H nana,* with cysticercoids derived from insects, has no developmental phase within the villi. Consequently, no strong immune response in humans results from an insect-derived infection. An initial infection with cysticercoids formed in insects may therefore produce worms whose eggs are free to hatch in the gut without leaving the host and produce an internal autoreinfection. This may be responsible for occasional cases, especially in children, of massive infections with several thousand worms. Other than these instances of extremely heavy infection, disease caused by these worms is limited to minor intestinal disturbance.

The third category of cestodes is distinctive morphologically and epidemiologically. *D latum,* the broad fish tapeworm of humans (and many other fish-eating animals), reaches enormous size, sometimes exceeding 10 m long × 2 cm wide. It is unique among human tapeworms for its freshwater aquatic life cycle involving two intermediate hosts. The first is a copepod; the second, a fish (or series of fish). Eggs pass in great numbers in infected human stool. Portions of stool that reach fresh water dissipate and release eggs that hatch after a period of development. A ciliated swimming embryo, the **coracidium,** emerges from each egg. These are fed on by copepods, allowing the embryonic worms to change to a sausage-shaped **procercoid,** filling much of the body cavity of the copepod. Infected copepods ingested by minnows (or essentially any freshwater fish) permit the cycle to continue to the second, or **plerocercoid (sparganum),** stage, a nonencysted juvenile worm in the flesh of the fish. This stage has the ability to remain viable through a succession of piscivorous fish. With each host transfer, the plerocercoid migrates to the flesh of the new fish host. When a human or other mammal feeds on raw infected fish, the worm rapidly grows in the gut, develops a chain of segments, and within 3 months produces great numbers of eggs—up to 10^6/d. A tissue-infecting zoonosis of humans in Southeast Asia and North and South America called **sparganosis** develops by direct transfer of motile spargana (plerocercoids) of *Spirometra* and related tapeworms into a human sore or eye. The normal route of these tapeworms (related to but distinct from the human fish tapeworm, *Diphyllobothrium latum*) is from copepod to frog to water snake or rodent and to a cat or other carnivore. However, when infected frog or snake flesh is used as a poultice on a wound or injured eye, the larval cestode is attracted by the warmer temperature and crawls into the open tissue. No further development occurs, and inflammation and secondary infection are the usual outcome. Treatment is topical or surgical. Infection of human flesh is also reported by drinking water containing copepods infected with the procercoid larvae.

Disease caused by tapeworms is chiefly vague abdominal discomfort and loss of appetite, leading to weight loss. But *D latum* has an unusual capacity to absorb vitamin B_{12}, and among some groups—especially Finns—a vitamin B_{12} deficiency leading to various levels of pernicious anemia may rarely develop.

Treatment of infection with adult cestodes, as with trematodes, has been greatly simplified and improved with development of the drug praziquantel (Biltricide). However, chewable tablets of the drug niclosamide (Niclocide) are an equally effective alternative preferred by some practitioners.

A summary of basic information on the helminth parasites of humans is contained in Table 46–4.

REFERENCES

Beaver PC, Jung RC, Cupp EW: *Clinical Parasitology,* 9th ed. Lea & Febiger, 1984.

Bruckner DA: Amebiasis. Clin Microbiol Rev 1992;5:356.

Cox FEG (editor): *Modern Parasitology: A Textbook of Parasitology,* 2nd ed. Blackwell, 1993.

Drugs for parasitic infections. Med Lett Drugs Ther 1993; 35:111.

Garcia LS, Bruckner DA: *Diagnostic Medical Parasitology,* 2nd ed. American Society for Microbiology, 1993.

Genta RM: Diarrhea in helminthic infections. Clin Infect Dis 1993;16(Suppl 2):S122.

Gilles HM: *Management of Severe and Complicated Malaria. A Practical Handbook.* WHO, 1991.

Goldsmith RS: Infectious diseases: Protozoal, and Infectious diseases: Helminthic. In: Current Medical Diagnosis & Treatment 1995. Tierney LM Jr, McPhee SJ, Papadakis MA (editors). Appleton & Lange, 1995.

Goldsmith RS, Heyneman D (editors): *Tropical Medicine and Parasitology.* Appleton & Lange, 1989.

Gutierrez Y, Little MD (editors): Diagnosis of important parasitic diseases. Clin Lab Med 1991;11:811.

Jordan P, Webbe G, Sturrock RF (editors): *Human Schistosomiasis.* Univ Arizona Press, 1993.

MacLeod CL (editor): *Parasitic Infections in Pregnancy and the Newborn.* Oxford Univ Press, 1988.

Markell EK, Voge M, John DT: *Medical Parasitology,* 7th ed. Saunders, 1992.

McKerrow J, Heyneman D: Parasitic diseases. In: *Basic & Clinical Immunology,* 8th ed. Stites DP, Terr Al, Parslow TG (editors). Appleton & Lange, 1994.

Neafie RC, Marty AM: Unusual infections in humans. Clin Microbiol Rev 1993;6(1):34.

Ortega YR et al: *Cyclospora* species: A new protozoan pathogen of humans. N Engl J Med 1993;328:1308.

Peters W: *A Colour Atlas of Arthropods in Clinical Medicine.* Wolfe, 1992.

Peters W, Gilles HM: *A Colour Atlas of Tropical Medicine & Parasitology,* 3rd ed. Wolfe, 1989.

Pol S et al: Microsporidia infection in patients with the human immunodeficiency virus and unexplained cholangitis. N Engl J Med 1993;328:95.

Price DL: *Procedure Manual for the Diagnosis of Intestinal Parasites.* CRC Press, 1994.

Rusnak JM, Lucey DR: Clinical gnathostomiasis: Case report and review of the English-language literature. Clin Infect Dis 1993;16:3350.

Stephenson LS: The impact of helminth infections on human nutrition. In: *Schistosomes and Soil-Transmitted Helminths.* Taylor & Francis, 1987.

Sun T (editor): *Progress in Clinical Parasitology.* CRC Press, 1994.

Tanowitz HB et al: Chagas' disease. Clin Microbiol Rev 1992;5:400.

Voller A: Immunoassays for tropical parasitic infections. Trans R Soc Trop Med Hyg 1993;87:497.

Warren KS (editor): *Immunology and Molecular Biology of Parasitic Infections,* 3rd ed. Blackwell, 1993.

Wilson ME: *A World Guide to Infections, Diseases, Distribution, Diagnosis.* Oxford Univ Press, 1991.

World Health Organization: *Basic Laboratory Methods in Medical Parasitology.* WHO, 1991.

World Health Organization: Implementation of the global malaria control strategy. Report of a WHO Study Group on the Implementation of the Global Plan of Action for Malaria Control 1993–2000. WHO, 1993.

Wyler DJ: Malaria: Overview and update. Clin Infect Dis 1993;16:449.

Wyler DJ (editor): *Modern Parasite Biology. Cellular, Immunological, and Molecular Aspects,* 3rd ed. Blackwell, 1993.

Principles of Diagnostic Medical Microbiology

47

Diagnostic medical microbiology is concerned with the etiologic diagnosis of infection. Laboratory procedures used in the diagnosis of infectious disease in humans include the following:

(1) Morphologic identification of the agent in stains of specimens or sections of tissues (light and electron microscopy).

(2) Culture isolation and identification of the agent.

(3) Detection of antigen from the agent by immunologic assay (latex agglutination, EIA, etc) or by fluorescein-labeled (or peroxidase-labeled) antibody stains.

(4) DNA-DNA or DNA-RNA hybridization to detect pathogen-specific genes in patients' specimens.

(5) Demonstration of meaningful antibody or cell-mediated immune responses to an infectious agent.

In the field of infectious diseases, laboratory test results depend largely on the quality of the specimen, the timing and the care with which it is collected, and the technical proficiency and experience of laboratory personnel. Although physicians should be competent to perform a few simple, crucial microbiologic tests—make and stain a smear, examine it microscopically, and streak a culture plate—technical details of the more involved procedures are usually left to the bacteriologist or virologist and the technicians on the staff. Physicians who deal with infectious processes must know when and how to take specimens, what laboratory examinations to request, and how to interpret the results.

This chapter discusses diagnostic microbiology for bacterial, fungal, chlamydial, and viral diseases. The diagnosis of parasitic infections is discussed in Chapter 46.

COMMUNICATION BETWEEN PHYSICIAN & LABORATORY

Diagnostic microbiology encompasses the characterization of thousands of agents that cause or are associated with infectious diseases. The techniques used to characterize infectious agents vary greatly depending upon the clinical syndrome and the type of agent being considered, be it virus, bacterium, fungus, or other parasite. Because no single test will permit isolation or characterization of all potential pathogens, clinical information is much more important for diagnostic microbiology than it is for clinical chemistry or hematology. The clinician must make a tentative diagnosis rather than wait until laboratory results are available. When tests are requested, the physician should inform the laboratory staff of the tentative diagnosis (type of infection or infectious agent suspected). Proper labeling of specimens includes such clinical data as well as the requesting physician's name, address, and telephone number.

Many pathogenic microorganisms grow slowly, and days or even weeks may elapse before they are isolated and identified. Treatment cannot be deferred until this process is complete. After obtaining the proper specimens and informing the laboratory of the tentative clinical diagnosis, the physician should begin treatment with drugs aimed at the organism thought to be responsible for the patient's illness. As the laboratory staff begins to obtain results, they inform the physician, who can then reevaluate the diagnosis and clinical course of the patient and perhaps make changes in the therapeutic program. This "feedback" information from the laboratory consists of preliminary reports of the results of individual steps in the isolation and identification of the causative agent.

DIAGNOSIS OF BACTERIAL & FUNGAL INFECTIONS

Specimens

Laboratory examination usually includes microscopic study of fresh unstained and stained materials and preparation of cultures with conditions suitable for growth of a wide variety of microorganisms, including the type of organism most likely to be causative based on clinical evidence. If a microorganism is isolated, complete identification may then be pursued. Isolated microorganisms may be tested for susceptibility to antimicrobial drugs. When significant pathogens are isolated before treatment, follow-up laboratory examinations during and after treatment may be appropriate.

A properly collected specimen is the single most important step in the diagnosis of an infection, because the results of diagnostic tests for infectious diseases depend upon the selection, timing, and method of collection of specimens. Bacteria and fungi grow and die, are susceptible to many chemicals, and can be found at different anatomic sites and in different body fluids and tissues during the course of infectious diseases. Because isolation of the agent is so important in the formulation of a diagnosis, the specimen must be obtained from the site most likely to yield the agent at that particular stage of illness and must be handled in such a way as to favor the agent's survival and growth. For each type of specimen, suggestions for optimal handling are given in the following paragraphs and in the section on diagnosis by anatomic site, below.

Recovery of bacteria and fungi is most significant if the agent is isolated from a site normally devoid of microorganisms (a normally sterile area). Any type of microorganism cultured from blood, cerebrospinal fluid, joint fluid, or the pleural cavity is a significant diagnostic finding. Conversely, many parts of the body have a normal microbial flora (Chapter 11) that may be altered by endogenous or exogenous influences. Recovery of potential pathogens from the respiratory, gastrointestinal, or genitourinary tracts; from wounds; or from the skin must be considered in the context of the normal flora of each particular site. Microbiologic data must be correlated with clinical information in order to arrive at a meaningful interpretation of the results.

A few general rules apply to all specimens:

(1) The quantity of material must be adequate.

(2) The sample should be representative of the infectious process (eg, sputum, not saliva; pus from the underlying lesion, not from its sinus tract; a swab from the depth of the wound, not from its surface).

(3) Contamination of the specimen must be avoided by using only sterile equipment and aseptic precautions.

(4) The specimen must be taken to the laboratory and examined promptly. Special transport media may be helpful.

(5) Meaningful specimens to diagnose bacterial and fungal infections must be secured before antimicrobial drugs are administered. If antimicrobial drugs are given before specimens are taken for microbiologic study, drug therapy may have to be stopped and repeat specimens obtained several days later.

The type of specimen to be examined is determined by the presenting clinical picture. If symptoms or signs point to involvement of one organ system, specimens are obtained from that source. In the absence of localizing signs or symptoms, repeated blood samples for culturing are taken first, and specimens from other sites are then considered in sequence, depending in part upon the likelihood of involvement of a given organ system in a given patient and in part upon the ease of obtaining specimens.

Microscopy & Stains

Microscopic examination of stained or unstained specimens is a relatively simple and inexpensive but much less sensitive method than culture for detection of small numbers of bacteria. A specimen must contain at least 10^5 organisms per milliliter before it is likely that organisms will be seen on a smear. Liquid medium containing 10^5 organisms per milliliter does not appear turbid to the eye. Specimens containing 10^2–10^3 organisms per milliliter produce growth on solid media, and those containing ten or fewer bacteria per milliliter may produce growth in liquid media.

Gram staining is the single most useful procedure in diagnostic microbiology. Most specimens submitted when bacterial infection is suspected should be smeared on glass slides, Gram-stained, and examined microscopically. The materials and method for Gram staining are outlined in Table 47–1. On microscopic examination, the Gram reaction (purple-blue indicates gram-positive organisms; red, gram-negative) and morphology (shape: cocci, rods, fusiform, or other; see Chapter 2) of bacteria should be noted. The appearance of bacteria on Gram-stained smears does not permit identification of species. Reports of gram-positive cocci in chains are suggestive of, but not definitive for, streptococcal species; gram-positive cocci in clusters suggest a staphylococcal species. Gram-negative rods can be large, small, or even coccobacillary. Some non-

Table 47–1. Gram and acid-fast staining methods.

Gram stain
- (1) Fix smear by heat.
- (2) Cover with crystal violet.
- (3) Wash with water. Do not blot.
- (4) Cover with Gram's iodine.
- (5) Wash with water. Do not blot.
- (6) Decolorize for 10–30 seconds with gentle agitation in acetone (30 mL) and alcohol (70 mL).
- (7) Wash with water. Do not blot.
- (8) Cover for 10–30 seconds with safranin (2.5% solution in 95% alcohol).
- (9) Wash with water and let dry.

Ziehl-Neelsen acid-fast stain
- (1) Fix smear by heat.
- (2) Cover with carbolfuchsin, steam gently for 5 minutes over direct flame (or for 20 minutes over a water bath).
- (3) Wash with water.
- (4) Decolorize in acid-alcohol until only a faint pink color remains.
- (5) Wash with water.
- (6) Counterstain for 10–30 seconds with Loffler's methylene blue.
- (7) Wash with water and let dry.

Kinyoun carbolfuchsin acid-fast stain
- (1) Formula: Basic fuchsin, 4; phenol crystals, 8; alcohol (95%), 20; distilled water, 100.
- (2) Stain fixed smear for 3 minutes (no heat necessary) and continue as with Ziehl-Neelsen stain.

viable gram-positive bacteria can stain gram-negatively. Typically, bacterial morphology has been defined using organisms grown on agar. However, bacteria in body fluids or tissue can have highly variable morphology.

Specimens submitted for examination for mycobacteria should be stained for acid-fast organisms, using either Ziehl-Neelsen stain or Kinyoun stain (Table 47–1). An alternative fluorescent stain for mycobacteria, auramine-rhodamine stain, is more sensitive than other stains for acid-fast organisms but requires fluorescence microscopy and, if results are positive, confirmation of morphology with another acid-fast stain (see Chapter 24).

Immunofluorescent antibody staining (IF) is useful in the identification of many microorganisms. Such procedures are more specific than other staining techniques but also more cumbersome to perform. The fluorescein-labeled antibodies in common use are made from antisera produced by injecting animals with whole organisms or complex antigen mixtures. The resultant **polyclonal antibodies** may react with multiple antigens on the organism that was injected and may also cross-react with antigens of other microorganisms or possibly with human cells in the specimen. Quality control is important to minimize nonspecific IF staining. Use of **monoclonal antibodies** may circumvent the problem of nonspecific staining. IF staining is most useful in confirming the presence of specific organisms such as *Bordetella pertussis* or *Legionella pneumophila* in colonies isolated on culture media. The use of direct IF staining on specimens from patients is more difficult and less specific.

Stains such as calcafluor white, methenamine silver, and occasionally periodic acid-Schiff (PAS) and others are used for tissues and other specimens in which fungi or other parasites are present. Such stains are not specific for given microorganisms, but they may define structure so that morphologic criteria can be used for identification. Calcafluor white binds to cellulose and chitin in the cell walls of fungi and fluoresces under long wave length ultraviolet light. It may demonstrate morphology that is diagnostic of the species (eg, spherules with endospores in *Coccidioides immitis* infection). *Pneumocystis carinii* cysts are identified morphologically in silver-stained specimens. PAS is used to stain tissue sections when fungal infection is suspected. After primary isolation of fungi, stains such as lactophenol cotton blue are used to distinguish fungal growth and to identify organisms by their morphology.

Specimens to be examined for fungi can be examined unstained after treatment with a solution of 10% potassium hydroxide, which breaks down the tissue surrounding the fungal mycelia to allow a better view of the hyphal forms. Phase contrast microscopy is sometimes useful in unstained specimens. Darkfield microscopy is used to detect *Treponema pallidum* in material from primary or secondary syphilitic lesions.

Culture Systems

For diagnostic bacteriology, it is necessary to use several types of media for routine culture, particularly when the possible organisms include aerobic, facultatively anaerobic, and obligately anaerobic bacteria. The specimens and culture media used to diagnose the more common bacterial infections are listed in Table 47–2. The standard medium for specimens is blood agar, usually made with 5% sheep blood. Most aerobic and facultatively anaerobic organisms will grow on blood agar. Chocolate agar, a medium containing heated blood with or without supplements, is a second necessary medium; some organisms that do not grow on blood agar, including pathogenic *Neisseria* and *Haemophilus,* will grow on chocolate agar. A selective medium for enteric gram-negative rods (either MacConkey agar or eosin-methylene blue [EMB] agar) is a third type of medium used routinely. Specimens to be cultured for obligate anaerobes must be plated on at least two additional types of media, including a highly supplemented agar such as *Brucella* agar with hemin and vitamin K and a selective medium containing substances that inhibit the growth of enteric gram-negative rods and facultatively anaerobic or anaerobic gram-positive cocci.

Many other specialized media are used in diagnostic bacteriology; choices depend on the clinical diagnosis and the organism under consideration. The laboratory staff selects the specific media on the basis of the information in the culture request. Thus, freshly made Bordet-Gengou or charcoal-containing medium is used to culture for *B pertussis* in the diagnosis of whooping cough, and other special media are used to culture for *Vibrio cholerae, Corynebacterium diphtheriae, Neisseria gonorrhoeae,* and *Campylobacter* species. For culture of mycobacteria, Löwenstein-Jensen or other specialized solid and liquid media are commonly used. These media may contain inhibitors of other bacteria. Because many mycobacteria grow slowly, the cultures must be incubated and examined periodically for weeks (see Chapter 24).

Broth cultures in highly enriched media are important for back-up cultures of biopsy tissues and body fluids such as cerebrospinal fluid. Broth cultures may give positive results when there is no growth on solid media because of the small number of bacteria present in the inoculum (see above).

Many yeasts will grow on blood agar. Biphasic and mycelial phase fungi grow better on media designed specifically for fungi. Brain-heart infusion agar, with and without antibiotics, and inhibitory mold agar have largely replaced the traditional use of Sabouraud's dextrose agar to grow fungi. Media made with plant and vegetable materials, the natural habitats for many fungi, also grow many fungi that cause infections. Cultures for fungi are commonly done in paired sets, one set incubated at 25–30 °C and the other at 35–37 °C. Table 47–3 outlines specimens and other tests to be used for the diagnosis of fungal infections.

Table 47–2. Common localized bacterial infections: Agents, specimens, and diagnostic tests.

Disease	Specimen	Common Causative Agents	Usual Microscopic Findings	Culture Media	Comments
Cellulitis of skin	Swab	Group A β-hemolytic streptococci, *Staphylococcus aureus*, or both.	Occasionally gram-positive cocci.	Blood agar.	Aspirate from leading edge of infection may yield the organism.
Impetigo	Swab	As for cellulitis (above); rarely, *Corynebacterium diphtheriae*.	As for cellulitis (above) and pharyngitis (below).		
Skin ulcers	Swab	Mixed flora.	Mixed flora.	Blood, MacConkey, or EMB agar; anaerobic conditions.	Skin ulcers below the waist often contain aerobes and anaerobes like gastrointestinal flora.
Meningitis	CSF	*Neisseria meningitidis.*	Gram-negative intracellular or cell-associated diplococci.	Chocolate agar[1] and blood agar for CSF cultures.	Use latex agglutination to detect capsular polysaccharide antigens of serogroups A, C, Y, W135, and B.
		Haemophilus influenzae.	Small gram-negative coccobacilli.	Chocolate agar.[1]	Use latex agglutination to detect capsular polysaccharide antigen.
		Streptococcus pneumoniae.	Gram-positive cocci in pairs.	Blood agar.	Use latex agglutination to detect capsular polysaccharide antigen. Quellung reaction with pneumococcal omniserum.
		Group B streptococci.	Gram-positive cocci in pairs and chains.	Blood agar.	Use latex agglutination to detect capsular polysaccharide antigen.
		Escherichia coli and other Enterobacteriaceae.	Gram-negative rods.	Blood agar.	Mainly in newborns; no need for selective media in CSF culture.
		Listeria monocytogenes.	Gram-positive rods.	Blood agar.	β-Hemolytic and motile.
Brain abscess	Pus	Mixed infection; anaerobic gram-positive and gram-negative cocci and rods, aerobic gram-positive cocci.	Gram-positive cocci or mixed flora.	Blood agar, chocolate agar,[1] anaerobe media.	Specimen must be obtained surgically and transported under strict anaerobic conditions.
Perioral abscess	Pus	Mixed flora of mouth and pharynx.	Mixed flora.	Blood, MacConkey, or EMB agar; anaerobic conditions.	Usually mixed bacterial infection; rarely, actinomycosis.
Pharyngitis	Swab	Group A streptococci.	Not recommended.	Blood agar or selective medium.	β-Hemolytic.
		C diphtheriae.	Not recommended.	Löffler or Pai's medium, then cysteine-tellurite or Tinsdale's medium.	Granular rods in "Chinese character" patterns in smears from culture. Toxicity testing required.
Whooping cough (pertussis)	Swab	*Bordetella pertussis.*	Not recommended.	Regan-Lowe agar.	Fluorescent antibody test identifies organisms from culture and occasionally in direct smears.
Epiglottitis	Swab	*H influenzae.*	Usually not helpful.	Chocolate agar[1] (also use blood agar).	*H influenzae* is part of normal flora in nasopharynx.

(*continued*)

Table 47–2. Common localized bacterial infections: Agents, specimens, and diagnostic tests. (*Continued*)

Disease	Specimen	Common Causative Agents	Usual Microscopic Findings	Culture Media	Comments
Pneumonia	Sputum	*S pneumoniae.*	Many PMNs, gram-positive cocci in pairs or chains. Capsule swelling with omniserum.	Blood agar; also MacConkey, EMB, and chocolate agars.	*S pneumoniae* is part of normal flora in nasopharynx. Blood cultures specific (positive) in 10–20%.
		S aureus.	Gram-positive cocci in pairs, tetrads, and clusters.	Blood agar, also MacConkey, EMB, and chocolate agars.	Uncommon cause of pneumonia. Usually β-hemolytic, coagulase-positive.
		Enterobacteriaceae and other gram-negative rods.	Gram-negative rods.	Blood agar; MacConkey or EMB agar.	Uncommon causes of pneumonia.
		Mixed anaerobes and aerobes.	Mixed respiratory tract flora; sometimes many PMNs.	Blood, MacConkey or EMB agar; anaerobic medium.	Specimens must be obtained by bronchoscopy or transtracheal aspiration; expectorated sputum is unsatisfactory for anaerobes.
Chest empyema	Pus	Same as pneumonia, or mixed flora infection.	Mixed flora.	Blood, MacConkey, or EMB agar; anaerobic conditions.	Usually pneumonia; mixed aerobic and anaerobic flora derived from oropharynx.
Liver abscess	Pus	*E coli; Bacteroides fragilis*; mixed aerobic or anaerobic flora.	Gram-negative rods and mixed flora.	Blood, MacConkey, or EMB agar; anaerobic conditions.	Commonly enteric gram-negative aerobes and anaerobes; consider *Entamoeba histolytica* infection.
Cholecystitis	Bile	Gram-negative enteric aerobes, also *B fragilis.*	Gram-negative rods.	Blood, MacConkey, or EMB agar; anaerobic conditions.	Usually gram-negative rods from gastrointestinal tract.
Abdominal or perirectal abscess	Pus	Gastrointestinal flora.	Mixed flora.	Blood, MacConkey, or EMB agar; anaerobic conditions.	Aerobic and anaerobic bowel flora; often more than 5 species grown.
Enteric fever, typhoid	Blood, feces, urine	*Salmonella typhi.*	Not recommended.	MacConkey, Hektoen, bismuth sulfite agars; others.	Multiple specimens should be cultured; lactose-negative. H_2S produced.
Enteritis, enterocolitis, bacterial diarrheas, "gastroenteritis"	Feces	*Salmonella* species other than *S typhi.*	Gram stain or methylene blue stain may show PMNs.	MacConkey, Hektoen, bismuth sulfite agars; others.	Non-lactose-fermenting colonies onto TSI[2] slants: Nontyphoid salmonellae produce acid and gas in butt, alkaline slant, and H_2S.
		Shigella species.	Gram stain or methylene blue stain may show PMNs.	MacConkey, Hektoen, bismuth sulfite agars; others.	Non-lactose-fermenting colonies onto TSI[2] slants: Shigellae produce alkaline slant, acid butt without gas.
		Campylobacter jejuni.	"Gull wing-shaped" gram-negative rods and often PMNs.	Skirrow's or similar medium.	Incubate at 42 °C; colonies oxidase-positive; smear shows "gull wing-shaped" rods.
		Vibrio cholerae.	Not recommended.	Thiosulfate citrate bile salts sucrose agar; others. Taurocholate-peptone broth for enrichment.	Oxidase-positive colonies to Kligler iron agar slant: alkaline slant, acid butt without gas, no H_2S Serologic tests needed.

(*continued*)

Table 47–2. Common localized bacterial infections: Agents, specimens, and diagnostic tests. (*Continued*)

Disease	Specimen	Common Causative Agents	Usual Microscopic Findings	Culture Media	Comments
Enteritis, enterocolitis, bacterial diarrheas, "gastroenteritis" (*cont'd*)	Feces	Other vibrios.	Not recommended.	As for V *cholerae.*	Differentiate from *V cholerae* by biochemical and culture tests.
		Yersinia enterocolitica.	Not recommended.	MacConkey, CIN[2].	Enrichment at 4 °C helpful; incubate cultures at 25 °C.
Hemorrhagic colitis and hemolytic uremic syndrome	Feces	*E coli* O157:H7.	Not recommended.	Sorbitol MacConkey medium.	Look for sorbitol-negative colonies; type with antisera for O antigen 157 and flagellar antigen 7.
Urinary tract infection	Urine (clean-catch midstream specimen or one obtained by bladder catheterization or suprapubic aspiration)	*E coli;* Enterobacteriaceae; other gram-negative rods.	Gram-negative rods seen on stained smear of uncentrifuged urine indicate more than 10^5 organisms/mL.	Blood agar; MacConkey or EMB agar.	Gray colonies that are β-hemolytic and give a positive spot indole test are usually *E coli*; others require further biochemical tests.
Urethritis/cervicitis	Swab	*Neisseria gonorrhoeae.*	Gram-negative diplococci in or on PMNs. Specific for urethral discharge in men; less reliable in women.	Modified Thayer-Martin or similar antibiotic-containing selective medium.	Positive stained smear diagnostic in men. Culture needed in women. Gonococci are oxidase-positive.
		Chlamydia trachomatis.	PMNs with no associated gram-negative diplococci.	Culture in McCoy cells treated with cycloheximide.	Crescent-shaped inclusions in epithelial cells by stains or immunofluorescence. Direct EIA[3] or fluorescent antibody tests can be helpful.
Genital ulcers	Swab	*Haemophilus ducreyi* (chancroid).	Mixed flora.	Chocolate agar with IsoVitaleX and vancomycin.	Differential diagnosis of genital ulcers includes herpes simplex infection.
		Treponema pallidum (syphilis).	Darkfield or fluorescent antibody examination shows spirochetes.	None.	
	Pus aspirated from suppurating lymph nodes.	*C trachomatis* (lymphogranuloma venereum).	PMNs with no associated gram-negative diplococci.	Culture pus in cell culture (as for urethritis).	
Pelvic inflammatory disease	Cervical swab	*N gonorrhoeae.*	PMNs with associated gram-negative diplococci; mixed flora may be present.	Modified Thayer-Martin or similar antibiotic-containing selective medium.	Causative organisms may be gonococci, anaerobes, others. Anaerobes always present in endocervix; thus, endocervical specimen not suitable for anaerobic culture.
		C trachomatis.	See above.	Cell culture (as for urethritis).	

(*continued*)

Table 47–2. Common localized bacterial infections: Agents, specimens, and diagnostic tests. (*Continued*)

Disease	Specimen	Common Causative Agents	Usual Microscopic Findings	Culture Media	Comments
Pelvic inflammatory disease	Aspirate from cul de sac or by laparoscope	*N gonorrhoeae.*	Gram-negative diplococci in or on PMNs. Specific for urethral discharge in men; unreliable in women.	Modified Thayer-Martin medium.	
		C trachomatis.	See above.	Cell culture (as for urethritis).	
		Mixed flora.	Mixed flora.	Blood, MacConkey, or EMB agar, anaerobic medium.	Usually mixed anaerobic and aerobic bacteria.
Arthritis	Joint aspirate, blood	*S aureus.*	Gram-positive diplococci in pairs, tetrads, and clusters.	Blood agar; chocolate agar.[1]	Occurs in both children and adults; coagulase-positive; usually β-hemolytic.
		N gonorrhoeae.	Gram-negative diplococci in or on PMNs.	Modified Thayer-Martin medium.	
		Others.	Morphology depends upon organisms.	Blood agar, chocolate agar;[1] anaerobic medium.	Includes streptococci, gram-negative rods, and anaerobes.
Osteomyelitis	Pus or bone specimen obtained by aspiration or surgery	Multiple; often *S aureus.*	Morphology depends upon organisms.	Blood agar, MacConkey, EMB agar; anaerobic medium.	Usually aerobic organisms; *S aureus* is most common; gram-negative rods frequent; anaerobes less common.

[1]A chemical supplement such as IsoVitaleX enhances growth of *Haemophilus* and *Neisseria* species.
[2]TSI = triple sugar iron agar; CIN = Cefsuloain Irgasan Novobiocin medium.
[3]EIA = enzyme immunoassay.

Antigen Detection

Immunologic systems designed to detect antigens of microorganisms can be used in the diagnosis of specific infections. IF tests (direct and indirect fluorescent antibody tests) are one form of antigen detection and are discussed in separate sections in this chapter on the diagnosis of bacterial, chlamydial, and viral infections and in the chapters on the specific microorganisms.

Enzyme immunoassays (EIA), including **enzyme-linked immunosorbent assays (ELISA),** and agglutination tests are used to detect antigens of infectious agents present in clinical specimens. The principles of these tests are reviewed briefly here.

There are many variations of EIAs to detect antigens. One commonly used format is to bind a capture antibody, specific for the antigen in question, to the wells of plastic microdilution trays. The specimen containing the antigen is incubated in the wells followed by washing of the wells. A second antibody for the antigen, labeled with enzyme, is used to detect the antigen. Addition of the substrate for the enzyme allows detection of the bound antigen by colorimetric reaction. In some EIAs, the initial antibody is not necessary, because the antigen will bind directly to the plastic of the wells. EIAs are used to detect rotavirus in stool specimens (see Chapter 37), *Chlamydia trachomatis* (Chapter 28), and a few bacteria.

Another form of EIA, to detect antibody, is **immunoblotting ("Western blot"),** whereby defined antigens are placed on strips of nitrocellulose paper. Following incubation with the test antibody-containing specimen, the strip is further treated with an enzyme-labeled antibody, usually from another animal, against the test antibody. Addition of the substrate for the enzyme allows detection of the antigen-specific bound antibody by colorimetric reaction. Western blot tests are used as the specific tests for antibodies in HIV infection and Lyme disease.

In latex agglutination tests, an antigen-specific antibody (either polyclonal or monoclonal) is fixed to latex beads. When the clinical specimen is added to a suspension of the latex beads, the antibodies bind to the antigens on the microorganism forming a lattice structure, and agglutination of the beads occurs. Coagglutination is similar to latex agglutination except that staphylococci rich in protein A are used instead of latex particles; coagglutination is less useful for antigen detection compared with latex agglutination but is helpful when applied to identification of bacteria in cultures.

Latex agglutination tests are primarily directed at the detection of carbohydrate antigens of encapsulated microorganisms (Table 47–4). Antigen detection is used most often in the diagnosis of group A streptococcal pharyngitis, in the etiologic diagnosis of bac-

Table 47–3. Common fungal infections: Agents, specimens, and diagnostic tests.

	Specimen	Serologic and Other Tests	Comments
Invasive (deep-seated) mycoses			
Aspergillosis: *Aspergillus fumigatus,* other *Aspergillus* species			
Pulmonary	Respiratory secretions.	Immunodiffusion tests available; interpretation of results controversial.	Serology seldom useful.
Disseminated	Biopsy specimen, blood.		*Aspergillus* is difficult to grow from blood of patients with disseminated infection.
Blastomycosis: *Blastomyces dermatiditis*			
Pulmonary	Respiratory secretions.	Compliment fixation (CF).	CF test usually negative and therefore not very useful. Culture is the best diagnostic test; serology seldom done.
Oral and cutaneous ulcers	Biopsy or swab specimen.	CF.	
Bone	Bone biopsy.	CF.	
Coccidioidomycosis: *Coccidioides immitis*			
Pulmonary	Respiratory secretions.	CF, immunodiffusion, precipitation, latex agglutination, skin test with coccidioidin or spherulin.	*C immitis* will grow on routine blood agar cultures; positive cultures pose a serious hazard for laboratory workers. Serology often more useful than culture. Skin test does not alter results of serology. Skin test result may have prognostic implications.
Disseminated	Biopsy specimen from site of infection, eg, skin, bone, etc.	As above except that skin test with coccidioidin may be negative.	
Histoplasmosis: *Histoplasma capsulatum*			
Pulmonary	Respiratory secretions.	CF, immunodiffusion, skin test.	Serology very useful. Skin test can "boost" antibody titer and should not be done as a diagnostic test.
Disseminated	Bone marrow, blood, biopsy specimen from site of infection.	As above.	
Nocardiosis: *Nocardia asteroides*			
Pulmonary	Respiratory secretions.	Modified acid-fast stain.	*Nocardia* are bacteria that clinically behave like fungi. Weakly acid-fast, branching, filamenous gram-positive rods are *Nocardia*. Serology seldom used.
Subcutaneous	Aspirate or biopsy of abscess.		
Brain	Material from brain abscess.		
Paracoccidioidomycosis (South American blastomycosis): *Paracoccidioides brasiliensis*			
	Biopsy specimen from lesion.	Immunodiffusion, CF, skin test (paracoccidioidin).	Immunodiffusion test 95% sensitive and specific; CF test and skin test cross-react with histoplasmin. Positive skin test is of prognostic value.
Sporotrichosis: *Sporothrix schenckii*			
Skin and subcutaneous nodules	Biopsy specimen.	Agglutination.	
Disseminated	Biopsy specimen from infected site.	As above.	
Zygomycosis (phycomycosis, mucormycosis): *Rhizopus* species, *Mucor* species, others			
Nasal-ocular-cerebral	Nasal-orbital tissue.	None.	Nonseptate hyphae seen in microscopic sections.
Pulmonary and disseminated	Respiratory secretions, biopsy specimens.	None.	

(*continued*)

Table 47–3. Common fungal infections: Agents, specimens, and diagnostic tests. *(Continued)*

	Specimen	Serologic and Other Tests	Comments
Yeast infections			
Candidiasis: *Candida albicans* and similar yeasts (*Candida tropicalis, Candida parapsilosis,* other *Candida* species, *torulopsis glabrata*)			
Mucous membrane	Secretions.	KOH wet mount useful for microscopy in localized infection.	
Skin	Swab specimen.		
Systemic	Blood, biopsy specimen, urine.	Immunodiffusion, skin test.	Serology seldom helpful. Skin test used to screen for anergy, not to diagnose infection.
Cryptococcosis: *Cryptococcus neoformans*			
Pulmonary	Respiratory secretions.	Cryptococcal antigen rarely detected.	Antibodies to *C neoformans* rarely found.
Meningitis	CSF.	Latex agglutination for cryptococcal antigen is most useful.	Repeated examination of CSF may be necessary to diagnose meningitis.
Disseminated	Bone marrow, bone, blood, other.	Latex agglutination for cryptococcal antigen.	
Primary skin infections			
Dermatophytosis: *Microsporum* species, *Epidermophyton* species, *Trichophyton* species.			
	Hair, skin, nails from infected sites.	None.	

terial meningitis, and to a lesser extent in the diagnosis of lower respiratory tract infections, all in children. Detection of cryptococcal antigen is useful in the diagnosis of cryptococcal meningitis in patients with AIDS or other immunosuppressive diseases.

When latex agglutination tests are performed in the diagnosis of bacterial meningitis, the possible presence of interfering substances (eg, rheumatoid factor or other proteins) in the specimen must be taken into account. In general, it is important to boil the specimens briefly to denature interfering proteins and to analyze other controls in order to be certain that a positive test is truly specific and represents detection of the bacterial antigen.

The sensitivity of latex agglutination tests in the diagnosis of bacterial meningitis may not be better than that of Gram stain, which is approximately 100,000 bacteria per milliliter. Both tests can provide a rapid diagnosis. When Gram-stained smears are positive, agglutination tests can be used to identify the species; however, identification of the species may not allow modification of antimicrobial therapy, because susceptibility testing may be necessary to determine whether or not an organism, eg, *Haemophilus influenzae,* produces β-lactamase. Agglutination tests may be useful in the diagnosis of meningitis when a patient has received prior antimicrobial therapy and Gram stain and culture are negative.

Table 47–4. Commonly used antigen detection tests for bacterial and fungal infections.

Organism	Preferred Specimen	Comment
Lancefield group A streptococci (eg, *Streptococcus pyogenes*)	Throat swab	Antigen detection is 60–80% as sensitive as culture but is positive in most patients with streptococcal pharyngitis. Many commercial kits are available.
Lancefield group B streptococci (eg, *Streptococcus agalactiae*)	Urine (<2 weeks old CSF (>2 weeks old)	Can diagnose neonatal sepsis or meningitis when cultures are negative.
Streptococcus pneumoniae	CSF	Urine is not an acceptable specimen.
Haemophilus influenzae type b	CSF Urine (acceptable)	Common cause of meningitis in children.
Neisseria meningitidis (groups A, C, Y, W135, and B)	CSF	Separate tests are required for some of the groups (eg, B). Urine is not a good specimen.
Cryptococcus neoformans	CSF Serum	Antigen detection is much more sensitive than microscopy of an India ink preparation.

DNA Hybridization

The principle behind molecular diagnostics is the hybridization of a characterized **nucleic acid probe** to a specific nucleic acid sequence in a test specimen followed by detection of the paired hybrid. For example, single-stranded probe RNA or DNA is used to detect complementary RNA or denatured DNA in a test specimen. The nucleic acid probe typically is labeled with enzymes, antigenic substrates, chemiluminescent molecules, or radioisotopes to facilitate detection of the hybridization product. By carefully selecting the probe or making a specific **oligonucleotide** and performing the hybridization under conditions of high stringency, detection of the nucleic acid in the test specimen can be extremely specific. Use of the **polymerase chain reaction (PCR)** to amplify extremely small amounts of specific DNA present in a clinical specimen makes it possible to detect what were initially minute amounts of the DNA with a probe. There are many variations and increasingly complex molecular diagnostic methods for detection of microorganisms and diagnosis of infections. The field is changing very rapidly as new tests are described and marketed. The application of probe technology is likely to have a major impact in the future on diagnostic microbiology.

Nucleic acid probe technology is most cost-effective when used for identification of infectious agents that do not grow rapidly and to help make the diagnosis of infections in which the organisms are not easily cultured or cannot be cultured at all. For example, DNA hybridization technology makes it possible to rapidly identify *Mycobacterium tuberculosis, Mycobacterium avium-intracellulare, Mycobacterium kansasii* and *Mycobacterium gordonae* isolated in cultures, significantly reducing the time to reporting of the species of the isolate. Probe technology makes it possible to detect some pathogens directly in clinical specimens (though traditional methods may be less costly). Examples are *Neisseria gonorrhoeae* and *Chlamydia trachomatis.* With PCR and probe technology, it is also possible to detect specific markers in pathogens, such as genes coding for antimicrobial resistance. For example, PCR followed by probing with a specific oligonucleotide allows detection of the *mecA* gene coding for methicillin (and nafcillin and oxacillin) resistance in *Staphylococcus aureus* and *Staphylococcus epidermidis.* Some microorganisms for which molecular methods can be used for culture confirmation or identification—or for direct detection in a clinical specimen—are listed in Table 47–5. Many other organisms and tests are discussed in the literature of this subject.

DNA probe technology is changing rapidly, and DNA probe applications can be expected to continue to impact many aspects of diagnostic microbiology.

THE IMPORTANCE OF NORMAL BACTERIAL & FUNGAL FLORA

Organisms such as *Mycobacterium tuberculosis, Salmonella typhi,* and *Brucella* species are considered pathogens whenever they are found in patients. However, many infections are caused by organisms that are permanent or transient members of the normal flora. For example, *E coli* is part of the normal gastrointestinal flora and is also the most common cause of urinary tract infection. Similarly, the vast majority of mixed bacterial infections with anaerobes are caused by organisms that are members of the normal flora.

The relative numbers of specific organisms found in a culture are important when members of the normal flora are the cause of infection. When numerous gram-negative rods of species such as *Klebsiella pneumoniae* are found mixed with a few normal nasopharyngeal bacteria in a sputum culture, the gram-negative rods are strongly suspect as the cause of pneumonia, because large numbers of gram-negative rods are not normally found in sputum or in the nasopharyngeal flora; the organisms should be identified and reported. In contrast, abdominal abscesses commonly contain a normal distribution of aerobic, facultatively anaerobic, and obligately anaerobic organisms representative of the gastrointestinal flora. In such cases, identification of all species present is not warranted; instead, it is appropriate to report "normal gastrointestinal flora."

Yeasts in small numbers are commonly part of the normal microbial flora. However, other fungi are not normally present and therefore should be identified and reported. Viruses usually are not part of the normal flora as detected in diagnostic microbiology laboratories. However, some latent viruses, eg, herpes simplex, or live vaccine viruses such as poliovirus occasionally appear in cultures for viruses. In some parts of the world, stool specimens commonly yield

Table 47–5. Examples of microorganisms where molecular probes have been applied to diagnostic microbiology.

Culture Confirmation and Identification	Direct Detection in Clinical Specimens
Mycobacterium tuberculosis complex	*Mycobacterium tuberculosis*
Mycobacterium avium	
Mycobacterium avium complex	
Mycobacterium gordonae	
Mycobacterium kansasii	
Neisseria gonorrhoeae	*Neisseria gonorrhoeae*
Chlamydia trachomatis	*Chlamydia trachomatis*
Haemophilus influenzae	
Listeria monocytogenes	
Campylobacter species	*Legionella pneumophila*
Histoplasma capsulatum	
Coccidioides immitis	
Blastomyces dermatitidis	
Human papillomavirus	Human papillomavirus

evidence of parasitic infection. In such cases, it is the relative number of parasites correlated with the clinical presentation that is important. The presence of a few ova in a specimen should be noted but in itself does not mandate further diagnostic and therapeutic measures.

The organisms that comprise the normal flora of the human body are discussed more extensively in Chapter 11. Members of the normal anerobic flora that are most commonly present in patient specimens and that may be reported as "normal flora" are discussed in Chapter 22.

LABORATORY AIDS IN THE SELECTION OF ANTIMICROBIAL THERAPY

The antimicrobial drug used initially in the treatment of an infection is chosen on the basis of clinical impression after the physician is convinced that an infection exists and has made a tentative etiologic diagnosis on clinical grounds. On the basis of this "best guess," a probable drug of choice can be selected (see Chapter 10). Before this drug is administered, specimens are obtained for laboratory isolation of the causative agent. The results of these examinations may necessitate selection of a different drug. The identification of certain microorganisms that are uniformly drug-susceptible eliminates the necessity for further testing and permits the selection of optimally effective drugs solely on the basis of experience. Under other circumstances, tests for drug susceptibility of isolated microorganisms may be helpful (see Chapter 10).

The commonly performed **disk diffusion susceptibility test** must be used judiciously and interpreted with restraint. In general, only one member of each major class of drugs is represented. For staphylococci, penicillin G, nafcillin, cephalothin, erythromycin, gentamicin, and vancomycin are used. For gram-negative rods, ampicillin, and second- and third-generation cephalosporins, piperacillin and other "anti-pseudomonal penicillins," trimethoprim-sulfamethoxazole, quinolones, and the aminoglycosides (amikacin, tobramycin, gentamicin) are included. For urinary tract infections with gram-negative rods, nitrofurantoin, quinolones, and trimethoprim may be added. The choice of drugs to be included in a routine susceptibility test battery should be based on the susceptibility patterns of isolates in the laboratory, the type of infection (community-acquired or nosocomial), and cost-efficacy analysis for the patient population.

Isolates of *H influenzae* and *N gonorrhoeae* should be tested for β-lactamase production. Isolates of *B fragilis* and other anaerobic bacteria are seldom routinely tested for susceptibility to antimicrobials: The susceptibility test methods have been standardized only for reference laboratories; results from a laboratory using one method may differ widely from results from another laboratory using a different method on the identical strains; and correlations of susceptibility test results indicating clinical efficacy have not been done.

The sizes of zones of growth inhibition vary with the molecular characteristics of different drugs. Thus, the zone size of one drug cannot be compared to the zone size of another drug acting on the same organism. However, for any one drug the zone size can be compared to a standard, provided that media, inoculum size, and other conditions are carefully regulated. This makes it possible to define for each drug a minimum diameter of inhibition zone that denotes "susceptibility" of an isolate by the disk diffusion technique.

The disk test measures the ability of drugs to *inhibit* the growth of bacteria. The results correlate reasonably well with therapeutic response in those disease processes where body defenses can frequently eliminate infectious microorganisms.

In a few types of human infections, the results of disk tests are of little assistance (and may be misleading) because a *bactericidal* drug effect is required for cure. Outstanding examples are infective endocarditis, acute osteomyelitis, and severe infections in a host whose antibacterial defenses are inadequate, eg, persons with neoplastic diseases that have been treated with radiation and antineoplastic chemotherapy, or persons who are being given corticosteroids in high dosage and are immunosuppressed.

Instead of the disk test, a semiquantitative **minimum inhibitory concentration (MIC)** test procedure can be used. It measures more exactly the concentration of an antibiotic necessary to inhibit growth of a standardized inoculum under defined conditions. A semiautomated microtiter method is used in which defined amounts of drug are dissolved in a measured small volume of broth and inoculated with a standardized number of microorganisms. The end point, or minimum inhibitory concentration, is considered the last broth cup remaining clear, ie, free from microbial growth. The minimum inhibitory concentration provides a better estimate of the probable amount of drug necessary to inhibit growth in vivo and thus helps in gauging the dosage regimen necessary for the patient.

In addition, bactericidal effects can be estimated by subculturing the clear broth onto antibiotic-free solid media. The result, eg, a reduction of colony-forming units by 99.9% below that of the control, is called the **minimal bactericidal concentration (MBC).**

The selection of a bactericidal drug or drug combination for each patient can be guided by specialized laboratory tests. Such tests measure either the rate of killing or the proportion of the microbial population that is killed in a fixed time.

In urinary tract infections, the antibacterial activity of urine is far more important than that of serum. The disappearance of infecting organisms from the urine during treatment can serve as a partial drug level assay.

In persons with renal impairment who must receive nephrotoxic drugs and in other special clinical cases, the concentration of drug in serum can be estimated by an assay of serum against special test microorganisms or, even better, by chemical or EIA methods.

DIAGNOSIS OF INFECTION BY ANATOMIC SITE

Wounds, Tissues, Bones, Abscesses, Fluids

Microscopic study of smears and culture of specimens from wounds or abscesses may often give early and important indications of the nature of the infecting organism and thus help in the choice of antimicrobial drugs. Specimens from tissue biopsies obtained for diagnostic purposes should be submitted for bacteriologic as well as histologic examination. Such specimens for bacteriologic examination are kept away from fixatives and disinfectants, minced and finely ground, and cultured by a variety of methods.

The pus in closed, undrained soft tissue abscesses may contain only one organism as the causative agent—most commonly staphylococci, streptococci, or enteric gram-negative rods. The same is true in acute osteomyelitis, where the organisms can often be cultured from blood before the local lesion has become chronic. Because a multitude of microorganisms are frequently encountered in abdominal abscesses and abscesses contiguous with mucosal surfaces as well as in open wounds, it is difficult to decide which organisms are significant in such cases. When deep suppurating lesions drain onto exterior surfaces through a sinus or fistula, the flora of the surface through which the lesion drains must not be mistaken for that of the deep lesion.

Bacteriologic examination of pus from closed or deep lesions must include culture by anaerobic methods. Anaerobic bacteria (*Bacteroides,* streptococci) sometimes play an essential causative role, and mixtures of anaerobes are often present, whereas aerobes may represent surface contaminants. The typical wound infections due to clostridia are readily suspected in gas gangrene.

The methods used must be suitable for the semiquantitative recovery of common bacteria and also for recovery of specialized microorganisms including mycobacteria and fungi. Eroded skin and mucous membranes are frequently the sites of yeast or fungus infections. *Candida, Aspergillus,* and other yeasts or fungi can be seen microscopically in smears or scrapings from suspicious areas and can be grown in cultures.

Exudates that have collected in the pleural, peritoneal, or synovial spaces must be aspirated with meticulous aseptic technique to avoid superinfection. If the material is frankly purulent, smears and cultures are made directly. If the fluid is clear, it can be centrifuged at high speed for 10 minutes and the sediment used for stained smears and cultures. The culture method used must be suitable for the growth of organisms suspected on clinical grounds—eg, mycobacteria, anaerobic organisms, neisseriae—as well as the commonly encountered pyogenic bacteria. Although direct tests for causative microorganisms yield the most important information, tests on oxalated fluids are also helpful. The following results are suggestive of infection: specific gravity over 1.018; protein content over 3 g/dL, often resulting in clotting; and cell counts over 500–1000/μL. Polymorphonuclear leukocytes predominate in acute untreated pyogenic infections; lymphocytes or monocytes predominate in chronic infections. Transudates resulting from neoplastic growth may grossly resemble infectious exudates by appearing bloody or purulent and by clotting on standing. Cytologic study of smears or of sections of centrifuged cells may prove the neoplastic nature of the process.

Blood

Since bacteremia frequently portends life-threatening illness, its early detection is essential. Blood culture is the single most important procedure to detect systemic infection due to bacteria. It provides valuable information for the management of febrile, acutely ill patients with or without localizing symptoms and signs and is essential in any patient in whom infective endocarditis is suspected even if the patient does not appear acutely or severely ill. In addition to its diagnostic significance, recovery of an infectious agent from the blood provides invaluable aid in determining antimicrobial therapy. Every effort should therefore be made to isolate the causative organisms in bacteremia.

In healthy persons, properly obtained blood specimens are sterile. Although microorganisms from the normal respiratory and gastrointestinal flora occasionally enter the blood, they are rapidly removed by the reticuloendothelial system. These transients rarely affect the interpretation of blood culture results. If a blood culture yields microorganisms, this fact is of great clinical significance provided that contamination can be excluded. Contamination of blood cultures with normal skin flora is most commonly due to errors in the blood collection procedure. Therefore, proper technique in performing a blood culture is essential.

The following rules, rigidly applied, yield reliable results:

(1) Use only sterile equipment and strict aseptic technique.

(2) Apply a tourniquet and locate a fixed vein by touch.

(3) Prepare the skin by applying 2% tincture of iodine in widening circles, beginning with the site of proposed skin puncture. Remove iodine with 70% alcohol. After the skin has been prepared, do not touch it except with sterile gloves.

(4) Perform venipuncture and (for adults) withdraw approximately 20 mL of blood.

(5) Add the blood to aerobic and anaerobic blood culture bottles.

(6) Take specimens to the laboratory promptly, or place them in an incubator at 37 °C.

Several factors determine whether blood cultures will yield positive results: the volume of blood cultured, the dilution of blood in the culture medium, the use of both aerobic and anaerobic culture media, and the duration of incubation. For adults, a 20-mL blood sample is usually obtained, and half is placed in an aerobic blood culture bottle and half in an anaerobic one, with one pair of bottles comprising a single blood culture. However, different volumes of blood may be required for the many different blood culture systems that exist. One widely used blood culture system uses bottles that hold 5 mL rather than 10 mL of blood. An optimal dilution of blood in a liquid culture medium is 1:150–1:300; this minimizes the effects of the antibody, complement, and white blood cell antibacterial systems that are present. Because such large dilutions are impractical in blood cultures, most such media contain 0.05% sodium polyanethol sulfonate (SPS), which inhibits the antibacterial systems. However, SPS also inhibits growth of neisseriae, some anaerobic gram-positive cocci, and *Gardnerella vaginalis.* If any of these organisms are suspected, alternative blood culture systems without SPS should be used.

Blood cultures are incubated for 5–7 days unless it is specifically indicated by the physician that a slow-growing pathogen (eg, *Brucella*) might be present. In manual systems, the blood culture bottles are examined two or three times a day for the first 2 days and daily thereafter for 1 week. Automated blood culture systems use a variety of methods to detect positive cultures: detection of CO_2 by infrared spectroscopy, colorimetric detection of pH changes, fluorometric detection of metabolic products, and electronic detection of pressure changes. These automated methods allow frequent monitoring of the cultures and earlier detection of positive ones compared with manual methods. Many laboratories routinely subculture blood cultures to detect organisms that are not visible and have not been detected by the automated system.

The number of blood specimens that should be drawn for cultures and the period of time over which this is done depends in part upon the severity of the clinical illness. In hyperacute infections, eg, gram-negative sepsis with shock or staphylococcal sepsis, it is appropriate to culture two blood specimens obtained from different anatomic sites over a period of 10 minutes. In other bacteremic infections, eg, subacute endocarditis, three blood specimens should be obtained over 24 hours. A total of three blood cultures yields the infecting bacteria in more than 95% of bacteremic patients. If the initial three cultures are negative and occult abscess, fever of unknown origin, or some other obscure infection is suspected, additional blood specimens should be cultured before antimicrobial therapy is started.

Several types of blood culture bottles are available that contain resins which absorb most antimicrobial drugs and some antimicrobial host factors as well. Indications for the use of the resin-containing bottles include the following: a clinically septic patient receiving antimicrobial therapy who already had negative sets of blood cultures; a patient with clinical evidence of endocarditis and negative blood cultures and who is receiving antimicrobial therapy; a patient admitted to the hospital with sepsis who had been given antimicrobial therapy prior to admission. The resin-containing bottles should not be used to follow the effectiveness of therapy because the resin may absorb antimicrobials in the specimen and allow the culture to turn positive in spite of clinically efficacious therapy.

It is necessary to determine the significance of a positive blood culture. The following criteria may be helpful in differentiating "true positives" from contaminated specimens:

(1) Growth of the same organism in repeated cultures obtained at different times from separate anatomic sites strongly suggests true bacteremia.

(2) Growth of different organisms in different culture bottles suggests contamination but occasionally may follow clinical problems such as enterovascular fistulas.

(3) Growth of normal skin flora, eg, *Staphylococcus epidermidis,* diphtheroids (corynebacteria and propionibacteria), or anaerobic gram-positive cocci, in only one of several cultures suggests contamination. Growth of such organisms in more than one culture or from specimens from a patient with a vascular prosthesis enhances the likelihood that clinically significant bacteremia exists.

(4) Organisms such as viridans streptococci or enterococci are likely to grow in blood cultures from patients suspected to have endocarditis, and gram-negative rods such as *E coli* in blood cultures from patients with clinical gram-negative sepsis; therefore, when such "expected" organisms are found, they are more apt to be etiologically significant.

Virtually every species of bacteria has been grown in blood cultures at some time. The following are most commonly found: staphylococci, including *Staphylococcus aureus;* viridans streptococci; enterococci, including *Enterococcus faecalis;* gram-negative enteric bacteria, including *E coli, K pneumoniae,* and *Pseudomonas aeruginosa;* pneumococci; and *H influenzae. Candida* species, other yeasts, and some biphasic fungi such as *Histoplasma capsulatum* grow in blood cultures, but many fungi are rarely, if ever, isolated from blood. Cytomegalovirus and herpes simplex virus can occasionally be cultured from blood, but most viruses and rickettsiae and chlamydiae are not cultured from blood. Parasitic protozoa and helminths usually do not grow in routine blood cultures.

In most types of bacteremia, examination of direct blood smears is not useful. Diligent examination of Gram-stained smears of the buffy coat from anticoagulated blood will occasionally show bacteria in patients with *S aureus* infection, clostridial sepsis, or relapsing fever. In some microbial infections (eg, anthrax, plague, relapsing fever, rickettsiosis, leptospirosis, spirillosis, psittacosis), inoculation of blood into animals may give positive results more readily than does culture.

Urine

Bacteriologic examination of the urine is done mainly when signs or symptoms point to urinary tract infection, renal insufficiency, or hypertension. It should always be done in persons with suspected systemic infection or fever of unknown origin. It is desirable for women in the first trimester of pregnancy.

Urine secreted in the kidney is sterile unless the kidney is infected. Uncontaminated bladder urine is also normally sterile. The urethra, however, contains a normal flora, so that normal voided urine contains small numbers of bacteria. Because it is necessary to distinguish contaminating organisms from etiologically important organisms, only *quantitative* urine examination can yield meaningful results.

The following steps are essential in proper urine examination:

A. Proper Collection of Specimen: Proper collection of the specimen is the single most important step in a urine culture. Satisfactory specimens from males can usually be obtained by cleansing the meatus with soap and water and collecting midstream urine in a sterile container. Satisfactory midstream specimens from females can be obtained after spreading the labia and cleansing the vulva. Catheterization is sometimes unavoidable but it carries a risk of introducing microorganisms into the bladder. Separate specimens from the right and left kidneys and ureters can be obtained by the urologist using a catheter at cystoscopy. When an indwelling catheter and closed collection system are in place, urine should be obtained by sterile aspiration of the catheter with needle and syringe, not from the collection bag. To resolve diagnostic problems, urine can be aspirated aseptically directly from the full bladder by means of suprapubic puncture of the abdominal wall.

For most examinations, 0.5 mL of ureteral urine or 5 mL of voided urine is sufficient. Because many types of microorganisms multiply rapidly in urine at room or body temperature, urine specimens must be delivered to the laboratory rapidly or refrigerated not longer than overnight.

B. Microscopic Examination: Much can be learned from simple microscopic examination of urine. A drop of fresh uncentrifuged urine placed on a slide, covered with a coverglass, and examined with restricted light intensity under the high-dry objective of an ordinary clinical microscope can reveal leukocytes, epithelial cells, and bacteria if more than 10^5/mL are present. Finding 10^5 organisms/mL in a properly collected and examined urine specimen is strong evidence of active urinary tract infection. A Gram-stained smear of uncentrifuged midstream urine that shows gram-negative rods is diagnostic of urinary tract infection.

Brief centrifugation of urine readily sediments pus cells, which may carry along bacteria and thus may help in microscopic diagnosis of infection. The presence of other formed elements in the sediments—or the presence of proteinuria—is of little direct aid in the specific identification of active urinary tract infection. Pus cells may be present without bacteria, and, conversely, bacteriuria may be present without pyuria. The presence of many squamous epithelial cells, lactobacilli, or mixed flora on culture suggests improper urine collection.

Some urine dipsticks contain leukocyte esterase and nitrite, measurements of polymorphonuclear cells and bacteria, respectively, in the urine. Positive reactions are strongly suggestive of bacterial urinary tract infection.

C. Culture: Culture of the urine, to be meaningful, must be performed quantitatively. Properly collected urine is cultured in measured amounts on solid media, and the colonies that appear after incubation are counted to indicate the number of bacteria per milliliter. The usual procedure is to spread 0.01–0.1 mL of undiluted urine on blood agar plates and other solid media for quantitative culture. All media are incubated overnight at 37 °C; growth density is then compared to photographs of different densities of growth for similar bacteria, yielding semiquantitative data.

In active pyelonephritis, the number of bacteria in urine collected by ureteral catheter is relatively low. While accumulating in the bladder, bacteria multiply rapidly and soon reach numbers in excess of 10^5/mL—far more than could occur as a result of contamination by urethral or skin flora or from the air. Therefore, it is generally agreed that if more than 10^5 colonies/mL are cultivated from a properly collected and properly cultured urine specimen, this constitutes strong evidence of active urinary tract infection. The presence of more than 10^5 bacteria of the same type per milliliter in two consecutive specimens establishes a diagnosis of active infection of the urinary tract with 95% certainty. If fewer bacteria are cultivated, repeated examination of urine is indicated to establish the presence of infection.

The presence of fewer than 10^4 bacteria/mL, including several different types of bacteria, suggests that organisms come from the normal flora and are contaminants, usually from an improperly collected specimen. The presence of 10^4/mL of a single type of enteric gram-negative rod is strongly suggestive of urinary tract infection, especially in men. Occasionally, young women with acute dysuria and urinary tract infection will have 10^2–10^3/mL. If cultures are negative but clinical signs of urinary tract infection are present, "urethral syndrome," ureteral obstruction, tuberculosis of the bladder, or other disease must be considered.

Cerebrospinal Fluid

Meningitis ranks high among medical emergencies, and early, rapid, and precise diagnosis is essential. Diagnosis of meningitis depends upon maintaining a high index of suspicion, securing adequate specimens properly, and examining the specimens promptly. Because the risk of death or irreversible damage is great unless treatment is started immediately, there is rarely a second chance to obtain pretreatment specimens, which are essential for specific etiologic diagnosis and optimal management.

The most urgent diagnostic issue is the differentiation of acute purulent bacterial meningitis from "aseptic" and granulomatous meningitis. The immediate decision is usually based on the cell count and the glucose and protein content of cerebrospinal fluid (Table 47–6) and the results of microscopic search for microorganisms. The initial impression is modified by the results of culture, serologic tests, and other laboratory procedures. In evaluating the results of cerebrospinal fluid glucose determinations, the simultaneous blood glucose level must be considered. In some central nervous system neoplasms, the cerebrospinal fluid glucose level is low. In bacterial and fungal meningitis, the cerebrospinal fluid lactic acid level is often above 35 mg/dL.

A. Specimens: As soon as infection of the central nervous system is suspected, blood samples are taken for culture, and cerebrospinal fluid is obtained. To obtain cerebrospinal fluid, perform lumbar puncture with strict aseptic technique, taking care not to risk compression of the medulla by too rapid withdrawal of fluid when the intracranial pressure is markedly elevated. Cerebrospinal fluid is usually collected in 3–4 portions of 2–5 mL each, in sterile tubes. This permits the most convenient and reliable performance of tests to determine the several different values needed to plan a course of action.

B. Microscopic Examination: Smears are made from fresh uncentrifuged cerebrospinal fluid that appears cloudy or from the sediment of centrifuged cerebrospinal fluid. Smears are stained with Gram's stain and occasionally with Ziehl-Neelsen stain. Study of stained smears under the oil immersion objective may reveal intracellular gram-negative diplococci (meningococci), intra- and extracellular lancet-shaped gram-positive diplococci (pneumococci), or small gram-negative rods (*H influenzae* or enteric gram-negative rods).

C. Antigen Detection and Counterimmunoelectrophoresis: If stained smears fail to reveal the presence of a microorganism, specific antisera against important central nervous system pathogens can be used in latex particle agglutination or coagglutination tests. Agglutination suggests the causative organism and can help in the selection of early specific treatment. Cryptococcal antigen in cerebrospinal fluid may be detected by a latex agglutination test.

D. Culture: The culture methods used must favor the growth of microorganisms most commonly encountered in meningitis. Sheep blood and chocolate agar together grow almost all bacteria and fungi that cause meningitis. The diagnosis of tuberculous meningitis requires cultures on special media (see Table 47–2 and Chapter 24). Virus isolation can be attempted in aseptic meningitis or meningoencephalitis. The virus can be successfully isolated from the cerebrospinal fluid in infections caused by mumps virus, echoviruses, or coxsackieviruses.

Table 47–6. Typical cerebrospinal fluid findings in various central nervous system diseases.

Diagnosis	Cells (per μL)	Glucose (mg/dL)	Protein (mg/dL)	Opening Pressure	Remark Below
Normal	0–5 lymphocytes	45–85	15–45	70–180 mm H_2O	1
Purulent meningitis (bacterial)	200–20,000 PMNs	Low (<45)	High (>50)	++++	2
Granulomatous meningitis (mycobacterial, fungal)	100–1000, mostly lymphocytes	Low (<45)	High (>50)	+++	2, 3
Aseptic meningitis, viral or meningoencephalitis	100–1000, mostly lymphocytes	Normal	Moderately high (>50)	Normal to +	3, 4
Spirochetal meningitis (syphilis, leptospirosis)	25–2000, mostly lymphocytes	Normal or low	High (>50)	+	3
"Neighborhood" reaction	Variably increased	Normal	Normal or high	Variable	5

1. CSF glucose level must be considered in relation to blood glucose level. Normally, CSF glucose level is 20–30 mg/dL lower than blood glucose level, or 50–70% of blood glucose normal value.
2. Organisms in smear or culture of CSF.
3. PMNs may predominate early.
4. Virus isolation from CSF early; antibody titer rise in paired specimens of serum.
5. May occur in mastoiditis, brain abscess, epidural abscess, sinusitis, septic thrombus, brain tumor, CSF culture usually negative.

E. Follow-Up Examination of Cerebrospinal Fluid: The return of the cerebrospinal fluid glucose level and cell count toward normal is good evidence of adequate therapy. The clinical response is of paramount importance.

Respiratory Secretions

Symptoms or signs often point to involvement of a particular part of the respiratory tract, and specimens are chosen accordingly. In interpreting laboratory results, it is necessary to consider the normal microbial flora of the area from which the specimen was collected.

A. Specimens:

1. Throat–Most "sore throats" are due to viral infection. Only 5–10% of "sore throats" in adults and 15–20% in children are associated with bacterial infections. The finding of a follicular yellowish exudate or a grayish membrane must arouse the suspicion that Lancefield group A β-hemolytic streptococcal, diphtherial, fusospirochetal (Vincent's), or candidal infection exists; such signs may also be present in infectious mononucleosis and herpesvirus, adenovirus, and other virus infections.

Throat swabs are taken from each tonsillar area and from the posterior pharyngeal wall. The normal throat flora includes an abundance of viridans streptococci, neisseriae, diphtheroids, staphylococci, small gram-negative rods, and many other organisms. Microscopic examination of smears from throat swabs is of little value in streptococcal infections, because all throats harbor a predominance of streptococci.

Cultures of throat swabs are most reliable if inoculated promptly after collection. Media selective for streptococci can be used to culture for group A organisms. In streaking selective media for streptococci or blood agar culture plates, it is essential to spread a small inoculum thoroughly and avoid overgrowth by normal flora. This can be done readily by touching the throat swab to one small area of the plate and using a second, sterile applicator (or sterile bacteriologic loop) to streak the plate from that area. Detection of β-hemolytic colonies is facilitated by slashing the agar (to provide reduced oxygen tension) and incubating the plate for 2 days at 37 °C.

Laboratory reports on throat culture should state the types of prevalent organisms. If potential pathogens (eg, β-hemolytic streptococci) are found on cultures, their approximate number is important. In "strep throat," group A streptococci prevail. A few colonies of β-hemolytic streptococci may well represent only "transients" in the throat and have no pathogenic meaning. Group A β-hemolytic streptococci often are present in cultures when patients have diseases such as diphtheria or infectious mononucleosis.

2. Nasopharynx–Specimens from the nasopharynx are studied infrequently because special techniques must be used to obtain them. (See Diagnosis of Viral Infections, below.) Whooping cough is diagnosed by culture of *B pertussis* from nasopharyngeal or nasal washings.

3. Middle ear–Specimens are rarely obtained from the middle ear because puncture of the drum is necessary. In acute otitis media, 30–50% of aspirated fluids are bacteriologically sterile. The most frequently isolated bacteria are pneumococci, *H influenzae, Moraxella catarrhalis,* and hemolytic streptococci.

4. Lower respiratory tract–Bronchial and pulmonary secretions of exudates are often studied by examining sputum. The most misleading aspect of sputum examination is the almost inevitable contamination with saliva and mouth flora. Thus, finding *Candida, S aureus,* or even *Streptococcus pneumoniae* in the sputum of a patient with pneumonitis has no etiologic significance unless supported by the clinical picture. Meaningful sputum specimens should be expectorated from the lower respiratory tract and should be grossly distinct from saliva. The presence of many squamous epithelial cells suggests heavy contamination with saliva; a large number of polymorphonuclear leukocytes (PMNs) suggests a purulent exudate. Sputum may be induced by the inhalation of heated hypertonic saline aerosol for several minutes. In pneumonia accompanied by pleural fluid, the pleural fluid may yield the causative organisms more reliably than does sputum. Most community-acquired bacterial pneumonias are caused by pneumococci. In suspected tuberculosis or fungal infection, gastric washings (swallowed sputum) may yield organisms when expectorated material fails to do so.

5. Transtracheal aspiration, bronchoscopy, lung biopsy, bronchoalveolar lavage–The flora in such specimens often reflects accurately the events in the lower respiratory tract. Specimens obtained by bronchoscopy may be necessary in the diagnosis of *Pneumocystis* pneumonia or infection due to *Legionella* or other organisms.

B. Microscopic Examination: Smears of purulent flecks or granules from sputum stained by Gram's stain or acid-fast methods may reveal causative organisms and PMNs. Some organisms (eg, *Actinomyces*) are best seen in unstained wet preparations. A direct "quellung" test for pneumococci can be performed with polyvalent serum on fresh sputum.

C. Culture: The media used for sputum cultures must be suitable for the growth of bacteria (eg, pneumococci, *Klebsiella*), fungi (eg, *Coccidioides immitis*), mycobacteria (eg, *M tuberculosis*), and other organisms. Specimens obtained by bronchoscopy and lung biopsy should also be cultured on other media (eg, for anaerobes, *Legionella,* and others). The relative prevalence of different organisms in the specimen must be estimated. Only a finding of one predominant organism or the simultaneous isolation of an organism from both sputum and blood can clearly establish its role in a pneumonic or suppurative process.

Gastrointestinal Tract Specimens

Acute symptoms referable to the gastrointestinal tract, particularly nausea, vomiting, and diarrhea, are commonly attributed to infection. In reality, most such attacks are caused by intolerance to food or drink, enterotoxins, drugs, or systemic illnesses. *Helicobacter pylori* is associated with peptic ulcer disease.

Many cases of acute infectious diarrhea are due to viruses. On the other hand, many viruses (eg, adenoviruses, enteroviruses) can multiply in the gut without causing gastrointestinal symptoms. Similarly, some enteric bacterial pathogens may persist in the gut following an acute infection. Thus, it may be difficult to assign significance to a bacterial or viral agent cultured from the stool, especially in subacute or chronic illness.

These considerations should not discourage the physician from attempting laboratory isolation of enteric organisms but should constitute a warning of some common difficulties in interpreting the results.

The lower bowel has an exceedingly large normal bacterial flora. The most prevalent organisms are anaerobes (*Bacteroides,* gram-positive rods, and gram-positive cocci), gram-negative enteric organisms, and *S faecalis.* Any attempt to recover pathogenic bacteria from feces involves separation of pathogens from the normal flora, usually through the use of differential selective media and enrichment cultures. Important causes of acute gastrointestinal upsets include viruses, toxins (of staphylococci, clostridia, vibrios, toxigenic *E coli*), invasive enteric gram-negative rods, slow lactose fermenters, shigellae and salmonellae, and campylobacteria. The relative importance of these groups of organisms differs greatly in various parts of the world.

A. Specimens: Feces and rectal swabs are the most readily available specimens. Bile obtained by duodenal drainage may reveal infection of the biliary tract. The presence of blood, mucus, or helminths must be noted on gross inspection of the specimen. Leukocytes seen in suspensions of stool examined microscopically are a useful means of differentiating invasive from noninvasive infectious diarrheas. Special techniques must be used to search for parasitic protozoa and helminths and their ova. Stained smears may reveal a prevalence of leukocytes and certain abnormal organisms, eg, *Candida* or staphylococci, but they cannot be used to differentiate enteric bacterial pathogens from normal flora.

B. Culture: Specimens are suspended in broth and cultured on ordinary as well as differential media (eg, MacConkey agar, EMB agar) to permit separation of non-lactose-fermenting gram-negative rods from other enteric bacteria. If *Salmonella* infection (typhoid fever or paratyphoid fever) is suspected, the specimen is also placed in an enrichment medium (eg, selenite F broth) for 18 hours before being plated on differential media (eg, Hektoen enteric or *Shigella-Salmonella* agar). *Yersinia enterocolitica* is more likely to be isolated after storage of fecal suspensions for 2 weeks at 4 °C, but it can be isolated on *Yersinia* or *Shigella-Salmonella* agar incubated at 25 °C. Vibrios grow best on thiosulfate citrate bile salts sucrose agar. Campylobacteria are isolated on Campy agar or Skirrow's selective medium incubated at 40–42 °C in 10% CO_2 with greatly reduced O_2 tension. Bacterial colonies are identified by standard bacteriologic methods. Agglutination of bacteria from suspect colonies by pooled specific antiserum is often the fastest way to establish the presence of salmonellae or shigellae in the intestinal tract.

Gastric washings represent swallowed sputum and may be cultured for tubercle bacilli and other mycobacteria on special media (see Chapter 24). For virus isolation, fecal specimens are submitted; paired serum specimens can be submitted later.

Intestinal parasites and their ova are discovered by repeated microscopic study of fresh fecal specimens. The specimens require special handling in the laboratory (see Chapter 46).

Genital Lesions

Gonorrhea, nongonococcal urethritis (chlamydial or mycoplasmal), and herpes simplex are prominent among the infections associated with local lesions of the external genitalia, discharge, and regional adenopathy. Syphilis, chancroid, lymphogranuloma venereum, and granuloma inguinale are less common but important diseases. Each has a characteristic natural history and evolution of lesions, but one can mimic another. The laboratory diagnosis of most of these infections is covered elsewhere in this book. A few diagnostic tests are listed below and outlined in Table 47–2.

A. Gonorrhea: A stained smear of urethral or cervical exudate shows intracellular gram-negative diplococci. Exudate, rectal swab, or throat swab must be plated promptly on special media to yield *N gonorrhoeae.* Serologic tests are not helpful.

B. Chlamydial Genital Infections: See section on the diagnosis of chlamydial infections, below.

C. Herpes Progenitalis: See Chapter 33 and the section on the diagnosis of viral infections, below.

D. Syphilis: Darkfield or immunofluorescence examination of tissue fluid expressed from the base of the chancre may reveal typical *T pallidum.* Serologic tests for syphilis become positive 3–6 weeks after infection. A positive flocculation test (eg, VDRL or RPR) requires confirmation. A positive immunofluorescent treponemal antibody test (eg, FTA-ABS, MHATP; see Chapter 25) proves syphilitic infection.

E. Chancroid: Smears from a suppurating lesion usually show a mixed bacterial flora. Swabs from lesions should be cultured on two or three media that are selective for *Haemophilus ducreyi.* Serologic tests are not helpful.

F. Granuloma Inguinale: *Calymmatobacterium (Donovania) granulomatis,* the causative agent of this hard, granulomatous, proliferating lesion, can be grown in complex bacteriologic media, but this is rarely attempted in practice. Histologic demonstration of intracellular "Donovan bodies" in biopsy material most frequently supports the clinical impression. Serologic tests are not helpful.

G. Vaginitis: Vaginitis (bacterial vaginosis) associated with *G vaginalis* or *Mobiluncus* (see Chapter 22) is diagnosed in the examining room by inspection of the vaginal discharge; the discharge (1) is grayish and sometimes frothy, (2) has a pH above 4.6, (3) has an amine ("fishy" odor when alkalinized with potassium hydroxide, and (4) contains "clue cells," large epithelial cells covered with gram-negative or gram-variable rods. Similar observations are used to diagnose *Trichomonas vaginalis* (see Chapter 46) infection; the motile organisms can be seen in wet-mount preparations or cultured from genital discharge. *Candida albicans* vaginitis is diagnosed by finding pseudohyphae in a potassium hydroxide preparation of the vaginal discharge or by culture.

ANAEROBIC INFECTIONS

A large majority of the bacteria that make up the normal human flora are anaerobes. When displaced from their normal sites into tissues or body spaces, anaerobes may produce disease. Certain characteristics are suggestive of anaerobic infections: (1) They are often contiguous with a mucosal surface. (2) They tend to involve mixtures of organisms. (3) They tend to form closed-space infections, either as discrete abscesses (lung, brain, pleura, peritoneum, pelvis) or by burrowing through tissue layers. (4) Pus from anaerobic infections often has a foul odor. (5) Most of the pathogenetically important anaerobes except *Bacteroides* are highly susceptible to penicillin G. (6) Anaerobic infections are favored by reduced blood supply, necrotic tissue, and a low oxidation-reduction potential—all of which also interfere with delivery of antimicrobial drugs. (7) It is essential to use special collection methods, transport media, and sensitive anaerobic techniques and media to isolate the organisms. Otherwise, bacteriologic examination may be negative or yield only incidental aerobes.

The following are sites of important anaerobic infections.

Respiratory Tract

Periodontal infections, perioral abscesses, sinusitis, and mastoiditis may involve predominantly *Prevotella melaninogenica, Fusobacterium,* and peptostreptococci. Aspiration of saliva (containing up to 10^2 of these organisms) may result in necrotizing pneumonia, lung abscess, and empyema. Antimicrobial drugs and postural or surgical drainage are essential for treatment.

Central Nervous System

Anaerobes rarely produce meningitis but are common causes of brain abscess, subdural empyema, and septic thrombophlebitis. The organisms usually originate in the respiratory tract via extension or hematogenous spread.

Intra-abdominal & Pelvic Infections

The flora of the colon consists predominantly of anaerobes, 10^{11} per gram of feces. *B fragilis,* clostridia, and peptostreptococci play a main role in abscess formation originating in perforation of the bowel. *Prevotella bivia* and *Prevotella disiens* are important in abscesses of the pelvis originating in the female genital organs. Like *B fragilis,* these species are often relatively resistant to penicillin; therefore, clindamycin, metronidazole, or another effective agent should be used.

Skin & Soft Tissue Infections

Anaerobes and aerobic bacteria often join to form synergistic infections (gangrene, necrotizing fasciitis, cellulitis). Surgical drainage, excision, and improved circulation are the most important forms of treatment, while antimicrobial drugs act as adjuncts. It is usually difficult to pinpoint one specific organism as being responsible for the progressive lesion, since mixtures of organisms are usually involved.

DIAGNOSIS OF CHLAMYDIAL INFECTIONS

Although *Chlamydia trachomatis, Chlamydia pneumoniae* (TWAR), and *Chlamydia psittaci* are bacteria, they are obligate intracellular parasites. Cultures and other diagnostic tests for *Chlamydia* require procedures much like those used in diagnostic virology laboratories rather than those used in bacteriology and mycology laboratories. Thus, the diagnosis of chlamydial infections is discussed in a separate section of this chapter.

Specimens

For *C trachomatis* oculogenital infections, the specimens for direct examination of culture must be collected from infected sites by vigorous swabbing or scraping of the involved epithelial cell surface. Cultures or purulent discharges are not adequate, and purulent material should be cleaned away before the specimen is obtained. Thus, for inclusion conjunctivitis, a conjunctival scraping is obtained; for urethritis, a swab specimen is obtained from several centimeters into the urethra; for cervicitis, a specimen is obtained from the columnar cell surface of the endocervical canal. When upper genital tract infection is suspected in women, scrapings of the endometrium provide a good sample. Fluid obtained by culdocentesis or aspiration of the uterine tube has a low yield for *C trachomatis* on culture. Biopsy of the uterine tube for diagnostic culture is a research tool rather than a routine procedure.

For *C pneumoniae,* use nasopharyngeal (not throat) swab specimens.

For lymphogranuloma venereum, aspirates of buboes or fluctuant nodes provide the best specimen for culture.

For psittacosis, culture of sputum, blood, or biopsy material may yield *C psittaci.*

Swabs, scrapings, and tissue specimens should be placed in transport medium. A useful medium has 0.2 mol/L sucrose in 0.02 M phosphate buffer, pH 7.0–7.2, with 5% fetal calf serum. Other transport media may be equally suitable. The transport medium should contain antibiotics to suppress bacteria other than *Chlamydia* species. Gentamicin, 10 μg/mL, vancomycin, 100 μg/mL, and amphotericin B, 4 μg/mL, can be used in combination since they do not inhibit *Chlamydia.* If specimens cannot be processed rapidly, they can be refrigerated for 24 hours; otherwise, they should be frozen at −60 °C or colder until processed.

Microscopy & Stains

Cytologic examination is important and useful only in the examination of conjunctival scrapings to diagnose inclusion conjunctivitis and trachoma caused by *C trachomatis.* Typical intracytoplasmic inclusions can be seen, classically with Giemsa-stained specimens. A search for inclusions is not sufficiently sensitive to be of diagnostic value in chlamydial infections at anatomic sites other than the conjunctiva.

Fluorescein-conjugated monoclonal antibodies are widely used for direct examination of specimens from the genital tract, particularly when chlamydial cultures are not available (direct fluorescent antibody, or DFA). Commercially available kits provide slides, reagents, and instructions. An experienced microscopist is important, because it can be difficult on DFA stain to recognize the small extracellular elementary bodies present in the specimen. The tests are less sensitive than culture (70–90%) but are much more rapid than culture and can be performed in laboratories that do not have tissue culture facilities.

Lymphogranuloma venereum, *C pneumoniae* infection, and psittacosis are rarely diagnosed by direct microscopy, and the procedure is not recommended for these diseases.

Culture

Although egg inoculation can be used, cell culture techniques are recommended for the isolation of *Chlamydia* species. Cell culture for *C trachomatis* and *C psittaci* usually involves inoculation of the clinical specimens onto cycloheximide-treated McCoy cells, whereas *C pneumoniae* requires HeLa 229 (or HL or HEp−2) cells pretreated with diethylamino dextran. One technique uses a confluent growth of McCoy cells on 13 mm cover slips in small disposable vials. The inoculum is placed in duplicate vials and centrifuged onto the monolayers at approximately 3000 × *g* at 35 °C for 48–72 hours and stained. To detect *C trachomatis,* immunofluorescence, Giemsa's stain, or iodine stain is used to search for intracytoplasmic inclusions. Immunofluorescent techniques are the most sensitive of the three stains but require special IF reagents and microscopy. Giemsa is more sensitive than iodine, but the microscopy is more difficult. The iodine stain is easiest to use for specimens from oculogenital infections and provides a sensitivity of approximately 90% in comparison with immunofluorescent staining of the primary culture coupled with immunofluorescent staining of the blind subculture of the duplicate vial.

A second culture technique uses McCoy cells in 96-well microdilution plates and either iodine or fluorescent antibody staining. Because the surface area of the monolayer is less and the inoculum is smaller, the microdilution plate method is less sensitive than the cover slip-vial technique. The microdilution plate method coupled with fluorescent antibody staining is 70–80% as sensitive as the cover slip-vial technique. When iodine staining is used, the sensitivity drops to 50–60%. Differences between the sensitivity of the cover slip-vial technique and that of the microdilution plate technique occur with specimens in which there is a relatively low number of chlamydiae in the inoculum and the number of inclusions formed in the monolayer is less than ten.

Inclusions of *C trachomatis* stain with iodine, but inclusions of *C pneumoniae* and *C psittaci* do not. These two species are distinguished from *C trachomatis* by their different responses to iodine staining and by their susceptibility to sulfonamide. *C pneumoniae* in culture can be detected by using a genus-specific monoclonal antibody or, even better, a species-specific monoclonal antibody. Serologic techniques for species differentiation are not practical, though *C trachomatis* can be typed by the microimmunofluorescent method.

Antigen Detection & Nucleic Acid Hybridization

Enzyme immunoassays (EIAs) are used for detecting chlamydial antigens in genital tract specimens from patients with sexually transmitted disease. Compared with the more sensitive culture techniques for *Chlamydia* (see above), the EIA has a sensitivity of about 90% and a specificity of about 97% when used in populations with a moderate to high prevalence of infection (5–20%). In this setting, the sensitivity, specificity, and positive predictive values are roughly comparable to those for the DFA test. The utility of EIA in the diagnosis of chlamydial infections in a population with a low prevalence of infection (1–4%) is less clear, because as few as 40–50% of the positive tests could represent true chlamydial infections. Both EIA and DFA tests are useful in laboratories where cell culture facilities are not available. EIA is most useful when the laboratory processes a large enough number of specimens that there is benefit from batch processing; DFA is best applied in laboratories where there is a small number of specimens. Neither EIA, DFA, nor culture is needed in the diagnosis of symptomatic urethritis in the male, for which a Gram stain showing polymorphonuclear cells (with or without gram-negative intracellular diplococci indicating gonorrhea) is highly cost-effective and sufficient to indicate the need for treatment of *Chlamydia* infection.

Commercial kits with nonradioisotopic molecular probes for *C trachomatis* 16S RNA sequences have been marketed for direct detection of *C trachomatis* in clinical specimens. The test has a sensitivity of about 90% and a specificity of >99% when compared with culture. A high-quality culture system is estimated to detect about 90% of truly infected patients, and for that reason the molecular probe test may actually be positive for infected patients with negative cultures. A diagnostic test based on PCR also is available and shows promise of high sensitivity and specificity.

Serology

The complement fixation (CF) test is widely used to diagnose psittacosis and other chlamydial infections. A fourfold rise in CF titer in convalescent serum compared with acute serum is diagnostic, whereas a single titer of greater than 1:64 strongly suggests that clinical diagnosis of psittacosis is correct. The CF test cannot differentiate between *C pneumoniae, C psittaci,* and the chlamydiae of lymphogranuloma venereum and is less sensitive than the microimmunofluorescent test.

The microimmunofluorescence method is more sensitive than CF for measuring antichlamydial antibodies. The titer of IgG antibodies can be diagnostic when fourfold titer rises are seen in acute and convalescent sera. However, it may be difficult to show a rise in the IgG titer because of high background titers in the sexually active population. The measurement of IgM antibodies is particularly useful in the diagnosis of *C trachomatis* pneumonia in neonates. Babies born to mothers with chlamydial infections have serum IgG antichlamydial antibodies from the maternal circulation. Babies with ocular or upper respiratory tract infections have low titers of antichlamydial IgM, whereas babies with chlamydial pneumonia have antichlamydial IgM titers of 1:32 or greater.

DIAGNOSIS OF VIRAL INFECTIONS

Diagnostic virology requires communication between the physician and the laboratory and depends on the quality of specimens and information supplied to the laboratory.

The choice of methods for laboratory confirmation of a viral infection depends upon the stage of the illness (Table 47–7). Antibody tests require samples taken at appropriate intervals, and the diagnosis often is not confirmed until convalescence. Antibody tests can be performed only for those illnesses for which the causative viruses have been grown in the laboratory or for which special sources of antigen become available (eg, hepatitis B or human immunodeficiency viruses). Virus isolation is required (1) when new epidemics occur, as with influenza; (2) when serologic tests are not useful; and (3) when the same clinical illness may be caused by many different agents. For example, aseptic (nonbacterial) meningitis may be caused by many different viruses; similarly, respiratory disease syndromes may be caused by many viruses as well as by mycoplasmas and other agents.

Diagnostic methods based on nucleic acid amplification techniques will soon replace some but not all virus culture approaches. However, the need for appropriate sample collection and test interpretation will not change. Furthermore, there will be times when recovery of the infectious agent is desired.

Isolation of a virus may not establish the cause of a given disease. Many other factors must be considered. Some viruses persist in human hosts for long periods of time, and therefore the isolation of herpesviruses, poliovirus, echoviruses, or coxsackieviruses from a patient with an undiagnosed illness does not prove that the virus is the cause of the disease. A consistent clinical and epidemiologic pattern must be established before it can be determined that a particular agent is responsible for a specific clinical picture.

Table 47–7. Relation of stage of illness to presence of virus in test materials and to appearance of specific antibody.

Stage or Period of Illness	Virus Detectable in Test Materials	Specific Antibody Demonstrable[1]
Incubation	Rarely	No
Prodrome	Occasionally	No
Onset	Frequently	Occasionally
Acute phase	Frequently	Frequently
Recovery	Rarely	Usually
Convalescence	Very rarely	Usually

[1]Antibody may be detected very early in previously vaccinated persons.

Dual infections may occur. Different viruses may have the same seasonal and geographic occurrence. Enteroviruses and arboviruses sometimes occur simultaneously in communities. Thus, in one summer a patient may have inapparent infection with one virus and clinical infection with the other. If the clinical infection is mild, the syndrome (eg, aseptic meningitis) may have been produced by either virus. Antibody studies must be made for both viruses or the diagnosis may be missed altogether.

Isolation of active virus requires proper collection of appropriate specimens. All specimens must be safely contained for transport to the laboratory. Each specimen must be clearly labeled and should be accompanied by relevant information. Specimens must be preserved en route to and in the laboratory.

Many viruses are most readily isolated during the first few days of illness. The specimens to be used in virus isolation attempts are listed in Table 47–8. Tissues obtained at autopsy may also serve this purpose. A correlation of virus isolation and antibody presence helps in making the diagnosis (Table 47–9).

Specimens can be refrigerated for up to 24 hours before virus cultures are done, with the exception of respiratory syncytial and certain other viruses. Otherwise, material should be frozen (preferably at −60 °C or colder) if there is a delay in bringing it to the laboratory. A frozen specimen can be transported in a large wide-mouthed thermos jar or insulated carton, half-filled with pieces of solid CO_2 (dry ice). Specimens that should not be frozen include (1) whole blood drawn for antibody determination, from which the serum must be separated before freezing; and (2) tissue for organ or cell culture, which should be kept at 4 °C and taken to the laboratory promptly.

In general, virus is present in respiratory illnesses in pharyngeal or nasal secretions. Virus can be demonstrated in the fluid and scrapings from the base of vesicular rashes. In eye infections, virus is detectable in conjunctival swabs or scrapings and in tears. Encephalitides are usually diagnosed more readily by serologic means. Arboviruses and herpesviruses are not usually recovered from spinal fluid, but brain tissue from patients with viral encephalitis may yield the causative virus. In illnesses associated with enteroviruses, such as central nervous system disease, acute pericarditis, and myocarditis, viruses can be isolated from feces, throat swabs, or cerebrospinal fluid.

Direct Examination of Clinical Material: Microscopy & Stains

Viral diseases for which direct microscopic examination of imprints or smears has proved useful include rabies, herpes simplex infection, varicella-zoster infection, respiratory syncytial virus infection, and influenza A and is the method of choice for detection of many of these viruses..

Staining of viral antigens by immunofluorescence in a brain smear and corneal impressions from the rabid animal and from humans is the method of choice for routine diagnosis of rabies. The procedure is carried out as follows: Two impression smears on a glass slide are made with the suspect brain. The slide is fixed in acetone at −20 °C. One smear (control) is flooded with fluorescein-labeled antirabies globulin mixed with mouse brain containing rabies virus. The other smear (test) is flooded with the same fluorescein-labeled antirabies globulin mixed with normal mouse brain. The slide is incubated at 37 °C for 30 minutes in a moist chamber, then washed for 10 minutes in buffered saline, air dried, mounted, and examined. The positive test smear gives bright fluorescence, whereas the control smear gives no fluorescence because specifically labeled antibodies have been bound by the rabies antigen added in mouse brain.

The same principle of identifying viral antigens using immunofluorescence is useful in rapid diagnosis of (1) certain respiratory virus diseases (eg, respiratory syncytial disease, in which the virus is labile under ordinary laboratory conditions and cannot withstand freezing and thawing, and also influenza and parainfluenza) by examining smeared epithelial cells from the nasopharynx; and (2) herpetic lesions by examining cells scraped from the base of the lesion. Immunofluorescence microscopy is also used for detection of adenovirus, mumps, measles, varicella-zoster, and cytomegalovirus in appropriate clinical specimens.

Cytologic examination of urinary sediment may help make a presumptive diagnosis of congenital cytomegalovirus infection. Cytomegalic cells are characterized by their large size, scanty cytoplasm, and a large nucleus containing a prominent basophilic inclusion surrounded by a clear halo. However, cytologic study is insensitive and not pathognomonic for cytomegalovirus; it may detect about 50% of symptomatic congenital cytomegalovirus infections.

Virus Culture

A. Preparation of Inocula: Bacteria-free fluid materials such as cerebrospinal fluid, whole blood, plasma, or white blood cell buffy coat layer may be inoculated into cell cultures, animals, or eggs directly or after dilution with buffered phosphate solution (pH 7.6).

Tissue is washed in media or sterile water, minced into small pieces with scissors, and ground to make a homogeneous paste. Diluent is added in amounts sufficient to make a concentration of 10–20% (weight/volume). This suspension can be centrifuged at low speed (not >2000 rpm) for 10 minutes to sediment insoluble cellular debris. The supernatant fluid may be inoculated; if bacteria are present, they are eliminated as discussed below.

Tissues may also be trypsinized, and the resulting cell suspension may be (1) inoculated on an existing tissue culture cell monolayer or (2) cocultivated with another cell suspension of cells known to be virus-free.

Table 47–8. Viral infections: Agents, specimens, and diagnostic tests.

Syndrome and Virus	Specimen	Detection System[1,2]	Comments[2]
Respiratory diseases			
Influenza viruses	Nasopharyngeal washings or swab, sputum.	Cell culture (PMK, MDCK), embryonated eggs. Direct fluorescent antibody.	Virus detected by hemadsorption of guinea pig erythrocytes in 2–4 days. HI or IF used to identify virus.
Parainfluenza viruses	Nasopharyngeal washings or swab, sputum.	Cell culture (PMK, LLC-MK_2). Direct fluorescent antibody.	Virus detected by hemadsorption of guinea pig erythrocytes in 4–7 days. HI, IF, and HAI used to identify virus.
Respiratory syncytial virus	Nasopharyngeal washings.	Cell culture (HEL, HeLa, HEp-2). Direct fluorescent antibody.	CPE usually visible in 1–7 days. Detect antigen by EIA.
Adenovirus	Nasopharyngeal washings or swab, feces, conjunctival swab.	Cell culture (HEp-2, HEK).	CPE usually visible in 3–7 days. IF used to identify virus.
Rhinoviruses	Nasopharyngeal washings or swab.	Cell culture (HEL).	
Enteroviruses	Nasopharyngeal washings or swab, feces.	Cell culture (PMK, HEL), suckling mice.	Serologic tests are best done with virus isolated from patients; coxsackievirus A rarely grows in tissue culture.
Febrile diseases			
Dengue, other arboviruses	Serum, CSF, autopsy specimens, vector (*Aedes* mosquito).	Suckling mice, cell culture (Vero).	Many viruses in this group are highly infectious and easily transmissible to laboratory personnel. Some should only be studied in self-contained laboratories with controlled access. Use serology.
Hemorrhagic fevers			
See Chapter 38.	Serum, blood.	Suckling mice, cell culture (Vero).	See comment for Febrile Diseases.
Lymphocytic choriomeningitis (LCM)			
LCM virus	Blood, CSF.	Cell culture (Vero, BHK), suckling mice.	IF and neutralization in mice used for identification of virus.
Lassa fever			
Lassa virus	Blood, nasopharyngeal swab, exudates.	Cell culture (Vero, BHK).	Lassa virus isolation is restricted to self-contained laboratories with controlled access.
Encephalitis			
Arboviruses	Serum, CSF, nasopharyngeal swab.	Suckling mice, cell culture (Vero).	See comment for Febrile Diseases.
Enteroviruses	Feces, throat swab, CSF.	Cell culture (PMK, HEL).	
Rabies virus	Saliva, brain biopsy.	Suckling mice, direct IF.	Direct IF is preferable because speed of diagnosis is important for effective treatment.
Herpesvirus	Brain biopsy.	Cell culture (Vero, HFF), direct IF.	CPE usually visible in 24–72 hours.
Meningitis			
Enterovirus	Feces, CSF.	Cell culture (PMK, HEL).	
Mumps virus	CSF, nasopharyngeal swab, urine.	Cell culture (PMK).	Virus detected by hemadsorption of guinea pig erythrocytes in 4–7 days. HAI and IF used to identify virus in culture.
Infectious mononucleosis			
Epstein-Barr (EB) virus	Blood, nasopharyngeal swab.	Lmyphoid cell culture.	Culture of EB virus not performed routinely in clinical virology laboratories.

(*continued*)

Table 47–8. Viral infections: Agents, specimens, and diagnostic tests. (*Continued*)

Syndrome and Virus	Specimen	Detection System[1,2]	Comments[2]
Cytomegalovirus	Blood, urine, throat swab.	Cell culture (HFF); shell vial culture	Tissue culture tubes should be held 4 weeks; shell vial 24 hours.
Hepatitis (See Chapter 37 for available and indicated tests.)			
Hepatitis A virus	Serum, feces.	IEM.	
Hepatitis B virus	Serum.	EIA, RIA.	
Hepatitis C virus	Serum.	EIA, RIA, PCR.	
Hepatitis D virus	Serum.	EIA.	
Enteritis			
Rotavirus	Feces.	EIA.	
Norwalk agent, caliciviruses, astroviruses	Feces.	IEM.	
Enterovirus	Feces.	Cell culture (HEL, PMK).	Neutralization rarely done; usually requires paired sera and virus isolate from patient.
Exanthems			
Varicella-zoster virus	Vesicle fluid.	Cell culture (HEK). Direct fluorescent antibody is most sensitive.	CPE usually visible in 4 days to 2 weeks.
Measles (rubeola) virus	Nasopharyngeal swab, blood, urine.	Cell culture (PMK, HEK). Direct fluorescent antibody.	CPE usually visible in 2–3 weeks.
Rubella virus	Nasopharyngeal swab, blood, urine.	Cell culture (AGMK, Vero).	
Monkeypox, cowpox, vaccinia, and tanapoxviruses	Vesicle fluid.	Embryonated eggs, electron microscopy.	
Herpes simplex virus	Vesicles, usually oral or genital.	Cell culture (HFF, Vero).	Cultures usually become positive in 24–72 hours; direct IF is rapid.
Parotitis			
Mumps virus	Nasopharyngeal swab, urine.	Cell culture (PMK).	See comment for Meningitis, above.
Congenital anomalies			
Cytomegalovirus	Urine, throat swab.	See Infectious Mononucleosis, above.	
Rubella	Throat swab, CSF, blood.	See Exanthems, above.	
Conjunctivitis			
Herpes simplex Herpes zoster	Conjunctival swabs, tears.	See Exanthems, above.	
Adenovirus Enterovirus		See Respiratory Diseases, above.	
AIDS (acquired immunodeficiency syndrome)			
Human immunodeficiency virus	Blood, particularly leukocytes.	Cell culture patient's PBC.	Antibody by EIA, confirmed by Western blot. Virus almost always detectable in PBC even when serum antibodies present.
Papovavirus infections			
Human papovavirus JC Human papovavirus BK	Brain, urine, tissue specimens, biopsies, warts.	Cell culture (HFF), EM.	
Papillomaviruses		DNA, IF.	

[1]AGMK, African green monkey kidney; BHK, baby hamster kidney; HEK, human embryonic kidney; HEL, human embryonic lung; HEp-2, human epithelial cell line; PMK, primary monkey kidney; HeLa, human epithelial cell line; LLC-MK_2 and Vero, monkey kidney cell lines; MDCK, dog kidney cell line; HFF, human foreskin fibroblasts.

[2]A variety of tests using patients' sera and known viral antigens are used for diagnosis. Similar tests using the virus isolated from the patient and known antisera are used to identify the infecting agent. These tests include neutralization of viral replication (inhibition of cytopathic effect, CPE); CF, complement fixation; EIA, enzyme immunoassay; HAI, hemadsorption inhibition; HI, hemagglutination inhibition; IF, immunofluorescent antibody; RIA, radioimmunoassay; IEM, immune electron microscopy; PBC, peripheral blood cells; PCR, polymerase chain reaction.

Table 47–9. Laboratory aids in viral diagnoses.

Viral Antigen or Virus Isolation	Viral Antibody[1]	Neutralizing (Nt) Antibody	Antibody of IgM Class	Interpretation of Infection
–	–	–	–	None
+	– or +	–	–	Early
+	+	+	+	Current
–	+	+	+	Recent
–	– or +	+	–	Old
– or +	+	+	+	Persistent

[1]Antibody to viral antigens, either structural or nonstructural, can be detected by a variety of methods, eg, ELISA, RIA, CF, HI.

If the material to be tested contains bacteria (throat washings, stools, urine, infected tissue, or insects), they must be inactivated or removed before inoculation.

1. Bactericidal agents–

a. Antibiotics–Antibiotics are commonly employed in combination with differential centrifugation (see below).

b. Ether–If it is not harmful to the virus in question (eg, enteroviruses, vaccinia), ether may be added in concentrations of 10–15%.

2. Mechanical methods–

a. Filters–Millipore-type membrane filters of cellulose acetate or similar inert material are preferred. Earthenware and porcelain filters reduce virus concentration by adsorption and are therefore not recommended.

b. Differential centrifugation–This is a convenient method for removing many bacteria from heavily contaminated preparations of small viruses. Bacteria are sedimented at low speeds that do not sediment the virus, and high-speed centrifugation then sediments the virus. The virus-containing sediment is then resuspended in a small volume.

B. Cultivation in Cell Culture: Cell culture techniques are the most widely used for isolating viruses from clinical specimens. When viruses multiply in cell culture, they produce biologic effects (eg, cytopathic changes, viral interference, production of a hemagglutinin) that permit identification of the agent.

Test tube cultures are prepared by adding cells suspended in 1–2 mL of nutrient fluid that contains balanced salt solutions and various growth factors (usually serum, glucose, amino acids, and vitamins). Cells of fibroblastic or epithelial nature attach and grow on the wall of the test tube, where they may be examined with the aid of a low-power microscope.

With many viruses, growth of the agent is paralleled by degeneration of these cells (Figure 47–1). Some viruses produce characteristic cytopathic effect, commonly called CPE, in cell culture, making a rapid presumptive diagnosis possible when the clinical syndrome is known. For example, measles, mumps, parainfluenza, and respiratory syncytial viruses characteristically produce multinucleated giant cells, whereas adenoviruses produce grape-like clusters of large round cells, rhinoviruses produce focal areas of rounding and dendritic forms, and herpes simplex virus produces diffuse uniform rounding of cells.

Some viruses (eg, rubella virus) produce no direct cytopathic changes but can be detected by their interference with the cytopathic effect of a second challenge virus (viral interference).

Influenza viruses and some paramyxoviruses may be detected within 24–48 hours if erythrocytes are added to infected cultures. Viruses maturing at the cell membrane produce a hemagglutinin that enables the erythrocytes to adsorb at the cell surface (hemadsorption).

Organ cultures of ferret and human tracheal epithelium may support the growth of many viruses that cause upper respiratory tract disease, including some viruses that do not grow in conventional cell cultures (eg, coronaviruses). Viruses may cause general or focal necrosis of the ciliated epithelial cells or may be detected by a decline in ciliary movement.

The identity of a virus isolate is established with type-specific antiserum, which inhibits virus growth or which reacts with viral antigens in the tests described below (eg, complement fixation CF, hemagglutination inhibition HI).

C. Shell Vial Cultures: This method allows for rapid detection of viruses in clinical specimens. It has been adapted for several viruses, including cytomegalovirus and varicella-zoster virus. It is the preferred detection method for viruses that grow slowly. For example, CMV can be detected in 18–24 hours, compared with 2–4 weeks for classic cell culture; the sensitivities of shell vial and classic cell cultures for CMV are comparable. Monolayers of the appropriate cell line (eg, MRC-5 cells for CMV) are grown in monolayers on coverslips in 15 × 45 mm shell vials. After inoculation with the specimen, the vials are centrifuged at 700 × *g* for 40 minutes at room temperature. The vials are incubated at 37 °C for 16–24 hours, fixed, and reacted with a monoclonal antibody specific for a CMV nuclear protein that is present very early in the culture; several such antibodies are commercially

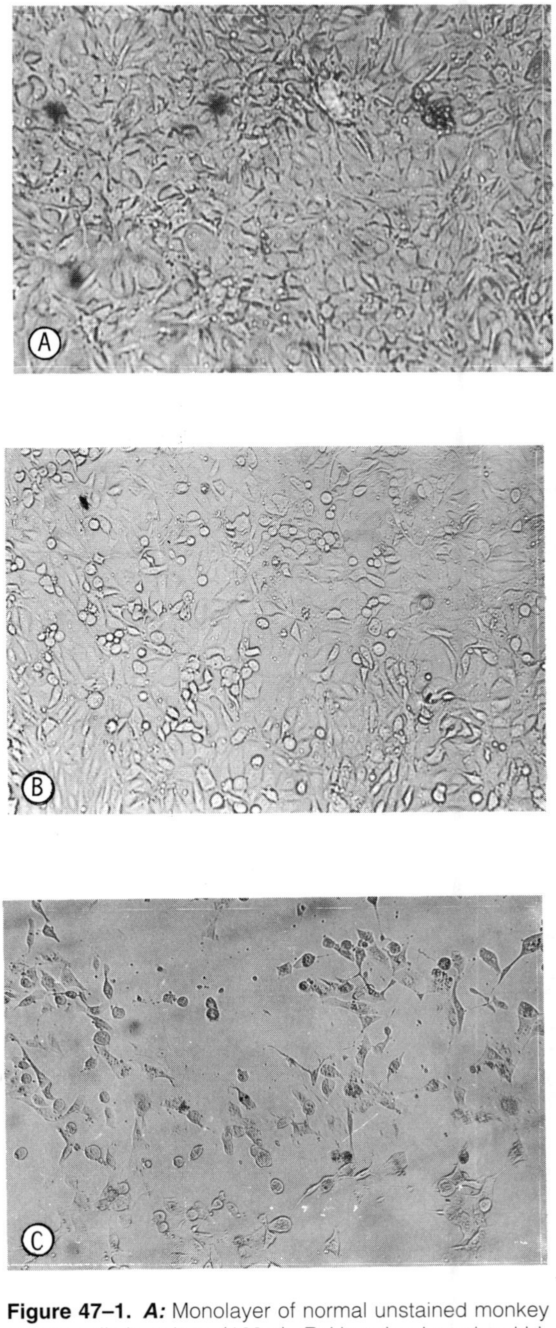

Figure 47–1. ***A:*** Monolayer of normal unstained monkey kidney cells in culture (120×). ***B:*** Unstained monkey kidney cell culture showing early stage of cytopathic effects typical of enterovirus infection (120×). Approximately 25% of the cells in the culture show cytopathic effects indicative of viral multiplication (1+ cytopathic effects). ***C:*** Unstained monkey kidney cell culture illustrating more advanced enteroviral cytopathic effect (3+ to 4+ cytopathic effects) (120×). Almost 100% of the cells are affected, and most of the cell sheet has come loose from the wall of the culture tube.

available. Direct or indirect antibody staining methods and fluorescence microscopy are used to determine positive shell vial cultures. Positive and negative control vials are included in each test run. Isolates are not obtained using the shell vial technique. If isolates are needed for susceptibility testing for antiviral drugs, the classic cell culture technique should be used.

D. Embryonated Eggs: Embryonated eggs in various stages of development can be inoculated by one of several routes. After inoculation, the eggs are reincubated and examined daily for viability. Standardized methods permit inoculation of the chorioallantoic membrane, the amniotic sac, the allantoic sac, the yolk sac, or the embryo. After suitable incubation, fluid or tissue is removed and examined for viral growth or lesions.

E. Animal Inoculation: Only relatively few specialized laboratories perform animal work. The laboratory animals employed include mice, hamsters, cotton rats, guinea pigs, rabbits, and monkeys. In some cases, infant mice (<48 hours old) are used. Intracerebral and intranasal inoculation are employed, particularly in mice; these routes require the special experience, skill, and methods available in public health or research laboratories that work with animals. The inoculated animals are observed for signs of illness and then killed, and their tissues are examined.

Antigen Detection

The recognition of hepatitis A virus and rotavirus by direct examination of fecal specimens led to the development of sensitive solid-phase immunoassays (enzyme immunoassay, EIA) for detection of the two viruses—inasmuch as these important pathogens are not readily grown in cell culture.

EIA for viral diagnosis consists of the following essential steps, which are similar to those used in EIA for bacterial infections:

(1) A specific antibody is adsorbed onto the wells in a plastic microdilution plate.

(2) The material to be tested is added. If the viral antigen is present, it will combine with the antibody. The excess is washed off.

(3) A conjugate consisting of antiviral antibody linked to an enzyme is added. If virus has been fixed to the plate, the antibody portion of the conjugate will attach. Unbound conjugate is washed off.

(4) A substrate for the enzyme is added, and the colored product is measured in a spectrophotometer. The resulting reading is proportionate to the amount of enzyme bound to the plate, which in turn is related to the quantity of virus antigen in the sample.

A more sensitive technique of antigen detection involves the use of a second specific antibody derived from a different animal species than the one used for preparing the coating antibody. The second antibody is reacted with viral antigen (in the clinical specimen) that has been bound to the original coating antibody.

A third antibody conjugated with enzyme is added; this antibody is directed against the immunoglobulin of the animal species used to prepare the second specific antibody. Again, the amount of antibody bound, determined by the enzyme activity, is a function of antigen concentration.

Nucleic Acid Hybridization

Nucleic acid hybridization to detect viruses is highly sensitive and specific. The specimen is spotted on a nitrocellulose membrane, and viral nucleic acid present in the sample is bound; it is then denatured with alkali in situ, hybridized with a labeled viral nucleic acid fragment, and the hybridized products detected. For rotavirus, which contains double-stranded RNA, the dot hybridization method is even more sensitive than EIA. RNA in heat-denatured fecal samples containing rotavirus is immobilized as above, and in situ hybridization is carried out with labeled single-stranded probes obtained by in vitro transcription of rotavirus. Complementary probes to enteroviruses may also be labeled and used in the dot hybridization method.

Dot hybridization is increasingly being used to detect viral nucleic acid sequences in tissue samples not only from patients with acute infection but also from those with chronic diseases from which virus is not readily isolated. The latter include chronic hepatitis and primary hepatocellular carcinoma (hepatitis B virus DNA probe), latent varicella-zoster in sensory ganglia (varicella-zoster virus DNA probe), acquired immunodeficiency syndrome (human immunodeficiency virus complementary [cDNA] probe), cervical neoplasms (cloned papillomavirus DNA probe), and nasopharyngeal carcinoma and Burkitt's lymphoma (cloned EB virus DNA probe).

Serology

Typically, a virus infection elicits immune responses directed against one or more viral antigens. Both cellular and humoral immune responses usually develop, and measurement of either may be used to diagnose a viral infection. Cellular immunity may be assessed by dermal hypersensitivity, lymphocyte transformation, and cytotoxicity tests. Humoral immune responses are of major diagnostic importance. Antibodies of the IgM class appear initially and are followed by IgG antibodies. The IgM antibodies disappear in several weeks, whereas the IgG antibodies persist for many years. Establishing the diagnosis of a viral infection is accomplished serologically by demonstrating a rise in antibody titer to the virus or by demonstrating antiviral antibodies of the IgM class.

Procedures for quantifying antibodies in viral diseases are based on classic antigen-antibody reactions (see Chapter 8), with some modifications for certain viruses. Commonly used methods include EIA, the neutralization (Nt) test, the complement fixation (CF) test, the hemagglutination inhibition (HI) test, and the immunofluorescence (IF) test. Less commonly used methods include passive hemagglutination, immunodiffusion and EIA. Tests available for viruses are listed in Table 47–9.

Measurement of antibodies by different methods does not necessarily give parallel results. Antibodies detected by the CF test are present during an enterovirus infection and in the convalescent period, but they do not persist. Antibodies detected by the Nt test also appear during infection and persist for many years. Assessment of antibodies by several methods in individuals or groups of individuals provides diagnostic information as well as information about epidemiologic features of the disease.

A. Collection of Blood Specimens: Serial samples of serum are essential for diagnostic purposes if antibodies are to be adequately tested and evaluated. In general, the first sample should be collected as soon as possible after the onset of the illness; the second, 2–3 weeks after onset. A third sample may be required later. Antibodies appear earlier in some viral infections than in others, and so the times of collecting specimens must be varied.

Blood specimens should be drawn with aseptic precautions and without anticoagulants and the serum separated and stored at 4 °C or −20 °C. Before performing serologic tests, it may be necessary to heat the serum (56 °C for 30 minutes) to remove nonspecific interfering or inhibiting substances and complement. This is essential for CF tests and also, with certain viruses, for Nt tests.

B. IgM Antibodies: If paired sera are not available, a presumptive diagnosis can sometimes be made by demonstrating IgM antibodies to the virus, even in the first serum sample taken. IgM antibodies may be detected by sensitivity to 2-mercaptoethanol or by immunofluorescence.

IgM antibodies develop simultaneously with or even before IgG antibodies but then disappear more quickly. However, IgM antibodies remain longer in persistent infections. In congenital infections, IgM antibody detection is of singular value, because IgM does not cross the placenta as does IgG. Thus, finding IgM antibodies to viruses in the serum of a newborn indicates that the child was infected in utero.

C. Neutralization (Nt) Tests: Virus-neutralizing antibodies are measured by adding serum containing these antibodies to a suspension of virus and then inoculating the mixture into susceptible cell cultures. The presence of neutralizing antibodies is demonstrated if the cell cultures fail to develop cytopathic effects (CPE) while control cell cultures, which have received virus plus a serum free of antibody, develop cytopathic effects. In some instances, the virus-antiserum mixture may be inoculated into susceptible experimental animals (as with type A coxsackieviruses) or embryonated eggs (as with mumps virus). The protection of the host from viral effects demonstrates neutralizing antibody.

To establish a diagnosis, one looks for a significant rise in antibody titer—fourfold or greater is desirable—during the course of the infection. In recurrent infections, eg, herpes simplex, high antibody titers are commonly detected in serial serum samples; the diagnostic rise between acute and convalescent sera is not registered. A positive test in a single sample of serum is not of diagnostic value in acute infections unless the antibody belongs to the IgM class. Neutralizing antibodies can persist for years, and their presence may indicate a past infection.

Although simple in principle, Nt tests are expensive in time and materials and must be standardized for each viral agent.

1. Nt test in cell culture–The details of this test vary in different laboratories, but the same principle underlies all of them: The viral antibody specifically neutralizes the cytopathogenic effects of the virus.

With each series of Nt tests, control titrations of virus are made. The highest concentration of each serum used is tested for possible nonspecific cell toxicity. A few tubes are left uninoculated to serve as cell controls. Typical results of sera obtained from a patient infected with type 1 poliovirus are shown in Table 47–10. The cultures were incubated at 36 °C for 3 days and then examined microscopically. At the end of that time, the virus titration showed that 100 $TCID_{50}$ doses had been added to each serum.

For viruses such as herpes or polio, which produce plaques on cell sheets, neutralization may be measured by comparing the number of plaques produced by the virus alone with the number produced in the presence of the serum. Such plaque reduction techniques are used where greater accuracy of quantitation is required.

2. Nt tests in eggs–The embryonated egg may be inoculated and used as an indicator system in virus Nt tests. With influenza and mumps viruses, the end point is measured by determining whether viral hemagglutinins have developed in the allantoic fluid. With herpes simplex virus and the poxviruses, neutralizing antibody prevents the production of characteristic pocks in the chorioallantoic membrane (pock-reduction test).

3. Nt test in mice–Mice of known uniform susceptibility and standard age are inoculated by a standard route with the virus-serum mixture. They are observed daily for signs of illness, such as weakness or paralysis, to establish specificity of the deaths. Illness and deaths are recorded daily for 21 days. Deaths within 24 hours after inoculation are attributed to traumatic or nonviral causes.

4. Interpretation of Nt tests–Since neutralizing antibodies for viruses persist for years, it is customary to demonstrate a rise in titer in sequential sera in order to establish current or recent infection by the virus. A fall in titer in the third (late) serum sample and unusually high titers can be significant.

D. Complement Fixation (CF) Tests: The principles underlying CF tests are described in Chapter 8. Because antiviral sera fix complement in the presence of the homologous antigens, such CF tests are employed in the diagnosis of many viral infections (Table 47–8). As in all CF tests, strictly standardized procedures must be employed. The main problem in viral CF tests is the preparation of specific antigens that are stable and not anticomplementary. Most antigens are derived from viral cell cultures (fluids or disrupted cells), embryonated eggs (fluids or tissues), or extracted tissues of infected animals (eg, mouse brains extracted with acetone for diagnosis of arbovirus infections).

In some instances, viruses may have two types of antigens: one associated with the virus particle (V) and the other a separate small "soluble" entity (S). Antibodies against different antigens may appear at different times during viral infection, as illustrated in mumps (see p 525). The interpretation of CF results depends on the antigen employed in the test and on the antibody titer rise observed.

Table 47–10. Cell culture neutralization (Nt) test with paired sera of patient infected with type 1 poliovirus.

Virus[1]	Serum (Day After Onset)	Cellular Degeneration (Cytopathic Effect) Final Serum Dilution					50% Serum Titer	
		1:2	1:10	1:50	1:250	1:1250	Logarithm	Antilog
Type 1	1	000	+++	+++	+++	+++	0.7	5
	20	000	000	000	00+	+++	2.5	320
Type 2	1	000	+++	+++	+++	+++	0.7	5
	20	000	000	0++	+++	+++	1.5	32
Type 3	1	+++	+++	+++	+++	+++	0	0
	20	+++	+++	+++	+++	+++	0	0
None	1	000						
	20	000						

[1]100 $TCID_{50}$ doses of each virus used in test. Three cultures were inoculated with each virus-serum mixture. + indicates cytopathic change in a culture because of virus growth. 0 indicates no growth of virus. ($TCID_{50}$ = 50% tissue culture infectious dose.) The patient was infected with type 1 poliovirus.

E. Hemagglutination Inhibition (HI) Test: Many viruses agglutinate erythrocytes, and this reaction may be specifically inhibited by immune or convalescent sera. This reaction forms the basis of many diagnostic tests for viral infections.

Diseases in which an antibody response may be demonstrated by the HI test are listed below:

- Influenza
- Rubella
- Mumps
- Measles
- Newcastle disease
- Variola
- Vaccinia
- California virus encephalitis
- St. Louis encephalitis
- Western equine encephalitis
- Japanese B encephalitis
- West Nile fever
- Dengue
- Adenovirus infections
- Reovirus infections
- Some enterovirus infections

The same general principles apply for HI tests used with various viral agents. However, a distinct species of erythrocytes may be necessary to agglutinate certain viruses—eg, some adenovirus types agglutinate only rat erythrocytes.

To be useful for diagnostic purposes, the erythrocyte suspension must be standardized and the viral antigen standardized and titrated. Positive and negative controls should be included in each test (Figure 47–2). The results are read as follows:

(1) Positive agglutination is indicated by a red, granular, diffused lining on the bottom of the tube.

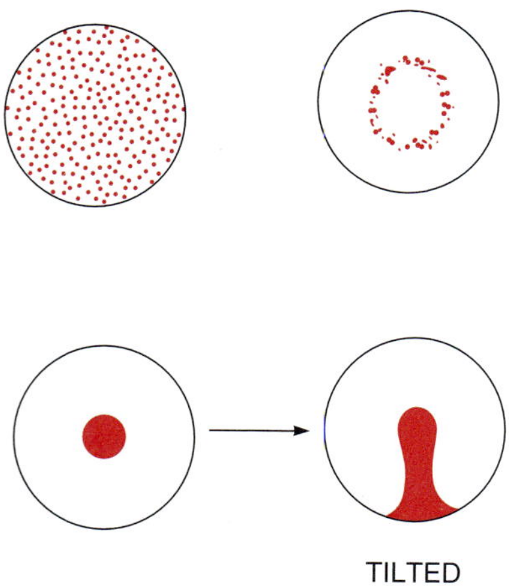

Figure 47–2. Patterns of positive (top) and negative (bottom) hemagglutination. When the tube is tilted, only nonagglutinated cells (bottom row) slide down the tube.

(2) Absence of agglutination is indicated by the formation of a compact red button at the bottom of the tube that slides when the tube is tilted.

(3) Partial agglutination is indicated by something in between a diffused lining on the bottom of the tube and a red button and takes the form of a ring with a hollow center.

Specific antiviral antibody inhibits the agglutination of red cells by virus suspensions. This principle is used to quantify the antibody level, to demonstrate rises in titer, and to establish the type-specific nature of the antibody rise in viral infections. Two serum specimens are needed from the patient, and these are taken at an interval of 2–3 weeks. The first specimen should be obtained as promptly as possible after the onset of illness. Serial dilutions of the sera are made in diluent, a standard amount (usually 4 hemagglutinating units) of virus suspension is added, and after thorough mixing the red cell suspension is added. Incubation is often at room temperature for 60 minutes. Care must be taken not to disturb the mixtures. The test is then read by the criteria outlined above. The highest dilution of serum that inhibits hemagglutination under standard conditions is considered the HI titer (Table 47–11). A fourfold or greater increase in antibody titer during a 2- to 3-week period is considered proof of active viral infection.

F. Immune Electron Microscopy: Viruses not detectable by conventional techniques may be observed by immune electron microscopy (IEM). Antigen-antibody complexes or aggregates formed between virus particles in suspension are caused by the presence of antibodies in added antiserum and are detected more readily and with greater assurance than individual virus particles.

With the IEM technique, the sample is first clarified by centrifugation and then mixed with specific or convalescent serum. Following incubation, the complexes formed are sedimented by centrifugation; the supernatant is discarded, and the pellet is suspended in distilled water, mixed with 3% phosphotungstic acid, and examined by electron microscopy.

The IEM technique may permit the use of convalescent sera from patients with fever of undetermined ori-

Table 47–11. An example of a hemagglutination inhibition (HI) test response.

Time of Taking Serum	Serum Dilution						Titer
	1:8	1:16	1:32	1:64	1:128	1:256	
Acute phase	0	+	+	+	+	+	1:8
Recovery phase	0	0	0	+	+	+	1:32
Convalescent	0	0	0	0	0	+	1:128

+ = Agglutination.
0 = No agglutination.

gin to construct antigen-antibody complexes with virus particles in acute-phase serum or in other specimens (eg, feces) obtained during the acute phase and thus to determine if infective agents were associated with the illness. This technique may sometimes offer a sensitive method of identifying new agents and subsequently determining their role in infectious disease.

Skin Tests

When available, tests for dermal hypersensitivity offer certain advantages in easily and quickly determining prior exposure to infectious agents. Tests have been described for mumps, herpes simplex, western equine encephalitis, and vaccinia. The skin test may lead to an increase in antibodies, eg, in the CF test.

The skin test antigen (0.1 mL) is injected intradermally into the flexor surface of one arm and the control material into the other arm. The sites of injection are examined after 12–48 hours. The mean diameter of erythematous reaction and induration is measured and compared to the control. A positive reaction is taken to indicate resistance to infection with some viruses.

REFERENCES

Balows A et al (editors): *Manual of Clinical Microbiology,* 5th ed. American Society for Microbiology, 1991.

Baron EJ, Finegold SM: *Bailey and Scott's Diagnostic Microbiology,* 9th ed. Mosby, 1994.

Campbell MC, Steward JL: *The Medical Mycology Handbook.* Wiley, 1980.

Fields BN et al (editors): *Fields Virology,* 2nd ed. Raven Press, 1990.

Finegold SM, George WL (editors): *Anaerobic Infections in Humans.* Academic Press, 1989.

Haley LD, Callaway CS: *Laboratory Methods in Medical Mycology,* 4th ed. Centers for Disease Control, US Department of Health, Education, and Welfare Publication No. CDC 78-8361, 1978.

Koneman EW et al: *Color Atlas and Textbook of Diagnostic Microbiology.* Lippincott, 1992.

Krieg NR, Holt JG (editors): *Bergey's Manual of Systematic Bacteriology,* Vol 1. Williams & Wilkins, 1984.

Kunin CM: *Detection, Prevention and Management of Urinary Tract Infections,* 4th ed. Lea & Febiger, 1987.

Lennette EH, Halonen P, Murphy FA (editors): *Laboratory Diagnosis of Infectious Diseases: Principles and Practice,* Vol 2: *Viral, Rickettsial, and Chlamydial Diseases.* Springer, 1988.

Lorian V (editor): *Antibiotics in Laboratory Medicine,* 2nd ed. Williams & Wilkins, 1986.

MacFaddin J: *Biochemical Tests for Identification of Medical Bacteria,* 2nd ed. Williams & Wilkins, 1980.

McFaddin JF: *Media for Isolation-Cultivation-Identification-Maintenance of Medical Bacteria,* Vol 1. Williams & Wilkins, 1985.

Persing DH et al: *Diagnostic Molecular Microbiology.* American Society for Microbiology, 1993.

Rippon JW: *Medical Mycology,* 3rd ed. Saunders, 1988.

Rose NR et al: *Manual of Clinical Laboratory Immunology,* 4th ed. American Society for Microbiology, 1992.

Schmidt NJ, Emmons R (editors): *Diagnostic Procedures for Viral, Rickettsial and Chlamydial Infections,* 6th ed. American Public Health Association, 1989.

Sneath PHA et al (editors): *Bergey's Manual of Systematic Bacteriology,* Vol 2. Williams & Wilkins, 1986.

Staley JT et al (editors): *Bergey's Manual of Systematic Bacteriology,* Vol 3. Williams & Wilkins, 1989.

Williams ST, Sharpe ME, Holt JG (editors): *Bergey's Manual of Systematic Bacteriology,* Vol 4. Williams & Wilkins, 1989.

48 Clinical Correlations

The diagnosis and management of infectious diseases requires an understanding of the presenting clinical manifestations and a knowledge of microbiology. Bacteria are frequent causes of acute life-threatening infections. Many viral, fungal, and parasitic infections present with constellations of focal and systemic signs and symptoms which in typical cases are highly suggestive of the diagnosis. However, some viruses, fungi, and parasites can cause severe acute diseases with signs and symptoms different from their classic presentations—eg, varicella-zoster virus typically involves the skin and mucous membranes, whereas *Histoplasma capsulatum* and *Coccidioides immitis* infect the lungs, but each can cause rapidly progressive disseminated disease with protean manifestations. This chapter presents ten cases and brief discussions illustrating the consequences of infections of the organ system involved by some common infectious causes.

Space considerations preclude complete descriptions of the infections for each anatomic site as well as discussion of all anatomic sites. The reader is referred to earlier chapters of this book for characterizations of the organisms; to Chapter 47 for information about diagnostic microbiology tests; and to textbooks of medicine and infectious diseases for more complete information about the clinical entities. One book that is very useful is Tierney LM Jr, McPhee SF, Papadakis MA (editors): *Current Medical Diagnosis and Treatment,* updated annually in January.

CENTRAL NERVOUS SYSTEM

CASE 1: MENINGITIS

A 3-year-old girl was brought to the emergency room by her parents because of fever and loss of appetite for the past 24 hours and difficulty in arousing her for the past 2 hours. The developmental history had been normal since birth. She attended a day care center and had a history of several episodes of presumed viral infections similar to those of other children at the center. Her childhood immunizations were up to date.

Clinical Features

Temperature was 39.5 °C, pulse 130/min, and respirations 24/min. Blood pressure was 110/60 mm Hg.

Physical examination showed a well-developed and well-nourished child of normal height and weight who was somnolent. When her neck was passively flexed, her legs also flexed (positive Brudzinski sign, suggesting irritation of the meninges). Funduscopic examination showed no papilledema, indicating that there had been no long-term increase in intracranial pressure. The remainder of her physical examination was normal

Laboratory Findings

Minutes later, blood was obtained for culture and other laboratory tests, and an intravenous line was placed. Lumbar puncture was performed less than 30 minutes after the patient arrived in the emergency room. The opening pressure was 350 mm of CSF (elevated). The fluid was cloudy. Several tubes of CSF were collected for culture, cell counts, and chemistry tests. One tube was taken immediately to the laboratory for Gram staining. The stain showed many polymorphonuclear (PMN) cells with cell-associated (intracellular) gram-negative diplococci suggestive of *Neisseria meningitidis.*

Blood chemistry tests were normal. The hematocrit was normal. The white blood cell count was 25,000/μL (markedly elevated), with 88% PMN forms and an absolute count of 22,000/μL (markedly elevated), 6% lymphocytes, and 6% monocytes. The CSF had 5000 PMNs/μL (normal, 0–5 lymphocytes/μL). The CSF protein was 100 mg/dL (elevated), and the glucose was 15 mg/dL (low, termed hypoglycorrhachia)—all consistent with bacterial meningitis. Cultures of blood and CSF grew serogroup B *N meningitidis.*

Treatment

Intravenous cefotaxime therapy was started within 35–40 minutes of the patient's arrival; dexamethasone was also given. The patient was treated with the antibiotic for 14 days and recovered without obvious sequelae. Further neurologic examinations and hearing tests are planned for the future. Rifampin prophylaxis was given to the other children who attended the day care center.

Comment

Bacterial meningitis usually presents with fever, headache, vomiting, photophobia, altered mental status ranging from sleepiness to coma, and neurologic signs ranging from abnormalities of cranial nerve function to seizures. However, subtle signs such as fever and lethargy are consistent with meningitis. Meningitis is considered to be acute with signs and symptoms of less than 24 hours' duration and subacute when signs and symptoms have been present for 1–7 days. Lumbar puncture with examination of the CSF is indicated whenever there is any suspicion of meningitis.

Acute meningitis is most often caused by bacteria of a few species: (Table 48–1) Lancefield serogroup B streptococci *(Streptococcus agalactiae)* and *Escherichia coli* in neonates; *Haemophilus influenzae* in children between the ages of 4–6 months and 6 years; *N meningitidis* in children and young adults; and *Streptococcus pneumoniae* occasionally in children and increasing in incidence in middle-aged and elderly persons. Many other species of microorganisms less commonly cause meningitis. *Listeria monocytogenes* causes meningitis in immunosuppressed patients and normal persons. The yeast *Cryptococcus neoformans* is the most common cause of meningitis in AIDS patients and can cause meningitis also in other immunosuppressed patients as well as in normal persons. Meningitis due to *Listeria* or *Cryptococcus* can be acute or insidious in onset. Gram-negative bacilli cause meningitis in acute head trauma and neurosurgical patients. *S pneumoniae* is found in recurrent meningitis in patients with basilar skull fractures. *Mycobacterium tuberculosis* can have a slow onset (chronic; >7 days) in immunologically normal persons but progresses more rapidly (subacute) in immunosuppressed persons such as AIDS patients. *Naegleria* species, free-living amebas, occasionally cause meningitis in persons with a recent history of swimming in warm fresh water. Viruses usually cause milder meningitis than bacteria. The viruses that most commonly cause meningitis are the enteroviruses (echoviruses and coxsackieviruses) and mumps virus.

The diagnosis of meningitis requires a high degree of suspicion when appropriate signs and symptoms are observed plus lumbar puncture without delay followed by examination of CSF. Findings in the spinal fluid typically include white blood cells in hundreds to thousands per microliter (PMNs for acute bacterial meningitis and lymphocytes for tuberculous and viral meningitis); glucose of <40 mg/dL, or less than 50% of the serum concentration; and protein of >100 mg/dL. In bacterial meningitis, Gram's stain of centrifuged sediment of CSF shows PMNs and bacterial morphology consistent with the species subsequently cultured: *N meningitidis,* intracellular gram-negative diplococci; *H influenzae,* small gram-negative coccobacilli; serogroup B streptococci and pneumococci; and gram-positive cocci in pairs and chains. Blood cultures should be done along with the CSF cultures.

Acute bacterial meningitis is fatal if untreated. Initial therapy should include parenteral antibiotics known to be effective against the suspected organisms, including penicillin G or ampicillin for serogroup B streptococci, pneumococci, and meningococci; third-generation cephalosporin for *H influenzae* and *E coli.* When selecting initial antibiotic therapy, it is important to take into account that pneumococci resistant to penicillin G are increasingly common, and meningococci relatively resistant to penicillin G have been reported; initial therapy with drugs other than the traditional penicillin G may be appropriate, switching then to penicillin G when the bacteria are known to be susceptible. Initial therapy with ampicillin for *H influen-*

Table 48–1. Common causes of meningitis.

Organism	Age Group	Comment	Chapter
Serogroup B streptococci *(Streptococcus agalactiae)*	Neonates to age 3 months	As many as 25% of mothers have vaginal carriage of serogroup B streptococci. Ampicillin prophylaxis during labor of women at high risk (prolonged rupture of membranes, fever, etc) or of known carriers reduces the incidence of infection in babies.	15
Escherichia coli	Neonates	Commonly have the K1 antigen.	16
Haemophilus influenzae	Children 6 months to 5 years	Widespread use of vaccine greatly reduces incidence of *H influenzae* meningitis in children.	19
Neisseria meningitis	Infants to 5 years and young adults	Polysaccharide vaccines against serogroups A, C, Y, and W135 are used in epidemic areas and in association with outbreaks.	21
Streptococcus pneumoniae	All age groups; highest incidence in the elderly	Often occurs with pneumonia; also with mastoiditis, sinusitis, and basilar skull fractures.	15
Cryptococcus neoformans	AIDS patients	Frequent cause of meningitis in AIDS patients.	45

zae is not recommended, because a significant proportion of these bacteria produce beta-lactamase.

CASE 2: BRAIN ABSCESS

A 57-year-old man presented to the hospital with seizures. Three weeks earlier he had developed bifrontal headaches that were relieved by aspirin. The headaches recurred several times, including the day prior to admission. On the morning of admission he was noted to have focal seizures with involuntary movements of the right side of his face and arm. While in the emergency room, he had a generalized seizure that was controlled by intravenous diazepam, phenytoin, and phenobarbital. Additional history from the patient's wife indicated that he had had a dental extraction and bridge work approximately 5 weeks earlier. He did not smoke, drank only socially, and took no medications. The remainder of his history was not helpful.

Clinical Features

The temperature was 37 °C, the pulse 110/min, and respirations 18/min. The blood pressure was 140/80 mm Hg.

On physical examination, the patient was sleepy and had a decreased attention span. He moved all his extremities, though the right arm moved less than the left. There was slight blurring of the left optic disk, suggesting possible increased intracranial pressure. The remainder of his physical examination was normal.

Laboratory Findings & Imaging

Laboratory tests were all normal, including hemoglobin and hematocrit, white blood cell count and differential, serum electrolytes, blood urea nitrogen, serum creatinine, urinalysis, chest x-ray, and ECG. Lumbar puncture was not done and cerebrospinal fluid was not examined because of possible increased intracranial pressure due to a mass lesion. Blood cultures were negative. CT scan of the patient's head showed a 1.5 cm localized ring-enhancing lesion in the left parietal hemisphere suggestive of brain abscess.

Treatment

The patient had a neurosurgical procedure with biopsy of the lesion, which was completely removed. Culture of necrotic material from the lesion yielded *Prevotella melaninogenica* and *Streptococcus anginosus.* Pathologic examination of the tissue suggested that the lesion was several weeks old. The patient received antibiotic therapy for 4 weeks. He had no more seizures and no subsequent neurologic deficits. One year later, anticonvulsant medications were discontinued and a follow-up CT scan was negative.

Comment

A brain abscess is a localized pyogenic bacterial infection within the brain parenchyma. The major clinical manifestations are related to the presence of a space-occupying mass in the brain rather than the classic signs and symptoms of infection. Thus, patients commonly present with headache and a change in mental status from normal to lethargy or coma. Focal neurologic findings related to location of the abscess occur in less than half of patients; one-third have seizures; less than half have fever. Occasionally, patients present with signs and symptoms suggesting acute meningitis. Initially, the clinician must differentiate brain abscess from other central nervous system processes, including primary or metastatic cancers, subdural or epidural abscesses, viral infections (herpes simplex encephalitis), meningitis, stroke, and a variety of other diseases.

Significant predisposing factors for brain abscess include distant site infections with bacteremia, such as endocarditis, lung infections, or other occult infections. Many patients have had relatively recent dental work. Brain abscess can also occur via spread from contiguous sites of infection such as in the middle ear, mastoid, or sinuses or following penetrating trauma. However, 20% of patients with brain abscesses have no discernible predisposing factors.

Brain abscess can be caused by a single species of bacteria, but more than one species are often isolated—in general, an average of two species. Of the facultative and aerobic bacteria, the viridans streptococci (including nonhemolytic and alpha-hemolytic stains, *S anginosus, S mitis,* etc; see Chapter 15) are most common, occurring in one-third to one-half of patients. *Staphylococcus aureus* (Chapter 14) is isolated in 10–15% and when present is often the only isolate found. Enteric gram-negative rods occur in about 25%, often in mixed cultures. Many other facultative or aerobic bacteria (eg, *S pneumoniae, Nocardia asteroides,*) also occur in brain abscesses. Anaerobic bacteria are found in 50% or more of cases (Chapter 22). *Peptostreptococcus* is most common, followed by *Bacteroides* and *Prevotella. Fusobacterium, Actinomyces,* and *Eubacterium* are less common, followed by other anaerobes. Many fungi and parasites can cause brain abscesses or infection in the central nervous system. In immunosuppressed patients, particularly AIDS patients, the list of predominant causes of brain abscesses expands to include *Toxoplasma gondii, Cryptococcus neoformans, Mycobacterium tuberculosis,* and atypical mycobacteria.

Lumbar puncture to obtain CSF is generally not indicated in patients with brain abscess (or other mass lesions in the brain). The increased intracranial pressure makes the procedure life-threatening, because herniation of the brain through the tentorium cerebelli results in midbrain compression. The findings in CSF are not specific for brain abscess: white blood cells, predominantly mononuclear cells, are often present; the glucose level may be moderately low and the protein concentration elevated. Thus, when fever and signs suggesting acute meningitis are absent and brain abscess is suspected, the clinician should obtain a CT scan. Brain abscesses typically show ring-enhanced uptake of contrast material on CT scan, though similar findings can be found in patients with brain tumors and other diseases. MRI may be helpful in differentiating brain abscesses from tumors. Technetium 99 and indium 111 scans also have been used. Definitive differentiation between brain abscess and tumor is done by pathologic examination and culture of tissue from the lesion obtained by a neurosurgical procedure.

Untreated brain abscesses are fatal. Surgical excision provides the initial therapy as well as the diagnosis of brain abscess. Needle aspiration using stereotactic technique is an alternative to surgical excision. Antibiotic therapy should be parenteral and should include high-dose penicillin G for streptococci and many anaerobes, metronidazole for anaerobes resistant to penicillin G, plus a third-generation cephalosporin for enteric gram-negative rods. Vancomycin or another drug specific for *S aureus* should be included in the initial therapy if the patient has endocarditis, is known to have staphylococcal bacteremia, or the abscess yields staphylococci. Initial therapy with antibiotics rather than surgery can be instituted in some patients whose brain abscesses are small (< 2 cm), multiple, or difficult to reach surgically, but deteriorating neurologic functions indicate the need for surgery. Once culture results from the abscess material are known, initial antibiotic therapy should be modified to be specific for the bacteria isolated from the lesion. Antibiotic therapy should be continued for at least 3–4 weeks when surgical excision has been done or for 8 weeks or longer when there has been no surgery. Nonbacterial causes of brain abscesses require definitive diagnoses and specific therapy; for example, in AIDS patients, toxoplasmosis of the brain is diagnosed by biopsy and treated with sulfadiazine and pyrimethamine. Steroids to decrease swelling should be used only when there is mass effect.

CHEST

CASE 3: PNEUMONIA

A 35-year-old man came to the emergency room because of fever and pain in his left chest when he coughed. Five days earlier he had developed signs of a viral upper respiratory infection with sore throat, runny nose, and increased cough. The day before presentation he developed left lateral chest pain when he coughed or took a deep breath. Twelve hours before coming to the emergency room he was awakened with a severe shaking chill and sweating. Further history taking disclosed that the patient drank moderate to heavy amounts of alcohol and had smoked one package of cigarettes daily for about 17 years. He worked as an automobile repair man. He had a history of two prior hospitalizations—4 years ago for alcohol withdrawal and 2 years ago for acute bronchitis.

Clinical Features

Temperature was 39 °C, pulse 130/min and respirations 28/min. Blood pressure was 120/80 mm Hg.

Physical examination showed a slightly overweight man who was coughing frequently and holding his left chest when he coughed. He produced very little thick rusty-colored sputum. His chest examination showed normal movement of the diaphragm. There was dullness to percussion of the left lateral posterior chest, suggesting consolidation of the lung. Tubular (bronchial) breath sounds were heard in the same area along with dry crepitant sounds (rales), consistent with lung consolidation and viscous mucus in the airway. The remainder of his physical examination was normal

Laboratory Findings & Imaging

Chest films showed a dense left lower lobe consolidation consistent with bacterial pneumonia. The hematocrit was 45% (normal). The white blood cell count was 16,000/μL (markedly elevated) with 80% PMN forms with an absolute PMN count of 12,800/μL (markedly elevated), 12% lymphocytes, and 8% monocytes. Blood chemistry tests, including electrolytes, were normal. Sputum was thick, yellow to rusty colored and purulent in appearance. Gram's stain of the sputum showed many PMN cells and lancet-shaped gram-positive diplococci. Twenty-four hours later, the blood cultures were positive for *Streptococcus pneumoniae.* Cultures of sputum grew numerous *S pneumoniae* and a few colonies of *Haemophilus influenzae.*

Treatment

The initial diagnosis was bacterial pneumonia, probably pneumococcal. Parenteral aqueous penicillin G therapy was begun, and the patient was given parenteral fluids. Within 48 hours, his temperature was normal and he was coughing up large amounts of purulent sputum. Penicillin G was continued for 7 days. At follow-up 4 weeks after admission to the hospital, the lung consolidation had cleared.

Comment

Acute bacterial pneumonia commonly presents with an abrupt onset of chills and fever, cough, and often **pleuritic chest pain.** The cough frequently is productive of **purulent sputum,** but many patients with pneumonia are not adequately hydrated and do not produce sputum until they receive fluids, as in this case. Pleuritic chest pain occurs when the inflammatory process of the pneumonia involves the pleural lining of the lung and chest cavity; movement of the pleura, as occurs with coughing or deep breathing, yields localized pain. Patients with acute pneumonia appear ill and usually have tachypnea (rapid breathing) and tachycardia (rapid heart rate). Many patients with pneumonia have predisposing factors (congestive heart failure, chronic obstructive pulmonary disease, etc) which become exacerbated before or in association with the pneumonia.

The findings on physical examination are those associated with **consolidation of the lung tissue,** purulent mucus **(sputum)** in the airway, and, in some patients, fluid in the chest cavity. On percussion, there is dullness over the area of consolidation (or fluid). When consolidation occurs, the small airways are closed, leaving only the large airways open; on auscultation, there are tubular breath sounds over the area. If all the airways are blocked, no breath sounds are audible. Dry crepitant sounds (rales) or crackling sounds on auscultation indicate fluid or mucus in the airways; these sounds may change when the patient coughs.

The most common causes of **community-acquired pneumonia** are *S pneumoniae, Mycoplasma pneumoniae* (**atypical pneumonia** in young persons), and *Legionella pneumophila* (Table 48–2); collectively, these pathogens may cause as many as 75% of cases of community-acquired pneumonia. *H influenzae* pneumonia is common in association with chronic cardiopulmonary disease. Other causes include *Chlamydia pneumoniae* (as much as 10% of community-acquired pneumonia), *Staphylococcus aureus* in association with influenza virus infections, and *Klebsiella pneumoniae* in chronic alcoholics. Other gram-negative bacilli are uncommon causes of community-acquired pneumonia. **Pleural pulmonary infections with mixed anaerobic bacteria** are associated with predisposing factors such as periodontal disease, seizure disorders, stupor or coma, and aspiration of oropharyngeal bacteria into the lung. Pneumonia, lung abscesses, and infection of the pleural space (**empyema,** or pus in the chest cavity) occur with mixed anaerobic infections.

Hospital-acquired (nosocomial) pneumonia is frequently caused by enteric gram-negative bacilli such as *Escherichia coli, Pseudomonas aeruginosa, S aureus,* and *Legionella.* Fungi, including *Histoplasma capsulatum, Coccidioides immitis,* and *Cryptococcus neoformans* cause **community-acquired** pneumonia; *Candida* and *Aspergillus* species are more likely to cause nosocomial infections. Viruses that commonly cause pneumonia in children are respiratory syncytial virus, parainfluenza viruses, and influenza A virus. In adults, the viruses that are likely to cause pneumonia are the influenza viruses and certain adenoviruses. The clinician should keep in mind, however, that any microorganism can cause pneumonia; the organisms mentioned here are a short list of the most common pathogens.

Blood counts in patients with pneumonia usually show leukocytosis with increased polymorphonuclear cells. Chest radiography shows segmental or lobar infiltrates. Cavities may be seen especially with mixed anaerobic infections or pneumonia due to *S aureus* or group A streptococci. Pleural effusions may also be found and, if present, may call for thoracentesis to obtain fluid for cell counts and culture. Blood cultures should be done in all patients with acute pneumonia. Sputum should be cultured as well.

Most patients with bacterial pneumonia and many patients with pneumonia due to other causes have mucopurulent sputum. Rusty-colored sputum suggests alveolar involvement and is associated with pneumococcal pneumonia but occurs with other organisms also. Foul-smelling sputum suggests mixed anaerobic infection. A purulent portion of the sputum should be chosen for Gram's stain and microscopic examination; an adequate sputum specimen will have over 25 polymorphonuclear cells and fewer than 10 epithelial cells per low-power field (100 × magnification). Traditionally, microscopic examination of the sputum has been used to help determine the cause of pneumonia; however, it may be difficult to differentiate organisms that are part of the normal oropharyngeal flora from those that are causing the pneumonia. The finding of numerous lancet-shaped gram-positive diplococci strongly suggests *S pneumoniae,* but streptococci that are part of the oropharyngeal flora can have the same appearance. The major value of stained sputum smears is when organisms that would not be expected are found (eg, numerous gram-negative bacilli suggesting enteric bacilli or *Pseudomonas,* numerous gram-positive cocci in clusters suggesting staphylococci). Sputum cultures have many of the same drawbacks as smears; it may be difficult to differentiate normal flora or colonizing bacteria from the cause of the pneumonia.

True demonstration of the cause of pneumonia comes from a limited set of specimens: a positive blood culture in a pneumonia patient with no confounding infections; a positive pleural fluid or direct lung aspirate culture; and detection of circulating antigen of a specific organism with no confounding infection. A positive culture of sputum obtained by transtracheal aspiration is very helpful. Cultures of fluid obtained at bronchoscopy also can strongly suggest the cause of pneumonia, but a small amount of normal oropharyngeal flora usually are present in such cultures.

Three of the primary causes of community-acquired pneumonia—*S pneumoniae, Mycoplasma,* and *Legionella*—as well as *Chlamydia pneumoniae* are typically susceptible to erythromycin. Thus, erythromycin can be used to treat most community-acquired pneumonia. Penicillin G is the drug of choice if pneumococcal pneumonia is diagnosed; however, pneumococci can be resistant to penicillin G and occasionally erythromycin. *H influenzae* is not susceptible to erythromycin. Other causes of pneumonia should be treated with antibiotics demonstrated to be active against them.

Table 48–2. Characteristics and treatment of selected pneumonias.

Organism	Clinical Setting	Gram-Stained Smears of Sputum	Chest Radiograph[1]	Laboratory Studies	Complications	Preferred Antimicrobial Therapy[2]	Chapter
Streptococcus pneumoniae (pneumococcus)	Chronic cardiopulmonary disease; follows upper respiratory tract infections.	Gram-positive diplococci.	Lobar consolidation.	Gram-stained smear of sputum; culture of blood, pleural fluid.	Bacteremia, meningitis, endocarditis, pericarditis, empyema.	Penicillin G (or V, oral).	15
Haemophilus influenzae	Chronic cardiopulmonary disease; follows upper respiratory tract infection.	Small gram-negative coccobacilli.	Lobar consolidation.	Culture of sputum, blood, pleural fluid.	Empyema, endocarditis.	Ampicillin (or amoxicillin). Cefotaxime or ceftriaxone for severe infections.	19
Staphylococcus aureus	Influenza epidemics; nosocomial.	Gram-positive cocci in clumps.	Patchy infiltrates.	Culture of sputum, blood, pleural fluid.	Empyema, cavitation.	Nafcillin.[3]	14
Klebsiella pneumoniae	Alcohol abuse, diabetes mellitus; nosocomial.	Gram-negative encapsulated rods.	Lobar consolidation.	Culture of sputum, blood, pleural fluid.	Cavitation, empyema.	A cephalosporin for severe infection, a cephalosporin plus gentamicin,tobramycin, or amikacin.	16
Escherichia coli	Nosocomial; rarely, community-acquired.	Gram-negative rods.	Patchy infiltrates, pleural effusion.	Culture of sputum, blood, pleural fluid.	Empyema.	Aminoglycoside or a cephalosporin.	16
Pseudomonas aeruginosa	Nosocomial; cystic fibrosis.	Gram-negative rods.	Patchy infiltrates, cavitation.	Culture of sputum, blood.	Cavitation.	Aminoglycoside plus anti-*Pseudomonas* penicillin, eg, ticarcillin, piperacillin.	17
Anaerobes	Aspiration, periodontitis.	Mixed flora.	Patchy infiltrates in dependent lung zones.	Culture of pleural fluid or of material obtained by transtracheal or transthoracic aspiration.	Necrotizing pneumonia, abscess, empyema.	Clindamycin.	11, 48
Mycoplasma pneumoniae	Young adults; summer and fall.	PMNs and monocytes; no bacterial pathogens.	Extensive patchy infiltrates.	Complement fixation titer.[4] Cold agglutinin serum titers are not helpful as they lack sensitivity and specificity.	Skin rashes, bullous myringitis; hemolytic anemia.	Erythromycin.	26
Legionella species	Summer and fall; exposure to contaminated construction site, water source, air conditioner; community-acquired or nosocomial.	Few PMNs; no bacteria.	Patchy or lobar consolidation.	Direct immunofluorescent examination of sputum or tissue; immunofluorescent antibody titer,[4] culture of sputum or tissue.[5]	Empyema, cavitation, endocarditis, pericarditis.	Erythromycin, with or without rifampin.	23
Chlamydia pneumoniae	Clinically similar to *M pneumoniae,* but prodromal symptoms last longer (up to 2 weeks). Sore throat with hoarseness common. Mild pneumonia in teenagers and young adults.	Nonspecific.	Subsegmental infiltrate, less prominent than in *M pneumoniae* pneumonia. Consolidation rare.	Isolation of the organism is very difficult. Serologic studies include microimmunofluorescence with TWAR antigen and a nonspecific complement fixation antibody test.	Reinfection in older adults with underlying COPD or heart failure may be severe or even fatal.	Tetracycline, erythromycin, clarithromycin.	28
Moraxella catarrhalis	Preexisting lung-disease; elderly; corticosteroid or immunosuppressive therapy.	Gram-negative diplococci.	Patchy infiltrates; occasional lobar consolidation.	Gram stain and culture of sputum or bronchial aspirate.	Rarely, pleural effusions and bacteremia.	Trimethoprim-sulfamethoxazole or amoxicillin-clavulanic acid.	21
Pneumocystis carinii	AIDS, immunosuppressive or cytotoxic drug therapy, cancer.	Not helpful in diagnosis.	Diffuse interstitial and alveolar infiltrates; apical or upper lobe infiltrates in patients on aerosolized pentamidine.	Cysts and trophozoites of *P carinii* on methenamine silver or Giemsa stains of sputum or bronchoalveolar lavage fluid.	Pneumothorax, respiratory failure, ARDS,[6] death.	Trimethoprim-sulfamethoxazole, pentamidine isethionate.	45

[1] X-ray findings lack specificity.
[2] Antimicrobial susceptibility should guide therapy.
[3] Methicillin-resistant *S aureus* infections are treated with vancomycin.
[4] Fourfold rise in titer is diagnostic.
[5] Selective media are required.
[6] Adult Respiratory Distress Syndrome

HEART

CASE 4: ENDOCARDITIS

A 45-year-old woman was admitted to the hospital because of fever, shortness of breath, and weight loss. Chills, sweats, and anorexia started 6 weeks before admission and increased in severity until admission. Persistent back pain developed 4 weeks prior to admission. Her shortness of breath on exertion increased to one block from her usual three blocks of walking. At the time of admission, she reported a 10-pound weight loss.

Rheumatic fever had been diagnosed in childhood, when she had swollen joints and fever and was confined to bed for 3 months. Subsequently, a heart murmur was heard.

Clinical Features

Temperature was 38 °C, pulse 90/min, and respirations 18/min. Blood pressure was 130/80 mm Hg.

Physical examination showed a moderately overweight woman who was alert and oriented. She became short of breath while walking up two flights of stairs. Examination of her eyes showed a Roth spot (a round white spot surrounded by hemorrhage) in the retina of her right eye. Petechiae were seen in the conjunctiva of both eyes. Her head and neck were otherwise normal. Splinter hemorrhages were seen under two fingernails of her right hand and one finger of the left hand. Osler's nodes (tender, small, raised, red or purple lesions of the skin) were seen in the pads of one finger and one toe. Her heart size was normal to percussion. On auscultation, a low-pitched diastolic murmur consistent with mitral valve stenosis was heard at the apex; a loud mitral valve opening snap was heard over the left chest. Examination of her abdomen was difficult because of obesity; one observer felt an enlarged spleen. The remainder of her physical examination was normal

Laboratory Findings & Imaging

The films from a chest x-ray showed a normal heart size and normal lungs. The ECG showed a normal sinus rhythm with broad P waves (atrial conduction). Echocardiography showed an enlarged left atrium, thickened mitral valve leaflets, and a vegetation on the posterior leaflet. The hematocrit was 29% (low). The white blood cell count was 9800/μL (high normal), with 68% PMNs (high), 24% lymphocytes, and 8% monocytes. The erythrocyte sedimentation rate was 68 mm/h (high). Blood chemistry tests, including electrolytes and tests of renal function, were normal. Three blood cultures were obtained on the day of admission; 1 day later, all three were positive for gram-positive cocci in chains that were viridans streptococci and subsequently identified as *Streptococcus sanguis.*

Treatment

Endocarditis of the mitral valve was diagnosed. Intravenous penicillin G and gentamicin was begun and continued for 2 weeks. The patient was afebrile within 3 days after starting therapy. Following the successful treatment of her endocarditis, she was referred for long-term management of her heart disease.

Comment

The symptoms and signs of **endocarditis** are quite varied because any organ system can be secondarily (or primarily) involved. Fever occurs in 80–90% of patients, chills in 50%, anorexia and weight loss in about 25%, skin lesions in about 25%. Nonspecific symptoms such as headache, backache, cough, and arthralgia are very common. Up to 25% of endocarditis patients present with neurologic signs or strokes secondary to emboli from **heart valve vegetations.** Backache, chest pain, and abdominal pain occur in 10–20% of the patients. Physical findings typically include fever in 90–95%, a **heart murmur** in 80–90% with a new or changing heart murmur in about 15%, and splenomegaly and skin lesions in about 50% of patients. Many other symptoms and physical findings are directly related to the complications of metastatic infection and embolization from the vegetation.

Streptococci cause about 70% of endocarditis cases. Viridans streptococci of several species (eg, *S sanguis, S salivarius, S mutans, S bovis*; Chapter 15) are most common, followed by enterococci (eg, *E faecalis*) and other streptococci. The streptococci usually cause endocarditis on abnormal heart valves. *S aureus* causes 20–25% and *Staphylococcus epidermidis* about 5% of endocarditis (Chapter 14). *S aureus* can infect normal heart valves, is common in intravenous drug abusers, and produces more rapidly progressive disease than the streptococci. *S epidermidis* is a cause of endocarditis on prosthetic valves and only rarely infects native valves. Gram-negative bacilli occur in about 5% and yeasts such as *Candida albicans* in about 3% of cases. Many other bacteria—indeed any species—can cause endocarditis; a small percentage are culture-negative.

The history and physical examination are important diagnostic procedures. The diagnosis is strongly suggested by repeatedly positive blood cultures with no other site of infection. Echocardiography can be a very helpful adjunctive procedure.

Antibiotics are the basis of therapy because untreated endocarditis is fatal. Bactericidal drugs should be used. The choice of antibiotics depends upon the infecting organism: penicillin G plus gentamicin for 2 weeks for viridans streptococci and for 4 weeks for enterococci; *S aureus* is treated with a penicillinase-resistant penicillin (eg, nafcillin), often with addition of gentamicin or rifampin, usually for 4 weeks; vancomycin is an alternative drug to penicillin G and nafcillin for the streptococci and staphylococci; bacteria other than the streptococci and staphylococci are treated with antibiotics of demonstrated activity. Surgery with valve replacement is sometimes necessary when valvular regurgitation (eg, aortic regurgitation) results in acute heart failure even when active infection is present. Surgery is required for fungal endocarditis and with failure of medical therapy; frequently necessary with gram-negative endocarditis; and important when the infection involves the sinus of Valsalva or produces septal abscesses and when embolization recurs.

ABDOMEN

CASE 5: PERITONITIS & ABSCESSES

An 18-year-old male student was admitted to the hospital because of fever and abdominal pain. He had been well until 3 days prior to admission, when he developed diffuse abdominal pain and vomiting following the evening meal. The pain persisted through the night and was worse the following morning. He was seen in the emergency room, where abdominal tenderness was noted; X-rays of the chest and abdomen were normal; the white blood cell count was 24,000/μL; other laboratory tests, including tests of liver, pancreas, and renal function, were normal. The patient returned home, but the abdominal pain and intermittent vomiting persisted and fever to 38 °C developed. The patient was admitted to the hospital on the third day of illness.

There was no history of use of medication, drug or alcohol abuse, trauma, or infections, and the family history was negative.

Clinical Features

The temperature was 38 °C, the pulse 100/min, respirations 24/min. The blood pressure was 110/70 mm Hg.

Physical examination showed a normally developed young man who appeared acutely ill and complained of diffuse abdominal pain. The chest and heart examinations were normal. The abdomen was slightly distended. There was diffuse periumbilical and right lower quadrant tenderness to palpation with guarding (muscle rigidity with palpation). There was a suggestion of a right lower quadrant mass. Bowel sounds were infrequent.

Laboratory Findings & Imaging

The hematocrit was 45% (normal), and the white blood cell count was 20,000/μL (markedly elevated) with 90% polymorphonuclear cells (markedly elevated) and 12% lymphocytes. The serum amylase (a test for pancreatitis) was normal. Electrolytes and tests of liver and renal function were normal. X-ray films of the chest and abdomen were normal, though several distended loops of small bowel were seen. CT scan of the abdomen showed a fluid collection in the right lower quadrant with extension into the pelvis.

Treatment

The patient was taken to the operating room. At surgery, a perforated appendix with a large periappendiceal abscess extending into the pelvis was found. The appendix was removed, About 300 mL of foul-smelling abscess fluid was evacuated, and drains were placed. The patient was treated with gentamicin, ampicillin, and metronidazole for 2 weeks. The drains were advanced daily and totally removed 1 week after surgery. Culture of the abscess fluid revealed at least six species of bacteria, including *Escherichia coli, Bacteroides fragilis,* viridans streptococci, and enterococci (normal gastrointestinal flora). The patient recovered uneventfully.

Comment

Pain is the usual primary manifestation of **peritonitis** and **intra-abdominal abscess** formation. The localization and intensity of the pain are related to the primary disease of the abdominal viscera. Perforation of a peptic ulcer quickly yields epigastric pain that rapidly spreads throughout the abdomen with the spillage of gastric contents. A ruptured appendix or sigmoid colon diverticulum often produces more localized right or left lower quadrant pain, respectively, associated with the focal peritonitis and abscess formation. Nausea, vomiting, anorexia, and fever accompany the pain.

The signs and symptoms following acute spillage of bowel contents into the abdomen tend to take two phases. The first is the peritonitis stage, with acute pain associated with infection by *E coli* and other facultative anaerobic bacteria; this occurs over the first 1–2 days and if untreated is associated with a high mortality rate. The second stage is abscess formation associated with infection with *B fragilis* and other obligately anaerobic bacteria.

Physical examination during the acute phase shows abdominal rigidity and diffuse or local tenderness. Often the tenderness is pronounced when palpation of the abdomen is released, termed **rebound tenderness.** Later, abdominal distention and loss of bowel motility **(paralytic ileus)** occur.

The bacteria that make up the **normal gastrointestinal flora** (Chapter 11) are the causes of acute peritonitis and abscesses associated with bowel rupture: *E coli* and other enteric gram-negative rods, enterococci, viridans streptococci, *B fragilis* and other anaerobic gram-negative rods, and anaerobic gram-positive cocci and rods of many species.

The history and physical examination are the important initial steps in the diagnosis, to determine the acuteness and localization of the problem. Laboratory tests, such as white blood cell counts, yield nonspecific abnormal results or help rule out diseases such as pancreatitis, as in this case. X-ray films of the abdomen are very useful diagnostic adjuncts and may show gas and fluid collections in the large and small bowel. Much definitive information indicating focal abnormalities is obtained using CT scans. When fluid is present, needle aspiration and culture yield a diagnosis of infection but do not define the underlying disease process.

Surgery may be necessary to obtain a definitive diagnosis, while at the same time it provides the definitive step in therapy. The underlying disease process, such as a gangrenous bowel or ruptured appendix, can be corrected and the localized infection drained. Antimicrobial drugs are important adjunctive therapy. The selection of drugs might include an antimicrobial active against the enteric gram-negative rods, one active against the enterococci and streptococci, and a third against the anaerobic gram-negative rods that are often resistant to penicillin G. Many regimens have been described; one regimen includes gentamicin, ampicillin, and metronidazole.

CASE 6: GASTROENTERITIS (Invasive Enteric Infections)

Four members of a migrant farm worker family came to the hospital because of diarrhea and fever starting 6–12 hours earlier. The father was 28, the mother 24, and the children 6 and 4 years of age. The previous day, the family had a meal of mixed green salad, ground meat, beans, and tortillas prepared by another person in the encampment. Another child in the family, 8 months old, had not eaten the same meal and remained well. Approximately 24 hours after the meal, the children developed abdominal cramps, fever, and watery diarrhea. These symptoms had persisted for the preceding 12 hours, and in both children the diarrhea had become bloody. The parents had developed similar symptoms 6 and 8 hours earlier but did not have blood visible in their stools.

The parents stated that several other people in the camp had similar illnesses during the previous 2 weeks. The sanitation facilities in the camp were primitive.

Clinical Features

On physical examination, the children had temperatures of 39–39.5 °C and the parents 38 °C. All had tachycardia (rapid heart rates) and appeared acutely ill. Both children appeared dehydrated.

White blood cell counts ranged from 12,000 to 16,000/μL, with 55–76% polymorphonuclear cells. Multiple white blood cells were seen in the fecal wet mounts. Stool from the children was grossly bloody and mucoid. Cultures of the stools from each of the patients subsequently grew *Shigella flexneri.*

Treatment

Both children were admitted to the hospital and given intravenous fluids and ampicillin. The parents were treated as outpatients, with oral fluids and oral ciprofloxacin. All recovered uneventfully. Public health follow-up led to improved sanitation conditions at the camp.

Comment

Nausea, vomiting, abdominal pain, diarrhea, and fever are the major clinical findings in gastrointestinal infections. The predominant symptoms are dependent upon the etiologic agent and whether it is toxigenic or invasive or both. When preformed toxins are in food, they often are associated with nausea and vomiting. For example, *S aureus* and *Bacillus cereus* produce **enterotoxins** in food; nausea and vomiting—and to a much lesser extent diarrhea—occur a few hours following ingestion of the food. Organisms that produce enterotoxins affect the proximal small bowel and tend to cause **watery diarrhea** (eg, enterotoxigenic *E coli, Vibrio cholerae*). Agents such as rotaviruses, Norwalk virus, and *Giardia lamblia* cause watery diarrhea through the mechanism of mucosal irritation or destruction. Invasive or cytotoxin-producing bacteria infect the colon and cause abdominal pain, frequent diarrhea often with blood and mucus, fever, and dehydration, as in this case; this group of signs and symptoms is called **dysentery.** Organisms that cause dysentery include *Salmonella* of many serotypes, *Shigella, Campylobacter jejuni,* enteroinvasive *E coli, Clostridium difficile,* and *Entamoeba histolytica.* **Enteric fever** is a life-threatening infection characterized by fever, headache, and variable abdominal symptoms; *Salmonella typhi* (and also *S paratyphi* A and B, and *S choleraesuis*) and *Yersinia enterocolitica* cause enteric fever. The agents that commonly cause toxin-induced gastroenteritis and gastrointestinal infections are listed in Table 48-3.

Gastrointestinal infections are very common, especially in developing countries, where the associated mortality rate is high in infants and young children. Public health prevention through fostering good hygiene and providing sanitary water and food supplies is of the utmost importance.

In only a small percentage of cases is the etiologic agent demonstrated by means of stool culture or immunoassay. Finding white blood cells on fecal wet mounts is highly suggestive of infection

Maintaining adequate hydration is the most important feature of treatment, especially in infants and children. Antimicrobial therapy is necessary in treatment of enteric fever **(typhoid fever)** and shortens the duration of symptoms in *Shigella, Campylobacter,* and *V cholerae* infections, but it prolongs the symptoms and fecal shedding of *Salmonella.*

There is no specific therapy for infection due to rotaviruses, the most common viral cause of diarrhea.

Table 48–3. Agents that commonly cause toxin-induced gastroenteritis and gastrointestinal infections.

Organism	Typical Incubation Period	Signs and Symptoms	Epidemiology	Pathogenesis	Clinical Features	Chapter
Staphylococcus aureus	1–8 hours (rarely, up to 18)	Nausea and vomiting	Staphylococci grow in meats, dairy, and other foods and produce enterotoxin.	Enterotoxin acts on receptors in the gut that transmit impulse to medullary centers that control vomiting.	Very common, abrupt onset, intense vomiting for up to 24 hours, regular recovery in 24–48 hours. Occurs in persons eating the same food. No treatment usually necessary except to restore fluids and electrolytes.	14
Bacillus cereus	2–16 hours	Vomiting or diarrhea	Reheated fried rice is common vehicle.	Enterotoxin formed in food or in gut from growth of *B cereus*.	With incubation period of 2–8 hours, mainly vomiting. With incubation period of 8–16 hours, mainly diarrhea.	12
Clostridium perfringens	8–16 hours	Watery diarrhea	Clostridia grow in rewarmed meat dishes. Huge numbers ingested.	Enterotoxin produced during sporulation in gut, causes hypersecretion.	Abrupt onset of profuse diarrhea; vomiting occasionally. Recovery usual without treatment in 1–4 days. Many clostridia in cultures of food and feces of patients.	12
Clostridium botulinum	18–24 hours	Paralysis	*C botulinum* grow in anaerobic food and produce toxin.	Toxin absorbed from gut blocks acetylcholine at neuromuscular junction.	Diplopia, dysphagia, dysphonia, difficulty breathing. Treatment requires ventilatory support and antitoxin. Diagnosis confirmed by finding toxin in blood or stool.	12
Escherichia coli (enterogenic; ETEC)	24–72 hours	Watery diarrhea	Most common cause of "traveler's diarrhea."	ETEC in the gut produce heat-labile (HL) or heat-stable (HS) enterotoxins. Toxins[1] cause hypersecretion in small intestine.	Usually abrupt onset of diarrhea; vomiting rare. A serious infection in newborns. In adults, usually self-limiting in 1–3 days.	9, 16
Escherichia coli (enteroinvasive; EIEC)	48–72 hours	Dysentery	Occasional outbreaks of dysentery; infrequent cause of sporadic infection.	Inflammatory invasion of the colonic mucosa; similar to shigellosis. EIEC are closely related to *Shigella*.	Acute bloody diarrhea with malaise, headache, high fever, and abdominal pain. Severe disease in poorly nourished children. WBC present in stool.	9, 16
Escherichia coli (enterohemorrhagic; EHEC)	24–72 hours	Watery, bloody diarrhea	Bloody diarrhea associated with undercooked hamburgers in fast-food restaurants.	EHEC produces vero toxin (Shiga-like toxin). Often serotype O157:H7.	Causes bloody diarrhea, hemorrhagic colitis, and the majority of cases of hemolytic-uremic syndrome. Culture stool for sorbitol-negative *E coli* and serotype isolates with antisera for O157:H7.	9, 16

(*continued*)

Table 48–3. Agents that commonly cause toxin-induced gastroenteritis and gastrointestinal infections. *(Continued)*

Organism	Typical Incubation Period	Signs and Symptoms	Epidemiology	Pathogenesis	Clinical Features	Chapter
Escherichia coli (enteropathogenic; EPEC)	Slow in onset	Watery diarrhea	Common cause of diarrhea in neonates in developing countries. Classically, cause of epidemic diarrhea in newborn nurseries with high mortality rates; less common now in developed countries.	EPEC attach to mucosal epithelial cells and produce cytoskeletal changes; may invade cells. Different from other *E coli* that are enteroadherent or enteroaggregative and cause diarrhea.	Insidious onset over 3–6 days with listlessness, poor feeding, and diarrhea.Usually lasts 5–15 days. Dehydration, electrolytic imbalance, and other complications may cause death. Antimicrobial therapy is important.	9,16
Vibrio parahaemolyticus	6–96 hours	Watery diarrhea	Organisms grow in seafood and in gut and produce toxin, or invade.	Toxin causes hypersecretion; vibrios invade eithelium; stools may be bloody.	Abrupt onset of diarrhea in groups consuming the same food, especially crabs and other seafood. Recovery is usually complete in 1–3 days. Food and stool cultures are positive.	18
Vibrio cholerae	24–72 hours	Watery diarrhea	Organisms grow in gut and produce toxin.	Toxin[1] causes hypersecretion in small intestine. Infective dose $> 10^5$ organisms.	Abrupt onset of liquid diarrhea in endemic area. Needs prompt replacement of fluids and electrolytes IV or orally. Stool cultures positive.	9, 18
Shigella species (mild cases)	24–72 hours	Dysentery	Organism grow in superficial gut epithelium.	Organisms invade epithelial cells; blood, mucus, and PMNs in stools. Infective dose $< 10^3$ organisms.	Abrupt onset of diarrhea; can have blood and pus in stools, cramps, tenesmus, and lethargy. WBC in stool. Stool cultures are positive. Often mild and self-limiting. Restore fluids.	16
Shigella dysenteriae type 1 (Shiga's bacillus)	24–72 hours	Dysentery, bloody diarrhea	Causes outbreaks in developing countries.	Produces cytotoxin and neurotoxin.	Severe bloody diarrhea in children in developing countries; high fatality rate. Rare in the United States.	16
Salmonella species	8–48 hours	Dysentery	Organisms grow in gut. Do not produce toxin.	Superficial infection of gut, little invasion. Infective dose $> 10^5$ organisms.	Gradual or abrupt onset of diarrhea and low-grade fever. WBC in stool. Stool cultures are positive. No antimicrobials unless systemic dissemination is suspected. Prolonged carriage is frequent.	16
Clostridium difficile	Days to weeks after antibiotic therapy	Dysentery	Antibiotic-associated pseudomembranous colitis.	Makes enterotoxin and cytotoxin, which cause diarrhea and epithelial cell necrosis.	Abrupt onset of bloody diarrhea and fever. Toxin in stool. Patients typically received antibiotics in previous days to weeks.	12
Campylobacter jejuni	2–10 days	Dysentery	Infection via oral route from food, pets. Organisms grow in small intestine.	Invasion of mucous membrane. Toxin production uncertain.	Fever, diarrhea; PMNs, and fresh blood in stool, especially in children. Usually self-limited. Special media needed for culture at 42° C. Patients usually recovery in 5–8 days.	18

(continued)

Rotavirus	48–96 hours	Watery diarrhea	Virus is the major cause of diarrheal disease in infants and young children worldwide.	Induces histopathologic changes in intestinal mucosal cells.	Fever and vomiting usually precede abdominal distress and diarrhea. Death in infants in developing countries follows dehydration and electrolyte imbalance. Typical course is 3–9 days. Diagnosis by immunoassay detection of rotavirus antigen in stool.	37
Giardia lamblia	1–2 weeks	Watery diarrhea	Most commonly identified intestinal parasite. Frequent pathogen in outbreaks of waterborne diarrhea.	Complex and poorly understood interaction of parasite with mucosal cells and patient's immune response.	Diarrhea self-limited in 1–3 weeks; chronic symptoms of intermittent diarrhea, malabsorption, and weight loss may last 6 months. Diagnosis by finding trophozoites or cysts in stool or duodenal contents, or by immunoassay detection of *Giardia* antigen in stool.	46
Entamoeba histolytica	Gradual onset 1 3 wooko	Dysentery	Highest prevalence in developing countries; 10% of world's population may be infected.	Invades colonic mucosa and lyses cells, including leukocytes.	Diarrhea, abdominal pain, weight loss, and fever are common. Can give rise to many complications, including fulminant colitis, perforation, and liver abscess. Diagnosis by finding trophozoites or cysts in stool.	46
Salmonella typhi (*S paratyphi* A and B; *S cholaeraesuis*)	10–14 days	Enteric fever	Humans are the only reservoir for *S typhi.*	Invade intestinal mucosa and multiply in macrophages in intestinal lymph follicles; enter mesenteric lymph glands to blood and dissemination.	Insidious onset of malaise, anorexia, myalgias, and headache; high remittent fever; may have constipation or diarrhea. Hepatosplenomegaly in about 50% of patients. Diagnosis by culture of *S typhi* from blood, stool, or other site. Antibiotic therapy is important.	16
Yersinia enterocolitica	4–7 days	Enteric fever	Fecal-oral transmission. Foodborne. Animals infected.	Gastroenteritis or mesenteric adenitis. Occasional bacteremia. Toxin produced occasionally.	Severe abdominal pain, diarrhea, fever; PMNs and blood in stool; polyarthritis, erythema nodosum, especially in children. Keep stool specimen at 4° C before culture.	20

[1] Cholera toxin and *E coli* heat-labile toxin stimulate adenylyl cyclase activity, increasing cAMP concentration in gut, yielding secretion of chloride and water, and reduced reabsorption of sodium. *E coli* heat-stable toxin activates intestinal guanylyl cyclase and results in hypersecretion.

URINARY TRACT

CASE 7: ACUTE UNCOMPLICATED BLADDER INFECTION (Cystitis)

A 21-year-old woman presented to the university student health service with a 2-day history of increasing urinary frequency along with urgency and dysuria. Her urine had been pink or bloody for about 12 hours. She had no history of prior urinary tract infection. The patient had recently become sexually active and was using a diaphragm and spermicide.

Clinical Features

The temperature was 37.5 °C, pulse 105/min, and respirations 18/min. The blood pressure was 105/70 mm Hg.

On physical examination, the only abnormal finding was mild tenderness to deep palpation in the suprapubic area.

Laboratory Findings

Laboratory tests showed a slightly elevated white blood cell count of 10,500/μL; 66% were PMNs, also elevated. Blood urea nitrogen, serum creatinine and glucose, and serum electrolytes were normal. The urine sediment contained innumerable white cells, moderate numbers of red cells, and many bacteria suggestive of urinary tract infection. Culture yielded more than 10^5 colony-forming units (CFU)/mL of *E coli* (diagnostic of a urinary tract infection). Antimicrobial susceptibility tests were not done.

Treatment

The patient was cured by 3 days of oral sulfamethoxazole-trimethoprim therapy.

Comment

See below.

CASE 8: COMPLICATED URINARY TRACT INFECTION

A 67-year-old man developed fever and shock 3 days after a transurethral resection of his prostate gland. Two weeks earlier he had urinary obstruction with retention secondary to the enlargement; benign prostatic hypertrophy had been diagnosed. Urinary bladder catheterization had been necessary. Following the surgery, an indwelling urinary bladder catheter attached to a closed drainage system was left in place. Two days after surgery, the patient developed fever to 38 °C; on the third postoperative day, he became confused and disoriented and had a shaking chill.

The temperature was 39 °C, the pulse was 120/min, and the respirations were 24/min. The blood pressure was 90/40 mm Hg.

On physical examination, the patient knew his name but was disoriented to time and place. His heart, lungs, and abdomen were normal. There was mild costovertebral tenderness over the area of the left kidney.

Laboratory tests showed a normal hematocrit and hemoglobin but an elevated white blood cell count of 18,000/μL; 85% were PMNs (markedly elevated). Blood urea nitrogen, serum creatinine, serum glucose, and electrolytes were normal. Urine was obtained from the catheter port using a needle and syringe. The urine sediment contained innumerable white cells, a few red blood cells, and numerous bacteria, indicating a urinary tract infection. Urine culture yielded more than 10^5 CFU/mL of *Klebsiella pneumoniae,* confirming the diagnosis of urinary tract infection. Blood culture also yielded the *K pneumoniae,* which was susceptible to third-generation cephalosporins, gentamicin, and tobramycin.

The patient had urinary tract infection associated with the bladder catheter. The left kidney was presumed to be involved based on the left costovertebral angle tenderness. He also had secondary bacteremia with shock (sometimes termed gram-negative sepsis and shock). He was treated with intravenous fluids and antibiotics and recovered. The same strain of *Klebsiella pneumoniae* had been isolated from other patients in the hospital, indicating nosocomial spread of the bacteria.

Comment

Urinary tract infections may involve just the lower tract or both the lower and upper tracts. **Cystitis** is the term used to describe infection of the bladder signs and symptoms including dysuria, urgency, and frequency as in Case 7. **Pyelonephritis** is the term used to describe upper tract infection often with flank pain and tenderness, dysuria, urgency, and frequency, as in Case 8. Cystitis and pyelonephritis often present as acute diseases, but recurrent or chronic infections occur frequently.

It is generally accepted that 10^5 of more bacteria or CFU/mL of urine is significant bacteriuria, though the patients may be symptomatic or asymptomatic. Some young women have dysuria and other symptoms of cystitis with less than 10^5 CFU/mL of urine; in these women, as few as 10^3 CFU/mL of a gram-negative rod may be significant bacteriuria.

The prevalence of bacteriuria is 1–2% in school-age girls, 1–3% in nonpregnant women, and 4–7% during pregnancy. The prevalence of bacteriuria increases with age, and the sex ratio of infections becomes nearly equal. Over the age of 70 years, 20–30% or more of women and 10% or more of men have bacteriuria. Upper urinary tract infections routinely occur in patients with indwelling catheters even with optimal care and closed drainage systems: 50% after 4–5 days, 75% after 7–9 days, and 100% after 2 weeks. Sexual activity and use of spermicides increase the risk for UTIs in young women.

E coli (Chapter 16) causes 80–90% of acute uncomplicated bacterial upper tract infections (cystitis) in young women. Other enteric bacteria and *Staphylococcus saprophyticus* cause most of the other culture-positive bladder infections in this patient group. Some young women with acute dysuria suggesting cystitis have negative urine cultures for bacteria. In these patients, selective cultures for *Neisseria gonorrhoeae* and *Chlamydia trachomatis,* and evaluation for herpes simplex infection should be considered.

In complicated upper tract infections, in the setting of anatomic abnormality or chronic catheterization, the spectrum in infecting bacteria is larger than in uncomplicated cases. *E coli* is frequently present, but other gram-negative rods of many species (eg, *Klebsiella, Proteus,* and *Enterobacter* [Chapter 16] and *Pseudomonas* species [Chapter 17]), enterococci, and staphylococci are also common. Often two or more species are present, and frequently the bacteria are resistant to antimicrobials given in association with prior therapy.

The presence of white blood cells in urine is highly suggestive but not specific for bacterial upper tract infections. White blood cells can be detected by microscopic examination of urine sediment or, indirectly, by dipstick detection of leukocyte esterase. The presence of red blood cells also is found on microscopy of the urine sediment, or indirectly by dipstick detection of hemoglobin. Proteinuria also is detected by dipstick. The presence of bacteria on Gram's stain of noncentrifuged urine is strongly suggestive of 10^5 or more bacteria per milliliter of urine.

The presence of bacteriuria is confirmed by quantitative culture of the urine by any one of several methods. One frequently used method is to culture urine using a bacteriologic loop calibrated to deliver 0.01 or 0.001 mL followed by counting the number of colonies that grow.

Acute uncomplicated cystitis is usually caused by *E coli* susceptible to readily achievable urine concentrations of antibiotics appropriate for treatment of urinary tract infections. Thus, in the setting of the first such infection in a young woman, definitive identification and susceptibility testing of the bacteria are seldom necessary. Such cases can be treated by a single dose of appropriate antibiotic, but a 3-day course of therapy yields a lower relapse rate. Pyelonephritis is treated with 10–14 days of antibiotic therapy. Recurrent or complicated upper tract infections are best treated with antibiotics shown to be active against the infecting bacteria; definitive identification and susceptibility testing is indicated. Therapy for 14 days is appropriate and for 14–21 days if there is recurrence. Patients with complicated upper tract infections should have evaluations for anatomic abnormalities, stones, etc.

BONE & SOFT TISSUE

CASE 9: OSTEOMYELITIS

A 34-year-old man suffered an open fracture of the middle third of his tibia when his motorized three-wheel vehicle tipped over in a field and fell on him. He was taken to a hospital and promptly to the operating room. The wound was cleaned and debrided, the fracture was reduced, and the bone aligned. Metal plates were placed to span the fracture, align it, and hold it in place. Pins were placed through the skin and bone proximal and distal to the fracture to allow splinting and immobilization of the leg. One day after surgery, the leg remained markedly swollen; a moderate amount of serous drainage was present on the dressings. Two days later, the leg remained swollen and red, requiring opening of the surgical wound. Cultures of pus in the wound grew *Staphylococcus aureus* resistant to penicillin G but susceptible to nafcillin. The patient was treated with intravenous nafcillin for 10 days, and the swelling and redness decreased. Three weeks later, pus began to drain from a small opening in the wound. Cultures again grew *S aureus.* Exploration of the opening showed a sinus tract to the site of the fracture. An x-ray film of the leg showed poor alignment of the fracture. Osteomyelitis was diagnosed, and the patient was returned to the operating room, where the fracture site was debrided of necrotic soft tissue and dead bone; the pins and plates were removed. Bone grafts were placed. The fracture was immobilized by external fixation. Cultures obtained during surgery grew *S aureus.* The patient was treated with intravenous nafcillin for 1 month followed by oral dicloxacillin for 3 additional months. The wound and fracture slowly healed. After 6 months, there was no x-ray evidence of further osteomyelitis, and the patient was able to bear weight on the leg.

Comment

Osteomyelitis follows **hematogenous spread** of pathogenic bacteria from a distant site of infection to bone or, as in this case, direct inoculation of the bone and soft tissue, as can occur with an open fracture or from a contiguous site of soft tissue infection. The primary symptoms are fever and pain at the infected site; swelling, redness, and occasionally drainage can be seen, but the physical findings are highly dependent upon the anatomic location of the infection. For example, osteomyelitis of the spine may present with fever, back pain, and signs of a paraspinous abscess; infection of the hip may show as fever with pain on movement and decreased range of motion. In children, the onset of osteomyelitis following hematogenous spread of bacteria can be very sudden, while in adults the presentation may be more indolent. Sometimes osteomyelitis is considered to be chronic or of long standing, but the clinical spectrum of osteomyelitis is broad, and the distinction between acute and chronic may not be clear either clinically or on morphologic examination of tissue.

S aureus (Chapter 14) is the primary agent of osteomyelitis in 60–70% of cases (90% in children). *S aureus* causes the infection after hematogenous spread or following direct inoculation. Streptococci cause osteomyelitis in about 10% of cases, enteric gram-negative rods (eg, *E coli*) and other bacteria such as *Pseudomonas aeruginosa* in 20–30%. Anaerobic bacteria (eg, *Bacteroides* species) are also common, particularly in osteomyelitis of the bones of the feet associated with diabetes and foot ulcers. Any bacteria that cause infections in humans has been associated with osteomyelitis.

Definitive diagnosis of the etiology of osteomyelitis requires culture of a specimen obtained at surgery or by needle aspiration of bone or periosteum through uninfected soft tissue. Culture of pus from the opening of a draining sinus tract or superficial wound associated with the osteomyelitis commonly yields bacteria that are not present in the bone. Blood cultures are often positive when systemic symptoms and signs (fever, weight loss, elevated white blood cell count, high erythrocyte sedimentation rate) are present.

Early in the course of osteomyelitis, x-ray films of the infected site are negative. The initial findings noted radiologically usually are soft tissue swelling, loss of tissue planes, and demineralization of bone; 2–3 weeks after onset, bone erosions and evidence of periostitis appear. Bone scans with radionuclide imaging are very sensitive. They become positive within a few days after onset and are particularly helpful in localizing the site of infection and determining if there are multiple sites of infection; however, bone scans do not differentiate between fractures, bone infarction (as occurs in sickle cell disease), and infection. CT and MRI also are sensitive and especially helpful in determining the extent of soft tissue involvement.

Antimicrobial therapy and surgical debridement are the mainstays of treatment of osteomyelitis. The specific antimicrobial should be selected after culture of a properly obtained specimen and susceptibility tests and continued for 6–8 weeks or longer, depending on the infection. Surgery should be done to remove any dead bone and sequestra that are present. Immobilization of infected limbs and fixation of fractures are important features of competent care.

CASE 10: GAS GANGRENE

A 22-year-old man fell while riding his new motorcycle and suffered an open fracture of his left femur and severe lacerations and crushing injury to the thigh and less extensive soft tissue injuries to other parts of his body. He was rapidly transported to the hospital and immediately taken to the operating room, where the fracture was reduced and the wounds debrided. At admission, results of his blood tests included a hematocrit of 45% and a hemoglobin of 15 g/dL. The immediate postoperative course was uneventful, but 24 hours later pain developed in the thigh. Fever was noted. Pain and swelling of the thigh increased rapidly.

The temperature was 40 °C, the pulse 150/min, and respirations 28/min. The blood pressure was 80/40 mm Hg.

Physical examination showed an acutely ill young man who was in shock and delirious. The left thigh was markedly swollen and cool to touch. Large ecchymotic areas were present near the wound, and there was a serous discharge from the wound. Crepitus was felt, indicative of gas in the tissue of the thigh. An x-ray film also showed gas in the tissue planes of the thigh. Gas gangrene was diagnosed, and the patient was taken to the operating room for emergency extensive debridement of necrotic tissue. At the time of surgery, his hematocrit had fallen to 27% and his hemoglobin to 9 g/dL; his serum was red-brown in color, indicating hemolysis with free hemoglobin in his circulation. Anaerobic cultures of the specimen obtained at surgery grew *Clostridium perfringens*. The patient developed renal failure and heart failure, and died 3 days after his injury.

Comment

Case 10 illustrates a classic case of clostridial gas gangrene. *Clostridium perfringens* (or occasionally other *Clostridium* species) are inoculated into the traumatic wound from the environment; the clostridia are discussed in Chapter 12. The presence of necrotic tissue and foreign body material provides a suitable anaerobic environment for the organisms to multiply. After an incubation period usually of 2–3 days but sometimes only 8–12 hours, there is acute onset of pain, which rapidly increases in intensity associated with shock and delirium. The extremity or wound shows tenderness, tense swelling, and a serosanguineous discharge. Crepitus is often present. The skin near the wound is pale but rapidly becomes discolored, and fluid-filled blebs form in the nearby skin. Skin areas of black necrosis appear. In severe cases, there is rapid progression.

In patients such as this one, Gram's stain of fluid from a bleb or of a tissue aspirate shows large gram-positive rods with blunt ends and is highly suggestive of clostridial infection. Anaerobic culture provides the definitive laboratory confirmation. The differential diagnosis of clostridial gas gangrene includes anaerobic streptococcal myonecrosis, synergistic necrotizing myonecrosis, and necrotizing fasciitis. These clinically overlapping diseases can be differentiated from clostridial gas gangrene by Gram's stain and cultures of appropriate specimens.

X-ray films of the infected site show gas in the fascial planes. Laboratory tests include hematocrit, which is often low. The hemoglobin may be low or normal even when the hematocrit is low, consistent with hemolysis and cell-free circulating hemoglobin. Leukocytosis is usually present.

Extensive surgery with removal of all the dead and infected tissue is necessary as a lifesaving procedure. Penicillin G is the antibiotic of choice. Antitoxin is of no help. When shock and circulating free hemoglobin are present, renal failure and other complications are common and the prognosis is poor.

Index

NOTE: Page numbers in **boldface** type indicate a major discussion. A *t* following a page number indicates tabular material and an *i* following a page number indicates an illustration.

Other subgroups
Phlebovirus
Sandfly fever viruses
Rift Valley fever virus
Nairovirus
Crimean-Congo hemorrhagic fever virus
Other serogroups
Hantavirus
Korean hemorrhagic fever
Hantavirus pulmonary syndrome
Retroviridae
Mammalian type C oncovirus
Human T-cell lymphotropic viruses 1 and 2
Lentivirus
Human immunodeficiency viruses 1 and 2
Arenaviridae
Arenavirus
Lymphocytic choriomeningitis virus
Lassa fever virus
Junin virus
Machupo virus
DNA VIRUSES
Parvoviridae
Parvovirus
Human parvovirus B19
Papovaviridae
Papillomavirus
Papilloma viruses
Polyomavirus
BK and JC viruses
Adenoviridae
Mastadenovirus
Adenoviruses
Hepadnaviridae
Orthohepadnavirus
Hepatitis B virus
Herpesviridae
Alphaherpesvirinae
Simplexvirus
Herpes simplex viruses 1 and 2
Varicellovirus
Varicella-zoster virus
Betaherpesvirinae
Cytomegalovirus
Cytomegalovirus
Gammaherpesvirinae
Lymphocryptovirus
Epstein-Barr virus
Human herpesviruses 6 and 7
Poxviridae
Orthopoxvirus
Vaccinia virus
Smallpox virus (variola)
Monkeypox virus
Cowpox virus
Parapoxvirus
Orf virus
Virus of milker's nodule
Yatapoxvirus
Yabapox and tanapox viruses
Molluscipoxvirus
Molluscum contagiosum virus
UNCONVENTIONAL AGENTS
Creutzfeldt-Jakob virus

IV. Fungi

DERMATOPHYTES
Epidermophyton floccosum
Microsporum audouinii
Microsporum canis
Microsporum species
Trichophyton mentagrophytes
Trichophyton rubrum
Trichophyton tonsurans
Trichophyton species
YEASTS
Candida albicans
Candida krusei
Candida parapsilosis
Candida tropicalis
Candida species
Cryptococcus neoformans
Geotrichum species
Malassezia furfur
Rhodotorula species
Torulopsis glabrata
Trichosporon species
Pneumocystis carinii
DIMORPHIC FUNGI
Blastomyces dermatitidis
Coccidioides immitis
Histoplasma capsulatum
Paracoccidioides brasiliensis
Sporothrix schenckii
FILAMENTOUS MOLDS
Acremonium species
Aspergillus flavus
Aspergillus fumigatus
Aspergillus niger
Aspergillus species
Fusarium species
Penicillium species
Pseudallescheria boydii
DEMATIACEOUS FUNGI
Alternaria species
Aureobasidium species
Bipolaris species
Cladosporium species
Exerohilum species
Exophiala species
Fonsecaea species
Phialophora species
Wangiella species
AGENTS OF ZYGOMYCOSIS
Absidia species
Mucor species
Rhizopus species

V. Parasites

PROTOZOA
Amebae
Acanthamoeba species
Endolimax nana
Entamoeba histolytica
Entamoeba species
Hartmanella species
Iodamoeba bütschlii
Naegleria fowleri
Ciliates
Balantidium coli
Flagellates
Chilomastix mesnili
Dientomoeba fragilis
Enteromonas hominis
Giardia lamblia
Leishmania species
Retortamonas intestinalis
Trichomonas vaginalis
Trichomonas species
Trypanosoma brucei gambiense
Trypanosoma brucei rhodesiense
Trypanosoma cruzi
Sporozoa
Babesia species
Cryptosporidium parvum
Isospora belli
Plasmodium falciparum
Plasmodium malariae
Plasmodium ovale
Plasmodium vivax
Sarcocystis species
Toxoplasma gondii
Uncertain Classification
Blastocystis hominis
MICROSPORIDA
Cyclospora species
Encephalitozoon hellum
Enterocytozoon bineusi
Nosema corneum
Pleistophora species
Septata intestinalis
HELMINTHS
Cestodes
Diphyllobothrium latum
Dipylidium caninum
Echinococcus granulosus
Echinococcus multilocularis
Echinococcus species
Hymenolepis diminuta
Hymenolepis nana
Multiceps multiceps
Taenia saginata
Taenia solium
Taenia species
Nematodes
Ancylostoma duodenale
Ancylostoma species
Angiostrongylus species
Anisakis species
Ascaris lumbricoides
Brugia malayi
Capillaria species
Dirofilaria species
Dracunculus medinensis
Enterobius vermicularis
Gnathostoma spinigerum
Loa loa
Mansonella species
Necator americanus
Onchocerca volvulus
Strongyloides stercoralis
Toxocara species
Trichostrongylus species
Trichuris trichiura
Trichinella spiralis
Wuchereria bancrofti
Trematodes
Clonorchis sinensis
Dicrocoelium dendriticum
Fasciola hepatica
Fasciolopsis buski
Echinostoma species
Gastrodiscoides hominis
Heterophyes heterophyes
Metagonimus yokogawai
Nanophyetus salmincola
Opisthorchis viverrini
Paragonimus westermani
Paragonimus species
Schistosoma mansoni
Schistosoma haematobium
Schistosoma japonicum
Schistosoma species